Pain Management in Veterinary Practice

Pain Management in Veterinary Practice

Editors

Christine M. Egger

Lydia Love

Tom Doherty

WILEY Blackwell

This edition first published 2014 © 2014 by John Wiley & Sons, Inc.

Editorial offices: 1606 Golden Aspen Drive, Suites 103 and 104, Ames, Iowa 50010, USA
The Atrium, Southern Gate, Chichester, West Sussex, PO19 8SQ, UK
9600 Garsington Road, Oxford, OX4 2DQ, UK

For details of our global editorial offices, for customer services and for information about how to apply for permission to reuse the copyright material in this book please see our website at www.wiley.com/wiley-blackwell.

Library of Congress Cataloging-in-Publication Data

Pain management in veterinary practice / editors, Christine M. Egger, Lydia Love, Tom Doherty.
    pages ; cm
  Includes bibliographical references and index.
   ISBN 978-0-8138-1224-3 (pbk. : alk. paper) – ISBN 978-1-118-76133-5 (emobi) – ISBN 978-1-118-76134-2 (epdf) –
ISBN 978-1-118-76160-1 (epub)   1. Pain in animals–Treatment.   I. Egger, Christine M., editor of compilation.
II. Love, Lydia, editor of compilation.   III. Doherty, T. J. (Tom J.), editor of compilation.
  [DNLM: 1. Pain Management–veterinary.   2. Veterinary Medicine–methods. SF 925]
  SF910.P34P35 2014
  636.089′60472–dc23
                                                                                    2013024797

A catalogue record for this book is available from the British Library.

Wiley also publishes its books in a variety of electronic formats. Some content that appears in print may not be available in electronic books.

Cover images: Front cover, Top and Bottom Left: Gregory Hirshoren, University of Tennessee CVM; Back Cover, Left: Kristie Mozzachio
            and Valarie V. Tynes; Middle and Right: Gregory Hirshoren
Cover design by Modern Alchemy LLC

Set in 9.5/11.5 pt Times by Aptara® Inc., New Delhi, India

1   2014

Contents

Contributors

Henry S. Adair, DVM, MS, CERP, DACVS, DACVSMR
Associate Professor, Equine Surgery
Director of Equine Performance and Rehabilitation
Department of Large Animal Clinical Sciences
College of Veterinary Medicine
University of Tennessee
Knoxville, TN

Alvin J. Beitz, BS, PhD
Professor and Chair
Distinguished Teacher
Department of Veterinary and Biomedical Sciences
College of Veterinary Medicine, University of Minnesota
St. Paul, MN

Mona Boudreaux DVM, CVA, MMQ
Owner
A Time To Heal
Wonder Lake, IL

Shauna Cantwell, DVM, MVSc, CVA, CVSMT, DACVAA
Courtesy Professor
University of Florida
Medicine Wheel Veterinary Services, Inc.
Ocala, FL

Sathya K. Chinnadurai, DVM, MS, DACZM, DACVAA
Associate Veterinarian
Chicago Zoological Society/Brookfield Zoo
Brookfield, IL

Stuart Clark-Price, DVM, MS, DACVIM-LA, DACVAA
Assistant Professor, Anesthesia and Analgesia
Head, Anesthesia Clinical Service
Department of Veterinary Clinical Medicine
College of Veterinary Medicine
University of Illinois
Urbana, IL

Alice Crook, BSc, DVM
Coordinator
Sir James Dunn Animal Welfare Centre
Adjunct Professor
Department of Companion Animals
Atlantic Veterinary College
University of Prince Edward Island
Charlottetown, Canada

Lowri Davies, BVSc, MRCVS, CVA, CCRP
The SMART Veterinary Clinic Ltd
Weigbridge Referral Center
Swansea, Wales, UK

Lisa DiBernardi, DVM, DACVIM (Oncology), DACVR (Radiation Oncology)
Animal Specialty Hospital of Florida
Naples, FL
Palm Beach Veterinary Specialists
West Palm Beach, FL

Robin Downing, DVM, CVPP, CCRP, DAAPM
Hospital Director
The Downing Center for Animal Pain Management, LLC
Windsor, CO

Bernd Driessen, DVM, PhD, DACVAA, DECVPT
Professor, Anesthesiology
School of Veterinary Medicine
University of Pennsylvania
New Bolton Center
Kennett Square, PA

Tanya Duke-Novakovski, BVetMed, MSc, DVA, DACVAA, DECVAA
Professor, Veterinary Anesthesiology and Analgesia
Department of Small Animal Clinical Sciences
Western College of Veterinary Medicine
University of Saskatchewan
Saskatoon, Canada

Lynelle Graham, DVM, MS, DACVAA
Clinical Professor of Anesthesia
Veterinary Clinical Sciences
University of Minnesota
St. Paul, MN

Cheryl B. Greenacre, DVM, DABVP (Avian), DABVP (Exotic Companion Mammal)
Professor, Avian and Zoological Medicine
Department of Small Animal Clinical Sciences
College of Veterinary Medicine
University of Tennessee
Knoxville, TN

Tamara Grubb, DVM, PhD, DACVAA
Assistant Clinical Professor, Anesthesia and Analgesia
Veterinary Clinical Sciences
Washington State University
Pullman, WA

Anna Hielm-Björkman, DVM, PhD, CVA (IVAS)
Assistant Professor
Department of Equine and Small Animal Medicine
Pain and Rehabilitation Clinic and Research Center
Faculty of Veterinary Medicine
Helsinki University
Helsinki, Finland

Jacob A. Johnson, DVM, DACVAA
Assistant Professor, Anesthesia and Pain Management
Auburn University College of Veterinary Medicine
Auburn, AL

Keri Jones, DVM, CVPP
Medical Director
Homeward Bound Animal Hospital
Arvada, CO

Martin W. Kaufmann, ABC, c-PED
OrthoPets
Center for Animal Pain Management and Mobility Solutions
Denver, CO

Kip A. Lemke, BS, DVM, MS, DACVAA
Professor, Anesthesiology
Chief of Anesthesiology Service
Department of Companion Animals
College of Veterinary Medicine
University of Prince Edward Island
Charlottetown, Canada

Emma Love, BVMS, PhD, DVA, DECVAA, MRCVS, FHEA, RCVS
Senior Teaching Fellow in Veterinary Anaesthesia
University of Bristol
Bristol, UK

Lydia Love, DVM, DACVAA
Director of Anesthesia and Pain Management
Animal Emergency and Referral Associates
Fairfield, NJ

Karen L. Machin, DVM, PhD
Associate Professor
Department of Veterinary Biomedical Sciences
Western College of Veterinary Medicine
University of Saskatchewan
Saskatoon, Canada

Steve Marsden, DVM, ND, MSOM, Lac, Dipl.CH, CVA
Director
College of Integrative Veterinary Therapies
Edmonton, Canada

Patrice M. Mich, DVM, MS, DABVP, DACVAA, CCRT
Medical Director
OrthoPets
Center for Animal Pain Management and Mobility Solutions
Denver, CO

Kristie Mozzachio, DVM, DACVP
Mozzachio Mobile Veterinary Services
Hillsborough, NC
Adjunct faculty
North Carolina State University College of Veterinary Medicine
Raleigh, NC

Arthur I. Ortenburger, DVM, MS
Associate Professor of Surgery
Department of Health Management
University of Prince Edward Island
Charlottetown, Canada

Cholawat Pacharinsak, DVM, MS, PhD, DACVAA
Assistant Professor
Director of Anesthesia, Pain Management, and Surgery
School of Medicine
Stanford University
Stanford, CA

Peter J. Pascoe, BVSc, DVA, DACVAA, DECVAA
Professor, Veterinary Anesthesia and Critical Patient Care
Department of Surgical and Radiological Sciences,
School of Veterinary Medicine
University of California
Davis, CA

Lysa Pam Posner, DVM, DACVAA
Associate Professor Anesthesiology
Director of Anesthesia Services
College of Veterinary Medicine
North Carolina State University
Raleigh, NC

Bruno H. Pypendop, DrMedVet, DrVetSci, DACVAA
Professor, Veterinary Anesthesia and Critical Patient Care
Department of Surgical and Radiological Sciences
School of Veterinary Medicine
University of California
Davis, CA

Jane Quandt, DVM, MS, DACVAA, DACVECC
Associate Professor, Anesthesiology
College of Veterinary Medicine
University of Georgia
Athens, GA

Jessica K. Rychel, DVM, CVMA, CCRP
Veterinary Emergency and Rehabilitation Hospital
Fort Collins, CO

Reza Seddighi, DVM, MS, PhD, DACVAA
Assistant Professor, Anesthesia and Analgesia
Department of Large Animal Clinical Sciences
College of Veterinary Medicine
University of Tennessee
Knoxville, TN

Kersti Seksel, BVSc (Hons), MRCVS, MA (Hons), FACVSc,
DACVB, CMAVA, DECVBM-CA
Registered Veterinary Specialist, Behavioral Medicine
Sydney Animal Behavior Service
Seaforth, Australia

Yael Shilo, DVM, DACVAA
Senior Anesthesiologist,
Anesthesia Department
Veterinary Teaching Hospital
Koret School of Veterinary Medicine
The Hebrew University of Jerusalem
Rehovot, Israel

Lesley J. Smith, DVM, DACVAA
Clinical Professor of Anesthesiology and Pain Management
Department of Surgical Sciences
School of Veterinary Medicine
University of Wisconsin
Madison, WI

Kevin J. Stafford, MVB, MSc, PhD, FRCVS, FANZCVSc
Professor
Institute of Veterinary Animal and Biomedical Sciences
Massey University
Palmerston North, New Zealand

Dave Thompson, DVM
Clyde Park Veterinary Clinic
Wyoming, MI

Lesa Thompson, MA, BVM&S, DZooMed
(Mammalian), MSc, MRCVS, RCVS
Tokyo, Japan

Valarie V. Tynes, DVM, DACVB
Premier Veterinary Behavior Consulting
Sweetwater, TX

Alexander Valverde, DVM, DVSc, DACVAA
Associate Professor, Anesthesiology
Department of Clinical Studies
Ontario Veterinary College
University of Guelph
Guelph, Canada

Rick Wall, DVM, CCRP, DAAPM
Certified Myofascial Trigger Point Therapist
Center for Veterinary Pain Management and Rehabilitation
The Woodlands, TX

Kate L. White, MA, Vet MB, DVA, DECVAA, MRCVS
Clinical Associate Professor, Anesthesia
Head of Division of Medicine
College of Veterinary Medicine
University of Nottingham
Sutton Bonington Campus
Loughborough, UK

Bonnie Wright, DVM, DACVA, CVMA, CVPP, CCRP
Veterinary Emergency and Rehabilitation Hospital
Fort Collins, CO

Laura Zarucco, DMV, PhD
Associate Professor of Surgery
Dipartimento di Scienze Veterinarie
Scuola di Agraria e Medicina Veterinaria
Università degli Studi di Torino
Grugliasco, Italy

Preface

New analgesics and new formulations of old analgesics are constantly being introduced to the veterinary market, yet the ability to recognize and quantify pain in veterinary species remains a challenge. Pain assessment and scoring systems are being validated in many veterinary species, but clinically relevant, objective methods of assessment of all types of pain in all species remain elusive. Ultimately, it is left to the caregiver to decide if analgesic therapy is indicated, and this requires empathy and logic. The purpose of this book is to provide the reader with easily accessible, evidence-based information to aid in the recognition and treatment of pain in veterinary species.

ORGANIZATION AND FEATURES OF THE BOOK

Section I begins with an introductory chapter discussing welfare issues associated with pain and its management in veterinary species. The chapters that follow provide a review of the current understanding of the physiology and pathophysiology of acute pain, chronic pain, and cancer pain.

Section II provides extensive information about the pharmacology of opioids, nonsteroidal anti-inflammatory drugs, alpha-2 adrenoreceptor agonists, local anesthetics, and non-traditional analgesics (e.g., anti-epileptic drugs, NMDA receptor antagonists, and nutritional supplements). Novel methods of drug delivery and the pharmacokinetics of continuous rate infusions are also discussed.

The non-pharmacological management of pain, including physical therapy, orthotics and prosthetics, myofascial trigger point therapy, acupuncture, chiropractic, herbal therapy, and homeopathy are discussed in Section III. These chapters are not intended to provide expert training in these areas. They are meant to provide a basic explanation of some techniques that can be easily incorporated into daily practice and to discuss scientific evidence, or lack thereof, supporting these modalities.

The recognition and treatment of acute and chronic pain in dogs, cats, small exotic mammals, birds, reptiles, amphibians, fish, camelids, ruminants, pigs, and horses is discussed in Section IV. Chapters on the treatment of cancer pain and the recognition and treatment of pain in intensive care patients are also included. The chapters in this section discuss pharmacological and non-pharmacological strategies for use in each species to provide a balanced pain management protocol. Much of the information from these chapters is summarized in tables to allow easy access to information.

The fifth and final section includes a chapter describing strategies for incorporating pain management into veterinary practice, including some economic and legal considerations, and a final chapter discussing veterinary hospice and palliative care.

ACKNOWLEDGMENTS

The authors wish to thank the staff of Wiley for their support and encouragement. This work would not have been possible without the contributions of the authors who come from academic, research, and clinical practice backgrounds in the USA, Canada, Great Britain, Europe, New Zealand, and Australia. A feature common to all is the desire to improve the recognition, prevention, and treatment of pain in animals. We hope that this book contributes significantly to that endeavor.

Christine M. Egger
Lydia Love
Tom Doherty

Section 1
Introduction and Anatomy, Physiology, and Pathophysiology of Pain

Pain Management in Veterinary Practice, First Edition. Edited by Christine M. Egger, Lydia Love and Tom Doherty.
© 2014 John Wiley & Sons, Inc. Published 2014 by John Wiley & Sons, Inc.

1
Introduction: Pain: An Issue of Animal Welfare

Alice Crook

There has been considerable progress since the early 1990s in pain research in animals and in our understanding of related physiology and pharmacology, enabling great strides to be made in pain management. But pain is still a huge welfare issue for animals: farm animals are routinely subjected to painful husbandry procedures with no anesthesia or analgesia; perioperative pain management in small and exotic animals is inconsistent; and management of cancer-related and chronic pain remains a challenge. Pain can diminish animal well-being substantially due to its aversive nature, the distress arising from the inability to avoid such sensations, and the secondary effects that may adversely affect the animal's quality of life (QOL). Pain may affect an animal's appetite, sleep habits (e.g., fatigue), grooming (e.g., self-mutilation), ability to experience normal pleasures (e.g., reduced play and social interaction), personality and temperament, and intestinal function (e.g., constipation), and may prolong the time needed for recovery from the underlying condition (ACVA, 1998; McMillan, 2003). Untreated pain may also result in systemic problems; for example, hepatic lipidosis in cats as a result of inappetance and inadequate caloric intake (Mathews, 2000).

Much is known about the recognition and assessment of pain in animals; however, more work is needed to develop valid and reliable pain scoring systems for all species that are practical in real-life situations. Perception of animal pain directly affects analgesic usage, and there is a wide range in attitudes among veterinarians, farmers, and pet owners. This can best be addressed through education. There are also economic, regulatory, and other constraints to effective pain management, particularly in large animals.

RECOGNITION AND ASSESSMENT OF PAIN IN ANIMALS

Pain is an unpleasant sensory and emotional experience associated with actual or potential tissue damage, or described in terms of such damage (IASP, 1994). The experience of pain is always subjective. Self-reporting is the gold standard in people, yet how can we know the experience of animals?

Three approaches are used in the recognition and measurement of pain in animals. The first approach includes measures of general body function or productivity (e.g., food and water intake, weight gain) that are relatively easy to quantify; such measures reflect what was happening to the animal over the period between observations. The second approach includes physiological measures (such as changes in heart rate or cortisol concentrations) that are widely used in studies assessing pain in animals (Stafford & Mellor, 2005; Vickers et al., 2005; Whay et al., 2005) and are, in principle, particularly useful in prey species that are considered stoic and therefore unlikely to show pronounced behavioral responses until injuries are advanced (Phillips, 2002; Rutherford, 2002). However, the physical restraint required to obtain such measurements may itself be stressful and confound the results (Weary et al., 2006). Also, while cortisol measurements are useful for comparing treatments and controls, they are not useful in assessing the degree of pain an individual animal is experiencing (Rutherford, 2002).

Behavioral measures—the third approach—represent a way in which animals can "self-report." Weary (2006) provides a comprehensive review of the ways such measures are used to recognize and quantify animal pain, and discusses the evidence necessary to ensure that the measures are valid (i.e., that the measure provides useful information about the pain the animal is experiencing) and reliable (i.e., repeatable). The three main classes of behavior used in pain assessment are pain-specific behaviors (e.g., gait impairment in lame dairy cows (Flower et al., 2008) or head shaking and rubbing in dehorned dairy calves (Vickers et al., 2005)); a decline in frequency or magnitude of certain behaviors (e.g., locomotory behaviors in rats postoperatively) (Roughan & Flecknell, 2003); and choice or preference testing (e.g., hens' responses to different concentrations of carbon dioxide used in stunning) (Webster & Fletcher, 2004). Rutherford (2002) discusses the usefulness of behaviors associated with acute, subacute, and longer-lasting pain in assessing the experience of pain in animals, including specific parameters that may be useful for veterinarians in clinical assessment of pain and by scientists studying pain in animals. These include simple and more complex behavioral responses, both qualitative and quantitative, which may or may not be adaptive, such as behaviors associated with escape or avoidance, guarding or protection (e.g., postural changes), and depression or "learned helplessness."

Pain Management in Veterinary Practice, First Edition. Edited by Christine M. Egger, Lydia Love and Tom Doherty.
© 2014 John Wiley & Sons, Inc. Published 2014 by John Wiley & Sons, Inc.

Pain Recognition Tools

Pain researchers and clinicians alike agree that there is a need for sensitive and specific measures that are practical for real-time assessments in a variety of animal settings including farms, veterinary clinics, and laboratories (Viñuela-Fernández et al., 2007). Multidimensional pain scales that integrate objective and subjective behavioral observations with various other measures can be used to characterize an individual animal's experience of pain (Rutherford, 2002). Another approach is to develop questionnaires for use by animal owners that can be used in the assessment of pain and its impact on QOL (McMillan, 2003; Wiseman-Orr et al., 2004; Yazbek & Fantoni, 2005). Wiseman-Orr (2006) provides a thorough discussion of the approaches and potential pitfalls of designing and validating questionnaires where self-reporting is not possible and the questionnaires are designed for use by a proxy, as in the case of animals. Work continues in the development of scientifically validated pain recognition tools for veterinarians for clinical assessment of pain and for scientists studying pain in large, small, exotic, and laboratory animals (Roughan & Flecknell, 2003; Wiseman-Orr et al., 2004; Yazbek & Fantoni, 2005; Morton, 2005; Wojciechowska et al., 2005; Föllmi et al., 2007; Flecknell et al, 2007; Weary & Fraser, 2008).

PAIN AND CONSCIOUSNESS

Pain is always subjective and psychological variables such as past experience, attention, and other cognitive activities affect the individual's experience of pain (Melzack, 1993). Self-reporting is the gold standard in people and, because of the subtlety of communication possible with language, the understanding of pain has been greatly advanced through human subjects' descriptions of pain and the effects of different modalities of analgesia (Johnson, 2008). However, "The inability to communicate verbally does not negate the possibility that an individual is experiencing pain and is in need of appropriate pain-relieving treatment" (IASP, 1994).

If we cannot know the subjective emotional experiences of other human beings, how can we possibly know the emotional experience of animals? For most people, the evidence that animals have nociceptive receptors and pathways, physiological responses, and behavioral reactions to pain similar to that of people, is sufficient to accept that animals experience pain and suffer as a result. However, some scientists, surprisingly, suggest that animals are not capable of experiencing pain. Psychologist Bermond (2001), for example argues that animals other than anthropoid apes have an "irreflexive consciousness" (a consciousness without past or future) due to the lack of a well-developed prefrontal cortex, and that reflection is a requirement to experience suffering and pain as unpleasant. Therefore, he distinguishes between "the registration of pain as a stimulus, which does not induce feelings of suffering and the experience of pain as an emotion, which does induce suffering" (Bermond, 2001).

What kind of observations can provide evidence for or against the experience of pain and other affective states in animals? The neurophysiologist Gentle (2001) carried out an elegant series of studies to provide information on cognitive perception of pain in chickens by looking at the effect of selective attention on pain-related behavior. Noting that the human experience of pain can be modulated by shifts in attention through such modalities as relaxation training, hypnosis, and other therapies, he reasoned that if a chicken's response to a painful event was simply an unconscious automatic reaction the response would not be influenced by shifting the bird's attention. On the other hand, if the bird actually felt the pain as an unpleasant experience, redirecting its attention might reduce the signs of pain, as in people (e.g., installation of overhead television screens in dental offices). In his work, Gentle induced gout in one leg of chickens by injecting sodium urate crystals. Chickens kept in barren cages avoided placing weight on the affected leg and, if encouraged to walk, did so with a limp. These pain-related behavioral signs were greatly reduced or eliminated in chickens given a variety of motivational changes including nesting, feeding, exploration, and social interaction. The shifts in attention not only reduced pain but also reduced peripheral inflammation.

This work has far-reaching consequences. The evidence that motivational changes, by altering the birds' attention, significantly altered pain-related behaviors, and hence probably the pain experience for the animal, indicates a cognitive component of pain in the chicken and provides evidence of consciousness. On a practical level, these results also reinforce the importance of environmental enrichment, which will promote shifts in attention and, thereby, potentially improve the welfare of birds suffering pain under commercial conditions. Strategies, such as distraction and refocusing attention through positive interaction, are very familiar to veterinarians and animal health technicians as adjuncts to pain management in small animals in clinical settings.

ATTITUDES TOWARD ANIMAL PAIN

"Freedom from pain, injury, or disease (by prevention or rapid diagnosis and treatment)" is one of the Five Freedoms widely accepted as the major components of good animal welfare (Farm Animal Welfare Council, 2009). The recognition and effective treatment of pain is central to animal welfare (Rutherford, 2002). There is a strong emphasis on pain among animal welfare researchers, with the number of pain-related articles in scientific journals considerably outweighing articles on the other Freedoms (freedom to behave normally, freedom from fear and distress, freedom from hunger and thirst, and freedom from discomfort) (Phillips, 2008).

National animal welfare advisory bodies in Australia, New Zealand, and the European Union have recommended steps to avoid or minimize animal pain and associated suffering, and the World Organization for Animal Health (OIE) produced a special edition in its Technical Series on "Scientific assessment and management of animal pain" (Mellor et al., 2008). Veterinary associations commonly have positions or policies advocating the effective management of pain in animals (CVMA, 2007; AVMA, 2011).

In theory, then, we agree that animals should not be in pain, yet studies show that attitudes toward pain vary greatly among societal groups responsible for animal care, including veterinarians. Veterinary attitudes toward pain and pain management in companion and production animals have been studied in Canada (Dohoo & Dohoo, 1996; Hewson et al., 2006b, 2007a, 2007b), the United States (Hellyer et al., 1999), the United Kingdom (Lascelles et al., 1999; Capner et al., 1999; Huxley, 2006), Finland (Raekallio et al., 2003), Scandinavia (Thomsen et al., 2010), Europe (Hugonnard et al., 2004; Guatteo et al., 2008), and New Zealand (Laven et al., 2009). Other surveys have looked at the attitudes of veterinary and animal science students (Levine et al., 2005; Heleski & Zanella, 2006; Kielland et al., 2009).

These studies reveal some common themes. Considerable variation in clinical recognition and treatment of pain exists in both companion and production animal practice. A perception that an animal is in pain is a decisive factor in the provision of analgesia, yet there is great variation in pain ratings among veterinarians. Women and more recent graduates generally tended to rate pain more highly and treat it more frequently (Dohoo & Dohoo, 1996; Lascelles et al., 1999; Raekallio et al., 2003; Williams et al., 2005; Huxley, 2006; Laven et al., 2009) and increased usage of analgesics among newer veterinarians may well be due to the changes in emphasis of the treatment of pain that have taken place in veterinary medicine during the past 10–15 years (Thomsen et al., 2010). Although the vast majority of respondents generally agree that provision of analgesia is beneficial, and that animals recover more quickly postoperatively if analgesia is provided, the myth still persists that postoperative pain provides some benefit in preventing animals from being too active (Raekallio et al., 2003; Guatteo et al., 2008), even among veterinarians who graduated in the 2000s (Thomsen et al., 2010)—despite the position, held since 1998, of the American College of Veterinary Anesthesiologists that unrelieved pain provides no benefits to animals (ACVA, 1998). Even where a large majority of respondents agree about the importance of treating pain, there is much variation in the circumstances under which pain is treated (Hellyer et al., 1999; Hugonnard et al., 2004; Whay & Huxley, 2005).

Data from repeat Canadian surveys were somewhat encouraging. A 1994 survey showed that approximately 50% of Canadian veterinarians did not use analgesics postoperatively in dogs and cats (Dohoo & Dohoo, 1996). Usage among the other 50% varied with the procedure, and opioids were used almost exclusively, predominantly butorphanol. A similar survey in 2001 showed a marked increase in analgesic usage, with only about 12% of Canadian veterinarians not using analgesics (Hewson et al., 2006b). Given, however, the low usage of perioperative analgesics for many surgeries, together with a continued overreliance on weak opioids (e.g., butorphanol, meperidine) and under usage of strong opioids and NSAIDs, it was evident that postoperative pain was not being managed effectively much of the time.

In the 1994 survey, pain perception scores attributed to different surgical procedures were one of two primary factors affecting analgesic usage (the second was concern about the use of potent opioid agonists in the postoperative period) (Dohoo & Dohoo, 1996). Perception of pain was also a strong predictor of postoperative analgesic usage in 2001 (Hewson et al., 2006a); ratings of pain caused by different surgeries had increased markedly since 1994. In both surveys, veterinarians identified lectures and seminars at the regional level, as well as review articles, as the preferred way to receive continuing education regarding pain and analgesia.

PAINFUL HUSBANDRY PRACTICES IN FARM ANIMALS

The use of at least some degree of perioperative analgesia is fairly widespread in small animal practice (Lascelles et al., 1999; Hugonnard et al., 2004; Hewson et al., 2006b), even if consistency is lacking and there is much room for improvement to provide truly effective, multimodal analgesia. The same cannot be said with large animals, where it remains customary to perform many procedures without anesthesia or analgesia, particularly in North America (Hewson et al., 2007b; Fulwider et al., 2008). However, in some countries analgesia is legally required when carrying out certain husbandry procedures. For example, all the Scandinavian countries now have regulations governing the use of anesthesia and analgesia for procedures such as dehorning and castrating calves (Thomsen et al., 2010). In New Zealand, analgesia is required for castration of cattle over 6 months and for dehorning in those over 9 months (Laven et al., 2009).

Surveys that have compared attitudes toward, and frequency of, pain alleviation in different species pointed out large differences among different animal species undergoing similar operations and among clinical conditions that received equal pain ratings (Hellyer et al., 1999; Raekallio et al., 2003). Even though there is no physiological basis for this differentiation, the discrepancy between practice in companion and production animals is pronounced (Stookey, 2005).

Roadblocks to Treating Pain in Farm Animals

There are many practices carried out routinely in the management of livestock and poultry that cause pain and distress (e.g., castration, tail docking, dehorning, branding, beak trimming). Many of these husbandry procedures are carried out on very young animals (e.g., tail docking in piglets and lambs, beak trimming in poultry); yet there is mounting evidence that such tissue damage early in life may program the animal to a lasting state of somatosensory sensitization and increased pain (Viñuela-Fernández et al., 2007).

Cost–benefit analyses of performing such procedures as an aid to management have too often ignored the costs to the animals themselves in terms of pain and suffering (Hewson, 2006). Increasingly, the public expects pain relief to be provided to farm animals (Phillips et al., 2009; Whay & Main, 2009), yet there are economic, practical, and regulatory constraints, such as the cost of treatment relative to the monetary value of the individual animal, limited availability of licensed analgesic drugs in food animals, and concern about drug residues and food safety (Viñuela-Fernández et al., 2007; Mellor et al., 2008a).

In considering a harm/benefit analysis of husbandry procedures, we should first attempt to minimize the harm (Weary et al., 2006) by asking questions such as:

1. Is the procedure necessary? Is it justified in terms of direct benefit to the animals and/or to the farming enterprise? For example hot iron branding is a cause of avoidable pain to animals and yet, since 2005, a US trade rule has required that all feeder cattle entering the United States from Canada be branded, despite the fact that Canadian cattle for export already bear an ear tag traceable to the farm of origin through the Canadian Cattle Identification infrastructure (Whiting, 2005). Is there another way of achieving the same end, for example, the development of polled breeds to eliminate the need for dehorning calves or immunocastration in calves, piglets, and lambs (Stafford & Mellor, 2009)?

2. What harms are caused, how bad are they, can they be avoided or reduced (e.g., through treatment of pain)?

3. What are the availability, cost, effectiveness, and ease of administration of pain-relieving drugs? Are there adverse effects or residues? Is administration by a veterinarian required?

Husbandry practices with no benefits for animals or farmers may become entrenched. For example, studies have shown no benefits of tail docking in dairy cows, and yet this practice, which has been shown to cause acute and chronic pain, as well as increased fly numbers, and to which the American and Canadian Veterinary Medical Associations are officially opposed (AVMA, 2009, CVMA, 2010), is still widespread in the United States (Fulwider et al., 2008).

The recognition of pain in species such as cattle and sheep may be more difficult because, as prey species, there was strong evolutionary pressure to mask signs of pain and associated weakness (Phillips, 2002; Rutherford, 2002). A large European survey describing pain management practices in cattle (Guatteo et al., 2008) showed very high variability among veterinarians in the knowledge of and sensitivity to pain in cattle. Again, awareness of and ability to assess an animal's pain were critical to the decision on whether to treat pain. In a similar survey in the United Kingdom, cattle practitioners who did not use analgesics assigned significantly lower pain scores to painful procedures or conditions (Huxley, 2006).

In such studies, veterinarians expressed the concern that producers would be unwilling to pay additional costs of providing analgesia (Whay et al., 2005; Huxley, 2006; Hewson et al., 2007a; Guatteo et al., 2008). However, a follow-up study (Huxley & Whay, 2007) showed that, for a significant minority of cattle farmers, the cost of providing analgesia may not be a barrier. For castration and dehorning, for example, 40% and 25% of respondents, respectively, were prepared to pay additional fees sufficient to cover the cost of appropriate analgesic drugs (local anesthesia and NSAIDs). Fifty-three percent of farmers surveyed agreed with the statement "Veterinary surgeons do not discuss controlling pain in cattle with farmers enough."

As well, there are costs to NOT providing analgesia. Apart from causing animal suffering, pain can cause significant economic losses (Denaburski & Tworkowska, 2009; Whay & Main, 2009; Grandin, 2009). Yet, a UK study (Leach et al., 2010) showed that, despite a high prevalence of lameness in dairy cows (36% in farms surveyed in 2006–2007), the majority of farmers did not perceive lameness to be a problem on their farm, and underestimated the cost of pain to production.

Management of pain is dependent on the stockperson (or animal caregiver) and the veterinarian. Effective pain management requires recognition of the pain, provision of an environment where the animal can recover, and knowledge about and provision of appropriate analgesic drugs. The ways in which an animal is handled and cared for can exacerbate or mitigate pain and distress. Studies in all major farm animal species have confirmed a strong relationship between the methods used in handling animals, the degree of fear the animals show toward people, and the productivity of the farm (Rushen & Passillé, 2009). For example, a large study of US dairy farms showed lower somatic cell counts in the milk and tendencies to lower percentages of lame cows and shorter calving intervals on farms where the cows were more willing to approach the observer (Fulwider et al., 2008).

A special issue of *Applied Animal Behaviour Science*, "Pain in Farm Animals," summarizes current knowledge about addressing many of the major causes of such pain, for example, disbudding and dehorning in cattle (Stafford & Mellor, 2011a), castration in pigs and other livestock (Sutherland & Tucker, 2011), identification and prevention of intra- and postoperative pain (Walker et al., 2011), and pain issues in poultry (Gentle, 2011).

THE WAY FORWARD

There have been many advances in the understanding of and ability to treat pain in animals in recent decades. We have the knowledge to effectively manage perioperative pain through multimodal analgesia and there are practical resources available to assist veterinarians to do so (Tranquilli et al., 2004; Cracknell, 2007; Flecknell et al., 2007; Lemke & Crook, 2011). There are published recommendations for managing painful procedures in large animals (Lemke et al., 2008; Stafford & Mellor, 2011b), although there are still many constraints. The management of chronic pain continues to present a challenge.

The widespread finding that a veterinarian's perception of pain is a significant predictor of analgesic usage is a major concern, especially considering pain ratings vary so markedly. A persuasive case is made in pediatric medicine against allowing personal beliefs about the experience of pain to prevent "optimal recognition and treatment of pain for all children" (Hagen et al., 2001). Veterinary practitioners must adopt the same approach for animals.

Veterinarians commonly feel their knowledge of issues related to recognition and management of pain is inadequate, and are interested in continuing education opportunities to address this lack. There is a great deal of information available on assessment and management of pain, which needs to be better communicated to veterinary students and veterinarians.

So what can veterinarians do to better manage pain in animals? Veterinarians working with all species should avail themselves of continuing education regularly to ensure they have current knowledge about recognizing, assessing, and managing pain. Veterinarians working with large animals should ensure that they inform farmers of the strategies available to mitigate pain associated with production practices and with chronic conditions, and of the resulting benefits to the animal and to the bottom line. And veterinarians, as a profession, can work with other stakeholders, as expected of them by society as advocates for animals, to address regulatory, technological, and economic constraints.

REFERENCES

ACVA (1998) American college of veterinary anesthesiologists' position paper on the treatment of pain in animals. *Journal of the American Veterinary Medical Association*, 213(5), 628–630.

AVMA (2009) *Tail Docking of Cattle* [Homepage of the American Veterinary Medical Association], http://www.avma.org/issues/policy/animal_welfare/tail_docking_cattle.asp (accessed July 24, 2013).

AVMA (2011) *Animal Welfare Policies* [Homepage of the American Veterinary Medical Association], https://www.avma.org/KB/Policies/Pages/Pain-in-Animals.aspx (accessed July 24, 2013).

Bermond, B. (2001) A neuropsychological and evolutionary approach to animal consciousness and animal suffering. *Animal Welfare*, 10, S47–S62.

Capner, C.A., Lascelles, B.D.X., & Watermann-Pearson, A. (1999) Current British veterinary attitudes to perioperative analgesia for dogs. *Veterinary Record*, 145(4), 95–99.

Cracknell, J. (2007) *Analgesia in Exotics: A Review and Update*, British Veterinary Zoological Society, Romford, UK.

CVMA (2010) *Tail Docking of Dairy Cattle* [Homepage of the Canadian Veterinary Medical Association], http://www.canadianveterinarians.net/documents/tail-docking-of-dairy-cattle#.UfANWG0U0ms (accessed July 24, 2013).

CVMA (2007) *Pain Control in Animals* [Homepage of the Canadian Veterinary Medical Association], http://www.canadianveterinarians.net/documents/pain-control-in-animals#.UfAN3W0U0ms (accessed July 24, 2013).

Denaburski, J. & Tworkowska, A. (2009) The problem of pain in farm animals and its effects on animal welfare and certain economic results. *Polish Journal of Veterinary Sciences*, 12(1), 123–131.

Dohoo, S.E. & Dohoo, I.R. (1996) Postoperative use of analgesics in dogs and cats by Canadian veterinarians. *The Canadian Veterinary Journal. La Revue Vétérinaire Canadienne*, 37(9), 546–551.

Farm Animal Welfare Council (2009) *Five Freedoms* [Homepage of FAWC], http://www.fawc.org.uk/freedoms.htm (accessed July 24, 2013).

Flecknell, P., Gledhill, J., & Richardson, C. (2007) Assessing animal health and welfare and recognising pain and distress. *ALTEX*, 24, Spec No 82–83.

Flower, F.C., Sedlbauer, M., Carter, E., von Keyserlingk, M.A., Sanderson, D.J., & Weary, D.M. (2008) Analgesics improve the gait of lame dairy cattle. *Journal of dairy science*, 91(8), 3010–3014.

Föllmi, J., Steiger, A., Walzer, C., et al. (2007) A scoring system to evaluate physical condition and quality of life in geriatric zoo mammals. *Animal Welfare*, 16(3), 309–318.

Fulwider, W.K., Grandin, T., Rollin, B.E., Engle, T.E., Dalsted, N.L., & Lamm, W.D. (2008) Survey of dairy management practices on one hundred thirteen north central and northeastern United States dairies. *Journal of dairy science*, 91(4), 1686–1692.

Gentle, M.J. (2001) Attentional shifts alter pain perception in the chicken. *Animal Welfare*, 10, S187.

Gentle, M.J. (2011) Pain issues in poultry. *Applied Animal Behaviour Science*, 135(3), 252–258.

Grandin, T. (2009) *The Importance of Measurement to Improve the Welfare of Livestock, Poultry and Fish*, CABI, Wallingford, UK.

Guatteo, R., Holopherne, D., Whay, H.R., & Huxley, J.N. (2008). Attitudes et pratiques actuelles des vétérinaires praticiens dans la prise en charge de la douleur des bovins [Attitudes and practices of veterinary practitioners in the management of pain in cattle]. *Bulletin des GTV*, 44, 57–64.

Hagen, J.F., Coleman, W.L., Foy, J.M., et al. (2001) The assessment and management of acute pain in infants, children, and adolescents. *Pediatrics*, 108(3), 793.

Heleski, C.R. & Zanella, A.J. (2006) Animal science student attitudes to farm animal welfare. *Anthrozoös*, 19(1), 3–16.

Hellyer, P.W., Frederick, C., Lacy, M., Salman, M.D., & Wagner, A.E. (1999) Attitudes of veterinary medical students, house officers, clinical faculty, and staff toward pain management in animals. *Journal of the American Veterinary Medical Association*, 214(2), 238–244.

Hewson, C.J. (2006) "Eat well, spend less." The costs of cheap food to animals and humans. *Canadian Veterinary Journal*, 47(1), 38–41.

Hewson, C.J., Dohoo, I.R., & Lemke, K.A. (2006a) Factors affecting the use of postincisional analgesics in dogs and cats by Canadian veterinarians in 2001. *Canadian Veterinary Journal*, 47(5), 453–459.

Hewson, C.J., Dohoo, I.R., & Lemke, K.A. (2006b) Perioperative use of analgesics in dogs and cats by Canadian veterinarians in 2001. *Canadian Veterinary Journal*, 47(4), 352–359.

Hewson, C.J., Dohoo, I.R., Lemke, K.A., & Barkema, H.W. (2007a) Factors affecting Canadian veterinarians' use of analgesics when dehorning beef and dairy calves. *Canadian Veterinary Journal*, 48(11), 1129–1136.

Hewson, C.J., Dohoo, I.R., Lemke, K.A., & Barkema, H.W. (2007b) Canadian veterinarians' use of analgesics in cattle, pigs, and horses in 2004 and 2005. *The Canadian Veterinary Journal. La Revue Vétérinaire Canadienne*, 48(2), 155–164.

Hugonnard, M., Leblond, A., Keroack, S., Cadore, J., & Troncy, E. (2004) Attitudes and concerns of French veterinarians towards pain and analgesia in dogs and cats. *Veterinary Anaesthesia & Analgesia*, 31(3), 154–163.

Huxley, J.N. & Whay, H.R. (2006) Current attitudes of cattle practitioners to pain and the use of analgesics in cattle. *The Veterinary Record*, 159(20), 662–668.

Huxley, J.N. & Whay, H.R. (2007) Attitudes of UK veterinary surgeons and cattle farmers to pain and the use of analgesics in cattle. *Cattle Practice*, 15(2), 189–193.

IASP (1994) Pain terms, a current list with definitions and notes on usage in *Classification of Chronic Pain*, 2nd edn (eds H. Merskey & N. Bogduk), IASP Press, Seattle, WA, pp. 209–214.

Johnson, C.B. (2008) Lessons learned from pain management in humans, in *Scientific Assessment and Management of Animal Pain*, (eds D.J. Mellor, P.M. Thornber, D. Bayvel, et al.), OIE (World Organisation for Animal Health), Paris, pp. 184–194.

Kielland, C., Skjerve, E., & Zanella, A.J. (2009) Attitudes of veterinary students to pain in cattle. *Veterinary Record*, 165(9), 254–258.

Lascelles, B.D.X., Capner, C.A., & Watermann-Pearson, A. (1999) Current British veterinary attitudes to perioperative analgesia for cats and small mammals. *Veterinary Record*, 145(21), 601–604.

Laven, R.A., Huxley, J.N., Whay, H.R., & Stafford, K.J. (2009) Results of a survey of attitudes of dairy veterinarians in New Zealand regarding painful procedures and conditions in cattle. *New Zealand Veterinary Journal*, 57(4), 215–220.

Leach, K.A., Whay, H.R., Maggs, C.M., et al. (2010) Working towards a reduction in cattle lameness: 1. Understanding barriers to lameness control on dairy farms. *Research in Veterinary Science*, 89(2), 311–317.

Lemke, K.A. & Crook, A.D. (2011) *Examples of Anaesthetic and Pain Management Protocols for Healthy Cats and Dogs*, 2nd edn [Homepage of the Canadian Veterinary Medical Association], http://www.upei.ca/awc/files/awc/English%20poster%20indiv.panels_0.pdf (accessed July 24, 2013).

Lemke, K.A., Hewson, C.J., & Crook, A.D. (2008) *Examples of Anaesthetic and Pain Management Protocols for Large Animals* [Homepage of the Canadian Veterinary Medical Association], http://www.upei.ca/awc/files/awc/Poster%20ENG%203%20Sep%20Pages.pdf (accessed July 24, 2013).

Levine, E.D., Mills, D.S., & Houpt, K.A. (2005) Attitudes of veterinary students at one US college toward factors relating to farm animal welfare. *Journal of Veterinary Medical Education*, 32(4), 481–490.

Mathews, K.A. (2000) Pain assessment and general approach to management. *The Veterinary Clinics Of North America Small Animal Practice*, 30(4), 729.

McMillan, F.D. (2003) Maximizing quality of life in ill animals. *Journal of the American Animal Hospital Association*, 39(3), 227–235.

Mellor, D.J., Fisher, M.W., & Stafford, K.J. (2008) *A Cost-benefit Analysis of Pain Relief for Farm Animals*, in *Scientific Assessment and Management of Animal Pain*, (eds D.J. Mellor, P.M. Thornber, D. Bayvel, et al.), OIE (World Organisation for Animal Health), Paris, pp. 47–55.

Mellor, D.J., Thornber, P.M., Bayvel, D., & Kahn, S. (2008) *Scientific Assessment and Management of Animal Pain*, OIE (World Organisation for Animal Health), Paris.

Melzack, R. (1993) Pain: past, present and future. *Canadian Journal of Experimental Psychology*, 47(4), 615.

Morton, C.M. (2005) Application of a scaling model to establish and validate an interval level pain scale for assessment of acute pain in dogs. *American Journal of Veterinary Research*, 66(12), 2154–2166.

Phillips, C. (2008) *Pain As An Animal Welfare Issue*, in *Scientific Assessment and Management of Animal Pain*, (eds D.J. Mellor, P.M. Thornber, D. Bayvel, et al.), OIE (World Organisation for Animal Health), Paris, pp. 38–46.

Phillips, C. (2002) Environmental perception and cognition in *Cattle Behaviour and Welfare*, 2nd edn (ed. C. Phillips), Blackwell Science, Oxford, pp. 49–61.

Phillips, C.J., Wojciechowska, J., Meng, J., & Cross, N. (2009) Perceptions of the importance of different welfare issues in livestock production. *Animal*, 3(8), 1152–1166.

Raekallio, M., Heinonen, K.M., Kuussaari, J., & Vainio, O. (2003) Pain alleviation in animals: attitudes and practices of Finnish veterinarians. *Veterinary Journal*, 165(2), 131–135.

Roughan, J.V. & Flecknell, P.A. (2003) Evaluation of a short duration behaviour-based post-operative pain scoring system in rats. *European Journal of Pain (London, England)*, 7(5), 397–406.

Rushen, J. & Passillé, A.M.D. (2009) *The Importance of Good Stockmanship and Its Benefits for the Animals*, CABI, Wallingford, UK.

Rutherford, K.M.D. (2002) Assessing pain in animals. *Animal Welfare*, 11, 31–53.

Stafford, K.J. & Mellor, D.J. (2009) *Painful Husbandry Procedures in Livestock and Poultry*, CABI, Wallingford, UK.

Stafford, K.J. & Mellor, D.J. (2005) The welfare significance of the castration of cattle: a review. *New Zealand Veterinary Journal*, 53(5), 271–278.

Stafford, K.J. & Mellor, D.J. (2011) Addressing the pain associated with disbudding and dehorning in cattle. *Applied Animal Behaviour Science*, 135(3), 226–231.

Stookey, J.M. (2005) The veterinarian's role in controlling pain in farm animals. *The Canadian Veterinary Journal. La Revue Vétérinaire Canadienne*, 46(5), 453.

Sutherland, M.A. & Tucker, C.B. (2011) The long and short of it: a review of tail docking in farm animals. *Applied Animal Behaviour Science*, 135(3), 179–191.

Thomsen, P.T., Gidekull, M., Herskin, M.S., et al. (2010) Scandinavian bovine practitioners' attitudes to the use of analgesics in cattle. *Veterinary Record*, 167(7), 256–258.

Tranquilli, W.J., Grimm, K.A., & Lamont, L.A. (2004) *Pain Management for the Small Animal Practitioner*, 2nd edn, Teton NewMedia, Jackson, WY.

Vickers, K.J., Niel, L., Kiehlbauch, L.M., & Weary, D.M. (2005) Calf response to caustic paste and hot-iron dehorning using sedation with and without local anesthetic. *Journal of Dairy Science*, 88(4), 1454–1459.

Viñuela-Fernández, I., Jones, E., Welsh, E.M., & Fleetwood-Walker, S.M. (2007) Pain mechanisms and their implication for the management of pain in farm and companion animals. *Veterinary Journal* 174(2), 227–239.

Walker, K.A., Duffield, T.F., & Weary, D.M. (2011) Identifying and preventing pain during and after surgery in farm animals. *Applied Animal Behaviour Science*, 135(3), 259–265.

Weary, D.M. & Fraser, D. (2008) *Identifying Pain in Farm Animals*, in *Scientific Assessment and Management of Animal Pain*, (eds D.J. Mellor, P.M. Thornber, D. Bayvel, et al.), OIE (World Organisation for Animal Health), Paris, pp. 157–171.

Weary, D.M., Niel, L., Flower, F.C., & Fraser, D. (2006) Identifying and preventing pain in animals. *Applied Animal Behaviour Science*, 100(1–2), 64–76.

Webster, A.B. & Fletcher, D.L. (2004) Assessment of the aversion of hens to different gas atmospheres using an approach-avoidance test. *Applied Animal Behaviour Science*, 88(3), 275–287.

Whay, H.R., Webster, A.J., & Waterman-Pearson, A.E. (2005) Role of ketoprofen in the modulation of hyperalgesia associated with lameness in dairy cattle. *Veterinary Record*, 157(23), 729–733.

Whay, H.R. & Huxley, J.N. (2005) Pain relief in cattle: a practitioner's perspective. *Cattle Practice*, 13(2), 81–85.

Whay, H.R. & Main, D.C.J. (2009) *Improving Animal Welfare: Practical Approaches for Achieving Change*, CABI, Wallingford, UK.

Whiting, T.L. (2005) Hot iron branding - not a reasonable requirement for international trade in live ruminants. *Canadian Veterinary Journal*, 46(11), 1042–1046.

Williams, V.M., Lascelles, B.D.X., & Robson, M.C. (2005) Current attitudes to, and use of, peri-operative analgesia in dogs and cats by veterinarians in New Zealand. *New Zealand Veterinary Journal*, 53(3), 193–202.

Wiseman-Orr, M., Nolan, A.M., Reid, J., & Scott, E.M. (2004) Development of a questionnaire to measure the effects of chronic pain on health-related quality of life in dogs. *American Journal of Veterinary Research*, 65(8), 1077–1084.

Wiseman-Orr, M., Scott, E.M., Reid, J., et al. (2006) Validation of a structured questionnaire as an instrument to measure chronic pain in dogs on the basis of effects on health-related quality of life. *American Journal of Veterinary Research*, 67(11), 1826–1836.

Wojciechowska, J.I., Hewson, C.J., Stryhn, H., Guy, N.C., Patronek, G.J, Timmons, V. (2005) Development of a discriminative questionnaire to assess nonphysical aspects of quality of life of dogs. *American Journal of Veterinary Research*, 66(8), 1453–1460.

Yazbek, K.V.B. & Fantoni, D.T. (2005) Validity of a health-related quality-of-life scale for dogs with signs of pain secondary to cancer. *Journal of the American Veterinary Medical Association*, 226(8), 1354–1358.

2

Anatomy, Physiology, and Pathophysiology of Pain

Yael Shilo and Peter J. Pascoe

Pain in animals has been defined as "an aversive sensory and emotional experience representing an awareness by the animal of damage or threat to the integrity of its tissues; it changes the animal's physiology and behavior to reduce or avoid damage, to reduce the likelihood of recurrence, and to promote recovery" (Molony & Kent, 1997).

The ability to react to environmental change is crucial for the survival of an organism, and an essential prerequisite is the capacity to detect and respond to aversive stimuli. Primary afferent nerve fibers provide information to the central nervous system (CNS) about the environment and also about the state of the organism itself. Incoming non-noxious input from the periphery is important for discerning fine discriminative touch, pressure, and position in space. Most animals have dedicated sensory afferents that respond to noxious stimuli. These nociceptive afferents are described by the International Association for the Study of Pain (IASP) as "preferentially sensitive to a noxious stimulus or to a stimulus which would become noxious if prolonged" (Wall et al., 2006; Smith & Lewin, 2009). Information about a noxious event in the periphery can initiate a protective reflexive withdrawal event (Westlund, 2005; Smith & Lewin, 2009).

Nociception, derived from the Latin *nocere* meaning "to hurt/harm," is the name given to the process by which organisms detect potentially or actually damaging stimuli and the transmission of that information to the brain. It is important to differentiate nociception from pain, which always encompasses an emotional component. Nociceptor activation in and of itself does not necessarily result in pain (Julius & Basbaum, 2001; Muir & Woolf, 2001; Smith & Lewin, 2009; Basser, 2012).

Noxious input is transmitted to the brain through specialized receptors, fibers, and neurons, and processing occurs at many levels (Figure 2.1). Sensory processing includes

Transduction: the conversion of noxious stimuli into an action potential at the level of the specialized receptors or free nerve endings.
Transmission: the propagation of the action potentials by primary afferent neurons to the spinal cord.
Modulation: the process by which nociceptive information is augmented or inhibited.

Projection : the conveyance of nociceptive information through the spinal cord to the brain (to the brainstem and thalamus and then to the cortex).
Perception: the integration of the nociceptive information by the brain, or, in other words, the overall conscious, emotional experience of pain (Muir & Woolf, 2001; Westlund, 2005; Muir, 2009).

NOCICEPTORS

Activation of nociceptors requires that adequate stimuli depolarize peripheral terminals (producing a receptor potential) with sufficient amplitude and duration. This ensures that despite any attenuation and slowing of the action potential (by passive propagation), information such as stimulus intensity will be encoded in the resulting train of impulses (Dubin & Patapoutian, 2010).

Nociceptive neurons that detect chemical stimuli have a distinct expression of ion channel systems or transduction channels, including transient receptor potential (TRP) ion channels, acid-sensing ion channels (ASIC), purinoceptors, serotonin receptors, and sodium, calcium, and potassium channels (Wall et al., 2006). Agents such as protons or capsaicin directly depolarize nociceptive neurons by triggering the opening of cation channels permeable to sodium and/or calcium. In contrast, agents such as bradykinin and nerve growth factor (NGF) act on G protein-coupled receptors and receptor tyrosine kinase, respectively, to initiate intracellular signaling cascades that, in turn, sensitize depolarizing cation channels to their respective physical or chemical regulators. Other agents, such as glutamate, acetylcholine (ACh), and adenosine triphosphate (ATP), activate ion channels and G-protein-coupled receptors to produce a spectrum of direct and indirect effects on nociceptor membrane potentials (Caterina et al., 2005). This chapter will focus on several important transduction channels; however, it is beyond the scope of this chapter to discuss all of these.

Transient Receptor Potential Ion Channel

The TRPs have emerged as a family of principal transducing channels on sensory neurons, and are classified according to their primary amino acid sequence (rather than according to their selectivity or ligand affinity), as their properties are heterogeneous and their

Pain Management in Veterinary Practice, First Edition. Edited by Christine M. Egger, Lydia Love and Tom Doherty.
© 2014 John Wiley & Sons, Inc. Published 2014 by John Wiley & Sons, Inc.

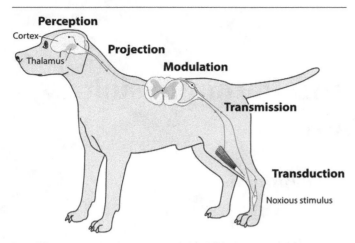

Figure 2.1. Pathways involved in nociception. Noxious stimuli (mechanical, chemical, thermal) are transduced into electrical signals that are transmitted to the spinal cord, where they are modulated before being relayed (projected) to the brain for final processing and awareness (Reprinted from Muir, W.W., 3rd. (2009). Physiology and Pathophysiology of Pain, in: J.S. Gaynor & W. W. Muir, 3rd (eds). *Handbook of Veterinary Pain Management*, p. 14. Copyright MOSBY Elsevier (2009). Reproduced with permission from Elsevier.

regulation is complex. The transient receptor potential vanilloid (TRPV) channels were first named vanilloid receptors after the active vanillyl structure in the family of compounds that activate these channels. The TRPV1 is a ligand-gated, nonselective cation channel with a preference for Ca^{2+}, which is also activated by noxious stimuli including heat ($>43°C$), protons, pH < 5.9, and various peptides. Upon opening, Transient Receptor Ion Channel (in particular, Ca^{2+}) flow into the cell and depolarize it. The TRPV1 receptor is predominantly expressed in sensory neurons, and is believed to play a crucial role in temperature sensing and nociception (Caterina et al., 2000; Wall et al., 2006; Rohacs et al., 2008; Vriens et al., 2009; Chung et al., 2011; Schaible et al., 2011). Disruption of the TRPV1 gene in mice eliminates or severely reduces the responses to vanilloid compounds, acid, and heat ($>43°C$) (Caterina et al., 2000). Thermosensitive TRP channels respond to a wide range of ambient temperatures and may account for the detection of all commonly encountered thermal stimuli, from noxious cold to noxious heat. For example, TRPA1 is sensitive to temperatures less than $17°C$, TRPM8 to temperatures of $8°C–26°C$, TRPV4 to temperatures over $27°C$, TRPV3 to temperatures over $31°C$, TRPV1 to temperatures over $43°C$, and TRPV2 to temperatures over $52°C$ (Wall et al., 2006).

Capsaicin, the hydrophobic compound that lends "hot" capsicum peppers their pungency, is one of a family of structurally related compounds isolated from plants and animals that are essentially sensitizers at TRPV1 because they act by decreasing the thermal "physiological" activation threshold of TRPV1. Nevertheless, because these compounds bind directly to TRPV1 they are considered agonists or direct activators of this channel, resulting in pain sensation when administered subcutaneously. However, TRPV1-containing neurons can be rendered insensitive to further painful stimuli through receptor desensitization in response to capsaicin,

which can result in a generalized lack of responsiveness of this receptor to further noxious stimuli (Caterina et al., 2005; Vyklicky et al., 2008; Vriens et al., 2009; Rosenbaum et al., 2010; Chung et al., 2011). This is the rationale for the topical application of capsaicin and other vanilloids in the treatment of some painful conditions, as capsaicin causes persistent functional desensitization of polymodal primary nociceptors after repeated or prolonged application. This desensitization is suggested to have multiple mechanisms of action and likely involves increasing intracellular free Ca^{2+} concentrations. The Ca^{2+} influx activates Ca^{2+}-sensitive phospholipase C (PLC), leading to depletion of phosphatidylinositol 4,5-bisphosphate (PIP_2), which leads to diminished channel activity. The calcium sensor calmodulin has also been implicated in desensitization, directly and indirectly, by activating the protein phosphatase calcineurin. ATP may also play a role in this complex process. This TRPV1 desensitization depends on the channel concentration and duration of exposure to capsaicin, and may represent a feedback mechanism protecting the cell from toxic Ca^{2+} overload (Leffler et al., 2008; Rohacs et al., 2008; Vyklicky et al., 2008).

Although the role of TRPV1 has been primarily studied in cutaneous pain models, it is evident that TRPV1 is involved in nociception not only in skin but also in musculoskeletal and visceral tissues. Expression of TRPV1 has also been demonstrated in the spinal cord, mainly laminae I and II of the dorsal horn (Caterina et al., 2000; Rohacs et al., 2008; Chung et al., 2011).

Sensory Neuronal Sodium Channel

When noxious stimuli result in adequate depolarization, voltage-gated sodium channels open and action potentials are generated. Voltage-gated sodium channels (Na_v) are complex transmembrane proteins that allow the rapid influx of sodium underlying the depolarizing upstroke of action potentials in excitable cells. Na_v typically open (activate) within a millisecond in response to membrane depolarizations, leading to a regenerative all-or-none depolarization typical of action potentials in neurons (Cummins et al., 2007; Schaible et al., 2011).

Nine distinct Na_v α-subunits (Na_v 1.1–1.9) have been cloned from mammals. Many of the Na_v 1 α-subunits have specific developmental, tissue, or cellular distributions: Na_v 1.4 is almost exclusively expressed in skeletal muscle; Na_v 1.5 is predominantly expressed in cardiac muscle; Na_v 1.3 is predominantly expressed in immature neurons and is normally found at very low concentrations in adult neurons. However, under certain conditions Na_v 1.3 expression is upregulated in adult neurons, and this may play a role in altered pain sensation. Adult CNS neurons may express combinations of Na_v 1.1, Na_v 1.2, and Na_v 1.6. Adult dorsal root ganglia (DRG) sensory neurons can express combinations of Na_v 1.1, Na_v 1.6, Na_v 1.7, Na_v 1.8, and Na_v 1.9, and peripheral primary sensory afferents express Na_v 1.7, Na_v 1.8, and Na_v 1.9 (Cummins et al., 2007; Qi et al., 2011).

Tetrodotoxin (TTX), a toxin found in the liver of the puffer fish, is a highly selective blocker of CNS and skeletal muscle sodium currents but a relatively weak blocker of cardiac muscle sodium currents, emphasizing that distinct proteins generate the sodium currents in different tissues. While CNS neurons express relatively homogeneous currents exhibiting rapid activation, rapid inactivation, and high sensitivity to TTX, DRG neurons express more complex currents that contain both rapidly inactivating TTX-sensitive (TTX-S) components and slowly inactivating TTX-resistant (TTX-R) components. The slower TTX-R currents are thought to prolong the duration of the action potentials, thereby modulating neurotransmitter release at the nerve terminals. The sodium channels Na_v 1.1, Na_v 1.3, Na_v 1.6, and Na_v 1.7 are TTX-S, whereas Na_v 1.8 and Na_v 1.9 are TTX-R (Cummins et al., 2007; Schaible et al., 2011).

The resting potential of DRG neurons is about −60 mV. After small depolarizations (at −50 to −40 mV), Na_v 1.7 opens and this initial Na^+ influx brings the neuron closer to the membrane potential for elicitation of an action potential. The Na_v 1.8, which is expressed only in sensory neurons and largely restricted to nociceptive neurons, opens at −30 to −20 mV, that is, when the cell has been predepolarized (e.g., by Na_v 1.7), and provides about 80% of the inward current of the upstroke of the action potential in DRG neurons. In particular, Na_v 1.8 is located primarily on the terminals and the cell body, suggesting a role in action potential initiation at the sensory terminal of nociceptive neurons. It also mediates repetitive action potentials during persistent membrane depolarization (e.g., in the presence of inflammatory mediators). While Na_v 1.7 and Na_v 1.8 are directly involved in the generation of the action potential, Na_v 1.9 influences the threshold for action potentials. The channel opens around −60 mV and conducts persistent Na^+ currents at voltages below the threshold for action potential generation, thus regulating the distance between membrane potential and threshold; it does not contribute to the upstroke of the action potential (Schaible et al., 2011).

Acid-sensing Ion Channel

Nociceptive neurons can also be activated by reductions in extracellular pH, as is often observed in tissue injury, inflammation, or ischemia. One group of ion channels implicated in acid-evoked nociception is the ASIC family of proteins, which are highly selective Na^+ channels expressed in DRG neurons. It is believed that ASICs are most important in skeletal muscle and the heart, in which impaired circulation causes immediate pain (Caterina et al., 2005; Schaible et al., 2011).

NOCICEPTIVE AFFERENTS

The cell bodies of nociceptive afferents are located in the DRG and the trigeminal ganglion and extend central axonal endings into the spinal gray matter to communicate with second-order neurons in the dorsal horn (terminating predominantly in laminae I, II, and V) or the trigeminal subnucleus caudalis (Vc) in the caudal medulla, respectively (Westlund, 2005; Smith & Lewin, 2009; Dubin & Patapoutian, 2010).

Nociceptive afferents may be subclassified with respect to the presence or absence of myelination, the modalities of stimulation that evoke a response (i.e., thermal, mechanical, or chemical), the response characteristics (rapid versus slow response), and the distinctive chemical markers (e.g., receptors expressed on the membrane). The most common means of classification of primary sensory neurons is based on the conduction velocity of their peripheral axons, which is directly related to the axon diameter and the degree of axonal myelination. Based on peripheral conduction velocities, primary sensory neurons are routinely divided into different groups: Aβ, Aδ, and C (Table 2.1) (Caterina et al., 2005; Wall et al., 2006; Dubin & Patapoutian, 2010).

Nociceptive afferents responding to thermal (heat, H and cold, C), mechanical (M), and chemical stimuli (polymodal) are the most common C-fiber type observed in fiber recordings (C-MH, C-MC, C-MHC). C fibers responsive to noxious heat (C-H; ~10% of C-nociceptors) play a major role in heat sensation. A-δ fiber

Table 2.1. Primary afferent axons

Fiber type	Diameter[a]	Myelination	Conduction velocity	Stimuli	Innervation	Activation result/signaling
Aβ fibers	Large diameter	Thick myelin sheath	Very rapid >10 m/s	Detecting non-noxious mechanical stimuli, proprioception	Variety of defined structures in the hair and skin, such as hair follicles and Meissner corpuscles	Pleasant touch and position in space
Aδ fibers	Medium diameter	Lightly myelinated	Medium conduction 2–10 m/s	Nociceptors activated by high-intensity, noxious stimuli	Lose their myelin and terminate as free endings in the epidermis	Fast pricking or sharp pain
C fibers	Small diameter	Unmyelinated	Slow conduction <1.5 m/s	Polymodal nociceptors activated by noxious stimuli. Some have low-threshold properties and are activated by innocuous stimuli	Terminate in the skin as free nerve endings	Slow burning, aching pain

[a]Specific diameter changes with animal size.
Sources: Julius & Basbaum, 2001; Wall et al., 2006; Smith & Lewin, 2009.

nociceptors are predominantly heat- and/or mechanosensitive (A-MH, A-H, A-M); however, sensitivity to noxious cold is also observed (Smith & Lewin, 2009; Dubin & Patapoutian, 2010). See Table 2.1 for detailed comparison among fiber types (Julius & Basbaum, 2001; Smith & Lewin, 2009).

Approximately half of Aδ-fiber nociceptors and 30% of C-fiber nociceptors have very high mechanical thresholds (>6 bar = 600 kPa = 60 g/mm^2) or are unresponsive to mechanical stimuli. This class of nociceptors is termed "mechanically insensitive afferents," or "silent nociceptors." However, after exposure to inflammatory mediators, some of these insensitive fibers become responsive to mechanical and/or heat stimuli, a process known as sensitization (Wall et al., 2006; Smith & Lewin, 2009; Dubin & Patapoutian, 2010).

Primary sensory neurons are often classified according to their expression of molecular markers, and two broad categories of unmyelinated nociceptors (C fibers) have emerged: peptidergic cells that express calcitonin gene-related peptide (CGRP) and substance P (SP), and are sensitive to neural cell derived-NGF; and nonpeptidergic cells that lack these peptides but express the receptor tyrosine kinase, have binding sites for the plant isolectin B4, and are responsive to glial cell line-derived neurotrophic factor. The central projections of these two nociceptor types are segregated in different laminae of the dorsal horn. Peptidergic neurons are thought to be involved with inflammatory pain and release SP and CGRP from their sensory endings, inducing vasodilation, plasma extravasation, and other effects, thus producing a "neurogenic inflammation" (Julius & Basbaum, 2001; Golden et al., 2010; Schaible et al., 2011). The nonpeptidergic neurons may be involved in neuropathic pain, that is, pain that arises from damage to the CNS or peripheral nervous system (Willcockson & Valtschanoff, 2008; Golden et al., 2010).

SPINAL CORD

A transverse section of the spinal cord shows a central canal filled with cerebrospinal fluid (CSF) surrounded by the gray matter—a region containing mainly the cell bodies of neurons and also dendrites, axons, and glial cells and the peripheral white matter—a region containing mostly axons and also glial cells (Figure 2.2).

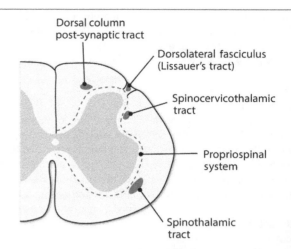

Figure 2.3.   The main ascending nociception pathways of the spinal cord in animals.

White Matter

The white matter is divided into three columns (or funiculi) by the horns of the gray matter: dorsal, lateral, and ventral (Figure 2.2). Ascending or descending axons that have a common function typically travel together and are identified as a tract, which is usually named for its origin and termination. The main ascending tracts associated with nociception in animals are the spinothalamic, the spinocervicothalamic (also termed spinocervical), and the postsynaptic dorsal column (Figure 2.3). The relative importance of these nerve tracts in transmitting noxious sensory information to the brain varies among species. For example, the spinothalamic pathway, which is the major ascending nociceptive pathway in rodents and primates, is thought to be less important in carnivores; however, the spinocervicothalamic tract is regarded as the dominant nociceptive pathway in carnivores (Fletcher, 1993). The postsynaptic dorsal column conveys information about visceral pain.

The propriospinal system (Figure 2.3) projects throughout the white matter and for varied distances both rostrally and caudally. Included are propriospinal fibers that travel between cervical and lumbosacral cord enlargements, long descending propriospinal tract (LDPT) axons, as well as short propriospinal tract axons that either ascend or descend for a few segments throughout the length of the cord. The propriospinal system is important in mediating reflex control in response to noxious stimuli, and in coordination during locomotion (Conta & Stelzner, 2004).

The dorsolateral fasciculus or the tract of Lissauer is situated between the dorsal horn and the surface of the spinal cord (Figure 2.3). It consists of overlapping ascending and descending axonal branches of small, primary afferent neurons, which respond to noxious, thermal, or tactile stimuli (Fletcher, 1993).

The Gray Matter

The gray matter is divided into three main zones: the dorsal horn, the ventral horn, and the lateral horn or intermediolateral column. The dorsal horn is comprised of sensory nuclei that receive and process incoming somatosensory information. The lateral horn is limited to the thoracic and upper two lumbar spinal cord segments. It contains preganglionic sympathetic neurons whose axons exit the spinal

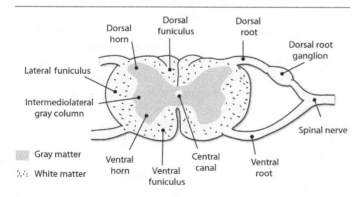

Figure 2.2.   A transverse section of the spinal cord.

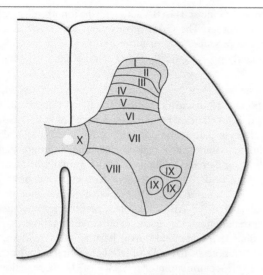

Figure 2.4. The Rexed laminae distinguish 10 different layers in the spinal gray matter on the basis of the characteristics of their neurons. The dorsal horn contains laminae I–VI, while the ventral horn, comprising the motor neurons, contains laminae VII–IX. Lamina X surrounds the central canal.

cord via the ventral roots. Preganglionic parasympathetic neurons are located in a comparable region of the gray matter at the S2–S4 levels of the spinal cord. The ventral horn comprises motor neurons that innervate skeletal muscle (Figure 2.2) (Goshgarian, 2003; Watson & Kayalioglu, 2009).

The distribution of cells and fibers within the gray matter of the spinal cord exhibits a pattern of lamination, which led Rexed in 1952 to propose a new classification based on 10 layers (laminae) (Figure 2.4). This classification is useful because it is related more accurately to function than the previous classification scheme, which was based on major nuclear groups. In general, the first six laminae compose the dorsal horn.

Lamina I, also known as the marginal layer, forms a thin sheet covering the dorsal aspect of the dorsal horn and contains projection neurons, with axons that travel rostrally in the white matter and convey information to various parts of the brain, and interneurons, with axons that remain in the spinal cord and contribute to local neuronal circuits. The projection cells are generally larger than the interneurons and a few particularly large projection neurons are known as giant marginal cells of Waldeyer.

Lamina II is known as the substantia gelatinosa because the lack of myelinated fibers within it gives it a translucent appearance in unstained sections. Virtually all of the neurons in this lamina are small interneurons and these are particularly densely packed in its outer part.

Lamina III also contains a high density of neurons. Most are small interneurons, which are generally somewhat larger than those of lamina II, but scattered large projection neurons are also present in this lamina.

Laminae IV–VI are more heterogeneous, with neurons of various sizes, some of which are projection cells. The borders between these

laminae are difficult to place with certainty. (Goshgarian, 2003; Wall et al., 2006).

Lamina VII contains all visceral motor neurons, whose axons extend to autonomic ganglia.

Laminae VIII and IX are in the ventral horn. Lamina VIII is composed of interneurons, whereas lamina IX is comprised of individual clusters of α motor neurons. The axons of these neurons innervate mainly skeletal muscle.

Lamina X is comprised of small neurons surrounding the central canal and contains neuroglia (Goshgarian, 2003; Watson & Kayalioglu, 2009).

C fibers and Aδ fibers convey nociceptive information principally to the superficial (laminae I/II) and deep (V/VI) laminae of the dorsal horn as well as to the circumcanular lamina X. Aβ fibers transmit non-noxious information to laminae III–VI (Millan, 2002).

DORSAL HORN NEURONS

The cell bodies of primary sensory neurons that innervate the limbs and trunk are located in the DRG. Their axons bifurcate within the ganglion and give rise to a peripheral branch that innervates various tissues, and a central branch that travels through a dorsal root to enter the dorsal horn of the spinal cord, where it forms synapses with second-order neurons.

These second-order neurons include projection cells, interneurons, and propriospinal neurons. Propriospinal neurons transfer inputs from one segment of the spinal cord to another. Although their role in nociception is poorly understood, propriospinal neurons act as a multisynaptic pathway transferring information to the brain, and, in addition, have a major role in controlling locomotion and organizing coordinated reflex responses (Sandkuhler et al., 1993; Wall et al., 2006; Cowley et al., 2008).

Interneurons make up the great majority of the neuronal population in the dorsal horn, and can be divided into two main morphological classes: the islet cells are found throughout lamina II and are thought to be inhibitory interneurons, which use γ-aminobutyric acid (GABA) and/or glycine as a transmitter, and the stalked cells that are found primarily at the junction between laminae I and II and are reported to serve as either inhibitory interneurons or excitatory interneurons, which use glutamate. Interneurons play a critical role in modulating nociceptive signals from the primary afferents and conveying the information to projection neurons (Todd & Ribeiro-Da-Silva, 2005; Wall et al., 2006; Maxwell et al., 2007). The projection neurons and the interneurons that encode nociceptive information can be divided into two major classes: wide dynamic range neurons (WDR; also called "convergent"), which are activated by weak mechanical stimuli but respond with increasing discharge frequencies as the intensity of the mechanical stimulus increases, and nociceptive-specific neurons, that respond only to intense noxious forms of mechanical, thermal, or chemical stimuli (Millan, 2002; Todd & Ribeiro-Da-Silva, 2005; Wall et al., 2006). The WDR neurons are important substrates for the expression of descending controls, and their sensitization by repetitive, nociceptive stimulation plays a key role in the induction of long-term inflammatory and/or neuropathic pain states (Millan, 2002).

DORSAL HORN SYNAPTIC TRANSMISSION

Dorsal horn nociceptive neurons possess a rich diversity of receptors whose activation regulates neurotransmitter release and subsequent activation of second order neurons. Excitatory receptors include the α-amino-3-hydroxy-5-methyl-4-isoxazolepropionic acid (AMPA) and N-methyl-D-aspartate (NMDA) classes of ionotropic glutamate receptors and the metabotropic glutamate receptors. These receptors act via multiple intracellular mechanisms including the activation of G-proteins, which activates PLC, resulting in suppression of K^+ currents and enhancement of Ca^{2+} currents.

The neurokinin-1 (NK1) receptor is another excitatory receptor present throughout the dorsal horn, with the highest concentration in lamina I. The excitatory influence of NK1 receptors upon neuronal activity is due to the activation of G-proteins and PLC, resulting in suppression of K^+ currents and enhancement of Ca^{2+} currents. SP is probably released from primary afferents at extrasynaptic sites and acts on NK1 receptors on the projection neurons through "volume transmission." Volume transmission involves activation of receptors via extrasynaptic diffusion of neurotransmitter, allowing amplification of the signal by transmission to multiple neurons (Zoli et al., 1999; Millan, 2002; Wall et al., 2006; Rice & Cragg, 2008).

Within the dorsal horn the terminal of the primary afferent neuron synapses with a dorsal horn neuron and, depending on the intensity of stimulation, this may be sufficient to produce a postsynaptic output. Like the vast majority of fast excitatory synapses throughout the CNS, most presynaptic excitatory terminals in the dorsal horn release glutamate, which activates ionotropic AMPA, kainate, and NMDA receptors, and the G-protein-coupled metabotropic family of receptors on the postsynaptic neurons. The excitatory postsynaptic potentials (EPSPs) resulting from single presynaptic action potentials are caused primarily by activation of the AMPA and kainate subtypes of the ionotropic glutamate receptor, and typically last for only a few milliseconds. This type of fast excitatory synaptic transmission occurs even at synapses of "slow" nociceptor C-fiber primary afferents. With low-frequency activation of nociceptors produced by mild noxious stimuli, these EPSPs signal to dorsal horn neurons the onset, duration, intensity, and location of noxious stimuli in the periphery.

GABA receptors are also expressed by sensory neurons, and play a crucial and complex role in inhibition of nociceptive processing. These receptors are mainly located in the superficial laminae, and include two classes of receptors: $GABA_A$ receptors are concentrated on the postsynaptic membrane of inhibitory synapses, are comprised of pentameric ion channels, and exert their inhibitory action by increasing permeability to chloride anions. $GABA_B$ receptors are localized to presynaptic terminals and are heterodimers that inhibit adenylyl cyclase (AC) via G-protein activation, resulting in increased K^+ currents and suppression of Ca^{2+} currents (Millan, 2002; Wall et al., 2006).

The three main opioid receptors (μ, δ, and κ) are located on primary sensory neurons, and α-2 adrenergic receptors are localized at the central terminals of peptidergic fibers. Activation of opioid receptors and α-2 receptors inhibits AC, which enhances K^+ currents and suppresses Ca^{2+} currents, thus inhibiting neuronal excitability (Millan, 2002; Wall et al., 2006). A coexpression of δ-opioid receptors and α-2A adrenergic receptors on SP-expressing primary afferent fibers was shown in rat dorsal horn and skin. This may underlie the mechanism of the synergistic interaction observed *in vivo* when agonists of both receptors are coadministered spinally (Riedl et al., 2009).

Fast inhibitory postsynaptic potentials (IPSPs) hyperpolarize the postsynaptic membrane and are produced by chloride currents mediated by glycine and GABA acting on the ionotropic glycine and $GABA_A$ receptors. The $GABA_B$ receptor is a G-protein-coupled receptor and produces slower-onset and longer-lasting inhibition, predominantly presynaptically (Wall et al., 2006).

GLIAL AND IMMUNOCOMPETENT CELLS IN THE DORSAL HORN

It is important to discuss the influence of non-neuronal units in the dorsal horn. These include resident glial cells (astrocytes, oligodendrocytes, and immunocompetent microglia) and immigrant immunocompetent T cells, which may infiltrate the dorsal horn following damage to the spinal cord, primary afferent fibers, or peripheral tissue, and subsequent loss of blood–brain barrier integrity. The function of glial cells is subject to modulation by glutamate, ACh, SP, GABA, serotonin, norepinephrine, adenosine, and other transmitters originating in descending pathways, primary afferent fiber terminals, and dorsal horn neurons (Millan, 2002). Of particular note is the role of glial membrane transporters in regulating the accumulation or reuptake of the three major amino acid neurotransmitters in the CNS: glutamate, GABA, and glycine. This function of glial cells suggests their involvement in the regulation of synaptic activity. Glial transporters regulate the clearance of neurotransmitters released by neurons (e.g., glial transporters play a critical role in protecting neurons from glutamate-induced neurotoxicity), and also release neuroactive compounds in response to multiple stimuli (Gadea and Lopez-Colome, 2001a; Gadea and Lopez-Colome, 2001b; Gadea and Lopez-Colome, 2001c; Millan, 2002).

Glial cells regulate neuronal cholinergic transmission via secretion of an ACh-binding protein, and control glutamatergic function by modification of the subunit composition of NMDA receptors on neurons. Glial and immunocompetent cells generate a plethora of factors which can influence nociceptive processing in the dorsal horn, notably, cytokines (such as interleukins, neurotrophins, and tissue necrosis factor α (TNF-α)), nitric oxide (NO), prostaglandins, histamine, ATP, glycine, and glutamate (Millan, 2002).

Modulation of Nociception

THE GATE CONTROL THEORY

The dorsal horn of the spinal cord is the location of the first synapse in nociceptive pathways and, as such, is a powerful target for regulation of nociceptive transmission by both local segmental and supraspinal mechanisms. The existence of a specific pain modulatory system was first described by Melzack and Wall (1965) in the gate control theory of pain. It was proposed that inhibitory interneurons located in the substantia gelatinosa play a crucial role in controlling incoming sensory information before it is transmitted to the brain through ascending pathways. Inputs to the dorsal horn that originate from large myelinated peripheral nerves (e.g., Aβ fibers) activate inhibitory interneurons, which result in the inhibition of the projection of the information to the brain. An inhibition of the inhibitory interneurons occurs by small fibers (e.g., C fibers) and results in exaggeration of the arriving impulses and thus increased projection to the brain. Although the gate control theory has undergone modifications and corrections in the light of new information, it has had an important impact on the science of pain, and led researchers to regard the brain and spinal cord as active and dynamic systems (Melzack, 1999).

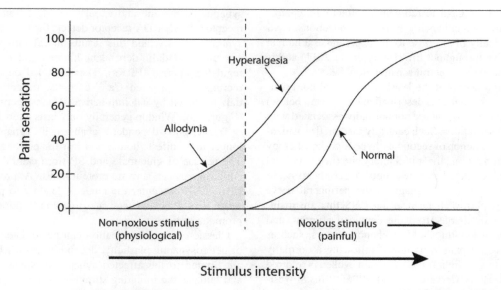

Figure 2.5. The pain-response curve. This diagram illustrates the changes in pain sensation induced by injury. The normal relationship between stimulus intensity and the magnitude of pain sensation is represented by the curve at the right-hand side of the figure. Pain sensation is only evoked by stimulus intensities in the noxious range (the vertical dotted line indicates the pain threshold). Injury provokes a leftward shift in the curve relating stimulus intensity to pain sensation. Under these conditions, innocuous stimuli evoke pain (allodynia) (Reprinted from: Cervero, F. & Laird, J.M.A. (1996) Mechanisms of touch-evoked pain. *Pain*, 68, 3–23. This figure has been reproduced with permission of the International Association for the Study of Pain® (IASP®). The figure may not be reproduced for any other purpose without permission).

PERIPHERAL SENSITIZATION

Differences in processing of acute and prolonged nociceptive stimulation provide the physiological basis for two major characteristics of clinical pain: hyperalgesia and allodynia (Figure 2.5). An acute stimulus triggers a series of events leading to excitatory nociceptive signals reaching the brain via the spinal cord. As the stimulus is short lived, so is the neuronal response. However, given a higher intensity and/or chronic stimulus, sensitization may occur at the peripheral and/or the central level. Hyperalgesia is defined as an increase in the painfulness of a noxious stimulus and a reduced threshold for pain. Primary hyperalgesia occurs in the peripheral tissues at the site of injury due to localized inflammation causing hyperexcitability of nociceptors via a reduction in threshold and increased responsiveness to noxious stimuli. This peripheral sensitization is the result of inflammatory mediators (e.g., prostaglandins, cytokines, ATP, H$^+$) that affect existing proteins in the cell membrane and change the expression of membrane proteins.

Inflammation may modulate TRPV1 in a number of ways. First, phosphorylation, following the activation of various kinases, enhances the functional competence of the receptor by increasing the affinity to capsaicin or by reducing the temperature threshold of activation so that TRPV1 can be activated at or near body temperature. Second, phosphorylation and NGF induce upregulation of the TRPV1 receptor. Lastly, inflammatory mediators may enhance TRPV1 activity by reversing the inhibition of TRPV1 by phosphatidylinositol 4,5-biphosphate (Chung et al., 2011).

Inflammatory mediators, such as prostaglandin E$_2$ (PGE$_2$), bradykinin, serotonin, and adenosine, modulate neuronal TTX-R sodium channels (Na$_v$1.8 and Na$_v$1.9), thus increasing the development of inflammatory hyperalgesia. This modulation is manifested by the phosphorylation of the channel through activation of cyclic AMP-dependent protein kinase and results in increased conduction, increased activation, and a depolarizing shift in the voltage-dependence of activation. These changes will eventually lower the action potential threshold and decrease the magnitude of the generator potential necessary to evoke an action potential. During inflammation there is also an increase in the expression of neuronal TTX-R sodium channels, which contributes to the maintenance of hyperalgesia and nociceptor sensitization (Caterina et al., 2005; Schaible et al., 2011).

Cytokines can also induce long-lasting effects on the excitability of neurons through regulation of receptor expression. During the acute phase of inflammation, macrophages invade the DRG of the segments that innervate an inflamed organ and directly sensitize primary afferent cell bodies through release of TNF-α (Schaible et al., 2011). In a mouse model of immune-mediated arthritis, it was demonstrated that there is a correlation between mechanical hypernociception and the production of TNF-α and inflammatory interleukins by neutrophil infiltrates in the joint (Sachs et al., 2011).

There are a few specific agonists at peripheral receptors that have an inhibitory action on nociception. The endogenous opioid peptides β-endorphin, enkephalin, and dynorphin produce profound antinociception at peripheral and central opioid receptors. Another emerging field of interest is the cannabinoid receptors, which produce antinociception when activated by their endogenous ligands, anandamide and 2-arachidonoylglycerol, or by exogenous cannabinoids (Bushlin et al., 2010).

CENTRAL SENSITIZATION AND PLASTICITY

Synaptic processing in the spinal cord is not fixed or hardwired but, instead, is subject to diverse forms of plasticity. CNS plasticity refers to the ability of the CNS to reorganize, effecting a change in input to output ratio and enhancing synaptic connections. CNS plasticity occurs normally in response to the experiences a human or an animal will have throughout life (Henry et al., 2011) and is the underlying mechanism of central sensitization.

Central sensitization occurs at the level of the dorsal horn neuron. Amplification mechanisms (as described in more detail below) enable the peripheral neurons that are not normally associated with pain to evoke painful sensations. Such centrally mediated sensitization underlies the phenomenon of secondary hyperalgesia, whereby mechanical stimulation around the initial injury site (i.e., in normal skin) produces pain. A related manifestation of peripheral nerve and tissue injury is seen when damage to the peripheral nerve and/or tissue induces plastic changes in the CNS that are maintained by continuing discharge from the damaged afferent, and result in recruitment of low-threshold mechanoreceptors, such as Aβ fibers. Here, because pain is produced following a normally nonpainful stimulus (e.g., a light brush), the pain evoked is referred to as allodynia (Figure 2.5) (Cervero & Laird, 1996; Willis & Westlund, 1997; Brooks & Tracey, 2005, Wall et al., 2006; Lee et al., 2011).

Some forms of activity-dependent plasticity are very brief; others relatively long-lasting, involving changes in protein phosphorylation and altered gene expression; and some irreversible, with a loss of neurons and the formation of new synapses. Structural plasticity (including the recruitment of microglia, alterations in synaptic contacts, and loss of inhibitory interneurons) plays a major role in producing the increase in pain sensitivity in neuropathic pain. This form of plasticity involves structural reorganization of the synaptic circuitry of the system. Neurons may die, axonal terminals may degenerate or atrophy, new axonal terminals may appear, and the structural contact between cells at the synapses is modified. This may result in the loss of normal connections, formation of novel abnormal connections, and an alteration in the normal balance between excitation and inhibition. Such changes typically occur after injury to the peripheral CNS, and are responsible for a range of sensory abnormalities including reduced tactile sensibility, paresthesia, and pain. Structural reorganization within the dorsal horn and its functional sequelae can last long after the initial injury has healed, representing a persistent change in dorsal horn sensory processing.

Different forms of plasticity are now considered to constitute the general phenomenon of central sensitization.

Windup is an activity-dependent progressive increase in the response of neurons over the course of a train of inputs. Repetitive discharge of primary afferent nociceptors results in glutamate vesicle release (in response to a greater influx of calcium in the presynaptic terminal), which then causes a release of the neuropeptides SP and CGRP. These neuropeptides activate postsynaptic G-protein-coupled receptors, which lead to slow postsynaptic depolarizations, and the resultant cumulative depolarization is boosted by the recruitment of NMDA receptor currents. While the AMPA receptor is responsible for the baseline response to noxious stimuli, the NMDA receptor contributes little to the responses to single presynaptic action potentials because NMDA receptors are tonically suppressed by extracellular Mg^{2+}, which blocks the central cation selective channel. Sustained or intense nociceptive signaling from primary afferents leads to increased glutamate release, which in turn partially depolarizes the post-synaptic membrane and expels the Mg^{2+} ion from the NMDA receptor. The NMDA receptor detects the coincident pre-and post-synaptic activity, and this results in calcium influx, stimulating calcium/calmodulin-dependent kinases and extracellular signal-regulated kinases (ERKs). The sustained depolarization further recruits voltage-gated Ca^{2+} currents, triggering plateau potentials mediated by calcium-activated nonselective cation channels (Figure 2.6). Windup generally only lasts a few seconds.

Transcription-dependent changes in synaptic function take longer to manifest (hours) and last for prolonged periods (days). The release of glutamate and SP from central nociceptive afferent terminals can activate protein kinase A, protein kinase C, and ERK. ERK can enter the nucleus, leading to phosphorylation of serine-133, which can activate gene transcription by binding to the promoter regions of genes.

Classic central sensitization can be initiated by homosynaptic or heterosynaptic plasticity, depending upon whether the changes are limited to the affected synapse or spread to adjacent ones, and outlasts the initiating stimulus for tens of minutes. Homosynaptic potentiation is the simplest means to sensitize central pain transmission neurons by increasing the efficacy of the excitatory primary afferent inputs to these neurons. It is elicited by brief duration, high-frequency inputs (long-term potentiation) and it is induced by a cascade of NMDA receptor activation with a dramatic enhancement of calcium influx leading to activation of calcium/calmodulin-dependent kinase II and phosphorylation of the AMPA receptor, which causes AMPA channels to open in a high-conductance state. Heterosynaptic activity-dependent plasticity allows for an increase in synaptic efficacy in dorsal horn neurons not directly activated by the conditioning or initiating stimulus, such as the low-threshold mechanosensitive Aβ fibers. Heterosynaptic plasticity also results in an increase in the responsiveness of dorsal horn neurons, and an expansion of the receptive fields of dorsal horn neurons. Calcium influx through the NMDA ion channel is the major way that heterosynaptic potentiation is induced; however, other ways, such as activation of voltage-gated calcium channels or release of cytokines (e.g., TNF-α) from glial cells, are described.

Loss of inhibition occurs by two mechanisms: an activity-dependent decrease in synaptic input to inhibitory interneurons (due to substantial loss of inhibitory currents, particularly those mediated by GABA), and a loss or death of these neurons (mainly a selective death of GABAergic inhibitory interneurons following nerve injury) (Woolf & Salter, 2000; Kawasaki et al., 2004; McMahon & Priestley, 2005; Salter & Woolf, 2005; Wall et al., 2006; Basser, 2012).

Central sensitization is characterized by diffuse pain sensitivity and increased pain severity during and after repeated stimuli. Individuals with central sensitization have low thermal and mechanical thresholds in a diffuse pattern, reflecting enlargement of the spinal cord neuron receptive fields. Repeated stimulation results in painful after-sensations that persist after a stimulus is withdrawn, as well as enhanced temporal summation of pain such that the pain rating for the last stimulus is greater than the pain rating for the first stimulus, even though the stimuli are exactly the same (Woolf & Salter, 2000; Lee et al., 2011). The receptive field of a somatic sensory neuron assigns a specific topographic location to sensory information, and each receptor responds only to stimulation within its receptive field. A characteristic feature of central

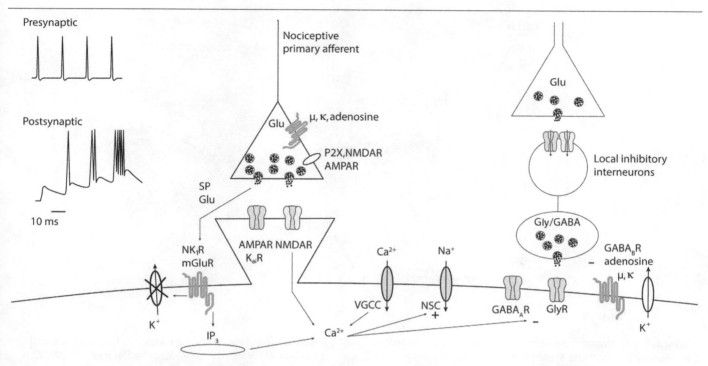

Figure 2.6. Slow synaptic responses and wind-up. Rapid action potential discharge rate in primary afferent nociceptors leads to release of transmitters, such as SP, in addition to glutamate, which generate slow excitatory postsynaptic potentials (EPSPs). Postsynaptically, fast and slow EPSPs summate temporally and initiate postsynaptic signaling, which leads to enhanced discharge of dorsal horn neurons. IP3, inositol trisphosphate; P2X, purinoreceptor; SP, substance P (Reprinted from: Woolf, C.J., and Salter, M.W. (2006) Plasticity and pain: role of the dorsal horn, in S. McMahon and M. Koltzenburg (eds). *Wall and Melzack's Textbook of Pain*, p. 14. Copyright Elsevier/Churchill Livingstone (2006). Reproduced with permission from Elsevier).

sensitization is an expansion of receptive fields. This reorganization of the sensory body maps occurs from the spinal dorsal horns through to the somatosensory cortex (Basser, 2012).

SUPRASPINAL CENTERS

Nociceptive signaling initiated in peripheral sensory neurons enters the spinal cord dorsal horn and is conveyed to supraspinal structures (Figure 2.7). The axons of the projection neurons synapse in the medulla, midbrain, and thalamus, which in turn project to the cortex to drive the three components of the pain experience: sensory-discriminative, motivational-affective, and evaluative-cognitive (Melzack, 1999; Treede et al., 1999; Dubin & Patapoutian, 2010; Zhuo et al., 2011). The sensory-discriminative component refers to the basic sensory information, such as the location, quality, and the intensity of pain. The motivational-affective component determines the approach-avoidance behavior of the individual, and includes the emotional reaction to pain. And the evaluative-cognitive component includes the learned behavior and the past experience of pain of an individual, and it may influence (e.g., block or enhance) the perception of pain (Melzack, 1999; Treede et al., 1999; Hofbauer et al., 2001; Masedo & Esteve, 2002; Melzack & Katz, 2002; Gustin et al., 2011).

Perception

Advances in functional imaging techniques have contributed to the body of knowledge of the pain system, especially the role of supraspinal processing. New discoveries have pointed to the presence of a pain "matrix", a group of cortical regions consistently activated by the pain experience (Heinricher et al., 2009; Basser, 2012). The pain matrix generally is thought to include the primary (S1) and secondary (S2) somatosensory cortices, the insular cortex, the anterior cingulate cortex (ACC), the amygdala, and the thalamus (Hofbauer et al., 2001; Brooks & Tracey, 2005; Henry et al., 2011) (Figure 2.7). Activations in and around S2 and the insula are of particular interest, as these regions are the most robustly activated in response to noxious and innocuous stimuli, and are the only cortical areas in which direct electrical stimulation produces a perception of pain (Peyron et al., 2000; Ostrowsky et al., 2002; Brooks & Tracey, 2005).

Modulation also occurs at supraspinal sites, and forebrain areas are involved in both opiate- and nonopiate-mediated modulation. Although peripheral and spinal actions of opiates are important for analgesia, receptors in the ACC may be particularly important for opiate-related changes in the emotional aspects of pain. Other chemicals in the brain, such as dopamine, also play a role in pain modulation. Modulation of pain by psychological factors, such as attention, emotional state, or expectation is manifested by changes in pain-evoked activity in the cerebral cortex, and most

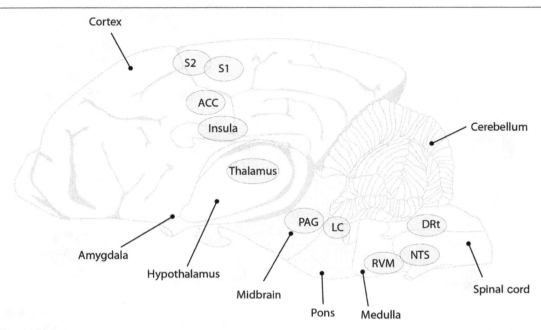

Figure 2.7. Supraspinal centers involved in pain sensation. ACC, anterior cingulate cortex; S1 and S2, first and second somatosensory cortical areas; PAG, periaqueductal gray; LC, locus coeruleus; RVM, rostral ventromedial medulla; NTS, nucleus tractus solitarius; DRt, dorsal reticular nucleus.

likely involves intrinsic descending modulatory circuits (Wall et al., 2006). Activation of the insula, S1, S2, and the lateral thalamus are thought to be related to the sensory-discriminative aspects of pain processing, whereas the ACC, reticular, and limbic structures appear to participate in the motivational-affective component of pain sensation, or in other words, the perception of pain as an unpleasant experience. The posterior parietal cortex, and the ACC appear to be involved in cognitive processes, such as attention, and in memory networks activated by noxious stimuli (Hofbauer et al., 2001; Melzack & Katz, 2002; Brooks & Tracey, 2005).

Descending Modulatory Pathways

The descending modulation of spinal nociceptive processing can be either inhibitory (antinociceptive) or facilitatory (pronociceptive) (Table 2.2; Figure 2.8). The relative activity of these opposing mechanisms controls the output of second order nociceptive neurons that project to more rostral brain sites, and thus eventually contributes to the prioritization of pain perception relative to other competing behavioral needs and homeostatic demands (Millan, 2002; Gebhart & Proudfit, 2005; Heinricher et al., 2009; Dubin & Patapoutian, 2010; Henry et al., 2011). Under extreme conditions, pain may be subjugated temporarily in favor of emergency fight-or-flight behavior. Such an endogenous analgesia-producing system is an adaptive response, which optimizes the chances of survival in a life-threatening environment (Melzack et al., 1982; Lovick & Bandler, 2005; Wagner, 2010). Descending facilitation occurs after suspension of conflict and disengagement from potentially dangerous conditions, and may be regarded as a homeostatic mechanism for a return to equilibrium in the transmission of nociceptive input (Millan, 2002; Heinricher et al., 2009). A shift toward descending facilitation can also be seen with inflammation, nerve

injury, systemic illness, and chronic opioid administration (Heinricher et al., 2009).

Several areas in the brainstem (e.g., periaqueductal gray) can produce either inhibition or facilitation of spinal nociceptive transmission depending on the intensity of the stimulation or, under experimental conditions, the concentration of microinjected agonist drugs (e.g., cholinergic agonists, GABA receptor agonists, glutamate, and opioid agonists). In general, facilitation is produced by low intensities of electrical stimulation or low concentrations of agonist drugs, whereas inhibition is produced by greater intensities of stimulation or greater concentrations of those drugs (Gebhart & Proudfit, 2005).

Table 2.2. The neurotransmitters involved in descending modulation of spinal nociceptive processing.

Inhibition
  Norepinephrine
  Serotonin
  Dopamine
  Opioids
  GABA
  Cannabinoids
  Adenosine
Facilitation
  Substance P
  Glutamate
  Nerve growth factor
  Cholecystokinin

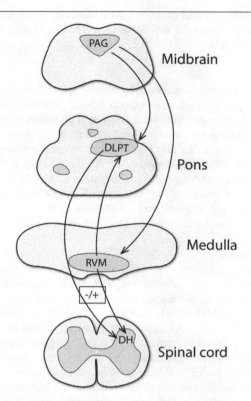

Figure 2.8. A simplified model of the brainstem descending modulation pathways. Neurons in the periaquaductal gray (PAG) modulate the activity of neurons in the dorsolateral pontine tegmentum (DLPT) and in the rostral ventromedial medulla (RVM), which in turn can inhibit or facilitate second order nociceptive neurons in the dorsal horn that project nociceptive information to more rostral brain sites.

The descending modulatory system receives input from the ACC, the anterior insular cortex, and the amygdala, allowing influence by affective and cognitive processes. For example, simple manipulations of attention alter the subjective pain experience as well as the corresponding pattern of activation during painful stimulation. The main effect of distracting subjects during pain appears to be increased activity within the orbitofrontal and rostral cingulate cortices and a corresponding reduction in activation in the thalamus and insula (Brooks & Tracey, 2005; Henry et al., 2011).

Descending control (Figure 2.8) arises from the midbrain periaqueductal gray (PAG), the rostral ventromedial medulla (RVM), the dorsal reticular nucleus (DRt), the nucleus raphe magnus (NRM), and the ventrolateral medulla (VLM) (Willis & Westlund, 1997; Millan, 2002; Heinricher et al., 2009). Areas in the pons (locus coeruleus, subcoeruleus, and Kölliker-Fuse nuclei), and several nuclei of the reticular formation are also involved. In addition, structures at higher levels of the nervous system, including the cerebral cortex, and various limbic structures, including the hypothalamus, contribute to analgesia (Willis & Westlund, 1997; Brooks & Tracey, 2005; Lovick & Bandler, 2005; Basser, 2012). These pathways utilize several different neurotransmitter systems, primarily opioidergic, but also nonopioid systems, including dopaminergic,

serotonergic, cannabinergic, and monoaminergic (Willis & Westlund, 1997; Kut et al., 2011). The major descending systems are reviewed in the following sections.

PERIAQUEDUCTAL GRAY

The PAG is the source of a number of descending pathways that exert powerful modulatory influences on the transmission of afferent impulses from nociceptors to the dorsal horn (Figure 2.8). It is organized functionally into four longitudinal columns of neurons. Two distinct forms of analgesia arise from location-specific activation of the PAG. Activation of the ventrolateral area induces long-acting, opioid-mediated analgesia, which results in passive-coping or conservation-withdrawal reactions. This activation is typically seen in response to extreme, inescapable physical stress, including traumatic injury, and functions to promote recovery and healing. In contrast, activation of the dorsolateral or lateral areas induces a short-acting, nonopioid-mediated analgesia, which results in active-coping or defensive reaction. This activation is typically seen in response to an escapable threat or stress. Originally, production of endogenous analgesia was attributed to the action of neurons in the PAG that project directly to the spinal cord, however, most of the connections between the PAG and the spinal cord are indirect; e.g., the PAG projects to the RVM and adjacent reticular formation and to several nuclei in the parabrachial area, including the locus coeruleus (Stamford, 1995; Willis & Westlund, 1997; Millan, 2002; Gebhart & Proudfit, 2005; Lovick & Bandler, 2005).

MEDULLA

The RVM is a heterogeneous region incorporating several nuclei, each of which provides descending pathways to superficial and deep dorsal horn laminae. It contains a large number of serotonin-containing neurons, located primarily in the NRM, that project to the spinal cord (Willis & Westlund, 1997; Gebhart & Proudfit, 2005). The PAG has excitatory connections with the NRM, suggesting that the antinociceptive effects of stimulation in the PAG are mediated by the NRM. Those antinociceptive effects have been attributed to the inhibition of nociceptive dorsal horn neurons, including spinothalamic tract cells. Neurotransmitters involved in the antinociceptive actions of the pathway from the PAG through the NRM and adjacent reticular formation include endogenous opiates, serotonin, and norepinephrine (Stamford, 1995; Willis & Westlund, 1997; Millan, 2002).

Inhibitory control from the PAG–RVM system preferentially suppresses nociceptive inputs mediated by C fibers, preserving sensory-discriminative information conveyed by more rapidly conducting A fibers (Heinricher et al., 2009).

The DRt, which is situated in the dorsolateral quadrant of the medulla, receives somatic and visceral nociceptive input from spinal projections. It has communications with the PAG and the RVM as well as with the thalamus, amygdala, and some cortical sites, and it sends modulatory projections to the superficial and deep laminae of the dorsal horn. Thus, the DRt forms a part of a spinal–supraspinal–spinal feedback loop that modulates pain. The mechanisms originating in the DRt appear to mediate either descending facilitation or inhibition (Millan, 2002; Ossipov et al., 2010).

PONS

Stimulation in the dorsolateral pons is reported to produce noradrenergic antinociception. Noradrenergic projections to all regions of the spinal cord arise almost entirely from the dorsolateral pontine catecholamine cell groups A5, A6, and A7, which include the locus coeruleus, the subcoeruleus, and the Kölliker-Fuse nucleus (Stamford, 1995; Willis & Westlund, 1997; Gebhart & Proudfit, 2005; Basser, 2012).

Electrical or chemical stimulation of the dorsolateral pons produces analgesic effects, which were thought to be mediated by α-2 adrenoceptors; however, more recent findings indicate that the analgesic effects may be attributable to an I_2 imidazoline receptor (Willis & Westlund, 1997).

The parabrachial nucleus (PBN), which is situated within the dorsolateral pontine tegmentum, mimics the hypothalamus in playing a major role in the integration of autonomic and somatosensory information, in being interlinked with higher structures involved in the emotional and cognitive dimension of pain, and in receiving nociceptive (in particular, visceral) information directly from the dorsal horn. Various subdivisions of the PBN project to the nucleus tractus solitarius (NTS), RVM, and dorsal horn. Pathways emanating from the PBN predominantly target neurons localized in superficial dorsal horn laminae. Stimulation of the PBN suppresses the response of dorsal horn neurons to both nociceptive and non-nociceptive input (Millan, 2002).

NUCLEUS TRACTUS SOLITARIUS

The NTS is the first relay station to receive visceral and taste afferents and it relays viscerosensory information to central autonomic regions, both directly and via the PBN. It receives major input from the vagus nerve, as well as afferents from superficial and deep dorsal horn neurons. Stimulation of the NTS can elicit antinociception. On the other hand, several studies have focused on vagal input to the NTS and potential mechanisms of triggering descending facilitation via the RVM (Millan, 2002; Benarroch, 2006).

THALAMUS

Stimulation of the ventral posterior lateral (VPL) or the ventral posterior medial (VPM) thalamic nuclei results in a reduction in pain. Stimulation in the VPL nucleus causes inhibition of primate spinothalamic tract neurons. The inhibition is suggested to result from antidromic activation of the axons of spinothalamic tract neurons that send collaterals to such brainstem nuclei as the PAG or the NRM. Neurons in the NRM are activated when stimuli are applied in the VPL nucleus, with subsequent release of serotonin in the spinal cord. Alternatively, the spinal cord inhibition resulting from stimulation in the VPL nucleus may occur through a cortical loop (Willis & Westlund, 1997; Brooks & Tracey, 2005).

CEREBRAL CORTEX

The cognitive and emotional dimensions of pain are of special importance with regard to the animal's experience and clinical management. Stimulation of the S1, insular, and ventro-orbital cortices can evoke antinociception via relays in other supraspinal structures such as the PAG. On the other hand, stimulation of the ACC, a region involved in the "aversiveness" of pain, can elicit pronociception in the rat, and stimulation of the motor cortex excites spinothalamic tract cells. The frontal cortex projects strongly to the NRM and other regions of the RVM, while frontocortical, somatosensory,

and parietal regions of the cortex are a source of direct projections terminating throughout the dorsal horn (Millan, 2002, Willis & Westlund, 1997).

LIMBIC STRUCTURES

Pain is quite often accompanied by motivational-affective and autonomic responses, including increased heart rate and blood pressure, neuroendocrine activation, increased attention, arousal, and anxiety. The neural pathways that mediate these changes likely parallel those relaying information about somatic pain sensations, but include additional structures of the limbic system. Much of the information about painful experiences may be relayed through spinoreticular inputs to the brainstem. Some of these brainstem sites then project to higher centers where they affect hypothalamic, limbic, and neocortical function (Willis & Westlund, 1997).

HYPOTHALAMUS

The hypothalamus plays an important role in coordinating autonomic and sensory information. The hypothalamus has well-documented nociceptive afferent and efferent projections to brainstem centers (NTS, PAG, and RVM), as well as corticolimbic structures. It receives nociceptive information from the dorsal horn, through the spinohypothalamic tract, and it is considered to be active in nociceptive processing and descending controls. Several hypothalamic nuclei have been implicated in this process. Stimulation of the medial preoptic nucleus inhibits the response of spinal neurons to noxious stimuli, stimulation of the anterior hypothalamus suppresses the response of WDR neurons in the dorsal horn to noxious stimuli, and stimulation of the lateral hypothalamus elicits antinociception via relays to the PAG and RVM. Lesions in the medial hypothalamus can result in hyperalgesia, however (Millan, 2002; Jaggi & Singh, 2011).

The ventromedial and dorsomedial hypothalamus provide an intense input to the PAG and also project to the NTS and amygdala. Antinociception elicited from the amygdala (which only minimally projects to the spinal cord) seems to involve a PAG link to the brainstem (Willis & Westlund, 1997; Millan, 2002; Brooks & Tracey, 2005).

VISCERAL PAIN

Visceral pain results from the activation of nociceptors of organs in the thoracic, abdominal, or pelvic cavities, and it is usually described as a deep, dull sensation. Visceral pain differs from somatic pain in several important ways. Adequate stimuli for production of visceral pain include distension of hollow organs, traction on the mesentery, ischemia, and endogenous chemicals typically associated with inflammatory processes. However, cutting or burning stimuli of the hollow organs will not be associated with pain unless there is already an insult, such as inflammation or distension. Visceral tissues like that of the lungs, liver, or kidneys are insensitive to any form of stimulation (although, the capsules of the kidneys and liver do contain nociceptors sensitive to inflammatory mediators and distension) (Cervero, 1994; Hobson & Aziz, 2003; Ness & Gebhart, 2005).

Visceral pain is diffuse and poorly localized and several factors contribute to this. Visceral afferent innervation is sparse relative to somatic innervation, and, at the level of the spinal cord, termination of visceral afferents on neurons in laminae I, II, V, and X is spread over several segments rostral and caudal to the spinal segment of entry, and may decussate to the contralateral side. In addition, these spinal neurons also receive convergent input from somatic structures, providing the structural basis for referred pain (see next paragraph). Finally, the viscera are unique in that thoracic, abdominal, and pelvic viscera receive dual extrinsic innervation. Each organ receives innervation from two sets of nerves: either vagal and spinal nerves or pelvic and spinal nerves. Autonomic input to the medulla is amplified by the branching and widespread distribution of afferent terminals (Gebhart, 2000b; Hobson & Aziz, 2003; Laird & Schaible, 2005; Ness & Gebhart, 2005; Wall et al., 2006; Sengupta, 2009; Romero et al., 2011). An older terminology described the spinal innervation of the viscera as sympathetic or parasympathetic. However, this terminology has been questioned due to the lack of correlation between pathways of projection and functional role; thus, visceral afferent fibers are best described by nerve name to avoid assumed functions (Cervero, 1994; Gebhart, 2000b).

Visceral pain is often referred and not felt at the source. The term referred pain is used to describe pain localized not in the site of its origin but in areas that may be adjacent to or at a distance from the location of the affected organ, typically somatic sites (e.g., skin, subcutaneous tissue, and muscle) (Figure 2.9a and b). Referred pain from visceral organs is important from a clinical point of view. This type of pain is observed especially when an algogenic process affecting a viscus is intense and long lasting or recurs frequently. Different pathogeneses may be involved in the onset of referred pain, including convergence of impulses in the CNS and reflexes inducing muscle contraction, sympathetic activation, and antidromic activation of afferent fibers (Weber et al., 1982; Cervero et al., 1992; Procacci & Maresca, 1999; Laird & Schaible, 2005; Sengupta, 2009).

Visceral pain is associated with strong emotional and autonomic responses, and can be accompanied by pallor, sweating, nausea, vomiting, and changes in blood pressure and heart rate (Cervero, 1994; Hobson & Aziz, 2003; Laird & Schaible, 2005; Romero et al., 2011).

Visceral pain is not necessarily linked to visceral injury; that is, in many cases it is not associated with obvious pathology (e.g., irritable bowel syndrome) (Laird & Schaible, 2005; Christianson & Davis, 2010), and there may be a poor correlation between the amount of visceral pathology and the intensity of pain (e.g., ulcerative colitis or gastric perforation may produce little or no pain in some individuals).

Visceral Nociception

With the exception of a small number of Aβ fibers associated with Pacinian corpuscles in the mesentery, the overwhelming majority of visceral afferent fibers are thinly myelinated Aδ fibers or unmyelinated C fibers. It is assumed that most peripheral visceral afferent terminals are unencapsulated, "free" nerve endings (Gebhart, 2000b; Wall et al., 2006). Most of the information transferred from the viscera to the CNS (e.g., responses to intraluminal nutrients, baroreceptor input, and normal gastrointestinal motility) is rarely perceived. Accordingly, the principal conscious sensations that arise from the viscera are discomfort and pain (Gebhart, 2000a; 2000b).

The cell bodies of visceral afferent neurons are located in the cranial ganglia and DRG; the exception is the nodose ganglion, which contains the cell bodies of vagal sensory neurons. However, the route visceral afferent neurons take to the spinal cord typically involves passage through or near prevertebral ganglia, where they can give off collateral axons to influence autonomic ganglion

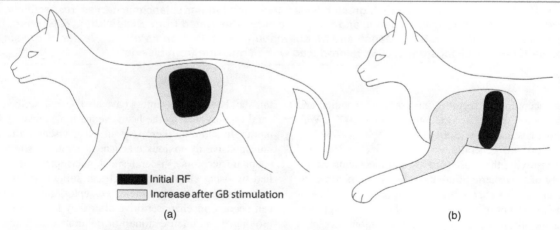

Initial RF

Increase after GB stimulation

(a)   (b)

Figure 2.9. Referred pain. (a) Increases in the size of the somatic receptive field (RF) of a GB+ neuron following repeated gall bladder distension. The initial receptive field is shown in black (Reprinted from Cervero et al. 1992. Selective changes of receptive field properties of spinal nociceptive neurones induced by noxious visceral stimulation in the cat. *Pain*, 51, 335–342. This figure has been reproduced with permission of the International Association for the Study of Pain® (IASP®). The figure may not be reproduced for any other purpose without permission). (b) Visceral and somatic inputs converging on the same spinal neuron. Bradykinin was injected into the heart via a cannula placed in the left atrium. There was a response when the skin of the blackened area was pinched. The stippled area is a composite of the locations of somatic receptive fields for all cells mapped with cardiac visceral overlap. This pattern is similar to that seen in humans with angina (Reprinted from Weber et al. 1982. Effects of cardiac administration of bradykinin on thoracic spinal neurons in the cat. *Experimental Neurology* 78, 703–715. Copyright Elsevier (1982). Reproduced with permission from Elsevier).

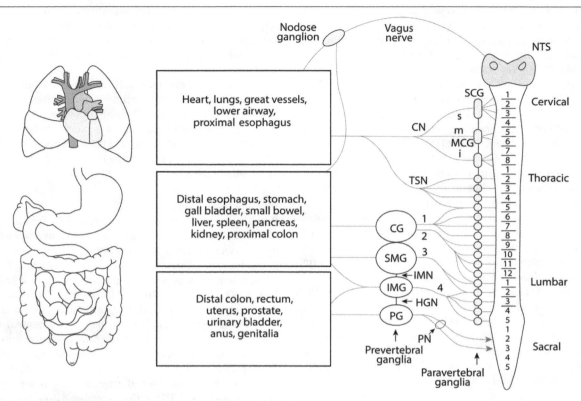

Figure 2.10. Visceral innervations. The vagus nerve, with cell bodies in the nodose ganglion and central terminals in the nucleus tractus solitarii (NTS), innervates organs in the thoracic and abdominal cavities. Afferent nerves with terminals in the spinal cord innervate the same thoracic and abdominal organs as well as those in the pelvic floor. Visceral spinal afferents pass through pre- and/or paravertebral ganglia en route to the spinal cord; their cell bodies are located in dorsal root ganglia (not illustrated). Prevertebral ganglia: CG, celiac ganglion; SMG and IMG, superior and inferior mesenteric ganglia, respectively, and PG, pelvic ganglion. Paravertebral ganglia: SCG and MCG, superior and middle cervical ganglia, respectively; and S, stellate ganglion. Nerves: CN, cardiac nerves (s, m and i, superior, middle, and inferior, respectively); TSN, thoracic splanchnic nerves; 1, 2, 3, and 4, greater, lesser, least and lumbar splanchnic nerves, respectively; IMN, intermesenteric nerve; HGN, hypogastric nerve; and PN, pelvic nerve (Reprinted from: Bielefeldt, K. & Gebhart, G.F. (2006) Visceral pain: basic mechanisms, in S. McMahon and M. Koltzenburg (eds). *Wall and Melzack's Textbook of Pain*, p 722. Copyright Elsevier/Churchill Livingstone (2006). Reproduced with permission from Elsevier).

cell bodies and, accordingly, secretory and motor functions, and paravertebral ganglia (Figure 2.10) (Gebhart, 2000a; 2000b; Wall et al., 2006; Christianson & Davis, 2010).

Visceral receptors are generally polymodal in character, and exhibit chemosensitivity, thermosensitivity, and mechanosensitivity. The majority of mesenteric afferents (afferent fibers innervating hollow organs) are mechanosensitive, and have either low or high thresholds for response to mechanical distension. Approximately 25% of the mechanosensitive fiber population have high thresholds for response (>30 mm Hg), and likely represent a group of visceral nociceptors. The remaining 75% of the mechanosensitive population have thresholds for response in the physiological range; most respond to distending stimuli between 1 and 5 mm Hg. Unlike low-threshold cutaneous mechanoreceptors, low-threshold mechanosensitive visceral afferent fibers encode distending pressures into the noxious range and, as a group, give greater magnitude responses throughout the noxious range of distending pressures than do the high-threshold visceral afferent fibers (Gebhart, 2000a; Sengupta, 2009; Christianson & Davis, 2010). High-

threshold mechanoreceptors have also been described in other visceral organs, such as the heart, veins, lungs, urinary bladder, and uterus. In addition, there is a subset of visceral afferents that are unresponsive to noxious mechanical stimulus similar to somatic silent nociceptors. Visceral silent nociceptors have been identified by using chemical or electrical stimuli or brief episodes of ischemia. These visceral silent nociceptors are chemosensitive, but can become mechanosensitive after they have been sensitized by prolonged and intense stimuli or inflammation (Laird & Schaible, 2005; Sengupta, 2009).

It is currently accepted that visceral pain is primarily signaled by spinal afferents, and vagal afferents signal non-painful sensations such as hunger, satiety, fullness, and nausea; moreover, several human and animal studies have documented that vagal nerve stimulation attenuates somatic and visceral pain. The analgesic effect of vagal activation could be related to its descending inhibitory influence on responses of spinal dorsal horn neurons or via the release of catecholamines from the adrenal medullae (Sengupta, 2009).

Visceral Sensitization and Hyperalgesia

Like somatic nociceptors, visceral nociceptors become sensitized. An injury to visceral tissue produces areas equivalent to areas of primary and secondary hyperalgesia seen after cutaneous injury. Primary visceral hyperalgesia occurs in the damaged area, as for the skin, and secondary visceral hyperalgesia similarly includes adjacent, undamaged regions of the same viscus. However, visceral damage may also result in hypersensitivity in other, undamaged organs, and this phenomenon is termed viscero-visceral hyperalgesia. Furthermore, visceral lesions may also give rise to hyperalgesia in the area to which the visceral pain is referred (i.e., on the body wall), and this is known as referred hyperalgesia (Gebhart, 2000a; Laird and Schaible, 2005; Wall et al. 2006; Sengupta, 2009).

Visceral hypersensitivity can occur due to (1) sensitization of primary sensory afferents innervating the viscera, (2) hyperexcitability of spinal ascending neurons (central sensitization) receiving synaptic input from the viscera, and (3) dysregulation of descending pathways that modulate spinal nociceptive transmission (Sengupta, 2009).

Central Processing of Visceral Pain

Visceral sensation is primarily represented in S2, whereas its representation in S1 is diffuse. This difference could account for the poor localization of visceral sensation compared with somatic sensation. When visceral pain is experienced, the hypothalamus, PAG, thalamus, and various limbic cortical regions (e.g., ACC, insular, anterior cingulate, and prefrontal cortices) are activated. This pattern of activation is consistent with the strong affective and cognitive components of visceral sensation (Hobson & Aziz, 2003; Laird & Schaible, 2005).

NEUROPATHIC PAIN

Neuropathic pain has been defined by the Neuropathic Pain Special Interest Group of the IASP as "pain arising as a direct consequence of a lesion or disease affecting the somatosensory system" (Merskey & Bogduk, 1994; Koltzenburg, 2005; Jensen et al., 2011). Neuropathic pain is a chronic pain state resulting from peripheral or central nerve injury either due to acute events (e.g., amputation, spinal cord injury) or systemic disease (e.g., diabetes, viral infection, cancer) (Merskey & Bogduk, 1994; Scholz & Woolf, 2005; Zhuo et al., 2011). It has more recently been considered a syndrome, which manifests a variety of symptoms and signs, rather than a disease, and mechanisms underlying this syndrome are multiple, and mainly unknown (Jensen et al., 2011).

Plastic changes take place in peripheral nociceptors, spinal dorsal horn synapses, and subcortical and cortical nuclei that are involved in the processing of noxious information and it is believed that neuropathic pain is due to these long-term plastic changes. It is likely that synaptic potentiation in the spinal cord and cortical areas together with abnormal peripheral neuronal activity after the injury contribute to neuropathic pain (Zhuo et al., 2011).

Changes in the activity of spared sensory afferents after nerve injury can result from several mechanisms. Neurotrophic factors, such as NGF, have increased expression and are released from Schwann cells and keratinocytes at the injury site. In the DRG, neurotrophic factors are synthesized and enhance the expression of SP in nociceptors. Cytokines (primarily TNF-α) derived from Schwann and immune cells at the site of the nerve lesion and from macrophages and T-cell lymphocytes invading the DRG lead to increased excitability of intact sensory afferents. The membrane excitability of spared afferents is also increased by a redistribution of Na$_v$ 1.8 and upregulation of TRPV1. In addition, sympathetic fibers sprout into the DRG and can further sensitize intact neurons through the release of norepinephrine (Scholz & Woolf, 2005). NMDA-receptor-dependent synaptic plasticity at the spinal and cortical levels is believed to contribute to enhanced sensory responses after injury. Glial cells, including astrocytes and microglia, have recently been implicated in neuropathic pain. These glial cells form close interactions with neurons and thus, may modulate nociceptive transmission under pathological conditions (Scholz & Woolf, 2005; Austin & Moalem-Taylor, 2010; Zhuo et al., 2011).

Among the most important pathophysiological changes underlying the development of neuropathic pain is the electrical hyperexcitability and ectopic electrogenesis (abnormal impulse generation) that occurs in injured primary sensory neurons. Ectopia involves spontaneous firing in some neurons, and abnormal responsiveness to mechanical, thermal, and chemical stimuli in many more. Major sources of ectopic firing include neuroma endbulbs, regenerating or collateral sprouts, cell bodies in the DRG, and patches of demyelinated axons. The cellular mechanism that appears to underlie ectopic hyperexcitability is the remodeling of voltage-sensitive ion channels, transducer molecules, and receptors in the cell membrane. Specific Na$^+$ and K$^+$ channels appear to be primary players, as they are the most directly involved in the repetitive firing process (Koltzenburg, 2005; Wall et al., 2006).

Phantom Pain

Phantom limb pain is a complex neuropathic pain syndrome associated with direct nerve injury as a result of limb amputation. Phantom limb pain is described in 60–80% of human patients following amputation (Wall et al., 2006; Ramchandran & Hauser, 2010; Vase et al., 2011), and has been reported in animals (Eicher et al., 2006; O'Hagan, 2006; Forster et al., 2010). The term phantom limb has been used to define the illusory sensation that an amputated limb is still present. Phantom limb pain is reported as originating from a nonexistent limb. Phantom limb sensation is defined as any perception that is interpreted as coming from an amputated limb (Ramchandran & Hauser, 2010; Pereira & Alves, 2011). Phantom limb pain is distinct from pain at the actual site of the amputation (stump pain). In people, it is most commonly seen after limb amputation, but similar syndromes can occur with the removal of other body parts including breasts, testicles, eyes, and tongue, and it may also be present in animals after amputation of the tail (Bennett & Perini, 2003; Eicher et al., 2006). Some retrospective studies have pointed to preamputation pain as a risk factor for phantom pain. The hypothesis is that preoperative pain may sensitize the nervous system (O'Hagan, 2006; Wall et al., 2006). In most veterinary amputations a preexisting painful condition, such as a fracture or cancer, is likely to have been present; thus, it would be expected that the incidence of phantom limb pain would be quite high (O'Hagan, 2006).

The mechanisms underlying phantom limb pain are not completely understood, but it is thought to be mediated via both central and peripheral mechanisms (Ramchandran & Hauser, 2010; Vase et al., 2011). The formation of neuromas is very common after cutting a nerve and such neuromas show spontaneous and abnormal evoked activity, which is assumed to be the result of an increased and also novel expression of sodium channels (Wall et al., 2006; Vase et al., 2011). Amputation triggers an inflammatory process and subsequent healing affects peripheral innervation. The affected nerve pathways exhibit injuries of the epineurium, perineurium, endoneurium, and Schwann cells. In addition to the injury, the myelin of the axons also suffers inflammatory damage and much of it is lost. Nevertheless, a large number of free nerve endings remain viable at the ends of the nerves in the stump of the amputated limb (Pereira & Alves, 2011). In the DRG, cell bodies show similar abnormal spontaneous activity and increased sensitivity to mechanical and neurochemical stimulation. Dorsal root ganglion cells exhibit major changes in the expression of sodium channels with an altered expression pattern of other channel types. Spinal plasticity and increase in the general excitability of spinal cord neurons occur as well. The sympathetic nervous system may also play an important role in generating and maintaining phantom pain. Sympatholytic blocks can abolish neuropathic pain, whereas application of norepinephrine or activation of the postganglionic sympathetic fibers can provoke this pain. Following limb amputation there is a reorganization of the primary somatosensory cortex, which may be, at least in part, the consequence of alterations at the level of the thalamus and also at the brain stem or spinal cord (Wall et al., 2006).

AUTONOMIC SYSTEM AND PAIN

The nociceptive and autonomic systems interact at multiple levels, including the periphery, dorsal horn, brain stem, and forebrain (Benarroch & Sandroni, 2005). Pain causes strong negative emotional reactions and stimulates autonomic nervous system responses ranging from vagally mediated bradycardia to sympathetic nervous system activation resulting in hypertension and tachycardia. Whereas nociceptive inputs may trigger autonomic response via the NTS, PBN, amygdala, hypothalamus, and VLM, noxious stimuli also have direct access to effector preganglionic autonomic neurons. Nociceptive afferents activate neurons in the dorsal horn, which project monosynaptically to preganglionic sympathetic neurons at the same spinal segment. This provides the basis for segmental somatosympathetic and viscerosympathetic reflexes (Benarroch, 2006; Griffis et al., 2006).

Inflammation and nerve injury may produce sympathetically maintained pain through coupling of the sensory nociceptive and sympathetic efferent components of the peripheral nervous system (Wall et al., 2006). After partial nerve injury, injured and uninjured C and Aβ fibers upregulate expression of α-adrenoreceptors. This renders nociceptive axons sensitive to norepinephrine release from postganglionic sympathetic terminals, as well as to circulating catecholamines. Additionally, after injury sympathetic fibers sprout into the DRG and form "baskets" predominantly around large Aβ neuronal cell bodies. This sprouting is mediated by NGF and, overall, it is thought that these baskets may have a functional role in amplifying sensory inflow (Benarroch & Sandroni, 2005).

IMMUNE SYSTEM AND PAIN

Interactions between the immune and peripheral nervous systems may contribute to the generation of inflammatory and neuropathic pain (Wall et al., 2006; Austin & Moalem-Taylor, 2010). Various cytokines (in particular, TNFα and interleukins 1 and 6), produced by immunocompetent cells and Schwann cells following injury, can cause peripheral and central hyperalgesia (Benarroch & Sandroni, 2005; Leung & Cahill, 2010; Phillips & Clauw, 2011). Cytokines can also induce sympathetic sprouting in the DRG (Benarroch & Sandroni, 2005).

Pain has deleterious effects on immune function through the stress-response and activation of neuroendocrine pathways (Page & Ben-Eliyahu, 1997; Kremer, 1999; Page, 2000; Yardeni et al., 2009). It can influence immune variables including the number and functional capacity of natural killer cells (NK) and other lymphocytes (Griffis et al., 2006; Snyder & Greenberg, 2010), and the synthesis and release of certain cytokines. A decrease in the production of cytokines that favor cellular-mediated immunity, such as IL-2, IL-12, and IFN-γ, and an increase in the production of cytokines, such as IL-10, that interfere with cell-mediated immunity, occurs (Sommer & Kress, 2004; Yardeni et al., 2009; Snyder & Greenberg, 2010).

An emerging field of interest is the effect of pain on NK cells, which play a key role in controlling metastatic processes. Low NK activity during the perioperative period is associated with higher rates of cancer recurrence and mortality in humans with certain types of cancer. Pain-relieving treatment was shown to attenuate surgery-induced decreases in host resistance against metastasis in a rat model (Page, 2000; Snyder & Greenberg, 2010).

SUMMARY

The pain pathway allows detection and reaction to stimuli that pose a threat to the integrity, and potentially survival, of an organism. The anatomy and physiology underpinning the processing of pain are complex and current understanding is evolving. Multiple steps, from the periphery to higher order brain centers, are involved in the generation, transmission, modification, and perception of pain. Knowledge of the various components and processes will allow a more thorough approach to the prevention and treatment of pain and resultant suffering in veterinary patients.

REFERENCES

Austin, P.J. & Moalem-Taylor, G. (2010) The neuro-immune balance in neuropathic pain: involvement of inflammatory immune cells, immune-like glial cells and cytokines. *Journal of Neuroimmunology*, 229, 26–50.

Basser, D.S. (2012) Chronic pain: a neuroscientific understanding. *Medical Hypotheses*, 78, 79–85.

Benarroch, E.E. (2006) Pain-autonomic interactions. *Neurological Sciences*, 27, S130–S133.

Benarroch, E.E. & Sandroni, P. (2005) Pain and the autonomic nervous system, in *The Neurobiological Basis of Pain*, (ed. M. Pappagallo), McGraw-Hill Professional, New York.

Bennett, P.C. & Perini, E. (2003) Tail docking in dogs: a review of the issues. *Australian Veterinary Journal*, 81, 208–218.

Brooks, J. & Tracey, I. (2005) From nociception to pain perception: imaging the spinal and supraspinal pathways. *Journal of Anatomy*, 207, 19–33.

Bushlin, I., Rozenfeld, R., & Devi, L.A. (2010) Cannabinoid-opioid interactions during neuropathic pain and analgesia. *Current Opinions in Pharmacology*, 10, 80–86.

Caterina, M.J., Gold, M.S., & Meyer, R.A. (2005) Molecular biology of nociception, in *The Neurobiology of Pain* (eds S.P. Hunt & M. Koltzenburg), Oxford University Press, New York.

Caterina, M.J., Leffler, A., Malmberg, A.B., et al. (2000) Impaired nociception and pain sensation in mice lacking the capsaicin receptor. *Science*, 288, 306–313.

Cervero, F. (1994) Sensory innervation of the viscera: peripheral basis of visceral pain. *Physiological Reviews*, 74, 95–138.

Cervero, F. & Laird, J.M. (1996) Mechanisms of touch-evoked pain (allodynia): a new model. *Pain*, 68, 13–23.

Cervero, F., Laird, J.M., & Pozo, M.A. (1992) Selective changes of receptive field properties of spinal nociceptive neurones induced by noxious visceral stimulation in the cat. *Pain*, 51, 335–342.

Christianson, J.A. & Davis, B.M. (2010) The role of visceral afferents in disease, in *Translational Pain Research: From Mouse to Man* (eds L. Kruger, & A.R. Light), CRC Press, Boca Raton, FL.

Chung, M.K., Jung, S.J., & Oh, S.B. (2011) Role of TRP channels in pain sensation. *Advances in Experimental and Medical Biology*, 704, 615–636.

Conta, A.C. & Stelzner, D.J. (2004) Differential vulnerability of propriospinal tract neurons to spinal cord contusion injury. *Journal of Comparative Neurology*, 479, 347–359.

Cowley, K.C., Zaporozhets, E., & Schmidt, B.J. (2008) Propriospinal neurons are sufficient for bulbospinal transmission of the locomotor command signal in the neonatal rat spinal cord. *Journal of Physiology*, 586, 1623–1635.

Cummins, T.R., Sheets, P.L., & Waxman, S.G. (2007) The roles of sodium channels in nociception: Implications for mechanisms of pain. *Pain*, 131, 243–257.

Dubin, A.E. & Patapoutian, A. (2010) Nociceptors: the sensors of the pain pathway. *Journal of Clinical Investigation*, 120, 3760–3772.

Eicher, S.D., Cheng, H.W., Sorrells, A.D., & Schutz, M.M. (2006) Short communication: behavioral and physiological indicators of sensitivity or chronic pain following tail docking. *Journal of Dairy Science*, 89, 3047–3051.

Fletcher, T.F. (1993) Spinal cord and meninges, in *Miller's Anatomy of the Dog*, 3rd edn (ed. H.E. Evans), Saunders, Philadelphia, PA.

Forster, L.M., Wathes, C.M., Bessant, C., & Corr, S.A. (2010) Owners' observations of domestic cats after limb amputation. *Veterinary Record*, 167, 734–739.

Gadea, A. & Lopez-Colome, A.M. (2001a) Glial transporters for glutamate, glycine and GABA I. Glutamate transporters. *Journal of Neuroscience Research*, 63, 453–460.

Gadea, A. & Lopez-Colome, A.M. (2001b) Glial transporters for glutamate, glycine, and GABA III. Glycine transporters. *Journal of Neuroscience Research*, 64, 218–222.

Gadea, A. & Lopez-Colome, A.M. (2001c) Glial transporters for glutamate, glycine, and GABA: II. GABA transporters. *Journal of Neuroscience Research*, 63, 461–468.

Gebhart, G.F. (2000a) Pathobiology of visceral pain: molecular mechanisms and therapeutic implications IV. Visceral afferent contributions to the pathobiology of visceral pain. *American Journal of Physiology. Gastrointestinal and Liver Physiology*, 278, G834–G838.

Gebhart, G.F. (2000b) Visceral pain-peripheral sensitisation. *Gut*, 47(S4), iv54–iv55; discussion iv58.

Gebhart, G.F. & Proudfit, H.K. (2005) Descending control of pain processing, in *The Neurobiology of Pain* (eds S.P. Hunt, & M. Koltzenburg), Oxford University Press, New York.

Golden, J.P., Hoshi, M., & Nassar, M.A., (2010) RET signaling is required for survival and normal function of nonpeptidergic nociceptors. *Journal of Neuroscience*, 30, 3983–3994.

Goshgarian, H.G. 2003. Anatomy and Function of the Spinal Cord, in *Spinal Cord Medicine: Principles and Practice* (eds V. Lin, D. Cardenas & N.E.A. Cutter), Demos Medical Publishing, New York.

Griffis, C.A., Compton, P., & Doering, L. (2006) The effect of pain on leukocyte cellular adhesion molecules. *Biological Research for Nursing*, 7, 297–312.

Gustin, S.M., Wilcox, S.L., Peck, C.C., Murray, G.M., & Henderson, L.A. (2011) Similarity of suffering: equivalence of psychological and psychosocial factors in neuropathic and non-neuropathic orofacial pain patients. *Pain*, 152, 825–832.

Heinricher, M.M., Tavares, I., Leith, J.L., & Lumb, B.M. (2009) Descending control of nociception: Specificity, recruitment and plasticity. *Brain Research Reviews*, 60, 214–225.

Henry, D.E., Chiodo, A.E., & Yang, W. (2011) Central nervous system reorganization in a variety of chronic pain states: a review. *Physical Medicine & Rehabilitation: the journal of injury, function, and rehabilitation*, 3, 1116–1125.

Hobson, A.R. & Aziz, Q. (2003) Central nervous system processing of human visceral pain in health and disease. *News in Physiological Sciences*, 18, 109–114.

Hofbauer, R.K., Rainville, P., Duncan, G.H., & Bushnell, M.C. (2001) Cortical representation of the sensory dimension of pain. *Journal of Neurophysiology*, 86, 402–411.

Jaggi, A.S. & Singh, N. (2011) Role of different brain areas in peripheral nerve injury-induced neuropathic pain. *Brain Research*, 1381, 187–201.

Jensen, T.S., Baron, R., Haanpaa, M., et al. (2011) A new definition of neuropathic pain. *Pain*, 152, 2204–2205.

Julius, D. & Basbaum, A.I. (2001) Molecular mechanisms of nociception. *Nature*, 413, 203–210.

Kawasaki, Y., Kohno, T., Zhuang, Z.Y., et al. (2004) Ionotropic and metabotropic receptors, protein kinase A, protein kinase C, and Src contribute to C-fiber-induced ERK activation and cAMP response element-binding protein phosphorylation in dorsal horn neurons, leading to central sensitization. *Journal of Neuroscience*, 24, 8310–8321.

Koltzenburg, M. (2005) Mechanisms of peripheral neuropathic pain, in *The Neurobiology of Pain* (eds S.P. Hunt, & M. Koltzenburg), Oxford University Press, New York.

Kremer, M.J. (1999) Surgery, pain, and immune function. *The Clinical Forum for Nurse Anesthetists*, 10, 94–100.

Kut, E., Candia, V., von Overbeck, J., Pok, J., Fink, D., & Folkers, G. (2011) Pleasure-related analgesia activates opioid-insensitive circuits. *The Journal of Neuroscience*, 31, 4148–4153.

Laird, J.M.A. & Schaible, H.G. (2005) Visceral and deep somatic pain, in *The Neurobiology of Pain* (eds S.P. Hunt, & M. Koltzenburg), Oxford University Press, New York.

Lee, Y.C., Nassikas, N.J., & Clauw, D.J. (2011) The role of the central nervous system in the generation and maintenance of chronic pain in rheumatoid arthritis, osteoarthritis and fibromyalgia. *Arthritis Research and Therapy*, 13, 211.

Leffler, A., Fischer, M.J., Rehner, D., et al. (2008) The vanilloid receptor TRPV1 is activated and sensitized by local anesthetics in rodent sensory neurons. *Journal of Clinical Investigation*, 118, 763–776.

Leung, L. & Cahill, C.M. (2010) TNF-alpha and neuropathic pain–a review. *Journal of Neuroinflammation*, 7, 27.

Lovick, T. & Bandler, R. (2005) The organization of the midbrain periaqueductal grey and the integration of pain behaviours in *The Neurobiology of Pain* (eds S.P. Hunt & M. Koltzenburg), Oxford University Press, New York.

Masedo, A.I. & Esteve, R. (2002) On the affective nature of chronic pain. *Psicothema*, 14, 511–515.

Maxwell, D.J., Belle, M.D., Cheunsuang, O., Stewart, A., & Morris, R. (2007) Morphology of inhibitory and excitatory interneurons in superficial laminae of the rat dorsal horn. *Journal of Physiology*, 584, 521–533.

McMahon, S.B. & Priestley, J.V. (2005) Nociceptor plasticity, in *The Neurobiology of Pain* (eds S.P. Hunt& M. Koltzenburg), Oxford University Press, New York.

Melzack, R. (1999). From the gate to the neuromatrix. *Pain*, S6, S121–S126.

Melzack, R. & Katz, J. (2002) The problem of pain: measurement in clinical settings, in *Surgical Management of Pain* (ed. K. Burchiel), Thieme Medical Publishers, Inc., New York.

Melzack, R. & Wall, P.D. (1965) Pain mechanisms: a new theory. *Science*, 150, 971–979.

Melzack, R., Wall, P.D., & Ty, T.C. (1982) Acute pain in an emergency clinic: latency of onset and descriptor patterns related to different injuries. *Pain*, 14, 33–43.

Merskey, H. & Bogduk, N. (1994) Part III: Pain terms, a current list with definitions and notes on usage, in *Classification of Chronic Pain*, 2nd edn (eds H. Merskey & N. Bogduk), IASP Press, Seattle.

Millan, M.J. (2002) Descending control of pain. *Progress in Neurobiology*, 66, 355–474.

Molony, V. & Kent, J.E. (1997) Assessment of acute pain in farm animals using behavioral and physiological measurements. *Journal of Animal Science*, 75, 266–272.

Muir, W.W. 3rd (2009) Physiology and pathophysiology of pain, in *Handbook of Veterinary Pain Management*, 2nd edn (eds J.S. Gaynor & W.W. Muir 3rd), Mosby Elsevier, St. Louis, MO.

Muir, W.W. 3rd & Woolf, C.J. (2001) Mechanisms of pain and their therapeutic implications. *Journal of the American Veterinary Medical Association*, 219, 1346–1356.

Ness, T.J. & Gebhart, G.F. (2005) Mechanisms of visceral pain, in *The Neurobiological Basis of Pain* (ed. M. Pappagallo), McGraw-Hill Professional, New York.

O'Hagan, B.J. (2006) Neuropathic pain in a cat post-amputation. *Australian Veterinary Journal*, 84, 83–86.

Ossipov, M.H., Dussor, G.O., & Porreca, F. (2010) Central modulation of pain. *Journal of Clinical Investigation*, 120, 3779–3787.

Ostrowsky, K., Magnin, M., Ryvlin, P., Isnard, G., Guenot, M., & Mauguiere, F. (2002) Representation of pain and somatic sensation in the human insula: a study of responses to direct electrical cortical stimulation. *Cerebral Cortex*, 12, 376–385.

Page, G.G. (2000) The immune-suppressive effects of pain, in *Madame Curie Bioscience Database* [Internet], Landes Bioscience, Austin, TX.

Page, G.G. & Ben-Eliyahu, S. (1997) The immune-suppressive nature of pain. *Seminars in Oncology Nursing*, 13, 10–15.

Pereira, J.C. Jr. & Alves, R.C. (2011) The labelled-lines principle of the somatosensory physiology might explain the phantom limb phenomenon. *Medical Hypotheses*, 77, 853–856.

Peyron, R., Laurent, B. & Garcia-Larrea, L. (2000) Functional imaging of brain responses to pain. A review and meta-analysis. *Neurophysiologie Cliniques*, 30, 263–288.

Phillips, K. & Clauw, D.J. (2011) Central pain mechanisms in chronic pain states–maybe it is all in their head. Best Practice & Research. *Clinical Rheumatology*, 25, 141–154.

Procacci, P. & Maresca, M. (1999) Referred pain from somatic and visceral structures. *Current Reviews in Pain*, 3, 96–99.

Qi, F.H., Zhou, Y.L., & Xu, G.Y. (2011) Targeting voltage-gated sodium channels for treatment for chronic visceral pain. *World Journal of Gastroenterology*, 17, 2357–2364.

Ramchandran, K. & Hauser, J. (2010) Phantom limb pain. *Journal of Palliative Medicine*, 13, 1285–1286.

Rice, M.E. & Cragg, S.J. (2008) Dopamine spillover after quantal release: rethinking dopamine transmission in the nigrostriatal pathway. *Brain Research Reviews*, 58, 303–313.

Riedl, M.S., Schnell, S.A., Overland, A.C., et al. (2009) Coexpression of alpha 2A-adrenergic and delta-opioid receptors in substance P-containing terminals in rat dorsal horn. *Journal of Comparative Neurology*, 513, 385–398.

Rohacs, T., Thyagarajan, B., & Lukacs, V. (2008) Phospholipase C mediated modulation of TRPV1 channels. *Molecular Neurobiology*, 37, 153–163.

Romero, R., Sauzdalnitski, D., & Banack, T. (2011) Ischemic and visceral pain, in *Essentials of Pain Management* (eds N. Vadivelu, R.D. Urman, & R.L. Hines), Springer Science, New York .

Rosenbaum, T., Simon, S.A., & Islas, L.D. (2010) Ion channels in analgesia research. *Methods in Molecular Biology*, 617, 223–236.

Sachs, D., Coelho, F.M., Costa, V.V., et al. (2011) Cooperative role of tumour necrosis factor-alpha, interleukin-1beta and neutrophils in a novel behavioural model that concomitantly demonstrates articular inflammation and hypernociception in mice. *British Journal of Pharmacology*, 162, 72–83.

Salter, M.W. & Woolf, C.J. (2005) Cellular and molecular mechanisms of central sensitization, in *The Neurobiology of Pain* (eds S.P. Hunt & M. Koltzenburg), Oxford University Press, New York.

Sandkuhler, J., Stelzer, B., & Fu, Q.G. (1993) Characteristics of propriospinal modulation of nociceptive lumbar spinal dorsal horn neurons in the cat. *Neuroscience*, 54, 957–967.

Schaible, H.G., Ebersberger, A., & Natura, G. (2011) Update on peripheral mechanisms of pain: beyond prostaglandins and cytokines. *Arthritis Research and Therapy*, 13, 210.

Scholz, J. & Woolf, C.J. (2005) Mechanisms of neuropathic pain, in *The Neurobiological Basis of Pain* (ed. M. Pappagallo), McGraw-Hill Professional, New York.

Sengupta, J.N. (2009) Visceral pain: the neurophysiological mechanism. *Handbook of Experimental Pharmacology*, 194, 31–74.

Smith, E.S. & Lewin, G.R. (2009) Nociceptors: a phylogenetic view. *Journal of comparative physiology. A, Neuroethology, sensory, neural, and behavioral physiology*, 195, 1089–1106.

Snyder, G.L. & Greenberg, S. (2010) Effect of anaesthetic technique and other perioperative factors on cancer recurrence. *British Journal of Anaesthesia*, 105, 106–115.

Sommer, C. & Kress, M. (2004) Recent findings on how proinflammatory cytokines cause pain: peripheral mechanisms in inflammatory and neuropathic hyperalgesia. *Neuroscience Letters*, 361, 184–187.

Stamford, J.A. (1995) Descending control of pain. *British Journal of Anaesthesia*, 75, 217–227.

Todd, A.J. & Ribeiro-Da-Silva, A. (2005) Molecular architecture of the dorsal horn, in *The Neurobiology of Pain* (eds S.P. Hunt& M. Koltzenburg), Oxford University Press, New York.

Treede, R.D., Kenshalo, D.R., Gracely, R.H., & Jones, A.K. (1999) The cortical representation of pain. *Pain*, 79, 105–111.

Vase, L., Nikolajsen, L., Christensen, B., et al. (2011) Cognitive-emotional sensitization contributes to wind-up-like pain in phantom limb pain patients. *Pain*, 152, 157–162.

Vriens, J., Appendino, G., & Nilius, B. (2009) Pharmacology of vanilloid transient receptor potential cation channels. *Molecular Pharmacology*, 75, 1262–1279.

Vyklicky, L., Novakova-Tousova, K., Benedikt, J., Samad, A., Touska, F., Vlachova, V. (2008) Calcium-dependent desensitization of vanilloid receptor TRPV1: a mechanism possibly involved in analgesia induced by topical application of capsaicin. *Physiological Research*, 57(S3), S59–S68.

Wagner, A.E. (2010) Effects of stress on pain in horses and incorporating pain scales for equine practice. *Veterinary Clinics of North America: Equine Practice*, 26, 481–492.

Wall, P.D., McMahon, S.B., & Koltzenburg, M. (2006) *Wall and Melzack's Textbook of Pain*, Elsevier/Churchill Livingstone, Philadelphia, PA.

Watson, C.A. & Kayalioglu, G. (2009) The organization of the spinal cord, in *The Spinal Cord: A Christopher and Dana Reeve Foundation Text and Atlas* (eds C. Watson, G.A. Paxinos, & G. Kayalioglu), Academic Press Elsevier, London.

Weber, R.N., Blair, R.W., & Foreman, R.D. (1982) Effects of cardiac administration of bradykinin on thoracic spinal neurons in the cat. *Experimental Neurology*, 78, 703–715.

Westlund, K.N. (2005) Neurophysiology of nociception in *The Neurobiological Basis of Pain* (ed. M. Pappagallo), McGraw-Hill Professional, New York.

Willcockson, H. & Valtschanoff, J. (2008) AMPA and NMDA glutamate receptors are found in both peptidergic and non-peptidergic primary afferent neurons in the rat. *Cell and Tissue Research*, 334, 17–23.

Willis, W.D. & Westlund, K.N. (1997) Neuroanatomy of the pain system and of the pathways that modulate pain. *Journal of Clinical Neurophysiology*, 14, 2–31.

Woolf, C.J. & Salter, M.W. (2000) Neuronal plasticity: increasing the gain in pain. *Science*, 288, 1765–1769.

Yardeni, I.Z., Beilin, B., Mayburd, E., Levinson, Y., & Bessler, H. (2009) The effect of perioperative intravenous lidocaine on postoperative pain and immune function. *Anesthesia and Analgesia*, 109, 1464–1469.

Zhuo, M., Wu, G. & Wu, L.J. (2011) Neuronal and microglial mechanisms of neuropathic pain. *Molecular Brain*, 4, 31.

Zoli, M., Jansson, A., Sykova, E., Agnati, L.F., & Fuxe, K. (1999) Volume transmission in the CNS and its relevance for neuropsychopharmacology. *Trends in Pharmacological Sciences*, 20, 142–150.

3
Mechanisms of Cancer Pain

Cholawat Pacharinsak and Alvin J. Beitz

The life expectancy for cancer patients has increased dramatically due to knowledge gained from translational research and technological developments in cancer detection and therapy. However, the increase in life expectancy resulting from these technological breakthroughs has raised important issues related to quality of life, in that cancer patients may experience pain for a much longer period of time. Among human patients, 6.6 million people die from cancer each year, and pain can occur at any time during cancer development and progression (IASP, 2009). The treatment of human patients with cancer pain is typically suboptimal (Fine et al., 2004), because available therapeutics are often aimed at symptom management rather than targeting the multiple mechanisms underlying the generation and propagation of cancer-associated pain. The present review is focused on neurobiological mechanisms of cancer pain.

PREVALENCE OF CANCER PAIN

The prevalence of cancer pain is difficult to estimate due to a lack of validated methods to effectively assess pain, the variability in the pain experience that occurs among cancer patients, genetic covariants of pain severity, such as those associated with cytokine gene polymorphisms (Reyes-Gibby et al., 2009), and factors associated with clinician intention to address diverse aspects of pain (Shugarman et al., 2010). While it is difficult to gauge the exact prevalence of cancer pain in human patients, it is more challenging in veterinary medicine. A 1998 study based on postmortem examination, reported that 47% of dogs and 32% of cats died from cancer (Morris Animal Foundation, 1998). These data are consistent with a study of 2002 dogs, which reported that cancer accounted for 20% and 40–45% of the deaths for 5-year-old and 10- to 16-year-old dogs, respectively (Bronson, 1982). In a recent extensive survey of purebred dogs, it was established that the most common cause of death was cancer (27%) (Adams et al., 2010). The survey also found that cancers of the mammary glands, testicles, gastrointestinal tract, lungs, and soft tissue sarcomas are the most common neoplasms of older dogs. Cancer is also a major cause of death in cats and a 2010 survey of juvenile cats in the United Kingdom revealed that 70% of feline neoplasms were malignant or potentially would become malignant. The same study reported that the most common tumors in cats were lymphoma (22%) and soft tissue sarcomas (15%) (Schmidt et al., 2010b).

Collectively, these data support the concept that cancer is a major cause of death in cats and dogs, and one would anticipate that cancer, and the subsequent treatments, might have a dramatic impact on their quality of life. Unfortunately, there are no reliable data on the number of animals that suffer from cancer pain. It is likely that many animals are undertreated for cancer-associated pain due to a lack of recognition of pain and suffering, and the lack of baseline and follow-up assessments.

CAUSES OF CANCER PAIN

In human patients, tumor metastasis is the most common cause of pain associated with cancer (Coleman, 2000; 2001; 2006; Jimenez-Andrade et al., 2011). Veterinary cancer patients with advanced disease, particularly those with bone metastasis, also appear to experience significant pain, and it appears that the pain intensity is related to the degree of bone destruction. Cancer patients experience both persistent pain and breakthrough pain and the latter represents a distinct clinical entity (Caraceni & Portenoy, 1999; Caraceni & Weinstein, 2001). Pain can also be associated with cancer invasion of adjacent tissues, particularly peripheral nerves, adverse affects of treatment (e.g., radiation burns), and concurrent disease (e.g., osteoarthritis) (Caraceni & Weinstein, 2001; Fox, 2010).

MECHANISMS OF CANCER PAIN

While there have been attempts to develop a more comprehensive understanding of the underlying mechanisms of cancer pain over the past decade, the cancer pain process has proved to be multifaceted, uncovering the biochemical details has been challenging, and providing a simplistic neurobiological explanation seems unlikely. Cancer pain is a dynamic, complicated process and involves significant plasticity in both the peripheral and central nervous systems (Gordon-Williams & Dickenson, 2007). A number of different mediators, including endothelin-1 (ET-1), bradykinin, and calcitonin gene-related peptide (CGRP) are released peripherally and cause various physiological changes in the spinal cord during the course of cancer development. In addition, cancer can induce different types of pain depending upon the type and location of primary and secondary (metastasized) cancer (Schmidt et al., 2010a). Therefore, the pain caused by cancer can be classified into two

Pain Management in Veterinary Practice, First Edition. Edited by Christine M. Egger, Lydia Love and Tom Doherty.

categories—cancer-related pain and cancer-unrelated pain. Cancer-related pain can be classified into cancer-induced pain, pain due to cancer invasion or metastasis, cancer-induced peripheral neuropathy, chemotherapy- and radiotherapy-related peripheral neuropathy, and pain due to surgery. Cancer-unrelated pain can be classified into pain due to infection and inflammation, concurrent disorders, and psychological pain.

MECHANISMS OF CANCER-RELATED PAIN

Developing more effective treatments for tumor-induced pain requires a better knowledge of the mechanisms responsible for generating this type of nociception. In the past two decades, a number of animal models have been developed to study many types of complicated pain syndromes, for example, inflammatory pain, neuropathic pain, and cancer pain (Ma, 2007). Rodents are the most commonly used animal models of cancer pain. The first animal model of cancer pain was developed in 1998 (Wacnik et al., 1998). Additional animal models of cancer pain have since been developed in mice (Wacnik et al., 2000), rats (Medhurst et al., 2002; Pacharinsak & Beitz, 2008), and dogs (Brown et al., 2005).

While our knowledge is far from complete, the complexity of the biological events and mediators that trigger cancer pain are starting to be understood (Table 3.1; Figure 3.1). In the following sections, we will first summarize current knowledge related to peripheral mechanisms of cancer pain, and then provide an overview of the central mechanisms, particularly at the level of the spinal cord, that contribute to this chronic pain state.

Peripheral Mechanisms of Cancer Pain

Several peripheral mechanisms for the generation of cancer pain have been suggested, including ectopic impulse generation (Yaari & Devor, 1985), spontaneous discharge and decreased noxious stimulation threshold (Xiao & Bennett, 2008), and nociceptor sensitization (Hamamoto et al., 2008). Implantation of fibrosarcoma cells into rodent calcaneus bone results in the development of pain-related behaviors and mechanical hyperalgesia (Cain et al., 2001). Electrophysiological recording revealed that 34% of C-fibers developed tumor-induced spontaneous activity and decreased thermal thresholds for activation, suggesting that the developing tumor causes C-fiber activation and sensitization (Cain et al., 2001). This is partially dependent on the release of ET-1 at the tumor site (Hamamoto et al., 2008) and noradrenergic receptor activation (Paice, 2003). The following section summarizes some of the peripheral mediators released at the tumor site that are responsible for cancer pain.

ENDOTHELIN-1

ET-1 is a vasoactive peptide that acts at peripheral sites via the G-protein-coupled receptors ET-A and ET-B. Endothelin-A receptors are implicated in the development of acute pain, vasoconstriction, and bronchoconstriction, and ET-B receptors are associated with inflammatory pain and vasodilation (Bagnato & Natali, 2004). Both receptor types are found on dorsal root ganglion neurons (DRGs) and ET-B is also found on Schwann cells.

ET-1 injection excites nociceptors and enhances tumor-induced pain. Part of this hyperalgesic effect appears to occur via potentiation of transient receptor potential vanilloid subtype 1 (TRPV1)

Table 3.1. Neurochemical mediators and electrophysiological changes that contribute to cancer pain

Peripheral sensitization
ET-1
Bradykinin
NGF
Cytokines: TNF-α, IL-1β, IL-6, G-CSF, GM-CSF
ASIC
TRPV1
Osteoclasts
Others: prostanoids, COX, PAR-2
Central sensitization
Dynorphin
Substance P
CGRP
Glutamate/aspartate
c-Fos expression
Astrocyte hypertrophy
ATP (P_2X_3)
TRPV1
NGF (TrkA receptors)
Electrophysiology findings
↑ WDR neuron responses
↑ Receptive field size
↑ NS neuron responses to non-noxious stimuli
Alter NS:WDR neurons ratio

ASIC, acid-sensing ion channels; ATP, adenosine triphosphate; CGRP, calcitonin gene-related peptide; COX, cyclooxygenase; ET, endothelin; G-CSF, granulocyte colony-stimulating factor; GM-CSF, granulocyte-macrophage colony-stimulating factor; IL, interleukin; NS, nonspiking; NGF, nerve growth factor; PAR-2, protease-activated receptor 2; TNFα, tumor necrosis factor alpha; TRPVI, transient receptor potential vanilloid subtype 1; WDR, wide dynamic range.

receptors located on nociceptive fibers (Wacnik et al., 2000; Pomonis et al., 2001; Peters et al., 2004). ET-1 is found in a number of different tumor types including prostatic (Yuyama et al., 2004), oral squamous cell carcinoma (Schmidt et al., 2007), melanoma (Schmidt et al., 2007), and renal, ovarian, and breast carcinoma (Bagnato & Natali, 2004). Additionally, even though ET-1 is not produced by all tumor types it is often present at the tumor site, and may contribute to the nociceptive process induced by the tumor (Kurbel et al., 1999; Asham et al., 2001; Davar, 2001; Wacnik et al., 2001; Zhou et al., 2001; Pickering et al., 2008). Increased concentrations of ET-1 and concomitant activation of primary afferent fibers were observed in a fibrosarcoma bone tumor model, but not in a control melanoma bone tumor model, where ET-1 concentrations were undetectable (Wacnik et al., 2001). In addition, hyperalgesia was only observed in fibrosarcoma-implanted mice, and this hyperalgesia was significantly reduced by administration of an ET-A antagonist (Wacnik et al., 2001; Hasue et al., 2004; Peters et al., 2004).

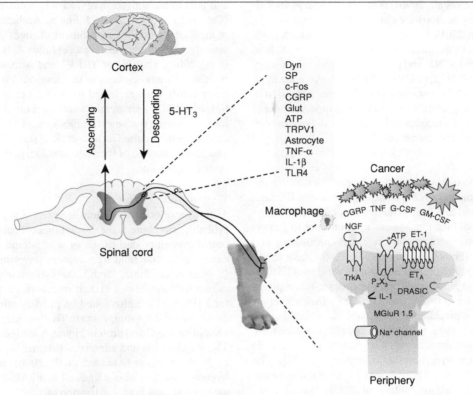

Figure 3.1. The crucial components for inducing and maintaining cancer pain occur both peripherally and centrally. At the injury site, cancer cells release substances such as CGRP, tumor necrosis factor alpha (TNF-α), and granulocyte and granulocyte-macrophage colony-stimulating factors (G-CSF and GM-CSF). In addition, there are other substances released in the area such as nerve growth factor (NGF; binding to TrkA receptors), ATP (binding to P_2X_3 receptors), and ET-1 (binding to ET-A receptors). Centrally, several substances are involved and receptors expressed, including dynorphin (Dyn), substance P (SP), c-Fos expression, CGRP, glutamate (Glut), ATP, transient receptor potential vanilloid 1 (TRPV1) receptor expression, astrocyte migration, tumor necrosis factor (TNF-α), interleukin-1 β (IL-1β), and toll-like receptor 4 (TLR4) expression. While pain perception is propagated to the higher brain levels via ascending pathways, the spinal cord also receives descending facilitation from the brain known to involve serotonin (5-HT₃). Courtesy of Janis Atuk-Jones.

ET-1 causes excitation of C and A-δ fibers via ET-A receptors (Gokin et al., 2001), but a large dose of ET-1 can actually produce antinociception via ET-B receptors (Piovezan et al., 2000). Moreover, ET-A antagonists decreased mechanical hyperalgesia and ongoing pain behaviors, and ET-B antagonists enhanced these behaviors (Peters et al., 2004). Mechanical hyperalgesia, induced by prostatic cancer, can be attenuated by oral administration of an ET-A antagonist (Yuyama et al., 2004; Russo et al., 2010). Thus, it seems that antinociception in the periphery can be induced by administration of either ET-A antagonists or ET-B agonists (Gokin et al., 2001; Khodorova et al., 2002; Quang & Schmidt, 2010). Endothelin-B agonists can significantly reduce pain for up to 3 hours after administration, and this effect is attenuated by administration of a μ opioid receptor antagonist, suggesting that it is mediated by endogenous opioids (Quang & Schmidt, 2010). Interestingly, ET-B receptors are upregulated in certain types of cancers (melanoma, ovarian, and breast cancer) (Wulfing et al., 2003; Grimshaw et al., 2004), but downregulated in other types (squamous cell carcinoma, prostatic, colorectal, and bladder cancer) (Jeronimo et al., 2003; Quang & Schmidt, 2010). Thus, the role of these

receptors in tumor-induced nociception may differ depending on the tumor type.

BRADYKININ

Bradykinin is produced by melanoma cells, and is another vasoactive peptide with potent algogenic properties that appears to be involved in cancer pain. Bradykinin was shown to act on kinin B1 and B2 receptors on primary afferent neurons in a mouse model of skin cancer (Fujita et al., 2010). The release of bradykinin at the tumor site stimulates nerve fibers that innervate the tumor, and both bone-cancer-induced ongoing and movement-evoked nocifensive behaviors are reduced when the bradykinin B1 receptor is blocked (Sevcik et al., 2005). Additional information related to bradykinin and its interaction with ET-1 to cause pain can be found in the recent review by Schmidt et al. (2010a).

NERVE GROWTH FACTOR

NGF is involved in the regulation of neuronal function, synaptic plasticity, prevention of programmed cell death, and modulation and promotion of local growth and survival of sensory afferent neurons (Levi-Montalcini et al., 1996). With many cancers, including bone cancer, sensory neurons are chronically exposed to NGF (Jankowski & Koerber, 2010; Pantano et al., 2011), which leads to a number of changes in the microenvironment that contribute to pain. NGF binds directly to TRK and p75NTR receptors on primary sensory neurons. Mantyh et al. (2010) and Jimenez-Andrade et al. (2011) have shown that early, sustained administration of anti-NGF blocks the pathological sprouting of sensory and sympathetic nerve fibers and the formation of neuroma-like structures in bone cancer, inhibiting the development of cancer pain.

CYTOKINES

It is likely that tumor-associated pain is, in part, driven by the inflammatory cascade and the release of various cytokines. Immune cells at the tumor site and tumor cells themselves release a number of cytokines and chemokines that appear to contribute to tumor-induced pain. Numerous cytokines are released from tumor cell lines including IL-1β (Fonsatti et al., 1997), IL-6 (Nasu et al., 1998), IL-8 (Nasu et al., 1998), tumor necrosis factor alpha (TNF-α) (Basolo et al., 1993), and granulocyte and granulocyte-macrophage colony stimulating factor (G-CSF and GM-CSF) (Schweizerhof et al., 2009). TNF-α is a proinflammatory cytokine released at the tumor site by various cell types, including mast cells, macrophages, endothelial cells, and fibroblasts, which stimulates immune cells and generates mechanical hyperalgesia (Wacnik et al., 2005). The TNF-α receptors, TNFR1 and TNFR2, may be involved in maintaining thermal hyperalgesia (Constantin et al., 2008). Wacnik et al., (2005) demonstrated that fibrosarcoma-implanted animals exhibit an increased concentration of TNF-α at the tumor site. Administration of TNF-α causes mechanical hyperalgesia in naive animals and increased hyperalgesia in animals with fibrosarcoma (Wacnik et al., 2005). In addition, administration of a TNF-α antagonist attenuated TNF-α associated thermal hyperalgesia without affecting the tumor size (Constantin et al., 2008).

OSTEOCLASTS

Bone metastases are the most common cause of cancer-associated pain. Bone destruction caused by metastatic lesions occurs due to an increased rate of bone turnover in the absence of a complementary increase in bone formation. Osteoclast activity is crucial for bone resorption (Mantyh, 2004); thus, if osteoclast activity could be inhibited, the resulting cancer-induced pain should be relieved (Clohisy & Ramnaraine, 1998; Honore et al., 2000). This can be accomplished with intravenous bisphosphonates, but the next generation of bone metastasis treatments is in clinical development, and among them, the most advanced drug is denosumab. Denosumab is a human monoclonal antibody that inhibits osteoclast maturation and activation, and functions by binding to a receptor activator of nuclear factor κ B ligand, with the final result being a reduced rate of bone resorption (Castellano et al., 2011).

ACID-SENSING ION CHANNELS AND TRANSIENT RECEPTOR POTENTIAL VANILLOID SUBTYPE I RECEPTORS

Acid-sensing ion channels (ASIC) (Mantyh et al., 2002; Garber, 2003; Sabino & Mantyh, 2005) and TRPV1 receptors (Asai et al., 2005; Ghilardi et al., 2005; Shinoda et al., 2008; Niiyama et al., 2009; Kawamata et al., 2010; Lotsch & Geisslinger, 2011) have been implicated in cancer pain. The presence of protons and an acidic environment (pH < 6) are a distinctive feature of cancer,

and lead to the activation of TRPV1 receptors and ASIC channels (Caterina & Julius, 2001; Julius & Basbaum, 2001). The development of an acidic environment changes ASIC expression and sensitizes peripheral nociceptors (Julius & Basbaum, 2001; Nagae et al., 2007). The role of TRPV1 and ASICs as well as the acidic bone cancer environment in the development of bone cancer pain has recently been reviewed by Yoneda et al. (2011). Administration of a TRPV1 antagonist attenuated tumor-induced pain behaviors, suggesting that selective blockade of TRPV1 channels reduces cancer-induced pain (Ghilardi et al., 2005). Thus, TRPV1 and ASIC antagonists may be of therapeutic value, particularly with regard to bone cancer pain.

OTHER MEDIATORS

A number of other mediators are present at many tumor sites, and probably contribute to the development of cancer pain. Prostanoids, proinflammatory derivatives of arachidonic acid, are released by cancer cells and bind to receptors on primary afferent neurons (Sabino et al., 2002; Urch, 2004). Similarly, proteases, secreted during inflammation, and their receptors, protease-activated receptor 2 (PAR-2), are also found on primary afferent neurons. PAR-2 causes thermal hyperalgesia via TRPV1 receptors. The blockade of protein kinase C and protein kinase A abolishes the sensitization of TRPV1 channels and attenuates thermal hyperalgesia precipitated by PAR activation (Amadesi et al., 2006). In addition to thermal hyperalgesia, it is also suggested that PAR-2 may cause mechanical hyperalgesia via the activation of TRPV4 channels (Grant et al., 2007).

Central Mechanisms of Cancer Pain

WINDUP AND CENTRAL SENSITIZATION

Nociceptive input from the periphery reaches spinal cord neurons, where it is modified, and then carried by ascending pathways (the spinothalamic and spinocervicothalamic tracts) to supraspinal sites (Simone et al., 1991; Willis et al., 1999). Nociceptor inputs can trigger a prolonged but reversible increase in the excitability and synaptic efficacy of neurons in central nociceptive pathways, a phenomenon termed central sensitization (Woolf, 2011). The presence of either hyperalgesia or allodynia in a patient with cancer pain who has "spontaneous or ongoing" pain is highly indicative of central pain mechanisms. Part of this sensitization process involves "windup" which is caused by repeated stimulation of peripheral nerve fibers, leading to progressively increasing electrical response in the corresponding spinal dorsal horn neurons. Windup has been proposed to be due to gradual recruitment of N-methyl-D-aspartate (NMDA) receptor activity, to summation of slow excitatory potentials mediated by substance P (SP) (and related peptides), and/or to facilitation of slow calcium channels by metabotropic glutamate receptors (Baranauskas & Nistri, 1998). The basis for central sensitization and the mechanisms underlying this phenomenon has recently been reviewed by Woolf (2011), and are discussed more fully in Chapter 2.

Bone cancer pain is one of the most painful types of tumor-induced pain (Medhurst et al., 2002; Vermeirsch et al., 2004). Profound neurochemical changes, reorganization of the spinal cord, and resulting widespread spinal sensitization may be the underlying mechanisms responsible for the development of chronic bone cancer pain (Schwei et al., 1999; Honore et al., 2000; Honore et al.,

2000; Luger et al., 2001). Prostate cancer can induce upregulation of spinal cord IL-1β expression (Zhang et al., 2005). Electrophysiological studies in prostate cancer reveal an increased responsiveness of wide dynamic range (WDR) neurons in the spinal cord in terms of spontaneous activity and responses to mechanical and thermal stimuli (Khasabov et al., 2005). The responses of superficial WDR neurons, generally stimulated by non-noxious and noxious input, are dramatically enhanced, while deeper WDR neurons showed minimal changes, suggesting involvement of ascending and descending facilitation pathways (Urch et al., 2003; Urch et al., 2005). A recent study in a mouse model of bone cancer pain has shown that substantia gelatinosa neurons in the spinal cord dorsal horn exhibited spontaneous excitatory postsynaptic currents (EPSCs) in tumor-bearing mice (Yanagisawa et al., 2010). The amplitudes of spontaneous EPSCs were significantly larger in cancer-bearing compared to control mice, without any changes in passive membrane properties of substantia gelatinosa neurons. The α-amino-3-hydroxy-5-methyl-4-isoxazole-propionic acid (AMPA)- and NMDA-mediated ESPCs were also enhanced in mice with cancer. This study, as well as others, indicates that widespread spinal sensitization may be one of the underlying mechanisms for the development of chronic bone, and other types of cancer pain.

GLIA

A remarkable finding in animals with tumors is the development of a massive astrocyte hypertrophy in the ipsilateral spinal cord, which can be identified with glial fibrillary acidic protein (GFAP) immunostaining. Astrocyte hypertrophy occurs during cancer-induced bone destruction (Schwei et al., 1999; Zhang et al., 2005). Evidence suggests that the activation of glia contributes to central sensitization in the spinal cord (Watkins et al., 2001; Sessle, 2007; Watkins et al., 2007). The astrocyte hypertrophy observed in animal models of cancer pain is uncommonly seen with inflammatory or neuropathic pain and, therefore, represents a unique signature of cancer pain. This GFAP expression is evident as early as day 17 after tumor inoculation (Medhurst et al., 2002). Exceptionally large astrocyte hypertrophy is obvious in bone cancer models, and is believed to partly play a role in cancer pain development and maintenance (Watkins et al., 2001).

Bone Metastasis

Bone metastasis is a serious complication of many neoplastic diseases such as breast, prostate, and lung cancer and a significant contributor to cancer pain.

Pain due to Cancer Invasion of Neural Tissues

Cancer invasion of surrounding tissues can occur during cancer progression, and has been reported in human patients with pancreatic cancer (Zhu et al., 1999) and with vertebral metastasis (Zhu et al., 1999; Shimoyama et al., 2002). Invasion of neural tissue can lead to a neuropathic pain syndrome. Fibrosarcoma cells implanted near the sciatic nerve caused perineural invasion leading to the development of mechanical allodynia (Wacnik et al., 2000). Animals implanted with sarcoma cells in close proximity to the sciatic nerves also demonstrate signs of spontaneous pain, for example, lifting and guarding of the painful area, as well as thermal allodynia and hyperalgesia (Shimoyama et al., 2002). Mechanical allodynia also occurs, and transitions into mechanical hypersensitivity after

2 weeks. Cancer-induced nerve invasion causes damage to myelinated and nonmyelinated nerve fibers that is more extensive than damage caused by nerve ligation, suggesting that neoplastic nerve invasion may involve a mechanism other than direct nerve damage.

Chemotherapy- and Radiotherapy-Related Peripheral Neuropathy

Chemotherapy-induced peripheral neuropathies are dose-limiting adverse effects of many anticancer drugs. Vincristine, paclitaxel, and cisplatin produce chemotherapeutic-induced neuropathic pain in 30–70% of human patients undergoing chemotherapy (Polomano & Bennett, 2001; Vadalouca et al., 2012). The underlying cause of this chemotherapy-induced neuropathy remains unclear. However, it seems that the degree of chemotherapy-induced neuropathy varies with dose, treatment duration, and pre-existing conditions of the patient. Insight into neurotoxic mechanisms is critical to the development of new treatment and prevention strategies for chemotherapy-induced peripheral neuropathies.

Vincristine, a vinca alkaloid, is one of the most commonly used chemotherapeutic agents, and is reported to cause mechanical hyperalgesia (Authier et al., 1999; Higuera & Luo, 2004). This mechanical hyperalgesia developed as early as 2 weeks after intravenous injection in rats, and ceased when vincristine was discontinued (Aley et al., 1996). Vincristine was also reported to produce greater mechanical hyperalgesia in female rats (Joseph & Levine, 2003). Interestingly, a continuous rate infusion of vincristine dose-dependently produced mechanical hyperalgesia, but not thermal hyperalgesia (Nozaki-Taguchi et al., 2001). This mechanical hyperalgesia could be attenuated by morphine or lidocaine administration (Nozaki-Taguchi et al., 2001), but not by μ opioid antagonists (Aley et al., 1996). A recent comparison of vincristine-induced peripheral neuropathy and that induced by another anticancer agent, bortezomib, using gene expression profiling, suggests that the factors involved in the development of peripheral neuropathy are distinct, and involve different molecular mechanisms (Richardson, 2010).

Paclitaxel is commonly used to treat solid tumors, and its adverse effects include myelosuppression and peripheral neuropathy (Polomano & Bennett, 2001). In addition, human patients who received paclitaxel complained of numbness and burning pain (Polomano & Bennett, 2001). Paclitaxel-induced neuropathy lasts for several weeks and is limited to peripheral nerves, with the animals showing no systemic toxicity or axonal degeneration (Cavaletti et al., 1995; Polomano & Bennett, 2001; Xiao & Bennett, 2008). Behavioral signs include mechanical hyperalgesia and thermal hyperalgesia without motor deficits (Polomano & Bennett, 2001).

Cisplatin causes peripheral neuropathy and mechanical hyperalgesia (Authier et al., 2000) by affecting large myelinated axons, but has no effect on nonmyelinated axons. In addition, cisplatin decreases nerve conduction velocity of peripheral sensory nerves, but not motor nerves (de Koning et al., 1987a; de Koning et al., 1987b; Authier et al., 2003).

POTENTIAL FUTURE TREATMENTS

TRPV1 is a nonselective cation channel that is found on primary afferent neurons. It plays an important role in pain sensitivity of sensory neurons in the periphery (Premkumar & Sikand, 2008). Ablating the DRG neurons expressing TRPV1 receptors may be an effective treatment for controlling chronic cancer pain, while leaving other sensory functions intact (Karai et al., 2004; Ghilardi et al., 2005). Dogs with spontaneous bone cancer developed profound analgesia for up to 3.5 months after intrathecal treatment with the capsaicin analog resiniferatoxin, a potent TRPV1 agonist (Brown et al., 2005).

The concept of selective DRG neuron ablation has been used by some laboratories for targeting other neurons, for example, neurons expressing NK-1 receptors. These approaches have shown no adverse effects in either rat or dog models (Khasabov et al., 2005; Allen et al., 2006).

ALLEVIATION OF CANCER PAIN

Cancer-pain treatment guidelines provided by the World Health Organization (WHO) include the use of opioids, nonsteroidal anti-inflammatory drugs (NSAIDs), corticosteroids, local anesthetics, antidepressants, and anticonvulsants, either alone or in combination. These current conventional therapies may not be effective in controlling cancer pain, and they may have significant adverse effects. One of the contributing factors making cancer pain difficult to treat is that it is a mixed-pain syndrome having nociceptive, inflammatory, and neuropathic components (Paice, 2003). Therefore, a combination of treatment approaches is warranted.

The development and maintenance of cancer pain is a dynamic process. Alleviation of cancer pain may have to be based on disease progression. At the early stage of tumor growth, as tumors start to proliferate, pronociceptive factors (PGE_2 and ET) are released. Therefore, COX inhibitors or ET antagonists may be effective treatments during this period. In later stages, when tumors are growing and compressing surrounding nerve bundles, neuropathic pain medications may provide better pain control. When tumors fill the intramedullary canal and dead tumor cells produce an acidic environment, TRPV1 or ASIC receptor antagonists may be beneficial in controlling pain. Once bone destruction becomes evident, ATP antagonists (ATP, present during cancer growth, is an endogenous ligand for P2X (membrane ion channel) receptors) may block movement-related pain (Mantyh, 2004; Mantyh & Hunt, 2004). Interesting therapeutic options also include targets on nociceptive afferents that innervate the bone, such as TRPV1, Trk, and cannabinoid receptors. Newly discovered therapeutic treatments developed based on our current understanding of these mechanisms, such as resiniferatoxin or SP-saporin (SP-SAP; causing ablation of SP-expressing cells by conjugating a toxin, saporin, into SP), may yield promising results.

The newly developed gene database based on the knockout of individual mouse genes allows investigators to study pain-related phenotypes associated with specific genes, generating a better understanding of the roles that these genes and their protein products have in pain processing and modulation. This information will be crucial to developing novel therapeutic drugs targeting specific genes for particular types of cancer pain (Lacroix-Fralish et al., 2007). See Chapter 27 for discussion of treatment of cancer pain.

SUMMARY

Cancer pain mechanisms are complicated. Cancer itself can induce pain both peripherally and centrally. There are many substances or mediators released during cancer growth that induce and maintain cancer pain. In addition, cancer pain may occur indirectly via chemotherapy, and coexisting painful conditions may be present. Understanding these complex mechanisms is necessary to effectively control and manage pain. Further studies are required to better understand the distinctive molecular mechanisms of cancer pain in order to target specific sites or mechanistic pathways with pharmacological agents.

ACKNOWLEDGMENT

We thank Janis Atuk-Jones for her image production assistance.

REFERENCES

Adams, V.J., Evans, K.M., Sampson, J., & Wood, J.L. (2010) Methods and mortality results of a health survey of purebred dogs in the UK. *The Journal of Small Animal Practice*, 51, 512–524.

Aley, K.O., Reichling, D.B., & Levine, J.D. (1996) Vincristine hyperalgesia in the rat: a model of painful vincristine neuropathy in humans. *Neuroscience*, 73, 259–265.

Allen, J.W., Mantyh, P.W., Horais, K., et al. (2006) Safety evaluation of intrathecal substance P-saporin, a targeted neurotoxin, in dogs. *Toxicological Sciences*, 91, 286–298.

Amadesi, S., Cottrell, G.S., Divino, L., et al. (2006) Protease-activated receptor 2 sensitizes TRPV1 by protein kinase C-, epsilon- and A-dependent mechanisms in rats and mice. *The Journal of Physiology*, 575, 555–571.

Asai, H., Ozaki, N., Shinoda, M., et al. (2005) Heat and mechanical hyperalgesia in mice model of cancer pain. *Pain*, 117, 19–29.

Asham, E., Shankar, A., Loizidou, M., et al. (2001) Increased endothelin-1 in colorectal cancer and reduction of tumour growth by ET(A) receptor antagonism. *British Journal of Cancer*, 85, 1759–1763.

Authier, N., Coudore, F., Eschalier, A., & Fialip, J. (1999) Pain related behaviour during vincristine-induced neuropathy in rats. *Neuroreport*, 10, 965–968.

Authier, N., Fialip, J., Eschalier, A., & Coudoré, F. (2000) Assessment of allodynia and hyperalgesia after cisplatin administration to rats. *Neuroscience Letters*, 291, 73–76.

Authier, N., Gillet, J.P., Fialip, J., Eschalier, A., & Coudore, F. (2003) An animal model of nociceptive peripheral neuropathy following repeated cisplatin injections. *Experimental Neurology*, 182, 12–20.

Bagnato, A. & Natali, P.G. (2004) Endothelin receptors as novel targets in tumor therapy. *Journal of Translational Medicine*, 2, 16.

Baranauskas, G. & Nistri, A. (1998) Sensitization of pain pathways in the spinal cord: cellular mechanisms. *Progress in Neurobiology*, 54, 349–365.

Basolo, F., Conaldi, P.G., Fiore, L., Calvo, S., & Toniolo, A. (1993) Normal breast epithelial cells produce interleukins 6 and 8 together with tumor-necrosis factor: defective IL6 expression in mammary carcinoma. *International Journal of Cancer (Journal International Du Cancer)*, 55, 926–930.

Bronson, R.T. (1982) Variation in age at death of dogs of different sexes and breeds. *American Journal of Veterinary Research*, 43, 2057–2059.

Brown, D.C., Iadarola, M.J., Perkowski, S.Z., et al. (2005) Physiologic and antinociceptive effects of intrathecal resiniferatoxin in a canine bone cancer model. *Anesthesiology*, 103, 1052–1059.

Cain, D.M., Wacnik, P.W., Eikmeier, L., Beitz, A., Wilcox, G.L., & Simone, D.A. (2001) Functional interactions between tumor and peripheral nerve in a model of cancer pain in the mouse. *Pain Medicine*, 2, 15–23.

Caraceni, A. & Portenoy, R.K. (1999) An international survey of cancer pain characteristics and syndromes. IASP Task Force on Cancer Pain. International Association for the Study of Pain. *Pain*, 82, 263–274.

Caraceni, A. & Weinstein, S.M. (2001) Classification of cancer pain syndromes. *Oncology (Williston Park)*, 15, 1627–1640, 1642.

Castellano, D., Sepulveda, J.M., Garcia-Escobar, I., Rodriguez-Antolín, A., Sundlöv, A., & Cortes-Funes, H. (2011) The role of RANK-ligand inhibition in cancer: the story of denosumab. *Oncologist*, 16, 136–145.

Caterina, M.J. & Julius, D. (2001) The vanilloid receptor: a molecular gateway to the pain pathway. *Annual Review of Neuroscience*, 24, 487–517.

Cavaletti, G., Tredici, G., Braga, M., & Tazzari, S. (1995) Experimental peripheral neuropathy induced in adult rats by repeated intraperitoneal administration of taxol. *Experimental Neurology*, 133, 64–72.

Clohisy, D.R. & Ramnaraine, M.L. (1998) Osteoclasts are required for bone tumors to grow and destroy bone. *Journal of Orthopaedic Research*, 16, 660–666.

Coleman, R.E. (2000) Management of bone metastases. *Oncologist*, 5, 463–470.

Coleman, R.E. (2001) Metastatic bone disease: clinical features, pathophysiology and treatment strategies. *Cancer Treatment Reviews*, 27, 165–176.

Coleman, R.E. (2006) Clinical features of metastatic bone disease and risk of skeletal morbidity. *Clinical Cancer Research*, 12, 6243s–6249s.

Constantin, C.E., Mair, N., Sailer, C.A., et al. (2008) Endogenous tumor necrosis factor alpha (TNFalpha) requires TNF receptor type 2 to generate heat hyperalgesia in a mouse cancer model. *The Journal of Neuroscience*, 28, 5072–5081.

Davar, G. (2001) Endothelin-1 and metastatic cancer pain. *Pain Medicine*, 2, 24–27.

de Koning, P., Neijt, J.P., Jennekens, F.G., & Gispen, W.H. (1987a) Evaluation of cis-diamminedichloroplatinum (II) (cisplatin) neurotoxicity in rats. *Toxicology and Applied Pharmacology*, 89, 81–87.

de Koning, P., Neijt, J.P., Jennekens, F.G., & Gispen, W.H. (1987b) Org.2766 protects from cisplatin-induced neurotoxicity in rats. *Experimental Neurology*, 97, 746–750.

Fine, P.G., Miaskowski, C., & Paice, J.A. (2004) Meeting the challenges in cancer pain management. *The Journal of Supportive Oncology*, 2, 5–22.

Fonsatti, E., Altomonte, M., Coral, S., et al. (1997) Tumour-derived interleukin 1alpha (IL-1alpha) up-regulates the release of soluble intercellular adhesion molecule-1 (sICAM-1) by endothelial cells. *British Journal of Cancer*, 76, 1255–1261.

Fox, S.M. (2010) *Chronic Pain in Small Animal Medicine*, Manson Publishing Ltd., London.

Fujita, M., Andoh, T., Ohashi, K., Akira, A., Saiki, I., & Kuraishi, Y. (2010) Roles of kinin B1 and B2 receptors in skin cancer pain produced by orthotopic melanoma inoculation in mice. *European Journal of Pain*, 14, 588–594.

Garber, K. (2003) Why it hurts: researchers seek mechanisms of cancer pain. *Journal of the National Cancer Institute*, 95, 770–772.

Ghilardi, J.R., Rohrich, H., Lindsay, T.H., et al. (2005) Selective blockade of the capsaicin receptor TRPV1 attenuates bone cancer pain. *The Journal of Neuroscience*, 25, 3126–3131.

Gokin, A.P., Fareed, M.U., Pan, H.L., Hans, G., Strichartz, G.R., & Davar, G. (2001) Local injection of endothelin-1 produces pain-like behavior and excitation of nociceptors in rats. *The Journal of Neuroscience*, 21, 5358–5366.

Gordon-Williams, R.M. & Dickenson, A.H. (2007) Central neuronal mechanisms in cancer-induced bone pain. *Current Opinion of Supportive and Palliative Care*, 1, 6–10.

Grant, A.D., Cottrell, G.S., Amadesi, S., et al. (2007) Protease-activated receptor 2 sensitizes the transient receptor potential vanilloid 4 ion channel to cause mechanical hyperalgesia in mice. *The Journal of Physiology*, 578, 715–733.

Grimshaw, M.J., Hagemann, T., Ayhan, A., Gillett, C.E., Binder, C., & Balkwill, F.R. (2004) A role for endothelin-2 and its receptors in breast tumor cell invasion. *Cancer Research*, 64, 2461–2468.

Hamamoto, D.T., Khasabov, S.G., Cain, D.M., & Simone, D.A. (2008) Tumor-evoked sensitization of C nociceptors: a role for endothelin. *Journal of Neurophysiology*, 100, 2300–2311.

Hasue, F., Kuwaki, T., Yamada, H., Fukuda, Y., & Shimoyama, M. (2004) Inhibitory actions of endothelin-1 on pain processing. *Journal of Cardiovascular Pharmacology*, 44, S318–S320.

Higuera, E.S. & Luo, Z.D. (2004) A rat pain model of vincristine-induced neuropathy. *Methods in Molecular Medicine*, 99, 91–98.

Honore, P., Luger, N.M., Sabino, M.A., et al. (2000) Osteoprotegerin blocks bone cancer-induced skeletal destruction, skeletal pain and pain-related neurochemical reorganization of the spinal cord. *Nature Medicine*, 6, 521–528.

Honore, P., Schwei, J., Rogers, S.D., et al. (2000) Cellular and neurochemical remodeling of the spinal cord in bone cancer pain. *Progress in Brain Research*, 129, 389–397.

International Association for the Study of Pain IASP (2009) March 2009. Pain Clinical Update: Cancer Pain Management in Developing Countries.

Jankowski, M.P. & Koerber, H.R. (2010) Neurotrophic factors and nociceptor sensitization, in *Translational Pain Research: from Mouse to Man*, (eds L. Kruger & A.R. Light), CRC Press, Boca Raton, FL.

Jeronimo, C., Henrique, R., Campos, P.F., et al. (2003) Endothelin B receptor gene hypermethylation in prostate adenocarcinoma. *Journal of Clinical Pathology*, 56, 52–55.

Jimenez-Andrade, J.M., Ghilardi, J.R., Castaneda-Corral, G., Kuskowski, M.A., & Mantyh, P.W. (2011) Preventive or late administration of anti-NGF therapy attenuates tumor-induced nerve sprouting, neuroma formation, and cancer pain. *Pain*, 152, 2564–2574.

Joseph, E.K. & Levine, J.D. (2003) Sexual dimorphism for protein kinase c epsilon signaling in a rat model of vincristine-induced painful peripheral neuropathy. *Neuroscience*, 119, 831–838.

Julius, D. & Basbaum, A.I. (2001) Molecular mechanisms of nociception. *Nature*, 413, 203–210.

Karai, L., Brown, D.C., Mannes, A.J., et al. (2004) Deletion of vanilloid receptor 1-expressing primary afferent neurons for pain control. *The Journal of Clinical Investigation*, 113, 1344–1352.

Kawamata, T., Niiyama, Y., Yamamoto, J., & Furuse, S. (2010) Reduction of bone cancer pain by CB1 activation and TRPV1 inhibition. *Journal of Anesthesia*, 24, 328–332.

Khasabov, S.G., Ghilardi, J.R., Mantyh, P.W., & Simone, D.A. (2005) Spinal neurons that express NK-1 receptors modulate descending controls that project through the dorsolateral funiculus. *Journal of Neurophysiology*, 93, 998–1006.

Khodorova, A., Fareed, M.U., Gokin, A., Strichartz, G.R., & Davar, G. (2002) Local injection of a selective endothelin-B receptor agonist inhibits endothelin-1-induced pain-like behavior and excitation of nociceptors in a naloxone-sensitive manner. *The Journal of Neuroscience*, 22, 7788–7796.

Kurbel, S., Kurbel, B., Kovacic, D., et al. (1999) Endothelin-secreting tumors and the idea of the pseudoectopic hormone secretion in tumors. *Medical Hypotheses*, 52, 329–333.

Lacroix-Fralish, M.L., Ledoux, J.B., & Mogil, J.S. (2007) The pain genes database: an interactive web browser of pain-related transgenic knockout studies. *Pain*, 131, 3–4.

Levi-Montalcini, R., Skaper, S.D., Dal, T.R., Petrelli, L., & Leon, A. (1996) Nerve growth factor: from neurotrophin to neurokine. *Trends in Neuroscience*, 19, 514–520.

Lotsch, J. & Geisslinger, G. (2011) Pharmacogenetics of new analgesics. *British Journal of Pharmacology*, 163, 447–460.

Luger, N.M., Honore, P., Sabino, M.A., et al. (2001) Osteoprotegerin diminishes advanced bone cancer pain. *Cancer Research*, 61, 4038–4047.

Ma, C. (2007) Animal models of pain. *International Anesthesiology Clinics*, 45, 121–131.

Mantyh, P.W. (2004) A mechanism-based understanding of bone cancer pain. *Novartis Foundation Symposium*, 261, 194–214 discussion 214–19, 256–61.

Mantyh, P.W., Clohisy, D.R., Koltzenburg, M., & Hunt, S.P. (2002) Molecular mechanisms of cancer pain. *Nature Review Cancer*, 2, 201–209.

Mantyh, P.W. & Hunt, S.P. (2004) Mechanisms that generate and maintain bone cancer pain. *Novartis Foundation Symposium*, 260, 221–238; discussion 238–40, 277–9.

Mantyh, W.G., Jimenez-Andrade, J.M., Stake, J.I., et al. (2010) Blockade of nerve sprouting and neuroma formation markedly attenuates the development of late stage cancer pain. *Neuroscience*, 171, 588–598.

Medhurst, S.J., Walker, K., Bowes, M., et al. (2002) A rat model of bone cancer pain. *Pain*, 96, 129–140.

Morris Animal Foundation (1998)—Animal Health Survey. *Companion Animal News*, Englewood, CO.

Nagae, M., Hiraga, T., & Yoneda, T. (2007) Acidic microenvironment created by osteoclasts causes bone pain associated with tumor colonization. *Journal of Bone and Mineral Metabolism*, 25, 99–104.

Nasu, K., Matsui, N., Narahara, H., Tanaka, Y., & Miyakawa, I. (1998) Effects of interferon-gamma on cytokine production by endometrial stromal cells. *Human Reproduction (Oxford England)*, 13, 2598–2601.

Niiyama, Y., Kawamata, T., Yamamoto, J., Furuse, S., & Namiki, A. (2009) SB366791, a TRPV1 antagonist, potentiates analgesic effects of systemic morphine in a murine model of bone cancer pain. *British Journal of Anaesthesia*, 102, 251–258.

Nozaki-Taguchi, N., Chaplan, S.R., Higuera, E.S., Ajakwe, R.C., & Yaksh, T.L. (2001) Vincristine-induced allodynia in the rat. *Pain*, 93, 69–76.

Pacharinsak, C.F. & Beitz, A. (2008) Animal models of cancer pain. *Comparative Medicine*, 58, 220–233.

Paice, J.A. (2003) Mechanisms and management of neuropathic pain in cancer. *The Journal of Supportive Oncology*, 1, 107–120.

Pantano, F., Zoccoli, A., Iuliani, M., et al. (2011) New targets, new drugs for metastatic bone pain: a new philosophy. *Expert Opinion on Emerging Drugs*, 16, 403–405.

Peters, C.M., Lindsay, T.H., Pomonis, J.D., et al. (2004) Endothelin and the tumorigenic component of bone cancer pain. *Neuroscience*, 126, 1043–1052.

Pickering, V., Jay, G.R., Quang, P., Jordan, R.C., & Schmidt, B.L. (2008) Effect of peripheral endothelin-1 concentration on carcinoma-induced pain in mice. *European Journal of Pain (London, England)*, 12, 293–300.

Piovezan, A.P., D'Orleans-Juste, P., Souza, G.E., & Rae, G.A. (2000) Endothelin-1-induced ET(A) receptor-mediated nociception, hyperalgesia and oedema in the mouse hind-paw: modulation by simultaneous ET(B) receptor activation. *British Journal of Pharmacology*, 129, 961–968.

Polomano, R.C. & Bennett, G.J. (2001) Chemotherapy-evoked painful peripheral neuropathy. *Pain Medicine*, 2, 8–14.

Pomonis, J.D., Rogers, S.D., Peters, C.M., Ghilardi, J.R., & Mantyh, P.W. (2001) Expression and localization of endothelin receptors: implications for the involvement of peripheral glia in nociception. *The Journal of Neuroscience*, 21, 999–1006.

Premkumar, L.S. & Sikand, P. (2008) TRPV1: a target for next generation analgesics. *Current Neuropharmacology*, 6, 151–163.

Quang, P.N. & Schmidt, B.L. (2010) Peripheral endothelin B receptor agonist-induced antinociception involves endogenous opioids in mice. *Pain*, 149, 254–262.

Reyes-Gibby, C.C., Shete, S., Yennurajalingam, S., et al. (2009) Genetic and nongenetic covariates of pain severity in patients with adenocarcinoma of the pancreas: assessing the influence of cytokine genes. *Journal of Pain and Symptom Management*, 38, 894–902.

Richardson, P.G. (2010) Towards a better understanding of treatment-related peripheral neuropathy in multiple myeloma. *The Lancet Oncology*, 11, 1014–1016.

Russo, A., Bronte, G., Rizzo, S., et al. (2010) Anti-endothelin drugs in solid tumors. *Expert Opinion on Emerging Drugs*, 15, 27–40.

Sabino, M.A., Ghilardi, J.R., Jongen, J.L., et al. (2002) Simultaneous reduction in cancer pain, bone destruction, and tumor growth by selective inhibition of cyclooxygenase-2. *Cancer Research*, 62, 7343–7349.

Sabino, M.A. & Mantyh, P.W. (2005) Pathophysiology of bone cancer pain. *The Journal of Supportive Oncology*, 3, 15–24.

Schmidt, B.L., Hamamoto, D.T., Simone, D.A., & Wilcox, G.L. (2010a) Mechanism of cancer pain. *Molecular Interventions*, 10, 164–178.

Schmidt, B.L., Pickering, V., Liu, S., et al. (2007) Peripheral endothelin A receptor antagonism attenuates carcinoma-induced pain. *European Journal of Pain (London, England)*, 11, 406–414.

Schmidt, J.M., North, S.M., Freeman, K.P., & Ramiro-Ibañez, F. (2010b) Feline paediatric oncology: retrospective assessment of 233 tumours from cats up to one year (1993 to 2008). *Journal of Small Animal Practice*, 51, 306–311.

Schwei, M.J., Honore, P., Rogers, S.D., et al. (1999) Neurochemical and cellular reorganization of the spinal cord in a murine model of bone cancer pain. *The Journal of Neuroscience*, 19, 10886–10897.

Schweizerhof, M., Stosser, S., Kurejova, M., et al. (2009) Hematopoietic colony-stimulating factors mediate tumor-nerve interactions and bone cancer pain. *Nature Medicine*, 15, 802–807.

Sessle, B.J. (2007) Glia: non-neural players in orofacial pain. *Journal of Orofacial Pain*, 21, 169–170.

Sevcik, M.A., Ghilardi, J.R., Halvorson, K.G., Lindsay, T.H., Kubota, K., & Mantyh, P.W. (2005) Analgesic efficacy of bradykinin B1 antagonists in a murine bone cancer pain model. *The Journal of Pain*, 6, 771–775.

Shimoyama, M., Tanaka, K., Hasue, F., & Shimoyama, N. (2002) A mouse model of neuropathic cancer pain. *Pain*, 99, 167–174.

Shinoda, M., Ogino, A., Ozaki, N., et al. (2008) Involvement of TRPV1 in nociceptive behavior in a rat model of cancer pain. *The Journal of Pain*, 9, 687–699.

Shugarman, L.R., Asch, S.M., Meredith, L.S., et al. (2010) Factors associated with clinician intention to address diverse aspects of pain in seriously ill outpatients. *Pain Medicine (Malden, Mass.)*, 11, 1365–1372.

Simone, D.A., Sorkin, L.S., Oh, U., et al. (1991) Neurogenic hyperalgesia: central neural correlates in responses of spinothalamic tract neurons. *Journal of Neurophysiology*, 66, 228–246.

Urch, C.E. (2004) The pathophysiology of cancer-induced bone pain: current understanding. *Palliative Medicine*, 18, 267–274.

Urch, C.E., Donovan-Rodriguez, T., & Dickenson, A.H. (2003) Alterations in dorsal horn neurones in a rat model of cancer-induced bone pain. *Pain*, 106, 347–356.

Urch, C.E., Donovan-Rodriguez, T., Gordon-Williams, R., Bee, L.A., & Dickenson, A.H. (2005) Efficacy of chronic morphine in a rat model of cancer-induced bone pain: behavior and in dorsal horn pathophysiology. *Journal of Pain*, 6, 837–845.

Vadalouca, A., Raptis, E., Moka, E., Zis, P., Sykioti, P., & Siafaka, I. (2012) Pharmacological treatment of neuropathic cancer pain: a comprehensive review of the current literature. *Pain Practice*, 12, 219–251.

Vermeirsch, H., Nuydens, R.M., Salmon, P.L., & Meert, T.F. (2004) Bone cancer pain model in mice: evaluation of pain behavior, bone destruction and morphine sensitivity. *Pharmacology, Biochemistry, and Behavior*, 79, 243–251.

Wacnik, P.W., Eikmeier, L.J., Ruggles, T.R., et al. (2001) Functional interactions between tumor and peripheral nerve: morphology, algogen identification, and behavioral characterization of a new murine model of cancer pain. *The Journal of Neuroscience*, 21, 9355–9366.

Wacnik, P.W., Eikmeier, L.J., Simone, D.A., Wilcox, G.L., & Beitz, A.J. (2005) Nociceptive characteristics of tumor necrosis factor-alpha in naive and tumor-bearing mice. *Neuroscience*, 132, 479–491.

Wacnik, P.W., Stool, L., Lauretti, G.R., et al. (1998) Animal model of cancer pain: comparing different hind limb sites of melanoma cell implantation. *Society of Neuroscience*, 24, 628.

Wacnik, P.W., Wilcox, G.L., Clohisy, D.R., et al. (2000) Cancer pain mechanisms and animal models of cancer pain. Proceeding of the 9th World Congress on Pain, Progress in Pain Research and Management, Vienna, Austria, pp. 615–637.

Watkins, L.R., Hutchinson, M.R., Ledeboer, A., Wieseler-Frank, J., Milligan, E.D., & Maier, S.F. (2007) Norman Cousins Lecture. Glia as the "bad guys": implications for improving clinical pain control and the clinical utility of opioids. *Brain, Behavior, and Immunity*, 21, 131–146.

Watkins, L.R., Milligan, E.D., & Maier, S.F. (2001) Glial activation: a driving force for pathological pain. *Trends in Neurosciences*, 24, 450–455.

Willis, W.D., Al-Chaer, E.D., Quast, M.J., & Westlund, K.N. (1999) A visceral pain pathway in the dorsal column of the spinal cord. *Proceedings of the National Academy of Sciences of the United States of America*, 96, 7675–7679.

Woolf, C.J. (2011) Central sensitization: implications for the diagnosis and treatment of pain. *Pain*, 152, S2–S15.

Wulfing, P., Diallo, R., Kersting, C., et al. (2003) Expression of endothelin-1, endothelin-A, and endothelin-B receptor in human breast cancer and correlation with long-term follow-up. *Clinical Cancer Research*, 9, 4125–4131.

Xiao, W.H. & Bennett, G.J. (2008) Chemotherapy-evoked neuropathic pain: abnormal spontaneous discharge in A-fiber and C-fiber primary afferent neurons and its suppression by acetyl-L-carnitine. *Pain*, 135, 262–270.

Yaari, Y. & Devor, M. (1985) Phenytoin suppresses spontaneous ectopic discharge in rat sciatic nerve neuromas. *Neuroscience Letters*, 58, 117–122.

Yanagisawa, Y., Furue, H., Kawamata, T., et al. (2010) Bone cancer induces a unique central sensitization through synaptic changes in a wide area of the spinal cord. *Molecular Pain*, 6, 38.

Yoneda, T., Hata, K., Nakanishi, M., et al. (2011) Involvement of acidic microenvironment in the pathophysiology of cancer-associated bone pain. *Bone*, 48(1), 100–105.

Yuyama, H., Koakutsu, A., Fujiyasu, N., et al. (2004) Inhibitory effects of a selective endothelin-A receptor antagonist YM598 on endothelin-1-induced potentiation of nociception in formalin-induced and prostate cancer-induced pain models in mice. *Journal of Cardiovascular Pharmacology*, 44(Suppl. 1), S479–S482.

Zhang, R.X., Liu, B., Wang, L., et al. (2005) Spinal glial activation in a new rat model of bone cancer pain produced by prostate cancer cell inoculation of the tibia. *Pain*, 118, 125–136.

Zhou, Q.L., Strichartz, G., & Davar, G. (2001) Endothelin-1 activates ET(A) receptors to increase intracellular calcium in model sensory neurons. *Neuroreport*, 12, 3853–3857.

Zhu, Z., Friess, H., diMola, F.F., et al. (1999) Nerve growth factor expression correlates with perineural invasion and pain in human pancreatic cancer. *Journal of Clinical Oncology*, 17, 2419–2428.

Section 2
Pharmacology of Analgesic Drugs

4
Opioids

Tanya Duke-Novakovski

Morphine was first isolated in 1804 by the German pharmacist, Friedrich Sertürner, who also reported its respiratory depressant effects. Codeine was isolated in 1832 and papaverine in 1848. Although it is possible to synthesize morphine, it is easier to derive it from the dried latex obtained from the opium poppy (*Papaver somniferum*). Legal production is controlled by the United Nations Single Convention on Narcotic Drugs and other international drug treaties. Innovative ways to extract morphine from the poppy developed during World War II due to demands for potent analgesics. Morphine remains the opioid to which all others are compared.

TERMINOLOGY

"Opium" is derived from Greek and means "juice." The poppy plant is a source of 20 alkaloids of opium and contains up to 12% morphine. Other naturally occurring alkaloids include codeine, thebaine, papaverine, and noscapine. An "opiate" is derived from opium. An "opioid" refers to all exogenous substances whether natural or synthetic that can bind to opioid receptors and produce a morphine-like effect. Opioids can produce analgesia without loss of touch, proprioception, or consciousness. Opioids are commonly classified into opioid agonists, agonist–antagonists, and antagonists (Figure 4.1).

STRUCTURE OF OPIOIDS

Two distinct chemical classes exist: phenanthrenes and benzylisoquinolines. The phenanthrene group includes morphine, codeine, and thebaine, and other clinically useful opioids. There is a close relationship between the stereochemical structure and the potency of opioids and, in most cases, it is the levorotatory isomer that is most active.

Semisynthetic opioids are based on morphine. Substitution of a hydroxyl group for a methyl group on carbon 3 results in methylmorphine or codeine. Substitution of acetyl groups on carbons 3 and 6 results in diacetylmorphine (heroin). Thebaine does not have much opioid activity, but is the precursor for etorphine.

Synthetic opioids contain the phenanthrene nucleus but are not derived from opium. These include levorphanol, methadone derivatives, benzomorphan derivatives (pentazocine), and phenylpiperidine derivatives (meperidine (pethidine), fentanyl). The main differences among these drugs are potency and rate of equilibration between the plasma and the site of drug effect (biophase).

OPIOID RECEPTORS

Opioid receptors belong to the large guanine (G) protein-coupled receptor family, which also includes muscarinic, adrenergic, gamma-aminobutyric acid (GABA$_B$), and somatostatin receptors. Opioid G-protein receptors consist of seven transmembrane units, with the inner end of the protein unit connected to cell signaling cascades that close voltage-sensitive calcium channels, stimulate potassium efflux, and reduce cyclic adenosine monophosphate production. These actions generally decrease neuronal excitability through hyperpolarization of the cell, and inhibit release of neurotransmitters, including acetylcholine, dopamine, norepinephrine, substance P, and GABA.

Opioid receptors have been subclassified into μ or OP3 or MOP receptors, κ or OP2 or KOP receptors, δ or OP1 or DOP receptors, and nociceptin/orphanin FQ peptide receptors (FQ or NOP), also referred to as ORL-1 receptors. These different classifications arise from traditional pharmacology nomenclature (Greek symbols), International Union of Pharmacology Recommendations (OP 1–3 classification) and molecular biology nomenclature (MOP, KOP, DOP, NOP). The Greek names will be used to describe receptor types throughout this chapter.

The opioid receptor system is integral to regulation of appetite, thermoregulation, stress responses, respiratory control, and pain (Pattinson, 2008). Endogenous endorphins activate the μ-opioid receptor, enkephalins activate the μ- and δ-opioid receptors, dynorphins activate κ-receptors, and nociceptin/orphanin peptides activate the FQ/ORL-1 receptor.

The μ-opioid receptors are principally involved in spinal (substantia gelatinosa) and supraspinal (periaqueductal gray area, amygdala, corpus striatum, and hypothalamus) analgesia. Activation of $μ_1$ is speculated to produce profound analgesia, whereas stimulation of $μ_2$ receptors results in respiratory depression (hypoventilation), vagal effects (bradycardia), and physical dependence. Sedation is also a prominent effect of μ-opioid receptor activation and can be useful for premedication, chemical restraint/immobilization techniques, and for providing postoperative sedation. Common exogenous μ-opioid agonists used in veterinary medicine include

Pain Management in Veterinary Practice, First Edition. Edited by Christine M. Egger, Lydia Love and Tom Doherty.
© 2014 John Wiley & Sons, Inc. Published 2014 by John Wiley & Sons, Inc.

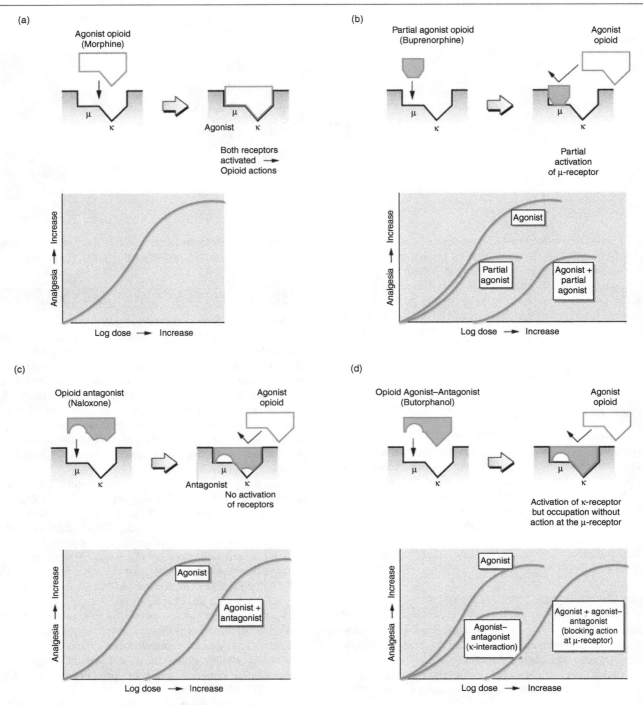

Figure 4.1. Opioid receptor interactions. A lock-and-key analogy is used to illustrate different drug interactions at μ- and κ-receptors. A relative dose–response curve for analgesic potency is diagrammed. (a) An opioid agonist stimulates both μ- and κ-receptors, resulting in increased analgesic effect with increased dose. (b) A partial agonist weakly stimulates the μ-receptor to achieve a reduced maximum analgesic effect compared with a full agonist. A large dose of a partial agonist will block the receptor actions of the full agonist and this moves its dose–response curve to the right and depresses the maximal analgesic response. Buprenorphine, a commonly used partial agonist, has very strong receptor binding so that even with very large doses of an agonist, the limited analgesic effect of buprenorphine predominates. (c) Complete opioid antagonists possess no intrinsic activity but block the μ- and κ-receptors. Because of the competitive nature of the binding at the receptors, more agonist is required in the presence of antagonist to produce its full analgesic effect. (d) Agonist–antagonists have mixed activity at the two receptor types. Most, such as nalbuphine or butorphanol, have agonist activity at κ-receptors and antagonist activity at μ-receptors. In the presence of a full μ-agonist, these opioids tend to act as antagonists and increase the dose of full agonist required to achieve maximum analgesic effect. (Modified from Maddison. J., Page, S., and Church, D. *Small Animal Clinical Pharmacology,* Elsevier 2008, p. 312. with permission.)

morphine, L-methadone, meperidine (pethidine), fentanyl, sufentanil, alfentanil, remifentanil, etorphine, and carfentanil. Buprenorphine is a partial μ-agonist, occupying but not fully activating the receptor. Naloxone is a specific antagonist with high affinity for the μ-opioid receptor, but with no intrinsic activity. Naltrexone also has antagonist activity, but with a longer duration compared to naloxone.

κ-Receptors mediate spinal analgesia, mild sedation, and miosis, and cause less respiratory depression and vagally mediated bradycardia than μ-receptor activation. Dysphoria and diuresis may occur through activation of calcium-channel-linked receptors. κ-opioid agonists are usually reserved for mild to moderate pain. κ-agonists may not be as useful as μ-opioid agonists for controlling severe forms of pain, but can help to alleviate visceral pain (Kalpravidh et al., 1984a, 1984b; Muir & Robertson, 1985; Houghton et al., 1991; Ide et al., 2008). Opioid agonist–antagonists stimulate κ-opioid receptors, are antagonistic to the μ-opioid receptor and, in veterinary medicine, include pentazocine, nalbuphine, and butorphanol. Buprenorphine exhibits antagonism at κ-receptors.

δ-Receptors may modulate μ-opioid receptors. There are no specific δ-opioid agonists in use in veterinary medicine.

The function of the FQ peptide/ORL-1 receptor is still under intense research (Chiou et al., 2007). Spinally localized antinociceptive and supraspinally mediated pronociceptive effects have been documented (Rizzi et al., 2006).

PERIPHERAL OPIOID EFFECTS

Peripheral analgesic effects of opioids may be due to activation of opioid receptors located on primary afferent neurons. Inflammation increases synthesis, axonal transport, and expression of opioid receptors on nociceptive afferents. Activation of these receptors decreases the release of excitatory neurotransmitters.

BASIC OPIOID PHARMACOKINETICS

Opioids are generally metabolized through the hepatic microsomal enzyme system, and metabolites are eliminated through biliary or renal excretion. There are differences in the metabolism of opioids among species, and some metabolites are active.

The lungs play an important role in the pharmacokinetics of opioids and may act as a "sink" or play an active role in metabolism. Most drugs handled by the lungs are basic amines with a pKa greater than 8. Opioids taken up by the lungs include fentanyl, sufentanil, alfentanil, meperidine, methadone, morphine, and codeine. The first pass uptake of fentanyl and sufentanil into the lungs is large, with 75% and 61% of the administered dose of fentanyl and sufentanil remaining in the lungs, respectively. Pulmonary uptake of alfentanil is around 10% of the administered dose (Boer, 2003). Morphine is taken up and bound in very limited amounts, but not metabolized. Meperidine and methadone are significantly taken up into the lungs, but meperidine is not metabolized, and methadone metabolism is minimal.

Buprenorphine, butorphanol, alfentanil, sufentanil, and methadone pharmacokinetics do not appreciably change in humans with renal failure, but hydromorphone can accumulate and toxicity has been reported. Tramadol and sufentanil are reportedly safe to administer to patients with renal dysfunction, but respiratory depression from tramadol accumulation was observed in a human

patient with renal failure. Fentanyl may accumulate in critically ill patients, but appears to be safe in patients with mild renal impairment. Patients with renal failure may be more prone to the respiratory depressant effects of potent opioids, with the exception of remifentanil. Metabolism of morphine is altered in patients with renal failure, resulting in accumulation of morphine-3-glucuronide (M3G) and morphine-6-glucuronide (M6G); thus, care should be taken with repeat dosing of morphine. Meperidine is not affected by renal failure, but the metabolite normeperidine is not excreted as efficiently and is proconvulsant.

Age-related changes in opioid metabolism occur, and meperidine elimination half-life increases in dogs older than 10 years of age (63 minutes compared to 37 minutes, after IV injection; 146 minutes compared to 51 minutes, after intramuscular (IM) injection) (Waterman & Kalthum, 1989, 1992).

SIDE EFFECTS OF OPIOIDS

Opioids are widely used in pain management regimens, but they do have side effects that may require attention. Some side effects could be considered useful, such as sedation in the perioperative period. Drug-specific side effects will be discussed in the individual drug sections.

Respiratory System

Dose-dependent respiratory center depression is observed with μ-opioid agonists in particular. The μ$_2$-opioid receptors decrease the responsiveness of neurons in the medullary respiratory center to carbon dioxide, and the corresponding decrease in pH and hypercapnia results. Coadministration of opioids with other anesthetic agents and sedatives can compound the depressant effects to the point where hypoventilation occurs or ventilation ceases. Patients may require artificial ventilatory support and oxygen therapy. Stimulation of κ-opioid receptors does not have as profound an effect on the respiratory system (MacCrackin et al., 1994). Humans are more susceptible to opioid-induced respiratory depression compared to animals (Pattinson, 2008). Veterinarians must be aware of the sensitivity of humans to respiratory depression when sending patients home with fentanyl patches (Martin et al., 2006; Schmiedt & Bjorling, 2007), or when other opioid medications are prescribed for owners to administer to their pets (Lust et al., 2011; George et al., 2010; Haymarle et al., 2010).

Pain stimulates the respiratory center and can offset the respiratory depression caused by opioids. If breakthrough pain is controlled using another drug or technique, concurrent opioid-induced respiratory depression becomes more evident and should be anticipated. An excellent review of the effects of opioids and details of their action on the respiratory center is available (Pattinson, 2008).

Cardiovascular System

Opioids are often used in patients with cardiovascular instability as these drugs, at clinical doses, have minimal effects on cardiac output, cardiac rhythm, and arterial blood pressure. The μ-opioid agonists cause bradycardia through stimulation of the vagal nucleus, and this is the most noticeable clinical effect. The increased vagal tone can be reversed with anticholinergic drugs. Rapid IV administration of high doses of morphine, and especially meperidine, will cause histamine release, vasodilation, and hypotension (Kalthum & Waterman, 1988). Potent μ-opioid agonists can be used in some clinical situations to decrease heart rate and ventricular arrhythmogenicity.

Gastrointestinal System and Emesis

μ-Agonist opioids cause emesis by direct stimulation of dopamine receptors in the chemoreceptor trigger zone (CRTZ), located outside the blood–brain barrier in the area postrema of the medulla. Apomorphine acts at this site and dopamine antagonists can help prevent emesis. More lipid-soluble opioids are thought to act on the vomiting center inside the blood–brain barrier and have an inhibitory effect (Blancquaert et al., 1986). There is individual variability in the emetic response and species differences exist. Horses, rabbits, ruminants, and swine do not vomit after μ-opioid agonist administration. Cats and dogs do vomit, but dogs appear to be more sensitive to opioid-induced emesis. Interestingly, dogs usually do not vomit when opioids are administered IV or when μ-opioid agonists are administered to dogs in pain. Whether or not emesis occurs is the final result of excitatory actions on the CRTZ and inhibitory actions on the vomiting center, and is related to the dose and lipophilicity of the drug. High doses of morphine and clinical doses of fentanyl do not produce emesis in dogs, whereas clinical doses of morphine do cause emesis (Blancquaert et al., 1986). The use of antidopaminergic drugs, such as acepromazine, prior to administration of opioids decreases the incidence of vomiting (Valverde et al., 2004). There are also differences among individual opioids in dogs. Morphine and hydromorphone appear to cause emesis more often compared to meperidine, methadone, tramadol, and fentanyl (Valverde et al., 2004; Monteiro et al., 2008, 2009).

Other gastrointestinal effects are mediated through μ- and δ-opioid receptors located within the mesenteric plexus of the gastrointestinal tract (GIT). Stimulation of these receptors causes defecation in dogs, and occasionally causes defecation in cats. Following this initial effect, there is reduced propulsion that can lead to ileus and constipation. Horses and ruminants are particularly sensitive to these effects, and this has led to reluctance to use opioids for postoperative analgesia in these species. Some studies indicate that morphine administration increases the risk of ileus, but other studies do not support the correlation (Doherty, 2009). It appears that using morphine infusions intra-operatively does not increase the risk of postoperative colic in horses, although administration for longer than 24 hours may do so (Boscan et al., 2006a). Dogs and cats appear to succumb to the GIT effects with longer-term opioid treatment regimens and side effects may be managed with stool softeners and, if possible, physical activity such as walking. Acute postoperative ileus in cats and dogs can be managed with drugs, such as metoclopramide (Graves et al., 1989), that stimulate propulsion. In horses, methylnaltrexone, a peripherally acting opioid antagonist, reversed the effects of morphine on gut motility, but does not have prokinetic effects *per se* (Boscan et al., 2006b).

In humans, morphine and fentanyl increase the tone of the sphincter of Oddi, leading to increased bile duct pressure ranging from 99% with fentanyl to 53% with morphine and 61% with meperidine. The incidence of clinical problems in humans is 3% with use of fentanyl (Radnay et al., 1980). There are anatomical differences among species that may complicate the extrapolation of findings in studies using primates to canines or felines. In humans, denial of potent analgesics for fear of promoting pancreatitis or cholangitis is now considered unwise. It is also unknown how the effects on bile duct pressure relate to the pancreatic duct (Thompson, 2001). Despite no proof that μ-opioid agonists aggravate pancreatitis in veterinary medicine, there are still reports that morphine should be avoided and meperidine or buprenorphine used instead (Zoran, 2006). In treating severe pain from pancreatitis, potent opioids should not be withheld (Dyson, 2008).

μ- Opioid-induced increased pyloric sphincter tone may create problems during endoscopy or foreign body removal, though this is anecdotal. One study evaluated ease of passage of the endoscope into the duodenum with hydromorphone or butorphanol in cats, and found no differences between opioids (Smith et al., 2004a). Butorphanol can be used to reverse the μ-opioid effects during the procedure if problems are observed (MacCrackin et al., 1994).

In dogs, gastroesophageal reflux under anesthesia can cause postoperative esophageal strictures (Wilson & Walshaw, 2004) or lead to aspiration if the airway is unprotected (Java et al., 2009). Meperidine was shown to reduce the incidence of gastroesophageal reflux compared to morphine (Wilson et al., 2007). If regurgitation occurs, esophageal lavage should be performed and the airway protected.

Thermoregulatory Center

Opioids act at the thermoregulatory center in the hypothalamus and effects on thermoregulation are clinically observable. Hyperthermia after opioid administration has been reported in cats (Wesley & Cumby, 1978; Posner et al., 2010), horses (Carregaro et al., 2006; Thomasy et al., 2006), swine (Bossone & Hannon, 1991), and ruminants (Caulkett et al., 2000; Uhrig et al., 2007), and may be partly linked to increased locomotor activity in these species. In one study, the resulting hypermetabolic state was probably due to using greater doses of morphine than are used clinically (Bossone & Hannon, 1991).

In cats, the increase in body temperature is normally mild (Gellasch et al., 2002) but recently, hydromorphone was implicated in an increase in temperature greater than 41.7°C (107°F) (Niedfeldt & Robertson, 2006; Posner et al., 2007). A controlled study examined these effects in more detail and found that all μ-opioid agonists and partial μ-opioid agonists can produce a mild to moderate increase in body temperature, which did not appear to be dose dependent. The authors caution that greater doses than those studied may still have a significant effect (Posner et al., 2010). Sedative doses of ketamine may also increase body temperature, but ketamine did not appear to exaggerate the effects of the coadministered opioid (Posner et al., 2010).

Panting is a well-recognized side effect of administration of μ-opioid agonists to dogs, due to lowering of the thermoregulatory set point, and the incidence can be reduced by 20–30% with coadministration of acepromazine (Smith et al., 2001; Monteiro et al., 2008). Hypothermia appears to be more common than hyperthermia in canines with administration of opioids, and the combination of opioid and acepromazine can further promote the decrease in body temperature (Monteiro et al., 2008, 2009).

Shivering

Opioid receptors appear to be involved in the act of shivering. IV administration of μ-opioid agonists, such as low-dose meperidine and tramadol, have been used to limit postoperative shivering unrelated to hypothermia in patients where the subsequent increased metabolic demand may give cause for concern (Mohta et al., 2009). Human patients are more likely to shiver with the sudden withdrawal of remifentanil, and pre-emptive ketamine administration can prevent this (Nakasuji et al., 2010). No reports on these effects of remifentanil have been published in the veterinary literature.

Antitussive Actions

Depression of the cough reflex is an effect of opioid administration. Vagal afferent information is normally processed in the brainstem, and the cough reflex is coordinated through efferent nerve activity. The presence of a true cough reflex center is in dispute, but stimulation of the medulla or nucleus tractus solitarius can elicit a cough. Opioids, such as morphine, suppress these areas. Butorphanol was originally marketed as an antitussive in dogs before it became popular as an analgesic, and is still used for this purpose (Cavanagh et al., 1976; Westermann et al., 2005). Butorphanol has 100 times the antitussive effect of codeine and 4 times that of morphine (Cavanagh et al., 1976). Codeine and hydrocodone are used specifically for suppression of the cough reflex in humans, but 0.6 mg/kg codeine had no antitussive effect in horses when given orally (Westermann et al., 2005).

Euphoria and Dysphoria

Sedation is the typical response to opioids observed in pain-free dogs, monkeys, and humans, but excitement or euphoria can be observed in pain-free mice, cats, horses, goats, sheep, pigs, and cows. Euphoria, in dogs, is described as excessive wakefulness and vocalization; whereas, in cats, euphoria causes rolling, "kneading," and extreme friendliness. Dysphoria in dogs causes agitation, excitement, restlessness, excessive vocalization, and disorientation. In cats, dysphoria causes fearful and apparent hallucinatory behavior, open-mouth breathing, agitation, vocalization, and pacing.

The use of opioids for pain control has been limited in species that exhibit dysphoria. Pain-free horses have increased locomotor activity and an excited look about them when given potent opioids (Pascoe et al., 1991). The dysphoric or euphoric response may not be observed if the patient was in pain before opioid administration. The final response may be linked with the distribution of μ-, δ-, and κ-opioid receptors and subtypes within the central nervous system. Interestingly, within the species that are normally expected to respond to opioids with excitement are individuals that do not respond at all and appear normal. This has been observed with mice, cats, and horses. Stimulation of the κ-opioid receptor is known to produce dysphoria in most species.

Central dopamine release has been linked with increased opioid-induced locomotor activity in horses, and can be reversed using dopamine antagonists such as acepromazine (Tobin, 1978). A study investigating individual D_1 and D_2 receptor antagonists in horses treated with alfentanil failed to reduce locomotor activity and, in fact, the dopamine antagonists, including azaperone, also stimulated increased locomotor activity (Pascoe & Taylor, 2003). The authors concluded that opioid-induced dopamine release did not cause the excitatory behavior observed in horses. However, the general sedative effects of acepromazine and α-2-adrenergic agonists have been used successfully with μ- and κ-opioid agonists in clinical situations to provide chemical restraint in horses and cats without producing excitement.

Opioids stimulate the oculomotor nucleus leading to miosis. Species that respond to opioids with sedation will exhibit miosis, but the release of catecholamines in species which respond to opioids with excitement tends to override the stimulation of the oculomo-

tor center, and mydriasis is the final effect observed (Wallenstein & Wang, 1979).

Urinary System

μ-opioid agonists cause inhibition of sacral parasympathetic nervous system outflow. This inhibition causes detrusor muscle relaxation, an increase in bladder capacity, and urinary retention, and this is especially evident when opioids are used spinally or epidurally. Increased antidiuretic hormone and plasma natriuretic peptide concentrations with μ-agonists can cause decreased urine production. κ-opioid agonists can decrease antidiuretic hormone release and cause diuresis.

Immunomodulatory Effects

Immunosuppressive properties of opioids are related more to their molecular structure than their antinociceptive potency. Morphine, fentanyl, codeine, and methadone are more immunosuppressive than hydromorphone, tramadol, oxycodone, and hydrocodone. Buprenorphine and μ-opioid antagonists may enhance the immune system or have no effect. The μ-opioid receptor modifies central actions of the neuroendocrine axis, leading to a reduction in natural killer T-cell activity, lymphocyte proliferation, and interferon activity. Direct stimulation of μ-opioid and δ-opioid receptors on B lymphocytes, monocytes, and macrophages is primarily responsible for peripheral immunosuppression. Opioids generally induce the release of catecholamines that act on primary and secondary lymphoid organs to depress cell function. Morphine generally increases proinflammatory cytokine and decreases anti-inflammatory cytokine production in a dose-dependent manner. However, opioids should be used if analgesic effects are required, because ongoing, untreated pain will detrimentally modulate the immune system more significantly than do opioids (Odunayo et al., 2010).

SPECIFIC μ-AGONISTS

Studies examining the pharmacokinetics of opioids in cats, dogs, and horses are summarized in Tables 4.1, 4.2, 4.3, and 4.4.

Morphine

Morphine has a pKa of 7.9, with 23% in the nonionized form at pH 7.4, and is approximately 30–40% protein bound. Morphine is a full agonist and acts at μ-, δ-, and κ-opioid receptors. Due to its relative hydrophilicity, morphine makes a slow transition into the central nervous system; however, the lag time is clinically not a deterrent and morphine has an action of 3–4 hours duration.

Generally, morphine is conjugated to M3G and M6G, although there may be alternative pathways in cats, possibly forming ethereal sulfates (Taylor et al., 2001). M6G has similar properties as morphine and contributes to analgesia, whereas M3G has little affinity for μ-opioid receptors and can produce excitatory effects. In dogs, concentrations of M6G after IV injection of morphine are much lower than those in humans (KuKanich et al., 2005a). Because M6G likely does not contribute significantly to the analgesic effects in dogs, the question arises as to the correct dosing schedule for dogs, and this has not yet been ascertained. To maintain the known analgesic plasma concentrations of morphine for humans (20 ng/mL) the dosing schedule of 0.5 mg/kg given IV or IM every 2 hours was

Table 4.1. Summary of studies examining the pharmacokinetics of opioids in the cat. Further details can be obtained from the references used (some data expressed with standard deviation where available)

Drug	Dose (mg/kg)	Route	T_{max} (min)	Clearance mL/min/kg	Volume of distribution at steady state (L/kg)	Mean elimination half-life (h or min)	Bioavailability (%)	Reference
Alfentanil	0.05	IV	NA	11.6 ± 3.2	4.9 ± 1.6	2.0 h	NA	Pascoe et al., 1993a
Buprenorphine	0.01	IV	NA	16.7	7.1	7.0 h	NA	Taylor et al., 2001
Buprenorphine	0.01	IM	3.0	23.7	8.9	6.3 h	NA	Taylor et al., 2001
Buprenorphine	0.02	IV	NA	9.3	4.8	6.2 h	NA	Robertson et al., 2005b
Buprenorphine	0.02	Buccal	30.0	NA	NA	NA	116.3	Robertson et al., 2005b
Butorphanol	0.4	IM	21.0	12.9 ± 5	7.6 ± 6.3	6.3 ± 2.3 h	NA	Wells et al., 2008
Butorphanol	0.4	Buccal	66.0	35.3 ± 6.5	15.6 ± 4.7	5.2 ± 5.7 h	37.2	Wells et al., 2008
Fentanyl	0.0072 ± 0.0012	IV	NA	19.8 ± 2.7	2.6 ± 0.3	2.4 ± 0.6 min	NA	Lee, 2000
Fentanyl	0.01	IV	2.0	NA	NA	NA	NA	Robertson et al., 2005a
Hydromorphone	0.1	IV	NA	24.6	3.0	1.7 h	NA	Wegner et al., 2004
Meperidine	5.0	IM	10.0	20.8	5.2	3.6 h	NA	Taylor et al., 2001
Morphine	0.2	IV	NA	24.1	2.6	1.3 h	NA	Taylor et al., 2001
Morphine	0.2	IM	15.0	13.9	1.7	1.6 h	NA	Taylor et al., 2001
Remifentanil	1.0 μg/kg/min	Infusion	5.0	766	7.63	17.4 min	NA	Pypendop et al., 2008a
Tramadol	2.0	IV	NA	20.8 ± 3.2	3.3 ± 0.13	2.2 ± 0.3 h	NA	Pypendop & Ilkiw, 2007
Tramadol	5.0	Oral	40 ± 14	NA	NA	3.4 ± 0.1 h	93 ± 7	Pypendop & Ilkiw, 2007
Tramadol	2.0	IV	NA	14.9 ± 6.1	1.9 ± 0.4	1.9 ± 0.7 h	NA	Cagnardi et al., 2011

NA, not available or applicable; IV, intravenous; IM, intramuscular.

Table 4.2. Summary of studies examining the pharmacokinetics of opioids in the dog. Further details can be obtained from the references used (some data expressed with standard deviation where available)

Drug	Dose (mg/kg)	Route	T_{max}	Clearance (mL/min/kg)	Volume of distribution at steady state (L/kg)	Elimination half-life	Bioavailability (%)	Reference used
Alfentanil	1.6 mg/kg/min	Infusion	NA	29.8 ± 14.5	0.56 ± 0.2	19.9 ± 0.9 min	NA	Hoke et al., 1997
Buprenorphine	0.015	IV	2 (2–5) min	5.4 ± 1.9	1.6 ± 0.3	4.5 ± 2.2 h	NA	Krotscheck et al., 2008
Buprenorphine	0.02	IV	NA	~23.5	~6.0	4.4 ± 1.4 h	NA	Andaluz et al., 2009a
Buprenorphine	0.02	IV	NA	22.2±0.3	0.42 ± 0.2	17.3 ± 0.8 min	NA	Pieper, 2011
Butorphanol	0.25	SC	28.7 ± 13 min	5.83 ± 2.2	8.4 ± 3.1	1.7 ± 0.4 h	NA	Pfeffer et al., 1980
Butorphanol	0.25	IM	42.2 ± 13 min	5.68 ± 1.5	7.5 ± 2.4	1.5 ± 0.2 h	NA	Pfeffer et al., 1980
Butorphanol	0.25	Epidural	13.9 min	33.7	4.39	3.2 h	NA	Troncy et al., 1996
Codeine	0.734	IV	NA	30	3.2	NA	NA	KuKanich, 2009
Codeine	1.43	Oral	55.0 min	NA	NA	NA	4.0	KuKanich, 2009
Fentanyl	0.01	IV	NA	77.9	5.0	45.7 min	NA	Sano et al., 2006
Hydromorphone	0.1	IV	NA	106.28	4.24	0.33 min	NA	KuKanich et al., 2008a
Hydromorphone	0.1	SC	11.4 min	57.4	3.29	0.40 min	NA	KuKanich et al., 2008a
Methadone	0.4	IV	NA	27.9 ± 7.3	9.2 ± 3.3	3.9 ± 1.0 h	NA	Ingvast-Larsson et al., 2010
Methadone	0.5	IV	NA	56.0 ± 9.4	7.8 ± 1.9	1.5 ± 0.2 h	NA	KuKanich & Borum, 2008c
Methadone	0.4	SC	1.26 ± 1.2 h	NA	NA	10.7 ± 4.3 h	79 ± 22	Ingvast-Larsson et al., 2010
Meperidine	2.0	IV	NA	77 ± 8.3	3.1 ± 0.6	36.6 ± 6.0 min	NA	Kalthum & Waterman, 1988
Meperidine	2.0	SC	20.0 min	NA	NA	57.6 ± 7.6 min	0.11–0.13	Waterman & Kalthum, 1989
Morphine	0.5	IV	NA	85.2	7.2	1.6 h	NA	Barnhart et al., 2000
Morphine	1.0	IM	5.0 min	91.2	6.8	1.4 h	119	Barnhart et al., 2000
Morphine	2.0	Rectal	5.0 min	88.4	6.1	1.1 h	16.5	Barnhart et al., 2000
Morphine	0.5	IV	NA	62.5 ± 10.4	4.6 ± 0.2	1.2 ± 0.2 h	NA	KuKanich et al., 2005a
Oxymorphone	0.1	IV	NA	52.3	4.1	0.48 min	NA	KuKanich et al., 2008b
Oxymorphone	0.1	SC	13 min	48.3	4.2	0.59 min	NA	KuKanich et al., 2008b
Remifentanil	0.5 µg/kg/min	Infusion	NA	63.1 ± 18.1	0.22 ± 0.1	5.6 ± 0.6 min	NA	Hoke et al., 1997
Tramadol	4.4	IV	NA	54.6 ± 8.2	3.8±0.9	0.8 ± 1.2 h	NA	KuKanich & Papich, 2004
Tramadol	11.0	Oral	1.04 ± 0.5 h	52.3 ± 24	NA	1.7 ± 0.12 h	65 ± 38	KuKanich & Papich, 2004
Tramadol	4.0	IV	NA	35.6 ± 3.0	3.4 ± 0.5	1.4 ± 0.4 h	NA	McMillan et al., 2008

NA, not available or applicable; IV, intravenous; IM, intramuscular; SC, subcutaneous.

Table 4.3. Summary of studies examining the pharmacokinetics of opioids in the horse. Further details can be obtained from the references used (some data expressed with standard deviation where available)

Drug	Dose (mg/kg)	Route	T_{max} (minutes; unless hours specified)	Clearance (mL/min/kg)	Volume of distribution at steady state (L/kg)	Mean elimination half-life	Bioavailability (%)	Reference used
Alfentanil	0.04	IV	NA	14.1 ± 0.7	0.34 ± 0.053	21.7 ± 4.0 min	NA	Pascoe et al., 1991
Buprenorphine	0.01	IV	NA	18.5	3.0	3.3 h	NA	Davis et al., 2012
Butorphanol	0.08	IV	NA	4.6 ± 1.7	1.13 ± 0.92	7.8 ± 5.1 h	NA	Sellon et al., 2008
Butorphanol	0.08	IM	19.2	12.4 ± 3.9	0.62 ± 0.26	34.3 ± 24.6 min	37.3 ± 6.1	Sellon et al., 2008
Butorphanol Foals 3–12 days old	0.05	IV	NA	31.4 ± 4.4	5.5 ± 3.0	2.1 ± 1.4 h	NA	Arguedes et al., 2008
Butorphanol Foals 3–12 days old	0.05	IM	6.0 ± 2.4	NA	NA	0.9 ± 0.3 h	66.1 ± 12.0	Arguedes et al., 2008
Fentanyl	~0.004	IV	NA	5.9 ± 1.3	0.68 ± 0.17	130 ± 30 min	NA	Maxwell, 2003
Fentanyl	0.004	IV	NA	9.2 ± 1.7	0.37 ± 0.09	60.0 ± 28.0 min	NA	Thomasy et al., 2007
Meperidine	1.0	IV	NA	17.7		57.7 min	NA	Waterman & Amin, 1992
Methadone	0.1	Oral	22.5 ± 8.6	17.3 ± 3.5	3.1 ± 0.7	2.2 ± 35.6 h	NA	Linardi et al., 2009
Methadone	0.2	Oral	37.5 ± 15.0	13.5 ± 5.2	1.2 ± 0.2	1.3 ± 46.1 h	NA	Linardi et al., 2009
Methadone	0.4	Oral	30.0 ± 21.2	15.8 ± 3.2	2.0 ± 0.7	1.5 ± 40.8 h	NA	Linardi et al., 2009
Morphine	0.1	IV				1.6 h		Combie et al., 1983
Morphine	0.05	Intra-articular	120.0	NA	0.18 ± 0.08	2.6 ± 0.2 h	NA	Lindegaard et al., 2010
Tramadol	2.0	IV	NA	26.0 ± 3.0	2.2 ± 0.5	1.4 ± 0.2 h	NA	Shilo et al., 2007
Tramadol	2.0	IM	20.0 ± 6.0	NA	NA	1.5 ± 0.2 h	111 ± 39	Shilo et al., 2007
Tramadol	2.0	Oral	50.0 ± 18.0	NA	NA	NA	3.0 ± 2.0	Shilo et al., 2007
Tramadol	5.0	IV	NA	1.16 ± 0.1	1.42 ± 0.08	41.4 ± 6.0 min	NA	Giorgi et al., 2007
Tramadol Slow release	5.0	Oral	4.46 ± 0.6 h	NA	NA	3.43 ± 0.5 h	10.5 ± 2.4	Giorgi et al., 2007
Tramadol	2.0	Oral	35.4 ± 10.8	55.6 ± 13.0	NA	10.1 ± 4.2 h	NA	Cox et al., 2010
Tramadol	2.0	IV	NA	20.4 ± 5.7	2.5 ± 0.7	2.1 ± 0.9 h	NA	Dhanjal et al., 2009

NA, not available or applicable; IV, intravenous; IM, intramuscular.

Table 4.4. Summary of studies examining the pharmacokinetics of slow-release opioids in the dog. Further details can be obtained from the references used (some data expressed with standard deviation where available)

Drug	Dose (mg/kg)	Route	T_{max} (Min)	Clearance (mL/min/kg)	Volume of distribution at steady state (L/kg)	Mean elimination half-life (h)	Bioavailability (%)	Reference used
Hydromorphone	1.0	SC	16.2	NA	NA	5.22	NA	Smith et al., 2008
Hydromorphone	2.0	SC	10.8	NA	NA	31.9	NA	Smith et al., 2008
Hydromorphone	3.0	SC	13.2	NA	NA	24.1	NA	Smith et al., 2008
Morphine	~1.4	Oral	85.0 ± 51.7	NA	NA	8.1 ± 70	21.2 ± 4.4	Dohoo et al., 1994
Morphine	~2.7	Oral	50.0 ± 11.0	NA	NA	10.4 ± 14.0	19.8 ± 7.0	Dohoo et al., 1994
Morphine	~1.6	Oral	105.0	~55.0	3.52	1.6	15.1	Dohoo & Taskar, 1997
Morphine	1.2	SC	55 ±11.2	281 ± 20.1	4.77 ± 1.2	1.8 ± 0.4	NA	Tasker et al., 1997
Morphine	1.0	Oral	338.4 ± 323.4	~150.0	NA	14.7 ± 4.4	NA	Aragon et al., 2008
Morphine	2.0	Oral	171.6 ± 94.2	~90.0	NA	42.9 ± 40.2	NA	Aragon et al., 2008
Oxymorphone	0.5 & 1.0	SC	~30.0	NA	NA	NA	NA	Smith et al., 2004b

NA, not available or applicable;
SC, subcutaneous.

recommended in dogs (KuKanich et al., 2005a). Morphine infusions have become popular and have mild analgesic effects at a rate of 0.17 mg/kg/h with mild to moderate analgesic effects at a rate of 0.34 mg/kg/h. Both infusion rates provided plasma concentrations of morphine well in excess of the 20 ng/mL target defined in humans (Guedes et al., 2007a).

The analgesic effect of morphine has been demonstrated in many species, but difficulty arises with excitatory effects in species such as horses (Clark et al., 2005; Love et al., 2006). Another limitation of using morphine in horses is the concern for postoperative ileus. General thoughts are inclined toward provision of analgesia with morphine, as evidence shows that short-term morphine administration to painful horses may be well tolerated (Andersen et al., 2006; Boscan et al., 2006a) and ileus treatable (Boscan et al., 2006b).

Intra-articular administration of morphine has been developed to circumnavigate the potential problems of systemic administration of morphine to horses undergoing joint surgery. Intra-articular morphine in ponies produced detectable, albeit low, concentrations in plasma 30 minutes after administration, and morphine did not cause problems in normal joints (Raekallio et al., 1996). Intra-articular morphine (120 mg) alleviated pain in a lipopolysaccharide model of joint inflammation in horses (van Loon et al., 2010).

In cats, morphine is efficacious in painful conditions and in nonpainful situations for sedation (Stanway et al., 2002; Steagall et al., 2006), but there are no clinical studies evaluating appropriate analgesic doses and dosing intervals.

Morphine does not sensitize the heart to circulating catecholamines if oxygen and carbon dioxide partial pressure are in the normal range. Cardiac arrhythmias were observed in one dog after a high-dose of morphine was given IV (Guedes et al., 2007b). Histamine release, and the possibility of hypotension, occurs after IV injection of morphine at doses of 0.5 mg/kg and 1.0 mg/kg given over 15 seconds, especially with the higher dose (Guedes et al., 2007b).

Oral slow-release formulations are now available and have been evaluated in dogs and rats (Dohoo et al., 1994; Tasker et al., 1997; Aragon et al., 2008; Leach et al., 2010). The rapid hepatic first pass effect when oral formulations are used is a limitation in animal species.

Meperidine (Pethidine)

Meperidine is a synthetic derivative of phenylpiperidine, is structurally similar to atropine, and possesses a clinically useful antispasmodic effect. It is 65–75% protein bound, has a pKa of 8.5, and 7% is in the nonionized form at pH 7.4. It is an agonist at μ- and κ-opioid receptors, and the principal effects are similar to morphine. Meperidine has a tenth of the potency of morphine, but at equipotent doses, produces a similar degree of sedation, nausea, and ventilatory depression. At clinical doses, meperidine sedation is not as profound in dogs, and the dose of induction drug is not reduced as much, when compared to the use of morphine (Wilson et al., 2007). Meperidine is associated with a lower incidence of gastroesophageal reflux when compared to morphine. However, combining meperidine with acepromazine appears to increase the incidence of reflux (Wilson et al., 2007).

IV injection of meperidine causes vasodilation, hypotension, and bradycardia (Kalthum & Waterman, 1988). Dose-dependent histamine release causes the observed hemodynamic changes, as the decrease in arterial pressure is dependent on plasma histamine concentration (Thompson & Walton, 1964). Thus, IV administration is not recommended.

Elimination of meperidine, after IV injection, is rapid in dogs, with an elimination half-life of 37 minutes (Kalthum & Waterman, 1988; Waterman & Kalthum, 1989). Plasma meperidine concentrations are not detectable at 90 minutes (Kalthum & Waterman, 1988). Clearance can be prolonged by concurrent use of inhalational anesthetics, which reduce hepatic blood flow (Kalthum & Waterman, 1988). The elimination half-life for meperidine given IM is 51 minutes with an estimated bioavailability of 86% (Waterman & Kalthum, 1989). Administration of meperidine using subcutaneous routes is not recommended due to poor bioavailability and rapid elimination (Waterman & Kalthum, 1989). Resedation is possible in humans as meperidine can be ion-trapped in gastric juices and reabsorbed into the circulation once passed into the small intestine (Trudnowski & Gessner, 1979); this effect is also suspected to occur in dogs (Kalthum & Waterman, 1988). Dogs with portosystemic shunts had an elimination half-life of about 76 minutes after IV injection and 108 minutes after IM injection (Waterman & Kalthum, 1990). Clearance of meperidine and normeperidine through the kidneys appears to be minimal in dogs (Kalthum & Waterman, 1990), and 58 ± 13% of meperidine is cleared through the lung (Kramer et al., 1985).

In cats, IM meperidine, at a dose of 5 mg/kg, did not cause dysphoria and had an elimination half-life of 216.4 ± 122.6 minutes (Taylor et al., 2001).

Meperidine undergoes N-demethylation to the convulsant, normeperidine. Normeperidine has less analgesic effect, but a longer elimination compared to the parent drug. Normeperidine can be detected 1 hour after injection in cats (Taylor et al., 2001). Normeperidine production in dogs is low, but can reach convulsant concentrations with accidental overdose (Golder et al., 2010). Treatment is with conventional anticonvulsants, as naloxone will not reverse the convulsive effects of normeperidine.

In horses, the redistribution half-life of IV meperidine is 3 minutes and the elimination half-life is 57 minutes. It is suggested that a plasma concentration of 0.4 μg/mL is analgesic (Waterman & Amin, 1992).

Hydromorphone

Hydromorphone is a hydrogenated ketone derivative and a pure μ-opioid agonist, and is 20% protein bound. It is about 5–10 times more potent than morphine, and appears to be equal in potency to oxymorphone (Pettifer & Dyson, 2000). It has largely superseded oxymorphone in veterinary practice in North America because it is less expensive and has similar properties. Hydromorphone is metabolized through conjugation in a similar manner to the structurally related drug morphine, producing 3-O-glucuronide metabolites (Wright et al., 2001). In humans, the metabolite can accumulate in the presence of renal insufficiency and can produce neuroexcitatory behaviors (Wright et al., 2001). Hydromorphone produces sedation, respiratory depression, bradycardia, and potent analgesia, but only slightly increases plasma histamine concentrations after IV injection (Pettifer & Dyson, 2000; Campbell et al., 2003; Guedes et al., 2007b). In dogs, it causes panting, defecation, and vomiting. The incidence of vomiting can be reduced to 18% with administration of acepromazine 15 minutes before injection of IM hydromorphone, compared to an incidence of 45% when the drugs are simultaneously injected (Valverde et al., 2004). In common with other opioids, vomiting is not often observed with IV injection, as the inhibitory effects on the vomiting center preside (Robertson et al., 2009). A 2-hourly IV dosing interval (0.1 mg/kg) or an infusion rate of 0.03 mg/kg/h is recommended for dogs (KuKanich et al., 2008a).

A long-acting formulation of hydromorphone is available, that can be injected subcutaneously, has a rapid onset, and provides antinociception for up to 4 days at a dosage of 3 mg/kg (Smith et al., 2008) (Chapter 9). This long-acting formulation can produce respiratory depression during the first 6 hours after administration (Wunsch et al., 2010).

In cats, hydromorphone is an effective analgesic, although the occasional cat will become dysphoric, especially if not in pain. After an IV dose of 0.1 mg/kg, the plasma concentration of hydromorphone was below limits of quantification by 6 hours, although antinociceptive effects were evident by 15 minutes after administration and lasted for 7.5 hours (Wegner et al., 2004). A follow-up study examining different doses of IV hydromorphone in cats found that 0.1 mg/kg produced a rapid onset of antinociception that lasted for 3.3 hours (Wegner & Robertson, 2007). The IM administration of 0.1 mg/kg produced emesis in some cats, but no dysphoria (Lascelles & Robertson, 2004a). Onset of antinociception was rapid and lasted 5.5 hours (Lascelles & Robertson, 2004a). Subcutaneous administration of 0.1 mg/kg hydromorphone to cats is not as efficacious as IV or IM routes (Robertson et al., 2009). These authors found a slower onset (just less than 2 hours) and shorter duration of antinociception (3.5 hours), with adverse effects of hyperthermia, dysphoria, and emesis (Robertson et al., 2009).

Oxymorphone

Oxymorphone is a μ-opioid agonist with ten times the potency of morphine, and is not reported to release histamine in dogs (Robinson et al., 1988). Dogs typically pant with oxymorphone and may show signs of dysphoria. Bradycardia and sedation are also typical responses (Haskins et al., 1991; KuKanich et al., 2008b). IV injection causes bradycardia and an increase in arterial blood pressure through increased systemic vascular resistance, even in hypovolemic dogs (Haskins et al., 1991). Increased respiratory rate and decreased alveolar ventilation mildly increases $PaCO_2$ and decreases PaO_2 (Haskins et al., 1991). Oxymorphone is rapidly absorbed from subcutaneous sites, and is rapidly eliminated in dogs, with an elimination half-life of 49 minutes after IV injection, and 59 minutes after subcutaneous injection (KuKanich et al., 2008b). Maintenance of serum oxymorphone concentrations greater than 4 ng/mL, a concentration considered to be effective for analgesia in humans, would require dosing intervals of every 2–3 hours at a dose of 0.1 mg/kg (KuKanich et al., 2008b). Alternatively, these authors recommend an IV infusion of oxymorphone (12 μg/kg/h) to achieve the same serum concentration (KuKanich et al., 2008b).

Methadone

Methadone has been used, in Europe, for many years for analgesia and sedation. Methadone is now becoming popular for veterinary use in countries where it is available as either a racemic mixture or the more active (R) or l-isomer (Monteiro et al., 2008; Credie et al., 2010). Methadone has a higher intrinsic efficacy for the μ-opioid receptor than morphine (Selley et al., 2001). Methadone is antagonistic at the N-methyl-D-aspartate receptor, and is a norepinephrine and serotonin uptake inhibitor (Codd et al., 1995). Methadone has

a half-life of 3.9 $\pm$ 1 hours after IV injection in healthy dogs (Ingvast-Larsson et al., 2010). After subcutaneous injection, the time to peak plasma concentration is 1.26 $\pm$ 1.04 hours, bioavailability is 79 $\pm$ 22%, and elimination half-life is 10.7 $\pm$ 4.3 hours (Ingvast-Larsson et al., 2010). It is recommended to start analgesia regimens with an IV loading dose and to follow with subcutaneous administration, rather than start with the latter route. These authors did not notice whining in dogs with a dose of 0.4 mg/kg, but no other signs of agitation or vomiting. Other reports have described panting and defecation as side effects in dogs, but no vomiting (KuKanich & Borum, 2008c). Methadone is cleared rapidly through hepatic metabolism with little excreted as the parent compound in bile or urine (Garrett et al., 1985). Greyhounds require a more frequent dosing regimen of 1.0–1.5 mg/kg every 3–4 hours because of a greater volume of distribution and faster clearance compared to Beagles (KuKanich & Borum, 2008c). Oral bioavailability is poor in dogs (KuKanich et al., 2005b).

In cats, methadone is a proven analgesic, and does not provoke emesis or cause excitement at dosages of 0.5 mg/kg using the IM route (Steagall et al., 2006). Methadone is also used to sedate and provide analgesia in other species. Its usefulness with α_2-adrenergic agonists and/or acepromazine to sedate horses has been recognized for decades (Nolan & Hall, 1984; Clarke & Paton, 1988; Nilsfors et al., 1988). In horses, oral methadone administered at doses of 0.1, 0.2, and 0.4 mg/kg did not produce signs of excitement or changes in gut motility. Serum methadone was detectable 15 minutes after administration and for 12 hours afterward (Linardi et al., 2009). Analgesic serum concentrations have not been evaluated for horses, but concentrations after oral administration were similar to those known to be analgesic in humans. Differences in absorption among species may be explained through differences in the anatomy of the GIT and, possibly, absorption through buccal mucosa (Linardi et al., 2009).

Fentanyl

The phenylpiperidine derivative fentanyl is highly lipophilic and is 75–125 times more potent than morphine. Fentanyl is a weak base with a pKa of 8.4, and 8.5% is in the nonionized form at pH 7.4. Fentanyl is 80–85% protein bound, and takes 6–8 minutes to equilibrate with the biophase.

Fentanyl has a more rapid action and elimination compared to morphine, due to its lipophilic nature. It has a pulmonary first pass effect and 75% is taken up into the lungs and stored. With frequent dosing or long-term infusions these sites become saturated, and the plasma concentration of fentanyl does not decrease as rapidly, reflected in long context-sensitive half-times. Fentanyl accumulation does not appear to occur in dogs after a 4-hour infusion (10 μg/kg/h), although long-term use for postoperative analgesia might result in accumulation (Sano et al., 2006). Fentanyl is metabolized by N-demethylation to norfentanyl, which is similar to normeperidine. Norfentanyl has less analgesic potency than fentanyl.

The optimal analgesic plasma concentration in cats is considered to be greater than 1.07 ng/mL (Robertson et al., 2005a). Plasma fentanyl concentrations greater than 0.95 ng/mL are analgesic in dogs (Robinson et al., 1999). A serum fentanyl concentration of 7.82 ng/mL appears to provide some somatic analgesia in horses, but fentanyl does not have any effect on visceral nociception (Sanchez et al., 2007). Transdermal fentanyl augmented the analgesic effects of phenylbutazone or flunixin meglumine in horses, but seemed to be more effective in relieving soft tissue pain than orthopedic pain (Thomasy et al., 2004).

Fentanyl infusions have been successfully used in cats at a rate of 6 μg/kg/h, and decreased the amount of propofol required to maintain anesthesia (Mendes & Selmi, 2003). An alternative method of fentanyl delivery has been investigated in cats that could replace fentanyl patches in some situations (Sykes et al., 2009). Osmotic pumps have been developed for continual release of fentanyl, and produced greater serum fentanyl concentrations in cats, without a lag period, and with a similar duration as transdermal fentanyl patches (Sykes et al., 2009).

Remifentanil

Remifentanil is an ultrashort-acting μ-agonist with 70% protein binding. Remifentanil has a pKa of 7.3, and 58% is nonionized at a pH of 7.4. It takes 1.1 minutes for remifentanil to equilibrate with the biophase, and it has a context-sensitive half-time of 4 minutes after a 4 hour infusion in humans. Recovery from a bolus dose is through rapid metabolism rather than redistribution. The ester side chain is metabolized by blood and tissue nonspecific esterases to a less active compound. Because of this unique metabolism and small volume of distribution, remifentanil does not accumulate with prolonged infusions or repeat doses. Pseudocholinesterase does not appear to metabolize remifentanil, therefore, plasma cholinesterase depletion does not affect elimination.

Remifentanil is a μ-opioid agonist similar in potency to fentanyl, although in dogs it may have only half the potency (Michelsen et al., 1996). Peak analgesic effects are observed within 1–3 minutes of IV injection and last approximately 10 minutes. It is mainly used as an infusion, although repeat bolus doses can be used. In propofol-anesthetized cats, analgesic effects were evident during surgery at an infusion rate of 18 μg/kg/h (Correa et al., 2007). Cats, similar to other species, also exhibit rapid recovery from remifentanil, although clearance can be delayed by concurrent use of isoflurane through reduction of blood flow to vessel-rich organs (Pypendop et al., 2008a).

Pharmacokinetics do not vary with dose, and there is little remifentanil found in liver and kidney tissues of dogs given infusions of 22 μg/kg/h and 2.2 mg/kg/h (Chism & Rickert, 1996). Dosing should be based on lean body mass in very obese patients, but normal dosages can be used in patients with renal or hepatic disease (Egan et al., 1998). Conscious cats can become dysphoric at infusion rates greater than 60 μg /kg/h (Brosnan et al., 2009).

There are few published reports of remifentanil use in horses, but the author has used infusion rates of 3 μg /kg/h in research horses and in clinical cases (Benmansour & Duke-Novakovski, 2013). A rapid bolus of 2 μg /kg can cause profound bradycardia, and bolus doses should be administered slowly.

In humans, remifentanil infusion appears to produce a greater incidence of respiratory depression than fentanyl, when used for postoperative analgesia (Dahan et al., 2010). Postoperative shivering is reported to occur in 40% of human patients, and may be due to stimulation of N-methyl-D-aspartate receptors after sudden drug withdrawal (Nakasuji et al., 2010).

Alternative analgesic techniques or drugs are required immediately after stopping the administration of remifentanil because of its rapid removal or it can be used as a postoperative analgesic at low infusion rates, as long as the respiratory system is monitored.

Remifentanil is 300–1000 times more potent than its metabolite, GR90291, which is renally excreted in rats and cats (Hoke et al., 1997; Brosnan et al., 2009). Pharmacokinetics of remifentanil and GR90291 follow a two-compartment model with remifentanil and GR90291 elimination half-lives of 6 minutes and 19 minutes, respectively (Hoke et al., 1997).

Sufentanil

Sufentanil is a short-acting μ-agonist that is 10–15 times more potent than fentanyl. It is very lipid soluble and equilibrates between the blood and brain tissue in 6.2 minutes. Sufentanil has a shorter elimination half-life than fentanyl because it is mainly nonionized at plasma pH (80%) and has higher protein binding (93%), mainly to α_1-acid glycoprotein. Sufentanil has a context-sensitive half-time of 30 minutes after a 4 hour infusion in humans. Hepatic metabolism involves N-dealkylation and O-demethylation in humans, but there are no details of its metabolism in dogs and cats.

In common with potent μ-opioid agonists, sufentanil causes profound respiratory depression, which may require patient ventilation. Sufentanil produces hemodynamic stability with mild vasodilatory effects, but bradycardia can be profound with the higher doses used during induction in dogs (3–5 μg/kg, IV) and an anticholinergic may be required. It can be administered systemically and spinally, although its action is short, by either route, unless administered as an infusion.

Like fentanyl, sufentanil can be used as a bolus for short-term blunting of response to intense noxious stimulation. It can also be used at low infusion rates postoperatively for pain control in conscious dogs, but will produce some sedation and respiratory depression (Latasch & Freye, 2002). Large doses (20 μg/kg) administered to dogs decrease cerebral blood flow alongside a reduction in cerebral metabolism, without altering intracranial pressure (Werner et al., 1991).

Alfentanil

Alfentanil is a short-acting, rapid onset μ-opioid agonist. It is not as potent as fentanyl, but ten times more potent than morphine. Alfentanil is a weaker base than fentanyl, and is unique in having a pKa of 6.5; therefore, 89% is in the nonionized form at plasma pH. The different pKa and its lipid solubility allow alfentanil to rapidly cross the blood–brain barrier, and alfentanil produces effects within 1 minute after IV injection, including sedation and respiratory depression. Alfentanil is 92% bound to plasma proteins, mainly to α_1-acid glycoprotein, and is eliminated from the body faster than fentanyl through N-dealkylation and O-demethylation in the liver to inactive metabolites (Mather, 1983).

Alfentanil pharmacokinetics has been studied in cats (Pascoe et al., 1993a) after a dose of 50 μg/kg IV. At this dose, cats exhibited brief and transient excitement, mydriasis, a slight increase in systemic blood pressure, and approximately 20 minutes of analgesia, with sedation in some cats. Alfentanil has a rapid redistribution phase and slower elimination phase, similar to humans. Alfentanil elimination half-life is longer in cats (112 minutes) (Pascoe et al., 1993a) than dogs (19 minutes) (Hoke et al., 1997). Alfentanil has a context-sensitive half-time of 60 minutes after a 4 hour infusion in humans. After an 8-hour long infusion, alfentanil has a longer context-sensitive half-time than sufentanil due to the rapid equilibration of alfentanil into plasma after discontinuation of the infusion (Hughes et al., 1992).

Alfentanil allows for hemodynamic stability and produces mild decreases in systemic blood pressure, but heart rate can profoundly decrease. Alfentanil has been used as an induction agent in dogs, as part of a balanced anesthesia approach, and for postoperative analgesia.

Intense muscle rigidity has been reported in some humans and dogs (Benthuysen et al., 1986). Alfentanil can increase intracranial pressure in humans with brain tumors, unlike fentanyl, although the increase may be insignificant if $PaCO_2$ is controlled.

Tramadol

Tramadol is classified as an atypical μ-opioid agonist that also inhibits serotonin and norepinephrine uptake, and is 20% protein bound. Tramadol exists as a racemic mixture, and (+)tramadol interacts with opiate, $α_2$-adrenergic, and serotonin receptors, and (-)tramadol interacts with $α_2$-adrenergic receptors (KuKanich & Papich, 2004). Tramadol has a tenth of the potency of morphine, and may be most suited for the treatment of mild to moderate pain (Mastrocinque & Fantoni, 2003). It has few respiratory, cardiovascular, and gastrointestinal effects, can be used as an antitussive, and has slight sedative properties (Monteiro et al., 2009).

Tramadol has active metabolites such as O-desmethyltramadol (M1) with avid affinity for the μ-opioid receptor but weak intrinsic activity. The metabolite also exists as two stereoisomers, (+)M1 acts on μ-opioid receptors, while (−)M1 interacts with $α_2$-adrenergic receptors (KuKanich & Papich, 2004). The production of M1 from tramadol is slower than its elimination, but M1 production is considered to be low in dogs (McMillan et al., 2008). N-desmethyltramadol (M2) is inactive, and can be metabolized to mainly inactive N-N didesmethyltramadol (M3) and N-N-O tridesmethyltramadol (M4), and N-O didesmethyltramadol (M5) (Giorgi et al., 2009). The metabolite M5 has affinity for the μ-opioid receptor, but does not effectively cross the blood–brain barrier. The elimination of tramadol and M1 after oral dosing in dogs is faster than in humans (KuKanich & Papich, 2004).

No side effects were noticed after oral administration of 4 mg/kg of tramadol to dogs, it took 9.5 minutes for tramadol to be detected in the plasma, 1.5 hours before peak tramadol plasma concentration was reached, and tramadol was detectable for 5–10 hours (Giorgi et al., 2009). Low concentrations of M1 were detected, but high concentrations of M2 and M5 were present. Tramadol, M3 and M5 were detected in urine, but no M1 was detected (Giorgi et al., 2009).

In cats, IV and oral administration resulted in a slower clearance than observed in dogs, with good bioavailability (93%) after oral administration, although the authors caution that this may be erroneously high (Pypendop & Ilkiw, 2007). Time to reach peak concentration after oral administration is similar to that found in dogs (Pypendop & Ilkiw, 2007). It appears that M1 is the principle product in the metabolism of tramadol in the cat (Pypendop & Ilkiw, 2007; Cagnardi et al., 2011).

The IV dose of 2 mg/kg appears to have postoperative analgesic effects after castration or spay in cats, with little effect on the respiratory or cardiovascular system (Cagnardi et al., 2011). A dosing schedule of 4 mg/kg every 6 hours was recommended in order to maintain analgesic effects in cats (Pypendop et al., 2009).

In horses, tramadol has been studied after IV injection and after administration of immediate- and slow-release tramadol formulations orally (Giorgi et al., 2007). The M2 metabolite appeared to be the product of tramadol metabolism, with low amounts of M1 and

M5. Peak concentrations of tramadol were observed in 2–3 hours after oral administration (Giorgi et al., 2007). Another study found peak tramadol concentrations in 1 hour after 2 mg/kg of an oral formulation. Metabolites M1 and M5 were the main metabolites in that study. The authors caution that IV tramadol at the same dose produced adverse effects of sweating and ataxia 15 minutes after injection (Cox et al., 2010). Giorgi et al. (2007) gave 5 mg/kg of tramadol IV to horses and also reported agitation and tachycardia 3–5 minutes following injection. These effects peaked at 15–20 minutes and resolved by the second hour after administration. Incremental IV doses of tramadol were given to horses and the antinociceptive properties examined (Dhanjal et al., 2009). After a cumulative dose of 3.1 mg/kg horses became visibly agitated with head bobbing and trembling. No antinociception was detected with a dose of 2 mg/kg.

Tapentadol

Tapentadol Immediate Release received FDA approval in 2008 and is available in 50, 75, and 100 mg tablets for treatment of moderate to severe pain. It is also available as an extended release formulation. Like tramadol, it is a μ-opioid agonist and norepinephrine uptake inhibitor, but unlike tramadol, the effects are from the parent compound as metabolism is not required for the effect (Heitz et al., 2009; Frampton, 2010). In humans, there are fewer adverse effects of nausea, vomiting, constipation, and pruritus. Animal trials have been performed in mice, rats, rabbits, and dogs where it was administered IV, intraperitoneally, intrathecally, and by the oral route. Rats have an extensive first pass metabolism and orally administered tapentadol was found to be ineffective; oral bioavailability is low in the dog but pharmacodynamic studies are needed to assess clinical effects (Giorgi et al., 2012). Patients with mild renal or hepatic dysfunction can still receive tapentadol.

OPIOID AGONIST–ANTAGONISTS

Butorphanol

Butorphanol is a synthetic agonist–antagonist that is extensively used in veterinary medicine. It is an agonist at κ-opioid receptors and is antagonistic at μ-opioid receptors. Butorphanol is best reserved for mild to moderate pain and can provide some visceral analgesia lasting 30 minutes in cats and dogs (Kalpravidh et al., 1984a, 1984b; Muir & Robertson, 1985; Houghton et al., 1991; Lascelles & Robertson, 2004b). The effects can be poor or short-lived (30–90 minutes), and the patient must be monitored for signs of breakthrough pain (Jochle et al., 1989; Love et al., 2009).

Increased locomotor activity can be observed in nonpainful horses, but ponies given "rescue" analgesia after castration did not become agitated (Nolan et al., 1994; Love et al., 2009). Administering butorphanol as an infusion (13 μg/kg/h) avoids problems with its short duration of action, and proved beneficial for treatment of pain in horses after abdominal surgery (Sellon et al., 2004). The horse should be monitored for decreased gastrointestinal activity, but effects tend to be mild and short-lived. The pharmacokinetics of butorphanol after IM injection dictate that a dosing schedule of 0.08 mg/kg every 3 hours may be necessary to maintain a concentration above 10 ng/mL (Sellon et al., 2008). Updated analytical techniques enabled better detection of lower concentrations of butorphanol, and the recommended infusion rate may be decreased from 13 μg/kg/h, although further studies are required to confirm this statement (Sellon et al., 2008).

Butorphanol produces minimal sedation and can potentially cause dysphoria (Sawyer & Rech, 1986). It is often used with a tranquilizer or sedative to provide more reliable sedation and allow most noninvasive procedures (Clarke & Paton, 1988; Dyson & Atilola, 1992; Bartram et al., 1994). Butorphanol does not release histamine on IV injection and has few effects on the respiratory or cardiovascular system.

Butorphanol has been used in many species, and is especially useful in birds, although its metabolism is rapid, and a liposome-encapsulated formulation may have greater benefit (Sladky et al., 2006; Riggs et al., 2008).

Buprenorphine

Buprenorphine is a semisynthetic, highly lipophilic, partial μ-opioid agonist. It is 96% protein bound, mainly to globulins. Buprenorphine avidly binds to the μ-opioid receptor with an affinity 1000 times that of morphine, but dissociates slowly and does not exert a maximal response. The half-life of dissociation from the μ-opioid receptor is 166 minutes, compared to 7 minutes with fentanyl, resulting in a long duration of action. The long duration of action is also attributed to slow equilibration with the biophase.

Buprenorphine has a weaker affinity for the δ-opioid receptor with antagonistic effects, and recently was found to act at the ORL-1 receptor. It is a weak antagonist at κ-opioid receptors (Lutfy & Cowan, 2004; Mégabane et al., 2006). Buprenorphine appears to have a ceiling effect or bell-shaped dose–response curve, whereby supraclinical doses do not increase the effect. This is thought to be due to partial agonist actions at μ-opioid receptors and antagonistic actions at κ-opioid receptors with higher doses, and is termed "autoinhibition." Other mechanisms are also thought to play a role, and may involve the ORL-1 receptor (Lutfy & Cowan, 2004).

A dose of 15 μg/kg administered IV has similar pharmacokinetics in dogs and cats. It is recommended that this dose be given every 3–4 hours to maintain analgesic effects (Taylor et al, 2001; Krotscheck et al., 2008). Bioavailability from IM injection was good in cats (Taylor et al., 2001). Buccal absorption is also good in cats, and is discussed later.

Analgesia was assessed in dogs after lateral thoracotomy, and 10 μg/kg buprenorphine IV every 6 hours appeared to provide reasonable analgesia, although dogs had higher pain scores than those that received intrapleural bupivacaine (Conzemius et al., 1994). Higher doses of buprenorphine are currently recommended for dogs. Postoperative analgesia was assessed after using IV, IM, subcutaneous, and buccal administration of buprenorphine (10 μg/kg) in cats that had been spayed (Giordano et al., 2010). More rescue analgesia was required in cats receiving buprenorphine through the subcutaneous and buccal routes. The subcutaneous route of administration was not recommended by the authors to treat pain in cats, and this was also reported in earlier studies examining thermal nociceptive threshold and postoperative pain scores (Gassel et al., 2005; Steagall et al., 2006). The dose for the buccal administration group may have been too low. A previous study also reported that transmucosal buprenorphine (10 μg/kg) was not reliably effective after surgery in cats (Gassel et al., 2005). A pharmacokinetic study in cats assessed a dose of 20 μg/kg (Robertson et al., 2005b).

A dose-related response to nociceptive testing could not be confirmed after IV doses of 10, 20, and 40 μg/kg buprenorphine in cats

(Steagall et al., 2009a). Considering the mild effects on the respiratory and cardiovascular systems (Scott et al., 1980; Jacobson et al., 1994; Martinez et al., 1997), few other adverse effects, and very high median lethal dose in dogs (79 mg/kg), higher doses of buprenorphine may, and can, be administered, if necessary (Krotscheck et al., 2008). Pre-emptive administration of buprenorphine (60 μg/kg IV) to rabbits in a visceral pain model helped to attenuate cardiovascular responses to colon distension (Shafford & Schadt, 2008).

Buprenorphine is rapidly metabolized through the liver in humans to inactive conjugates such as buprenorphine-3-glucuronide. *N*-dealkylation produces norbuprenorphine, which has analgesic activity (Huang et al., 2001), but formation of this metabolite appears to be low in dogs (Garrett & Chandran, 1990).

Cardiovascular effects of buprenorphine (16 μg/kg IV) in dogs include mild decreases in systemic arterial blood pressure, cardiac index, and heart rate (Martinez et al., 1997). In horses, buprenorphine (10 μg/kg IV) caused increased systemic arterial blood pressure, heart rate, and cardiac output due to sympathetic stimulation; arterial blood gases did not change. Gastrointestinal motility was decreased for 4 hours, but horses did not show signs of colic (Carregaro et al., 2006).

It appears buprenorphine causes an excitatory effect, similar to the action of other opioids, in horses, and lower doses of buprenorphine (3 μg/kg) do so in pain-free horses (Szöke et al., 1998). After administering a dose of 5 μg/kg buprenorphine IV, signs of excitement were observed within 5–10 minutes, and spontaneous locomotor activity was significant from 1 to 6 hours, and from 15 minutes to 14 hours after a dose of 10 μg/kg buprenorphine (Carregaro et al., 2007). Only the higher dose (10 μg/kg) had antinociceptive effects for 1–6 hours after administration (Carregaro et al., 2007). Horses sedated with α_2-adrenergic agonists or acepromazine did not show signs of excitement when buprenorphine (4 μg/kg and 6 μg/kg) was administered IV (Nolan & Hall, 1984; van Dijk et al., 2003).

Serious respiratory depression has been reported in humans with accidental overdose alongside other sedative drugs; however, respiratory depression at clinical doses in veterinary patients appears to be mild or nonexistent.

OPIOID ANTAGONISTS

Antagonists have high affinity for opioid receptors but little or no intrinsic activity. They are titrated to reverse undesirable effects of agonists or to completely reverse all effects. Research continues into obtaining more specific opioid receptor antagonists such as a δ-opioid receptor antagonist, naltrindole, and a pure μ-opioid receptor antagonist, β-funaltrexamine (Latasch & Freye, 2002).

Naloxone

Naloxone is an antagonist to μ-opioid agonists. It was first synthesized in 1960, and found to be antagonistic at μ-, δ-, and κ-receptors (Dahan et al., 2010). As for all true antagonists, naloxone produces a shift to the right for agonist dose–response curves. Orally administered naloxone is effectively metabolized through the hepatic first pass effect to inactive naloxone-3-glucuronide. In rats and humans, 30% of naloxone is excreted unchanged through the kidneys. The higher the dose of agonist used, the higher the required dose of naloxone needed to reverse the effects. Naloxone can be titrated to reverse respiratory depression because more agonist receptor occupation is required for respiratory depression than for analgesia. This does not apply to continuous infusions of agonists such as sufentanil. Because of naloxone's short duration of action (30–40 minutes) one dose of nalaxone during sufentanil infusion will only temporarily reverse respiratory depression. In order to prevent reoccurrence of undesirable opioid-agonist effects naloxone can be administered as an infusion (4–8 µg/kg/h). Remifentanil appears to have strong affinity for the µ-opioid receptor and high doses of naloxone are required to compete for the receptor; however, remifentanil is rapidly metabolized such that decreasing or stopping remifentanil infusion is often sufficient and pharmacological reversal is not required.

Naloxone is required in high doses to reverse the long-acting partial µ-opioid agonist buprenorphine. Infusions are also required because of the slower dissociation kinetics from receptors of buprenorphine. Naloxone can have a bell-shaped curve in its actions to reverse buprenorphine in humans, with little effect at normal clinical doses (~10 µg/kg), complete reversal at doses of ~30 µg/kg, and doses of approximately 85 µg/kg cause a decline in reversal. The cause for the bell-shaped dose–response curve to reverse buprenorphine-induced respiratory depression remains unknown (Dahan et al., 2010).

Reversal of analgesia in the face of severe pain can precipitate cardiac arrest in humans. High doses of naloxone cause catecholamine-related cardiac arrhythmias and vasoconstriction, and the vasoconstriction may lead to pulmonary edema. Use of lower doses in a titratable manner appears safe (Dahan et al., 2010). The catecholamine release has been used to advantage in patients that are already in cardiac arrest or septic, but its routine use remains controversial (Martins et al., 2008). In order to prevent reversal of analgesia, other nonopioid drugs have been investigated to reverse respiratory depression and include 5-hydroxytryptamine (serotonin) agonists and ampakinines (Dahan et al., 2010).

Nalmefene

Nalmefene has been investigated as a behavioral modification drug to reduce vices in horses and has been used to treat tail chasing in a dog (Dodman, 1987; Schwartz, 1993). It is 45% protein bound and has a pKa of 7.6. Nalmefene has also been used to reverse opioids used in immobilization of wildlife (Kreeger et al., 1987). Nalmefene undergoes species-specific metabolism. *N*-dealkylation plays a strong role in metabolism of nalmefene in rats, whereas conjugation to nalmefene glucuronides occurs in the dog (Murthy et al., 1996). Nalmefene (0.03 mg/kg IV) completely reversed oxymorphone sedation in dogs, whereas low-dose naloxone treated dogs renarcotized, and butorphanol only partially reversed sedation (Dyson et al., 1990).

Naltrexone

Naltrexone is used in humans for treatment of opioid addiction (Dahan et al., 2010). It is 21% protein bound. In veterinary medicine, naltrexone is used to reverse the potent opioids used for immobilization of wildlife. The longer duration of action of naltrexone reduces the risk of renarcotization following reversal. Naltrexone has also been used intranasally to successfully reverse the effects of carfentanil (Shury et al., 2010).

Methylnaltrexone is a quarternary derivative of naltrexone. The addition of the methyl group increases polarity and lowers lipid solubility. Methylnaltrexone functions as a peripherally acting µ-opioid receptor antagonist that does not cross the blood–brain barrier, and therefore should not reverse centrally mediated analgesia. Methylnaltrexone has been investigated in horses for treatment of opioid-induced ileus (Boscan et al., 2006b). It has an elimination half-life of ~47 minutes at a dose of 1 mg/kg and, when given alone, no promotility effects on the GIT were observed. An IV dose of methylnaltrexone (0.75 mg/kg) decreased the effects of morphine (0.5 mg/kg IV) on gut motility (Boscan et al., 2006b).

Reversal of µ-Opioid Agonists with Agonist–Antagonists or Partial Agonists

The antagonist actions of agonist–antagonists, such as butorphanol, can be used to partially reverse the effects of pure µ-opioid agonists, while still providing some analgesia through κ-opioid receptors (Dyson et al., 1990; MacCrackin et al., 1994). Butorphanol has affinity for the µ-opioid receptor, but with no intrinsic activity, while it has high affinity and moderate intrinsic activity at κ-opioid receptors. It appears to have a "ceiling" effect with respect to respiratory depression, as high doses do not cause profound respiratory depression, unlike pure µ-opioid receptor agonists (Nagashima et al., 1976). The author has observed dysphoria unrelated to pain immediately after reversal of pure µ-opioid agonists with rapid administration of butorphanol, which is probably due to κ-opioid receptor stimulation (MacCrackin et al., 1994). The incidence appears much reduced when butorphanol (0.02–0.4 mg/kg IV) is administered over at least 60 seconds, and titrated to achieve the desired effect. Small volumes may be diluted prior to administration.

The interaction of buprenorphine with concurrently administered pure µ-opioid agonists is less well defined. One report indicates that premedication with buprenorphine increases the required sufentanil dose during surgery in dogs (Goyenechea Jaramillo et al., 2006). This is countered by a laboratory study indicating that buprenorphine does not affect the antinociceptive effects of drugs such as morphine, hydromorphone, and fentanyl, except when buprenorphine is given at higher dosages than are used clinically (Kögel et al., 2005). Doses of buprenorphine greater than those used clinically have been employed in monkeys to study receptor dissociation kinetics of pure µ-opioid agonists, such as alfentanil, by irreversibly and partially blocking µ-opioid receptors (Walker et al., 1995). Buprenorphine's slow dissociation–association receptor kinetics and lower intrinsic activity at the µ-opioid receptor accounted for reversal of morphine- and alfentanil-induced antinociception. Buprenorphine is considered to be pseudo-irreversible (noncompetitive antagonist), and is not easily displaced by increasing doses of a pure µ-opioid agonist. Other studies have reported that buprenorphine can enhance the antinociceptive effects of morphine, but this can depend on intensity of the stimulus and dosages used (Morgan et al., 1999). The different observed effects when buprenorphine is combined with drugs such as tramadol may be due to the complicated nature of these drug interactions. Butorphanol has been mixed with buprenorphine on the assumption that butorphanol will have a rapid onset of action, and buprenorphine will provide long-term analgesia. This theory was tested in cats using thermal nociception threshold assessment, and the combination was not found to be different from the use of buprenorphine alone (Johnson et al., 2007). If buprenorphine is to be reversed using naloxone, it is recommended that naloxone be given as a continuous infusion to cover the slow receptor kinetics of buprenorphine (Yassan et al., 2007).

OPIOIDS FOR ENTERAL ABSORPTION

Codeine

In humans, codeine is metabolized by the liver enzyme system CYP2D6 into many metabolites, including M6G and codeine-6-glucuronide. In addition to codeine, the metabolites M6G and codeine-6-glucuronide provide effective analgesia in humans, but in dogs the bioavailability of codeine after oral administration, and concentration of morphine product, is low. In a dental pulp stimulation model in dogs, the subcutaneous administration of codeine resulted in short-lived analgesia, even with increased dosage (Skingle & Tyers, 1980). Few studies have examined the utility of oral codeine in dogs. One study found that very little morphine was produced, and the bioavailability from orally administered codeine was 6–7%, which was considered an overestimate because of cross-reactivity error (Findlay et al., 1979). A later study examined the uptake and metabolism of a codeine (2 mg/kg) and acetaminophen combination after oral administration to Greyhounds (KuKanich, 2009). Bioavailability of oral codeine was 4% and peak plasma concentration occurred just under an hour after administration, but with rapid elimination. Most of the absorbed codeine was metabolized to codeine-6-glucuronide. The concentration of morphine was below the limits of quantification for the test used, and this may be due to the rapid hepatic conversion of morphine to glucuronides (KuKanich, 2009). Most opioids undergo high hepatic clearance in dogs and efficient first pass effects; therefore, oral bioavailability is often poor. The bioavailability of morphine (KuKanich et al., 2005a), methadone (KuKanich et al., 2005b), and oxycodone (Weinstein & Gaylord, 1979) are similar to that of codeine. It is unlikely that codeine-6-glucuronide is an effective analgesic in dogs, because the polar characteristics of the molecule make entry into the central nervous system difficult (KuKanich, 2009). Clinical use of codeine in cats has not been reported.

Morphine and Hydromorphone Slow Release

Slow-release oral formulations are often used to provide analgesia in humans for up to 12 hours. They are designed with controlled-release melt extrusion technology that encases the drug in granules. The coating of the granules slowly dissolves in the gut, releasing the enclosed drug. Cationic exchange resin technology is also used to bind the drug. The resin releases the drug as ion exchange occurs within the gut.

Slow-release hydromorphone contained within liposomes has been investigated as a subcutaneous injection in dogs, but there are currently no clinical studies investigating the use of slow-release or immediate-release oral formulations in dogs or cats. It is possible that slow-release formulations may not be effective in dogs due to rapid biotransformation of absorbed drug.

Preliminary studies have demonstrated that slow-release morphine (64 mg/kg) and hydromorphone (16 mg/kg) increase thermal nociception threshold in rats with few side effects apart from mild sedation (Leach et al., 2010). Rats had an increase in nociceptive threshold 1 hour after administration of hydromorphone, the threshold peaked at 3 hours and the effect was gone at 5 hours. Slow-release morphine produced antinociceptive effects for up to 11 hours after administration. To obtain the correct dosage of hydromorphone, the capsule was broken and the granules administered

to the rats. The authors postulate that damage to the granule coating may have been responsible for differences between hydromorphone and morphine (Leach et al., 2010).

Hydrocodone

Dihydrocodeinone (hydrocodone) is an analog of codeine and has 0.6 times the potency of morphine, and is mainly used as an antitussive in humans (Cone et al., 1978). There are few studies examining the effects of hydrocodone in dogs. A dose of 10 mg/kg subcutaneously was given to two dogs in order to study the metabolic pathway (Cone et al., 1978). Most metabolites have greater analgesic properties than the parent compound, and hydrocodone can be metabolized through O-demethylation to the more potent, hydromorphone (Cone et al., 1978). The production of hydromorphone in dogs is slightly greater than in humans, but not as great as in rabbits (Cone et al., 1978). Rapid metabolism of hydromorphone through the liver may, however, limit the effectiveness of hydrocodone in the clinical setting.

BUCCAL ABSORPTION OF OPIOIDS

Fentanyl and Sufentanil

Buccal absorption avoids the hepatic first pass effect and is ideal for drugs that are highly lipophilic and tasteless. Fentanyl lollipops have been used for some time to sedate young children prior to anesthesia (Zimmer & Ashburn, 2001). The onset of effects is usually about 20 minutes. Absorption of fentanyl across the buccal mucosa increases as the saliva pH increases, due to changes in drug ionization (Streisand et al., 1995). Sublingual fentanyl tablets are under investigation for breakthrough pain in humans. Effervescence from the tablets causes changes in buccal pH, which facilitates absorption (Cranwell-Bruce, 2007). The effects of fentanyl (50 μg/kg) in a carboxymethylcellulose gel applied to the buccal mucosa (pH 7) were investigated in dogs. Serum concentrations were found to be above 0.95 ng/mL at 5 minutes after application, and remained above this concentration for 236 ± 87 (mean ± SD) minutes, with a mean (± SD) bioavailability of 29 ± 10% (Little et al., 2008).

A device allowing a 2 day supply of sublingual sufentanil is under investigation in humans, but requires patient cooperation, therefore, its use may be limited in veterinary medicine (Heitz et al., 2009).

Buprenorphine

Enterally administered buprenorphine has a bioavailability of only 3–6% in dogs due to a rapid hepatic first pass effect (Garrett & Chandran, 1990). Buprenorphine is, however, a highly lipophilic drug and is a good candidate for absorption across mucosa. Sublingual sprays of buprenorphine (400 μg/100 μL in 30% ethanol) have been developed for use in humans, and show favorable absorption in dogs (McInnes et al., 2008). Bioavailability of buprenorphine after buccal application in dogs is 38 ± 12% for the commercial parenteral formulation at a dose of 20 μg/kg, and 47 ± 16% for a dose of 120 μg/kg (Abbo et al., 2008). Peak plasma concentration occurred at 42 ± 12 minutes and lasted for 8.0 ± 2.5 hours for the 20 μg/kg dose. Peak plasma concentration occurred at 30 ± 18 minutes and lasted for 20.0 ± 0 hours with a dose of 120 μg/kg (Abbo et al., 2008). Pharmacokinetics of buprenorphine (50 μg/kg) in a sodium carboxymethylcellulose gel formulation applied to the buccal mucosa of dogs was similar to buprenorphine (15 μg/kg) given IV (Krotscheck et al., 2010). The buccal pH of the dogs was 7 and peak plasma concentration was achieved in 38 minutes with a bioavailability of 63%. Clearly, this formulation holds promise for use in dogs (Krotscheck et al., 2010).

Buccal mucosal bioavailability of the commercial parenteral formulation of buprenorphine (20 μg/kg) is 116.3% in cats (Robertson et al., 2005b). Cats tend to have a higher saliva pH (pH 9.0) than dogs, and this enables more buprenorphine to exist in a nonionized form. The thermal threshold in cats increased from 30 minutes to 6 hours after transmucosal application and was as effective as IV buprenorphine (20 μg/kg) (Robertson et al., 2005b). In horses, sublingual buprenorphine (6 μg/kg) has a bioavailability of $138 \pm 72\%$, with a peak concentration reached after 43 ± 18 minutes, and may prove useful for treating pain in horses (Messenger et al., 2011).

The intranasal route of two different formulations of buprenorphine has also been explored in rabbits and sheep. Buprenorphine was rapidly absorbed, with bioavailability between 70% and 89% in sheep and 46% to 53% in rabbits (Lindhardt et al., 2000; Lindhardt et al., 2001).

TRANSDERMAL ROUTE

Absorption of drugs through the skin offers a unique route of administration that provides more sustained drug plasma concentrations, and avoids losing drug to hepatic first pass effects (Heitz et al., 2009). The stratum corneum, however, is selective, and only some drugs will pass through. There are also species differences in how the skin affects drug movement. Technological advances to improve skin absorption include the use of liposomes or nanoparticles, eutectic mixtures similar to that used for lidocaine and prilocaine, and prodrugs, which are converted to active drug. Active absorption techniques using ionotophoresis (fentanyl IONSYS™, Ortho-McNeil Inc.), or ultrasound technology are also under investigation. These technologies will allow more opioid analgesics to be used as transdermal applications (Heitz et al., 2009). A summary of studies examining transdermal applications in various species can be found in Table 4.5.

Fentanyl

Transdermal fentanyl has been successfully used for many years to provide postoperative pain relief in cats (Franks et al., 2000; Glerum et al., 2001; Gellasch et al., 2002), dogs (Robinson et al., 1999), pigs (Harvey-Clarke et al., 2000), and horses (Thomasy et al., 2004). Transdermal fentanyl is discussed in more detail in Chapter 9.

A long-acting transdermal solution of fentanyl (Recuvyra®) is approved in Europe and in the United States for use in dogs in the perioperative period. A single application of 2.6 mg/kg in the dorsal scapular area provides appropriate fentanyl plasma concentrations as well as analgesia over a 4 day period (Friese et al., 2012; Linton et al., 2012).

Buprenorphine

A transdermal matrix patch system has been developed for use in humans, and has been tested in cats (Murrell et al., 2007) and dogs (Andaluz et al., 2009b; Pieper et al., 2011). Results of these studies indicate that buprenorphine may have utility for treatment of pain in animal species. See Chapter 9.

NEURAXIAL OPIOIDS

Summaries of studies performed in conscious cats and dogs are presented in Tables 4.6 and 4.7.

Opioids are often used in the epidural or subarachnoid space to manage acute or chronic pain. Unlike the use of local anesthetics at this site, opioids do not produce motor weakness, disruption of the sympathetic nervous system, or loss of proprioception, and provide dose-related analgesia.

Although opioids are absorbed by epidural fat and can be taken up by blood circulating through the space, epidurally administered opioids must diffuse across the dura mater in order to reach the biophase. Molecular weight and fat solubility of the drug are important determinants of passage across the dura mater. Lipophilic drugs, such as fentanyl or sufentanil, follow similar pharmacokinetics as IV administration. Lumbosacral epidural injection of fentanyl in cats produced antinociception on the hindlimbs, but not on the forelimbs, indicating no cranial migration (Duke et al., 1994). Lipophilic hydromorphone injected at the lumbosacral epidural site produced analgesic effects detectable on the thoracic dermatomes within 15 minutes (due to systemic uptake), which peaked again 2–3 hours later (spinal effects) demonstrating some cranial migration (Ambros et al., 2009). Less lipophilic drugs, such as morphine, cross the dura mater slowly, but have a longer analgesic effect (Tung & Yaksh, 1982; Popilskis et al., 1993; Castro et al., 2009). L-Methadone appears to have similar onset and duration as hydromorphone, and meperidine has a duration of about 2 hours at a dose of 5 mg/kg in cats (Tung & Yaksh, 1982). Administration of morphine into the epidural space is commonly chosen in veterinary medicine because of its lasting effects (up to 12 hours).

Fentanyl and sufentanil rapidly cross the dura mater, and peak cerebrospinal fluid (CSF) concentrations are achieved within 20 minutes. In contrast, morphine concentrations peak in 1–4 hours and only about 3% of the dose reaches the CSF. Vascular absorption of epidurally administered drugs can be extensive, especially with lipophilic drugs. Fentanyl blood concentrations peak in 5–10 minutes, and blood concentrations of sufentanil can peak sooner. Morphine blood concentrations peak after 10–15 minutes. This is similar to the pharmacokinetics after IM administration. In cats, buprenorphine blood concentrations peak 15 minutes after epidural administration, similar to using the IM or buccal routes (Duke-Novakovski et al., 2011).

Placement of the drug into the subarachnoid space allows more immediate action, as the dura mater is no longer a barrier. Vascular absorption of opioids after subarachnoid administration is clinically insignificant. Dose–response curves have been obtained for spinal sufentanil (3–30 μg/kg), fentanyl (10–100 μg/kg), and morphine (30–300 μg/kg) in cats, using thermal nociception tests (Yaksh et al., 1986). No behavioral changes were observed at these stated doses, although high doses of sufentanil (300 μg/kg) did cause excitement, convulsions, and death (Yaksh et al., 1986).

In humans, cervical morphine concentrations increase 1–5 hours after lumbar intrathecal injection, and drug movement is influenced by bulk flow of CSF. In dogs receiving 0.1 mg/kg morphine into the lumbosacral epidural space, morphine was detected in the cisternal CSF by 1–3 hours. Lower concentrations of morphine were detected in serum between 1–5 minutes of epidural injection reflecting systemic uptake (Valverde et al., 1992).

Table 4.5. Summary of studies examining the pharmacokinetics of transdermal opioids. Further details can be obtained from the references used (some data expressed with standard deviation where available)

Drug	Dose (µg/h)	Species	T_{max} after patch application (h)	Mean elimination half-life (h)	Comment	Reference used
Buprenorphine	70.0	Dog	~36.0		13.8 ± 2.8 kg bodyweight Patch applied for 108 h	Andaluz et al., 2009b
Buprenorphine	52.5	Dog	54.9		12.7 ± 1.8 kg bodyweight Nociception thresholds increased 36 h after patch application until removal Patch applied for 72 h	Pieper et al., 2011
Buprenorphine	35.0	Cat	~34.0–78.0	~10.0	5.1–7.4 kg bodyweight Plasma concentrations increased after patch removal after 72 h No change in nociception threshold	Murrell et al., 2007
Fentanyl	50.0	Dog	~24	3.6 ± 1.2	19.9 ± 3.4 kg bodyweight Patches applied for 72 h	Egger, 1998
Fentanyl	75.0	Dog	~24	3.4 ± 2.7	As above	Egger, 1998
Fentanyl	100.0	Dog	~24	2.5 ± 2.0	As above Became sedated	Egger, 1998
Fentanyl	88.0 mg/kg	Dog	2.3		21.1–38.9 kg bodyweight Pluronic lecithin organogel formulation Fentanyl plasma concentration low	Krotscheck et al., 2004
Fentanyl	25.0	Cat	44.3		2.2–5.6 kg bodyweight 35.9% absorbed	Lee, 2000
Fentanyl	25.0	Cat	14.0 ± 1.9	4.5 ± 4.3	2.3–4.3 kg bodyweight Patch applied for 72 h	Egger, 2003
Fentanyl	25.0	Cat	24.0		1.3–4.3 kg bodyweight Cats underwent surgery 24 h after patch application	Davidson, 2004
Fentanyl	~200.0	Horse	8.0 ± 2.0		464–585 kg bodyweight 94 ± 31% bioavailability Patches applied for 48 h	Maxwell, 2003
Fentanyl	~300.0	Horse	26 ± 13		327 ± 118 kg bodyweight Pain scores decreased	Thomasy et al., 2004
Fentanyl	~300.0	Horse	11.4 ± 2.9		459–503 kg bodyweight Patches applied for 72 h Used three 100 mg/h patches	Orsini et al., 2006
Fentanyl	100.0	Foal	14.3 ± 7.6		4–8 days old 56–74 kg bodyweight Patches applied for 72 h Plasma fentanyl returned to baseline 12 h after patch removal	Eberspächer, 2008
Fentanyl	2.0 µg/kg/h	Sheep	12.0	15.6	63 ± 8.2 kg bodyweight Patches removed after 72 h	Ahern et al., 2010
Morphine	1670.0/kg	Dog	2.5		21.1–38.9 kg bodyweight Pluronic lecithin organogel formulation Plasma morphine concentration low	Krotscheck et al., 2004

Table 4.6. Summary of studies examining different opioids injected into the lumbosacral epidural space of the conscious cat. See references for further details

Opioid	Dosage (mg/kg)	Onset	Duration	Nociceptive test and adverse effects	Reference
Meperidine	5.0	Immediate	1–2 h	Thermal	Tung & Yaksh, 1982
Meperidine	10.0	Immediate	2–4 h	Thermal; Vomiting observed	Tung & Yaksh, 1982
L-methadone	1.0	10–30 min	1–2 h	Thermal	Tung & Yaksh, 1982
Fentanyl	0.004	Not tested	20 min	Electrical	Duke et al., 1994
Hydromorphone	0.05	15 min	5 h	Thermal; Euphoria, mydriasis	Ambros et al., 2009
Morphine	0.1	Not assessed	10 h	Thermal	Pypendop et al., 2008b
Morphine	0.1	Not assessed	>12 h	Mechanical	Castro et al., 2009
Morphine	1.0	30–60 min	5–6 h	Thermal	Tung & Yaksh, 1982
Buprenorphine	0.0125	Not assessed	16 h	Thermal	Pypendop et al., 2008b
Buprenorphine	0.02	<15 min	24 h	Thermal	Steagall, 2009b
Tramadol	1.0	Not assessed	6–8 h	Mechanical	Castro et al., 2009

Sustained-release-encapsulated morphine has also been administered neuraxially and results are promising (Yaksh et al., 2000).

Adverse Effects of Neuraxial Opioids

Most adverse effects are experienced whether the drug is in the CSF or systemic circulation.

PRURITUS

Pruritus is commonly reported in humans, especially in women undergoing childbirth. Histamine release does not appear to be the mechanism, but it may be due to opioid receptor stimulation in the trigeminal nucleus. The sedative effects of antihistamines have been found to be effective in providing relief, but naloxone reverses the pruritus. The incidence of pruritus is low in veterinary patients.

URINARY RETENTION

There have been several published reports documenting urinary retention when using opioids in the epidural space of canines (Herperger, 1998; Kona-Boun et al., 2003). Urinary retention appears to be more common with this route of administration compared to systemic routes. Opioids attach to opioid receptors located in the sacral spinal cord, which promote inhibition of sacral parasympathetic nervous system outflow. This inhibition causes detrusor muscle relaxation, an increase in bladder capacity, and urinary retention. In humans, the effects of morphine can persist for 16 hours, but can be reversed with naloxone in some cases. Stimulants of detrusor muscle function such as bethanechol may be effective (Kona-Boun et al., 2003). Patients receiving epidural opioids should have their bladders expressed in the recovery phase and should be checked for active urination for at least 24 hours afterward (Herperger, 1998).

DEPRESSION OF VENTILATION

Considered an adverse effect of spinal opioid use in humans, respiratory depression does not appear to be a major problem in veterinary medicine, probably because most of our patients receive single-dose morphine rather than spinal infusions of fentanyl or sufentanil. Severe respiratory depression in humans affects 1% of the population receiving neuraxial opioids, similar to systemic routes of administration, and can be detected by pulse oximetry. Most cases involve use of lipophilic opioids such as sufentanil, and may be due to systemic uptake, as well as some cranial migration to the ventral medulla. In humans, some ventilatory depression has been detected 6–12 hours after epidural single-dose morphine, but

Table 4.7. Summary of studies examining different opioids injected into the epidural space of the conscious dog. See references for further details

Opioid	Dosage (mg/kg)	Onset	Duration (h)	Route	Nociceptive test Adverse effects	Reference
Morphine	0.1	Not assessed	~12	LS epidural	Observation of clinical signs and pain scoring	Pascoe & Dyson, 1993b
Morphine	0.1	Not assessed	>6	LS epidural	Observation of clinical signs and pain scoring	Day et al., 1995
Oxymorphone	0.1	Not assessed	10	Thoracic epidural	Observation of clinical signs and pain scoring	Popilskis et al., 1993
Oxymorphone	0.05	Not assessed	~7	LS epidural	Observation of clinical signs and pain scoring	Vesal et al., 1996

no cases have been reported to occur after 24 hours after the administration. Arterial carbon dioxide partial pressure was not increased in dogs given epidural oxymorphone for postoperative analgesia during the 8-hour study period (Vesal et al., 1996).

SEDATION

Sedation is most commonly observed after the use of lipophilic drugs such as sufentanil. If sedation is evident after the use of neuraxial opioids, the patient should also be checked for ventilatory depression. Cats can appear euphoric within 15 minutes following lumbosacral epidural injection of buprenorphine or hydromorphone and this is thought to be due to systemic uptake of these lipophilic opioids (Ambros et al., 2009; Steagall et al., 2009b).

CENTRAL NERVOUS SYSTEM EXCITATION

Tonic skeletal muscle rigidity is an adverse effect of high doses of systemic opioids, and has also been observed in a dog given spinal preservative-free morphine (Kona-Boun et al., 2003). In this case, spasms became evident 90 minutes after spinal injection and persisted throughout the procedure. The dog was successfully treated with pentobarbital following recovery from isoflurane anesthesia. Cranial migration of the opioid and inhibition of glycine or GABA mediated inhibition in the brainstem or basal ganglia are the likely mechanism. Because nonopioid receptor mechanisms are involved, treatment with naloxone is often ineffective.

SPINAL CORD DAMAGE

Toxic preservatives in preparations not licensed for epidural or spinal use have been cited as the cause of motor or sensory dysfunction, myoclonic spasms, paresis, and paralysis. Low concentrations of chlorbutanol, sodium EDTA, sodium bisulfite, and metabisulfite appear neurologically safe in the epidural space, although may cause problems in the subarachnoid space (Kona-Boun et al., 2003). Preservative-free butorphanol given spinally to sheep caused muscle rigidity, irreversible paralysis (375 μg/kg), muscle weakness (75 μg/kg), and one death from respiratory depression, but these doses caused no problems when administered into the epidural space (Rawal et al., 1991). Large doses of sufentanil (7.5 μg/kg) also caused histopathological changes such as suppurative meningitis, but were less severe than those caused by butorphanol (Rawal et al., 1991).

SUMMARY

Recent pharmacokinetic/pharmacodynamic studies produce useful results, which can guide dosing regimens in clinical settings. For example, it should be emphasized that dogs rapidly metabolize opioids, and therefore currently used dosing regimens and routes of administration may not be adequate for pain control. Cats and horses should be able to receive opioids, if side effects can be anticipated and treated.

New and innovative technologies allow the use of alternative routes of administration for opioids, so pain control can be maintained for longer periods of time, without the necessity of prescribing controlled drugs to owners. On another note, the much longer-term effects of opioids in domestic animals have not been explored and may become important in the future as we develop treatment plans for chronic pain in cats and dogs.

REFERENCES

Abbo, L.A., Ko, J.C.H., Maxwell, L.K., et al. (2008) Pharmacokinetics of buprenorphine following intravenous and oral transmucosal administration in dogs. *Veterinary Therapeutics*, 9, 83–93.

Ahern, B.J., Soma, L.R., Rudy, J.A., Uboh, C.E., & Schaer, T.E. (2010) Pharmacokinetics of fentanyl administered transdermally and intravenously in sheep. *American Journal of Veterinary Research*, 71, 1127–1132.

Ambros, B., Steagall, P.V.M., Mantovani, F., Gilbert, P., & Duke-Novakovski, T. (2009) Antinociceptive effects of epidural administration of hydromorphone in conscious cats. *American Journal of Veterinary Research*, 70, 1187–1192.

Andaluz, A., Moll, X., Abellán, R., et al. (2009a) Pharmacokinetics of buprenorphine after intravenous administration of clinical doses to dogs. *The Veterinary Journal*, 181, 299–304.

Andaluz, A., Moll, X., Ventura, R., Abellán, R., Fresno, L., & García, F. (2009b) Plasma buprenorphine concentrations after the application of 70 μg/hr transdermal patch in dogs. *Journal of Veterinary Pharmacology and Therapeutics*, 32, 503–505.

Andersen, M.S., Clark, L., Dyson, S.J., & Newton, J.R. (2006) Risk factors for colic in horses after general anaesthesia for MRI or nonabdominal surgery: absence of evidence of effect from perianaesthetic morphine. *Equine Veterinary Journal*, 38, 368–374.

Aragon, C.L., Read, M.R., Gaynor, J.S., Barnhart, M.D, Wilson, D., & Papich, M.G. (2008) Pharmacokinetics of an immediate and extended release oral morphine formulation utilising the spheroidal oral drug absorption system in dogs. *Journal of Veterinary Pharmacology and Therapeutics*, 32, 129–136.

Arguedes, M.G., Hines, M.T., Papich, M.G., Farnsworth, K.D, & Sellon, D.C. (2008) Pharmacokinetics of butorphanol and evaluation of physiologic and behavioral effects after intravenous and intramuscular administration to neonatal foals. *Journal of Veterinary Internal Medicine*, 22, 1417–1426.

Barnhart, M.D., Hubbell, J.A.E., Muir, W.W., Sams, R.A., & Bednarski, R.M. (2000) Pharmacokinetics, pharmacodynamics, and analgesic effects of morphine after rectal, intramuscular, and intravenous administration in dogs. *American Journal of Veterinary Research*, 61, 24–28.

Bartram, D.H., Diamond, M.J., Tute, A.S., Trafford, A.W., & Jones, R.S. (1994) Use of medetomidine and butorphanol for sedation in dogs. *Journal of Small Animal Practice*, 35, 495–498.

Benmansour, P. & Duke-Novakovski, T. (2013) Prolonged anesthesia using sevoflurane, remifentanil and dexmedetomidine in a horse. *Veterinary Anaesthesia and Analgesia*. doi:10.1111/vaa.12048.

Benthuysen, J.L., Smith, N.T., Sanford, T.J., Head, N., & Dec-Silver, H. (1986) Physiology of alfentanil-induced rigidity. *Anesthesiology*, 64, 440–446.

Blancquaert, J.P., Lefebvre, R.A., & Willems, J.L. (1986) Emetic and antiemetic effects of opioids in the dogs. *European Journal of Pharmacology*, 128, 143–150.

Boer, F. (2003) Drug handling by the lungs. *British Journal of Anaesthesia*, 91, 50–60.

Boscan, P., van Hoogmoed, L.M., Farver, T.B., & Snyder, J.R. (2006a) Evaluation of the effects of the opioid agonist morphine on gastrointestinal tract function in horses. *American Journal of Veterinary Research*, 67, 992–997.

Boscan, P., van Hoogmoed, L.M., Pypendop, B.H., Farver, T.B, & Snyder, J.R. (2006b) Pharmacokinetics of the opioid antagonist N-methylnaltrexone and evaluation of its effects on gastrointestinal tract function in horses treated or not treated with morphine. *American Journal of Veterinary Research*, 67, 998–1004.

Bossone, C.A. & Hannon, J.P. (1991) Metabolic actions of morphine in conscious chronically instrumented pigs. *American Journal of Physiology*, 260, R1051–R1057.

Brosnan, R.J., Pypendop, B.H., Siao, K.T., & Stanley, S.D. (2009) Effects of remifentanil on measures of anesthetic immobility and analgesia in cats. *American Journal of Veterinary Research*, 70, 1065–1071.

Cagnardi, P., Villa, R., Zonca, A., et al. (2011) Pharmacokinetics, intraoperative effect and postoperative analgesia of tramadol in cats. *Research in Veterinary Science*, 90, 503–509.

Campbell, V.L., Drobatz, K.J., & Perkowski, S.Z. (2003) Postoperative hypoxemia and hypercarbia in healthy dogs undergoing routine ovariohysterectomy or castration and receiving butorphanol or hydromorphone for analgesia. *Journal of the American Veterinary Medical Association*, 222, 330–336.

Carregaro, A.B., Teixeira Neto, F.J., Beier, S.L., & Luna, S.P. (2006) Cardiopulmonary effects of buprenorphine in horses. *American Journal of Veterinary Research*, 67, 1675–1680.

Carregaro, A.B., Luna, S.P.L., Mataqueiro, M.I., &.de Queiroz-Neto, A. (2007) Effects of buprenorphine on nociception and spontaneous locomotor activity in horses. *American Journal of Veterinary Research*, 68, 246–250.

Castro, D.S., Silva, M.F.A., Shih, A.C., Motta, P.P, Pires, M.V, & Scherer, P.O. (2009) Comparison between the analgesic effects of morphine and tramadol delivered epidurally in cats receiving a standardized noxious stimulation. *Journal of Feline Medicine and Surgery*, 11, 948–953.

Caulkett, N.A., Cribb, P.H., & Haigh, J.C. (2000) Comparative cardiopulmonary effects of carfentanil-xylazine and medetomidine-ketamine used for immobilization of mule deer and mule deer/white-tailed deer hybrids. *Canadian Journal of Veterinary Research*, 64, 64–68.

Cavanagh, R.L., Gylys, J.A., & Bierwagen, M.E. (1976) Antitussive properties of butorphanol. *Archives Internationales de Pharmacodynamie et de Therapie*, 220, 258–268.

Chiou, L.C., Liao, Y.Y., Fan, P.C., et al. (2007) Nociceptin/orphanin FQ peptide receptors: pharmacology and clinical applications. *Current Drug Targets*, 8, 117–135.

Chism, J.P. & Rickert, D.E. (1996) The pharmacokinetics and extrahepatic clearance of remifentanil, a short-acting opioid agonist, in male beagle dogs during constant rate infusions. *Drug Metabolism and Disposition*, 24, 34–40.

Clarke, K.W. & Paton, B.S. (1988) Combined use of detomidine with opiates in the horse. *Equine Veterinary Journal*, 20, 331–334.

Clark, L., Clutton, R.E., Blissitt, K.J., & Chase-Topping, M.E. (2005) Effects of peri-operative morphine administration during halothane anaesthesia in horses. *Veterinary Anaesthesia and Analgesia*, 32, 10–15.

Codd, E.E., Shank, R., Schupsky, J.J., & Raffa, R.B. (1995) Serotonin and norepinephrine uptake inhibiting activity of centrally acting analgesics: structural determinants and role in antinociception. *Journal of Pharmacology and Experimental Therapeutics*, 274, 1263–1270.

Combie, J.D., Nugent, T.E., & Tobin, T. (1983) Pharmacokinetics and protein binding of morphine in horses. *American Journal of Veterinary Research*, 44, 870–874.

Cone, E.J., Darwin, W.D., Gorodetzky, C.W., & Tan, T. (1978) Comparative metabolism of hydrocodone in man, rat, guinea-pig, rabbit and dog. *Drug Metabolism and Disposition*, 6, 488–493.

Conzemius, M.G., Brockman, D.J., King, L.G., & Perkowski, S.Z. (1994) Analgesia in dogs after intercostal thoracotomy: a clinical trial comparing intravenous buprenorphine and interpleural bupivacaine. *Veterinary Surgery*, 23, 291–298.

Correa, Mdo,A., Aguiar, A.J., Teixeira Neto, F.J., Mendes Gda, M., Steagall, P.V.,& Lima, A.F. (2007) Effects of remifentanil infusion regimens on cardiovascular function and responses to noxious stimulation in propofol-anesthetized cats. *American Journal of Veterinary Research*, 68, 932–940.

Cox, S., Villarino, N., & Doherty, T. (2010) Determination of oral tramadol pharmacokinetics in horses. *Research in Veterinary Science*, 89, 236–241.

Cranwell-Bruce, L. (2007) Update on pain management: new methods of opiate delivery. *MedSurg Nursing*, 16, 333–335.

Credie, R.G., Teixeira Neto, F.J., Ferreira, T.H., Aguiar, A.J., Restitutti, F.C., & Corrente, J.E. (2010) Effects of methadone on the minimum alveolar concentration of isoflurane in dogs. *Veterinary Anaesthesia and Analgesia*, 37, 240–249.

Dahan, A., Aarts, L., & Smith, T.W. (2010) Incidence, reversal, and prevention of opioid-induced respiratory depression. *Anesthesiology*, 112, 226–238.

Davis, J.L., Messenger, K.M., LaFevers, D.H. et al. (2012) Pharmacokinetics of intravenous and intramuscular buprenorphine in the horse. *Journal of Veterinary Pharmacology and Therapeutics*, 35, 52–58

Davidson, C.D., Pettifer, G.R., Henry, J.D. Jr. (2004) Plasma fentanyl concentrations and analgesic effects during full or partial exposure to transdermal fentanyl patches in cats. *Journal of the American Veterinary Medicine Association*, 224(5), 700–705.

Day, T.K., Pepper, W.T., Tobias, T.A., Flynn, M.F., & Clarke, K.M. (1995) Comparison of intra-articular and epidural morphine for analgesia following stifle arthrotomy in dogs. *Veterinary Surgery*, 24, 522–530.

Dhanjal, J.K., Wilson, D.V., Robinson, E., Tobin, T.T, & Dirikolu, L. (2009) Intravenous Tramadol: effects, nociceptive properties, and pharmacokinetics in horses. *Veterinary Anaesthesia and Analgesia*, 36, 581–590.

Dodman, N.H., Shuster, L., Court, M.H., & Dixon, R. (1987) Investigation into the use of narcotic antagonists in the treatment of a stereotypic behavior pattern (crib-biting) in the horse. *American Journal of Veterinary Research*, 48, 311–319.

Doherty, T.J. (2009) Postoperative ileus: pathogenesis and treatment. *Veterinary Clinics of North America: Equine Practice*, 25, 351–362.

Dohoo, S., Taskar, R.A.R., & Donald, A. (1994) Pharmacokinetics of parenteral and oral sustained-release morphine sulphate in dogs. *Journal of Veterinary Pharmacology and Therapeutics*, 17, 426–433.

Dohoo, S.E. & Taskar, R.A.R. (1997) Pharmacokinetics of oral morphine sulphate in dogs: a comparison of sustained release and conventional formulations. *Canadian Journal of Veterinary Research*, 61, 251–255.

Duke, T., Komulainen-Cox, A.M., Remedios, A.M., & Cribb, P.H. (1994) The analgesic effects of administering fentanyl or medetomidine in the epidural space of cats. *Veterinary Surgery*, 23, 143–148.

Duke-Novakovski, T., Clark, C., Ambros, B., Gilbert, P., & Steagall, P.V. (2011) Plasma concentrations of buprenorphine after epidural administration in conscious cats. *Research in Veterinary Science*, 90, 480–483.

Dyson, D.H., Doherty, T., Anderson, G.I., & McDonell, W.N. (1990) Reversal of oxymorphone sedation by naloxone, nalmefene, and butorphanol. *Veterinary Surgery*, 19, 398–403.

Dyson, D.H. & Atilola, M. (1992) A clinical comparison of oxymorphone-acepromazine and butorphanol-acepromazine in dogs. *Veterinary Surgery*, 21, 418–421.

Dyson, D.H. (2008) Analgesia and chemical restraint for the emergent veterinary patient. *Veterinary Clinics of North America. Small Animal Practice*, 38, 1329–1352.

Eberspächer, E., Stanley, S.D., Rezende, M., et al. (2008) Pharmacokinetics and tolerance of transdermal fentanyl administration in foals. *Veterinary Anaesthesia and Analgesia*, 35(3), 249–255.

Egan, T.D., Huizinga, B., Gupta, S.K., et al. (1998) Remifentanil pharmacokinetics in obese versus lean patients. *Anesthesiology*, 89, 562–573.

Egger, C.M., Duke, T., Archer, J., et al. (1998) Comparison of plasma fentanyl concentrations by using three transdermal fentanyl patch sizes in dogs. *Veterinary Surgery*, 27(2), 159–166.

Egger, C.M., Glerum, L.E., Allen, S.W., & Haag, M. (2003) Plasma fentanyl concentrations in awake cats and cats undergoing anesthesia and ovariohysterectomy using transdermal administration. *Veterinary Anaesthesia and Analgesia*, 30(4), 229–236.

Findlay, J.W., Jones, E.C., & Welch, R.M. (1979) Radioimmunoassay determination of the absolute oral bioavailabilities and O-demethylation of codeine and hydrocodone in the dog. *Drug Metabolism and Disposition*, 7, 310–314.

Franks, J.N., Boothe, H.W., Taylor, L., et al. (2000) Evaluation of transdermal fentanyl patches for analgesia in cats undergoing onychectomy. *Journal of the American Veterinary Medical Association*, 217, 1013–1020.

Frampton, J.E. (2010) Tapentadol immediate release: a review of its use in the treatment of moderate to severe acute pain. *Drugs*, 70, 1719–1743.

Friese, K.J., Newbound, G.C., Tudan, C., & Clark, T.P. (2012) Pharmacokinetics and the effect of application site on a novel, long-acting transdermal fentanyl solution in healthy laboratory Beagles. *Journal of Veterinary Pharmacology and Therapeutics*, 35(Suppl. 2), 27–33.

Garrett, E.R., Derendorf, H., & Mattha, A.G. (1985) Pharmacokinetics of morphine and its surrogates. VII: High-performance liquid chromatographic analyses and pharmacokinetics of methadone and its derived metabolites in dogs. *Journal of Pharmaceutical Sciences*, 74, 1203–1214.

Garrett, E.R. & Chandran, V.R. (1990) Pharmacokinetics of morphine and its surrogates: analyses and pharmacokinetics of buprenorphine in dogs. *Biopharmaceutics and Drug Disposition*, 11, 311–350.

Gassel, A.D., Tobias, K.M., Egger, C.M., & Rohrbach, B.W. (2005) Comparison of oral and subcutaneous administration of buprenorphine and meloxicam for preemptive analgesia in cats undergoing ovariohysterectomy. *Journal of the American Veterinary Medical Association*, 227, 1937–1944.

Gellasch, K.L., Kruse-Elliott, K.T., Osmond, C.S., Shih, A.N, & Bjorling, D.E. (2002) Comparison of transdermal administration of fentanyl versus intramuscular administration of butorphanol for analgesia after onychectomy in cats. *Journal of the American Veterinary Medical Association*, 220, 1020–1024.

George, A.V., Lu, J.J., Pisano, M.V., Metz, J., & Erickson, T.B. (2010) Carfentanil – an ultra potent opioid. *American Journal of Emergency Medicine*, 28, 530–532.

Giordano, T., Steagall, P.V.M., Ferreira, T.H., et al. (2010) Postoperative analgesic effects of intravenous, intramuscular, subcutaneous, or oral transmucosal buprenorphine administered to cats undergoing ovariohysterectomy. *Veterinary Anaesthesia and Analgesia*, 37, 357–366.

Giorgi, M., Soldani, G., Manera, C., Ferrarini, P.L., Sgorbini, M., & Saccomanni, G. (2007) Pharmacokinetics of Tramadol and its metabolites, M1, M2, and M5 in horses following intravenous, immediate release (fasted/fed) and sustained release single dose administration. *Journal of Equine Veterinary Science*, 27, 481–488.

Giorgi, M., Del Carlo, S., Saccomanni, G., Łebkowska-Wieruszewska, B., & Kowalski, C.J. (2009) Pharmacokinetic and urine profile of tramadol and its major metabolites following oral immediate release capsules administration in dogs. *Veterinary Research and Communication*, 33, 875–885.

Giorgi, M., Meizler, A., & Mills, P.C. (2012) Pharmacokinetics of the novel atypical opioid tapentadol following oral and intravenous administration in dogs. *Veterinary Journal*, 194(3), 309–313.

Glerum, L.E., Egger, C.M., Allen, S.W., & Haag, M. (2001) Analgesic effect of the transdermal fentanyl patch during and after feline ovariohysterectomy. *Veterinary Surgery*, 30, 351–358.

Golder, F.J., Wilson, J., Larenza, P.M., & Fink, O.T. (2010) Suspected acute meperidine toxicity in a dog. *Veterinary Anaesthesia and Analgesia*, 37, 471–477.

Goyenechea Jaramillo, L.A., Murrell, J.C., & Hellebrekers, L.J. (2006) Investigation of the interaction between buprenorphine and sufentanil during anaesthesia for ovariectomy in dogs. *Veterinary Anaesthesia and Analgesia*, 33, 399–407.

Graves, G.M., Becht, J.L., & Rawlings, C.A. (1989) Metoclopramide reversal of decreased gastrointestinal myoelectric and contractile activity in a model of canine postoperative ileus. *Veterinary Surgery*, 18, 27–33.

Guedes, A.G.P., Papich, M.G., Rude, E.P., & Rider, M.A. (2007a) Pharmacological and physiological effects of two intravenous infusion rates of morphine in conscious dogs. *Journal of Veterinary Pharmacology and Therapeutics*, 30, 224–233.

Guedes, A.G.P., Papich, M.G., Rude, E.P., & Rider, M.A. (2007b) Comparison of plasma histamine levels after intravenous administration of hydromorphone or morphine in dogs. *Journal of Veterinary Pharmacology and Therapeutics*, 30, 516–522.

Harvey-Clarke, C.J., Gilespie, K., & Riggs, K.W. (2000) Transdermal fentanyl compared with parenteral buprenorphine in post-surgical pain in swine: a case study. *Laboratory Animals*, 34, 386–398.

Haskins, S.C., Copland, V.S., & Patz, J.D. (1991) The cardiopulmonary effects of oxymorphone in hypovolemic dogs. *Journal of Veterinary Emergency and Critical Care*, 1, 32–38.

Haymarle, A., Fahlman, Å., & Walzer, C. (2010) Human exposures to immobilising agents: results of an online survey. *Veterinary Record*, 167, 327–332.

Heitz, J.W., Witkowski, T.A., & Viscusi, E.R. (2009) New and emerging analgesics and analgesic technologies for acute pain management. *Current Opinion in Anaesthesiology*, 22, 608–617.

Herperger, L.J. (1998) Postoperative urinary retention in a dog following morphine with bupivacaine epidural anaesthesia. *Canadian Veterinary Journal*, 39, 650–652.

Hoke, F.J., Cunningham, F., James, M.K., Muir, K.T., & Hoffman, W.E. (1997) Comparative pharmacokinetics and pharmacodynamics of remifentanil, its principal metabolite (GR90291) and alfentanil in dogs. *Journal of Pharmacology and Experimental Therapeutics*, 281, 226–232.

Houghton, K.J., Rech, R.H., Sawyer, D.C., et al. (1991) Dose-response of intravenous butorphanol to increase visceral nociceptive threshold in dogs. *Proceedings of the Society for Experimental Biology and Medicine*, 197, 290–296.

Huang, P., Kehner, G.B., Cowan. A., & Liu-Chen, L.Y. (2001) Comparison of pharmacological activities of buprenorphine and norbuprenorphine: Norbuprenorphine is a potent opioid agonist. *Journal of Pharmacology and Experimental Therapeutics*, 297, 688–695.

Hughes, M.A., Glass, P.S., & Jacobs, J.R. (1992) Context-sensitive half-time in multicompartment pharmacokinetic models for intravenous anesthetic drugs. *Anesthesiology*, 76, 334–341.

Ide, S., Minami, M., Ishihara, K., et al. (2008) Abolished thermal and mechanical antinociception but retained visceral chemical antinociception induced by butorphanol in mu-opioid receptor knockout mice. *Neuropharmacology*, 54, 1182–1188.

Ingvast-Larsson, C., Holgersson, A., Bondesson, U., Lagerstedt, AS, & Olsson, K. (2010) Clinical pharmacology of methadone in dogs. *Veterinary Anaesthesia and Analgesia*, 37, 48–56.

Jacobson, J.D., McGrath, C.J., & Smith, E.P. (1994) Cardiorespiratory effects of four opioid-tranquilizer combinations in dogs. *Veterinary Surgery*, 23, 299–306.

Java, M.A., Drobatz, K.J., Gilley, R.S., Long, S.N, Kushner, L.I, & King, L.G. (2009) Incidence of and risk factors for postoperative pneumonia in dogs anesthetized for diagnosis or treatment of intervertebral disk disease. *Journal of the American Veterinary Medical Association*, 235, 281–287.

Jochle, W., Moore, J.N., Brown, J., et al. (1989) Comparison of detomidine, butorphanol, flunixin meglumine and xylazine in clinical cases of equine colic. *Equine Veterinary Journal: Supplement*, 7, 111–116.

Johnson, J.A., Robertson, S.A., & Pypendop, B.H. (2007) Antinociceptive effects of butorphanol, buprenorphine, or both, administered intramuscularly in cats. *American Journal of Veterinary Research*, 68, 699–703.

Kalpravidh, M., Lumb, W.V., Wright, M., & Heath, R.B. (1984a) Effects of butorphanol, flunixin, levorphanol, morphine, and xylazine in ponies. *American Journal of Veterinary Research*, 45, 217–223.

Kalpravidh, M., Lumb, W.V., Wright, M.,& Heath, R.B. (1984b) Analgesic effects of butorphanol in horses: dose-response studies. *American Journal of Veterinary Research*, 45, 211–216.

Kalthum, W. & Waterman, A.E. (1988) The pharmacokinetics of intravenous pethidine HCl in dogs: normal and surgical cases. *Journal of the Association of Veterinary Anaesthetists*, 15, 39–54.

Kalthum, W. & Waterman, A.E. (1990) The renal excretion of pethidine administered postoperatively to male dogs. *British Veterinary Journal*, 146, 243–248.

Kögel, B., Cristoph, T., Strassburger, W., & Friderichs, E. (2005) Interaction of mu-opioid receptor agonists and antagonists with the analgesic effect of buprenorphine in mice. *European Journal of Pain*, 9, 599–611.

Kona-Boun, J-J., Pibarot, P., & Quesnel, A. (2003) Myoclonus and urinary retention following subarachnoid morphine injection in a dog. *Veterinary Anaesthesia and Analgesia*, 30, 257–264.

Kramer, W.G., Gross, D.R., & Medlock, C. (1985) Contribution of the lung to total body clearance of meperidine in the dog. *Journal of Pharmaceutical Science*, 74, 569–571.

Kreeger, T.J., Plotka, E.D., & Seal, U.S. (1987) Immobilization of white-tailed deer by etorphine and xylazine and its antagonism by nalmefene and yohimbine. *Journal of Wildlife Diseases*, 23, 619–624.

Krotscheck, U., Boothe, D.M., & Boothe, H.W. (2004) Evaluation of transdermal morphine and fentanyl pluronic lecithin organogel administration in dogs. *Veterinary Therapeutics*, 5, 202–211.

Krotscheck, U., Boothe, D.M., & Little, A.A. (2008) Pharmacokinetics of buprenorphine following intravenous administration in dogs. *American Journal of Veterinary Research*, 69, 722–727.

Krotscheck, U., Boothe, D.M., & Little, A.A., et al. (2010) Pharmacokinetics of buprenorphine in a sodium carboxymethylcellulose gel after buccal transmucosal administration in dogs. *Veterinary Therapeutics*, 11, E1–E8.

KuKanich, B. & Papich, M.G. (2004) Pharmacokinetics of tramadol and the metabolite *O*-desmethyltramadol in dogs. *Journal of Veterinary Pharmacology and Therapeutics*, 27, 239–246.

KuKanich, B., Lascelles, B.D.X., & Papich, M.G. (2005a) Pharmacokinetics of morphine and plasma concentrations of morphine-6-glucuronide following morphine administration to dogs. *Journal of Veterinary Pharmacology and Therapeutics*, 28, 371–376.

KuKanich, B., Lascelles, B.D.X., Aman, A.M., Mealey, K.L, & Papich, M.G. (2005b) The effects of inhibiting cytochrome P450 3A, p-glycoprotein, and gastric acid secretion on the oral bioavailability of methadone in dogs. *Journal of Veterinary Pharmacology and Therapeutics*, 28, 461–466.

KuKanich, B., Hogan, B.K., Krugner-Higby, L.A. & Smith, L.J. (2008a) Pharmacokinetics of hydromorphone in healthy dogs. *Veterinary Anaesthesia and Analgesia*, 35, 256–264.

KuKanich, B., Schmidt, B.K., Krugner-Higby, L.A, Toerber, S., & Smith, L.J. (2008b) Pharmacokinetics and behavioral effects of oxymorphone after intravenous and subcutaneous administration to healthy dogs. *Journal of Veterinary Pharmacology and Therapeutics*, 31, 580–583.

KuKanich, B. & Borum, S.L. (2008c) The disposition and behavioral effects of methadone in Greyhounds. *Veterinary Anaesthesia and Analgesia*, 35, 242–248.

KuKanich, B. (2009) Pharmacokinetics of acetaminophen, codeine, and the codeine metabolites morphine and codein-6-glucuronide in healthy Greyhound dogs. *Journal of Veterinary Pharmacology and Therapeutics*, 13, 15–21.

Lascelles, B.D.X. & Robertson, S.A. (2004a) Antinociceptive effects of hydromorphone, butorphanol, or the combination in cats. *Journal of Veterinary Internal Medicine*, 18, 190–195.

Lascelles, B.D.X. & Robertson, S.A. (2004b) Use of thermal threshold response to evaluate the antinociceptive effects of butorphanol in cats. *American Journal of Veterinary Research*, 65, 1085–1089.

Latasch, L. & Freye, E. (2002) Sufentanil-related respiratory depression and antinociception in dogs. *Arzneimittel-Forschung*, 52, 870–876.

Leach, M.C., Bailey, H.E., Dickinson, A.L., Roughan, J.V, & Flecknell, P.A. (2010) A preliminary investigation into the practicality of use and duration of action of slow-release preparations of morphine and hydromorphone in laboratory rats. *Laboratory Animals*, 44, 59–65.

Lee, D.D., Papich, M.G., Hardie, E.M. (2000) Comparison of pharmacokinetics of fentanyl after intravenous and transdermal administration in cats. *American Journal of Veterinary Research*, 61(6), 672–677.

Linardi, R.L., Stokes, A.M., Barker, S.A., Short, C., Hosgood, G., & Natalini, C.C. (2009) Pharmacokinetics of the injectable formulation of methadone hydrochloride administered orally in horses. *Journal of Veterinary Pharmacology and Therapeutics*, 32, 492–497.

Lindegaard, C., Frost, A.B., Thomsen, M.H., Larsen, C., Hansen, S.H., & Andersen, P.H. (2010) Pharmacokinetics of intra-articular morphine in horses with lipopolysaccharide-induced synovitis. *Veterinary Anaesthesia and Analgesia*, 37, 186–195.

Lindhardt, K., Ravn, C., Gizurarson, S., et al. (2000) Intranasal absorption of buprenorphine – in vivo bioavailability in study in sheep. *International Journal of Pharmaceutics*, 205, 159–163.

Lindhardt, K., Baggar, M., Andreasen, K.H., & Bechgaard, E. (2001) Intranasal bioavailability of buprenorphine in rabbit correlated to sheep and man. *International Journal of Pharmaceutics*, 217, 121–126.

Little, A.A., Krotscheck, U., Boothe, D.M., & Erb, H.N. (2008) Pharmacokinetics of buccal mucosal administration of fentanyl in a carboxymethylcellulose gel compared with IV administration in dogs. *Veterinary Therapeutics*, 9, 201–211.

Linton, D.D., Wilson, M.G., Newbound, G.C., Freise, K.J., & Clark, T.P. (2012) The effectiveness of a long-acting transdermal fentanyl solution compared to buprenorphine for the control of postoperative pain in dogs in a randomized, multicentered clinical study. *Journal of Veterinary Pharmacology and Therapeutics*, 35(Suppl. 2), 53–64.

Love, E.J., Lane, G.J., & Murison, P.J. (2006) Morphine administration in horses anaesthetized for upper respiratory tract surgery. *Veterinary Anaesthesia and Analgesia*, 33, 179–188.

Love, E.J., Taylor, P.M., Clark, C., Whay, H.R., & Murrell, J. (2009) Analgesic of butorphanol in ponies following castration. *Equine Veterinary Journal*, 41, 552–556.

Lust, E.B., Barthold, C., Maleskar, M.A., & Wichman, T.O. (2011) Human health hazards of veterinary medications: information for emergency departments. *Journal of Emergency Medicine*, 40, 198–207.

Lutfy, K. & Cowan, A. (2004) Buprenorphine: a unique drug with complex pharmacology. *Current Neuropharmacology*, 2, 395–402.

MacCrackin, M.A., Harvey, R.C., Sackman, J.E., McLean, R.A., & Paddleford, R.R. (1994) Butorphanol tartrate for partial reversal of oxymorphone-induced postoperative respiratory depression in the dog. *Veterinary Surgery*, 23, 67–74.

Martin, T.L., Woodall, K.L., & MacLellan, B.A. (2006) Fentanyl-related deaths in Ontario, Canada: toxicological findings and circumstances of death in 112 cases (2002–2004). *Journal of Analytical Toxicology*, 30, 603–610.

Martinez, E.A., Hartsfield, S.M., Melendez, L.D., Matthews, N.S., & Slater, M.R. (1997) Cardiovascular effects of buprenorphine in anesthetized dogs. *American Journal of Veterinary Research*, 58, 1280–1284.

Martins, H.S., Silva, R.V., Bugano, D., et al. (2008) Should naloxone be prescribed in the ED management of patients with cardiac arrest? A case report and review of literature. *American Journal of Emergency Medicine*, 26, 113e5–113e8.

Mather, L.E. (1983) Clinical pharmacokinetics of fentanyl and its newer derivatives. *Clinical Pharmacokinetics*, 8, 422–446.

Mastrocinque, S. & Fantoni, D.T. (2003) A comparison of preoperative tramadol and morphine for control of early postoperative pain in canine ovariohysterectomy. *Veterinary Anaesthesia and Analgesia*, 30, 220–228.

Maxwell, L.K., Thomasy, S.M., Slovis, N., et al. (2003) Pharmacokinetics of fentanyl following intravenous and transdermal administration in horses. *Equine Veterinary Journal*, 35(5), 484–490.

McInnes, F., Clear, N., James, G., Stevens, H.N, Vivanco, U, & Humphrey, M. (2008) Evaluation of the clearance of a sublingual buprenorphine spray in the Beagle dog using gamma scintigraphy. *Pharmaceutical Research*, 25, 869–874.

McMillan, C.J., Livingston, A., Clark, C.R., et al. (2008) Pharmacokinetics of intravenous tramadol in dogs. *Canadian Journal of Veterinary Research*, 72, 325–331.

Mégabane, B., Hreiche, R., Pirnay, S., Marie, N., & Baud, F.J. (2006) Does high-dose buprenorphine cause respiratory depression?: possible mechanisms and therapeutic consequences. *Toxicological Reviews*, 25, 79–85.

Mendes, G.M. & Selmi, A.L. (2003) Use of a combination of propofol and fentanyl, alfentanil, or sufentanil for total intravenous anesthesia in cats. *Journal of the American Veterinary Medical Association*, 223(11), 1608–1613.

Messenger, K.M., Davis, J.L., Barlow, B.M., LaFevers, D.H., & Posner, L.P. (2011) Intravenous and sublingual buprenorphine in horses: pharmacokinetics and influence of sampling site. *Veterinary Anaesthesia and Analgesia*, 38(4), 374–384.

Michelsen, L.G., Salmenperä, M., Hug, C.C. Jr., Szlam, F., & Vander-Meer, D. (1996) Anesthetic potency of remifentanil in dogs. *Anesthesiology*, 84, 865–872.

Mohta, M., Kumari, N., Tyagi, A., Sethi, A.K., Agarwal, D., & Singh, M. (2009) Tramadol for prevention of postanaesthetic shivering: a randomised double-blind comparison with pethidine. *Anaesthesia*, 64, 141–146.

Monteiro, E.R., Figueroa, C.D.N., Choma, J.C., Campagnol, D., & Bettini, C.M. (2008) Effects of methadone, alone or in combination with acepromazine or xylazine, on sedation and physiologic values in dogs. *Veterinary Anaesthesia and Analgesia*, 35, 519–527.

Monteiro, E.R., Rodriguez Junior, A., Quirilos, H.M., Campagnol, D., & Quitzan, J.G. (2009) Comparative study on the sedative effects of morphine, methadone, butorphanol or tramadol, in combination with acepromazine, in dogs. *Veterinary Anaesthesia and Analgesia*, 36, 25–33.

Morgan, D., Cook, C.D., Smith, M.A., & Picker, M.J. (1999) An examination of the interactions between the antinociceptive effects of morphine and various mu-opioids: the role of intrinsic efficacy and stimulus intensity. *Anesthesia Analgesia*, 88, 407–413.

Muir, W.W. & Robertson, J.T. (1985) Visceral analgesia: effects of xylazine, butorphanol, meperidine, and pentazocine in horses. *American Journal of Veterinary Research*, 46, 2081–2084.

Murrell, J.C., Robertson, S.A., Taylor, P.M., McCown, J.L., Bloomfield, M., & Sear, J.W. (2007) Use of a transdermal matrix patch of buprenorphine in cats: preliminary pharmacokinetic and pharmacodynamic data. *Veterinary Record*, 160, 578–583.

Murthy, S.S., Mathur, C., Kvalo, L.T., Lessor, R.A., & Wilhelm, J.A. (1996) Disposition of the opioid antagonist, nalmefene, in rat and dog. *Xenobiotica*, 26, 779–792.

Nagashima, H., Karamanian, A., Malovany, R., et al. (1976) Respiratory and circulatory effects of intravenous butorphanol and morphine. *Clinical Pharmacology and Therapeutics*, 19, 738–745.

Nakasuji, M., Nakamuru, M, Imanaka, N., Tanaka, M., Nomura, M., & Suh, S.H. (2010) Intraoperative high-dose remifentanil increases post-anaesthetic shivering. *British Journal of Anaesthesia*, 105, 162–167.

Niedfeldt, R.L. & Robertson, S.A. (2006) Postanesthetic hyperthermia in cats: a retrospective comparison between hydromorphone and buprenorphine. *Veterinary Anaesthesia and Analgesia*, 33, 381–389.

Nilsfors, L., Kvart, C., Kallings, P., Carlsten, J., & Bondesson, U. (1988) Cardiorespiratory and sedative effects of a combination of acepromazine, xylazine and methadone in the horse. *Equine Veterinary Journal*, 20, 364–367.

Nolan, A.M. & Hall, L.W. (1984) Combined use of sedatives and opiates in horses. *Veterinary Record*, 114, 63–67.

Nolan, A.M., Besley, W., Reid, J., & Gray, G. (1994) The effects of butorphanol on locomotor activity in ponies: a preliminary study. *Journal of Veterinary Pharmacology and Therapeutics*, 17, 323–326.

Odunayo, A., Dodam, J.R., Kerl, M.E., & DeClue, A.E. (2010) Immunomodulatory effects of opioids. *Journal of Veterinary Emergency and Critical Care*, 20, 376–385.

Orsini, J.A., Moate, P.J., Kuersten, K., Soma, L.R, & Boston, R.C. (2006) Pharmacokinetics of fentanyl delivered transdermally in healthy adult horses – variability among horses and its clinical applications. *Journal of Veterinary Pharmacology and Therapeutics*, 29, 539–546.

Pascoe, P.J., Black, W.D., Claxton, J.M., & Sansom, R.E. (1991) The pharmacokinetics and locomotor activity of alfentanil in the horse. *Journal of Veterinary Pharmacology and Therapeutics*, 14, 317–325.

Pascoe, P.J., Ilkiw, J.E., Black, W.D., Claxton, J.M., & Suter, C.M, (1993a) The pharmacokinetics of alfentanil in healthy cats. *Journal of Veterinary Anaesthesia*, 20, 9–13.

Pascoe, P.J. & Dyson, D.H. (1993b) Analgesia after lateral thoracotomy in dogs. Epidural morphine vs intercostal bupivacaine. *Veterinary Surgery*, 22, 141–147.

Pascoe, P.J. & Taylor, P.M. (2003) Effects of dopamine antagonists on alfentanil-induced locomotor activity in horses. *Veterinary Anaesthesia and Analgesia*, 30, 165–171.

Pattinson, K.T.S. (2008) Opioids and the control of respiration. *British Journal of Anaesthesia*, 100, 747–758.

Pettifer, G. & Dyson, D. (2000) Hydromorphone: a cost-effective alternative to the use of oxymorphone. *The Canadian Veterinary Journal*, 41, 135–137.

Pfeffer, M., Smyth, R.D., Pittman, K.A., & Nardella, P.A. (1980) Pharmacokinetics of subcutaneous and intramuscular butorphanol in dogs. *Journal of Pharmaceutical Sciences*, 69, 801–803.

Pieper, K., Schuster, T., Levinnois, O., Matis, U., & Bergadano, A. (2011) Antinociceptive efficacy and plasma concentrations of transdermal buprenorphine in dogs. *The Veterinary Journal*, 187, 335–341.

Popilskis, S., Kohn, D.F., Laurent, L., & Danilo, P. (1993) Efficacy of epidural morphine versus intravenous morphine for post-thoracotomy pain in dogs. *Journal of Veterinary Anaesthesia*, 20, 21–25.

Posner, L.P., Gleed, R.D., Erb, H.N., & Ludders, J.W. (2007) Postanesthetic hyperthermia in cats. *Veterinary Anaesthesia and Analgesia*, 34, 40–47.

Posner, L.P., Pavuk, A.A., Rokshar, J.L., Carter, J.E., & Levine, J.F. (2010) Effects of opioids and anesthetic drugs on body temperature in cats. *Veterinary Anaesthesia and Analgesia*, 37, 35–43.

Pypendop, B.H. & Ilkiw, J.E. (2007) Pharmacokinetics of tramadol, and its metabolite *O*-desmethy-tramadol, in cats. *Journal of Veterinary Pharmacology and Therapeutics*, 31, 52–59.

Pypendop, B.H., Brosnan, R.J., Siao, K.T., & Stanley, S.D. (2008a) Pharmacokinetics of remifentanil in conscious cats and cats anesthetized with isoflurane. *American Journal of Veterinary Research*, 69, 531–536.

Pypendop, B.H., Siao, K.T., Pascoe, P.J., & Ilkiw, J.E. (2008b) Effects of epidurally administered morphine or buprenorphine on the thermal threshold in cats. *American Journal of Veterinary Research*, 69, 983–987.

Pypendop, B.H., Siao, K.T., & Ilkiw, J.E. (2009) Effects of tramadol hydrochloride on the thermal threshold in cats. *American Journal of Veterinary Research*, 70, 1465–1470.

Radnay, P.A., Brodman, E., Mankikar, D., & Duncalf, D. (1980) The effect of equi-analgesic doses of fentanyl, morphine, meperidine, and pentazocine on common bile duct pressure. *Anaesthetist*, 29, 26–29.

Raekallio, M., Taylor, P.M., Johnson, C.B., Tulamo, R.M., & Ruprah, M. (1996) The disposition and local effects of intra-articular morphine in normal ponies. *Journal of the Association of Veterinary Anaesthetists*, 23, 23–26.

Rawal, N., Nuutinen, L., Raj, P.P., et al. (1991) Behavioral and histopathologic effects following intrathecal administration of butor-

phanol, sufentanil, and nalbuphine in sheep. *Anesthesiology*, 75, 1025–1034.

Riggs, S.M., Hawkins, M.G., Craigmill, A.L., Kass, P.H., Stanley, S.D., & Taylor, I.T. (2008) Pharmacokinetics of butorphanol tartrate in red-tailed hawks (*Buteo jamaicensis*) and great horned owls (*Bubo virginianus*). *American Journal of Veterinary Research*, 69, 596–603.

Rizzi, A., Nazzaro, C., Marzola, G.G., et al. (2006) Endogenous nociceptin/orphanin FQ signalling produces opposite spinal antinociceptive and supraspinal pronociceptive effects in the mouse formalin test: pharmacological and genetic evidences. *Pain*, 124(1–2), 100–108.

Robertson, S.A., Taylor, P.M., Sear, J.W., & Keuhnel, G. (2005a) Relationship between plasma concentrations and analgesia after intravenous fentanyl and disposition after other routes of administration in cats. *Journal of Veterinary Pharmacology and Therapeutics*, 28, 87–93.

Robertson, S.A., Lascelles, B.D.X., Taylor, P.M., & Sear, J.W. (2005b) PK-PD modeling of buprenorphine in cats: intravenous and oral transmucosal administration. *Journal of Veterinary Pharmacology and Therapeutics*, 28, 453–460.

Robertson, S.A., Wegner, K., & Lascelles, B.D.X. (2009) Antinociceptive and side-effects of hydromorphone after subcutaneous administration in cats. *Journal of Feline Medicine and Surgery*, 11, 76–81.

Robinson, E.P., Faggella, A.M., Henry, D.P., & Russell, W.L. (1988) Comparison of histamine release induced by morphine and oxymorphone administration in dogs. *American Journal of Veterinary Research*, 49, 1699–1701.

Robinson, T.M., Kruse-Elliott, K.T., Markel, M.D., Pluhar, G.E., Massa, K., & Bjorling, D.E. (1999) A comparison of transdermal fentanyl versus epidural morphine for analgesia in dogs undergoing major orthopedic surgery. *Journal of the American Animal Hospital Association*, 35, 95–100.

Sanchez, L.C., Robertson, S.A., Maxwell, L.K., Zientek, K., & Cole, C. (2007) Effect of fentanyl on visceral and somatic nociception in conscious horses. *Journal of Veterinary Internal Medicine*, 21, 1067–1075.

Sano, T., Nishimura, R., Kanazawa, H., et al. (2006) Pharmacokinetics of fentanyl after single intravenous injection and constant rate infusion in dogs. *Veterinary Anaesthesia and Analgesia*, 33, 266–273.

Sawyer, D.C. & Rech, R.H. (1986) Analgesia and behavioral effects of butorphanol, nalbuphine and pentazocine in the cat. *Journal of the American Animal Hospital Association*, 23, 438–446.

Schmiedt, C.W. & Bjorling, D.E. (2007) Accidental prehension and suspected transmural or oral absorption of fentanyl from a transdermal patch in a dog. *Veterinary Anaesthesia and Analgesia*, 34, 70–73.

Schwartz, S. (1993) Naltrexone-induced pruritus in a dog with tail-chasing behavior. *Journal of the American Veterinary Medical Association*, 202, 278–280.

Scott, D.H., Arthur, G.R., & Scott, D.B. (1980) Haemodynamic changes following buprenorphine and morphine. *Anaesthesia*, 35, 957–961.

Selley, D.E., Cao, C.C., Sexton, T., Schwegel, J.A, Martin, T.J., & Childers, S.R. (2001) mu-Opioid receptor-mediated G-protein activation by heroin metabolites: evidence for greater efficacy of 6 monoacetylmorphine compared with morphine. *Biochemical Pharmacology*, 62, 447–455.

Sellon, D.C., Roberts, M.C., Bliksager, A.T., Ulibarri, C., & Papich, M.G. (2004) Effects of continuous rate infusion of butorphanol on physiologic and outcome variables in horses after celiotomy. *Journal of Veterinary Internal Medicine*, 18, 555–563.

Sellon, D.C., Papich, M.G., Palmer, L., & Remund, B. (2008) Pharmacokinetics of butorphanol in horses after intramuscular injection. *Journal of Veterinary Pharmacology and Therapeutics*, 32, 62–65.

Shafford, H.L. & Schadt, J.C. (2008) Effect of buprenorphine on the cardiovascular and respiratory response to visceral pain in conscious rabbits. *Veterinary Anaesthesia and Analgesia*, 35, 333–340.

Shilo, Y., Britzi, M., Eytan, B., Lifschitz, T., Soback. S., & Steinman, A. (2007) Pharmacokinetics of tramadol in horses after intravenous, intramuscular and oral administration. *Journal of Veterinary Pharmacology and Therapeutics*, 31, 60–65.

Shury, T.K., Caulkett, N.A., & Woodbury, M.R. (2010) Intranasal naltrexone and atipamezole for reversal of white-tailed deer immobilized with carfentanil and medetomidine. *Canadian Veterinary Journal* 51, 501–505.

Skingle, M. & Tyers, M.B. (1980) Further studies on opiate receptors that mediate antinociception: tooth pulp stimulation in the dog. *British Journal of Pharmacology*, 70, 323–327.

Sladky, K.K., Krugner-Higby, L., Meek-Walker, E., Heath, T.D., & Paul-Murphy, J. (2006) Serum concentrations and analgesic effects of liposome-encapsulated and standard butorphanol tartrate in parrots. *American Journal of Veterinary Research*, 67, 775–781.

Smith, L.J., Yu, J.K.A., Bjorling, D.E., & Waller, K. (2001) Effects of hydromorphone or oxymorphone, with or without acepromazine, on preanesthetic sedation, physiologic values, and histamine release in dogs. *Journal of the American Veterinary Medical Association*, 218, 1101–1105.

Smith, A.A., Posner, L.P., Goldstein, R.E., et al. (2004a) Evaluation of the effects of premedication on gastroduodenoscopy in cats. *Journal of the American Veterinary Medical Association*, 225, 540–544.

Smith, L.J., Krugner-Higby, L.A., Trepanier, L.A., Flaska, D.E., Joers, V., & Heath, T.D. (2004b) Sedative effects and serum drug concentrations of oxymorphone and metabolites after subcutaneous administration of a liposome-encapsulated formulation in dogs. *Journal of Veterinary Pharmacology and Therapeutics*, 27, 369–372.

Smith, L.J., KuKanich, B., Hogan, B.K., Brown, C., Heath, T.D., Krugner-Higby, L.A. (2008) Pharmacokinetics of a controlled-release liposome encapsulated hydromorphone administered to healthy dogs. *Journal of Veterinary Pharmacology and Therapeutics*, 31, 415–422.

Stanway, G.W., Taylor, P.M., & Brodbelt, D.C. (2002) A preliminary investigation comparing pre-operative morphine and buprenorphine for postoperative analgesia and sedation in cats. *Veterinary Anaesthesia and Analgesia*, 29, 29–35.

Steagall, P.V.M., Carnicelli, P., Taylor, P.M., Luna, S.P., Dixon, M., & Ferreira, T.H. (2006) Effects of subcutaneous methadone, morphine, buprenorphine or saline on thermal and pressure thresholds in cats. *Journal of Veterinary Pharmacology and Therapeutics*, 29, 531–537.

Steagall, P.V.M, Mantovani, F.B., Taylor, P.M., Dixon, M.J., & Luna, S.P. (2009a) Dose-related antinociceptive effects of intravenous buprenorphine in cats. *The Veterinary Journal*, 182, 203–209.

Steagall, P.V.M., Millette, V., Mantovani, F.B., Gilbert, P., Luna, S.P.L., & Duke-Novakovski, T. (2009b) Antinociceptive effects of epidural buprenorphine, or medetomidine, or the combination, in conscious cats. *Journal of Veterinary Pharmacology and Therapeutics*, 32, 477–484.

Streisand, J.B., Zhang, J., Niu, S., McJames, S., Natte, R., & Pace, N.L. (1995) Buccal absorption of fentanyl is pH-dependent in dogs. *Anesthesiology*, 82, 759–764.

Sykes, J.M., Cox, S., & Ramsay, E.C. (2009) Evaluation of an osmotic pump for fentanyl administration in cats as a model for nondomestic felids. *American Journal of Veterinary Research*, 70, 950–955.

Szöke, M.O., Blais, D., Cuvelliez, S.G., & Lavoie, J.P. (1998) Effects of buprenorphine on cardiovascular and pulmonary function in clinically normal horses and horses with chronic obstructive pulmonary disease. *American Journal of Veterinary Research*, 59, 1287–1291.

Tasker, R.A.R., Ross, S.J., Dohoo, S.E., & Elson, C.M. (1997) Pharmacokinetics of an injectable sustained-release formulation of morphine for use in dogs. *Journal of Veterinary Pharmacology and Therapeutics*, 20, 362–367.

Taylor, P.M., Robertson, S.A., Dixon, M.J., et al. (2001) Morphine, pethidine and buprenorphine disposition in the cat. *Journal of Veterinary Pharmacology and Therapeutics*, 24, 391–398.

Thomasy, S.M., Slovis, N., Maxwell, L.K., & Kollias-Baker, C. (2004) Transdermal fentanyl combined with nonsteroidal anti-inflammatory drugs for analgesia in horses. *Journal of Veterinary Internal Medicine*, 18, 550–554.

Thomasy, S.M., Steffey, E.P., Mama, K.R., Solano, A, Stanley, S.D. (2006) The effects of i.v. fentanyl administration on the minimum alveolar concentration of isoflurane in horses. *British Journal of Anaesthesia*, 97, 232–237.

Thomasy, S.M., Mama, K.R., Whitley, K., Steffey, E.P., & Stanley, S.D. (2007) Influence of general anaesthesia on the pharmacokinetics of intravenous fentanyl and its primary metabolite in horses. *Equine Veterinary Journal*, 39, 54–58.

Thompson, W.L. & Walton, R.P. (1964) Elevation of plasma histamine levels in the dog following administration of muscle relaxants, opiates, and macromolecular polymers. *Journal of Pharmacology Experimental Therapeutics*, 143, 131–136.

Thompson, D.R. (2001) Narcotic analgesic effects on the sphincter of Oddi: a review of the data and therapeutic implications in treating pancreatitis. *American Journal of Gastroenterology*, 96, 1266–1272.

Tobin, T. (1978) Pharmacology review: narcotic analgesics and the opiate receptor in the horse. *Journal of Equine Medicine and Surgery*, 2, 397–399.

Troncy, E., Besner, J.G., Charbonneau, R., Cuvelliez, S.G, & Blais, D. (1996) Pharmacokinetics of epidural butorphanol in isoflurane-anaesthetized dogs. *Journal of Veterinary Pharmacology and Therapeutics*, 19, 268–273.

Trudnowski, R.J. & Gessner, T. (1979) Gastric secretion of intravenously administered meperidine in surgical patients. *Anesthesia Analgesia*, 58, 88–92.

Tung, A.S. & Yaksh, T.L. (1982) The antinociceptive effects of epidural opiates in the cat: studies on the pharmacology and the effects of lipophilicity in spinal analgesia. *Pain*, 12, 343–356.

Uhrig, S.R., Papich, M.G., KuKanich, B., et al. (2007) Pharmacokinetics and pharmacodynamics of morphine in llamas. *American Journal of Veterinary Research*, 68, 25–34.

Valverde, A., Conlon, P.D., Dyson, D.H., & Burger, J.P. (1992) Cisternal CSF and serum concentrations of morphine following epidural administration in the dog. *Journal of Veterinary Pharmacology and Therapeutics*, 15, 91–95.

Valverde, A., Cantwell, S., Hornández, J., & Brotherson, C. (2004) Effects of acepromazine on the incidence of vomiting associated with opioid administration in dogs. *Veterinary Anaesthesia and Analgesia*, 31, 40–45.

van Dijk, P., Lankveld, D.P., Rijkenhuizen, A.B., & Jonker, F.H. (2003) Hormonal, metabolic and physiological effects of laparoscopic surgery using a detomidine-buprenorphine combination in standing horses. *Veterinary Anaesthesia and Analgesia*, 30, 72–80.

van Loon, J.P.A., de Grauw, J.C., van Dierendonck, M., L'ami, J.J., Back, W., & van Weeren, P.R. (2010) Intra-articular opioid analgesia is effective in reducing pain and inflammation in an equine LPS induced synovitis study. *Equine Veterinary Journal*, 42, 412–419.

Vesal, N., Cribb, P.H., & Frketic, M. (1996) Postoperative analgesic and cardiopulmonary effects in dogs of oxymorphone administered epidurally, and intramuscularly and medetomidine administered epidurally: a comparative clinical study. *Veterinary Surgery*, 25, 361–369.

Walker, E.A., Zernig, G., & Woods, J.H. (1995) Buprenorphine antagonism of Mu-opioids in the Rhesus monkey tail-withdrawal procedure. *Journal of Pharmacology and Experimental Therapeutics*, 273, 1345–1352.

Wallenstein, M.C. & Wang, S.C. (1979) Mechanism of morphine-induced mydriasis in the cat. *American Journal of Physiology*, 236, R292–296.

Waterman, A.E. & Kalthum, W. (1989) Pharmacokinetics of intramuscularly administered pethidine in dogs and the influence of anaesthesia and surgery. *Veterinary Record*, 124, 293–296.

Waterman, A.E. & Kalthum, W. (1990) The effect of clinical hepatic disease on the distribution and elimination of pethidine administered post-operatively to dogs. *Journal of Veterinary Pharmacology and Therapeutics*, 13, 137–147.

Waterman, A.E. & Kalthum, W. (1992) Pharmacokinetics of pethidine administered intramuscularly and intravenously to dogs over 10 years old. *Research in Veterinary Science*, 48, 245–248.

Waterman, A.E. & Amin, A. (1992) The influence of surgery and anaesthesia on the pharmacokinetics of pethidine in the horse. *Equine Veterinary Journal: Supplement*, 11, 56–58.

Wegner, K., Robertson, S.A., Kollias-Baker, C., Sams, R.A., & Muir, W.W. 3rd. (2004) Pharmacokinetic and pharmacodynamic evaluation of intravenous hydromorphone in cats. *Journal of Veterinary Pharmacology and Therapeutics*, 27, 329–336.

Wegner, K. & Robertson, S.A. (2007) Dose-related thermal antinociceptive effects of intravenous hydromorphone in cats. *Veterinary Anaesthesia and Analgesia*, 34, 132–138.

Weinstein, S.H. & Gaylord, J.C. (1979) Determination of oxycodone in plasma and identification of a major metabolite. *Journal of Pharmaceutical Sciences*, 68, 527–528.

Wells, S.M., Glerum, L.E., & Papich, M.G. (2008) Pharmacokinetics of butorphanol in cats after intramuscular and buccal transmucosal administration. *American Journal Veterinary Research*, 69, 1548–1554.

Werner, C., Hoffman, W.E., Baughman, V.L., Albrecht, R.F., & Schulte, J. (1991) Effects of sufentanil on cerebral blood flow, cerebral blood flow velocity, and metabolism in dogs. *Anesthesia Analgesia*, 72, 177–181.

Wesley, C.G. & Cumby, H.R. (1978) Hyperthermic responses to central and peripheral injections of morphine sulphate in the cat. *British Journal of Pharmacology*, 63, 65–71.

Westermann, C.M., Laan, T.T., Nieuwstadt, R.A., Bull, S., & Fink-Gremmels, J. (2005) Effects of antitussive agents administered before bronchoalveolar lavage in horses. *American Journal of Veterinary Research*, 66, 1420–1424.

Wilson, D.V. & Walshaw, R. (2004) Postanesthetic esophageal dysfunction in 13 dogs. *Journal of the American Animal Hospital Association*, 40, 455–460.

Wilson, D.V., Evans, A.T., & Mauer, W.A. (2007) Pre-anesthetic meperidine: associated vomiting and gastroesophageal reflux during the subsequent anesthetic in dogs. *Veterinary Anaesthesia and Analgesia*, 34, 15–22.

Wright, A.W.E., Mather, L.E., & Smith, M.T. (2001) Hydromorphone-3-glucuronide: a more potent neuro-excitant than its structural analogue, morphine-3-glucuronide. *Life Sciences*, 69, 409–420.

Wunsch, L.A., Schmidt, B.K., Krugner-Higby, L.A., & Smith, L.J. (2010) A comparison of the effects of hydromorphone HCl and a novel extended release hydromorphone on arterial blood gas values in conscious healthy dogs. *Research in Veterinary Science*, 88, 154–158.

Yaksh, T.L., Nouiehed, R.Y., & Durant, P.A.C. (1986) Studies of the pharmacology and pathology of intrathecally administered 4-anilinopiperidine analogues and morphine in the rat and cat. *Anesthesiology*, 64, 54–66.

Yaksh, T.L., Provencher, J.C., Rathbun, M.L., et al. (2000) Safety assessment of encapsulated morphine delivered epidurally in a sustained-release multivesicular liposome preparation in dogs. *Drug Delivery*, 7, 27–36.

Yassan, A., Olofsen, E., van Dorp, E., et al. (2007) Mechanism-based pharmacokinetic-pharmacodynamic modelling of the reversal of buprenorphine-induced respiratory depression by naloxone: a study in healthy volunteers. *Clinical Pharmacokinetics*, 46, 965–980.

Zimmer, R. & Ashburn, M.A. (2001) Noninvasive drug delivery. *Comprehensive Therapy*, 27, 293–301.

Zoran, D.L. (2006) Pancreatitis in cats: diagnosis and management of a challenging disease. *Journal of the American Animal Hospital Association*, 42, 1–9.

5

Nonsteroidal Anti-Inflammatory Drugs and Corticosteroids

Stuart Clark-Price

Nonsteroidal anti-inflammatory drugs (NSAIDs) are a class of drugs that produce anti-inflammatory and anti-nociceptive effects. NSAIDs are also anti-pyretic, anti-endotoxemic, and anti-neoplastic, and one of the fastest growing classes of drugs in veterinary medicine. Significant resources are being devoted to research and development, and veterinary practitioners can expect to see new and improved versions of NSAIDs in the future. When used properly, NSAIDs are a primary tool of the veterinarian for the management of pain.

HISTORY

NSAIDs are one of the oldest classes of analgesics, and their use is recorded as far back as the seventeenth century BCE. An ancient Egyptian surgical text, known as the Edwin Smith Papyrus, mentions the use of salicylate-containing plants to relieve pain. Hippocrates wrote about the medicinal uses of similar agents in the fifth century BCE. In 1763, Reverend Edward Stone described the medicinal properties of willow bark in a publication of the Royal Society of England. The active agent in willow bark is salicylic acid, first isolated and described in 1828 by Henry Leroux and Raffaele Piria. In 1897, Felix Hoffman, while working for the Bayer Chemical Company, synthesized acetylsalicylic acid, which was later renamed aspirin, the first commercially available NSAID. In 1971, Sir John Vane described the ability of aspirin-like drugs to inhibit the production of prostaglandins (Vane, 1971). It is now understood that NSAIDs mediate their effects via a number of mechanisms.

MECHANISMS OF ACTION

NSAIDs act primarily by inhibiting the production of inflammatory mediators synthesized from arachidonic acid (AA) (Figure 5.1). AA, a 20 carbon polyunsaturated fatty acid, is formed through the actions of the enzyme phospholipase on cellular membrane lipids in response to tissue damage or release of inflammatory mediators (Tizard, 2009). AA is derived from cellular membranes of phenotypically and functionally diverse cells, and the cell of origin determines the final disposition.

AA interacts with two enzymes, lipoxygenase (LOX) and cyclooxygenase (COX), and is oxidized to produce the eicosanoids

leukotrienes and prostaglandins (Higgins & Lees, 1984). Leukotrienes and prostaglandins influence numerous physiological systems. Leukotrienes formed from AA include B_4, A_4, C_4, D_4, and E_4. Leukotrienes mediate inflammation via inflammatory cell recruitment and activation (Tizard, 2009). Unlike prostaglandins, there are fewer clinical options for the manipulation of leukotriene concentrations for therapeutic purposes.

When presented with AA, the COX enzyme performs the first step in the synthesis of prostaglandins, cyclizing and adding a 15-hydroperoxy group to AA (Vane & Botting, 1998). This produces prostaglandin G_2, which is further modified by a peroxidase to form prostaglandin H_2 (Vane & Botting, 1998). Additional modification of prostaglandin H_2 forms a number of other prostaglandins and thromboxanes. Prostaglandins formed from AA include E_2, I_2, D_2, and $F_{2\alpha}$, each with different effects on biological systems.

Prostaglandins are important in homeostatic mechanisms necessary for normal organ function. When there is tissue damage, however, these same prostaglandins can incite inflammation, further tissue damage, and pain. Prostaglandin E_2 (PGE_2) is involved in the regulation of the reproductive, neurological, metabolic, and immune systems, bone formation and healing, temperature regulation, and vasomotor responses (Legler et al., 2010). PGE_2 is also a classic pro-inflammatory mediator, promoting redness, swelling, pain, and the development of hyperalgesia (Pratico & Dogne, 2009; Legler et al., 2010). Prostaglandin I_2 (PGI_2), or prostacyclin, is an important regulatory prostaglandin and a potent vasodilator and inhibitor of platelet aggregation (Pratico & Dogne, 2009). Prostaglandin D_2 (PGD_2), commonly derived from lipid membranes of mast cells and macrophages, causes bronchoconstriction (particularly in asthmatics and those with pulmonary inflammation), vasodilation, increased capillary permeability, and mucous production (Oguma et al., 2008). Prostaglandin $F_{2\alpha}$ ($PGF_{2\alpha}$) is important in luteolysis, normal ovarian function, luteal maintenance of pregnancy, and parturition, and is used therapeutically to manipulate reproductive function. Additionally, $PGF_{2\alpha}$ is an active player in acute and chronic inflammation, and in cardiovascular and rheumatic diseases (Basu, 2007).

Regulation of the COX enzyme is the main mechanism for the therapeutic effects of NSAIDs, and first-generation NSAIDs

Pain Management in Veterinary Practice, First Edition. Edited by Christine M. Egger, Lydia Love and Tom Doherty.
© 2014 John Wiley & Sons, Inc. Published 2014 by John Wiley & Sons, Inc.

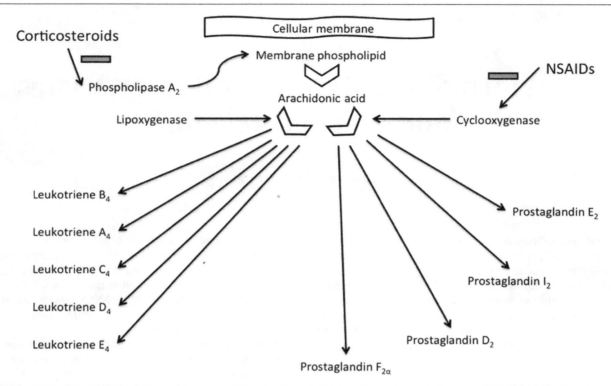

Figure 5.1. Prostaglandins and leukotrienes produced through the actions of phospholipase A_2, lipoxygenase, and cyclooxygenase enzymes on cellular membrane phospholipid. Dashes represent the inhibition of phospholipase A_2 by corticosteroids and cyclooxygenase by NSAIDs.

nonspecifically decreased the activity of the COX enzyme, thus suppressing all prostaglandin production. In the early 1990s, it was discovered that two isoforms of the COX enzyme exist (Xie et al., 1991) and that the second isoform was inducible with stimulating events, such as inflammation (Kujubu et al., 1991; Xie et al., 1991). The two isoforms, cyclooxygenase-1 (COX-1) and cyclooxygenase-2 (COX-2), are encoded by two separate genes (Warner & Mitchell, 2004). Both isoforms are membrane-bound proteins in the endoplasmic reticulum of cells, sharing approximately 60% homology of amino acid structure, including nearly identical amino acid conformation at their substrate-binding sites, and similarly catalyze AA to form prostaglandins (Warner & Mitchell, 2004). They differ, however, in the structure of their inhibitor-binding sites. For COX-1 and COX-2, AA and NSAIDs enter through a hydrophobic side channel (Khanapure et al., 2007) and NSAIDs compete with AA for this active site to inhibit production of prostaglandins. With COX-2 enzymes, valine-523 opens a "side pocket" next to the main channel, whereas in COX-1 enzymes, isoleucine-530 effectively eliminates a "side pocket" (Khanapure et al., 2007). This results in the COX-2 site being 25% larger, making COX-2 a better competitor for AA substrate (Warner & Mitchell, 2004). These differences in binding sites have been used to develop COX-2 selective inhibitors.

After the discovery of the COX-2 enzyme, it was postulated that COX-1 production of prostaglandins was constitutive and necessary for the normal functioning of organ systems. COX-2 was thought to be upregulated only during inflammation and other pathologi-

cal processes, and that control of inflammation and pain could be achieved with minimal side effects by suppressing COX-2. Numerous studies and reviews were published supporting the development of COX-2 selective/COX-1 sparing anti-inflammatory agents (Seibert et al., 1995; Seibert et al., 1997; FitzGerald & Patrono, 2001). However, more recent research and reports of adverse events in humans have forced reconsideration of the importance of the COX-1 versus the COX-2 enzyme. For example, in human patients the use of the COX-2 selective drug, rofecoxib significantly increased the risk of thrombotic cardiovascular events such as myocardial infarction, unstable angina, cardiac thrombus, and sudden death (Mukherjee et al., 2001). Likewise, in dogs, gastrointestinal perforation has been associated with the administration of deracoxib, a COX-2 selective drug, particularly when administered at high doses or when combined with other NSAIDs (Lascelles et al., 2005a). Based on this information, a COX-1 selective NSAID may cause more problems in certain circumstances than a COX-2 selective NSAID, and vice versa.

In 2002, a COX-3 enzyme isolated from the brains of dogs (Chandrasekharan et al., 2002) was determined to be a splice variant of the COX-1 enzyme, with identical mRNA except for a retained intron 1. COX-3 was selectively inhibited by acetaminophen (paracetamol), and this was thought to be the mechanism by which acetaminophen mediates analgesia. There is some debate about nomenclature and the role of COX-3, and some researchers have suggested that it be named COX-1b (Kis et al., 2005a; Simmons et al., 2005). The COX-3 mRNA in other species, such as humans and mice, encodes for a nonfunctional enzyme that does not play a role in prostaglandin-mediated fever (Kis et al., 2006). Prostaglandin production by rat cerebral endothelium is sensitive to acetaminophen, suggesting a central mechanism of action of the drug (Kis et al., 2005b). COX-3 mRNA has also been isolated from the human cerebral cortex and aorta, and rodent cerebral endothelium, heart, kidney, and neuronal tissue (Hersh et al., 2005). The role of COX-3 in inflammation, pain, and fever has yet to be completely elucidated and, to date, its clinical importance is unclear. However, synergism has been demonstrated between the COX-3 inhibitor acetaminophen and other COX isoform selective inhibitors, suggesting there may be benefits to the use of acetaminophen in combination with other NSAID therapy (Munoz et al., 2010).

Other Mechanisms of Action

The suppression of COX is the main mechanism by which NSAIDs exert their anti-inflammatory and analgesic effects; however, non-COX mediated mechanisms contribute to the analgesic and anti-inflammatory effects of NSAIDs.

Because NSAIDs tend to be lipophilic at low pH, some anti-inflammatory action appears to be due to the insertion of NSAIDs into the lipid bilayer of cell membranes and the physical disruption of cell signaling and protein-to-protein interactions (Dowling, 2010). This may result in decreased transmission of pain signals in the peripheral and central nervous systems.

Aspirin has been shown to have anti-inflammatory effects through inhibition of the kinase Erk, important in CD11b/CD18 integrin-dependent adhesiveness of neutrophils (Pillinger et al., 1998). This inhibition decreases neutrophil aggregation in areas of injury, reducing their inflammatory effects.

Other potential mechanisms of NSAID action include interaction with the endogenous opioid system, inhibition of nuclear factor κB, activation of the serotonergic bulbospinal pathway, involvement of the nitric oxide pathway, and an increase in cannabinoid/vanilloid tone (Mattia & Coluzzi, 2009; Fox, 2010). The interaction of NSAIDs with these and potentially other central nervous system receptors may be one of the reasons why human patients have a sense of well being while using these drugs.

CLASSIFICATION OF NSAIDs

No consensus currently exists on how NSAIDs should be classified, although several systems have been proposed. One method classifies NSAIDs based on their sequence of introduction to the market, similar to that used for antimicrobial agents (Fox, 2010). For example, first generation (e.g., aspirin, phenylbutazone, meclofenamic acid), second generation (e.g., carprofen, etodolac, meloxicam), third generation (e.g., tepoxalin, deracoxib, firocoxib), and so on. This method does not take into account different mechanisms of action within and among generations.

Chemical composition can be used to classify NSAIDs (Table 5.1). This method also does not consider the mechanism of action and provides little clinically useful information.

Another method of classification has been based on COX-2 inhibition, and divides NSAIDs into COX-2 inhibitors and nonspecific NSAIDs (Stoelting & Hillier, 2006). This method presents difficulties because it has been shown that although several of the newer NSAIDs, particularly the coxibs (Table 5.1), do possess very

Table 5.1. Nonsteroidal anti-inflammatory drugs used in veterinary medicine classified by chemical composition

Chemical Composition	NSAIDs
Salicylates	Aspirin
Benzones	Phenylbutazone
Propionic acid derivatives	Carprofen
	Flurbiprofen
	Ibuprofen
	Ketoprofen
	Naproxen
	Vedaprofen
Acetic acid derivatives	Diclofenac
	Etodolac
	Indomethacin
	Ketorolac
Enolic acid derivatives	Meloxicam
	Piroxicam
Fenamic acid derivatives	Meclofenamic acid
	Tolfenamic acid
Selective COX-2 inhibitors (coxibs)	Deracoxib
	Firocoxib
	Mavacoxib
	Robenacoxib
Miscellaneous	Flunixin
	Nimesulide
	Tepoxalin

strong suppression of COX-2, none of them has a complete absence of COX-1 suppression.

With the discovery of the COX-2 enzyme and the development of COX-2 preferential NSAIDs, currently the most popular method for classifying NSAIDs is based on their COX-1 versus COX-2 suppression profile, using the whole-blood assay as a gold standard. This profile is often expressed as a ratio (COX-1:COX-2) which is derived from the concentration of the NSAID necessary to inhibit 50% of the activity of the COX-1 enzyme (COX-1[IC_{50}]) and the concentration necessary to inhibit 50% of the activity of the COX-2 enzyme (COX-2[IC_{50}]). Therefore, the ratio can be written as COX-1 [IC_{50}]/COX-2 [IC_{50}], or simply COX-1/COX-2 (Papich, 2008). The greater the ratio is above 1.0, the more specific the NSAID is for the COX-2 enzyme. Using ratios derived from individual drugs, NSAIDs can be classified as COX-1 selective for ratios <1, COX-2 preferential for ratios >1–100, COX-2 selective for ratios >100–1000, and COX-2 specific for ratios >1000 (Fox, 2010) (Table 5.2). Published studies using different inhibition assays have given conflicting results, and it is now clear that differences in testing methods and species can result in different ratios for the same NSAID (Papich, 2008). In addition, using whole blood assay data from one species to predict suppression profiles in other species should be done cautiously. It is important to note that the COX-1/COX-2 profile of an NSAID does not predict its clinical efficacy, and one NSAID may be more effective than another in an individual patient.

Table 5.2. Nonsteroidal anti-inflammatory drugs classified by canine COX-1/COX-2 ratios

Category	NSAIDs (ratio)
COX-1 selective (COX-1/COX-2 ratio of <1)	Aspirin (0.4)
	Ketoprofen (0.88)
COX-2 preferential (COX-1/COX2 ratio of <1 to 100)	Carprofen (16.8)
	Deracoxib (48.5)
	Etodolac (6.6)
	Nimesulide (29.2)
	Meloxicam (7.3)
COX-2 selective (COX-1/COX-2 ratio of >100 to 1000)	Firocoxib (155)
	Robenacoxib (128.8)
COX-2 specific (COX-1/COX-2 ratio of >1000)	None commercially available

Sources: Streppa, H.K., Jones, C.J., & Budsberg, S.C. (2002) Cyclooxygenase selectivity of nonsteroidal anti-inflammatory drugs in canine blood. *American Journal of Veterinary Research,* 63, 91–94.; Li, J., Lynch, M.P., Demello, K.L., et al. (2005) In vitro and in vivo profile of 2-(3-di-fluoromethyl-5-phenylpyrazol-1-yl)-5-methanesulfonylpyridine, a potent, selective, and orally active canine COX-2 inhibitor. *Bioorganic & Medicinal Chemistry,* 13, 1805–1809.; King, J.N., Rudaz, C., Borer, L., et al. (2010) In vitro and ex vivo inhibition of canine cyclooxygenase isoforms by robenacoxib: a comparative study. *Research in Veterinary Science,* 88(3), 497–506.

ADVERSE EFFECTS AND CONTRAINDICATIONS

The adverse effects associated with the use of NSAIDs can be serious. There is a narrow therapeutic index for most NSAIDs, and a thorough knowledge of organ systems affected and associated clinical signs of toxicity is necessary for safe usage. The gastrointestinal, renal, and hepatic systems are most commonly associated with NSAID toxicity, but the coagulation, hematopoietic, and musculoskeletal systems can also be affected.

Effects on the Gastrointestinal Tract

In the gastrointestinal tract both COX-1 and COX-2 are necessary for proper function, maintenance, and repair of the mucosa. COX-1 related prostaglandins help regulate mucosal blood flow, secretion of buffers and mucous, and turnover of epithelial cells (Simmons et al., 2004). It was originally thought that COX-2 was not constitutively expressed and was only upregulated during inflammation; however, it is now known that COX-2 plays a role in mucosal protection and repair (Halter et al., 2001) and COX-1 may not be as important (Schmassmann et al., 2006). In a recent report of 27 clinically normal dogs not receiving NSAIDs, 22 had histopathological evidence of gastrointestinal inflammation or erosion even though none of the dogs had gross evidence of gastrointestinal disease, and when evaluated, COX-2 expression was increased compared to COX-1, indicating COX-2 is important for healing the mucosa (Wooten et al., 2010). Thus, it stands to reason that some dogs may have undetected gastrointestinal inflammation and that they

may be more prone to gastrointestinal adverse effects after COX-2 inhibition.

The gastrointestinal tract is by far the most common site of NSAID toxicity (DeNovo, 2003). Adverse gastrointestinal events reported in dogs, cats, and horses range from mild inflammation to catastrophic ulceration and death (Hough et al., 1999; Lascelles et al., 2005a; Lascelles et al., 2007). Because COX-2 is necessary for mucosal healing, the more specific a drug is for COX-2 the more likely it is to cause gastrointestinal ulceration and prevent healing of pre-existing lesions (Goodman et al., 2009). Gastrointestinal lesions caused by NSAIDs in dogs tend to be located in the pyloric antrum, and have a poor prognosis if not identified and treated early (Lascelles et al., 2005a). In horses, ulceration can occur anywhere along the gastrointestinal tract, including the colon; however, the right dorsal colon tends to be particularly sensitive to the toxic effects of NSAIDs (McConnico et al., 2008). Clinical signs of gastrointestinal erosions and ulcers include anorexia, depression, lethargy, diarrhea, vomiting, hematochezia, melena, abdominal pain, anemia, hypoproteinemia, leukocytosis or leukopenia, and increased blood urea nitrogen.

Effects on the Renal System

Prostaglandins regulate renal blood flow and glomerular filtration, especially during periods of systemic hypotension. Both COX-1 and COX-2 enzymes are required to maintain adequate renal perfusion (Fox, 2010). Renal prostaglandins work in concert with catecholamines to autoregulate renal blood flow and maintain renal perfusion when mean arterial pressure is between 60 and 150 mm Hg (Cohen et al., 1983). During conditions of hypovolemia, hypotension, or physiological stress, prostaglandins are upregulated in the kidneys to maintain adequate renal blood flow. Nonsteroidal anti-inflammatory suppression of renal prostaglandin production can disrupt autoregulation and result in renal ischemia. Acute renal failure, acute exacerbation of chronic renal failure, and renal papillary necrosis can result. Cats may be uniquely sensitive to NSAID toxicity because they possess approximately one-half the number of nephrons at birth compared to most species. Clearly, proper fluid balance and hydration are critically important when using NSAIDs, and their use should be avoided in patients with known or suspected renal disease.

Effects on the Hepatic System

NSAIDs have been implicated in hepatocellular damage and hepatic failure in several species. Acetaminophen toxicity is one of the leading causes of acute liver failure in humans (Bernal et al., 2010). NSAIDs are metabolized in the liver and excessive dosing can lead to hepatotoxicity. Hepatocellular toxicosis and death were reported in a dog after three different NSAIDs were administered over a 14-day period (Nakagawa et al., 2005). Idiosyncratic hepatocellular toxicosis with NSAIDs can also occur, as reported in a study in dogs treated with carprofen. Interestingly, Labrador Retrievers were overrepresented in that study (MacPhail et al., 1998). Liver disease from NSAIDs is not limited to small animal patients, and excessive dosing of phenylbutazone can produce hepatotoxicity in horses (Lees et al., 1983). Liver enzyme activity should be evaluated periodically in patients prescribed NSAIDs on a long-term basis, and a three- to fivefold increase in activity above baseline could indicate hepatotoxicity, especially if values return to normal after treatment is discontinued.

Effects on Platelet Function

Thromboxane is necessary for proper platelet function and is produced via the COX-1 enzyme. NSAIDs that strongly suppress COX-1 could have significant effects on platelets and clot formation. It is well known that aspirin can inhibit platelet aggregation and it is used therapeutically for that purpose (Smith et al., 2003; Brainard et al., 2007; Lamont & Mathews, 2007). In normal dogs, meloxicam had minimal effects on platelet function, whereas carprofen decreased clot strength and platelet aggregation (Brainard et al., 2007). It is not clear if the effect of carprofen on platelets is clinically significant. However, ketoprofen has been shown clinically to affect hemostasis, and should be avoided in cases where surgical bleeding may be difficult to control, such as in laparoscopic procedures (Lamont & Mathews, 2007). The coxib-type NSAIDs do not affect platelet function (Brainard et al., 2007).

Effects on Bone Healing

Bone healing after fracture or surgical osteotomy is a complex process that is affected by numerous variables including fracture gap, comminution, disturbance of blood flow, degree of soft tissue damage, mechanical stability, nutrition, and age (Pountos et al., 2012). Several drug classes slow or inhibit bone healing including corticosteroids, chemotherapeutics, and some antibiotics (Pountos et al., 2008; Pountos et al., 2011). Debate continues as to the effect of NSAIDs on bone healing, with several published studies supporting both sides of the argument. Prostaglandins play an important role in bone healing, directly induce osteogenesis, and help increase cortical and trabecular mass (Pountos et al., 2012). Physiologically, it makes sense to use NSAIDs judiciously in patients recovering from bone injury. However, the analgesic and anti-inflammatory properties of NSAIDs make them particularly useful in this set of patients. The use of NSAIDs for the treatment of bone pain has been demonstrated to be as effective as opioids, and some human studies have shown a greater reduction in pain scores (Camu et al., 2002; Monaon, 2010; Pountos et al., 2012). Currently, in human medicine, evidence suggests COX-2 inhibition may affect early fracture healing, but the evidence is not considered conclusive and therefore short term NSAID use is considered a safe and effective supplement for pain management (Kurmis et al., 2012). Studies in veterinary medicine regarding the use of NSAIDs and bone healing are sparse. One study demonstrated that long-term administration (120 days) of carprofen appeared to inhibit bone healing in dogs after tibial osteotomy (Ochi et al., 2011). Overall, the short-term use of NSAIDs after bone injury probably has minimal long-term effects on bone healing and should be considered in an analgesic plan in such patients.

CLINICAL USE OF NSAIDs

NSAIDs are one of the most commonly used classes of analgesics in veterinary medicine and are principally used to reduce effects of the primary disease, such as acute and chronic pain, inflammation, fever, endotoxemia, and hypercoagulability, but are also used to treat some neoplastic processes (Lascelles et al., 2005b). When NSAIDs are combined with other classes of drugs, such as opioids, there is a synergistic effect because each mediates anti-nociception via a different mechanism (Hellyer et al., 2007). Co-administration of NSAIDs with opioids enhances analgesia and reduces the dose of opioid required (Salerno & Hermann, 2006).

Care should be taken with patient selection when prescribing NSAIDs. In general, this class of drugs should be reserved for patients without renal, gastrointestinal, or hepatic dysfunction. In equine and bovine patients, however, NSAIDs may be used in conjunction with other treatments to relieve pain associated with gastrointestinal distress. NSAIDs should be avoided in immature animals in which organ maturation is not complete. General guidelines suggest that NSAIDs should be avoided in patients less than six weeks of age (Lamont & Mathews, 2007); however, many NSAIDs have not been evaluated in animals less than 1 year of age.

When prescribing NSAIDs, owner education regarding the signs of toxicity, such as vomiting, depression, or diarrhea, is critical. Followup physical examination and blood evaluation should continue on a regular basis, especially if treatment is prolonged.

Peri-operative use of NSAIDs requires careful consideration of not only the patient's preoperative physical status and history but also the nature and length of the general anesthetic event. Most anesthetic agents can affect cardiac output, blood pressure, and tissue perfusion. Consequently, the adverse effects of NSAIDs may be magnified in patients administered NSAIDs prior to anesthesia. Post-surgical administration of NSAIDs rather than preoperative administration may be more appropriate; that way, NSAIDs can be withheld from patients who experience hypotension, hypovolemia, or other adverse events that may exacerbate NSAID-induced adverse effects. If NSAIDs are used preoperatively, blood pressure monitoring and support is essential.

SELECTED NSAIDs

The following sections are general descriptions of the use of selected NSAIDs in dogs, cats, horses, and cattle. Detailed pharmacokinetic and pharmacodynamic data for many of the NSAIDs is available for several species and can be found in subsequent chapters. Several excellent reviews of NSAID use in dogs (Lascelles et al., 2005b; Papich, 2008; Sanderson et al., 2009), cats (Lascelles et al., 2007; Papich, 2008), horses (Goodrich & Nixon, 2006), and cattle (Smith et al., 2008) are available.

Acetaminophen (Paracetamol)

Although classified as an NSAID, acetaminophen may not impart its clinical effect through COX-1 or COX-2 inhibition. There is evidence that acetaminophen inhibits the COX-1 variant known as COX-3 (Chandrasekharan et al., 2002). It has been demonstrated that acetaminophen has minimal to no anti-inflammatory action because of its poor ability to inhibit COX in the presence of inflammatory mediators and byproducts of inflammation (Burk et al., 2006). One report demonstrated anti-inflammatory effects in dogs after orthopedic surgery, but the dose of acetaminophen used was higher than recommended (Mburu et al., 1988). Acetaminophen also has a disproportionate effect on COX in the brain, which may explain its strong anti-pyretic effects (Boutaud et al., 2002). Because acetaminophen has minimal effects on the gastrointestinal and renal systems when compared with classic NSAIDs, there are some who believe that acetaminophen works through non-COX pathways to provide analgesia (Papich, 2008). Acetaminophen has been used in dogs for analgesia and can be found in commercially available combinations with opioids, such as codeine, oxycodone, and hydrocodone. There is limited bioavailability of orally administered opioids in dogs, but there are anecdotal reports of efficacy of these combinations in some animals. Acetaminophen also has other uses. In dogs with certain ventricular arrhythmias, acetaminophen reduced the number of ectopic beats that developed during ischemia and reperfusion (Merrill et al., 2007). Acetaminophen has demonstrated anti-oxidant effects on low-density lipoproteins, also resulting in cardioprotection (Merrill & Goldberg, 2001; Chou & Greenspan, 2002).

There is the potential for serious adverse effects with the use of acetaminophen in veterinary patients. Acetaminophen is not approved for use in animals, and under no circumstances should acetaminophen be administered to a cat, domestic, exotic, or wild. A single 325 mg over-the-counter tablet may be lethal to the average domestic cat. Due to deficiencies in hepatic glucuronidation cats cannot metabolize acetaminophen in the liver with glucuronic acid. N-acetyl-p-benzoquinone forms and binds covalently to cellular molecules, ultimately resulting in hepatic necrosis. Other adverse effects that can occur in cats and dogs include methemoglobinemia and Heinz-body formation (McConkey et al., 2009). There is a case report of a dog that developed methemoglobinemia and Heinz-body hemolytic anemia after ingesting a toxic amount of acetaminophen. That dog was successfully treated with S-adenosyl-L-methionine and supportive care; thus, S-adenosyl-L-methionine may be an appropriate antidote for animals with acetaminophen toxicity (Wallace, 2002). There are minimal reports of the use of acetaminophen in horses, and its use in cattle is prohibited in the United States.

Aspirin

Aspirin is mainly a COX-1 inhibitor, and it irreversibly inactivates COX enzymes via acetylation (Dowling, 2010). This is distinct from other NSAIDs, and the duration of aspirin's effect is related to the turnover rate of the COX enzymes (Burk et al., 2006). Conversely, other NSAIDs work via competition with AA for binding sites, and their duration of action is related to drug concentration and disposition. Aspirin can be used as an analgesic for osteoarthritis in dogs (Lamont & Mathews, 2007), although it should be used cautiously as therapeutic concentrations are very close to toxic concentrations (Morton & Knottenbelt, 1989). Aspirin is associated with chondrodestruction, irreversible platelet dysfunction, and gastrointestinal bleeding and ulceration (Fox, 2010). Aspirin is also unique in that it induces the production of aspirin-triggered lipoxin (ATL) by the COX-2 enzyme in humans, and possibly in dogs (Papich, 2008). During chronic use of aspirin, ATL has a protective role in reducing inflammation and enhancing healing in the gastrointestinal tract (Papich, 2008). Production of ATL is thought to decrease the potential for further injury to the gastrointestinal tract with long-term use of aspirin (Souza et al., 2003). The addition of a stronger COX-2 inhibiting drug can result in loss of this adaptation and catastrophic ulceration. In cats, aspirin frequently causes gastric ulceration, does not predictably reduce thrombosis at therapeutic doses, and has not been evaluated for efficacy or safety for treatment of pain, fever, or inflammation (Lascelles et al., 2007). Aspirin has been used specifically for its effects on platelets in horses, and of all of the available NSAIDs, aspirin is the most effective for antiplatelet therapy (Cambridge et al., 1991). Suppression of COX-1 via aspirin also inhibits thromboxane A_2 production, which is necessary for platelet aggregation. In the equine, platelet thromboxane A_2 plays a minor role in aggregation of platelets, but aspirin still effectively abolishes aggregation (Heath et al., 1994). The antiplatelet effects of aspirin

have been used for the treatment of laminitis, disseminated intravascular coagulation, venous thrombosis, and equine verminous arteritis (Dowling, 2010). In cattle, aspirin has been used as an antipyretic and for inflammation associated with lower respiratory tract infections (Smith et al., 2008; Woolums et al., 2009). Aspirin has also been shown to reduce plasma cortisol concentrations in calves following castration (Coetzee et al., 2007). It is important to note that aspirin in not labeled for use in any animal in the United States, and its use in cattle is not recommended by the food animal residue avoidance and depletion (FARAD) program.

Carprofen

The use of carprofen in dogs was first reported in the early 1990s (Schmitt & Guentert, 1990; Nolan & Reid, 1993; Lascelles et al., 1994), and it is presently one of the most commonly used NSAIDs in dogs. Carprofen is the only NSAID licensed in the United States for dogs as both an oral and an injectable formulation, making it practical for perioperative use. In a review paper systematically evaluating study design, quality, criteria, consistency, relevance, and strength of evidence relating to management of canine osteoarthritis, the use of carprofen resulted in significant improvement and was supported by moderate evidence that the results could be extrapolated to the target population of dogs with osteoarthritis (Sanderson et al., 2009). Carprofen is considered more potent than aspirin or phenylbutazone for treatment of pain and inflammation, and may be safer than older NSAIDs (Fox & Johnston, 1997). The antithromboxane activity of carprofen appears to be minimal, suggesting that induced coagulopathy is less likely in patients with normal coagulation (Lamont & Mathews, 2007).

Shortly after carprofen was introduced there were several anecdotal reports of hepatic failure in dogs. Subsequently, a scientific report was published citing hepatocellular toxicosis in 21 dogs, 13 of which were Labrador Retrievers (MacPhail et al., 1998). It is believed that carprofen-associated hepatic toxicosis is idiosyncratic, and, when identified early, usually resolves after discontinuation of carprofen and administration of supportive care (MacPhail et al., 1998). It is recommended that dogs be prescreened for liver dysfunction prior to administration of carprofen, that owners be counseled as to clinical signs of toxicosis, and that carprofen be discontinued immediately if such signs are observed.

The use of carprofen in cats has been studied and pharmacokinetic data are available (Lascelles et al., 2007). Carprofen is labeled for single injection in cats in many European countries, Australia, and New Zealand. Carprofen is effective in cats for soft tissue and orthopedic pain (Al-Gizawiy & Rude, 2004; Mollenhoff et al., 2005). In healthy cats, a single dose of carprofen does not appear to cause gastrointestinal or renal lesions; however, toxicity is more likely with prolonged administration or in cats with concurrent systemic disease (Lascelles et al., 2007).

The use of carprofen in horses has been documented and it is licensed for use in horses in Europe. Pharmacokinetic and pharmacodynamic data for carprofen in horses are available (Lees et al., 1994). Carprofen is effective for treating visceral pain in horses (Schatzmann et al., 1992), and the duration of action is about 12 hours (Johnson et al., 1993). Carprofen may be most beneficial in the treatment of osteoarthritis (Clark-Price, 2009). When applied to chondrocytes, carprofen decreases production of inflammatory mediators, increases proteoglycan synthesis, and decreases glycosaminoglycan loss from cartilage (Armstrong & Lees, 1999;

Frean et al., 1999). In some European countries, carprofen is licensed for use in cattle for control of fever. In the United States, however, it would be difficult to justify its use over flunixin meglumine and, therefore, would most likely not be legal (Smith et al., 2008).

Deracoxib

Deracoxib was one of the first coxib-type drugs approved for veterinary use in the United States, and is approved as an oral formulation for control of postoperative and osteoarthritis pain in dogs. Deracoxib is effective in decreasing lameness and pain associated with synovitis, and pre-emptive administration decreased lameness scores in experimentally induced lameness in dogs (Millis et al., 2002). When first discovered, the coxib class of drugs was thought to have a decreased incidence of gastrointestinal adverse effects due to their relative COX-1 sparing effects. However, deracoxib has been associated with gastrointestinal perforation (Case et al., 2010), and it is recommended that deracoxib should only be used at approved dosages and never co-administered with corticosteroids or other NSAIDs (Lascelles et al., 2005a). The pharmacokinetics, but not clinical use, of deracoxib has been described in cats (Gassel et al., 2006).

Diclofenac

There are few publications describing the clinical use of diclofenac in dogs and cats, and with the approval of newer NSAIDs in these species, diclofenac is not commonly used. In the United States, diclofenac is approved for use in horses as a topically applied 1% liposomal cream. This formulation was developed for topical application to a localized area of inflammation, reducing frequency and severity of toxicity (Lynn et al., 2004); however, there is evidence of systemic absorption of the drug and the potential for systemic toxicity exists (Anderson et al., 2005). Diclofenac cream is efficacious for the treatment of osteoarthritis in horses (Frisbie et al., 2009), and may also be effective when applied over areas of soft tissue inflammation (Caldwell et al., 2004). It has also been used to decrease inflammation over catheter insertion sites (Levine et al., 2009). No formulation of diclofenac is approved for use in cattle in the United States.

Dipyrone

Dipyrone is thought to have a mechanism of action similar to acetaminophen. It is not approved for use in the United States; however, it is available by prescription in several European countries including Germany, Hungary, Italy, Portugal, and Spain. It is available as an over-the-counter preparation in Brazil, Bulgaria, Egypt, India, Israel, Mexico, Poland, Russia, and Turkey. Dipyrone is best used as an antipyretic, and is used in bacteremic neonatal foals. Dipyrone has been shown to induce blood dyscrasias in human patients, and should not be used in any animal that may enter the human food chain (Garbe, 2007).

Etodolac

Etodolac is labeled for use in dogs in the United States, and is effective for treatment of orthopedic conditions (Budsberg et al., 1999). Adverse effects of the drug appear to occur primarily in the gastrointestinal tract (Lamont & Mathews, 2007). Publications of use of etodolac in other veterinary species are sparse.

Firocoxib

Firocoxib is the only coxib-type NSAID approved for use in horses in the United States. It is available in tablet form for dogs and as an oral paste and intravenous injectable formulation for horses. Firocoxib is the most COX-1 sparing NSAID available in the United States for dogs. It is approved for osteoarthritis in dogs, and is effective in decreasing urate-induced synovitis, pain, inflammation, and lameness (Drag et al., 2007). In horses, the pharmacokinetics after single (Kvaternick et al., 2007) and multiple (Letendre et al., 2008) oral dosing have been described, and firocoxib is comparable in efficacy to phenylbutazone for treatment of osteoarthritis (Doucet et al., 2008). For horses with small intestinal colic, firocoxib may be preferred over flunixin meglumine, as it inhibits recovery of ischemia-injured mucosa to a lesser degree (Cook et al., 2009).

Flunixin Meglumine

Flunixin is considered moderately effective for the control of both soft tissue and orthopedic pain (Mathews et al., 1996), and decreases intraocular inflammation after ophthalmic surgery (Krohne & Vestre, 1987) in dogs. The systemic use of flunixin in dogs results in severe adverse effects including gastric ulceration, perforation, and peritonitis, increased plasma alanine aminotransferase activity and creatinine, and renal failure (Elwood et al., 1992; McNeil, 1992; Vonderhaar & Salisbury, 1993; Mathews et al., 1996). Flunixin meglumine has been used in cats and pharmacokinetic data are available (Lascelles et al., 2007); however, with the availability of safer NSAIDs approved for use in cats its use cannot be recommended. Flunixin is one of the more commonly used NSAIDs in horses (Hubbell et al., 2010), and can be administered orally, intravenously, or intramuscularly. Cases of myonecrosis have been reported with intramuscular use (Peek et al., 2003). Flunixin is efficacious for the treatment of osteoarthritic conditions (Goodrich & Nixon, 2006), and is comparable to phenylbutazone for the treatment of navicular syndrome (Erkert et al., 2005). When flunixin and phenylbutazone are combined, they are more effective in treating lameness than either NSAID administered alone (Keegan et al., 2008). Extreme caution should be used with concurrent administration as gastrointestinal ulceration and hypoproteinemia can result (Reed et al., 2006). Flunixin is mainly used for pain associated with gastrointestinal disease in the horse. In acute equine colic, flunixin provides less satisfactory analgesia than that obtained with the α-2 agonist detomidine (Jochle et al., 1989). Flunixin is currently the most commonly used NSAID in horses undergoing exploratory laparotomy for abdominal pain. There are conflicting reports of its effects on the intestinal mucosa after ischemic injury. One report demonstrated delayed recovery of the jejunal mucosa after ischemia and flunixin administration (Cook et al., 2009), whereas another study was not able to document an effect of flunixin on the recovery of colonic mucosa after ischemia (Matyjaszek et al., 2009). Concurrent administration of lidocaine ameliorated any inhibitory effects of flunixin meglumine on recovery of mucosa from ischemic injury, which may warrant the use of lidocaine as an adjunctive treatment to flunixin in horses with intestinal injury (Cook et al., 2008). Flunixin is also used in endotoxemic horses to decrease eicosanoid production. Administration of small doses of flunixin suppresses thromboxane B_2 and 6-keto-prostaglandin $F1_\alpha$ production associated with endotoxin administration, without masking the physical signs of endotoxemia that aid clinical evaluation of patient status (Semrad et al., 1987). In the United States, flunixin is the only NSAID labeled for use in cattle for treatment of pyrexia associated with respiratory tract disease, mastitis, and endotoxemia (Smith et al., 2008). Injections must be given intravenously, and administration by any other route is illegal.

Ketoprofen

Ketoprofen is a COX-1 selective NSAID that is effective in dogs for the treatment of orthopedic pain (Pibarot et al., 1997). Originally, ketoprofen was thought to inhibit LOX, but that has since been refuted (Goodrich & Nixon, 2006). Ketoprofen is only licensed for injection in horses in the United States. Ketoprofen has been used in dogs, but when compared with newer NSAIDs, such as carprofen, it has an increased incidence of adverse effects including prolonged bleeding times and gastric lesions (Luna et al., 2007). In fact, it is recommended that ketoprofen not be used when noncompressible bleeding may occur (Grisneaux et al., 1999), and that its use is restricted after laparotomy or thoracotomy until hemorrhage is no longer a concern (Lamont & Mathews, 2007). In a study using small doses of ketoprofen (0.25 mg/kg) in dogs, mild-to-moderate gastric lesions developed, although no adverse effects were noted on renal function or hemostasis (Narita et al., 2006). If ketoprofen is used in dogs, gastroprotectants should be coadministered (Lamont & Mathews, 2007). In cats, ketoprofen is effective in decreasing fever, and as an analgesic for acute surgical and chronic osteoarthritic pain (Lascelles et al., 2007). Excessive bleeding with ketoprofen administration does not seem to occur in cats (Slingsby & Waterman-Pearson, 1998), but renal insufficiency has been reported (Pages, 2005). In horses, ketoprofen has potent anti-inflammatory effects and accumulates in inflammatory exudates (Dowling, 2010) and inflamed joints (Owens et al., 1995). Ketoprofen is a good-to-excellent analgesic for musculoskeletal pain in horses (Goodrich & Nixon, 2006), and was superior to phenylbutazone for acute joint inflammation (Owens et al., 1996). Ketoprofen has a wider therapeutic index than phenylbutazone in the horse (Macallister et al., 1993), although oral bioavailability is poor (Dowling, 2010). Ketoprofen has been used in cattle, but its use has declined as it offers no benefit over flunixin meglumine, which is labeled for use in cattle in the United States (Smith et al., 2008).

Mavacoxib

Mavacoxib is a long-acting oral NSAID for dogs. The first two doses should be administered 14 days apart, and at 1-month intervals thereafter. The drug has a half-life of up to 38 days in dogs (Cox et al., 2010). Mavacoxib is available in many European countries, but is not available in the United States.

Meloxicam

Meloxicam is the only injectable NSAID approved for use in cats in the United States. It is available as an injectable formulation approved for use in dogs and for a single injection in cats, and also as an oral formulation approved for use in dogs only. Recently, the FDA announced a label change on the product and issued the following warning: "Repeated use of meloxicam in cats has been associated with acute renal failure and death. Do not administer additional injectable or oral meloxicam to cats." More information can be found at www.fda.gov. Interestingly, two recent retrospective studies found that long-term treatment with oral meloxicam did not appear to reduce the lifespan of cats with pre-existent stable chronic renal disease, nor did it worsen their renal disease (Gowan et al., 2011; Gowan et al., 2012). There is strong evidence that meloxicam provides a moderate level of analgesia in dogs with osteoarthritis (Sanderson et al., 2009). Long-term oral administration in dogs has been investigated and meloxicam was second only to carprofen in the lowest frequency of adverse gastrointestinal effects, followed by etodolac, flunixin, and ketoprofen (Luna et al., 2007). Additionally, meloxicam minimally affects hemostasis and is considered safe for perioperative use in dogs (Kazakos et al., 2005). Meloxicam may also have use as an antineoplastic agent (Wolfesberger et al., 2006). In horses, meloxicam has beneficial anti-inflammatory and analgesic effects when used as a treatment for acute synovitis (de Grauw et al., 2009). Although not approved for use in cattle in the United States, meloxicam decreases pain and distress after dehorning in dairy calves (Heinrich et al., 2010), and improves appetite and performance after a single injection at the onset of neonatal diarrhea complex (Todd et al., 2010).

Nimesulide

Nimesulide is a potent COX-2 preferential NSAID that is effective for the treatment of fever and lameness in dogs (Toutain et al., 2001). Nimesulide is available for use in dogs in France, but has been withdrawn from the market elsewhere due to serious hepatotoxicity and death in humans.

Phenylbutazone

Phenylbutazone is licensed for use in dogs in the United States but several safer NSAIDs are available and the use of phenylbutazone cannot be recommended. Adverse events associated with administration of phenylbutazone in dogs include gastrointestinal ulceration, gastroesophageal intussusception, pancytopenia, nonregenerative anemia, and thrombocytopenia (Watson et al., 1980; Badame et al., 1984; Lockwood et al., 2010). Similarly, phenylbutazone cannot be recommended for use in cats. Toxicity manifests as bone marrow suppression and gastrointestinal, renal, and hepatic injuries (Lascelles et al., 2007). The efficacy, availability, and affordability of phenylbutazone make it the most commonly used NSAID in horses (Goodrich & Nixon, 2006; Hubbell et al., 2010). It is available as parenteral and oral formulations. Care should be taken to avoid perivascular injection when administering phenylbutazone intravenously as it can result in tissue necrosis and sloughing (Dowling, 2010). Phenylbutazone is effective for the treatment of both soft tissue and bone pain in horses (Sanz et al., 2009; Foreman et al., 2008). Phenylbutazone has a prolonged half-life in horses and repeated dosing can extend the clinical efficacy well beyond the time when drug administration is discontinued, which could have implications for prepurchase examinations and competition (Dowling, 2010). Bioavailability after oral administration in the horse is high (~70%), and paste preparations may be more slowly absorbed, resulting in higher plasma concentrations after 24 hours (Tobin et al., 1986). Availability and ease of administration can lead to excessive dosing and toxic effects, particularly when horse owners, agents, and trainers have access to large quantities. Phenylbutazone has a narrow therapeutic index, particularly in very young, geriatric, and sick horses. It is imperative that veterinarians educate their clients about proper dosing and use of phenylbutazone. Reports of toxicity in horses include gastric ulceration, renal papillary necrosis, vascular thrombosis, oral ulceration, negative effects on bone healing, and right dorsal colitis (Gunson & Soma, 1983;

MacKay et al., 1983; MacAllister et al., 1993; Goodrich & Nixon, 2006; McConnico et al., 2008). More recently, the efficacy of suxibuzone, a prodrug of phenylbutazone, was evaluated (Sabate et al., 2009). It was shown to be a good alternative to phenylbutazone, as they were comparable in providing analgesia for lameness. It was thought that suxibuzone would have less irritating and ulcerogenic actions on the stomach than phenylbutazone, but that is not the case (Andrews et al., 2009). Use of phenylbutazone in cattle is illegal in the United States due to the potential for serious health hazards in humans (Smith et al., 2008).

Piroxicam

Piroxicam is not approved for use in veterinary patients and has little application as an analgesic as other NSAIDs with more favorable safety and efficacy profiles are available. Piroxicam has been used in dogs as a sole and adjunctive treatment for several different types of neoplasia that contain genes for expression of COX enzymes. Piroxicam, either combined with other chemotherapeutics or as a monotherapy in dogs, has been described for the treatment of transitional cell carcinoma (Knapp et al., 1994; Henry, 2003), mammary carcinoma (de M Souza et al., 2009), incompletely resected soft tissue sarcoma (Elmslie et al., 2008), and oral squamous cell carcinoma (Schmidt et al., 2001). There is the potential for gastric ulceration with the use of piroxicam and it is recommended that gastroprotectants be used concurrently (Knapp et al., 1994). In cats, piroxicam has been used in the treatment of similar neoplasias. There is a case report on the successful use of piroxicam for the treatment of squamous cell carcinoma in a horse (Moore et al., 2003).

Robenacoxib

Robenacoxib is a highly COX-2 selective coxib-type NSAID available in the United States and many European countries (King et al., 2010). It is licensed for dogs and cats, and is available as injectable and oral formulations in Europe. An oral formulation of robenacoxib has recently been approved for use in cats in the United States (Onsior®). It has high bioavailability after oral (84%) and subcutaneous administration (88%) in dogs (Jung et al., 2009). Robenacoxib improved weight bearing and decreased pain and swelling in an experimental model of joint inflammation in dogs (Schmid et al., 2010). Robenacoxib has demonstrated efficacy and tolerability in cats with signs of acute pain and inflammation associated with musculoskeletal disorders (Giraudel et al., 2010). Additionally, orally administered robenacoxib demonstrated no toxicological effects in cats, which may be related to the short residence time of the drug in the central compartment (King et al., 2012). There is no information available, to date, on use in other species.

Tepoxalin

Tepoxalin is unique in that it not only inhibits COX-1 and COX-2, but also LOX, thereby preventing synthesis of leukotrienes. Tepoxalin is approved for use in the United States for treatment of osteoarthritis in dogs and is administered as an oral wafer that dissolves in the mouth. Tepoxalin may also be more effective than carprofen or meloxicam for controlling uveitis in dogs (Gilmour & Lehenbauer, 2009). Dogs with atopic dermatitis had decreased pruritus when treated with tepoxalin (Horvath-Ungerboeck et al., 2009), and no adverse effects on hemostasis, renal, or hepatic function were noted after a single preoperative oral dose in healthy dogs undergoing anesthesia and surgery (Kay-Mugford et al., 2004).

NSAID USE IN BIRDS, EXOTIC, AND WILD ANIMALS

There is sparse information on the use of NSAIDs in nontraditional species, although individual case reports have described the use of NSAIDs in some. Information on NSAID use in birds is mostly extrapolated from studies in chickens (Machin, 2007) and can be found in the chapter on avian analgesia. A review on analgesia in exotic animals (Heard, 2001) is an excellent resource.

DOSAGES

Dosages of selected NSAIDS in dogs, cats, horses, and cattle can be found in the tables of this chapter (Tables 5.3–5.6). It is important to note that these are not recommended dosages, but what has been published in the literature or recommended by the manufacturer. A common recommendation is to use the lowest dose and least frequency of administration that is clinically effective. It is recommended that complete examination of all patients be performed prior to administration of NSAIDs or any other analgesic medication. The reader is referred to the references and species-specific chapters for dosages of NSAIDs used in other species.

CORTICOSTEROIDS

Corticosteroids are a class of steroid hormones that are produced in the adrenal cortex. They are involved in numerous physiological processes including the stress response, immune regulation, carbohydrate and protein metabolism, electrolyte balance, and

Table 5.3. Nonsteroidal anti-inflammatory drugs used in dogs

NSAID	Dosage
Acetaminophen	15 mg/kg PO, q8–12h
Aspirin	10 mg/kg PO, q12h
Carprofen	4.4 mg/kg PO, q24h
	2.2 mg/kg PO, q12–24h
	2.2 mg/kg SC, q12–24h
Deracoxib	1–2 mg/kg PO, q24h
Etodolac	10–15 mg/kg PO, q24h
Firocoxib	5 mg/kg, PO q24h
Ketoprofen	2 mg/kg IV, SC, IM once
	1 mg/kg IV, SC, IM q24h
Mavacoxib	2 mg/kg PO, q14d for 2 doses then
	2 mg/kg PO, q30d
Meloxicam	0.2 mg/kg IV, SC, PO once
	0.1 mg/kg IV, SC, PO, q24h
Nimesulide	5 mg/kg PO, q24h for up to 5 doses
Piroxicam	0.3 mg/kg q24h for 2 doses then q48h
Robenacoxib	1 mg/kg PO, q24h
Tepoxalin	10 mg/kg PO, q24h

Note: Use of some may be considered "off label". Approval of use varies depending on the country. Doses based on references in text. IM, intramuscular; IV, intravenous; PO, per os; SC, subcutaneous.

Table 5.4. Nonsteroidal anti-inflammatory drugs used in cats

NSAID	Dosage
Aspirin	10 mg/kg PO, q48h
Carprofen	4 mg/kg SC, once
Ketoprofen	2 mg/kg SC, q24h up to 3 doses
Meloxicam	0.3 mg/kg SC, once[a]
	0.1 mg/kg SC q24h up to 3 doses
Robenacoxib	1 mg/kg PO, q24h for 3–11 days (depends on the country)

Note: Use of some may be considered "off label". Approval of use varies depending on the country.

[a]Meloxicam approved for one-time use only in cats in the United States. Doses based on references in text. PO, per os; SC, subcutaneous.

modulation of inflammation. All corticosteroids have a similar four-ring structure composed of 17 carbon atoms. The main endogenous corticosteroid is cortisol, and it is the standard by which the potency of synthetic corticosteroids is compared. For example, dexamethasone is considered to be 25 times more potent and prednisone is considered to be four times more potent than cortisol (Schimmer & Parker, 2006). Corticosteroids are used clinically for a number of reasons. This discussion will be limited to the analgesic uses of this class of drugs.

Mechanism of Action

Corticosteroids have many effects on body systems through a myriad of mechanisms. They act on steroid-specific receptors and can upregulate or downregulate gene expression and protein synthesis (Schimmer & Parker, 2006). The main mechanism by which corticosteroids exert their analgesic effects is by decreasing inflammation. Corticosteroids inhibit phospholipase A2, which prevents

Table 5.5. Nonsteroidal anti-inflammatory drugs used in horses

NSAID	Dosage
Aspirin	10 mg/kg PO, q24h
Carprofen	0.7 mg/kg IV, q24h
Firocoxib	0.09 mg/kg IV, q24h up to 5 doses
	0.1 mg/kg PO, q24h for up to 14 days
Flunixin meglumine	1.1 mg/kg IV, q12–24h
	0.5 mg/kg IV, q12h
	0.25 mg/kg IV, q6–8h
	1.1 mg/kg PO, q12–24h
Ketoprofen	2–3 mg/kg IV, q24h
Phenylbutazone	2 mg/kg PO, q12h
	2 mg/kg IV, q12h

Note: Use of some may be considered "off label". Approval of use varies depending on the country. Doses based on references in text. PO, per os; IV, intravenous.

Table 5.6. Nonsteroidal anti-inflammatory drugs used in cattle

NSAID	Dosage
Aspirin	100 mg/kg PO, q12h
Flunixin meglumine	1 mg/kg IV, q12–24h
Ketoprofen	3 mg/kg IV, q24h

Note: Use of some may be considered "off label". Approval of use varies depending on the country. Doses based on references in text. IV, intravenous; PO, per os.

membrane phospholipid from entering the AA pathway, thereby inhibiting production of COX or LOX (Figure 5.1).

Caution must be used when administering corticosteroids as toxic effects can be profound. Adverse effects from inappropriate use of corticosteroids include impaired wound-healing, skin and connective tissue thinning, iatrogenic Cushing's disease (Salerno & Hermann, 2006), increased intraocular pressure and glaucoma (Francois, 1984), gastritis, intestinal ulceration and bleeding, fluid retention and hypertension (Jackson et al., 1981), decreased bone mineralization and osteonecrosis, and increased blood glucose and dysregulation of diabetes mellitus (Olefsky & Kimmerling, 1976). Most of these conditions have been described in humans, but can be expected to occur in veterinary patients as well. Of particular importance is the potential for severe gastrointestinal effects. Corticosteroids act synergistically with NSAIDs to increase the incidence of gastrointestinal events (Gabriel et al., 1991; Piper et al., 1991), and the combination should be avoided.

Clinical Use

Corticosteroids can be administered via almost any route. They are rapidly absorbed after oral administration with almost 100% bioavailability. Water-soluble formulations of corticosteroids can be given IV or IM to achieve high systemic concentrations quickly. Acetated formulations are insoluble in water, and are administered intramuscularly for slow absorption and prolonged duration of action (Salerno & Hermann, 2006). To reduce the risk of adverse effects associated with systemic administration of corticosteroids targeted therapy can be used. This includes depositing corticosteroids directly at the site of inflammation or pain. Intra-articular injection is commonly used for osteoarthritis therapy in horses (Goodrich & Nixon, 2006). Intra-articular injections in dogs have also been studied. Triamcinolone reduces the progression of osteoarthritis lesions in a ruptured cranial cruciate ligament model (Pelletier & Martel-Pelletier, 1991). Expression and synthesis of proteolytic enzymes is suppressed by injection of corticosteroids in experimental arthritis in dogs, and it has been suggested that intra-articular corticosteroids can be used both prophylactically and therapeutically (Pelletier et al., 1995). At least in humans, minimization of the frequency of intra-articular steroid injections is warranted, as repeated injection increases the incidence of painless joint destruction. It is recommended that intervals of at least 3 months be observed (Schimmer & Parker, 2006). Steroids administered via the epidural route in humans are efficacious for treatment of refractory back pain (Masini & Calaca, 2011) and lumbar disc prolapse (Singh et al., 2010). In dogs, epidural steroid application in cases of Hansen type II disc protrusion was similarly successful. Fluoroscopic-guided methylprednisolone acetate injection into the epidural space provided clinical outcomes similar to decompressive surgery, and may provide for a less invasive, alternative treatment (Janssens et al., 2009). Intrathecal injection may not have the same beneficial outcomes as epidural injection, as one study demonstrated histopathological changes that included inflammatory infiltrates, hemorrhage and necrosis in the spinal cord of dogs after betamethasone was injected intrathecally (Barros et al., 2007). Clearly, additional investigation into local application of steroids in spinal disease and pain are warranted.

SUMMARY

Inflammation is a key component in many acute and chronic pain states and anti-inflammatory drugs are central to appropriate multimodal analgesia. NSAIDs and corticosteroids are effective analgesic tools but must be used with consideration given to the patient's physiological status to avoid adverse effects.

REFERENCES

Al-Gizawiy, M.M. & Rude, E. (2004) Comparison of preoperative carprofen and postoperative butorphanol as postsurgical analgesics in cats undergoing ovariohysterectomy. *Veterinary Anaesthesia and Analgesia*, 31, 164–174.

Anderson, D., Kollias-Baker, C., Colahan, P., et al. (2005) Urinary and serum concentrations of diclofenac after topical application to horses. *Veterinary Therapeutics*, 6(1), 57–66.

Andrews, F.M., Reinemeyer, C.R., & Longhofer, S.L. (2009) Effects of top-dress formulations of suxibuzone and phenylbutazone on development of gastric ulcers in horses. *Veterinary Therapeutics*, 10(3), 113–120.

Armstrong, S. & Lees, P. (1999) Effects of R and S enantiomers and a racemic mixture of carprofen on the production and release of proteoglycan and prostaglandin E2 from equine chondrocytes and cartilage explants. *American Journal of Veterinary Research*, 60, 98–104.

Badame, F.G., Van Slyke, W., & Hayes, M.A. (1984) Reversible phenylbutazone-induces pancytopenia in a dog. *Canadian Veterinary Journal*, 25(6), 269–270.

Barros, G.A., Marques, M.E., & Ganem, E.M. (2007) The effects of intrathecal administration of betamethasone over the dogs' spinal cord and meninges. *Acta Cirurgica Brasileira*, 22(5), 361–365.

Basu, S. (2007) Novel cyclooxygenase-catalyzed bioactive prostaglandin $F_{2\alpha}$ from physiology to new principles in inflammation. *Medicinal Research Reviews*, 27(4), 435–468.

Bernal, W., Auzinger, G., Dhawan, A., et al. (2010) Acute liver failure. *Lancet*, 376(9736), 190–201.

Boutaud, O., Arnoff, D.M., Richardson, J.H., et al. (2002) Determinants of the cellular specificity of acetaminophen as an inhibitor of prostaglandin H(2) synthases. *Proceedings of the National Academy of Science USA*, 99(10), 7130–7135.

Brainard, B.M., Meredith, C.P., Callan, M.B., et al. (2007) Changes in platelet function, hemostasis, and prostaglandin expression after treatment with nonsteroidal anti-inflammatory drugs with various cyclooxygenase selectivities in dogs. *American Journal of Veterinary Research*, 68(3), 251–257.

Budsberg, S.C., Johnston, S.A., Schwarz, P.D., et al. (1999) Efficacy of etodolac for the treatment of osteoarthritis of the hip joints in dogs. *Journal of the American Veterinary Medical Association*, 214, 206–210.

Burk, A., Smyth, E., & FitzGerald, G.A. (2006) Analgesic-antipyretic agents; pharmacotherapy of gout in *Goodman and Gilman's the Pharmacologic Basis of Therapeutics*, 11th edn (eds L.L. Brunton, J.S. Lazo, & K.L. Parker), McGraw-Hill Companies, Inc., New York, pp. 671–715.

Caldwell, F.J., Mueller, P.O., Lynn, R.C., et al. (2004) Effect of topical application of diclofenac liposomal suspension on experimentally induced subcutaneous inflammation in horses. *American Journal of Veterinary Research*, 65(3), 271–276.

Cambridge, J., Lees, P., Hooke, R.E., et al. (1991) Antithrombotic actions of aspirin in the horse. *Equine Veterinary Journal*, 23, 123–127.

Camu, F., Beecher, T., Recker, D.P., et al. (2002) Valdecoxib, a COX-2 specific inhibitor, is an efficacious, opioid-sparing analgesic in patients undergoing hip arthroplasty. *American Journal of Therapeutics*, 9(1), 43–51.

Case, J.B., Fick, J.L., & Rooney, M.B. (2010) Proximal duodenal perforation in three dogs following deracoxib administration. *Journal of the American Animal Hospital Association*, 46, 255–258.

Chandrasekharan, N.V., Dai, H., Roos, K.L., et al. (2002) A cyclooxygenase-1 variant inhibited by acetaminophen and other analgesic/antipyretic drugs: cloning, structure, and expression. *Proceeding of the National Academy of Science USA*, 99(21), 13926–13931.

Chou, T.M. & Greenspan, P. (2002) Effect of acetaminophen in the myeloperoxidase-hydrogen peroxide-nitrate mediated oxidation of LDL. *Biochimica et Biophysica Acta*, 1581, 57–63.

Clark-Price, S.C. (2009) Intraarticular analgesia in the horse. Proceedings 15th International Veterinary Emergency and Critical Care Symposium, International Veterinary Emergency and Critical Care Society, Chicago, pp. 7–9.

Coetzee, J.F., Gehring, R., Bettenhausen, A.C., et al. (2007) Attenuation of acute plasma cortisol response in calves following intravenous sodium salicylate administration prior to castration. *Journal of Veterinary Pharmacology and Therapeutics*, 30(4), 305–313.

Cohen, H.J., March, D.J., & Kayser, B. (1983) Autoregulation in vasa recta of the rat kidney. *American Journal of Physiology*, 245, F32–F40.

Cook, V.L., Jones Shults, J., McDowell, M., et al. (2008) Attenuation of ischaemic injury in the equine jejunum by administration of systemic lidocaine. *Equine Veterinary Journal*, 40(4), 353–357.

Cook, V.L., Meyer, C.T., Campbell, N.B., et al. (2009) Effect of firocoxib or flunixin meglumine on recovery of ischemic-injured equine jejunum. *American Journal of Veterinary Research*, 70(8), 992–1000.

Cox, S.R., Lesman, S.P., Boucher, J.F., et al. (2010) The pharmacokinetics of mavacoxib, a long-acting COX-2 inhibitor, in young adult laboratory dogs. *Journal of Veterinary Pharmacology and Therapeutics*, 33(5), 461–470.

de Grauw, J.C., van de Lest, C.H., Brama, P.A., et al. (2009) In vivo effects of meloxicam on inflammatory mediators, MMP activity and cartilage biomarkers in equine joints with acute synovitis. *Equine Veterinary Journal*, 41(7), 693–699.

de M Souza, C.H., Toedo-Piza, E., Amorin, R., et al. (2009) Inflammatory mammary carcinoma in 12 dogs: clinical features, cyclooxygenase-2 expression, and response to piroxicam treatment. *Canadian Veterinary Journal*, 50(5), 506–510.

DeNovo, R.C. (2003) Diseases of the stomach, in *Handbook of Small Animal Gastroenterology*, 2nd edn (eds T.R. Tams), WB Saunders, Philadelphia, PA, pp. 160.

Doucet, M.Y., Bertone, A.L., Hendrickson, D., et al. (2008) Comparison of efficacy and safety of paste formulations of firocoxib and phenylbutazone in horses with naturally occurring osteoarthritis. *Journal of the American Veterinary Medical Association*, 232(1), 91–97.

Dowling, P.M. (2010) Nonsteroidal anti-inflammatory drugs, in *Equine Internal Medicine*, 3rd edn (eds A.M. Reed, W.M. Warwick, & D.C. Sellon), Saunders, St. Louis, MO, pp. 189–204.

Drag, M., Kunkle, B.N., Romano, D., et al. (2007) Firocoxib efficacy preventing urate-induced synovitis, pain, and inflammation in dogs. *Veterinary Therapeutics*, 8(1), 41–50.

Elmslie, R.E., Glawe, P., & Dow, S.W. (2008) Metronomic therapy with cyclophosphamide and piroxicam effectively delays tumor recurrence in dogs with incompletely resected soft tissue sarcomas. *Journal of Veterinary Internal Medicine*, 22(6), 1373–1379.

Elwood, C., Boswood, A., Simpson, K., et al. (1992) Renal failure after flunixin meglumine administration. *Veterinary Record*, 130(26), 582–583.

Erkert, R.S., MacAllister, C.G., Payton, M.E., et al. (2005) Use of force plate analysis to compare the analgesic effects of intravenous administration of phenylbutazone and flunixin meglumine in horses with navicular syndrome. *American Journal of Veterinary Research*, 66(2), 284–288.

FitzGerald, G.A. & Patrono, C. (2001) The coxibs, selective inhibitors of cyclooxygenase-2. *New England Journal of Medicine*, 345(6), 433–442.

Foreman, J.H., Barange, A., Lawrence, L.M., et al. (2008) Effects of single-dose intravenous phenylbutazone on experimentally induced, reversible lameness in the horse. *Journal of Veterinary Pharmacology and Therapeutics*, 31(1), 39–44.

Fox, S.M. (2010) Nonsteroidal anti-inflammatory drugs, in *Chronic Pain in Small Animal Medicine*, Manson Publishing, London, pp. 138–163.

Fox, S.M. & Johnston, S.A. (1997) Use of carprofen for the treatment of pain and inflammation in dogs. *Journal of the American Veterinary Medical Association*, 210(10), 1493–1498.

Francois, J. (1984) Corticosteroid glaucoma. *Ophthalmologica*, 188, 76–81.

Frean, S.P., Abraham, L.A., & Lees, P. (1999) In vitro stimulation of equine articular cartilage proteoglycan synthesis by hyaluronan and carprofen. *Research in Veterinary Science*, 67(2), 183–190.

Frisbie, D.D., McIlwraith, C.W., Kawcak, C.E., et al. (2009) Evaluation of topically administered diclofenac liposomal cream for treatment of horses with experimentally induced osteoarthritis. *American Journal of Veterinary Research*, 70(2), 210–215.

Gabriel, S.E., Jaakkimainen, L., & Bombardier, C. (1991) Risk for serious gastrointestinal complications related to use of nonsteroidal anti-inflammatory drugs. A meta-analysis. *Annuals of Internal Medicine*, 115, 787–796.

Garbe, E. (2007) Non-chemotherapy drug-induced agranulocytosis. *Expert Opinion on Drug Safety*, 6(3), 323–335.

Gassel, A.D., Tobias, K.M., & Cox, S.K. (2006) Disposition of deracoxib in cats after oral administration. *Journal of the American Animal Hospital Association*, 42(3), 212–217.

Gilmour, M.A. & Lehenbauer, T.W. (2009) Comparison of tepoxalin, carprofen, and meloxicam for reducing intraocular inflammation in dogs. *American Journal of Veterinary Research*, 70(7), 902–907.

Giraudel, J.M., Gruet, P., Alexander, D.G., et al. (2010) Evaluation of orally administered robenacoxib versus ketoprofen for treatment of acute pain and inflammation associated with musculoskeletal

disorders in cats. *American Journal of Veterinary Research*, 71(7), 710–719.

Goodman, L., Torres, B., Punke, J., et al. (2009) Effects of firoxocib and tepoxalin on healing in a canine gastric mucosal injury model. *Journal of Veterinary Internal Medicine*, 23(1), 56–62.

Goodrich, L.R. & Nixon, A.J. (2006) Medical treatment of osteoarthritis in the horse – A review. *Veterinary Journal*, 171, 51–69.

Gowan, R.A., Lingard, A.E., Johnston, L., et al. (2011) Retrospective case-control study of the effects of long-term dosing with meloxicam on renal function in aged cats with degenerative joint disease. *Journal of Feline Medicine and Surgery*, 13(10), 752–761.

Gowan, R.A., Baral, R.M., Lingard, A.E., et al. (2012) A retrospective analysis of the effects of meloxicam on the longevity of aged cats with and without overt chronic kidney disease. *Journal of Feline Medicine and Surgery*, 14(12), 876–881.

Grisneaux, E., Pibarot, P., Dupuis, J., et al. (1999) Comparison of ketoprofen and carprofen administered prior to orthopedic surgery for control of postoperative pain in dogs. *Journal of the American Veterinary Medical Association*, 215(8), 1105–1110.

Gunson, D.R. & Soma, L.R. (1983) Renal papillary necrosis in horses after phenylbutazone and water deprivation. *Veterinary Pathology*, 20, 603–610.

Halter, F., Tarnawski, A.S., Schmassmann, A., et al. (2001) Cyclooxygenase 2-implications on maintenance of gastric mucosal integrity and ulcer healing: controversial issues and perspectives. *Gut*, 49, 443–453.

Heard, D.J. (2001) Analgesia and anesthesia. *Veterinary Clinics of North America: Exotic Animal Practice*, 4(1), 83–117.

Heath, M.F., Evans, R.J., Poole, A.W., et al. (1994) The effects of aspirin and paracetamol on the aggregation of equine blood platelets. *Journal of Veterinary Pharmacology and Therapeutics*, 17(5), 374–378.

Heinrich, A., Duffield, T.F., Lissemore, K.D., et al. (2010) The effect of meloxicam on behavior and pain sensitivity of dairy calves following cautery dehorning with a local anesthetic. *Journal of Dairy Science*, 93(6), 2450–2457.

Hellyer, P.W., Roberston, S.A., Fails, A.D. (2007) Pain and its management, in *Lumb & Jones' Veterinary Anesthesia and Analgesia*, 4th edn (eds W.J. Tranquilli, J.C. Thurmon, & K.A. Crimm), Blackwell Publishing, Ames, IA, pp. 31–57.

Henry, C.J. (2003) Management of transitional cell carcinoma. *Veterinary Clinics of North America: Small Animal Practice*, 33(3), 597–613.

Hersh, E.V., Lally, E.T., & Moore, P.A. (2005) Update on cyclooxygenase inhibitors: has a third COX isoform entered the fray? *Current Medical Research and Opinion*, 21(8), 1217–1226.

Higgins, A.J. & Lees, P. (1984) The acute inflammatory process, arachidonic acid metabolism and the mode of action of anti-inflammatory drugs. *Equine Veterinary Journal*, 16(3), 163–175.

Horvath-Ungerboeck, C., Thoday, K.L., Shaw, D.J., et al. (2009) Tepoxalin reduces pruritus and modified CADESI-01 scores in dogs with atopic dermatitis: a prospective, randomized, double-blinded, placebo-controlled, cross-over study. *Veterinary Dermatology*, 20(4), 233–242.

Hough, M.E., Steel, C.M., Bolton, J.R., et al. (1999) Ulceration and stricture of the right dorsal colon after phenylbutazone administration in four horses. *Australian Veterinary Journal*, 77(12), 785–788.

Hubbell, J.A., Saville, W.J., Bednarski, R.M. (2010) The use of sedatives, analgesic and anaesthetic drugs in the horse: an electronic survey of members of the American Association of Equine Practitioners (AAEP). *Equine Veterinary Journal*, 42(6), 487–493.

Jackson, S.H., Beevers, D.G., & Myers, K. (1981) Does long-term low-dose corticosteroid therapy cause hypertension? *Clinical Science (London)*, 61 Supplement, 381s–383s.

Janssens, L., Beosier, Y., & Daems, R. (2009) Lumbosacral degenerative stenosis in the dog. The results of epidural infiltration with methylprednisolone acetate: a retrospective study. *Veterinary and Comparative Orthopaedics and Traumatology*, 22(6), 486–491.

Jochle, W., Moore, J.N., Brown, J., et al. (1989) Comparison of detomidine, butorphanol, flunixin meglumine and xylazine in clinical cases of equine colic. *Equine Veterinary Journal Supplement*, 7, 111–116.

Johnson, C.B., Taylor, P.M., Young, S.S., et al. (1993) Postoperative analgesia using phenylbutazone, flunixin or carprofen in horses. *Veterinary Record*, 133, 336–338.

Jung, M., Lees, P., Seewald, W., et al. (2009) Analytical determination and pharmacokinetics of robenacoxib in the dog. *Journal of Veterinary Pharmacology and Therapeutics*, 32(1), 41–48.

Kay-Mugford, P.A., Grimm, K.A., Weingarten, A.J., et al. (2004) Effect of preoperative administration of tepoxalin on hemostasis and hepatic and renal function in dogs. *Veterinary Therapy*, 5(2), 120–127.

Kazakos, G.M., Papazoglou, L.G., Rallis, T., et al. (2005) Effects of meloxicam on the haemostatic profile of dogs undergoing orthopaedic surgery. *Veterinary Record*, 157(15), 444–446.

Keegan, K.G., Messer, N.T., Reed, S.K., et al. (2008) Effectiveness of administration of phenylbutazone alone or concurrent administration of phenylbutazone and flunixin meglumine to alleviate lameness in horses. *American Journal of Veterinary Research*, 69(2), 167–173.

Khanapure, S.P., Garvey, D.S., Janero, D.R., et al. (2007) Eicosanoids in inflammation: biosynthesis, pharmacology, and therapeutic frontiers. *Current Topics in Medicinal Chemistry*, 7, 311–340.

King, J.N., Hotz, R., Reagan, E.L., et al. (2012) Safety of oral robenacoxib in the cat. *Journal of Veterinary Pharmacology and Therapeutics*, 35(3), 290–300.

King, J.N., Rudaz, C., Borer, L., et al. (2010) In vitro and ex vivo inhibition of canine cyclooxygenase isoforms by robenacoxib: a comparative study. *Research in Veterinary Science*, 88(3), 497–506.

Kis, B., Snipes, J.A., & Busija, D.W. (2005a) Acetaminophen and the cyclooxygenase-3 puzzle: sorting out facts, fictions, and uncertainties. *Journal of Pharmacology and Experimental Therapeutics*, 315(1), 1–7.

Kis, B., Snipes, J.A., Smandle, S.A., et al. (2005b) Acetaminophen-sensitive prostaglandin production in rat cerebral endothelial cells. *American Journal of Physiology - Regulatory, Integrative and Comparative Physiology*, 288(4), R897–R902.

Kis, B., Snipes, J.A., Gaspar, T., et al. (2006) Cloning of cyclooxygenase-1b (putative COX-3) in mouse. *Inflammation Research*, 55(7), 274–278.

Knapp, D.W., Richardson, R.C., Chan, T.C., et al. (1994) Piroxicam therapy in 34 dogs with transitional cell carcinoma of the urinary bladder. *Journal of Veterinary Internal Medicine*, 8, 273–278.

Krohne, S.D. & Vestre, W.A. (1987) Effects of flunixin meglumine and dexamethasone on aqueous protein values after intraocular surgery in the dog. *American Journal of Veterinary Research*, 48(3), 420–422.

Kujubu, D.A., Fletcher, B.S., Varnum, B.C., et al. (1991) TIS10, a phorbol ester tumor promoter-inducible mRNA from Swiss 3T3 cells, encodes a novel prostaglandin synthase/cyclooxygenase homologue. *The Journal of Biological Chemistry*, 266(20), 12866–12872.

Kurmis, A.P., Kurmis, T.P., O'Brien, J.X., et al. (2012) The effect of nonsteroidal anti-inflammatory drug administration on acute phase fracture healing: a review. *The Journal of Joint and Bone Surgery*, 94(9), 815–823.

Kvaternick, V., Pollmeier, M., Fischer, J., et al. (2007) Pharmacokinetics and metabolism of orally administered firocoxib, a novel second generation coxib, in horses. *Journal of Veterinary Pharmacology and Therapeutics*, 30(3), 208–217.

Lamont, L.A. & Mathews, K.A. (2007) Opioids, nonsteroidal anti-inflammatories, and analgesic adjuvants, in *Lumb & Jones' Veterinary Anesthesia and Analgesia*, 4th edn (eds W.J. Tranquilli, J.C. Thurmon, & K.A. Grimm), Blackwell Publishing, Ames, IA, pp. 241–271.

Lascelles, B.D., Butterworth, S.J., & Waterman, A.E. (1994) Postoperative analgesic and sedative effects of carprofen and pethidine in dogs. *Veterinary Record*, 134(8), 187–191.

Lascelles, B.D.X., Court, M.H., Hardie, E.M., et al. (2007) Nonsteroidal anti-inflammatory drugs in cats: a review. *Veterinary Anaesthesia and Analgesia*, 34, 228–250.

Lascelles, B.D., Blikslager, A.T., Fox, S.M., et al. (2005a) Gastrointestinal tract perforation in dogs treated with a selective cyclooxygenase-2 inhibitor: 29 cases (2002–2003). *Journal of the American Veterinary Medical Association*, 227(7), 1112–1117.

Lascelles, B.D.X., McFarland, M.J., & Swann, H. (2005b) Guidelines for safe and effective use of NSAIDs in dogs. *Veterinary Therapeutics*, 6(3), 237–251.

Lees, P., Creed, R.F., Gerring, E.E., et al. (1983) Biochemical and haematological effects of phenylbutazone in horses. *Equine Veterinary Journal*, 15(2), 158–167.

Lees, P., McKellar, Q., May, S.A., et al. (1994) Pharmacodynamics and pharmacokinetics of carprofen in the horse. *Equine Veterinary Journal*, 26, 203–208.

Legler, D.F., Bruckner, M., Uetz-von Allmen, E., et al. (2010) Prostaglandin E_2 at new glance: novel insights in functional diversity offer therapeutic chances. *The International Journal of Biochemistry & Cell Biology*, 42, 198–201.

Letendre, L.T., Tessman, R.K., McClure, S.R., et al. (2008) Pharmacokinetics of firocoxib after administration of multiple consecutive daily doses to horses. *American Journal of Veterinary Research*, 69(11), 1399–1405.

Levine, D.G., Epstein, K.L., Neelis, D.A., et al. (2009) Effect of topical application of 1% diclofenac sodium liposomal cream on inflammation in healthy horses undergoing intravenous regional limb perfusion with amikacin sulfate. *American Journal of Veterinary Research*, 70(11), 1323–1325.

Li, J., Lynch, M.P., Demello, K.L., et al. (2005) In vitro and in vivo profile of 2-(3-di-fluoromethyl-5-phenylpyrazol-1-yl)-5-methanesulfonylpyridine, a potent, selective, and orally active canine COX-2 inhibitor. *Bioorganic & Medicinal Chemistry*, 13, 1805–1809.

Lockwood, A., Radlinsky, M., & Crochik, S. (2010) Gastroesophageal intussusception in a German Shepherd. *Compendium Continuing Education for Veterinarians*, 32(7), E1–E4.

Luna, S.P.L., Basilio, A.C., Steagall, P.V.M., et al. (2007) Evaluation of adverse effects of long-term oral administration of carprofen, etodolac, flunixin meglumine, ketoprofen, and meloxicam in dogs. *American Journal of Veterinary Research*, 68(3), 258–264.

Lynn, R.C., Hepler, D.I., Kelch, W.J., et al. (2004) Double-blinded placebo-controlled clinical field trial to evaluate the safety and efficacy of topically applied 1% diclofenac liposomal cream for the relief of lameness in horses. *Veterinary Therapeutics*, 5(2), 128–138.

MacAllister, C.G., Morgan, S.J., Borne, A.T., et al. (1993) Comparison of adverse effects of phenylbutazone, flunixin meglumine, and ketoprofen in horses. *Journal of the American Veterinary Medical Association*, 202, 71–77.

Machin, K.L. (2007) Wildlife analgesia, in *Zoo Animal & Wildlife Immobilization and Anesthesia* (eds G. West, D. Heard, & N. Caulkett), Blackwell Publishing, Ames, IA, pp. 43–59.

MacKay, R.J., French, T.W., Nguyen, H.T., et al. (1983) Effects of large doses of phenylbutazone administration to horses. *American Journal of Veterinary Research*, 44, 774–780.

MacPhail, C.M., Lappin, M.R., Meyer, D.J., et al. (1998) Hepatocellular toxicosis associated with administration of carprofen in 21 dogs. *Journal of the American Veterinary Medical Association*, 212(12), 1895–1901.

Masini, M. & Calaca, A. (2011) Minimally invasive treatment for refractory low back pain, targeted by epidural endoscopy with $O(2)/O(3)$ and steroid therapy. *Acta Neurochirurgica Supplement*, 108, 33–37.

Mathews, K.A., Paley, D.M., Foster, R.A., et al. (1996) A comparison of ketorolac with flunixin, butorphanol, and oxymorphone in controlling postoperative pain in dogs. *Canadian Veterinary Journal*, 37(9), 557–567.

Mattia, C. & Coluzzi, F. (2009) What anesthesiologists should know about paracetamol (acetaminophen). *Minerva Anesthesiologica*, 75(11), 644–653.

Matyjaszek, S.A., Morton, A.J., Freeman, D.E., et al. (2009) Effects of flunixin meglumine on recovery of colonic mucosa from ischemia in horses. *American Journal of Veterinary Research*, 70(2), 236–246.

Mburu, D.N., Mbugua, S.W., Skoglund, L.A., et al. (1988) Effects of paracetamol and acetylsalicylic acid on the post-operative course after experimental orthopaedic surgery in dogs. *Journal of Veterinary Pharmacology and Therapeutics*, 11(2), 163–170.

McConkey, S.A., Grant, D.M., & Cribb, A.E. (2009) The role of para-aminophenol in acetaminophen-induced methemoglobinemia in dogs and cats. *Journal of Veterinary Pharmacology and Therapeutics*, 32(6), 585–595.

McConnico, R.S., Morgan, T.W., Williams, C.C., et al. (2008) Pathophysiologic effects of phenylbutazone on the right dorsal colon in horses. *American Journal of Veterinary Research*, 69(11), 1496–1505.

McNeil, P.E. (1992) Acute tubule-interstitial nephritis in a dog after halothane anaesthesia and administration of flunixin meglumine and trimethoprim-sulphadiazine. *Veterinary Record*, 131(7), 148–151.

Merrill, G.F. & Goldberg, E. (2001) Antioxidant properties of acetaminophen and cardioprotection. *Basic Research in Cardiology*, 96, 423–430.

Merrill, G.F., Merrill, J.H., Golfetti, R., et al. (2007) Antiarrhythmic properties of acetaminophen in the dog. *Experimental Biology and Medicine*, 232(9), 1245–1252.

Millis, D.L., Weigel, J.P., Moyers, T., et al. (2002) Effect of deracoxib, a new COX-2 inhibitor, on the prevention of lameness induced by chemical synovitis in dogs. *Veterinary Therapeutics*, 3(4), 453–464.

Mollenhoff, A., Nolte, I., & Kramer, S. (2005) Anti-nociceptive efficacy of carprofen, levomethadone and buprenorphine for pain relief in cats following major orthopaedic surgery. *Journal of Veterinary Medicine. A, Physiology, Pathology, Clinical Medicine*, 52, 186–198.

Monaon, D.G., Vazquez, J., Jauregui, J.R., et al. (2010) Pain treatment in post-traumatic hip fracture in the elderly: regional block vs. systemic non-steroidal analgesics. *International Journal of Emergency Medicine*, 3(4), 321–325.

Moore, A.S., Beam, S.L., Rassnick, K.M., et al. (2003) Long-term control of mucocutaneous squamous cell carcinoma and metas-

tases in a horse using piroxicam. *Equine Veterinary Journal*, 35(7), 715–718.

Morton, D.J. & Knottenbelt, D.C. (1989) Pharmacokinetics of aspirin and its application in canine veterinary medicine. *Journal of the South African Veterinary Association*, 60(4), 191–194.

Mukherjee, D., Nissen, S.E., & Topol, E.J. (2001) Risk of cardiovascular events associated with selective COX-2 inhibitors. *Journal of the American Medical Association*, 286(8), 954–959.

Munoz, J., Navarro, C., Noriega, V., et al. (2010) Synergism between COX-3 inhibitors in two animal models of pain. *Inflammopharmacology*, 18(2), 65–71.

Nakagawa, K., Yamagami, T., & Takemura, N. (2005) Hepatocellular toxicosis associated with the alternate administration of carprofen and meloxicam in a Siberian Husky. *Journal of Veterinary Medical Science*, 67(10), 1051–1053.

Narita, T., Sato, R., Tomizawa, N., et al. (2006) Safety of reduced-dosage ketoprofen for long-term oral administration in healthy dogs. *American Journal of Veterinary Research*, 67(7), 1115–1120.

Nolan, A. & Reid, J. (1993) Comparison of the postoperative analgesic and sedative effects of carprofen and papaveretum in the dog. *Veterinary Record*, 133(10), 240–242.

Ochi, H., Hara, Y., Asou, Y., et al. (2011) Effects of long-term administration of carprofen on healing of a tibial osteotomy in dogs. *American Journal of Veterinary Research*, 72(5), 634–641.

Oguma, T., Asano, K., & Ishizaka, A. (2008) Role of prostaglandin D_2 and its receptors in the pathophysiology of asthma. *Allergology International*, 57(4), 307–312.

Olefsky, J.M. & Kimmerling, G. (1976) Effects of glucocorticoids on carbohydrate metabolism. *American Journal of Medical Science*, 271(2), 202–210.

Owens, J.G., Kamerling, S.G., Barker, S.A., et al. (1995) Pharmacokinetics of ketoprofen in healthy horses and horses with acute synovitis. *Journal of Veterinary Pharmacology and Therapeutics*, 18, 187–195.

Owens, J.G., Kamerling, S.G., Stanton, S.R., et al. (1996) Effects of pretreatment with ketoprofen and PBZ on experimentally induced synovitis in horses. *American Journal of Veterinary Research*, 57, 866–874.

Pages, J.P. (2005) Nephropaties dues aux anti-inflammatoires non steroidiens (AINS) chez le Chat: 21 observations (1993–2001). *Pratique Medicale Et Chirurgicale De L'Anim Compagnie*, 40, 177–181.

Papich, M.G. (2008) An update on nonsteroidal anti-inflammatory drugs (NSAIDs) in small animals. *Veterinary Clinics of North America: Small Animal Practice*, 38(6), 1243–1266.

Peek, S.F., Semrad, S.D., & Perkins, G.A. (2003) Clostridial myonecrosis in horses (37 cases 1985–2000). *Equine Veterinary Journal*, 35, 86–92.

Pelletier, J.P., DiBattista, J.A., Raynauld, J.P., et al. (1995) The in vivo effects of intraarticular corticosteroid injections on cartilage lesions, stromelysin, interleukin-1, and oncogene protein synthesis in experimental osteoarthritis. *Laboratory Investigation*, 72(5), 578–586.

Pelletier, J.P. & Martel-Pelletier, J. (1991) In vivo protective effects of prophylactic treatment with tiaprofenic acid or intraarticular corticosteroids on osteoarthritic lesions in the experimental dog model. *Journal of Rheumatology Supplement*, 27, 127–130.

Pibarot, P., Dupuis, J., Grisneaux, E., et al. (1997) Comparison of ketoprofen, oxymorphone hydrochloride, and butorphanol in the treatment of postoperative pain in dogs. *Journal of the American Veterinary Medical Association*, 211(4), 438–444.

Pillinger, M.H., Capodici, C., Rosenthal, P., et al. (1998) Modes of action of aspirin-like drugs: salicylates inhibit Erk activation and integrin-dependent neutrophil adhesion. *Proceedings of the National Academy of Science of The United States of America*, 95, 14540–14545.

Piper, J.M., Ray, W.A., Daugherty, J.R., et al. (1991) Corticosteroid use and peptic ulcer disease: role of nonsteroidal anti-inflammatory drugs. *Annals of Internal Medicine*, 114, 735–740.

Pountos, I., Georgouli, T., Bird, H., et al. (2011) The effect of antibiotics on bone healing: current evidence. *Expert Opinion of Drug Safety*, 10(6), 935–945.

Pountos, I., Georgouli, T., Blokhuis, T.J., et al. (2008) Pharmacological agents and impairment of fracture healing: what is the evidence? *Injury*, 39(4), 384–394.

Pountos, I., Georgouli, T., Calori, G., et al. (2012) Do nonsteroidal anti-inflammatory drugs affect bone healing? A critical analysis. *The Scientific World Journal*, 2012;2012:606404 doi:10.1100/2012/606404.

Pratico, D. & Dogne, J. (2009) Vascular biology of eicosanoids and atherogenesis. *Expert Reviews in Cardiovascular Therapy*, 7(9), 1079–1089.

Reed, S.K., Messer, N.T., Tessman, R.K., et al. (2006) Effects of phenylbutazone alone or in combination with flunixin meglumine on blood protein concentrations in horses. *American Journal of Veterinary Research*, 76(3), 398–402.

Sabate, D., Homedes, J., Salichs, M., et al. (2009) Multicentre, controlled, randomized and blinded field study comparing efficacy of suxibuzone and phenylbutazone in lame horses. *Equine Veterinary Journal*, 41(7), 700–705.

Salerno, A. & Hermann, R. (2006) Efficacy and safety of steroid use for postoperative pain relief. Update and review of the medical literature. *Journal of Bone & Joint Surgery*, 88(6), 1361–1372.

Sanderson, R.O., Beata, C., Flipo, R-M., et al. (2009) Systematic review of the management of canine osteoarthritis. *Veterinary Record*, 164, 418–424.

Sanz, M.G., Sellon, D.C., Cary, J.A., et al. (2009) Analgesic effects of butorphanol tartrate and phenylbutazone administered alone and in combination in young horses undergoing routine castration. *Journal of the American Veterinary Medical Association*, 235(10), 1194–1203.

Schatzmann, U., Gugelmann, M., & Cranach, J. (1992) Visceral and peripheral pain detection models in the horse, using flunixin and carprofen, in *Animal Pain* (eds C.E. Short & A. Poznak), Saunders, pp. 411–420.

Schimmer, B.P. & Parker, K.L. (2006) Adrenocorticotropic hormone; adrenocortical steroids and their synthetic analogs; inhibitors of the synthesis and actions of adrenocortical hormones, in *Goodman and Gilman's the Pharmacologic Basis of Therapeutics*, 11th edn (eds L.L. Brunton, J.S. Lazo, & K.L. Parker), McGraw-Hill Companies, Inc., New York, pp. 1587–1612.

Schmassmann, A., Zoidl, G., Peskar, B.M., et al. (2006) Role of the different isoforms of cyclooxygenase and nitric oxide synthase during gastric ulcer healing in cyclooxygenase-1 and -2 knockout mice. *American Journal of Physiology – Gastrointestinal and Liver Physiology*, 290, G747–G756.

Schmid, V.B., Spreng, D.E., Seewald, W., et al. (2010) Analgesic and anti-inflammatory actions of robenacoxib in acute joint inflammation in dog. *Journal of Veterinary Pharmacology and Therapeutics*, 33(2), 118–131.

Schmidt, B.R., Glickman, N.W., DeNicola, D.B., et al. (2001) Evaluation of piroxicam for the treatment of oral squamous cell carcinoma in dogs. *Journal of the American Veterinary Medical Association*, 218(11), 1783–1786.

Schmitt, M. & Guentert, T.W. (1990) Biopharmaceutical evaluation of carprofen following single intravenous, oral, and rectal doses in dogs. *Biopharmaceutics & Drug Disposition*, 11(7), 585–594.

Seibert, K., Masferrer, J., Zhang, Y., et al. (1995) Medication of inflammation by cyclooxygenase-2. *Agents and Actions Supplement*, 46, 41–50.

Seibert, K., Zhang, Y., Leahy, K., et al. (1997) Distribution of COX-1 and COX-2 in normal and inflamed tissues. *Advances in Experimental Medicine and Biology*, 400A, 167–170.

Semrad, S.D., Hardee, G.E., Hardee, M.M., et al. (1987) Low dose flunixin meglumine: effects on eicosanoid production and clinical signs induced by experimental endotoxaemia in horses. *Equine Veterinary Journal*, 19(3), 201–206.

Simmons, D.L., Botting, R.M., & Hla, T. (2004) Cyclooxygenase isozymes: the biology of prostaglandin synthesis and inhibition. *Pharmacological Reviews*, 56(3), 387–437.

Simmons, D.L., Chandrasekharan, N.V., Hu, D., et al. (2005) Comments of "Acetaminophen and the cyclooosygenase-3 puzzle: sorting out facts, fictions, and uncertainties." *Journal of Pharmacology and Experimental Therapeutics*, 315(3), 1412–1414.

Singh, H., Kaur, M., Nagpal, S., et al. (2010) Role of caudal epidural steroid injections in lumbar disc prolapsed. *Journal of the Indian Medical Association*, 108(5), 287–288, 290–291.

Slingsby, L.S. & Waterman-Pearson, A.E. (1998) Comparison of pethidine, buprenorphine and ketoprofen for postoperative analgesia after ovariohysterectomy in the cat. *Veterinary Record*, 143, 185–189.

Smith, G.W., Davis, J.L., Tell, L.A., et al. (2008) Extra label use of nonsteroidal anti-inflammatory drugs in cattle. *Journal of the American Veterinary Medical Association*, 232(5), 697–701.

Smith, S.A., Tobias, A.H., Jacob, K.A., et al. (2003) Arterial thromboembolism in cats: acute crisis in 127 cases (1992–2001) and long-term management with low-dose aspirin in 24 cases. *Journal of Veterinary Internal Medicine*, 17(1), 73–83.

Souza, M.H., de Lima, O.M., Zamuner, S.R., et al. (2003) Gastritis increases resistance to aspirin-induced mucosal injury via COX-2-mediated lipoxin synthesis. *American Journal of Physiology – Gastrointestinal & Liver Physiology*, 285(1), G54–G61.

Stoelting, R.K. & Hillier, S.C. (2006) Cyclooxygenase-2 inhibitors and nonspecific nonsteroidal anti-inflammatory drugs, in *Pharmacology & Physiology in Anesthetic Practice*, 4th edn, Lippincott Williams & Wilkins, Philadelphia, PA, pp. 276–291

Streppa, H.K., Jones, C.J., & Budsberg, S.C. (2002) Cyclooxygenase selectivity of nonsteroidal anti-inflammatory drugs in canine blood. *American Journal of Veterinary Research*, 63, 91–94.

Tizard, I.R. (2009) How inflammation is triggered, in *Veterinary Immunology*, 8th edn, Saunders, St. Louis, MO, pp. 11–27.

Tobin, T., Chay, S., Kamerling, S., et al. (1986) Phenylbutazone in the horse: a review. *Journal of Veterinary Pharmacology and Therapeutics*, 9(1), 1–25.

Todd, C.G., Millman, S.T., McKnight, D.R., et al. (2010) Nonsteroidal anti-inflammatory drug therapy for neonatal calf diarrhea complex: Effects on calf performance. *Journal of Animal Science*, 88(6), 2019–2028.

Toutain, P.L., Cester, C.C., Haak, T., et al. (2001) A pharmacokinetic/pharmacodynamic approach vs. a dose titration for the determination of a dosage regimen: the case of nimesulide, a Cox-2 selective nonsteroidal anti-inflammatory drug in the dog. *Journal of Veterinary Pharmacology and Therapeutics*, 24(1), 43–55.

Vane, J.R. (1971) Inhibition of prostaglandin synthesis as a mechanism of action for aspiring-like drugs. *Nature: New Biology*, 231(25), 232–235.

Vane, J.R. & Botting, R.M. (1998) Anti-inflammatory drugs and their mechanism of action. *Inflammation Research*, 47(Suppl. 2), S78–S87.

Vonderhaar, M.A. & Salisbury, S.K. (1993) Gastroduodenal ulceration associated with flunixin meglumine administration in three dogs. *Journal of the American Veterinary Medical Association*, 203(1), 92–95.

Wallace, K.P., Center, S.A., Hickford, F.H., Warner, K. L., Smith, S. (2002) S-adenosyl-L-methionine (SAMe) for the treatment of acetaminophen toxicity in a dog. *Journal of the American Animal Hospital Association*, 38(3), 246–254.

Warner, T.S. & Mitchell, J.A. (2004) Cyclooxygenases: new forms, new inhibitors, and lesions from the clinic. *The FASEB Journal*, 18, 790–804.

Watson, A.D., Wilson, J.T., & Turner, D.M. (1980) Phenylbutazone-induced blood dyscrasias suspected in three dogs. *Veterinary Record*, 107(11), 239–241.

Wolfesberger, B., Walter, I., Hoelzl, C., et al. (2006) Antineoplastic effect of the cyclooxygenase inhibitor meloxicam on canine osteosarcoma cells. *Research in Veterinary Science*, 80(3), 308–316.

Woolums, A.R., Ames, T.R., & Baker, J.G. (2009) Lower respiratory tract diseases, in *Large Animal Internal Medicine*, 4th edn (ed B.P. Smith), Mosby, St. Louis, MO, pp. 601–643.

Wooten, J.G., Lascelles, B.D.X., Cook, V.L., et al. (2010) Evaluation of the relationship between lesions in the gastroduodenal region and cyclooxygenase expression in clinically normal dogs. *American Journal of Veterinary Research*, 71(6), 630–635.

Xie, W.L., Chipman, J.G., Robertson, D.L., et al. (1991) Expression of a mitogen-responsive gene encoding prostaglandin synthase is regulated by mRNA splicing. *Proceedings of the National Academy of Science of the United States of America*, 88(7), 2692–2696.

6

Local Anesthetics

Kip A. Lemke

Local and regional anesthetic techniques are gaining widespread acceptance in the management of pain in small and large animals (Lemke & Dawson, 2000; Anderson & Muir, 2005; Valverde & Gunkel, 2005). In recent years, a clearer understanding of the pathophysiology of pain has provided the conceptual framework for a more rational use of these techniques (Muir & Woolf, 2001; Lemke, 2004; Lamont, 2008; Lemke & Creighton, 2010). Tissue trauma and inflammation produce sensitization of the peripheral nervous system, and the subsequent barrage of nociceptive input produces sensitization of neurons in the dorsal horn of the spinal cord. Because local and regional anesthetic techniques are the only analgesic techniques that produce complete blockade of peripheral nociceptive input, they are the most effective way to prevent sensitization of the central nervous system (CNS) and the development of pathological or maladaptive pain. Lidocaine can also be administered systemically to reduce anesthetic requirements and to manage certain types of pain in veterinary species (Valverde et al., 2004; Robertson et al., 2005). The precise mechanism underlying the antinociceptive effects of systemically administered lidocaine is unclear, but peripheral and central neural mechanisms have been proposed (Cook & Blikslager, 2008).

STRUCTURE AND PHYSICAL PROPERTIES

Local anesthetics penetrate peripheral nerves and induce reversible blockade of impulse conduction in myelinated and unmyelinated nerve fibers by inhibiting voltage-gated sodium channels. These drugs are weak bases, and are classified as aminoesters (e.g., procaine) or amino amides (e.g., lidocaine or lignocaine) (Figure 6.1). All local anesthetics have an aromatic group that is connected to a tertiary amine group by either an ester (RCOOR') or an amide (RNHCOR') linkage. As a general rule, the structure of the aromatic group determines the lipid solubility of the drug, and the structure of the tertiary amine determines the water solubility of the drug.

At physiological pH (7.4), the tertiary amine group readily accepts protons and the local anesthetic molecule exists in equilibrium as a neutral, lipid-soluble base and as a positively charged, water-soluble acid. The dissociation constant, or pKa, is the pH at which concentrations of neutral base and positively charged acid are equal. Most local anesthetics have pKa values in the range

7.5–8.5. As the pKa value decreases, a greater fraction of the drug exists as neutral base and more molecules penetrate the lipid membranes, and the onset of action tends to be more rapid. Conversely, as the pKa value increases, a greater fraction of the drug exists as positively charged acid and fewer molecules penetrate the lipid membranes, and the onset of action tends to be slower.

The structure of the aromatic group determines the lipid solubility of local anesthetics as well as potency, duration of action, and binding to tissue and plasma proteins (Table 6.1). Drugs with low lipid solubility (procaine) tend to have low potency, a short duration of action, and limited protein binding. Drugs with intermediate lipid solubility (lidocaine) tend to have intermediate potency, an intermediate duration of action, and intermediate protein binding. Drugs with high lipid solubility (bupivacaine) tend to have high potency, a long duration of action, and high protein binding.

Some local anesthetics (mepivacaine, bupivacaine, ropivacaine) have an asymmetrical carbon atom, and exist in solution as paired stereoisomers or enantiomers. These enantiomers are mirror images of each other, and cannot be superimposed without breaking the chemical bonds. The physical properties of enantiomers are identical, but their biological activity can differ significantly. Enantiomers are classified based on their ability to rotate a plane of polarized light when dissolved in a specified solvent. Enantiomers that rotate polarized light to the right are designated dextrorotatory (d or +) isomers, and those that rotate polarized light to the left are designated levorotatory (l or −) isomers. Racemic mixtures contain equal amounts of both enantiomers. Mepivacaine and bupivacaine are supplied as racemic mixtures, and levobupivacaine and ropivacaine are supplied as the pure levorotatory enantiomer.

Another method of classification is based on unequivocal designation of molecular structure by assigning sequence priority to groups attached to a tetrahedral chiral center. A clockwise group sequence is designated as the R isomer, and a counterclockwise group sequence is designated as the S isomer. It should be noted that no fixed relationship between the d/l and R/S designations exists.

MECHANISM OF ACTION

Local anesthetics block the conduction of nerve impulses by inhibiting voltage-gated sodium channels in neuronal membranes. The

---

Pain Management in Veterinary Practice, First Edition. Edited by Christine M. Egger, Lydia Love and Tom Doherty.
© 2014 John Wiley & Sons, Inc. Published 2014 by John Wiley & Sons, Inc.

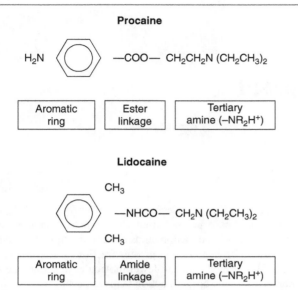

Figure 6.1. Chemical structure of aminoester (procaine) and aminoamide (lidocaine) local anesthetics. Procaine and lidocaine are the prototypical aminoester and aminoamide local anesthetics, respectively. All local anesthetics have an aromatic ring connected to a tertiary amine with either an ester or an amide linkage. The aromatic ring determines the lipid solubility and the tertiary amine determines the water solubility of the drug. Ester-linked local anesthetics are metabolized rapidly by plasma esterases, and amide-linked local anesthetics are metabolized more slowly by the liver.

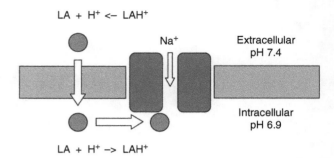

Figure 6.2. Diffusion and binding of local anesthetics to voltage-gated sodium channels. The binding site for local anesthetics is on the cytoplasmic or intracellular surface of the sodium channel. Neutral local anesthetic base diffuses across the lipid membrane. Once inside the cell, the tertiary amine group is protonated and local anesthetic binds to the sodium channel and stabilizes inactive conformational states. LA, neutral local anesthetic; LAH$^+$, protonated local anesthetic

binding site for local anesthetics is located on the cytoplasmic or intracellular surface of the sodium channel (Figure 6.2). The neutral base must diffuse across the lipid membrane and dissociate from the membrane to gain access to this site. Once inside the cell, the tertiary amine group is protonated and the charged acid binds to the sodium channel. Local anesthetics stabilize inactive conformational states of the sodium channel and delay reactivation of the channel rather than physically blocking the pore. Only

moderately lipid-soluble local anesthetics with pKa values close to physiological pH can penetrate the connective tissue sheaths and neuronal membranes, gain access to the cytoplasmic binding site, and inactivate sodium channels.

ANATOMY OF PERIPHERAL NERVES

Peripheral nerves are composed of different types of sensory, motor, and autonomic nerve fibers surrounded by connective tissue sheaths. Local anesthetics injected near peripheral nerves must penetrate these connective tissue sheaths before reaching the neuronal membrane. Diffusion of the local anesthetics away from the injection site is a function of tissue binding and uptake into the systemic circulation.

Sensory nerve fibers are classified by axon diameter, the presence or absence of myelination, and their response to mechanical, thermal, and chemical stimuli (Table 6.2). A-beta (Aβ) sensory fibers have large myelinated axons that conduct impulses at a velocity of

Table 6.1. Physical properties of local anesthetics

Drug	pKa	Onset of action (min)	Relative lipid solubility[a]	Relative potency[a]	Duration of action (min)	Plasma protein binding (%)
Low potency and short duration of action						
Procaine	8.9	10–20	1	1	30–60	6
Intermediate potency and duration of action						
Lidocaine	7.9	5–10	1.4	2	60–120	65
Mepivacaine	7.7	5–10	12.4	2	90–180	78
High potency and long duration of action						
Bupivacaine	8.1	10–20	204	4	180–360	95
Levobupivacaine	8.1	10–20	204	4	180–360	95
Ropivacaine	8.1	10–20	68	3	120–240	94

[a]Lipid solubility and potency are relative to procaine.

Table 6.2. Types of neurons blocked with local anesthetics

Neuron type	Function	Myelination	Order of blockade	Signs of blockade
A alpha	Motor skeletal muscle	Myelinated	Fifth	Loss of motor function
A beta	Sensory touch, pressure	Myelinated	Fourth	Loss of sensation to touch and pressure
A gamma	Motor muscle spindles, proprioception	Myelinated	Third	Loss of proprioception
A delta	Fast pain, temperature	Myelinated	Second	Pain relief, loss of temperature sensation
B	Autonomic, preganglionic sympathetic	Myelinated	First	Increased skin temperature
C	Slow pain, autonomic, postganglionic sympathetic, polymodal nociceptors	Unmyelinated	Second	Pain relief, loss of temperature sensation

greater than 30 m/s. The free nerve endings of these fibers respond to non-noxious mechanical stimuli (touch), but do not respond to noxious stimuli directly. A-delta (Aδ) nociceptive fibers have small myelinated axons that conduct impulses at a velocity of 10–30 m/s and carry the nociceptive input responsible for the fast sharp pain that occurs immediately after injury. The free nerve endings of these fibers contain membrane-bound receptors that respond primarily to intense mechanical and thermal stimuli and are called mechanothermal nociceptors. C-nociceptive fibers have small unmyelinated axons that conduct nerve impulses at a velocity of less than 3 m/s. The free nerve endings of these fibers contain membrane-bound receptors that respond to chemical as well as thermal and mechanical stimuli, and are called polymodal nociceptors. The nociceptive input responsible for the prolonged dull pain that occurs several seconds after a painful stimulus is carried by C fibers. Some local anesthetics (bupivacaine) preferentially block nociceptive Aδ and C fibers.

Motor and autonomic fibers are also blocked by local anesthetics. These fibers are also classified by axon diameter and the presence or absence of myelination. A-alpha (Aα) motor fibers directly innervate skeletal muscles and have large myelinated axons that conduct impulses at a velocity of greater than 70 m/s. A-gamma (Aγ) fibers control muscle spindle tone and have small myelinated axons that conduct impulses at a velocity of 10–30 m/s. The postganglionic autonomic fibers that regulate vascular smooth muscle tone are small unmyelinated C fibers. Blockade of these fibers is responsible for the decrease in blood pressure observed after epidural administration of local anesthetics.

The location of nerve bundles within large peripheral nerves, the presence or absence of myelination, and the discharge rate influence the onset and duration of neural blockade. Generally, nerve bundles innervating proximal regions are located more superficially in large peripheral nerves than those innervating distal regions. Local anesthetics penetrate superficial nerve bundles first and proximal areas are blocked sooner than more distal areas. The presence or absence of myelination also influences the uptake of local anesthetics by nerve fibers. As a general rule, small myelinated and unmyelinated nerve fibers are blocked before large myelinated fibers, and the con-

ventional understanding has been that small sensory fibers, specifically myelinated (Aδ) and unmyelinated (C) nociceptive fibers are blocked before larger sensory (Aβ) and motor (Aα) fibers. However, small unmyelinated (C) fibers are more resistant to blockade with local anesthetics than previously thought (Wildsmith et al., 1987). In certain circumstances, transmission mediated by unmyelinated C fibers can persist even after complete motor blockade has been established (Gokin et al., 2001). The discharge rate of the nerve fiber also influences the development of neural blockade. Local anesthetics have a higher binding affinity for open and inactivated sodium channels than they do for resting channels. Increased binding of local anesthetics to sodium channels at high discharge rates stabilizes inactive conformational states and enhances the development of neural blockade. This enhancement of neural blockade at high discharge rates is termed phasic or use-dependent blockade. A damaged nerve fiber may develop ectopic high-frequency impulse generation, and use-dependent blockade may allow for more effective analgesia at lower concentrations of local anesthetics (Brau et al., 2001; Hoffmann et al., 2008).

SYSTEMIC ABSORPTION AND METABOLISM

Systemic absorption of local anesthetics is determined by dose, volume, and route of administration. Absorption from mucosal, pleural, and peritoneal surfaces is rapid, and peak plasma concentrations are reached within 10 minutes. Plasma concentrations achieved after interpleural or intercostal administration are comparable to those achieved after intravenous administration. Local anesthetics are also absorbed quickly from epidural injection sites, and peak plasma concentrations are reached in approximately 30 minutes. Absorption from subcutaneous sites is slower, and peak plasma concentrations are approximately half of those achieved after interpleural or intercostal administration.

Binding of local anesthetics to tissue proteins and the vascularity of the injection site also influence systemic absorption of local anesthetic drugs. Moderately lipid-soluble drugs (e.g., lidocaine/lignocaine) do not bind extensively to tissue proteins and are absorbed rapidly, and highly lipid-soluble drugs (e.g., bupivacaine) bind extensively to tissue proteins and are absorbed more slowly. All commonly used local anesthetics cause vasodilation that accelerates systemic absorption of the drug. Vasoconstrictors (e.g., epinephrine) can be added to local anesthetic solutions to delay absorption and reduce systemic toxicity, but they can also cause localized ischemia. Epinephrine decomposes rapidly on exposure to air or light, thus antioxidants (metabisulfite) are added, and the pH of local anesthetic solutions containing epinephrine is decreased to prolong the shelf life. The pH of solutions containing epinephrine ranges from 3.0 to 4.5, while the pH of solutions without epinephrine ranges from 4.5 to 6.5. Although the addition of epinephrine delays systemic absorption, the decrease in pH also delays the onset of action. Epidural administration of acidic local anesthetic solutions containing antioxidants has also been associated with neurotoxicity (Ravindran et al., 1982). Historically, vasoconstrictors have been added to short-acting and intermediate-acting drugs (procaine, lidocaine); however, they have a limited effect on the duration of action and systemic absorption of long-acting drugs (bupivacaine). Given the potential for localized ischemia as well as the availability of long-acting local anesthetics with inherently slow systemic absorption, the addition of vasoconstrictors to local anesthetic solutions may have limited clinical utility.

Once absorbed into the systemic circulation, local anesthetics bind reversibly to plasma proteins (e.g., α-1 acid glycoprotein, albumin) and red blood cells. The degree of tissue and protein binding influences the onset and duration of action, as well as the toxicity of local anesthetic drugs. Consequently, doses of local anesthetics should be calculated carefully for patients with significant anemia and hypoproteinemia. Aminoesters tend to be less lipid-soluble and protein-bound, and therefore have a faster onset and shorter duration of action. Conversely, aminoamides tend to be more lipid-soluble and protein-bound, and as a result have a slower onset and longer duration of action.

Aminoesters and aminoamides are metabolized by distinctly different pathways and at very different rates. Aminoesters are rapidly hydrolyzed by the tissue and plasma esterases, and the metabolites are excreted by the kidneys. Aminoamides are metabolized primarily in the liver by cytochrome P450 enzymes at a relatively slow rate. Clearance of aminoamides is dependent on cardiac output and hepatic blood flow. In anesthetized animals, clearance of lidocaine decreases by approximately 50% and plasma concentrations double (Mather et al., 1986; Feary et al., 2005). The major routes of hepatic metabolism are hydroxylation, N-dealkylation, and hydrolysis, with subsequent elimination of metabolites by the kidneys. The lungs also temporarily sequester a significant amount of drug after systemic absorption of local anesthetics. Doses of aminoamides should be calculated carefully for patients with hypoproteinemia and delayed drug metabolism caused by advanced liver disease.

LOCAL TISSUE AND SYSTEMIC TOXICITY

Local anesthetics are safe drugs if they are used with reasonable care. Administration of an incorrect dose and inadvertent intravenous administration are probably the most common causes of systemic toxicity. Interpleural or intercostal administration of large doses is also a potential cause of systemic toxicity, especially in small animals. Toxicity of local anesthetics is additive,

and care should be taken when multiple routes of exposure (e.g., topical and regional), mixtures of local anesthetics, or repeated dosing are employed. Some aminoesters (procaine) are derivatives of para-aminobenzoic acid and have the potential to cause allergic reactions, but they are used infrequently in veterinary medicine. Conversely, allergic reactions to aminoamide local anesthetics are extremely rare, although some preservatives (methylparaben) can cause allergic reactions. Several veterinary species can develop methemoglobinemia after topical exposure to benzocaine, though cats are most susceptible and benzocaine-containing products including Cetacaine (a combination of benzocaine, butamben, and tetracaine) should be avoided in this species (Davis et al., 1993).

Most commonly used local anesthetic solutions cause some degree of local tissue irritation, and inappropriate administration of concentrated solutions causes local tissue toxicity and nerve damage. Application of 5% lidocaine to peripheral nerves causes irreversible conduction block within minutes. Even standard concentrations of commonly used local anesthetics (e.g., 2% lidocaine) produce localized tissue irritation and histological changes. Short-term in vitro exposure of articular chondrocytes to 2% lidocaine, 0.5% ropivacaine, or 0.5% bupivacaine also produces significant cytotoxicity, although the clinical significance of this is not known (Piper et al. 2011). Dilution of local anesthetics plays an important role in reducing local tissue toxicity. Preservatives are added to multi-dose local anesthetic solutions, and some of these preservatives are potentially allergenic (e.g., methylparaben) or neurotoxic (e.g., metabisulfite). To prevent neurotoxicity, only low concentrations (2% lidocaine, 0.5% bupivacaine) of single-dose preservative-free local anesthetic solutions should be administered by the intrathecal or epidural route. The relative potency and systemic toxicity of bupivacaine is approximately four times that of lidocaine. As a result, a 0.5% (5 mg/mL) solution of bupivacaine is equivalent to a 2% (20 mg/mL) solution of lidocaine in terms of potency and toxicity.

Systemic reactions to local anesthetics involve primarily the CNS, but the cardiovascular system can be affected if very large doses are given. Initial signs of CNS toxicity include sedation, disorientation, and ataxia. Muscle tremors, convulsions, and respiratory depression can occur after administration of large doses. Threshold plasma concentrations for CNS toxicity are approximately 5–10 mcg/mL for lidocaine and mepivacaine, and 2–4 mcg/mL for bupivacaine, levobupivacaine, and ropivacaine.

Cats and horses are more likely than other domestic species to develop signs of CNS toxicity after administration of local anesthetics. In horses, muscle tremors developed after intravenous administration of lidocaine at a dose of 4.9 mg/kg (1.5 mg/kg bolus followed by a 0.3 mg/kg/min infusion) (Meyer et al., 2001). The intravenous dose of lidocaine that produces convulsions in cats (12 mg/kg) is approximately 50% lower than that in dogs (22 mg/kg), and the intravenous dose of bupivacaine that produces convulsions in cats (3.8 mg/kg) is only 25% lower than that in dogs (5 mg/kg) (Liu et al., 1983; Chadwick, 1985). Initial signs of CNS toxicity (sedation, ataxia) become apparent after administration of approximately half of the convulsive dose. Furthermore, moderate respiratory acidosis ($PaCO_2 = 60$–80 mmHg) increases cerebral blood flow and the proportion of unbound free drug available for diffusion across neuronal membranes, decreasing the convulsive dose of lidocaine and bupivacaine by approximately 50% (Englesson, 1974). As a result, adequate ventilatory support, in addition to anticonvulsant therapy (e.g., diazepam), is critically important in the management of systemic toxicity.

Clinical signs of cardiovascular toxicity occur at doses that are approximately four times higher than those required to produce CNS toxicity. Local anesthetics produce direct effects on the heart and blood vessels, as well as indirect effects mediated by blockade of the autonomic nervous system. Toxic doses of local anesthetics depress myocardial contractility and cause peripheral vasodilation and profound hypotension. Conduction abnormalities and arrhythmias are rarely observed after administration of large doses of short-acting local anesthetics (e.g., lidocaine, mepivacaine). However, intravenous administration of large doses of long-acting local anesthetics (e.g., bupivacaine) can produce ventricular arrhythmias and cardiovascular collapse in animals (Feldman et al., 1989). Newer long-acting local anesthetics (e.g., ropivacaine, levobupivacaine) appear to be less cardiotoxic than bupivacaine at equipotent doses (McClure, 1996; Foster & Markham, 2000).

Intravenous administration of a lipid emulsion (i.e., 20% Intralipid) has been used to successfully treat bupivacaine toxicity in dogs (Weinberg et al., 2003). The emulsion may draw lipid-soluble local anesthetics from tissues and sequester them in the vascular compartment. Lipid-soluble local anesthetics also inhibit mitochondrial oxidation of free fatty acids that supply 70% of myocardial energy requirements. Lipid therapy may also restore normal mitochondrial function and myocardial energy production.

CLINICAL PHARMACOLOGY OF LOCAL ANESTHETICS

Articaine

The structure of articaine is unique among amide local anesthetics in that it contains an additional ester group, allowing for rapid metabolism by plasma esterases and a resultant short anesthetic time. In addition, the aromatic group is a thiophene ring instead of a benzene ring, thereby conferring increased lipid solubility and improving diffusion through tissues and possibly increasing efficacy (Katyal, 2010). The addition of epinephrine prolongs the duration of action of articaine, and this formulation (Septocaine®) has gained widespread popularity in human dental procedures. Although anecdotal reports of the use of Septocaine exist in veterinary dental procedures, no published data are available. The manufacturer recommends a maximum dose of 7 mg/kg for adults and children over 4 years of age.

Bupivacaine

In small animals, and to a more limited extent in large animals, perioperative use of bupivacaine has gained acceptance in recent years. The drug is a structural analog of mepivacaine and has a relatively long onset time (10–20 minutes) and duration of action (3–6 hours). The potency of bupivacaine is four times that of lidocaine and mepivacaine. The drug has a pKa of 8.1, and is highly lipid-soluble and protein-bound. Bupivacaine can be used for local infiltration as well as for peripheral and central (epidural) nerve blocks. It is also used to block digital nerves and manage pain in horses with acute laminitis. Bupivacaine is not approved for use in animals in North America. Several formulations are available including 0.5% (5 mg/mL) racemic solutions with and without preservative. Administration of less concentrated solutions (0.25%) may provide adequate sensory analgesia with limited motor blockade. The total dose of bupivacaine should not exceed 1.5–2 mg/kg in healthy dogs and cats. For example, a healthy 3 kg cat should not be given more than 1 mL of the 0.5% solution.

Levobupivacaine

Levobupivacaine is the "levo" enantiomer of bupivacaine, and is used to a limited extent in animals. Like bupivacaine, the drug has a relatively long onset time (10–20 minutes) and duration of action (3–6 hours). The pKa, potency, lipid-solubility, and degree of protein binding of levobupivacaine are identical to those of bupivacaine; however, the drug is less likely to produce cardiovascular toxicity than bupivacaine. Levobupivacaine can be used for local infiltration as well as for peripheral and central (epidural) nerve blocks. The drug is not approved for use in animals in North America. Several formulations are available including a 0.5% (5 mg/mL) solution.

Lidocaine/Lignocaine

Lidocaine is the most versatile and commonly used local anesthetic in veterinary medicine. The drug is an aminoamide with a relatively short onset time (5–10 minutes) and duration of action (1–2 hours). Lidocaine has a pKa of 7.9 and is moderately lipid-soluble and protein-bound. The drug is effective topically at high concentrations, and can be used for local infiltration as well as for peripheral and central (i.e., epidural) nerve blocks. Lidocaine is approved for use in small and large animals in North America. Several formulations are available including a 10% (100 mg/mL) topical spray and a 2% (20 mg/mL) solution. Topical gels, creams, and patches are also available, but the time required to desensitize intact skin is approximately 1 hour. The total dose of lidocaine should not exceed 6–8 mg/kg in healthy dogs and cats. For example, a healthy 3 kg cat should not be given more than 1 mL of the 2% solution, or 0.2 mL of the 10% spray. See Chapter 9 for further discussion of novel formulations of lidocaine.

INTRAVENOUS LIDOCAINE

Systemic administration of lidocaine can be used to reduce the minimum alveolar concentration (MAC) of inhalational anesthetics, provide analgesia, control ventricular arrhythmias, and prevent postoperative ileus (Muir et al., 2003). An intravenous loading dose of 1–2 mg/kg is appropriate for dogs. Intraoperatively, intravenous infusion rates for dogs are 50–100 mcg/kg/min. Postoperatively, lower intravenous infusion rates of 12–25 mcg/kg/min are used to provide analgesia and to improve gastrointestinal motility.

Objective clinical data on the use of intraoperative and postoperative lidocaine infusions in cats are limited. Intravenous lidocaine at the doses required to reduce the MAC of inhalational anesthetics in cats leads to greater cardiovascular depression than an equipotent dose of isoflurane alone (Pypendop & Ilkiw, 2005a; Pypendop & Ilkiw, 2005b). In addition, lidocaine infusions do not affect the thermal threshold in conscious cats (Pypendop et al., 2006). However, it should be noted that lidocaine may be more effective as an antihyperalgesic agent in conditions of central sensitization, rather than a primary antinociceptive agent. In addition, it is established that postoperative intestinal function is improved by perioperative lidocaine infusions in humans (McCarthy et al., 2010). Because this benefit may extend to veterinary species, including cats, selected feline patients undergoing abdominal surgeries may be considered for low-dose (~12 mcg/kg/min) perioperative intravenous lidocaine.

Systemic administration of lidocaine can be used intra- and postoperatively in horses to provide analgesia and to improve gastrointestinal motility (Malone et al., 2006) (Chapter 30). Rapid intravenous administration of lidocaine can cause muscle tremors and collapse in horses, and loading doses should be given slowly. An intravenous loading dose of 1–2 mg/kg, administered over 5–10 minutes, is appropriate for most healthy, awake patients. Lidocaine is administered intravenously at a rate of 2–3 mg/kg/h. Objective clinical data on the perioperative use of lidocaine infusions in ruminants and swine are limited.

Mepivacaine

Mepivacaine is another local anesthetic that is used commonly in small and large animals. It is an aminoamide with potency, toxicity, and onset of action comparable to lidocaine, but with a slightly longer duration of action. Mepivacaine has a pKa of 7.7, and is moderately lipid-soluble and protein-bound. The drug can be used for local infiltration and for peripheral and central (epidural) nerve blocks. Mepivacaine is approved for use in dogs and horses in North America. The drug produces limited local tissue inflammation, and is used frequently for diagnostic nerve blocks and intra-articular injections in horses. Mepivacaine is available as a 2% (20 mg/mL) racemic solution.

Proparacaine

Proparacaine is one of the few local ester anesthetics currently employed in clinical veterinary practice. It is a topical ophthalmic anesthetic agent widely used to desensitize the cornea for intraocular pressure measurements, collection of conjunctival samples, or minor corneal surgery. In cats and horses, maximal effect occurs within 5 minutes of administration and wanes by 25 minutes (Binder & Herring, 2006; Kalf et al., 2008). In dogs, the anesthetic effects appear to last much longer (~45 minutes) and can be extended by multiple applications (Herring et al., 2005).

Ropivacaine

Ropivacaine is a structural analog of bupivacaine. The drug is marketed as the pure "S" enantiomer, and is used to a limited extent in animals. Ropivacaine has a relatively long onset time (10–20 minutes) and duration of action (2–4 hours), and the drug is slightly less potent than bupivacaine. The pKa and protein binding of ropivacaine are similar to that of bupivacaine. The lipid solubility of ropivacaine is approximately half that of bupivacaine, and the drug is less likely to produce cardiovascular toxicity. Ropivacaine can be used for local infiltration and for peripheral and central nerve blocks. It is not approved for use in animals in North America. Several formulations are available, including a 0.75% (7.5 mg/mL) solution. Administration of less concentrated solutions (0.5%) may provide adequate sensory analgesia with limited motor blockade.

Mixtures of Local Anesthetics

Mixtures of a short-acting local anesthetic (e.g., lidocaine or mepivacaine) with a long-acting one (e.g., bupivacaine) have the potential advantage of producing a rapid onset with a prolonged duration of action. However, data from clinical studies in humans indicate that there is little change in onset time and there is a significant reduction in duration of action when the mixture is compared to the long-acting local anesthetic alone (Galindo & Witcher, 1980; Cuvillon et al., 2009). Because toxicity of local anesthetics is additive, administering mixtures of local anesthetics offers no advantage.

Methods for Potentiating Local Anesthesia

Bicarbonate can be added to local anesthetics to increase the pH and to reduce pain associated with injection (Hanna et al., 2009; Cepeda et al., 2010), although clinical results are inconsistent (Burns et al., 2006). Theoretically, alkalinization increases the amount of nonionized drug, resulting in a shorter onset time (Lee et al., 2012). However, data from clinical research with human subjects indicate that alkalinization of a local anesthetic solution produces an inconsistent effect on the time of onset (Candido et al., 1995). The ratio of bicarbonate to lidocaine or bupivacaine should be kept at 1:9 because higher ratios may cause precipitation. Bupivacaine in particular precipitates easily as the pH is adjusted upward.

Many commercially available formulations of local anesthetics contain epinephrine to counteract vasodilation and decrease the rate of vascular absorption. Alternatively, epinephrine can be added to make a 1:200,000 solution (0.1 mL epinephrine [1 mg/mL] added to 20 mL local anesthetic). Addition of epinephrine extends the duration of action of peripheral and central neural blockade with short-acting local anesthetics (e.g., lidocaine or mepivacaine), but it has a limited effect on the duration of action of long-acting local anesthetics (e.g., bupivacaine). Local anesthetic solutions that contain epinephrine can be applied to the surgical field to provide hemostasis, but these solutions can also produce localized ischemia. Local anesthetic solutions that contain epinephrine should not be injected in extremities (e.g., distal limbs and pinnae) as vasoconstriction can cause ischemic damage and subsequent tissue necrosis. Additionally, systemic absorption of epinephrine can precipitate cardiac arrhythmias and hypertension.

The α-2 agonist clonidine is used as an adjunct with local anesthetics to prolong the duration of neural blockade in human patients. Recently, dexmedetomidine, a more selective α-2 agonist, was used as an adjunct with levobupivacaine to prolong the duration of neural blockade of the brachial plexus in human patients (Esmaoglu et al., 2010). In dogs, either perineural or systemic administration of medetomidine (10 mcg/kg) with mepivacaine prolongs the duration of sensory and motor blockade of the radial nerve (Lamont & Lemke, 2008). Systemic adverse effects of α-2 agonists may occur even when administered perineurally at low doses; patients should be volume-replete and have normal cardiovascular function.

Opioids are often mixed with local anesthetics for epidural administration. Additionally, some opioids have been used to extend the duration of peripheral nerve blocks. In particular, the mixed agonist–antagonist opioid buprenorphine has been used in regional blocks for oral surgery (Modi et al., 2009). Many full μ agonists, including morphine and fentanyl, have also been used to extend the duration of a variety of central and peripheral nerve blocks; however, the results of studies designed to determine the efficacy of this adjunctive technique are mixed (Axelsson & Gupta, 2009).

Dexamethasone has been combined with a variety of local anesthetics to prolong the duration of peripheral nerve blockade (Yoshitomi et al. 2008; Parrington et al., 2010). Corticosteroids should be administered cautiously and avoided entirely if patients are receiving NSAIDs.

Though not an adjuvant, warming local anesthetics to body temperature may increase the amount of nonionized base, decrease onset time, and decrease pain on injection (Hogan et al., 2011). Warming local anesthetic solutions is easy and inexpensive, and should be considered for all peripheral nerve blocks in conscious patients.

SUMMARY

Local anesthetics can be used to manage pain safely and effectively in a variety of clinical settings. Peripheral and central neural blockade can be used to manage pain in surgical and nonsurgical patients. Local anesthetics can also be given systemically to manage perioperative pain and ileus. They are often used in combination with other classes of analgesic drugs as part of a multi-modal pain management strategy (Muir & Woolf, 2001; Lemke, 2004; Lamont & Lemke, 2008; Lemke & Creighton, 2010). Local anesthetics have the unique ability to produce complete blockade of peripheral nociceptive input, preventing the development of pathological pain as well as the stress response.

REFERENCES

Anderson, D.E. & Muir, W.W. (2005) Pain management in cattle. *The Veterinary Clinics of North America: Food Animal Practice*, 21(3), 623–635.

Axelsson, K. & Gupta, A. (2009) Local anaesthetic adjuvants: neuraxial versus peripheral nerve block. *Current Opinion in Anaesthesiology*, 22(5), 649–654.

Binder, D.R. & Herring, I.P. (2006) Duration of corneal anesthesia following topical administration of 0.5% proparacaine hydrochloride solution in clinically normal cats. *American Journal of Veterinary Research*, 67(10), 1780–1782.

Brau, M.E., Dreimann, M., Olschewski, A., Vogel, W., & Hempelmann, G. (2001) Effect of drugs used for neuropathic pain management on tetrodotoxin-resistant Na^+ currents in rat sensory neurons. *Anesthesiology*, 94(1), 137–144.

Burns, C.A., Ferris, G., Feng, C., Cooper, J.Z., & Brown, M.D. (2006) Decreasing the pain of local anesthesia: a prospective, double-blind comparison of buffered, premixed 1% lidocaine with epinephrine versus 1% lidocaine freshly mixed with epinephrine. *Journal of the American Academy of Dermatology*, 54(1), 128–131.

Candido, K.D., Winnie, A.P., Covino, B.G., Raza, S.M., Vasireddy, A.R., & Masters, R.W. (1995) Addition of bicarbonate to plain bupivacaine does not significantly alter the onset or duration of plexus anesthesia. *Regional Anesthesia*, 20(2), 133–138.

Cepeda, M.S., Tzortzopoulou, A., Thackrey, M., Hudcova, J., Arora, G.P., & Schumann, R. (2010) Adjusting the pH of lidocaine for reducing pain on injection. *Cochrane Database of Systematic Reviews*, (12), CD006581. doi: 10.1002/14651858.CD006581.pub2.

Chadwick, H.S. (1985) Toxicity and resuscitation in lidocaine- or bupivacaine-infused cats. *Anesthesiology*, 63(4), 385–390.

Cook, V.L. & Blikslager, A.T. (2008) Use of systemically administered lidocaine in horses with gastrointestinal tract disease. *Journal of the American Veterinary Medical Association*, 232(8), 1144–1148.

Cuvillon, P., Nouvellon, E., Ripart, J., et al. (2009) A comparison of the pharmacodynamics and pharmacokinetics of bupivacaine, ropivacaine (with epinephrine) and their equal volume mixtures with lidocaine used for femoral and sciatic nerve blocks: a double-blind randomized study. *Anesthesia & Analgesia*, 108(2), 641–649.

Davis, J.A., Greenfield, R.E., & Brewer, T.G. (1993) Benzocaine-induced methemoglobinemia attributed to topical application of the anesthetic in several laboratory animal species. *American Journal of Veterinary Research*, 54(8), 1322–1326.

Englesson, S. (1974) The influence of acid-base changes on central nervous system toxicity of local anaesthetic agents. I. An experimental study in cats. *Acta Anaesthesiologica Scandinavica*, 18(2), 79–87.

Esmaoglu, A., Yegenoglu, F., Akin, A., & Turk, C.Y. (2010) Dexmedetomidine added to levobupivacaine prolongs axillary brachial plexus block. *Anesthesia & Analgesia*, 111(6), 1548–1551.

Feary, D.J., Mama, K.R., Wagner, A.E., & Thomasy, S. (2005) Influence of general anesthesia on pharmacokinetics of intravenous lidocaine infusion in horses. *American Journal of Veterinary Research*, 66(4), 574–580.

Feldman, H.S., Arthur, G.R., & Covino, B.G. (1989) Comparative systemic toxicity of convulsant and supraconvulsant doses of intravenous ropivacaine, bupivacaine, and lidocaine in the conscious dog. *Anesthesia and Analgesia*, 69(6), 794–801.

Foster, R.H. & Markham, A. (2000) Levobupivacaine: a review of its pharmacology and use as a local anaesthetic. *Drugs*, 59(3), 551–579.

Galindo, A. & Witcher, T. (1980) Mixtures of local anesthetics: bupivacaine-chloroprocaine. *Anesthesia and Analgesia*, 59(9), 683–685.

Gokin, A.P., Philip, B., & Strichartz, G.R. (2001) Preferential block of small myelinated sensory and motor fibers by lidocaine: in vivo electrophysiology in the rat sciatic nerve. *Anesthesiology*, 95(6), 1441–1454.

Hanna, M.N., Elhassan, A., Veloso, P.M., et al. (2009) Efficacy of bicarbonate in decreasing pain on intradermal injection of local anesthetics: a meta-analysis. *Regional Anesthesia and Pain Medicine*, 34(2), 122–125.

Herring, I.P., Bobofchak, M.A., Landry, M.P., & Ward, D.L. (2005) Duration of effect and effect of multiple doses of topical ophthalmic 0.5% proparacaine hydrochloride in clinically normal dogs. *American Journal of Veterinary Research*, 66(1), 77–80.

Hoffmann, T., Sauer, S.K., Horch, R.E., & Reeh, P.W. (2008) Sensory transduction in peripheral nerve axons elicits ectopic action potentials. *Journal of Neuroscience*, 28(24), 6281–6284.

Hogan, M.E., vanderVaart, S., Perampaladas, K., Machado, M., Einarson, T.R., & Taddio, A. (2011) Systematic review and meta-analysis of the effect of warming local anesthetics on injection pain. *Annals of Emergency Medicine*, 58(1), 86–98.e1.

Kalf, K.L., Utter, M.E., & Wotman, K.L. (2008) Evaluation of duration of corneal anesthesia induced with ophthalmic 0.5% proparacaine hydrochloride by use of a Cochet-Bonnet anesthesiometer in clinically normal horses. *American Journal of Veterinary Research*, 69(12), 1655–1658.

Katyal, V. (2010) The efficacy and safety of articaine versus lignocaine in dental treatments: a meta-analysis. *Journal of Dentistry*, 38(4), 307–317.

Lamont, L.A. (2008) Multimodal pain management in veterinary medicine: the physiologic basis of pharmacologic therapies. *The Veterinary Clinics of North America: Small Animal Practice*, 38(6), 1173–1186.

Lamont, L.A. & Lemke, K.A. (2008) The effects of medetomidine on radial nerve blockade with mepivacaine in dogs. *Veterinary Anaesthesia and Analgesia*, 35(1), 62–68.

Lee, R., Kim, Y.M., Choi, E.M., Choi, Y.R., & Chung, M.H. (2012) Effect of warmed ropivacaine solution on onset and duration of axillary block. *Korean Journal of Anesthesiology*, 62(1), 52–56.

Lemke, K.A. (2004), Understanding the pathophysiology of perioperative pain. *The Canadian Veterinary Journal*, 45(5), 405–413.

Lemke, K.A. & Creighton, C.M. (2010) Analgesia for anesthetized patients. *Topics in Companion Animal Medicine*, 25(2), 70–82.

Lemke, K.A. & Dawson, S.D. (2000), Local and regional anesthesia. *The Veterinary Clinics of North America: Small Animal Practice*, 30(4), 839–857.

Liu, P.L., Feldman, H.S., Giasi, R., Patterson, M.K., & Covino, B.G. (1983) Comparative CNS toxicity of lidocaine, etidocaine, bupivacaine, and tetracaine in awake dogs following rapid intravenous administration. *Anesthesia and Analgesia*, 62(4), 375–379.

Malone, E., Ensink, J., Turner, T., et al. (2006) Intravenous continuous infusion of lidocaine for treatment of equine ileus. *Veterinary Surgery*, 35(1), 60–66.

Mather, L.E., Runciman, W.B., Carapetis, R.J., Ilsley, A.H., & Upton, R.N. (1986) Hepatic and renal clearances of lidocaine in conscious and anesthetized sheep. *Anesthesia and Analgesia*, 65(9), 943–949.

McCarthy, G.C., Megalla, S.A., & Habib, A.S. (2010) Impact of intravenous lidocaine infusion on postoperative analgesia and recovery from surgery: a systematic review of randomized controlled trials. *Drugs*, 70(9), 1149–1163.

McClure, J.H. (1996) Ropivacaine. *British Journal of Anaesthesia*, 76(2), 300–307.

Meyer, G.A., Lin, H.C., Hanson, R.R., & Hayes, T.L. (2001) Effects of intravenous lidocaine overdose on cardiac electrical activity and blood pressure in the horse. *Equine Veterinary Journal*, 33(5), 434–437.

Modi, M., Rastogi, S., & Kumar, A. (2009) Buprenorphine with bupivacaine for intraoral nerve blocks to provide postoperative analgesia in outpatients after minor oral surgery. *Journal of Oral & Maxillofacial Surgery*, 67(12), 2571–2576.

Muir, W.W., 3rd, Wiese, A.J., & March, P.A. (2003) Effects of morphine, lidocaine, ketamine, and morphine-lidocaine-ketamine drug combination on minimum alveolar concentration in dogs anesthetized with isoflurane. *American Journal of Veterinary Research*, 64(9), 1155–1160.

Muir, W.W., 3rd & Woolf, C.J. (2001) Mechanisms of pain and their therapeutic implications. *Journal of the American Veterinary Medical Association*, 219(10), 1346–1356.

Parrington, S.J., O'Donnell, D., Chan, V.W., et al. (2010) Dexamethasone added to mepivacaine prolongs the duration of analgesia after supraclavicular brachial plexus blockade. *Regional Anesthesia and Pain Medicine*, 35(5), 422–426.

Piper, S.L., Kramer, J.D., Kim, H.T., et al. (2011) Effects of local anesthetics on articular cartilage. *American Journal of Sports Medicine*, 39(10), 2245–2253.

Pypendop, B.H. & Ilkew, J.E. (2005a) The effects of intravenous lidocaine administration on the minimum alveolar concentration of isoflurane in cats. *Anesthesia and Analgesia*, 100(1), 97–101.

Pypendop, B.H. & Ilkiw, J.E. (2005b) Assessment of the hemodynamic effects of lidocaine administered IV in isoflurane-anesthetized cats. *American Journal of Veterinary Research*, 66(4), 661–668.

Pypendop, G.H., Ilkiw, J.E., & Robertson, S.A. (2006) Effects of intravenous administration of lidocaine on the thermal threshold in cats. *American Journal of Veterinary Research*, 67(1), 16–20.

Ravindran, R.S., Turner, M.S., & Muller, J. (1982) Neurologic effects of subarachnoid administration of 2-chloroprocaine-CE, bupivacaine, and low pH normal saline in dogs. *Anesthesia and Analgesia*, 61(3), 279–283.

Robertson, S.A., Sanchez, L.C., Merritt, A.M., & Doherty, T.J. (2005) Effect of systemic lidocaine on visceral and somatic nociception in conscious horses. *Equine Veterinary Journal*, 37(2), 122–127.

Valverde, A., Doherty, T.J., Hernandez, J., & Davies, W. (2004) Effect of lidocaine on the minimum alveolar concentration of isoflurane in dogs. *Veterinary Anaesthesia and Analgesia*, 31(4), 264–271.

Valverde, A. & Gunkel, C.I. (2005), Pain management in horses and farm animals. *Journal of Veterinary Emergency and Critical Care*, 15(4), 295–307.

Weinberg, G., Ripper, R., Feinstein, D.L., & Hoffman, W. (2003) Lipid emulsion infusion rescues dogs from bupivacaine-induced cardiac toxicity. *Regional Anesthesia and Pain Medicine*, 28(3), 198–202.

Wildsmith, J.A., Gissen, A.J., Takman, B., & Covino, B.G. (1987) Differential nerve blockade: esters v. amides and the influence of pKa. *British Journal of Anaesthesia*, 59(3), 379–384.

Yoshitomi, T., Kohjitani, A., Maeda, S., Higuchi, H., Shimada, M., & Miyawaki, T. (2008) Dexmedetomidine enhances the local anesthetic action of lidocaine via an α-2A adrenoceptor. *Anesthesia and Analgesia*, 107(1), 96–101.

7

α-2 Adrenoceptor Agonists

Reza Seddighi

α-2 adrenoceptor agonists, also referred to as α-2 agonists, provide dose-dependent sedation, analgesia, and muscle relaxation. These effects are primarily caused by stimulation of presynaptic α-2 adrenergic receptors resulting in a decrease in norepinephrine release, centrally and peripherally, and a subsequent reduction in central nervous system sympathetic outflow and circulating catecholamine concentrations (Berthelsen & Pettinger, 1977; Bylund & U'Prichard, 1983). Activation of α-2 adrenoreceptors in supraspinal and spinal sites produces antihyperalgesia, analgesia, and sedation (Yaksh & Reddy, 1981; Pertovaara et al., 1991; Molina & Herrero, 2006).

α-2 agonists are frequently used in veterinary patients for sedation prior to general anesthesia, and to reduce the dose of induction and maintenance agents (Gomez-Villamandos et al., 2006; Oku et al., 2011). α-2 agonists are often used in combination with other analgesics and anesthetics (e.g., opioids, ketamine), to attenuate the stress response associated with surgery or diagnostic procedures (Ethier et al., 2008; Jeong et al., 2009). The analgesic efficacy of α-2 agonists is enhanced by the concomitant use of opioids (Kuo & Keegan, 2004), and small doses of α-2 agonists provide sedation and analgesia postoperatively and facilitate a smooth recovery (Larenza et al., 2008; Valtolina et al., 2009; Valverde et al., 2010).

PHARMACOLOGY OF α-2 ADRENOCEPTOR AGONISTS

Adrenergic Receptors

Adrenergic receptors (or adrenoceptors) are targets for catecholamines, particularly norepinephrine (noradrenaline) and epinephrine (adrenaline), and are present in a variety of tissues. Adrenergic receptors are closely associated, structurally and functionally, with membrane-associated G proteins, which are responsible for initiating intracellular signaling cascades and, as such, are classified as G-protein-coupled receptors (GPCRs) (Hayashi & Maze, 1993; Westfall & Westfall, 2011).

CLASSIFICATION OF ADRENERGIC RECEPTORS

Early descriptions classified adrenergic receptors into two groups, those with activity that results in excitation, and those with activity that results in inhibition of the effector cells (Dale, 1906; Cannon,

1933). However, further experiments indicated that this classification scheme is overly simple, and each type may have either excitatory or inhibitory action (Ahlquist, 1948). Ahlquist proposed that catecholamines could be excitatory or inhibitory, and the variation in the adrenoceptors' physiological effects could be due to differences in the receptors involved and quantitative differences in potency. Thus, he tentatively classified adrenergic receptors into α- and β-adrenotropic receptors. With further studies on the function and anatomical location of adrenergic receptors, heterogeneity among α- and β-adrenergic receptors was recognized, and receptor subtypes were identified (Westfall, 1977). In an effort to refine the classification of α-adrenoceptors, a classification based on the synaptic location of these receptors (i.e., presynaptic α-2 and postsynaptic α-1) was proposed (Langer, 1974; Berthelsen & Pettinger, 1977). However, as postsynaptic and extrasynaptic (i.e., located in vascular endothelium and platelets) α-2 receptors were also found, a classification strictly based on anatomical location has proven to be untenable (Drew & Whiting, 1979; Stoelting & Hillier, 2006). Ultimately, with the development of more selective α-adrenoceptor antagonists, and investigations of their interaction with each adrenoceptor, the pharmacological basis for classification of α-adrenergic receptors was developed (Bylund & U'Prichard, 1983). For instance, based on pharmacological effects, α-1 receptors are those that are more sensitive to prazosin (a selective α-1 receptor antagonist), whereas yohimbine (an α-2 receptor antagonist) is more potent than prazosin at α-2 receptors (Hayashi & Maze, 1993).

α-2 ADRENOCEPTOR SUBTYPES

Receptor cloning has revealed additional heterogeneity of α-2 adrenergic receptors, and resulted in the classification of three distinct α-2 receptor subtypes (A, B, and C) (Bylund 1992)

α-2A subtype: Although the cellular distribution of the three subtypes is incompletely understood, it appears that subtype A is the predominant subtype in the central nervous system. *In situ* hybridization of receptor mRNA and receptor subtype-specific antibodies indicates that α-2A receptors in the brain may be either presynaptic or postsynaptic. α-2A receptors in the canine brain seem to mediate sedation, supraspinal antinociception, and hypothermia (Fagerholm et al., 2008). They provide centrally

Pain Management in Veterinary Practice, First Edition. Edited by Christine M. Egger, Lydia Love and Tom Doherty.
© 2014 John Wiley & Sons, Inc. Published 2014 by John Wiley & Sons, Inc.

mediated sympatholysis by inhibition of norepinephrine release from sympathetic nerve endings, and this results in bradycardia and hypotension (Philipp et al., 2002; Ma et al., 2004; Fagerholm et al., 2008; Westfall & Westfall, 2011). The α-2A adrenergic receptor is the primary mediator of spinal analgesia from endogenous norepinephrine as well as exogenous adrenergic agonists (Stone et al., 1997). This subtype, also located postsynaptically on pancreatic β cells, is responsible for hyperglycemia secondary to inhibition of insulin release (Angel et al., 1988, 1990).

α-2B subtype: The α-2B subtype is mainly found in the peripheral vasculature and it mediates the initial increase in systemic vascular resistance (vasoconstriction) that results in reflex bradycardia. It has also been reported that the α-2B receptor subtype is involved in spinal analgesia (Philipp et al., 2002). The antishivering properties of α-2 agonists in people are thought to be mediated via the α-2B receptor subtype (Stoelting & Hillier, 2006).

α-2C subtype: The α-2C subtype is located in the ventral and dorsal striatum and hippocampus, and inhibits the release of catecholamines from the adrenal medulla, modulates dopamine neurotransmission in the brain, and has a role in various behavioral responses (Hunter et al., 1997; Westfall & Westfall, 2011).

Molecular Basis of Adrenergic Receptor Function

Adrenergic receptors are GPCRs that convert a transmembrane signal to an effector mechanism that may include a transmembrane ion channel or generation of an intracellular second messenger cascade. There are more than 20 species of G proteins that are characterized by differences in the amino acid sequence of one of three subunits, the α subunit. Each major type of adrenergic receptor is associated with a particular class of G proteins (i.e., α-1 with G_q, α-2 with G_i, and β with G_s) (Westfall & Westfall, 2011), and these discrete differences in the α subunit provide the unique response mediated by each of the adrenergic receptors (Hayashi & Maze, 1993; Westfall & Westfall, 2011).

Inhibition of adenyl cyclase activity is the main pathway by which α-2 adrenergic receptors exert their effect. This inhibition results in a decrease in the accumulation of cAMP, and diminishes the stimulation of cAMP-dependent protein kinase and subsequent phosphorylation of target regulatory proteins. Efflux of K^+ via activation of G-protein-gated K^+ channels results in hyperpolarization of excitable membranes, and provides an effective means of suppressing neuronal firing. α-2 adrenoceptor stimulation also suppresses Ca^{2+} entry into the nerve terminals via inhibition of voltage-gated Ca^{2+} channels, which may be responsible for its inhibitory effect on the secretion of neurotransmitters. Other second-messenger systems linked to α-2 receptor activation include acceleration of Na^+/H^+ exchange, arachidonic acid mobilization, and increased phosphoinositide hydrolysis (Hayashi & Maze, 1993; Stoelting & Hillier, 2006; Westfall & Westfall, 2011).

Binding to spinal presynaptic α-2 receptors blocks the release of neurotransmitters and neuropeptides from C fibers terminating in the superficial laminae of the dorsal horn of the spinal cord (Buerkle & Yaksh, 1998). This occurs via activation of G_0 proteins, which results in a decrease in calcium flux and glutamate, substance P, neurotensin, calcitonin gene-related peptide, and vasoactive intestinal peptide release. Stimulation of spinal α-2 receptors located postsynaptically on wide-dynamic-range projection neurons results in hyperpolarization via G_i-protein-coupled potassium channels.

MECHANISMS OF ACTION OF α-2 ADRENOCEPTOR AGONISTS

The sedative and anxiolytic effects of α-2 agonists are mediated by decreased activity of ascending neural projections to the cerebral cortex and limbic systems via activation of supraspinal presynaptic or postsynaptic receptors located in the pontine locus coeruleus, an important modulator of vigilance (Stoelting & Hillier, 2006; Hellyer et al., 2007). Conversely, although the mechanism of α-2 agonist-mediated antinociception is not entirely understood, it appears that it is primarily the result of spinal α-2 receptor stimulation. α-2 adrenergic receptors are present in high density in the substantia gelatinosa and intermediolateral cell columns of the spinal cord and on primary afferent terminals, indicating a direct involvement of spinal α-2 receptors in antinociception (Yaksh, 1985; Yaksh et al., 1995). Stimulation of α-2 adrenergic receptors could suppress nociceptive signals at various points in the pain pathway via inhibition of neurotransmitter release from the primary afferent fibers in the dorsal horn. This affects pre- and postsynaptic modulation of nociceptive signals, influences descending modulatory systems from the brainstem, inhibits the release of substance P, and alters ascending modulation of nociceptive signals in the diencephalon and limbic areas (Kuraishi et al., 1985; Murrell & Hellebrekers, 2005).

Activation of supraspinal α-2 receptors within the pons plays an important role in the descending noradrenergic-serotonergic modulation of nociceptive input, resulting in analgesic and antihyperalgesic effects (Guo et al., 1996; Hellyer et al., 2007). It has been proposed that α-2 agonists not only mediate their analgesic action via stimulation of the spinal α-2 receptors but also directly suppress the locus coeruleus, which, in turn, increases spinal cord norepinephrine concentrations. This increase in spinal norepinephrine concentration activates spinal α-2 receptors and results in antinociception (Guo et al., 1996).

α-2 agonists may also attenuate or reverse allodynia in states of chronic pain via a spinally mediated antinociceptive effect. In a nerve ligation model in rats, lumbar intrathecal administration of α-2 agonists significantly reduced allodynia via activation of spinal α-2 receptors and decreased presynaptic sympathetic outflow (Yaksh et al., 1995).

The analgesic and antihyperalgesic effects of α-2 agonists are more pronounced during inflammation, although the effects depend on the stage of the inflammatory process. In a rat model, the antiallodynic and antihyperalgesic activities of medetomidine were greater in the middle phase of the inflammatory process than in the early or late phases (Molina & Herrero, 2006).

Clinically, the degree of sedation and analgesia produced by an α-2 agonist is related not only to the density, location, and type of α-2 adrenoceptors but also to the individual selectivity and affinity of the specific drug molecule for the α-1 and α-2 receptor binding sites (Sinclair, 2003). At least in the case of dexmedetomidine, it is known that the α-2 adrenoceptor selectivity is dose dependent. During administration of small to medium doses or slow infusion rates, a high degree of α-2 adrenoceptor selectivity is observed, and large doses or rapid infusion rates are associated with both α-1 and α-2 activation (Virtanen et al., 1988).

PHYSIOLOGICAL EFFECTS OF α-2 ADRENOCEPTOR AGONISTS

α-2 receptors are located in the peripheral and central nervous systems and in other tissues such as the liver, kidney, pancreas, eye, vascular smooth muscle, and platelets (Maze & Tranquilli, 1991). Thus, the physiological responses mediated by α-2 agonists depend on the location of the affected receptors, accounting for the diversity of their effects. Some drugs in this group (e.g., clonidine, medetomidine, and dexmedetomidine) also activate the nonadrenergic imidazoline receptors, and this may be responsible for the centrally mediated hypotensive and antiarrhythmic effects of these drugs (Tibirica et al., 1991; Noyer et al., 1994; Hieble & Ruffolo, 1995). Additionally, the net effect of α-2 agonists may be influenced by factors such as the receptor selectivity of the drug, the dosage used, concurrently administered drugs, species, health status, and environmental factors. The main effects of α-2 agonists on the function of different organ systems are described below.

Effects on the Cardiovascular System

The effects of α-2 adrenergic agents on the cardiovascular system can be significant, and include bradycardia, first- or second-degree atrioventricular (AV) blockade, decreased cardiac output, and an initial increase in peripheral vascular resistance followed by hypotension. The initial vasoconstriction results in an early hypertensive effect due to stimulation of postsynaptic α-2B receptors in arterial and venous vasculature (Ruffolo, 1985; Stoelting & Hillier, 2006). Currently, there is no strong evidence to support the existence of postsynaptic α-2 receptors in the myocardium; therefore, a direct effect of α-2 agonists on the myocardium is doubtful (Housmans, 1990; Hayashi & Maze, 1993). The decrease in heart rate is mainly due to the central sympatholytic effect of α-2 agonists and a reflex response to the increased peripheral vascular resistance. Anticholinergic agents (e.g., atropine) resolve the α-2 agonist-induced bradycardia; however, as the bradycardia is a physiological reflex and a protective response to the α-2 agonist-induced increase in peripheral vascular resistance, coadministration of an anticholinergic drug may further increase mean arterial blood pressure and heart rate, resulting in myocardial hypoxia and deleterious cardiac arrhythmias (Alibhai et al., 1996; Congdon et al., 2011).

The initial increase in peripheral vascular resistance and hypertension is followed by peripheral vasodilation and a decrease in arterial blood pressure. The latter changes primarily result from stimulation of inhibitory α-2 adrenergic receptors (principally α-2A) in the medullary vasomotor center, and result in decreased sympathetic nervous system outflow (Stoelting & Hillier, 2006). The decrease in systolic left ventricular pressure and plasma catecholamines in dogs after dexmedetomidine administration is attributed to this decrease in sympathetic outflow (Flacke et al., 1993). α-2 agonists may also potentiate parasympathetic activity via the nucleus tractus solitarius, which has an important role in modulation of autonomic control, especially vagal activity (Kubo & Misu, 1981). Although these cardiovascular effects appear to be dose dependent (Pypendop & Verstegen, 1998), infusion of dexmedetomidine, at rates as low as 1 μg/kg/h, decreased cardiac output in dogs (Carter et al., 2010).

The receptor selectivity of the particular α-2 agonist is another determinant of the magnitude of the cardiovascular effects of these drugs. The α-2 to α-1 adrenoceptor selectivity ratios reported for medetomidine and dexmedetomidine are much greater than those reported for detomidine, clonidine, and levomedetomidine (Virtanen et al., 1988; Scheinin et al., 1989). It is generally accepted that less selective α-2 adrenoceptor agonists (e.g., xylazine) cause more significant cardiovascular effects as, in addition to antagonizing the hypnotic responses (Guo et al., 1991), α-1 adrenoceptors may participate in the centrally mediated bradycardia and peripheral vasoconstriction (Xu et al., 1998). Medetomidine and dexmedetomidine are examples of α-2 agonists that have a very low affinity for α-1 adrenoceptors and which interact with central imidazoline receptors and, thus, are expected to have a better cardiovascular profile than less selective drugs such as xylazine (Murrell & Hellebrekers, 2005). However, in horses, the effects of medetomidine were similar to an equipotent dose of xylazine (Yamashita et al., 2002). In another study in horses, medetomidine induced dose-dependent cardiovascular effects similar to detomidine (AV blockade, decrease in cardiac index and stroke volume, and an initial hypertension); however, the cardiovascular effects of medetomidine and xylazine were not as prolonged as that of detomidine (Yamashita et al., 2000).

Although α-2 agonists may cause bradyarrhythmias, particularly first- and second-degree AV block, there is evidence that they may also have antiarrhythmogenic properties. For instance, dexmedetomidine increased the arrhythmogenic threshold of epinephrine necessary to induce ventricular fibrillation in a dose-dependent manner in dogs anesthetized with halothane (Hayashi et al., 1991). The antiarrhythmogenic effect of α-2 agonists is primarily due to an increase in parasympathetic tone and a decrease in sympathetic tone via stimulation of central α-2 (primarily α-2A) adrenergic receptors. In addition, imidazoline receptor activation, which results in reduction of sympathetic tone and the concentration of circulating catecholamines, may be involved in the antiarrhythmogenic effect of those α-2 agonists (e.g., dexmedetomidine) that have an affinity for imidazoline receptors (Kagawa et al., 2005; Chrysostomou et al., 2008).

In summary, although α-2 agonists may cause significant bradycardia and an increase in afterload resulting in reduced cardiac output, these effects are usually well tolerated in healthy animals (Lemke, 2007; Martinez, 2012). Lower doses of α-2 agonists (e.g., medetomidine at 2–10 μg/kg IM) were demonstrated to be safe in middle-aged and older dogs, provided cardiopulmonary function is closely monitored and supported during and after drug administration (Muir et al., 1999).

Effects on the Respiratory System

The main adverse effect of α-2 agonists on the respiratory system is hypoxemia, due to ventilation–perfusion mismatch and a decrease in the respiratory rate. Alveolar ventilation is usually not affected in healthy animals given clinical doses of α-2 agonists, and there is no significant increase in $PaCO_2$ (Bloor et al., 1989; Nguyen et al., 1992; Lamont et al., 2001). Nevertheless, with large doses, dark or cyanotic mucous membranes may be evident in dogs, in spite of a normal or near normal PaO_2. The peripheral cyanosis is believed to be the result of an increase in the concentration of desaturated hemoglobin in the mucous membranes, due to decreased perfusion of the peripheral tissues and increased oxygen extraction during capillary transit (Vaha-Vahe, 1989b; Sinclair, 2003). Although blood flow to the vital organs may not decrease to the same extent as it does in peripheral tissues, and the degree of mucous membrane cyanosis may not necessarily correlate with hypoxia of the vital organs, oxygen supplementation is recommended whenever α-2 agonists are used in animals already at risk for hypoxemia or when other respiratory depressant drugs (e.g., sedatives, opioids, anesthetics) are administered concurrently (Sinclair, 2003). Concurrent administration of L-methadone (Raekallio et al., 2009), butorphanol, or ketamine (Ko et al., 2000) significantly decreased the PaO_2 and increased the $PaCO_2$ when compared with medetomidine alone.

In horses, commonly used doses of xylazine and detomidine cause laryngeal relaxation and alteration of lung dynamic compliance and pulmonary vascular resistance (Reitemeyer et al., 1986; Lavoie et al., 1992b; McDonell & Kerr, 2007). The position of the head and neck is largely responsible for changes in respiratory mechanics in horses sedated with xylazine (Lavoie et al., 1992a). A decrease in PaO_2 of 10–20 mm Hg is commonly observed after administration of α-2 agonists to horses (Reitemeyer et al., 1986; Wagner et al., 1991; Lavoie et al., 1992a); however, an increase in $PaCO_2$ is uncommon (Wagner et al., 1991; Bettschart-Wolfensberger et al., 2005). Nevertheless, detomidine significantly increased $PaCO_2$ and decreased PaO_2 in horses secondary to ventilation–perfusion mismatch, and concurrent administration of butorphanol further increased $PaCO_2$ (Nyman et al., 2009).

Hypoxemia ($PaO_2 \leq 50$ mm Hg) is a prominent finding in sheep given clinically relevant sedative doses of α-2 agonists (Celly et al., 1997a, 1997b). The hypoxemia in sheep is mainly due to α-2 agonist activation of pulmonary intravascular macrophages, which results in bronchoconstriction and intra-alveolar edema and hemorrhage (Celly et al., 1999). Interestingly, there was no difference in the magnitude of the hypoxemia in sheep after administration of equipotent doses of xylazine, romifidine, detomidine, or medetomidine (Celly et al., 1997b).

Effects on the Renal System

α-2 agonists induce diuresis and changes in urine specific gravity and pH, plasma creatinine concentration and osmolality, and the concentrations of sodium, potassium, and chloride in urine and plasma (Burton et al., 1998; Saleh et al., 2005). Several mechanisms have been proposed for the diuretic effect of α-2 agonists. The increase in plasma glucose concentration and glucose excretion rate caused by α-2 agonist administration is not of sufficient magnitude to account for the diuresis observed (Miller et al., 2001). The primary mechanism responsible for diuresis relates to antidiuretic hormone (arginine vasopressin (AVP)). α-2 agonists inhibit secretion of AVP, and inhibit AVP-induced cAMP formation in the distal nephrons (Pettinger et al., 1987). α-2 agonists also cause an increase in the plasma concentration of atrial natriuretic peptide (ANP). In dogs, the increase in the plasma concentration of ANP was greater with medetomidine than with xylazine, and the diuretic effect of medetomidine was less dose dependent than that of xylazine (Talukder & Hikasa, 2009). Activation of imidazoline receptors also causes diuresis via an increase in ANP concentration (Mukaddam-Daher & Gutkowska, 2000; Greven & von Bronewski-Schwarzer, 2001), and the differences between the diuretic effect of xylazine and medetomidine could be due to differences in the action at imidazoline receptors, as only medetomidine activates imidazoline receptors (Talukder & Hikasa, 2009).

In addition to changes in plasma concentrations of AVP and ANP, other mechanisms may be involved in the diuretic response to α-2 agonists (Ruskoaho and Leppaluoto, 1989; Talukder & Hikasa, 2009). These may include increased glomerular filtration rate or decreased sodium reabsorption due to sympatholysis, and decreased renal sympathetic nerve influence on tubular sodium reabsorption (Kline & Mercer, 1990, Rouch et al., 1997; Leino et al., 2011). Although α-2 agonists have a strong diuretic effect, and should be used cautiously in animals with urethral obstruction, they may protect the kidneys by inhibiting renin release, increasing glomerular filtration, and increasing secretion of sodium and water (Gellai & Ruffolo, 1987; de Leeuw & Birkenhager, 1988). In animals with urinary blockage, the author reserves α-2 agonist administration for those with no significant electrolyte imbalance and that will soon have the obstruction relieved.

Effects on the Gastrointestinal System

α-2 adrenoceptors constitute the main receptor types on autonomic nerve terminals and cholinergic neurons of the myenteric plexus (DiJoseph et al., 1984). Prolongation of gastrointestinal transit time occurs after administration of α-2 agonists, and this is mediated via activation of α-2 adrenoceptors in the myenteric plexus, resulting in decreased gastrointestinal muscle contractions due to inhibition of acetylcholine release (Roger & Ruckebusch, 1987; Ross et al., 1990). In horses, clinically relevant doses of xylazine or detomidine significantly decreased duodenal motility (Merritt et al., 1998), and xylazine significantly increased gastric emptying time in ponies (Doherty et al., 1999). In dogs, decreased gastroesophageal sphincter pressure was associated with the administration of xylazine, which may result in reflux of gastric contents (Strombeck & Harrold, 1985). α-2 agonists may modulate the release of gastric acid (Berthelsen & Pettinger, 1977), yet no significant change in gastric pH was observed after administration of these drugs to humans (Orko et al., 1987). α-2 agonists decrease intestinal ion and water secretion in the large bowel, when administered orally, and are considered an effective treatment for watery diarrhea in humans (McArthur et al., 1982).

Nausea and vomiting are frequently observed after administration of α-2 agonists to dogs and cats (Vaha-Vahe, 1989a; Granholm et al., 2006); therefore, these drugs should be administered cautiously in animals prone to aspiration (e.g., brachycephalic animals) or those that may suffer from significant gastrointestinal disturbances. Although the involvement of α-1 adrenoceptors cannot be ruled out, α-adrenoceptor-mediated emesis appears to be mediated mainly by α-2 receptors in the dog (Hikasa et al., 1992).

Effects on the Hepatobiliary System

The cardiovascular effects induced by α-2 agonist administration may affect hepatic blood flow, and this suggests that these drugs should be used cautiously in animals with moderate to severe liver disease (Greene & Marks, 2007). In addition, as the elimination of α-2 agonists occurs mainly by biotransformation in the liver (Salonen, 1989), their clearance may be altered in animals with severe liver disease. However, in a study of human patients in early septic shock, a 24-hour continuous rate infusion of dexmedetomidine (0.2–2.5 μg/kg/h) did not affect hepatic blood flow (Memis et al., 2009). Moreover, the anti-inflammatory properties of dexmedetomidine had protective effects on the liver in a rat model of endotoxemia (Sezer et al., 2010). Thus, the consideration of α-2 agonists for sedation and analgesia in animals with liver disease should be based on the individual animal's health status, though lower doses are recommended.

Effects on the Ocular System

In dogs, xylazine alone did not decrease tear production, but it potentiated the effect of butorphanol in decreasing tear production (Dodam et al., 1998). An overall decrease in intraocular pressure (IOP) can be expected when an α-2 adrenergic agent is administered as a sole agent, as these agents commonly cause bradycardia and hypotension, a decrease in sympathetic activity, and possibly a decrease in aqueous production. A study of rabbit and cat nictitating membrane preparations showed that medetomidine decreases IOP, in part, by interacting with α-2 adrenoceptors located on sympathetic nerve endings. The effect of medetomidine on imidazoline receptors may also have some role in decreasing IOP (Potter & Ogidigben, 1991). However, because α-2 agonists may induce vomiting, these drugs should be used with caution in animals in which an increase in IOP would be deleterious to ocular health.

Pupil size may also be affected by α-2 agonists. Intravenous administration of medetomidine produced mydriasis in anesthetized rats (Potter et al., 1990); however, the clinical importance of this is unclear.

Metabolic Effects

α-2 agonists induce hyperglycemia through inhibition of insulin release secondary to stimulation of α-2 adrenoceptors on the β cells of the pancreas (Yamazaki et al., 1982; Hillaire-Buys et al., 1985). Conversely, imidazoline receptors may have the opposite role in increasing insulin release from β cells (Hirose et al., 1997). Thus, α-2 agonists with an affinity for imidazoline receptors (e.g., medetomidine and dexmedetomidine) (Hikasa et al., 1992; Kanda & Hikasa, 2008) may induce a different insulin response than α-2 agonists that lack imidazoline affinity, such as xylazine. Medetomidine and xylazine induced hyperglycemia and hypoinsulinemia and inhibited catecholamine release and lipolysis in dogs, but the hyperglycemic effect of medetomidine, in contrast to that of xylazine, was not dose dependent (Ambrisko & Hikasa, 2002). Medetomidine and xylazine induced a similar degree of hyperglycemia, suppression of epinephrine, norepinephrine, and insulin release, and inhibition of lipolysis in cats (Kanda & Hikasa, 2008). Interestingly, in the latter study, although the decrease in the plasma insulin concentration in cats was similar to that reported in dogs, the increase in plasma glucose concentration was considerably greater. The authors concluded that factors in addition to the effect of α-2 agonists on the plasma insulin concentration may be responsible for the observed difference in the hyperglycemic response between dogs and cats. Similar neurohormonal alterations after administration of α-2 agonists are reported in other species, including cattle and sheep (Gorewit, 1980; Ranheim et al., 2000). However, a study in neonatal foals demonstrated that, unlike in adult horses, intravenous xylazine (1.1 mg/kg) does not produce hypoinsulinemia and hyperglycemia, and that the process leading to inhibition of insulin release by xylazine is immature or absent in foals under 1 month of age (Robertson et al., 1990).

Effects on Other Body Systems

α-2 agonists affect thermoregulation. Administration of an α-2 agonist (mivazerol) selectively antagonized the early thermoregulatory responses to bacterial infection in rats (Tolchard et al., 2009). The authors of that study suggested that patients receiving α-2 agonists may not be capable of mounting a normal thermal response to infecting organisms, and monitoring the core temperature may not be as helpful in detection of infection in these patients. Rectal temperature decreased significantly by 30 minutes after administration of xylazine and was still decreased after 120 minutes in 10- and 28-day-old foals (Robertson et al., 1990). In rabbits, medetomidine markedly decreased body temperature and exhibited antipyretic and hypothermic effects (Szreder, 1993). The authors of the latter study claimed that these effects were associated with inhibition of the metabolic rate and/or redistribution of body heat to peripheral tissues and increased heat loss to the environment. A decrease in prostaglandin E_2 in the hypothalamus after administration of clonidine to Guinea pigs has also been reported (Feleder et al., 2004), and a similar mechanism may also be responsible for the antipyretic effect in febrile horses (Kendall et al., 2010).

ROUTES OF ADMINISTRATION OF α-2 AGONISTS

Systemic Administration

α-2 adrenoceptor agonists are administered systemically for sedation, as part of a premedication protocol (Maddern et al., 2010), or in the form of a constant rate infusion (CRI) during the maintenance of anesthesia in many species, including dogs (Ethier et al., 2008; Gomez-Villamandos et al., 2008) and horses (Solano et al., 2009; Valverde et al., 2010). Single dose and CRI administration of these drugs have also been successfully used during the recovery period to provide analgesia (Valtolina et al., 2009; van Oostrom et al., 2011). α-2 agonists interact synergistically with opioids to provide analgesia (Ambrisko et al., 2005).

Epidural Administration

Epidural administration of α-2 agonists blocks nociceptive pathways at the level of the spinal cord via activation of α-2 receptors (primarily α-2A). Epidurally administered α-2 agonists and opioids have synergistic analgesic effects because they act via similar mechanisms (Branson et al., 1993), and also because opioids induce changes in the α-2 adrenergic receptor density. Systemic daily administration of morphine in a rat model enhanced the analgesic effect of intrathecally administered dexmedetomidine via upregulation of the α-2A, α-2B, and α-2C receptor subtypes in the lumbar dorsal root ganglion and dorsal horn (Tamagaki et al., 2010).

In addition to spinally mediated analgesia, supraspinal analgesia, secondary to systemic absorption and cranial migration of drug, may contribute to the analgesic effects of epidurally or spinally administered α-2 agonists (Stone et al., 1997; Fairbanks et al., 2002; Virgin et al., 2010; Valverde et al., 2010).

Dose-dependent adverse cardiovascular and respiratory effects can be expected due to systemic absorption of epidurally and spinally administered α-2 agonists (Vesal et al., 1996; Seddighi, 2003). The onset and the extent of these effects are primarily affected by the lipid solubility of the drug. For instance, as dexmedetomidine is more rapidly absorbed than medetomidine, systemic effects can be expected sooner after epidural or spinal administration of dexmedetomidine (Kallio et al., 1989; Scheinin et al., 1989). In dogs, however, epidural administration of dexmedetomidine caused adequate neuroaxial analgesia with minimal cardiovascular and respiratory adverse effects, and systemic administration caused a hypnotic state with significant cardiorespiratory depression (Sabbe et al., 1994).

In horses, α-2 agonists are commonly injected at the caudal epidural space (S-C_1 or C_{1-2}). However, because the equine spinal cord terminates in the lumbosacral area, agents administered at more caudal spaces have to diffuse further cranially to reach the target receptors (Skarda & Tranquilli, 2007), and the resultant analgesic effect depends on the extent of cranial migration of the drug. Regardless, epidural xylazine in horses was shown to produce potent perineal analgesia without measurable cardiopulmonary effects (Leblanc & Eberhart, 1990). Ataxia and sedation due to the systemic absorption of epidurally administered α-2 agonists may limit their clinical application, especially when higher doses are used (Doria et al., 2008).

Intra-articular Administration

Although in humans the intra-articular administration of α-2 agonists, such as dexmedetomidine (Paul et al., 2010) and clonidine (Joshi et al., 2000; Tran et al., 2005), has significant synergistic effects with opioids and local anesthetics for pain control in knee surgery, currently, there are no reports of similar application of these drugs in animals.

α-2 Adrenoceptor Agonists and Local Nerve Blockade

α-2 adrenoceptor agonists have occasionally been used in humans, alone or in combination with local anesthetics, to improve analgesia and/or extend the duration of peripheral nerve conduction blockade in brachial plexus blocks (Singelyn et al., 1996), peribulbar blocks (Madan et al., 2001), intravenous regional blocks (Memis et al., 2004), spinal blocks with local anesthetics (Calasans-Maia et al., 2005; Kanazi et al., 2006), and intercostal nerve blocks (Tschernko et al., 1998). Although the exact mechanism of action of these drugs in enhancement of the local nerve blockade is not clear, several mechanisms have been proposed. One possible mechanism is that local vasoconstriction induced by these drugs leads to a delay in the absorption of the local anesthetic. Studies in laboratory animals have indicated other mechanisms of action for α-2 agonists in local nerve blockade. In a study of frog sciatic nerve blockade, dexmedetomidine produced nerve blockade that was resistant to α-2 antagonists (Kosugi et al., 2010). It was concluded that α-2 agonist inhibitory effects on nerve conduction are unlikely to be related to G-protein-coupled membrane receptors, such as α-2 adrenoceptors, or to imidazoline receptors. Other receptors that may be involved in nerve blockade by α-2 agonists are tetrodotoxin (TTX)-sensitive voltage-gated Na^+ channels and/or tetraethylammonium (TEA)-sensitive (delayed-rectifier) K^+ channels. Dexmedetomidine is more effective than clonidine, lidocaine, and cocaine and is similar to ropivacaine in its nerve conduction blocking effects (Kosugi et al., 2010). An inhibitory effect of dexmedetomidine on voltage-gated Na^+ channels in rat dorsal root ganglia has also been demonstrated (Oda et al., 2007), and this effect was not reversed with yohimbine administration. In laboratory animal models of nerve blockade, enhancement of the hyperpolarization-activated cation current, which prevents the nerve from returning from a hyperpolarized state to the resting membrane potential for subsequent firing, has also been shown to be responsible for the peripheral analgesic effects of dexmedetomidine and clonidine. This

mechanism is independent of the action of these drugs on α-2 receptors (Dale, 1906; Kroin et al., 2004; Brummett et al., 2011)

In summary, although incorporation of α-2 agonists into local nerve blocks appears to be promising based on preliminary data from laboratory animal studies, it has not been fully investigated in veterinary practice. The author occasionally includes an α-2 adrenoceptor agonist (e.g., dexmedetomidine, 1–2 µg/kg) in brachial plexus, sciatic, and femoral nerve blocks. However, objective evaluation of the benefits and any potential adverse effects from systemic absorption of these drugs in the clinical setting has yet to be determined.

SUMMARY

α-2 adrenoceptor agonists are sedative-analgesics commonly used in veterinary medicine. These drugs are administered systemically or in locoregional techniques to achieve sedation, analgesia, and muscle relaxation. Administration may cause adverse systemic effects, primarily cardiovascular in nature, in patients with cardiovascular instability or when used at higher doses. Careful patient selection is important, but many patients will benefit from the desirable clinical effects of these drugs.

REFERENCES

Ahlquist, R.P. (1948) A study of the adrenotropic receptors. *American Journal of Physiology*, 153, 586–600.

Alibhai, H.I., Clarke, K.W., Lee, Y.H., & Thompson, J. (1996) Cardiopulmonary effects of combinations of medetomidine hydrochloride and atropine sulphate in dogs. *Veterinary Record*, 138, 11–13.

Ambrisko, T.D. & Hikasa, Y. (2002) Neurohormonal and metabolic effects of medetomidine compared with xylazine in beagle dogs. *Canadian Journal of Veterinary Research*, 66, 42–49.

Ambrisko, T. D., Hikasa, Y., & Sato, K. (2005) Influence of medetomidine on stress-related neurohormonal and metabolic effects caused by butorphanol, fentanyl, and ketamine administration in dogs. *American Journal of Veterinary Research*, 66, 406–412.

Angel, I., Bidet, S., & Langer, S.Z. (1988) Pharmacological characterization of the hyperglycemia induced by alpha-2 adrenoceptor agonists. *Journal of Pharmacology and Experimental Therapeutics*, 246, 1098–1103.

Angel, I., Niddam, R., & Langer, S.Z. (1990) Involvement of alpha-2 adrenergic receptor subtypes in hyperglycemia. *Journal of Pharmacology and Experimental Therapeutics*, 254, 877–882.

Berthelsen, S. & Pettinger, W.A. (1977) A functional basis for classification of alpha-adrenergic receptors. *Life Sciences*, 21, 595–606.

Bettschart-Wolfensberger, R., Freeman, S.L., Bowen, I.M., et al. (2005) Cardiopulmonary effects and pharmacokinetics of i.v. dexmedetomidine in ponies. *Equine Veterinary Journal*, 37, 60–64.

Bloor, B.C., Abdul-Rasool, I., Temp, J., Jenkins, S., Valcke, C., & Ward, D.S. (1989) The effects of medetomidine, an alpha 2-adrenergic agonist, on ventilatory drive in the dog. *Acta Veterinaria Scandinavica Supplement*, 85, 65–70.

Branson, K.R., Ko, J.C., Tranquilli, W.J., Benson, J., & Thurmon, J.C. (1993) Duration of analgesia induced by epidurally administered morphine and medetomidine in dogs. *Journal of Veterinary Pharmacology and Therapeutics*, 16, 369–372.

Brummett, C.M., Hong, E.K., Janda, A.M., Amodeo, F.S., & Lydic, R. (2011) Perineural dexmedetomidine added to ropivacaine for sciatic nerve block in rats prolongs the duration of analgesia by blocking the hyperpolarization-activated cation current. *Anesthesiology*, 115, 836–843.

Buerkle, H. & Yaksh, T.L. (1998) Pharmacological evidence for different alpha 2-adrenergic receptor sites mediating analgesia and sedation in the rat. *British Journal of Anaesthesia*, 81, 208–215.

Burton, S., Lemke, K.A., Ihle, S.L., & Mackenzie, A.L. (1998) Effects of medetomidine on serum osmolality; urine volume, osmolality and pH; free water clearance; and fractional clearance of sodium, chloride, potassium, and glucose in dogs. *American Journal of Veterinary Research*, 59, 756–761.

Bylund, D.B. (1992) Subtypes of alpha 1- and alpha 2-adrenergic receptors. *Federation of American Societies for Experimental Biology Journal*, 6, 832–839.

Bylund, D.B. & U'Prichard, D.C. (1983) Characterization of alpha 1- and alpha 2-adrenergic receptors. *International Review of Neurobiology*, 24, 343–431.

Calasans-Maia, J.A., Zapata-Sudo, G. & Sudo, R.T. (2005) Dexmedetomidine prolongs spinal anaesthesia induced by levobupivacaine 0.5% in guinea-pigs. *Journal of Pharmacy and Pharmacology*, 57, 1415–1420.

Cannon, W.B. (1933) Chemical Mediators of Autonomic Nerve Impulses. *Science*, 78, 43–48.

Carter, J.E., Campbell, N.B., Posner, L.P., & Swanson, C. (2010) The hemodynamic effects of medetomidine continuous rate infusions in the dog. *Veterinary Anaesthesia and Analgesia*, 37, 197–206.

Celly, C.S., Atwal, O.S., McDonell, W.N., & Black, W.D. (1999) Histopathologic alterations induced in the lungs of sheep by use of alpha2-adrenergic receptor agonists. *American Journal of Veterinary Research*, 60, 154–161.

Celly, C.S., McDonell, W.N., Black, W.D., & Young, S.S. (1997a) Cardiopulmonary effects of clonidine, diazepam and the peripheral alpha 2 adrenoceptor agonist ST-91 in conscious sheep. *Journal of Veterinary Pharmacology and Therapeutics*, 20, 472–478.

Celly, C.S., McDonell, W.N., Young, S.S., & Black, W.D. (1997b) The comparative hypoxaemic effect of four alpha 2 adrenoceptor agonists (xylazine, romifidine, detomidine and medetomidine) in sheep. *Journal of Veterinary Pharmacology and Therapeutics*, 20, 464–471.

Chrysostomou, C., Beerman, L., Shiderly, D., Berry, D., Morell, V.O., & Munoz, R. (2008) Dexmedetomidine: a novel drug for the treatment of atrial and junctional tachyarrhythmias during the perioperative period for congenital cardiac surgery: a preliminary study. *Anesthesia & Analgesia*, 107, 1514–1522.

Congdon, J.M., Marquez, M., Niyom, S., & Boscan, P. (2011) Evaluation of the sedative and cardiovascular effects of intramuscular administration of dexmedetomidine with and without concurrent atropine administration in dogs. *Journal of American Veterinary Medical Association*, 239, 81–89.

Dale, H.H. (1906) On some physiological actions of ergot. *Journal of Physiology*, 34, 163–206.

de Leeuw, P.W. & Birkenhager, W.H. (1988) Alpha-adrenoceptors and the kidney. *Journal of Hypertension Supplement*, 6, S21–S24.

DiJoseph, J.F., Taylor, J.A., & Mir, G.N. (1984) Alpha-2 receptors in the gastrointestinal system: a new therapeutic approach. *Life Sciences*, 35, 1031–1042.

Dodam, J.R., Branson, K.R., & Martin, D.D. (1998) Effects of intramuscular sedative and opioid combinations on tear production in dogs. *Veterinary Ophthalmology*, 1, 57–59.

Doherty, T.J., Andrews, F.M., Provenza, M.K., & Frazier, D.L. (1999) The effect of sedation on gastric emptying of a liquid marker in ponies. *Veterinary Surgery*, 28, 375–379.

Doria, R.G., Valadao, C.A., Duque, J.C., Farias, A., Almeida, R.M., & Netto, A.C. (2008) Comparative study of epidural xylazine or clonidine in horses. *Veterinary Anaesthesia and Analgesia*, 35, 166–172.

Drew, G.M. & Whiting, S.B. (1979) Evidence for two distinct types of postsynaptic alpha-adrenoceptor in vascular smooth muscle in vivo. *British Journal of Pharmacology*, 67, 207–215.

Ethier, M.R., Mathews, K.A., Valverde, A., et al. (2008) Evaluation of the efficacy and safety for use of two sedation and analgesia protocols to facilitate assisted ventilation of healthy dogs. *American Journal of Veterinary Research*, 69, 1351–1359.

Fagerholm, V., Scheinin, M., & Haaparanta, M. (2008) Alpha2A-adrenoceptor antagonism increases insulin secretion and synergistically augments the insulinotropic effect of glibenclamide in mice. *British Journal of Pharmacology*, 154, 1287–1296.

Fairbanks, C.A., Stone, L.S., Kitto, K.F., Nguyen, H.O., Posthumus, I.J., & Wilcox, G.L. (2002) Alpha(2C)-Adrenergic receptors mediate spinal analgesia and adrenergic-opioid synergy. *Journal of Pharmacology and Experimental Therapeutics*, 300, 282–290.

Feleder, C., Perlik, V., & Blatteis, C.M. (2004) Preoptic alpha 1- and alpha 2-noradrenergic agonists induce, respectively, PGE2-independent and PGE2-dependent hyperthermic responses in guinea pigs. *American Journal of Physiology-Regululatory, Integrative and Comparative Physiology*, 286, R1156–R1166.

Flacke, W.E., Flacke, J.W., Bloor, B.C., McIntee, D.F., & Sagan, M. (1993) Effects of dexmedetomidine on systemic and coronary hemodynamics in the anesthetized dog. *Journal of Cardiothoracic and Vascular Anesthesia*, 7, 41–49.

Gellai, M. & Ruffolo, R.R. Jr. (1987) Renal effects of selective alpha-1 and alpha-2 adrenoceptor agonists in conscious, normotensive rats. *Journal of Pharmacology and Experimental Therapeutics*, 240, 723–728.

Gomez-Villamandos, R.J., Dominguez, J.M., Redondo, J.I., et al. (2006) Comparison of romifidine and medetomidine pre-medication in propofol-isoflurane anaesthetised dogs. *Journal of Veterinary Medicine. A, Physiology, Pathology, Clinical Medicine*, 53, 471–475.

Gomez-Villamandos, R.J., Palacios, C., Benitez, A., et al. (2008) Effect of medetomidine infusion on the anaesthetic requirements of desflurane in dogs. *Research in Veterinary Science*, 84, 68–73.

Gorewit, R.C. (1980) Effects of clonidine on glucose production and insulin secretion of cattle. *American Journal of Veterinary Research*, 41, 1769–1772.

Granholm, M., McKusick, B.C., Westerholm, F.C., & Aspegren, J.C. (2006) Evaluation of the clinical efficacy and safety of dexmedetomidine or medetomidine in cats and their reversal with atipamezole. *Veterinary Anaesthesia and Analgesia*, 33, 214–223.

Greene, S.A. & Marks, S.L. (2007) Hepatic disease, in *Lumb & Jones' Veterinary Anesthesia and Analgesia*, 4th edn (eds W.J. Tranquilli, J.C. Thurman, & K.A. Grimm), Blackwell Publishing, Ames, IA, pp. 921–926.

Greven, J. & von Bronewski-Schwarzer, B. (2001) Site of action of moxonidine in the rat nephron. *Naunyn-Schmiedeberg's Archives of Pharmacology*, 364, 496–500.

Guo, T.Z., Jiang, J.Y., Buttermann, A.E., & Maze, M. (1996) Dexmedetomidine injection into the locus ceruleus produces antinociception. *Anesthesiology*, 84, 873–881.

Guo, T.Z., Tinklenberg, J., Oliker, R., & Maze, M. (1991) Central alpha 1-adrenoceptor stimulation functionally antagonizes the hypnotic response to dexmedetomidine, an alpha 2-adrenoceptor agonist. *Anesthesiology*, 75, 252–256.

Hayashi, Y. & Maze, M. (1993) Alpha 2 adrenoceptor agonists and anaesthesia. *British Journal of Anaesthesia*, 71, 108–118.

Hayashi, Y., Sumikawa, K., Maze, M., et al. (1991) Dexmedetomidine prevents epinephrine-induced arrhythmias through stimulation of central alpha 2 adrenoceptors in halothane-anesthetized dogs. *Anesthesiology*, 75, 113–117.

Hellyer, P.W., Robertson, S.A. & Fails, A.D. (2007) Pain and its management, in *Lumb & Jones' Veterinary Anesthesia and Analgesia*, 4th edn (eds W.J. Tranquilli, J.C. Thurman, & K.A. Grimm), Blackwell Publishing, Ames, IA, pp. 31–57.

Hieble, J.P. & Ruffolo, R.R. Jr. (1995) Possible structural and functional relationships between imidazoline receptors and alpha 2-adrenoceptors. *Annals of the New York Academy of Sciences*, 763, 8–21.

Hikasa, Y., Ogasawara, S. & Takase, K. (1992) Alpha adrenoceptor subtypes involved in the emetic action in dogs. *Journal of Pharmacology and Experimental Therapeutics*, 261, 746–754.

Hillaire-Buys, D., Gross, R., Blayac, J.P., Ribes, G., & Loubatières-Mariani, M.M. (1985) Effects of alpha-adrenoceptor agonists and antagonists on insulin secreting cells and pancreatic blood vessels: comparative study. *European Journal of Pharmacology*, 117, 253–257.

Hirose, H., Seto, Y., Maruyama, H., Dan, K., Nakamura, K., & Saruta, T. (1997) Effects of alpha 2-adrenergic agonism, imidazolines, and G-protein on insulin secretion in beta cells. *Metabolism*, 46, 1146–1149.

Housmans, P.R. (1990) Effects of dexmedetomidine on contractility, relaxation, and intracellular calcium transients of isolated ventricular myocardium. *Anesthesiology*, 73, 919–922.

Hunter, J.C., Fontana, D.J., Hedley, L.R., et al. (1997) Assessment of the role of alpha2-adrenoceptor subtypes in the antinociceptive, sedative and hypothermic action of dexmedetomidine in transgenic mice. *British Journal of Pharmacology*, 122, 1339–1344.

Jeong, M.B., Narfstrom, K., Park, S.A., Park, S.A., Chae, J.M., & Seo, K.M. (2009) Comparison of the effects of three different combinations of general anesthetics on the electroretinogram of dogs. *Documenta Ophthalmologica*, 119, 79–88.

Joshi, W., Reuben, S.S., Kilaru, P.R., Sklar, J., & Maciolek, H. (2000) Postoperative analgesia for outpatient arthroscopic knee surgery with intraarticular clonidine and/or morphine. *Anesthesia & Analgesia*, 90, 1102–1106.

Kagawa, K., Hayashi, Y., Itoh, I., et al. (2005) Identification of the central imidazoline receptor subtype involved in modulation of halothane-epinephrine arrhythmias in rats. *Anesthesia & Analgesia*, 101, 1689–1694.

Kallio, A., Scheinin, M., Koulu, M., et al. (1989) Effects of dexmedetomidine, a selective alpha 2-adrenoceptor agonist, on hemodynamic control mechanisms. *Clinical Pharmacology & Therapeutics*, 46, 33–42.

Kanazi, G.E., Aouad, M.T., Jabbour-Khoury, S.I., et al. (2006) Effect of low-dose dexmedetomidine or clonidine on the characteristics of bupivacaine spinal block. *Acta Anaesthesiologica Scandinavica*, 50, 222–227.

Kanda, T. & Hikasa, Y. (2008) Neurohormonal and metabolic effects of medetomidine compared with xylazine in healthy cats. *Canadian Journal of Veterinary Research*, 72, 278–286.

Kendall, A., Mosley, C., & Brojer, J. (2010) Tachypnea and antipyresis in febrile horses after sedation with alpha-agonists. *Journal of Veterinary Internal Medicine*, 24, 1008–1011.

Kline, R.L. & Mercer, P.F. (1990) Contribution of renal nerves to the natriuretic and diuretic effect of alpha-2 adrenergic receptor activa-tion. *Journal of Pharmacology and Experimental Therapeutics*, 253, 266–271.

Ko, J.C., Fox, S.M., & Mandsager, R.E. (2000) Sedative and cardiorespiratory effects of medetomidine, medetomidine-butorphanol, and medetomidine-ketamine in dogs. *Journal of American Veterinary Medical Association*, 216, 1578–1583.

Kosugi, T., Mizuta, K., Fujita, T., Nakashima, M., & Kumamoto, E. (2010) High concentrations of dexmedetomidine inhibit compound action potentials in frog sciatic nerves without alpha(2) adrenoceptor activation. *British Journal of Pharmacology*, 160, 1662–1676.

Kroin, J.S., Buvanendran, A., Beck, D.R., Topic, J.E., Watts, D.E., & Tuman, K.J. (2004) Clonidine prolongation of lidocaine analgesia after sciatic nerve block in rats is mediated via the hyperpolarization-activated cation current, not by alpha-adrenoreceptors. *Anesthesiology*, 101, 488–494.

Kubo, T. & Misu, Y. (1981) Pharmacological characterisation of the alpha-adrenoceptors responsible for a decrease of blood pressure in the nucleus tractus solitarii of the rat. *Naunyn-Schmiedeberg's Archives of Pharmacology*, 317, 120–125.

Kuo, W.C. & Keegan, R.D. (2004) Comparative cardiovascular, analgesic, and sedative effects of medetomidine, medetomidine-hydromorphone, and medetomidine-butorphanol in dogs. *American Journal of Veterinary Research*, 65, 931–937.

Kuraishi, Y., Hirota, N., Sato, Y., Kaneko, S., Satoh, M., & Takagi, H. (1985) Noradrenergic inhibition of the release of substance P from the primary afferents in the rabbit spinal dorsal horn. *Brain Research*, 359, 177–182.

Lamont, L.A., Bulmer, B.J., Grimm, K.A., Tranquilli, W.J., & Sission, D.D. (2001) Cardiopulmonary evaluation of the use of medetomidine hydrochloride in cats. *American Journal of Veterinary Research*, 62, 1745–1749.

Lamont, L.A., Bulmer, B.J., Sisson, D.D., Grimm, K.A., & Tranquilli, W.J. (2002) Doppler echocardiographic effects of medetomidine on dynamic left ventricular outflow tract obstruction in cats. *Journal of the American Veterinary Medical Association*, 221, 1276–1281.

Langer, S.Z. (1974) Presynaptic regulation of catecholamine release. *Biochemical Pharmacology*, 23, 1793–1800.

Larenza, M.P., Althaus, H., Conrot, A., Balmer, C., Schaltzmann, U.,& Bettschart-Wolfensberger, R. (2008) Anaesthesia recovery quality after racemic ketamine or S-ketamine administration to male cats undergoing neutering surgery. *Schweizer Archiv für Tierheilkunde*, 150, 599–607.

Lavoie, J.P., Pascoe, J.R., & Kurpershoek, C.J. (1992a) Effect of head and neck position on respiratory mechanics in horses sedated with xylazine. *American Journal of Veterinary Research*, 53, 1652–1657.

Lavoie, J.P., Pascoe, J.R., & Kurpershoek, C.J. (1992b) Effects of xylazine on ventilation in horses. *American Journal of Veterinary Research*, 53, 916–920.

Leblanc, P.H. & Eberhart, S.W. (1990) Cardiopulmonary effects of epidurally administered xylazine in the horse. *Equine Veterinary Journal*, 22, 389–391.

Leino, K., Hynynen, M., Jalonen, J., Salmenpera, M., Scheinin, H., & Aantaa, R. (2011) Renal effects of dexmedetomidine during coronary artery bypass surgery: a randomized placebo-controlled study. *BMC Anesthesiology*, 11, 9.

Lemke, K.A. (2007) Anticholinergics and sedatives, in *Lumb & Jones' Veterinary Anesthesia and Analgesia*, 4th edn (eds W.J. Tranquilli, J.C. Thurman, & K.A. Grimm), Blackwell Publishing, Ames, IA, pp. 203–239.

Ma, D., Hossain, M., Rajakumaraswamy, N., et al. (2004) Dexmedetomidine produces its neuroprotective effect via the alpha

2A-adrenoceptor subtype. *European Journal of Pharmacology*, 502, 87–97.

Madan, R., Bharti, N., Shende, D., Khokhar, S.K., & Kaul, H.L. (2001) A dose response study of clonidine with local anesthetic mixture for peribulbar block: a comparison of three doses. *Anesthesia and Analgesia*, 93, 1593–1597.

Maddern, K., Adams, V.J., Hill, N.A., & Leece, N.A. (2010) Alfaxalone induction dose following administration of medetomidine and butorphanol in the dog. *Veterinary Anaesthesia and Analgesia*, 37, 7–13.

Martinez, E.A. (2012) Anesthetic agents, in *Small Animal Clinical Pharmacology & Therapeutics*, 2nd edn (ed. D.M. Boothe)., Elsevier, St. Louis, MO, pp. 887–893.

Maze, M. & Tranquilli, W. (1991) Alpha-2 adrenoceptor agonists: defining the role in clinical anesthesia. *Anesthesiology*, 74, 581–605.

McArthur, K.E., Anderson, D.S., Durbin, T.E., Orloff, M.J., & Dharmsathaphorn, K. (1982) Clonidine and lidamidine to inhibit watery diarrhea in a patient with lung cancer. *Annals of Internal Medicine*, 96, 323–325.

McDonell, W.N. & Kerr, C.L. (2007) Respiratory system, in *Lumb & Jones' Veterinary Anesthesia and Analgesia*, 4th edn (eds W.J. Tranquilli, J.C. Thurman, & K.A. Grimm), Blackwell Publishing, Ames, IA, pp. 117–151.

Memis, D., Kargi, M., & Sut, N. (2009) Effects of propofol and dexmedetomidine on indocyanine green elimination assessed with LIMON to patients with early septic shock: a pilot study. *Journal of Critical Care*, 24, 603–608.

Memis, D., Turan, A., Karamanlioglu, B., Pamukcu, Z., & Kurt, I. (2004) Adding dexmedetomidine to lidocaine for intravenous regional anesthesia. *Anesthesia & Analgesia*, 98, 835–840.

Merritt, A.M., Burrow, J.A., & Hartless, C.S. (1998) Effect of xylazine, detomidine, and a combination of xylazine and butorphanol on equine duodenal motility. *American Journal of Veterinary Research*, 59, 619–623.

Miller, J.H., McCoy, K.D., & Coleman, A.S. (2001) Renal actions of the alpha 2-adrenoceptor agonist, xylazine, in the anaesthetised rat. *New Zealand Veterinary Journal*, 49, 173–180.

Molina, C. & Herrero, J.F. (2006) The influence of the time course of inflammation and spinalization on the antinociceptive activity of the alpha 2-adrenoceptor agonist medetomidine. *European Journal of Pharmacology*, 532, 50–60.

Muir, W.W., 3rd, Ford, J.L., Karpa, G.E., Harrison, E.E., & Gadawski, J.E. (1999) Effects of intramuscular administration of low doses of medetomidine and medetomidine-butorphanol in middle-aged and old dogs. *Journal of the American Veterinary Medical Assocociation*, 215, 1116–1120.

Mukaddam-Daher, S. & Gutkowska, J. (2000) Atrial natriuretic peptide is involved in renal actions of moxonidine. *Hypertension*, 35, 1215–1220.

Murrell, J.C. & Hellebrekers, L.J. (2005) Medetomidine and dexmedetomidine: a review of cardiovascular effects and antinociceptive properties in the dog. *Veterinary Anaesthesia and Analgesia*, 32, 117–127.

Nguyen, D., Abdul-Rasool, I., Ward, D., et al. (1992) Ventilatory effects of dexmedetomidine, atipamezole, and isoflurane in dogs. *Anesthesiology*, 76, 573–579.

Noyer, M., de Laveleye, F., Vauquelin, G., Gobert, J., & Wulfert, E. (1994) Mivazerol, a novel compound with high specificity for alpha 2 adrenergic receptors: binding studies on different human and rat membrane preparations. *Neurochemistry International*, 24, 221–229.

Nyman, G., Marntell, S., Edner, A., Funkquist, P., Morgan, K., & Hedenstierna, G. (2009) Effect of sedation with detomidine and butorphanol on pulmonary gas exchange in the horse. *Acta Veterinaria Scandinavica*, 51, 22.

Oda, A., Iida, H., Tanahashi, S., Osawa, Y., Yamaguchi, S., & Dohi, S. (2007) Effects of alpha 2-adrenoceptor agonists on tetrodotoxin-resistant Na+ channels in rat dorsal root ganglion neurons. *European Journal of Anaesthesiology*, 24, 934–941.

Oku, K., Kakizaki, M., & Ohta, M. (2011) Clinical Evaluation of Total intravenous anesthesia using a combination of propofol and medetomidine following anesthesia induction with medetomidine, guaifenesin and propofol for castration in thoroughbred horses. *Journal of Veterinary Medical Sciences*, 73, 1639–1643.

Orko, R., Pouttu, J., Ghignone, M., & Rosenberg, P.H. (1987) Effect of clonidine on haemodynamic responses to endotracheal intubation and on gastric acidity. *Acta Anaesthesiologica Scandinavica*, 31, 325–329.

Paul, S., Bhattacharjee, D.P., Ghosh, S., Dawn, S., & Chatterjee, N. (2010) Efficacy of intra-articular dexmedetomidine for postoperative analgesia in arthroscopic knee surgery. *Ceylon Medical Journal*, 55, 111–115.

Pertovaara, A., Kauppila, T., Jyvasjarvi, E., & Kalso, E. (1991) Involvement of supraspinal and spinal segmental alpha-2-adrenergic mechanisms in the medetomidine-induced antinociception. *Neuroscience*, 44, 705–714.

Pettinger, W.A., Umemura, S., Smyth, D.D., et al. (1987) Renal alpha 2-adrenoceptors and the adenylate cyclase-cAMP system: biochemical and physiological interactions. *American Journal of Physiology*, 252, F199–F208.

Philipp, M., Brede, M., & Hein, L. (2002) Physiological significance of alpha(2)-adrenergic receptor subtype diversity: one receptor is not enough. *American Journal of Physiology-Regulatory, Integrative and Comparative Physiology*, 283, R287-R295.

Potter, D.E., Crosson, C.E., Heath, A.R., & Ogidigben, M.J. (1990) Functional evidence for heterogeneity of ocular alpha 2-adrenoceptors. *Proceedings of the Western Pharmacology Society*, 33, 257–260.

Potter, D.E. & Ogidigben, M.J. (1991) Medetomidine-induced alterations of intraocular pressure and contraction of the nictitating membrane. *Investigative Ophthalmology & Visual Science*, 32, 2799–2805.

Pypendop, B.H. & Verstegen, J.P. (1998) Hemodynamic effects of medetomidine in the dog: a dose titration study. *Veterinary Surgery*, 27, 612–622.

Raekallio, M.R., Raiha, M.P., Alanen, M.H., Saren, N.M., & Tuovia, T.A. (2009) Effects of medetomidine, L-methadone, and their combination on arterial blood gases in dogs. *Veterinary Anaesthesia and Analgesia*, 36, 158–161.

Ranheim, B., Horsberg, T.E., Søli, N.E., Ryeng, K.A., & Arnemo, J.M. (2000) The effects of medetomidine and its reversal with atipamezole on plasma glucose, cortisol and noradrenaline in cattle and sheep. *Journal of Veterinary Pharmacology and Therapeutics*, 23, 379–387.

Reitemeyer, H., Klein, H.J., & Deegen, E. (1986) The effect of sedatives on lung function in horses. *Acta Veterinaria Scandinavica Supplement*, 82, 111–120.

Robertson, S.A., Carter, S.W., Donovan, M., & Steele, C. (1990) Effects of intravenous xylazine hydrochloride on blood glucose, plasma insulin and rectal temperature in neonatal foals. *Equine Veterinary Journal*, 22, 43–47.

Roger, T. & Ruckebusch, Y. (1987) Colonic alpha 2-adrenoceptor-mediated responses in the pony. *Journal of Veterinary Pharmacology and Therapeutics*, 10, 310–318.

Ross, M.W., Cullen, K.K., & Rutkowski, J.A. (1990) Myoelectric activity of the ileum, cecum, and right ventral colon in ponies during interdigestive, nonfeeding, and digestive periods. *American Journal of Veterinary Research*, 51, 561–566.

Rouch, A.J., Kudo, L.H., & Hebert, C. (1997) Dexmedetomidine inhibits osmotic water permeability in the rat cortical collecting duct. *Journal of Pharmacology and Experimental Therapeutics*, 281, 62–69.

Ruffolo, R.R. Jr. (1985) Distribution and function of peripheral alpha-adrenoceptors in the cardiovascular system. *Pharmacology Biochemistry and Behavior*, 22, 827–833.

Ruskoaho, H. & Leppaluoto, J. (1989) The effect of medetomidine, an alpha 2-adrenoceptor agonist, on plasma atrial natriuretic peptide levels, haemodynamics and renal excretory function in spontaneously hypertensive and Wistar-Kyoto rats. *British Journal of Pharmacology*, 97, 125–132.

Sabbe, M.B., Penning, J.P., Ozaki, G.T.,& Yaksh, T.L. (1994) Spinal and systemic action of the alpha 2 receptor agonist dexmedetomidine in dogs. Antinociception and carbon dioxide response. *Anesthesiology*, 80, 1057–1072.

Saleh, N., Aoki, M., Shimada, T., Akiyoshi, H., Hassanin, A., & Ohashi, F. (2005) Renal effects of medetomidine in isoflurane-anesthetized dogs with special reference to its diuretic action. *Journal of Veterinary Medical Sciences*, 67, 461–465.

Salonen, J.S. (1989) Pharmacokinetics of medetomidine. *Acta Veterinaria Scandinavica Supplement*, 85, 49–54.

Scheinin, H., Virtanen, R., MacDonald, E., Lammintausta, R., Scheinin, M. (1989) Medetomidine–a novel alpha 2-adrenoceptor agonist: a review of its pharmacodynamic effects. *Progress in Neuropsychopharmacology and Biological Psychiatry*, 13, 635–651.

Seddighi, M. (2003) A comparison of the hemodynamic effects of epidurally administered medetomidine and xylazine in dogs [Abstract]. *Veterinary Anaesthesia and Analgesia*, 30, 98.

Sezer, A., Memis, D., Usta, U., Sut, N. (2010) The effect of dexmedetomidine on liver histopathology in a rat sepsis model: an experimental pilot study. *Ulusal Travma ve Acil Cerrahi Dergisi*, 16, 108–112.

Sinclair, M.D. (2003) A review of the physiological effects of alpha 2-agonists related to the clinical use of medetomidine in small animal practice. *Canadian Veterinary Journal*, 44, 885–897.

Singelyn, F.J., Gouverneur, J.M., & Robert, A. (1996) A minimum dose of clonidine added to mepivacaine prolongs the duration of anesthesia and analgesia after axillary brachial plexus block. *Anesthesia & Analgesia*, 83, 1046–1050.

Skarda, R.T. & Tranquilli, W.J. (2007) *Local and regional anesthetic and analgesic techniques: dogs*, in *Lumb & Jones' Veterinary Anesthesia and Analgesia*, 4th edn (eds W.J. Tranquilli, J.C. Thurman, & K.A. Grimm), Blackwell Publishing, Ames, IA, pp. 561–593.

Solano, A.M., Valverde, A., Desrochers, A., Nykamp, S., & Boure, L.P. (2009) Behavioural and cardiorespiratory effects of a constant rate infusion of medetomidine and morphine for sedation during standing laparoscopy in horses. *Equine Veterinary Journal*, 41, 153–159.

Stoelting, R.K. & Hillier, S.C. (2006) *Pharmacology & Physiology in Anesthetic Practice*, 4th edn, Lippincott Williams & Wilkins, Philadelphia.

Stone, L.S., MacMillan, L.B., Kitto, K.F., Limbird, L.E., & Wilcox, G.L. (1997) The alpha 2a adrenergic receptor subtype mediates spinal analgesia evoked by alpha 2 agonists and is necessary for spinal adrenergic-opioid synergy. *Journal of Neuroscience*, 17, 7157–7165.

Strombeck, D.R. & Harrold, D. (1985) Effects of atropine, acepromazine, meperidine, and xylazine on gastroesophageal sphincter pressure in the dog. *American Journal of Veterinary Research*, 46, 963–965.

Szreder, Z. (1993) Comparison between thermoregulatory effects mediated by alpha 1- and alpha 2-adrenoceptors in normothermic and febrile rabbits. *General Pharmacology*, 24, 929–941.

Talukder, M.H. & Hikasa, Y. (2009) Diuretic effects of medetomidine compared with xylazine in healthy dogs. *Canadian Journal of Veterinary Research*, 73, 224–236.

Tamagaki, S., Suzuki, T., Hagihira, S., Hayashi, Y., & Mashimo, T. (2010) Systemic daily morphine enhances the analgesic effect of intrathecal dexmedetomidine via up-regulation of alpha 2 adrenergic receptor subtypes A, B and C in dorsal root ganglion and dorsal horn. *Journal of Pharmacy and Pharmacology*, 62, 1760–1767.

Tibirica, E., Feldman, J., Mermet, C., Gonon, F., & Bousquet, P. (1991) An imidazoline-specific mechanism for the hypotensive effect of clonidine: a study with yohimbine and idazoxan. *Journal of Pharmacology and Experimental Therapeutics*, 256, 606–613.

Tolchard, S., Burns, P.A., Nutt, D.J., & Fitzjohn, S.M. (2009) Hypothermic responses to infection are inhibited by alpha 2-adrenoceptor agonists with possible clinical implications. *British Journal of Anaesthesia*, 103, 554–560.

Tran, K.M., Ganley, T.J., Wells, L., Ganesh, A., Minger, K.I., & Cucchiaro, G. (2005) Intraarticular bupivacaine-clonidine-morphine versus femoral-sciatic nerve block in pediatric patients undergoing anterior cruciate ligament reconstruction. *Anesthesia and Analgesia*, 101, 1304–1310.

Tschernko, E.M., Klepetko, H., Gruber, E., et al. (1998) Clonidine added to the anesthetic solution enhances analgesia and improves oxygenation after intercostal nerve block for thoracotomy. *Anesthesia and Analgesia*, 87, 107–111.

Vaha-Vahe, T. (1989a) The clinical efficacy of medetomidine. *Acta Veterinaria Scandinavica Supplement*, 85, 151–153.

Vaha-Vahe, T. (1989b) Clinical evaluation of medetomidine, a novel sedative and analgesic drug for dogs and cats. *Acta Veterinaria Scandinavica*, 30, 267–273.

Valtolina, C., Robben, J.H., Uilenreef, J., et al. (2009) Clinical evaluation of the efficacy and safety of a constant rate infusion of dexmedetomidine for postoperative pain management in dogs. *Veterinary Anaesthesia and Analgesia*, 36, 369–383.

Valverde, A., Rickey, E., Sinclair, M., et al. (2010) Comparison of cardiovascular function and quality of recovery in isoflurane-anaesthetised horses administered a constant rate infusion of lidocaine or lidocaine and medetomidine during elective surgery. *Equine Veterinary Journal*, 42, 192–199.

van Oostrom, H., Doornenbal, A., Schot, A., Stienen, P.J., & Hellebrekers, L.J. (2011) Neurophysiological assessment of the sedative and analgesic effects of a constant rate infusion of dexmedetomidine in the dog. *Veterinary Journal*, 190, 338–344.

Vesal, N., Cribb, P. H., & Frketic, M. (1996) Postoperative analgesic and cardiopulmonary effects in dogs of oxymorphone administered epidurally and intramuscularly, and medetomidine administered epidurally: a comparative clinical study. *Veterinary Surgery*, 25, 361–369.

Virgin, J., Hendrickson, D., Wallis, T., & Rao, S. (2010) Comparison of intraoperative behavioral and hormonal responses to noxious stimuli between mares sedated with caudal epidural detomidine hydrochloride or a continuous intravenous infusion of detomidine hydrochloride for standing laparoscopic ovariectomy. *Veterinary Surgery*, 39, 754–760.

Virtanen, R., Savola, J.M., Saano, V., & Nyman, L. (1988) Characterization of the selectivity, specificity and potency of medetomidine as an alpha 2-adrenoceptor agonist. *European Journal of Pharmacology*, 150, 9–14.

Wagner, A.E., Muir, W.W. 3rd, & Hinchcliff, K.W. (1991) Cardiovascular effects of xylazine and detomidine in horses. *American Journal of Veterinary Research*, 52, 651–657.

Westfall, T.C. (1977) Local regulation of adrenergic neurotransmission. *Physiological Review*, 57, 659–728.

Westfall, T.C. & Westfall, D.P. (2011) Neurotransmission: The autonomic and somatic motor nervous systems, in *Goodman & Gilman's The pharmacological Basis of Therapeutics*, 12th edn (ed. L. Brunton), McGraw-Hill Medical, New York, pp. 169–218.

Xu, H., Aibiki, M., Seki, K., Ogura, S., & Ogli, K. (1998) Effects of dexmedetomidine, an alpha2-adrenoceptor agonist, on renal sympathetic nerve activity, blood pressure, heart rate and central venous pressure in urethane-anesthetized rabbits. *Journal of Autonomic Nervous System*, 71, 48–54.

Yaksh, T.L. (1985) Pharmacology of spinal adrenergic systems which modulate spinal nociceptive processing. *Pharmacology Biochemistry and Behavior*, 22, 845–858.

Yaksh, T.L., Pogrel, J.W., Lee, Y.W., & Chaplan, S.R. (1995) Reversal of nerve ligation-induced allodynia by spinal alpha-2 adrenoceptor agonists. *Journal of Pharmacology and Experimental Therapeutics*, 272, 207–214.

Yaksh, T.L. & Reddy, S.V. (1981) Studies in the primate on the analgetic effects associated with intrathecal actions of opiates, alpha-adrenergic agonists and baclofen. *Anesthesiology*, 54, 451–467.

Yamashita, K., Muir, W.W. 3rd, Tsubakishita, S., et al. (2002) Clinical comparison of xylazine and medetomidine for premedication of horses. *Journal of the American Veterinary Medical Association*, 221, 1144–1149.

Yamashita, K., Tsubakishita, S., Futaok, S., et al. (2000) Cardiovascular effects of medetomidine, detomidine and xylazine in horses. *The Journal of Veterinary Medical Science*, 62, 1025–1032.

Yamazaki, S., Katada, T., & Ui, M. (1982) Alpha 2-adrenergic inhibition of insulin secretion via interference with cyclic AMP generation in rat pancreatic islets. *Molecular Pharmacology*, 21, 648–653.

8

Nontraditional Analgesic Agents

Lydia Love and Dave Thompson

Nontraditional analgesic agents are pain-relieving drugs other than opiates, nonsteroidal anti-inflammatory drugs (NSAIDs), and local anesthetics. The pharmacological mechanisms of nontraditional analgesic agents are diverse and are the focus of much current research activity. Many of these drugs are classified as adjuvant analgesics, used to potentiate the effect of traditional analgesics. As such, they may be employed in ambulatory surgical settings in order to decrease the dose of opioid, opioid-associated adverse effects, and time to discharge. Depending on the type of pain involved, some of the drugs in this group can be used as primary analgesic agents in the multimodal treatment of chronic pain.

The management of pain must be directed by the underlying mechanisms. Acute inflammatory pain is driven by cellular biochemical pathways that intersect with, but are distinct from, those of chronic neuropathic pain states. In addition, neuropathic pain can be divided into several different types, originating centrally or peripherally, and analgesic efficacy of adjunctive analgesics can vary accordingly. Most clinical studies of neuropathic pain have focused on humans with either peripheral diabetic neuropathy or postherpetic neuralgia. The diversity of underlying pain pathophysiology and dearth of veterinary-specific studies may delay understanding of the appropriate uses of adjunctive analgesics in the clinical veterinary setting.

The following review of nontraditional analgesics is arranged according to currently accepted pharmacological mechanisms, as opposed to susceptible pain states. In addition, certain drugs that could be considered nontraditional analgesics (e.g., α-2 agonists, tramadol) and novel applications of traditional agents (intravenous lidocaine) are considered in other chapters in this book. Finally, experimental evidence exists for the use of many different classes of drugs as analgesics, especially in neuropathic pain states. This review will focus on the classes of drugs currently used in clinical practice. Much of the information herein is extrapolated from human or experimental studies. When possible, veterinary studies are cited, but much work remains to be done to document the efficacy of these drugs in animal species.

ANTIEPILEPTIC DRUGS

Mechanism of Action

Since the 1960s, antiepileptic drugs (AEDs), including carbamazepine, gabapentin, and pregabalin, have been used to manage neuropathic pain in human patients (Alarcón-Segovia & Lazcono, 1968; Segal & Rordof, 1996; Hill et al., 2001). These AEDs act through various mechanisms to suppress seizure activity, and the same cellular processes are thought to be responsible for their analgesic efficacy.

Carbamazepine, a first-line treatment for trigeminal neuropathy (Zakrzewska, 2010), prevents activation of synaptosomal voltage-gated sodium channels (Sheets et al., 2008), thereby preventing conduction of neuronal action potentials and subsequent neurotransmitter release. Gabapentin and pregabalin (gabapentinoids) bind to the $\alpha 2\delta$ subunit of voltage-gated calcium channels (VGCC) (Field et al., 2000; Stahl, 2004) and appear to disrupt intracellular trafficking of these subunits (Tran-Van-Minh & Dolphin, 2010). Calcium influx activates multiple cellular processes, including release of neurotransmitters, regulation of gene expression, and alterations in cellular excitability (Cao, 2006). By binding to VGCC, gabapentinoids may interrupt some or all of these processes. Other cellular mechanisms may be important in the analgesia produced by the gabapentinoids, including upregulation of descending noradrenergic inhibition (Hayashida et al., 2008). Although many of the AEDs have been studied in human neuropathic pain states, gabapentin has received the most attention as a nontraditional analgesic in veterinary medicine, and the rest of this section will focus on the gabapentinoids.

Efficacy of Gabapentinoids in Acute Pain

The effectiveness of gabapentin has been established most strongly for neuropathic pain syndromes; however, several small randomized clinical human trials demonstrated efficacy in acute perioperative pain states, including arthroscopy (Bang et al., 2010), pediatric spinal fusion (Rusy et al., 2010), and after cesarean section (Moore et al., 2011). An interesting comparative study of oral gabapentin, ketamine infusion, or placebo demonstrated a decrease in pain scores and morphine consumption in the first 24 hours post hysterectomy in both the ketamine and gabapentin groups (Sen et al., 2009). Moreover, the gabapentin group reported a lower incidence of chronic pain and chronic incisional pain. Results of clinical trials are mixed, and although a recent Cochrane review (Straube et al., 2010) did identify an effective dose of gabapentin for established acute postoperative pain in adults, the number needed to treat (NNT) to have an effect in one person was 11; the authors concluded that this was too large to be clinically relevant.

Pain Management in Veterinary Practice, First Edition. Edited by Christine M. Egger, Lydia Love and Tom Doherty.
© 2014 John Wiley & Sons, Inc. Published 2014 by John Wiley & Sons, Inc.

Pregabalin is the structurally related successor to gabapentin, and is marketed in the United States as a Class V controlled drug, Lyrica®. Results of studies investigating the efficacy of pregabalin in acute pain settings are mixed, with some studies demonstrating a decrease in pain scores and/or opioid consumption (Hill et al., 2001; Kim et al., 2010; Durkin et al., 2010), while others have been unable to establish that pregabalin lessens acute perioperative pain (Paech et al., 2007).

Veterinary studies of gabapentin are limited in scope and nature, and the veterinary literature has been unable to demonstrate effectiveness of gabapentin in acute pain states. In experimental studies in awake cats, gabapentin at 5, 10, or 30 mg/kg did not affect thermal threshold (Pypendop et al., 2010), and plasma concentrations up to 20 μg/mL (equivalent to 13 mg/kg orally (Siao et al., 2010)) did not reduce the minimum alveolar concentration of isoflurane (Reid et al., 2010). Moreover, administration of oral gabapentin at 10 mg/kg prior to forelimb amputation in dogs followed by 5 mg/kg PO every 12 hours for three additional days, did not decrease pain scores during hospitalization or at home (Wagner et al., 2010). The authors concluded that gabapentin, at the given dose and frequency, did not provide a significant reduction in acute perioperative pain as part of a multimodal analgesic plan. More veterinary studies are needed to evaluate efficacy in different dosing scenarios and species, and to investigate the potential for decreasing chronic pain following acute nociceptive insults.

Efficacy of Gabapentinoids in Chronic Pain

In neuropathic pain states in humans, the gabapentinoids are widely accepted as a first-line treatment (Dworkin et al., 2010), with effectiveness demonstrated especially in peripheral diabetic neuropathy and post-herpetic neuralgia (Segal & Rordof, 1996; Ko et al., 2010). The efficacy of the gabapentinoids in neuropathic pain states is so well established that they are now used in comparative studies to investigate promising new pharmacotherapeutics (Sen et al., 2009; Amr, 2010). Some evidence exists that pregabalin may provide analgesic efficacy superior to that of gabapentin in peripheral neuropathies of humans (Toth, 2010).

Use of gabapentin in the treatment of neuropathic pain in veterinary species has been suggested (Robertson, 2005), but published studies are limited to case reports and case series. The first veterinary case report of the use of gabapentin for analgesia involved the treatment of a 24-year-old pregnant draft horse with signs of pain due to suspected femoral neuropathy after recovery from colic surgery (Davis et al., 2007). In 2009, a case series involving three dogs with chronic pain disorders, unresponsive to traditional analgesic agents, reported resolution of clinical signs in one of the dogs with gabapentin therapy (Cashmore et al., 2009). Also in 2009, a case report regarding the use of gabapentin in a prairie falcon, as part of a multimodal approach to suspected neuropathic pain, was published (Shaver et al., 2009). The authors are unaware of veterinary studies investigating gabapentin in comparison to placebo or traditional analgesics in neuropathic pain states.

Pharmacokinetics

In humans, gabapentin is slowly absorbed after oral administration and displays zero-order pharmacokinetics, that is, a constant amount of drug is eliminated per unit of time. In contrast, pregabalin is rapidly absorbed after oral dosing and is metabolized via first-order (or linear) processes (Bockbrader et al., 2010), wherein a fixed fraction of drug in the body is eliminated over time. Gabapentin and pregabalin are excreted intact via renal mechanisms, are not metabolized by hepatic microsomes, and are not highly protein bound; therefore, few clinically significant drug interactions occur. The most common side effects of short-term administration of the gabapentinoids are sedation and dizziness (Tiippana et al., 2007).

Pharmacokinetic (PK) data for gabapentin exists for dogs (Radulovic et al., 1995), greyhound dogs (KuKanich & Cohen, 2011), cattle (Coetzee et al., 2010), horses (Dirikolu et al., 2008; Terry et al., 2010), and cats (Siao et al., 2010). Rapid absorption and disposition of oral gabapentin occurs in dogs, with moderate hepatic transformation to N-methyl-gabapentin prior to renal elimination (Radulovic et al., 1995). Bioavailability is high in cats, and gabapentin exhibits a small volume of distribution with a moderately long half-life (Siao et al., 2010). Cattle demonstrate a long half-life after oral administration of gabapentin, leading the authors of one study to conclude that further evaluation of oral gabapentin for analgesia in cattle is warranted (Coetzee et al., 2010). In contrast to other species, bioavailability of oral gabapentin in horses is low but the half-life is long (Dirikolu et al., 2008). In addition, behavioral effects such as sedation and increased frequency of drinking were observed after oral administration of 20 mg/kg gabapentin to horses (Terry et al., 2010). Pregabalin studies in veterinary species are currently limited. A PK study in dogs demonstrated that 4 mg/kg orally resulted in plasma concentrations associated with analgesic efficacy in humans (Salazar et al., 2009). Similar results were reported for cats administered pregabalin at 4 mg/kg (Cautela et al., 2010).

Recommendations for Clinical Use

Of the currently available AEDs, gabapentin has the most experimental and anecdotal support for its use in veterinary species. In acute pain states, it is the authors' opinion that gabapentin may be useful as an adjunctive agent in multimodal analgesic protocols. In addition, the sedative and anxiolytic properties may be beneficial perioperatively. Finally, perioperative use may decrease the development of chronic pain, which can be very difficult to diagnose and treat in veterinary species. In neuropathic pain, it is quite likely that gabapentin and pregabalin may have beneficial effects, and can be used as first-line therapy or in addition to other analgesic agents. A suggested starting dose for gabapentin is 5–10 mg/kg every 8–12 hours. Because sedation can occur, especially in geriatric patients, owner compliance may be improved by beginning with once-daily dosing at night for a few days to allow acclimatization. In some instances the side effect of sedation is beneficial in painful patients with disrupted sleep patterns. When gabapentin is added to an analgesic regimen for patients with chronic pain the dose can be increased by 25–50% every week until an acceptable response occurs. One of the authors (DT) has used doses as high as 50–60 mg/kg every 8 hours in dogs with severe cancer pain, without adverse effect.

The use of pregabalin for neuropathic pain in veterinary species is limited to anecdotal reports and dosing is based on extrapolation from PK studies. For dogs, the suggested dose range is 2–4 mg/kg every 12 hours and for cats 1–2 mg/kg every 12 hours.

Gabapentin is currently available in 100 mg, 300 mg, and 400 mg capsules as well as 600 mg and 800 mg tablets. Liquid formulations can be compounded to specification by a licensed compounding pharmacy. The 50 mg/mL name brand liquid formulation,

Neurontin, contains 300 mg/mL xylitol, which can cause hypoglycemia in dogs at doses as low as 100 mg/kg and hepatotoxicity, and potentially death, at 500 mg/kg (Piscitelli et al., 2010). The toxic dose of xylitol in cats is unknown; to the authors' knowledge, no reports of feline xylitol toxicity exist. Pregabalin is available in a wide variety of capsules, ranging from 25 mg to 300 mg, and a 20 mg/mL oral solution.

NMDA RECEPTOR ANTAGONISTS

Mechanism of Action

The N-methyl-D-aspartate (NMDA) receptor is a nonselective cation channel that is located both pre- and postsynaptically throughout the CNS (Corlew et al., 2008). These receptors are widely distributed in the brain and spinal cord and are involved in many physiological functions (Corlew et al., 2008). Activation of the NMDA receptor contributes to development of hyperalgesia and chronic pain and is the basis of windup, long-term potentiation, and central sensitization (Zhuo, 2009; Tao, 2010). Interestingly, the NMDA receptor is implicated in conscious memory formation as well as central sensitization, which is essentially a "memory of pain."

The NMDA receptor is a molecular coincidence detector in that it is both ligand- and voltage-gated (Zhuo, 2009). Activation of the NMDA receptor is prevented under conditions of minimal nociceptive input by a magnesium (Mg^{2+}) ion block. High-frequency depolarization of the cell membrane causes expulsion of the Mg^{2+} ion. Concurrent binding of glutamate and glycine allows the NMDA receptor to conduct strong cation currents, including Na^+, K^+, and Ca^{2+}. The number and strength of postsynaptic currents increase, upregulating numerous protein kinases and causing adjustments in cellular enzyme products via transcriptional and posttranslational alterations (Zhuo, 2009). The result is both stimulus-independent firing of the second-order neuron and increased production and trafficking of excitatory glutamate receptors. These are the underlying cellular mechanisms of windup and central sensitization.

Antagonists of the NMDA receptor, such as the dissociative anesthetics ketamine and tiletamine, have traditionally been used in veterinary medicine as general anesthetics (Kaplan, 1972). However, there is a renewed interest in human and veterinary medicine in the use of NMDA antagonists as adjunctive analgesics in acute and chronic pain states. There are many drugs in current use that have antagonist activity at the NMDA receptor, including ketamine and tiletamine, amantadine, dextromethorphan, nitrous oxide, xenon, and some opioids, including methadone. This section will focus on ketamine and the oral NMDA antagonist amantadine, due to the large body of research available as well as ease of use in clinical veterinary medicine.

Efficacy in Acute Pain

Ketamine has been extensively researched for its analgesic and antihyperalgesic effects in the perioperative period (Figure 8.1). At subanesthetic doses ketamine is, by itself, a weak analgesic (Bergadano et al., 2009); however, low-dose perioperative ketamine improves opioid efficacy (Suzuki et al., 1999), decreases postoperative opioid requirements and side effects (Javery et al., 1996; Zakine et al., 2008), and decreases opioid-induced hyperalgesia (Minville et al.,

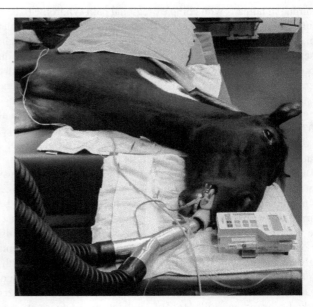

Figure 8.1. A continuous rate infusion of ketamine at a subanesthetic dose can be a useful adjunct to volatile anesthesia by providing additional analgesia.

2010). A Cochrane review established the efficacy and acceptability of perioperative ketamine in order to reduce opioid consumption in humans, although dosing strategies varied too widely to make a dose recommendation (Bell et al., 2006). Evidence exists that the development of chronic pain can be diminished by perioperative ketamine use (Remérand et al., 2009).

Perioperative ketamine infusions have been documented to decrease perioperative pain scores and increase activity in dogs undergoing forelimb amputation (Wagner et al., 2002). However, a similar small study in dogs demonstrated no decrease in opioid requirements in dogs postmastectomy (Sarrau et al., 2007). The latter study did find a significant increase in calorie consumption 2 days postoperatively in dogs given the highest ketamine infusion rates. Ketamine infusions are often used clinically to reduce perioperative or laminitic pain in horses, but published studies are limited to laboratory-based investigations. Ketamine reduces the withdrawal response to an electrical nociceptive stimulus in conscious horses (Peterbauer et al., 2008), whereas similar infusion rates do not decrease response to mechanical pain induced by hoof testers (Fielding et al., 2006).

The use of oral NMDA antagonists, such as amantadine, to decrease acute perioperative pain is not as well defined as administration of intravenous ketamine. A limited amount of data in humans indicates that multiple doses of amantadine before and after surgical intervention reduce pain scores and opioid consumption (Snijdelaar et al., 2004), whereas isolated preoperative administration does not (Gottschalk et al., 2001). To the authors' knowledge, no veterinary studies of perioperative amantadine use exist.

Efficacy in Chronic Pain

Ketamine may play a role in mitigating chronic pain states, especially that of neuropathic origin (Elsewaisy et al., 2010; Goldberg et al., 2010). Multi-day subanesthetic infusions of ketamine in humans with complex regional pain syndrome (CRPS) resulted in decreased pain scores (Sigtermans et al., 2009a; Dahan et al., 2011), although refractory CRPS may require a much higher dose (Kiefer et al., 2008). Oral NMDA antagonists have been disappointing in the treatment of established neuropathic pain, such as phantom limb pain (Maier et al., 2003). Conversely, some evidence exists that early or preventative treatment with oral NMDA antagonists may prevent development of chronic pain states (Schley et al., 2007; Hackworth et al., 2008). One study indicates that perioperative administration of amantadine decreases the development of postoperative chronic pain (Eisenberg et al., 2007).

Due to the lack of high-level evidence and potential psychotomimetic effects of ketamine, the use of NMDA antagonists for neuropathic pain in humans is not currently recommended as a first-line treatment, but can be considered in refractory cases. The veterinary literature concerning the use of NMDA antagonists for chronic pain states is limited. A case report of a cow tentatively diagnosed with CRPS reported successful treatment with a combination of extradural infusions of ketamine, detomidine, bupivacaine, and methadone (Bergadano et al., 2009). A randomized, masked, placebo-controlled trial of 31 client-owned dogs with signs of pelvic limb osteoarthritis (OA) pain despite NSAID therapy documented an increase in owner-scored activity with the addition of amantadine (Lascelles et al., 2008). Further research is necessary to define the role of NMDA antagonists in the treatment of chronic pain states in veterinary species.

Pharmacokinetics

A wide variety of PK data exists for ketamine, though most studies involve anesthetic doses. Analgesic effects may not correlate with plasma ketamine concentrations (Goldberg et al., 2010), and this may be due to effect site concentrations or downstream metabolites. In humans with CRPS, ketamine produced analgesia to acute experimental pain that correlated with detectable plasma concentrations; moreover, the study detected a decrease in pre-existing pain that persisted at least 5 hours beyond the ketamine infusion (Sigtermans et al., 2010). Although the racemic version is currently the only formulation available in the United States, the S(+) enantiomer is marketed in Europe and may be more a potent analgesic (Sigtermans et al., 2009b).

Human and canine PK data for amantadine indicate that it is highly absorbed after oral administration (Bleidner et al., 1965; Aoki & Sitar, 1988). In horses, bioavailability after oral administration is about 50% (Rees et al., 1997). One human study documented a decrease in morphine clearance in the group receiving oral amantadine, suggesting that PK mechanisms could be responsible for the reduction in opioid requirements (Snijdelaar et al., 2004). Amantadine is cleared by the kidneys in dogs and humans, with minimal hepatic transformation (Bleidner et al., 1965), and dose reductions should be considered in patients with renal disease.

Recommendations for Clinical Use

In acute pain states, including traumatic injury and surgical interventions, ketamine may be used as a constant rate infusion (CRI) to augment analgesia provided by traditional analgesics, decrease windup and central sensitization, and potentially decrease the development of chronic pain states. A dosing range of 2–20 μg/kg/min should provide NMDA receptor antagonism with minimal dissociative effects. For chronic pain, especially neuropathic pain states, ketamine CRIs may be useful in veterinary patients, though they

do require hospitalization. The authors have used this strategy most commonly in dogs with pain of neoplastic origin that may include a neuropathic component, often in combination with intravenous lidocaine and opioids. Amantadine may be most helpful in chronic and neuropathic pain states, and can be added to analgesic regimens at 3–5 mg/kg PO once daily. Rare side effects of amantadine include diarrhea and mild agitation. Amantadine is available in 100 mg capsules and a 10 mg/mL oral solution.

SEROTONIN AND NOREPINEPHRINE REUPTAKE INHIBITORS

Mechanism of Action

The neurotransmitters serotonin and norepinephrine (NE) are fundamental to many central nervous system activities, including vigilance, hunger, mood, and nociception (Arnold et al., 2008). Tricyclic antidepressants (TCAs) inhibit the reuptake transporters of serotonin and NE, thereby increasing concentrations in the CNS. TCAs have varying degrees of antagonist activity at histamine, α-adrenergic, muscarinic cholinergic, and serotonin receptors (Gillman, 2007). In addition, TCAs block voltage-gated sodium channels, which may contribute to their analgesic efficacy (Dick et al., 2007). Newer generation drugs that prevent the reuptake of serotonin and NE are known as dual reuptake inhibitors (SNRIs). Both TCAs and SNRIs are classified as antidepressants due to their mood elevating effects. However, analgesia provided by these drugs in chronic pain states appears to be independent of the mood-modulating effects (Bajwa et al., 2009). Mounting evidence indicates that NE systems may influence analgesia to a greater degree than serotonin pathways (Hall et al., 2011). Other analgesics also affect serotonin and NE reuptake, including tramadol and tapentadol. This section will focus on the TCA amitriptyline because of its widespread use in veterinary medicine. Clomipramine is another TCA that is used in veterinary medicine in the treatment of behavioral disorders, and there are reports in the human literature of its use in neuropathic pain syndromes. However, a high incidence of unpleasant side effects makes its use less attractive than amitriptyline or SNRIs. Because much attention has centered on the SNRI duloxetine for the management of chronic pain, relevant research will be reviewed. Tramadol and tapentadol are covered elsewhere in this book (see Chapter 4).

Efficacy in Acute Pain

Data for the efficacy of TCAs and SNRIs in acute pain states are very limited. Experimental evidence suggests that thermal nociception and hyperalgesia may be decreased by antidepressants that have strong NE reuptake inhibition (Bomholt et al., 2005; Jones et al., 2005). One recent placebo-controlled clinical trial demonstrated duloxetine decreased the requirement for opioids after total knee replacement, but no differences in pain scores or adverse events were detected (Ho et al., 2010).

Efficacy in Chronic Pain

TCAs have been used in the treatment of neuropathic pain states since the late 1950s (Bajwa et al., 2009), and are currently considered first-line therapy for neuropathic pain in humans (Dworkin et al., 2010). Amitriptyline is used in veterinary species for behavioral disorders, and has been investigated for treatment of pain associated with feline idiopathic cystitis. Short-term treatment with amitriptyline has not been effective in reducing signs or recurrence of idiopathic cystitis in cats (Kraijer et al., 2003; Kruger et al., 2003), but long-term therapy has been promising (Chew et al., 1998). A case series involving suspected neuropathic pain conditions in three dogs reported response to treatment with amitriptyline in two of the dogs (Cashmore et al., 2009).

The SNRIs, such as duloxetine, have garnered much interest in the treatment of chronic neuropathic pain because of the adverse effects associated with TCA therapy, including dry mouth and tachycardia due to antimuscarinic activity. A meta-analysis indicates that duloxetine is effective for the treatment of diabetic peripheral neuropathy and fibromyalgia in humans (Lunn et al., 2009). Duloxetine also appears to be effective in decreasing pain scores in humans with OA of the knee (Chappell et al., 2009). No veterinary studies concerning the efficacy of SNRIs in chronic or neuropathic pain were identified.

Pharmacokinetics

Amitriptyline is well absorbed from the gastrointestinal tract and undergoes moderate first-pass hepatic extraction, resulting in bioavailability ranging from 33% to 62% in man (Schulz et al., 1983). Bioavailability is similar in dogs (Kukes et al., 2009). Duloxetine is highly absorbed when administered orally to humans (Lantz et al., 2003). Both TCAs and SNRIs depend heavily on hepatic function for metabolism (Schulz et al., 1983; Lantz et al., 2003). PK studies of duloxetine in veterinary species are lacking.

Recommendations for Clinical Use

Amitriptyline may be most effective in the treatment of neuropathic pain states, and is administered at 0.5–3 mg/kg every 12–24 hours. Due to side effects, dose escalation should be gradual. Amitriptyline is available in a variety of tablet sizes, ranging from 10 mg to 150 mg. An effective and safe dose of duloxetine for veterinary species is unknown at this time.

Serotonin syndrome is reported in the veterinary literature and can involve changes in mentation, autonomic imbalance, including potentially fatal hyperthermia, and neuromuscular signs such as tremor (Crowell-Davis & Poggiagliolmi, 2008). Caution should be used when combining drugs that affect the serotonin system, including TCAs, SNRIs, tramadol, dextromethorphan, monoamine oxidase inhibitors (e.g., selegiline), certain opioids (e.g., meperidine and fentanyl), and selective serotonin reuptake inhibitors (e.g., fluoxetine).

DISEASE MODIFYING OSTEOARTHRITIS DRUGS

Mechanism of Action

Degenerative OA is a major cause of morbidity in aging veterinary populations, and can result in euthanasia due to poor quality of life. Disease modifying osteoarthritis drugs (DMOADs) are a diverse group of agents utilized in an attempt to modulate the pathological processes of OA. Alterations in the cartilage, synovial membrane, and subchondral bone are the result of the chronic and progressive nature of OA, and are driven by enzymatic and inflammatory mechanisms (Abramson & Attur, 2009). Existing research implicates matrix metalloproteinases (MMP) and inflammatory cytokines, including IL-1B, in the destruction of cartilage as well as the synovial membrane (Pelletier & Martel-Pelletier,

2007). Various DMOADs, including polysulfated glycosaminoglycans (PSGAGs), glucosamine, chondroitin sulfate, hyaluronic acid (HA), and omega-3 fatty acids, are utilized to counter the events of this degenerative cellular cascade.

PSGAGs, such as Adequan® and Cartrophen®, and oral chondroprotectives, including glucosamine and chondroitin, appear to inhibit degradation of cartilage (Fujiki et al., 2007; Scarpellini et al., 2008), decrease oxidative stress and inflammatory mediators (Tung et al., 2002; Calamia et al., 2010), and have been hypothesized to enhance chondrogenesis (Caron, 2005). HA is a nonsulfated glycosaminoglycan, which, like PSGAGs, appears to exert both anti-inflammatory activity and a direct chondroprotective effect (Greenberg et al., 2006; Kaplan et al., 2009). In addition, HA is theorized to improve the viscoelastic properties of synovial fluid.

Resolution of inflammation is an active process that is mediated by products of lipid metabolism. The omega-3 polyunsaturated fatty acids (PUFAs), docosahexenoic acid (DHA), and eicosapentanoic acid (EPA) offer an alternative substrate for cyclooxygenase and lipoxygenase enzymes, generating bioactive lipid mediators, including protectins and resolvins, that exert a direct anti-inflammatory effect (Serhan & Chiang, 2008), and reduce the production of MMP and other inflammatory mediators (Zainal et al., 2009; Wann et al., 2010). Additionally, resolvins may modulate synaptic plasticity at the level of the spinal cord (Xu et al., 2010).

Efficacy in Osteoarthritic Pain

Most evidence for the use of DMOADs in osteoarthritic pain is anecdotal or experimental in nature. In one small prospective study, lameness improved in 75% of dogs treated with intramuscular PSGAGs (Fujiki et al., 2007). In horses with induced OA, PSGAGs decreased joint effusion and histological markers of disease progression (Frisbie et al., 2009). Oral chondroprotectives are common in over-the-counter preparations for human OA pain, and several meta-analyses of their use have demonstrated modest effects that may not be clinically relevant, although this is debated intensely (Wandel et al., 2010). In canine OA patients, the combination of glucosamine and chondroitin sulfate (G/CS) has resulted in statistically significant improvements in pain scores and lameness, when compared with carprofen as a positive control (McCarthy et al., 2007). However, G/CS in combination with manganese did not improve force plate analysis scores or subjective assessment, when compared with carprofen or meloxicam in a separate canine study (Moreau et al., 2003). Reviews of the veterinary literature regarding glucosamine-based products in canine (Aragon et al., 2007) and equine (Pearson & Lindinger, 2009) patients indicate that the quality of evidence for the use of these nutraceuticals is questionable.

HA is used widely to treat horses with lameness due to OA. In experimentally induced OA, histological markers of disease progression were decreased by the intra-articular administration of HA, but no clinical improvement was noted (Frisbie et al., 2009). Intravenous HA also improved histological scores as well as clinical evaluation of lameness in experimentally induced OA of horses (Kawcak et al., 1997). As with horses, HA administered intravenously or intra-articularly has resulted in improvement in histological markers of canine OA, but has not consistently resulted in clinical improvement in either experimental or clinical models (Brandt et al., 2004; Canapp et al., 2005; Echigo et al., 2006).

Omega-3 fatty acid supplementation has been investigated in dogs with OA, and several small studies have documented improvements in owner evaluated clinical signs and weight bearing (Roush et al., 2010a, 2010b) as well as a reduction in carprofen dosage (Fritsch et al., 2010).

Recommendations for Clinical Use

Injectable PSGAGs are used widely in canine and equine OA. These products have an excellent safety profile and, although efficacy is debatable, may have some positive effects in specific patient populations and as a part of multimodal protocols. In the United States, Adequan® Canine is available as a 100 mg/mL solution, and is labeled for intramuscular use in dogs at 4 mg/kg twice weekly for 4 weeks. Anecdotal evidence indicates that the subcutaneous route may also be used, and owners can often be taught to give injections at home. Ongoing treatment at monthly, or more frequent intervals, is often recommended off-label for dogs and cats. An equine version of Adequan® is available in a dose pack of seven preservative-free vials, each containing 5 mL of 100 mg/mL solution. The labeled dose for horses is one 5 mL injection every 4 days for 28 days, although dosing is often extended in an off-label manner similar to dogs and cats.

Many oral OTC chondroprotectives are available, and dose recommendations are varied. The glucosamine dose in dogs ranges from 20 mg/kg to 100 mg/kg. Care should be taken to select a reputable manufacturer, as glucosamine/chondroitin content and quality may not correlate with label claims.

Legend® is a 10 mg/mL HA product that is labeled for intravenous use in horses, and is supplied in a box of six 4 mL vials. A 40 mg (4 mL) dose can be repeated weekly for three treatments. In an off-label manner, this product is also injected intra-articularly in horses, and intravenously or intra-articularly in dogs. Hylartin V (10 mg/mL) is marketed in the US for intra-articular injection in horses. In Canada and Europe, HY-50 (17 mg/mL) is approved for intra-articular or intravenous use in horses.

Many omega-3 fatty acid products are available and dosing is empirical and diverse. A common recommendation is to administer EPA at 36 mg/kg and DHA at 24 mg/kg.

BISPHOSPHONATES

Mechanism of Action

Bisphosphonates prevent resorption of bone by disrupting osteoclast function. These drugs localize to areas of active osteolysis by binding to Ca^{2+} and other divalent metal ions and cause apoptosis of osteoclasts (Roelofs et al., 2006). In addition, bisphosphonates have direct anti-inflammatory (Bianchi et al., 2008) and antineoplastic effects (Aft, 2011). Bisphosphonates are divided into nitrogen-containing and non-nitrogen-containing groups. Aminobisphosphonates contain nitrogen and are more potent. The aminobisphosphonates are commonly used in humans with metastatic bone disease to help manage pain as well as skeletal complications such as pathological fractures. In dogs with osteosarcoma undergoing palliative therapies, aminobisphosphonates reduce pain associated with skeletal neoplasia (Fan et al., 2007; Fan et al., 2009). For palliation of malignant bone pain, bisphosphonates are covered in more detail elsewhere in this book (see Chapter 27).

Efficacy in Osteoarthritic Pain

Because of their effects on bone remodeling, bisphosphonates have been investigated for the treatment of pain associated with OA in rats (Strassle et al., 2010), humans (Fujita et al., 2009), horses (Gough et al., 2010), and dogs (Moreau et al., 2011). In horses, tiludronate reduces lameness in navicular disease (Denoix et al., 2003), thoracolumbar OA (Coudry et al., 2007), and distal tarsal OA (Gough et al., 2010). Tiludronate is approved in Europe for the treatment of navicular disease and distal tarsal OA (or bone spavin).

Recommendations for Clinical Use

Tiludronate is available in Europe under the brand name Tildren. Formulated at a concentration of 5 mg/mL, the manufacturer recommends slow intravenous administration of 0.1 mg/kg every day for 10 days. Off-label uses include the administration of the total dose (1 mg/kg) over about 1 hour (Delguste et al., 2008), and as a regional limb perfusion. Tiludronate should not be used in horses under 3 years of age or those that are pregnant or lactating. Mild hypocalcemia can occur during injection and transient colic is occasionally reported.

It should be noted that long-term or high-dose bisphosphonate therapy has been linked to increased risk of osteonecrosis of the jaw in humans (Marx et al., 2007), and atypical femoral and pelvic fractures (Yli-Kyyny, 2011). Bisphosphonate-related osteonecrosis of the jaw has been experimentally reproduced in rats and dogs (Burr & Allen, 2009), and develops most commonly after oral surgery in humans. It is unknown if these conditions will occur in clinical veterinary patients.

EMERGING TREATMENTS

Many different classes of drugs hold promise for the treatment of pain and are currently being investigated. Among the most exciting are capsaicin and resiniferatoxin, which are agonists at transient receptor potential vanilloid type 1 (TRPV1) receptors. These are ligand-gated cation channels, expressed both centrally and peripherally, which respond to mechanical, thermal, and chemical stimuli, initiating action potentials along sensory neurons and ascending spinal tracts (Palazzo et al., 2010). Prolonged activation leads to downregulation of receptors and cytotoxicity of sensory neurons expressing TRPV1 channels. In one unblinded and uncontrolled study of dogs with naturally occurring bone cancers, significantly improved comfort levels were noted after intrathecal administration of resiniferatoxin (Brown et al., 2005). Other compounds of interest include VGCC blockers such as ziconotide. An FDA-approved treatment for refractory pain, ziconotide is derived from the venom of a predatory marine snail, genus *Conus* (Schmidtko et al., 2010). Limitations include side effects such as changes in mentation and nausea, and that it must be delivered intrathecally. Ongoing research is defining the analgesic profiles of many other classes of drugs, including cannabinoids, dopamine antagonists, novel anticonvulsants, astrocyte inhibitors, and immune-modulating drugs.

SUMMARY

Management of pain, acute or chronic, inflammatory or neuropathic, can be challenging. Often, pain is incompletely or ineffectively managed, and in veterinary species, pain that is not adequately controlled may affect quality of life to the extent that the patient may be euthanized. Nontraditional analgesics have expanded the veterinarian's armamentarium in the effort to offer appropriate analgesia, providing patients with relief of suffering and owners with peace of mind.

REFERENCES

Abramson, S.B. & Attur, M. (2009) Developments in the scientific understanding of osteoarthritis. *Arthritis Research and Therapy*, 11(3), 227–235.

Aft, R. (2011) Bisphosphonates in breast cancer: antitumor effects. *Clinical Advances in Hematology and Oncology*, 9(4), 292–299.

Alarcón-Segovia, D. & Lazcono, M.A. (1968) Carbamazepine for tabetic pain. *Journal of the American Medical Association*, 22(2), 107–119.

Amr, Y.M. (2010) Multi-day low dose ketamine infusion as adjuvant to oral gabapentin in spinal cord injury related chronic pain: a prospective, randomized, double blind trial. *Pain Physician*, 13(3), 245–249.

Aoki, F.Y. & Sitar, D.S. (1988) Clinical pharmacokinetics of amantadine hydrochloride. *Clinical Pharmacokinetics*, 14(1), 35–51.

Aragon, C.L., Hofmeister, E.H., & Budsberg, S.C. (2007) Systematic review of clinical trials of treatments for osteoarthritis in dogs. *Journal of the American Veterinary Medical Association*, 230(4), 514–521.

Arnold, L.M., Jain, R., & Glazer, W.M. (2008) Pain and the brain. *Journal of Clinical Psychiatry*, 69(9), e25.

Bajwa, Z.H., Simopoulos, T.T., Pal, J., et al. (2009) Low and therapeutic doses of antidepressants are associated with similar response in the context of multimodal treatment of pain. *Pain Physician*, 12(5), 893–900.

Bang, S.R., Yu, S.K., & Kim, T.H. (2010) Can gabapentin help reduce postoperative pain in arthroscopic rotator cuff repair? A prospective, randomized, double-blind study. *Arthroscopy*, 9, S106–S111.

Bell, R.F., Dahl, J.B., Moore, R.A., & Kalso, E. (2006) Perioperative ketamine for acute postoperative pain. *Cochrane Database of Systematic Reviews*, (1), CD004603.

Bergadano, A., Andersen, O.K., Arendt-Nielsen, L., Theurillat, R., Thormann, W., & Spadavecchia, C. (2009) Plasma levels of a low-dose constant-rate-infusion of ketamine and its effect on single and repeated nociceptive stimuli in conscious dogs. *Veterinary Journal*, 182(2), 252–260.

Bianchi, M., Franchi, S., Ferrario, P., Sotgiu, M.L., & Sacerdote, P. (2008) Effects of the bisphosphonate ibandronate on hyperalgesia, substance P, and cytokine levels in a rat model of persistent inflammatory pain. *European Journal of Pain*, 12(3), 284–292.

Bleidner, W.E., Harmon, J.B., Hewes, W.E., Lynes, T.E., & Hermann, E.C. (1965) Absorption, distribution and excretion of amantadine hydrochloride. *Journal of Pharmacology and Experimental Therapy*, 150(3), 484–490.

Bockbrader, H. N., Wesche, D., Miller, R., Chapel, S., Janiczek, N., & Burger, P. (2010) A comparison of the pharmacokinetics and pharmacodynamics of pregabalin and gabapentin. *Clinical Pharmacokinetics*, 49(10), 661–669.

Bomholt, S.F., Mikkelsen, J.D., & Blackburn-Munro, G. (2005) Antinociceptive effects of the antidepressants amitriptyline, duloxetine, mirtazapine and citalopram in animal models of acute, persistent and neuropathic pain. *Neuropharmacology*, 48(2), 252–263.

Brandt, K.D., Smith, G.N., & Myer, S.L. (2004) Hyaluronan injection affects neither osteoarthritis progression nor loading of the OA knee in dogs. *Journal of Rheumatology*, 28(6), 1341–1346.

Brown, D.C., Iadarola, M.J., Perkowski, S.Z., et al. (2005) Physiologic and antinociceptive effects of intrathecal resiniferatoxin in a canine bone cancer model. *Anesthesiology*, 103(5), 1052–1059.

Burr, D.B. & Allen, M.R. (2009) Mandibular necrosis in beagle dogs treated with bisphosphonates. *Orthodontics and Cravifacial Research*, 12(3), 221–228.

Calamia, V., Ruiz-Romero, C., Rocha, B. et al. (2010) Pharmacoproteomic study of the effects of chondroitin and glucosamine sulfate on human articular chondrocytes. *Arthritis Research & Therapy*, 12(4), R138.

Canapp, S.O., Cross, A.R., & Brown, M.P. (2005) Examination of synovial fluid and serum following intravenous injections of hyaluronan for the treatment of osteoarthritis in dogs. *Veterinary and Comparative Orthopaedics and Traumatology*, 18(3), 169–174.

Cao, Y.Q. (2006) Voltage-gated calcium channels and pain. *Pain*, 126, 5–9.

Caron, J. (2005) Intra-articular injections for joint disease in horses. *Veterinary Clinics of North America*, 21(3), 559–573.

Cashmore, R.G., Harcourt-Brown, T.R., Freeman, P.M., Jeffery, N.D., & Granger, N. (2009) Clinical diagnosis and treatment of suspected neuropathic pain in three dogs. *Australian Veterinary Journal*, 87(1), 45–50.

Cautela, M.A., Dewey, C.W., Schwark, W.S., et al (2010) Pharmacokinetics of oral pregabalin in cats after single dose administration. American College of Veterinary Internal Medicine Forum, Anaheim, California.

Chappell, A.S., Ossanna, M.J., Liu-Seifert, H., et al. (2009) Duloxetine, a centrally acting analgesic, in the treatment of patients with osteoarthritis knee pain: a 13-week, randomized, placebo-controlled trial. *Pain*, 146(3), 253–260.

Chew, D.J., Buffington, C.A., Kendall, M.S., DiBartola, S.P., & Woodworth, B.E. (1998) Amitriptyline treatment for severe recurrent idiopathic cystitis in cats. *Journal of the American Veterinary Medical Association*, 213(9), 1282–1286.

Coetzee, J. F., Mosher, R.A., Kohake, L.E., et al. (2010) Pharmacokinetics of oral gabapentin alone or co-administered with meloxicam in ruminant beef calves. *The Veterinary Journal*, 190(1), 98–102.

Corlew, R., Brasier, D.J., Feldman, D.E., & Philpot, B.D. (2008) Presynaptic NMDA receptors: newly appreciated roles in cortical synaptic function and plasticity. *Neuroscientist*, 14(6), 609–625.

Coudry, V., Thibaud, D., & Riccio, B. (2007) Efficacy of tiludronate in the treatment of horses with signs of pain associated with osteoarthritic lesions of the thoracolumbar vertebral column. *American Journal of Veterinary Research*, 68(3), 329–337.

Crowell-Davis, S.L. & Poggiagliolmi, S. (2008) Understanding behavior: serotonin syndrome. *Compendium on Continuing Education for Veterinarians*, 30(9), 490–493.

Dahan, A., Olofsen, E., Sigtermans, M., et al. (2011) Population pharmacokinetic-pharmacodynamic modeling of ketamine-induced pain relief of chronic pain. *European Journal of Pain*. 15(3), 258–267.

Davis, J.L., Posner, L.P., & Elce, Y. (2007) Gabapentin for the treatment of neuropathic pain in a pregnant horse. *Journal of the American Veterinary Medical Association*, 231(5), 755–758.

Delguste, C., Amory, H., Guyonnet, J., et al. (2008) Comparative pharmacokinetics of two intravenous administration regimens of tiludronate in healthy adult horses and effects on the bone resorption marker CTX-1. *Journal of Veterinary Pharmacology and Therapeutics*, 31(2), 108–116.

Denoix, J.M., Thibaud, D., Riccio, B. (2003) Tiludronate as a new therapeutic agent in the treatment of navicular disease: a double-blind placebo-controlled clinical trial. *Equine Veterinary Journal*, 35(4), 407–413.

Dick, I.E., Brochu, R.M., Purohit, Y., Kaczorowski, G.J., Martin, W.J., & Priest, B.T. (2007) Sodium channel blockade may contribute to the analgesic efficacy of antidepressants. *Journal of Pain*, 8(4), 315–324.

Dirikolu, L., Dafalla, A., Ely, K.J., et al. (2008) Pharmacokinetics of gabapentin in horses. *Journal of Veterinary Pharmacologic Therapy* 31(2), 175–177.

Durkin, B., Page, C., & Glass, P. (2010) Pregabalin for the treatment of postsurgical pain. *Expert Opinion in Pharmacotherapy*, 11(16), 2751–2758.

Dworkin, R.H., O'Connor, A.B., Audette, J., et al. (2010) Recommendations for the pharmacological management of neuropathic pain: an overview and literature update. *Mayo Clinic Proceedings*, 85(3), S3-S14.

Echigo, R., Mochizuki, M., & Nishimura, R. (2006) Suppressive effect of hyaluronan on chondrocyte apoptosis in experimentally induced acute osteoarthritis in dogs. *Journal of Veterinary Medical Science*, 68(8), 899–902.

Eisenberg, E., Pud, D., Koltun, L., & Loven, D. (2007) Effect of early administration of the N-methyl-d-aspartate receptor antagonist amantadine on the development of postmastectomy pain syndrome: a prospective pilot study. *Journal of Pain*, 8(3), 223–229.

Elsewaisy, O., Slon, B., & Monagle, J. (2010) Analgesic effect of subanesthetic intravenous ketamine in refractory neuropathic pain: a case report. *Pain Medicine*, 11(6), 946–950.

Fan, T.M., de Lorimer, L.P., O'Dell-Anderson, K., Lacoste, H.I, & Charney, S.C. (2007) Single-agent pamidronate for palliative therapy of canine appendicular osteosarcoma bone pain. *Journal of Veterinary Internal Medicine*, 21(3), 431–439.

Fan, T.M., Charney, S.C., de Lorimer, L.P., et al. (2009) Double-blind placebo-controlled trial of adjuvant pamidronate with palliative radiotherapy and intravenous doxorubicin for canine appendicular osteosarcoma bone pain. *Journal of Veterinary Internal Medicine*, 23(1), 152–160.

Field, M. J., Hughes, J., & Singh, L. (2000) Further evidence for the role of the α2δ subunit of voltage dependent calcium channels in models of neuropathic pain. *British Journal of Pharmacology*, 131, 282–286.

Fielding, C.L., Brumbaugh, G.W., Matthews, N.S., Peck, K.E, & Roussel, A.J. (2006) Pharmacokinetics and clinical effects of a subanesthetic continuous rate infusion of ketamine in awake horses. *American Journal of Veterinary Research*, 67(9), 1484–1490.

Frisbie, D.D., Kawcak, C.E, McIlwraith, C.W., & Werpy, N.M. (2009) Evaluation of polysulfated glycosaminoglycan or sodium hyaluronan intra-articularly for treatment of horses with experimentally induced osteoarthritis. *American Journal of Veterinary Research*, 70(2), 203–209.

Fritsch, D.A., Allen, T.A., Dodd, C.E., et al. (2010) A multicenter study of the effect of dietary supplementation with fish oil omega-3 fatty acids on carprofen dosage in dogs with osteoarthritis. *Journal of the American Veterinary Medical Association*, 236(5), 535–539.

Fujiki, M., Shineha, J., Yamanokuchi, K., Misumi, K., & Sakamoto, H. (2007) Effects of treatment with polysulfated glycosaminoglycans on serum cartilage oligomeric matrix protein and C-reactive protein concentrations, serum matrix metalloproteinase-2 and -9 activities, and lameness in dogs with osteoarthritis. *American Journal of Veterinary Research*, 68(8), 827–833.

Fujita, T., Ohue, M., & Fujii, Y., (2009) Comparison of the analgesic effects of bisphosphonates: etidronate, alendronate and risedronate

by electroalgometry utilizing the fall of skin impedance. *Journal of Bone and Mineral Metabolism*, 27(2), 234–239.

Gillman, P.K. (2007) Tricyclic antidepressant pharmacology and therapeutic drug interactions updated. *British Journal of Pharmacology*, 151(6), 737–748.

Goldberg, M.E., Torjman, M.C., Schwartzman, R.J., Mager, D.E., & Wainer, I.W. (2010) Pharmacodynamic profiles of ketamine (R)- and (S)- with five day inpatient infusion for the treatment of complex regional pain syndrome. *Pain Physician*, 13(4), 379–387.

Gottschalk, A., Schroeder, F., Ufer, M., Oncü, A., Buerkle, H., & Standl, T. (2001) Amantadine, a N-methyl-D-aspartate receptor antagonist, does not enhance postoperative analgesia in women undergoing abdominal hysterectomy. *Anesthesia & Analgesia*, 93(1), 192–196.

Gough, M.R., Thibaud, D., & Smith, R.K. (2010) Tiludronate infusion in the treatment of bone spavin: a double blind placebo-controlled trial. *Equine Veterinary Journal*, 42(5), 381–387.

Greenberg, D.D., Stoker, A., Kane, S., Cockrell, M., Cook, J.L. (2006) Biochemical effects of two different hyaluronic acid products in a co-culture model of osteoarthritis. *Osteoarthritis and Cartilage*, 14(8), 814–822.

Hackworth, R.J., Tokarz, K.A., Fowler, I.M., Wallace, S.C., & Stedje-Larsen, E.T. (2008) Profound pain reduction after induction of memantine treatment in two patients with severe phantom limb pain. *Anesthesia & Analgesia*, 107(4), 1377–1379.

Hall, F.S., Schwarzbaum, J.M., Perona, M.T., et al. (2011) A greater role for the norepinephrine transporter than the serotonin transporter in nociception. *Neuroscience*, 175, 315–327.

Hayashida, K., Obata, H., Nakajima, K., & Eisenach, J.C. (2008) Gabapentin acts within the locus coeruleus to alleviate neuropathic pain. *Anesthesiology*, 109(6), 1077–1084.

Hill, C.M., Balkenohl, M., Thomas, D.W., Walker, R., Mathé, H., & Murray, G. (2001) Pregabalin in patients with post-operative dental pain. *European Journal of Pain*, 5(2), 119–124.

Ho, K.Y., Tay, W., & Yeo, M.C. (2010) Duloxetine reduces morphine requirements after knee replacement surgery. *British Journal of Anaesthesia*, 105(3), 371–376.

Javery, K.B., Ussery, T.W., Steger, H.G., & Colclough, G.W. (1996) Comparison of morphine and morphine with ketamine for postoperative analgesia. *Canadian Journal of Anaesthesia*, 43(3), 212–215.

Jones, C.K., Peters, S.C., & Shannon, H.E. (2005) Efficacy of duloxetine, a potent and balanced serotonergic and noradrenergic reuptake inhibitor, in inflammatory and acute pain models in rodents. *Journal of Pharmacology and Experimental Therapeutics*, 312(2), 726–732.

Kaplan, B. (1972) Ketamine HCl anesthesia in dogs: observation of 327 cases. *Veterinary Medicine, Small Animal Clinician*, 67(6), 631–634.

Kaplan, L.D., Lu, Y., Snitzer, J., et al. (2009) The effect of early hyaluronic acid delivery in the development of an acute articular cartilage lesion in a sheep model. *American Journal of Sports Medicine*, 37(12), 2323–2327.

Kawcak, C.E., Frisbie, D.D., Trotter, G.W., et al. (1997) Effects of intravenous administration of sodium hyaluronate on carpal joints in exercising horses after arthroscopic surgery and osteochondral fragmentation. *American Journal of Veterinary Research*, 58(10), 1132–1140.

Kiefer, R.T., Rohr, P., Ploppa, A., et al. (2008) Efficacy of ketamine in anesthetic dosage for the treatment of refractory complex regional pain syndrome: an open-label phase II study. *Pain Medicine*, 9(8), 1173–1201.

Kim, S.Y., Jeong, J.J., Chung, W.Y., Kim, H.J., Nam, K.H., & Shim, Y.H. (2010) Perioperative administration of pregabalin for pain after robot-assisted endoscopic thyroidectomy: a randomized clinical trial. *Surgical Endoscopy*, 24(11), 2776–2781.

Ko, S. H., Kwon, H. S., Yu, J. M., et al. (2010) Comparison of the efficacy and safety of tramadol/acetaminophen combination therapy and gabapentin in the treatment of painful diabetic neuropathy. *Diabetes Medicine*, 27(9), 1033–1040.

KuKanich, B. & Cohen, R.L. (2011) Pharmacokinetics of oral gabapentin in greyhound dogs. *The Veterinary Journal*, 187(1), 133–135.

Kraijer, M., Fink-Gremmels, J., & Nickel, R.F. (2003) The short-term clinical efficacy of amitriptyline in the management of idiopathic feline lower urinary tract disease: a controlled clinical study. *Journal of Feline Medicine and Surgery*, 5(3), 191–196.

Kruger, J.M., Conway, T.S., Kaneene, J.B., et al. (2003) Randomized controlled trial of the efficacy of short-term amitriptyline administration for treatment of acute, nonobstructive, idiopathic lower urinary tract disease in cats. *Journal of the American Veterinary Medical Association*, 222(6), 749–758.

Kukes, V.G., Kondratenko, S.N., Savelyeva, M.I., Starodubtsev, A.K., & Gneushev, E.T. (2009) Experimental and clinical pharmacokinetics of amitriptyline: comparative analysis. *Bulletin of Experimental Biology and Medicine*, 147(4), 434–437.

Lantz, R.J., Gillespie, T.A., Rash, T.J., et al. (2003) Metabolism, excretion, and pharmacokinetics of duloxetine in healthy human subjects. *Drug Metabolism and Disposition*, 31(9), 1142–1150.

Lascelles, B.D., Gaynor, J.S., Smith, E.S., et al. (2008) Amantadine in a multimodal analgesic regimen for alleviation of refractory osteoarthritis pain in dogs. *Journal of Veterinary Internal Medicine*, 22(1), 53–59.

Lunn, M.P., Hughes, R.A., & Wiffen, P.J. (2009) Duloxetine for treating painful neuropathy or chronic pain. *Cochrane Database of Systematic Reviews*, 4, CD007115.

Maier, C., Dertwinkel, R., Mansourian, N., et al (2003) Efficacy of the NMDA-receptor antagonist memantine in patients with chronic phantom limb pain–results of a randomized double-blinded, placebo-controlled trial. *Pain*, 103(3), 277–283.

Marx, R.E., Cillo, J.E., & Ulloa, J.J. (2007) Oral bisphosphonate-induced osteonecrosis. *Journal of Oral and Maxillofacial Surgery* 65, 2397–2410.

McCarthy, G., O'Donovan, J., Jones, B., McAllister, H., Seed, M., & Mooney, C. (2007) Randomised double-blind, positive-controlled trial to assess the efficacy of glucosamine/chondroitin sulfate for the treatment of dogs with osteoarthritis. *Veterinary Journal*, 174(1), 54–61.

Minville, V., Fourcade, O., Girolami, J.P., & Tack, I. (2010) Opioid-induced hyperalgesia in a mice model of orthopaedic pain: preventive effect of ketamine. *British Journal of Anaesthesia*, 104(2), 231–238.

Moore, A., Costello, J., Wieczorek, P., Shah, V., Taddio, A., & Carvalho, J.C. (2011) Gabapentin improves postcesarean delivery pain management: a randomized, placebo-controlled trial. *Anesthesia and Analgesia*. 112(1), 167–173.

Moreau, M., Dupuis, J., Bonneau, N.H., & Desnoyers, M. (2003) Clinical evaluation of a nutraceutical, carprofen and meloxicam for the treatment of dogs with osteoarthritis. *Veterinary Record*, 152(11), 323–329.

Moreau, M., Rialland, P., Pelletier, J.P., et al. (2011) Tiludronate treatment improves structural changes and symptoms of osteoarthritis in the canine anterior cruciate ligament model. *Arthritis Research & Therapy*, 13(3), R98.

Paech, M.J., Goy, R., Chua, S., Scott, K., Christmas, T., & Doherty, D.A. (2007) A randomized, placebo-controlled trial of preoperative

oral pregabalin for postoperative pain relief after minor gynecological surgery. *Anesthesia & Analgesia*, 105(5), 1449–1453.

Palazzo, E., Luongo, L., de Novellis, V., Berrino, L., Rossi, F., Maione, S. (2010) Moving towards supraspinal TRPV1 receptors for chronic pain relief. *Molecular Pain*, 6, 66.

Pearson, W. & Lindinger, M. (2009) Low quality of evidence for glucosamine-based nutraceuticals in equine joint disease: review of in vivo studies. *Equine Veterinary Journal*, 41(7), 706–712.

Pelletier, J.P. & Martel-Pelletier, J. (2007) DMOAD developments: present and future. *Bulletin of the NYU Hospital for Joint Diseases*, 65(3), 242–248.

Peterbauer, C., Larenza, P.M., Knobloch, M., et al. (2008) Effects of a low dose infusion of racemic and S-ketamine on the nociceptive withdrawal reflex in standing ponies. *Veterinary Anaesthesia and Analgesia*, 35(5), 414–423.

Piscitelli, C., Dunayer, E., & Aumann, M. (2010) Xylitol toxicity in dogs. *Compendium on Continuing Education for Veterinarians*, 32(2), E1–E4.

Pypendop, B.H., Siao, K.T., & Ilkiw, J.E. (2010) Thermal antinociceptive effect of orally administered gabapentin in healthy cats. *American Journal of Veterinary Research*, 71(9), 1027–1032.

Radulovic, L.L., Türck, D., von Hodenberg, A., et al. (1995) Disposition of gabapentin (neurontin) in mice, rats, dogs, and monkeys. *Drug Metabolism and Disposition*, 23(4), 441–448.

Rees, W.A., Harkins, J.D., Woods, W.E., et al. (1997) Amantadine and equine influenza: pharmacology, pharmacokinetics and neurological effects in the horse. *Equine Veterinary Journal*, 29(2), 104–110.

Reid, P., Pypendop, B.H., & Ilkiw, J.E. (2010) The effects of intravenous gabapentin administration on the minimum alveolar concentration of isoflurane in cats. *Anesthesia & Analgesia*, 111(3), 633–637.

Remérand, F., Le Tendre, C., Baud, A. et al. (2009) The early and delayed analgesic effects of ketamine after total hip arthoplasty: a prospective, randomized, controlled, double-blind study. *Anesthesia & Analgesia*, 109(6), 1963–1971.

Robertson, S.A. (2005) Managing pain in feline patients. *Veterinary Clinic of North America Small Animal Practice*, 35(1), 129–146.

Roelofs, A.J., Thompson, K., Gordon, S, Rogers, M.J. (2006) Molecular mechanisms of action of bisphosphonates: current status. *Clinical Cancer Research*, 12(20 Suppl), 6222s–6230s.

Roush, J.K., Dodd, C.E., Fritsch, D.A., et al. (2010a) Multicenter veterinary practice assessment of the effects of omega-3 fatty acids on osteoarthritis in dogs. *Journal of the American Veterinary Medical Association*, 236(1), 59–66.

Roush, J.K., Cross, A.R., Renberg, W.C., et al. (2010b) Evaluation of the effects of dietary supplementation with fish oil omega-3 fatty acids on weight bearing in dogs with osteoarthritis. *Journal of the American Veterinary Medical Association*, 236(1), 67–73.

Rusy, L.M., Hainsworth, K.R., Nelson, T.J., et al. (2010) Gabapentin use in pediatric spinal fusion patients: a randomized, double-blind, controlled trial. *Anesthesia & Analgesia*, 110(5), 1393–1398.

Siao, K.T., Pypendop, B.H., & Ilkiw, J.E. (2010) Pharmacokinetics of gabapentin in cats. *American Journal of Veterinary Research*, 71(7), 817–821.

Salazar, V., Dewey, C.W., Schwark, W., et al. (2009) Pharmacokinetics of single-dose oral pregabalin administration in normal dogs. *Veterinary Anaesthesia and Analgesia*, 36(6), 574–580.

Sarrau, S., Jourdan, J., Dupuis-Soyris, F, & Verwaerde, P. (2007) Effects of postoperative ketamine infusion on pain control and feeding behaviour in bitches undergoing mastectomy. *Journal of Small Animal Practice*, 48(12), 670–676.

Schmidtko, A., Lötsch, J., Freynhagen, R., & Geisslinger, G. (2010) Ziconotide for treatment of severe chronic pain. *Lancet*, 375(9725), 1569–1577.

Segal, A.Z. & Rordof, G. (1996) Gabapentin as a novel treatment for post-herpetic neuralgia. *Neurology*, 46(4), 1175–1176.

Sen, H., Sizlan, A., Yanarates, O., et al. (2009) A comparison of gabapentin and ketamine in acute and chronic pain after hysterectomy. *Anesthesia & Analgesia*, 109(5), 1645–1650.

Scarpellini, M., Lurati, A., & Vignati, G. (2008) Biomarkers, type II collagen, glucosamine and chondroitin sulfate in osteoarthritis follow-up: the "Magenta osteoarthritis study". *Journal of Orthopaedics and Traumatology*, 9(2), 81–87.

Schley, M., Topfner, S., Wiech, K., et al. (2007) Continuous brachial plexus blockade in combination with the NMDA receptor antagonist memantine prevents phantom pain in acute traumatic upper limb amputees. *European Journal of Pain*, 11(3), 299–308.

Schulz, P., Turner-Tamiyasu, K., Smith, G., Giacomini, K.M., & Blaschke, T.F. (1983) Amitriptyline disposition in young and elderly normal men. *Clinical Pharmacology and Therapeutics*, 33(3), 360–366.

Serhan, C.N. & Chiang, N. (2008) Endogenous pro-resolving and anti-inflammatory lipid mediators: a new pharmacologic genus. *British Journal of Pharmacology*, 153(Suppl. 1), S200–S215.

Shaver, S. L., Robinson, N. G., Wright, B.D., Kratz, G.E., & Johnston, M.S. (2009) A multimodal approach to management of suspected neuropathic pain in a prairie falcon (*Falco mexicanus*). *Journal of Avian Medicine and Surgery*, 23(3), 209–213.

Sheets, P. L., Heers, C., Stoehr, T., & Cummins, T.R. (2008) Differential block of sensory neuronal voltage-gated sodium channels by lacosamide [(2R)-2-(acetylamino)-N-benzyl-3-methoxypropanamide], lidocaine, and carbamazepine. *The Journal of Pharmacology and Experimental Therapeutics* 326(1), 89–99.

Siao, K.T., Pypendop, B.H., & Ilkiw, J.E. (2010) Pharmacokinetics of gabapentin in cats. *American Journal of Veterinary Research*, 71(7), 817–821.

Sigtermans, M.J., van Hilten, J.J., Bauer, M.C., et al. (2009a) Ketamine produces effective and long-term relief in patients with Complex Regional Pain Syndrome Type I. *Pain*, 145(3), 304–311.

Sigtermans, M., Dahan A., Mooren, R., et al. (2009b) S(+)-ketamine effect on experimental pain and cardiac output. *Anesthesiology*, 111(4), 892–903.

Sigtermans, M., Noppers, I., Sarton, E., et al. (2010) An observational study on the effect of S+-ketamine on chronic pain versus experimental acute pain in Complex Regional Pain Syndrome type 1 patients. *European Journal of Pain*, 14(3), 302–307.

Snijdelaar, D.G., Koren, G., & Katz, J. (2004) Effects of perioperative oral amantadine on postoperative pain and morphine consumption in patients after radical prostatectomy: results of a preliminary study. *Anesthesiology*, 100(1), 134–141.

Stahl, S.M. (2004) Mechanism of action of alpha2delta ligands: voltage sensitive calcium channel (VSCC) modulators. *Journal of Clinical Psychiatry*, 65(8), 1033–1034.

Strassle, B.W., Mark, L., Leventhal, L., et al. (2010) Inhibition of osteoclasts prevents cartilage loss and pain in a rat model of degenerative joint disease. *Osteoarthritis and Cartilage*, 18(10), 1319–1328.

Straube, S., Derry, S., Moore, R.A., Wiffen, P.J., & McQuay, H.J. (2010) Single dose oral gabapentin for established acute postoperative pain in adults. *Cochrane Database of Systematic Reviews*, (5), CD008183.

Suzuki, M., Tsueda, K., Lansing, P.S., et al. (1999) Small-dose ketamine enhances morphine-induced analgesia after outpatient surgery. *Anesthesia & Analgesia*, 89(1), 98–103.

Tao, Y.X. (2010) Dorsal horn alpha-amino-3-hydroxy-5-methyl-4-isoxazolepropionic acid receptor trafficking in inflammatory pain. *Anesthesiology*, 112(5), 1259–1265.

Terry, R.L., McDonnell, S.M., Van Eps, A.W., et al. (2010) Pharmacokinetic profile and behavioral effects of gabapentin in the horse. *Journal of Veterinary Pharmacology and Therapeutics*, 33(5), 485–494.

Tiippana, E.M., Hamunen, K., Kontinen, V.K., & Kalso, E. (2007) Do surgical patients benefit from perioperative gabapentin/pregabalin? A systematic review of efficacy and safety. *Anesthesia and Analgesia*, 104(6), 1545–1556.

Toth, C. (2010) Substitution of gabapentin therapy with pregabalin therapy in neuropathic pain due to peripheral neuropathy. *Pain Medicine*, 11(3), 456–465.

Tran-Van-Minh, A. & Dolphin, A.C. (2010) The alpha2delta ligand gabapentin inhibits the Rab11-dependent recycling of the calcium channel subunit alpha2delta-2. *Journal of Neuroscience*, 30(38), 12856–12867.

Tung, J.T., Venta, P.J., & Caron, J.P. (2002) Inducible nitric oxide expression in equine articular chondrocytes: effects of anti-inflammatory compounds. *Osteoarthritis and Cartilage*, 10(1), 5–12.

Wagner, A.E., Walton, J.A., Hellyer, P.W., Gaynor, J.S., & Mama, K.R. (2002) Use of low doses of ketamine administered by constant rate infusion as an adjunct for postoperative analgesia in dogs. *Journal of the American Veterinary Medical Association*, 221(1), 72–75.

Wagner, A.E., Mich, P.M., Uhrig, S.R., & Hellyer, P.W. (2010) Clinical evaluation of perioperative administration of gabapentin as an adjunct for postoperative analgesia in dogs undergoing amputation of a forelimb. *Journal of the American Veterinary Medical Association*, 236(7), 751–756.

Wandel, S. Jüni, P., Tendal, B. et al. (2010) Effects of glucosamine, chondroitin, or placebo in patients with osteoarthritis of hip or knee: network meta-analysis. *British Medical Journal*, 341, c4675.

Wann, A.K.T., Mistry, J., Blain, E.J., Michael-Titus, A.T., & Knight, M.M. (2010) Eicosapentaenoic acid and docoasahexaenoic acid reduce interleukin-1β-mediated cartilage degradation. *Arthritis Research & Therapy*, 12, R207.

Xu, Z-Z., Zhang, L., Liu, T. et al. (2010) Resolvins RvE1 and RvD1 attenuate inflammatory pain via central and peripheral actions. *Nature Medicine*, 16(5), 592–597.

Yli-Kyyny, T. (2011) Bisphosphonates and atypical fractures of femur. *Journal of Osteoporosis*, 2011:754972.

Zainal, Z., Longman, A.J., Hurst, S., et al. (2009) Relative efficacies of omega-3 polyunsaturated fatty acids in reducing expression of key proteins in a model system for studying osteoarthritis. *Osteoarthritis and Cartilage*, 17(7), 896–905.

Zakine, J., Samarcq, D., Lorne, E., et al. (2008) Postoperative ketamine administration decreases morphine consumption in major abdominal surgery: a prospective, randomized, double-blind, controlled study. *Anesthesia & Analgesia*, 106(6), 1856–1861.

Zakrzewska, J.M. (2010) Medical management of trigeminal neuropathic pains. *Expert Opinions in Pharmacotherapy*, 11(8), 1239–1254.

Zhuo, M. (2009) Plasticity of NMDA receptor NR2B subunit in memory and chronic pain. *Molecular Brain*, 2(1), 4–15.

9

Novel Methods of Analgesic Drug Delivery

Lesley J. Smith

Beginning in January 2001, the United States Congress declared the Decade of Pain Control and Research. However, the undertreatment of hospitalized human patients remains a significant clinical problem (Taylor et al., 2008). This issue likely can be extrapolated to veterinary medicine as well. Barriers to effective analgesia are varied, and are probably more challenging in veterinary patients than in human patients due to the inability to offer patient-controlled analgesia (PCA) to the veterinary patient population.

An "ideal" analgesic would be effective against a broad range of pain types, have a rapid onset and controllable duration, be free of adverse effects such as respiratory depression and sedation, lack clinically problematic metabolites, and be readily accessible and cost-effective. Perhaps most importantly in veterinary medicine, the "ideal" analgesic would also be easy and safe to administer, with a dosing interval that is extended enough to be convenient for the practitioner as well as to the owner at home. Lastly, the "ideal" analgesic in veterinary medicine would be available in a formulation that prevents accidental access by children or illicit use by humans. Many of the currently available analgesics in the veterinary world meet some of these criteria, but no currently available analgesic meets all of the above stipulations.

One of the barriers to finding the "ideal" analgesic is a current deficiency in drug delivery technology. Many of the available analgesics are effective, for example, opioids, but are not formulated in delivery systems that provide steady-state analgesia or extended duration in veterinary patients. In the last decade, the pharmaceutical industry has made a focused effort to improve drug delivery systems by incorporating known analgesics, for example, morphine, into novel delivery matrices. This focus has been largely driven by the human analgesic market, and many of these technologies are essentially variations on PCA. Thus, many of the newly marketed novel delivery systems are not practical for use in veterinary medicine. This chapter will not review variations of PCA in novel delivery systems (e.g., iontophoretic transdermal self-delivery systems), because they are likely not practical or relevant to veterinary medicine.

This review will summarize the most relevant novel analgesic delivery systems or methods that are currently marketed for human application, with a focus on application in veterinary medicine, where appropriate. Some of the delivery systems that will be discussed are not yet commercially available, but show promise in research studies. Because this chapter is focused on delivery systems, the analgesic merit of the actual drugs incorporated into those delivery systems will not be covered in depth.

TOPICAL DRUG DELIVERY SYSTEMS

Topical analgesics deliver the drug locally when they are applied directly over the area of interest. In most cases, low to clinically insignificant serum concentrations of the drug are attained, making topical systems relatively free of adverse effects. Formulations have been developed to improve absorption across human skin using penetration enhancers (Brown et al., 2006). Because these topical agents are designed for penetration of human skin, their efficacy in veterinary patients is uncertain, and many products have yet to be tested or studied in the veterinary population.

Eutectic Mixture of Local Anesthetics

One product that has received acceptance in veterinary medicine as a topical local anesthetic is eutectic mixture of local anesthetics (EMLA) cream. This formulation is a eutectic mixture of lidocaine and prilocaine that is effective in facilitating catheter placement in pediatric and adult humans (Taddio, 2001). Application of EMLA cream to the skin allows for a high concentration of the local anesthetic drugs at the site of catheter placement without systemic absorption. Two studies have been reported in cats on the use of EMLA cream. In one study, healthy cats ($n = 10$) had 1 mL of EMLA cream applied to a shaved site over the jugular vein and wrapped with an occlusive bandage that was left in place for 1 hour (Gibbon et al., 2003). No cat in that study had measureable serum concentrations of local anesthetic and no methemoglobin was detected. Six cats were amenable to jugular catheter placement without sedation, and the other four cats required sedation, but had been apprehensive and difficult to handle prior to any intervention (Gibbon et al., 2003). In a second study, EMLA was assessed in clinically ill cats presented to a veterinary teaching hospital, and in need of jugular catheter placement (Wagner et al., 2006). EMLA was applied, as in the previous study, and 60% of cats had jugular catheters placed without sedation, whereas 38% required sedation. While these data did not reach statistical significance ($p = 0.06$) a larger number of animals may have been needed to demonstrate a positive effect of EMLA cream. In the author's experience,

Pain Management in Veterinary Practice, First Edition. Edited by Christine M. Egger, Lydia Love and Tom Doherty.
© 2014 John Wiley & Sons, Inc. Published 2014 by John Wiley & Sons, Inc.

application of EMLA to shaved skin of dogs, followed by a 20–30 minute period during which the area is covered with a simple occlusive dressing (e.g., Tegaderm® covered with Vetwrap®) in order to ensure continued contact of EMLA with the skin, substantially reduces struggling during catheter placement in unsedated or lightly sedated animals.

Needle-free Powder Lidocaine

A novel, needle-free powder lidocaine delivery system was recently developed for use in catheter placement in children. This prefilled system delivers dry powder lidocaine monohydrate through the epidermis by sealing the device against the skin and then pressing a button that releases pressurized helium from a microcylinder, causing a 0.5 mg cassette of lidocaine to rupture with velocities sufficient to penetrate the skin. In one study, the use of this device resulted in significant reductions in reported pain on venipuncture ($p < 0.001$), with no observable adverse effects on the overlying skin (Zempsky et al., 2008). While this system has potential application to veterinary patients, the company has since filed for bankruptcy, so a commercial product may not be forthcoming.

Lidocaine Patch

Like topical creams and gels, the concept behind the lidocaine patch is that the drug is absorbed across the skin for local delivery to a painful area, with minimal systemic uptake or risk of adverse effects. Lidocaine is a sodium channel blocker that is most effective against rapidly firing ectopic impulses that are generated from injured neurons. In neuropathic pain states, such as diabetic neuropathy or post-herpetic neuralgia, ectopic impulse generation from sensory nerves is a hallmark of the painful condition. The Lidoderm 5% patch® (Endo Pharmaceuticals, Newark, DE) was recently approved by the FDA for the treatment of post-herpetic neuralgia (Galer et al., 2002). A recent PubMed search by the author could not identify any studies on the analgesic efficacy of the lidocaine patch in companion animals. One study demonstrated a lack of systemic absorption of lidocaine (as measured by ELISA) after two lidocaine 5% patches were placed on the carpi of healthy horses, but analgesia was not evaluated in that study (Bidwell et al., 2007). Similarly, pharmacokinetic studies in dogs (Ko et al., 2007) and cats (Ko et al., 2008) indicate minimal systemic absorption from lidocaine patches.

Nonsteroidal Anti-inflammatory Drugs

Nonsteroidal anti-inflammatory drugs (NSAIDs) are commonly prescribed analgesics whose mechanism is to inhibit the cyclooxygenase (COX) class of enzymes, thereby reducing prostaglandin production and reducing inflammation at sites of tissue injury. Many topical NSAIDs have been developed in human medicine, and the primary advantage is that peak plasma concentrations of the drug are <10% of those that occur after oral intake of NSAIDs, therefore reducing the adverse effect profile associated with this class of drugs. Topical NSAIDs that have been developed in the form of cream, drops, foam, gel, ointments, patches, or sprays include diclofenac, ibuprofen, salicylic acid, ketorolac, flurbiprofen, felbinac, ketoprofen, indomethacin, and piroxicam (Stanos, 2009). In a review of 86 trials of topical NSAIDs, it was found that the treatment was superior to a placebo for the relief of acute musculoskeletal pain (Moore et al., 1998). In veterinary medicine, the only commercially available topical NSAID is Surpass® (Boerhinger Ingelheim Vetmedica, Saint Joseph, MO) (Figure 9.1). Surpass is a 1% diclofenac cream that has been shown to be effective against pain in horses with osteoarthritis when applied directly over the affected joint (Lynn et al., 2004). Other studies have confirmed the analgesic efficacy of Surpass® in experimentally induced osteoarthritis (Frisbie et al., 2009), and in horses with inflammation and undergoing regional limb perfusion (Levine et al., 2009). Application of Surpass® to the skin does result in measureable urinary and serum concentrations of diclofenac for up to 10 days; thus, its use should be undertaken with knowledge of the clearance times in horses that are in active competition (Anderson et al., 2005) and that may be tested for NSAID administration.

Topical Capsaicin Cream

Capsaicin, derived from red chili peppers, has long been reported to have analgesic properties (Turnbull, 1850). More recently, capsaicin has been shown to have analgesic benefits in various types of neuropathic pain states (The Capsaicin Study Group, 1991; Ellison et al., 1997). Capsaicin is an agonist at transient receptor potential vanilloid type 1 (TRPV1) receptors, which are ligand-gated cation channels, expressed both centrally and peripherally, that respond to mechanical, thermal, and chemical stimuli, initiating action potentials along sensory neurons and ascending spinal tracts (Palazzo et al., 2010). Prolonged activation leads to downregulation of receptors and cytotoxicity of sensory neurons expressing TRPV1 channels. Activation of TRPV1 receptors by capsaicin initially results in sensory neuronal depolarization, and the sensations of heat, burning, stinging, or itching. High concentrations of capsaicin or repeated applications, however, produce a persistent local effect on cutaneous nociceptors, described as defunctionalization, that results in reduced spontaneous activity and a loss of responsiveness to a wide range of sensory stimuli (Anand & Bley, 2011).

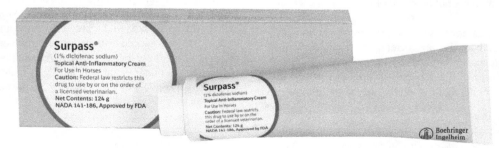

Figure 9.1.　Surpass, 1% topical diclofenac (With permission from Boehringer Ingelheim Vetmedica, Inc.)

In a review paper by Rains and Bryson (1995), depending on the methodology, 28–55% of people with osteoarthritis reported a reduction in the visual analogue scale pain score after capsaicin cream was applied topically 3–4 times daily to the arthritic area. Capsaicin cream (Equiblok®) has recently gained some popularity for the treatment of localized osteoarthritis in horses. The equine commercial capsaicin product contains 0.2% capsaicin, whereas the human product contains 0.075%. Despite being more concentrated, there is no evidence that the 0.2% capsaicin cream penetrates equine skin. Repeated topical application may cause skin irritation. Eye irritation can occur if the horse rubs its face near the area of application. There are no scientifically controlled published studies of the effectiveness of topical capsaicin cream for pain in horses with osteoarthritis.

TRANSDERMAL DELIVERY SYSTEMS

Unlike topical drug delivery systems, transdermal drug delivery centers on systemic uptake of the drug to create its analgesic effects. Because of systemic uptake, dose-dependent adverse effects are of similar concern as for intravenous or other parenteral routes of administration. However, transdermal delivery systems offer the advantages of convenient "at home" catheter-free drug delivery, as well as an extended duration of effective use.

Fentanyl Patch

Fentanyl is a potent μ agonist opioid that has a well-established place in treating moderate-to-severe pain. Some unique properties of fentanyl include its high lipophilicity, which allows for rapid penetration into the central nervous system (CNS) and, therefore, a rapid onset of effect. Because of its high lipophilicity, however, fentanyl is rapidly redistributed to muscle and fat, which act as storage sites for a later re-release back into the plasma. Like other μ opioids, fentanyl causes sedation in many veterinary patients, and dysphoria, nausea, constipation, urinary retention, and dose-dependent respiratory depression in some others. Fentanyl's high lipid solubility and low molecular weight make it ideal for transdermal delivery (Roy & Flynn, 1990). The traditional fentanyl patch, which is now available as a generic product in 12.5, 25, 50, and 100 μg/h delivery sizes of fentanyl, is a four-layer system. The outer layer is an impermeable polyester/ethylene coating that protects the patch, the second layer is the drug reservoir and contains fentanyl gelled in hydroxyethyl cellulose, the layer behind the drug reservoir is a rate-control membrane which is an ethylene-vinyl acetate copolymer that is more impermeable to fentanyl than skin and thus ensures the slow release of fentanyl across the membrane, and the last layer is a protective peel adhesive that is removed immediately prior to patch placement.

Recently, a novel matrix delivery system for fentanyl has been described that has release kinetics very similar to the reservoir system. In this system, fentanyl is incorporated directly into dipropylene glycol droplets that are within the adhesive coating (Sathyan et al., 2005). This more recent version of the fentanyl patch carries less likelihood for abuse due to the higher difficulty in accessing the fentanyl within the patch. In veterinary patients, however, the cost of this patch compared to the traditional reservoir system is likely to outweigh any theoretical advantages with respect to illicit use.

Many studies have been conducted on the efficacy and safety of the fentanyl patch in veterinary patients, and an exhaustive review of the literature is beyond the scope of this chapter. A few key points to mention are that systemic absorption of fentanyl from the patch varies with species, and effective plasma concentrations may not be reached for 6–24 hours (Egger et al., 2003; Hofmeister & Egger, 2004; Egger et al., 2007). Inter-individual absorption of fentanyl within species is also highly variable, so placement of a fentanyl patch does not guarantee that effective serum concentrations of fentanyl will be attained in that patient. Another point is that, at least in humans and cats, there is still a subcutaneous (SC) depot of fentanyl (approximately 30% of the total delivered dose) after the patch is removed that will continue to be absorbed for several hours (Portenoy et al., 1993; Lee et al., 2000). In addition, there is a risk of toxicity if a patch is ingested, and there is a case report describing profound sedation in a dog that ingested a fentanyl patch (Schmiedt & Bjorling, 2007).

There is a novel 'patchless' topical preparation of fentanyl (Recuvyra®) for application between the shoulder blades of dogs 2–4 hours prior to surgery. It is claimed that one application of Recuvyra® provides long-acting, continuous systemic delivery of fentanyl for up to 4 days (Linton et al., 2012). See Chapter 21 for further discussion of Recuvyra®.

Buprenorphine Patch

The buprenorphine patch has been evaluated to a limited extent in veterinary patients. This patch (Purdue Pharma, Cranberry NJ) was recently approved by the FDA for the treatment of moderate to severe pain in people. The patch is commercially available in sizes that deliver 35, 52.5, or 70 μg/h. Like the fentanyl patch, the buprenorphine patch should deliver drug at a relatively constant rate in a convenient formulation without the risk of first-pass metabolism. Buprenorphine is considered a partial μ agonist whose analgesic properties have been evaluated in dogs and cats; however, a review of this extensive body of literature is beyond the scope of this chapter. Murrell et al. (2007) evaluated serum concentrations and thermal threshold as an analgesic test in healthy cats that had a 35 μg /h buprenorphine patch placed on the shaved skin of their lateral thorax. In that study, they found that buprenorphine absorption was variable among cats, but all cats had measureable drug concentrations in serum by 6 hours after patch placement, accompanied by mild sedation or euphoria (Murrell et al., 2007). The mean peak buprenorphine concentration was 10 ng/mL, but several cats exceeded that peak at individual time points and buprenorphine concentrations remained well above zero for more than 24 hours after the patch was removed (Murrell et al., 2007). In the Murrell et al. (2007) study, despite buprenorphine drug concentrations in the therapeutic range, there was no analgesic effect as evidenced by thermal threshold testing. This may have been because the test model was not appropriate or it may be that release rates of buprenorphine from the patch are slow enough to delay transfer into the CNS for effective analgesia. A recent study in dogs also reported variable serum drug concentrations after a 70 μg/h buprenorphine patch was placed on a shaved area of the ventral abdomen in healthy beagles (Andaluz et al., 2009). In that study, drug concentrations increased during the first 36 hours after patch placement and peaked between 0.7 and 1.0 ng/mL (Figure 9.2). One dog had extremely low drug concentrations throughout the sampling period. These authors did not attempt to evaluate analgesia. From limited data available, it appears that the buprenorphine patch deserves further clinical investigation into its analgesic properties and assessment of inter-individual variability in drug absorption from the patch.

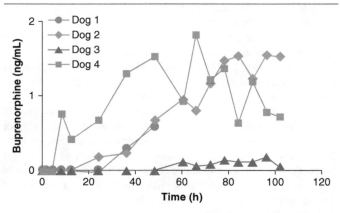

Figure 9.2. Plasma buprenorphine concentrations (ng/mL) in dogs after placement of a 70 μg/h transdermal buprenorphine patch (From Andaluz, A., Moll, X., Ventura, R., Abellán, R., Fresno, L., & García, F. (2009) Plasma buprenorphine concentrations after the application of a 70 μg/hour transdermal patch in dogs. Preliminary report. *Journal of Veterinary Pharmacology and Therapeutics*, 32(5), 503–505. With permission.)

TRANSMUCOSAL DRUG DELIVERY

Like transdermal delivery systems, transmucosal drug delivery offers ease of drug administration while achieving therapeutic serum concentrations of the drug. Therefore, adverse effects of systemic drug administration pertain to transmucosal routes of delivery. Of available analgesics perhaps fentanyl and buprenorphine have been the most intensively studied for transmucosal administration.

Oral Transmucosal Fentanyl

A fentanyl lozenge (Fentora®, Cephalon Inc., Frazer PA), which delivers 200, 400, 600, 800, 1200, or 1600 μg of fentanyl in a sugar base, has been developed for use in people. After the lozenge is placed in the mouth, approximately 25% of the total fentanyl available is absorbed almost immediately across the buccal mucosa, leading to a 10–15 minute onset of effect and peak plasma fentanyl concentrations. The remaining amount of the drug is swallowed with saliva, and is subsequently slowly absorbed from the GI tract to maintain fentanyl at therapeutic concentrations for about 2 hours (Zhang et al., 2002). This product has not been evaluated in companion animal patients, and is unlikely to be practical given the need for contact time between the lozenge and the oral mucosa, which is approximately 14–25 minutes, in order to completely dissolve the lozenge (Fentora Package Insert, December 2011).

Similarly, a fentanyl buccal tablet is newly available (Effentora®) that uses an effervescent technology to enhance fentanyl uptake by transiently changing oral pH. This product provides almost immediate therapeutic concentrations with a higher peak serum concentration of drug than achieved with the lozenge. Like the fentanyl lozenge, this product is not likely to be practical in veterinary species. Both the fentanyl buccal tablet and the fentanyl lozenge

are intended for use in severe breakthrough pain in people who are already on a background regular dose of an opioid.

Oral Transmucosal Buprenorphine

Buprenorphine has been extensively studied in cats as an oral transmucosal analgesic, but the studies in dogs are limited. Buprenorphine has close to 100% bioavailability when administered transmucosally to cats. Higher bioavailability in cats compared to other species is at least partially explained by differences in oral pH. Oral pH of cats has been reported to range from 8 to 9, whereas humans have an oral pH ranging from 5.4 to 7.5. Buprenorphine is a weak base with a pKa of 8.24. Therefore, a high percentage of the drug would exist in the unionized form in the feline oral cavity, enhancing its absorption.

The adverse effects (e.g., mania, excitement, hyperthermia) reported in cats treated with full μ opioid agonists are not as severe with buprenorphine. In cats, buprenorphine usually causes euphoria (purring, rolling, rubbing, and kneading with their forepaws) but rarely vomiting, nausea, or dysphoria (Robertson et al., 2003). Mild hyperthermia has been reported in cats after buprenorphine administration (Posner et al., 2010). Using a thermal and mechanical threshold-testing device, subcutaneous administration of buprenorphine resulted in slow onset, quick offset, and minimal antinociception in the cat (Steagall et al., 2007). Using the same thermal device method, Robertson et al. (2003) showed that oral transmucosal administration of buprenorphine in cats was as effective as the IV route (Robertson et al., 2003). In a clinical study of cats undergoing ovariohysterectomy, however, Giordano et al. (2010) showed that cats given buprenorphine by the IV and IM routes had significantly lower dynamic interactive visual analog scale pain scores than those given the drug by the SC and oral transmucosal routes. Also, in the latter two groups, there was a significantly higher incidence of treatment failure when compared with the IV and IM groups (Giordano et al., 2010). In the Giordano study (2010), cats were premedicated with medetomidine, and buprenorphine was administered soon after anesthetic induction. The absorption of a drug through the oral transmucosal route is dependent on the regional blood flow, local temperature, and mucosal integrity. It is possible that medetomidine could have caused local vasoconstriction, thereby contributing to poor systemic uptake of buprenorphine and therefore the poor analgesic effect observed after oral transmucosal administration. In that study, the dose of buprenorphine (0.01 mg/kg) was rather low, so it is possible that, had a larger dose been used, better analgesia would have been observed by the oral transmucosal route.

A recent study examined oral transmucosal buprenorphine in dogs (Abbo et al., 2008). In that study, 0.02 mg/kg or 0.12 mg/kg of buprenorphine were given by either the IV or oral transmucosal routes to healthy dogs. Bioavailability of buprenorphine after oral transmucosal administration was 38% + 12% after the 0.02 mg/kg dose, and 47% + 16% after the 0.12 mg/kg dose (Abbo et al., 2008). Peak plasma drug concentrations were similar between 0.02 mg/kg buprenorphine IV and 0.12 mg/kg buprenorphine transmucosal (Abbo et al., 2008). Given the relatively large volume of buprenorphine that would need to be administered to a dog to achieve a dose of 0.12 mg/kg transmucosally, and given the relatively low bioavailability reported in that study, oral transmucosal buprenorphine is probably not a practical or cost-effective analgesic option for dogs.

Oral Transmucosal Methadone

Methadone has physicochemical properties similar to buprenorphine, with a similar pK and, therefore, potentially similar bioavailability when administered via the oral transmucosal route. There are limited studies available as to the feasibility of using this opioid for analgesia via this route. One recent study demonstrated that methadone was indeed bioavailable after oral transmucosal administration in cats (Ferreira et al., 2011). These authors demonstrated that 0.6 mg/kg of oral transmucosal methadone resulted in peak plasma concentrations 2 hours after administration, with greater sedation as compared with a lower dose (0.3 mg/kg) given IV. The cats treated with oral transmucosal methadone were notably sedated for greater than 4 hours, and had evidence of analgesia for a similar time period, as assessed by mechanical pressure applied to the carpi. While these results are promising with respect to the use of methadone by this route in cats, further studies would be needed to prove that clinical analgesia (e.g., post-ovariohysterectomy) is achieved.

EXTENDED RELEASE ORAL OPIOIDS

Oral opioid formulations, both short- and long-acting forms, are the mainstay of pain medication for human beings. Some long-acting forms of morphine sulfate have been available in the United States for many years. The forms marketed as MS Contin® (Perdue Frederick, Stamford, CT) and Oramorph® (Roxane Pharmaceuticals, Columbus, OH) must be swallowed whole without being chewed or broken. If the pills are broken before reaching the stomach there is a potential for an overdose requiring treatment with reversal agents such as naloxone. This potentially makes dosing at appropriate mg/kg doses difficult in smaller veterinary patients.

Kapanol® (GlaxoSmithKline, Australia) is a long-acting, granular formulation of morphine developed for administration every 12–24 hours to humans. The Kapanol granules can be swallowed in a single dose within the gelatin capsule or the granules may be dispersed in liquid or semisolid food material, such as applesauce, and then swallowed without chewing (Broomhead et al., 1997). A dispersible granular formulation of a long-acting opioid medication could potentially be administered to veterinary patients in small amounts of highly palatable soft foods or Pill Pockets®; however, there is the risk that the animal may chew the granules and receive a very high dose. Currently, Kapanol is not available in the United States; however, two granular formulations of extended-release morphine sulfate have recently been approved for use by the FDA in the United States (Caldwell et al., 2002; Caldwell, 2004). Avinza® (Ligand Pharmaceuticals, San Diego, CA) is a novel morphine formulation that contains both immediate release granules and extended release granules. When extended release granules in Avinza come into contact with gastrointestinal fluid, they swell and release morphine into the gastrointestinal tract (Caldwell, 2004). Kadian®, another recently approved extended-release oral morphine product (Actavis Inc., Fort Lee, NJ), is similar to Kapanol in its extended release technology and its pharmacokinetics in human beings (Broomhead et al., 1997).

Most extended release oral opioid formulations have not been extensively studied in controlled clinical trials in veterinary patients. Although occasionally prescribed for post-operative or chronic pain in veterinary species, the actual efficacy of these oral formulations is questionable. In an early study using healthy bea-

gles, Dohoo & Tasker (1997) evaluated the pharmacokinetics of MS Contin as an oral sustained release morphine product. Dogs that were given 15 mg tablets of MS Contin (approximately a 1.5 mg/kg dose) attained serum concentrations that were approximately 3% of those attained after the same dose was administered IV (Dohoo & Tasker, 1997). In addition, the authors did not find a sustained serum concentration after MS Contin and drug concentrations tended to decrease well below non-therapeutic values by 200 minutes after drug administration (Dohoo & Tasker, 1997). The assay used in that study likely detected metabolites of morphine as well as the parent drug, so the relative area under the curve for morphine may have been falsely increased. The calculated bioavailability of MS Contin in dogs was 15%–17%, likely due to significant first-pass metabolism and large variability in absorption among individual animals. A similar study by KuKanich et al (2005) found that approximately 1.5 mg/kg of extended-release morphine administered orally to dogs resulted in very low serum concentrations of the drug that were nondetectable by 4 hours after drug administration (Figure 9.3). Differences between data in these two studies might be related to methodology in assaying morphine; however, both studies point to the impracticality and low therapeutic value in pursuing oral extended release morphine for analgesic purposes in dogs.

Avinza® oral pharmacokinetics has also been examined in dogs. Avinza®, as mentioned previously, has both immediate release and sustained release granules containing morphine. In a study using healthy Labrador dogs, this formulation of oral morphine was dosed at either 1 mg/kg or 2 mg/kg (Aragon et al., 2009). All dogs had detectable serum concentrations of morphine 3 hours after drug administration; however, 24 hours post-drug, only 5/14 dogs

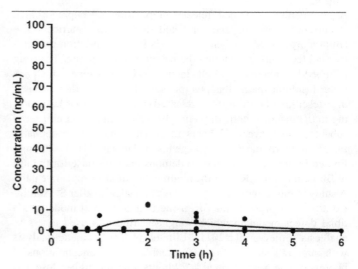

Figure 9.3. Plasma morphine concentrations (ng/mL) in dogs after oral administration of an extended release morphine sulphate preparation (From KuKanich, B., Lascelles, B.D.X., & Papich, M.G. (2005) Pharmacokinetics of morphine and plasma concentrations of morphine-6-glucuronide following morphine administration to dogs. *Journal of Veterinary Pharmacology and Therapeutics*, 28, 371–376. With permission.)

continued to have measureable serum morphine concentrations (Aragon et al., 2009). There was a large amount of variability among dogs with respect to serum concentration versus time curves, and the authors concluded that oral morphine in this formulation was poorly and unpredictably absorbed (Aragon et al., 2009). Again, this was likely due to first-pass metabolism, which is more prominent in dogs than in other species, including humans. In that study, because of the inconsistent nature of morphine's absorption and the low (below therapeutic) serum concentrations observed at many time points, the authors concluded that this oral morphine formulation was not useful for analgesic purposes in dogs. It is possible that veterinary species, other than dogs, with less first-pass metabolism may benefit from oral extended-release opioid formulations, but studies are lacking.

POLYMER GELS

Hydromorphone
Formulations of hydromorphone have been made using impregnation of the drug into water-soluble polymer gels that can be subcutaneously implanted for continuous drug delivery up to 4 weeks (Lesser et al., 1996). Drug formulations in polymerized gels have much longer kinetics (up to 4 weeks for rabbits *in vivo* for a hydromorphone preparation) than either traditional oral or parenteral forms of the same drugs (Lesser et al., 1996). These extremely long release kinetics are achieved at the cost of peak therapeutic concentrations in serum. Polymer gels also require minor surgery to place and replace the gel for animals undergoing treatment of chronic pain.

Buprenorphine
A commercial sustained release preparation of buprenorphine is currently available and marketed directly for veterinary use (Buprenorphine SR®). This product is likely a variation on polymer gel technology, although the patent is still pending. The drug is imbedded in a matrix of DL-lactide-co-caprolactone, which is a water-insoluble matrix that precipitates in body fluids thereby leaving a reservoir of the drug to be released (Dunn et al., 1996). According to the manufacturer, Buprenorphine SR® can be administered subcutaneously every 72 hours to provide analgesia (Zoopharm Inc., Buprenorphine SR® package insert, January 2012). Although limited in number, studies have demonstrated promise for the use of Buprenorphine SR® for the treatment of mild-to-moderate pain. A study in rats demonstrated 2–3 days of analgesia after SC administration of buprenorphine SR, using both a thermal model and a tibial defect model in which weight-bearing was used to assess analgesia (Foley et al., 2011). Limited pharmacokinetic analysis with three rats showed that measureable serum concentrations of buprenorphine were attained at 72 hours after the higher dose was administered (1.2 mg/kg). In a study of cats undergoing ovariohysterectomy, Catbagan et al. (2011) demonstrated similar analgesic efficacy of oral transmucosal buprenorphine (0.02 mg/kg) administered twice daily to Buprenorphine SR® administered once at premedication (0.12 mg/kg). Ten to 11 cats were studied in each group and side effects were similar. There was no difference between groups with respect to VAS score, Colorado State University Pain Score, or von Frey filament size threshold at any time point (Catbagan et al., 2011). All cats were also administered meloxicam,

so analgesia was not solely due to buprenorphine in either group. The analgesic use of Buprenorphine SR® in dogs or other species has not been examined in a controlled, nonbiased published study, but its use warrants further investigation. While Buprenorphine SR® holds promise as a viable and convenient extended-release opioid for use in veterinary medicine, this opioid is not considered to provide profound analgesia as may be necessary for major surgical pain.

LIPOSOME-ENCAPSULATED OPIOIDS

Encapsulation into liposomes is a method of preparing long-acting formulations of opioid drugs. Multivesicular liposome-encapsulated preparations of morphine produce significant blood concentrations for 6 days after a single SC injection in mice (Kim et al., 1993). Similar preparations have been shown to produce significant blood concentrations and analgesic effects after epidural administration in rats and dogs (Kim et al., 1996; Yaksh et al., 1999).

Liposomes release their contents in a number of ways, which may be broadly categorized as either release through efflux or release through liposome degradation in the biological milieu. Degradation of the liposome structure may occur through a number of mechanisms, such as lipases present in tissue fluid and uptake by phagocytic cells. Liposome degradation is affected by the lipid composition, the physical characteristics, and the method of manufacture. Efflux of liposome contents occurs directly through the liposome membrane without degradation of the membrane itself, and depends on the ability of the drug to partition through the membrane. This partitioning of the drug is primarily influenced by the polarity and molecular weight of the drug, and secondarily by the lipid composition and structure of the liposomes.

Epidural Administration
In 2004, the FDA approved an extended-release liposome-encapsulated formulation of morphine for epidural use in people (Depodur®, EKR Therapeutics Inc., Cedar Knolls NJ) (Figure 9.4). This technology utilizes a proprietary carrier, Depofoam®, that allows slow release of morphine across multiple lipid bilayers. Depodur® provides up to 48 hours of analgesia after epidural administration without the need for an indwelling epidural catheter. In a human clinical trial, people undergoing hip replacement were given 5 mg of standard morphine or 10, 15, 20, 25, or 30 mg doses of Depodur® epidurally prior to surgery, and their use of postoperative PCA with fentanyl was recorded (Viscusi et al., 2006). Patients that were given the epidural extended-release morphine had 3–6 times longer before first use of PCA, and lower overall fentanyl usage (Figure 9.5) (Viscusi et al., 2006). In a second trial, 200 patients undergoing hip arthroplasty were given epidural extended-release morphine at doses of 15, 20, or 30 mg or placebo (Viscusi et al., 2005). Intraoperative opioid dosing with fentanyl was standardized to 250μg. The mean time to the first request for additional analgesia was 21.1 hours in the patients that were given epidural extended-release morphine compared with 3.1 hours in those that received the placebo, and the cumulative fentanyl usage was significantly lower in all patients given the extended-release epidural morphine formulation (Viscusi et al., 2005). While Depodur® obviates the need for an indwelling epidural catheter, there are some disadvantages to its use including the current price of this product.

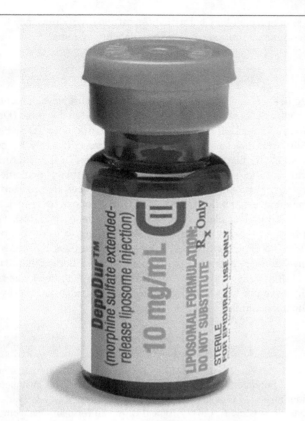

Figure 9.4. Depodur®, extended release liposomal morphine for epidural use (With permission from EKR Therapeutics.)

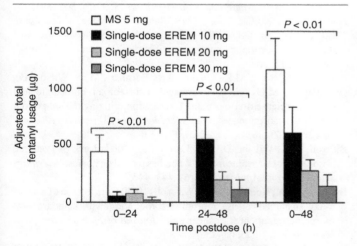

Figure 9.5. Total patient-controlled fentanyl use after hip arthroplasty in patients who received epidural morphine or epidural extended-release morphine (Depodur®) at 10, 20, or 30 mg (From Viscusi, E.R., Martin, G., Hartrick, C.T. Singla, N., Manvelian, G. & EREM Study Group. (2005) Forty-eight hours of postoperative pain relief after total hip arthroplasty with a novel, extended-release epidural morphine formulation. *Anesthesiology*, 102(5), 1014–1022. With permission.)

In conversations with MD anesthesiologists, there is also concern about the inability to "reverse" the extended-release product once it is administered epidurally in the event of an adverse reaction or a change in surgical planning. In veterinary medicine, the epidural route of administration of drugs is not routinely performed in dogs and cats, except in specialty practices. Therefore, Depodur® is not likely to gain wide acceptance as a novel analgesic delivery method in veterinary medicine.

Systemic Administration

The pharmacology laboratory at the University of Wisconsin has been working for a number of years on various types of liposome-encapsulated formulations of oxymorphone, hydromorphone, buprenorphine, and butorphanol for systemic administration to laboratory and companion animals for the purpose of providing extended durations of analgesia. In most of these studies, the liposome formulation was administered subcutaneously and no local skin reactions or infection at the site of injection have been observed. In early studies, in a rodent model of neuropathic pain and in a rodent model of visceral pain (Krugner-Higby et al., 2003; Clark et al., 2004; Smith et al., 2006), using a relatively "leaky" liposome made with egg phosphatidylcholine, encapsulated oxymorphone demonstrated prolonged and superior analgesia when compared with multiple doses of the standard formulation of oxymorphone. In these studies using the egg phosphatidylcholine liposomes, analgesia was maintained for approximately 48 hours. Later, the liposomes were synthesized to incorporate a different opioid, hydromorphone, using cholesterol and dipalmitoylphosphatidylcholine (DPPC-C) and the pharmacokinetics were evaluated in dogs (Smith et al., 2008). In that study, serum hydromorphone concentrations fluctuated around 4.0 ng/mL from 6–72 hours after 2.0 mg/kg, and mean concentrations remained above 4 ng/mL for 96 hours after 3.0 mg/kg DPPC-C hydromorphone (Smith et al., 2008) (Figure 9.6). In comparison, standard hydromorphone, when injected subcutaneously at 0.5 mg/kg, resulted in negligible serum concentrations 6 hours after administration (KuKanich et al., 2008). Two clinical studies, evaluating analgesia in a varied population of dogs after SC administration of DPPC-C hydromorphone, have been completed. In the first study in a shelter population of dogs undergoing ovariohysterectomy, preoperative DPPC-C hydromorphone provided analgesia equivalent to the standard of care premedication of acepromazine and morphine, based on dynamic Interactive visual analog scale (DIVAS) pain scoring by blinded observers (Krugner-Higby et al., 2011). Results of a clinical trial of client-owned dogs undergoing amputation suggested that DPPC-C hydromorphone given subcutaneously prior to surgery resulted in fewer treatment failures than a continuous intravenous fentanyl infusion for the first 24 hours after surgery (Smith et al., 2013). With both the egg phosphatidylcholine and the DPPC-C formulations of hydromorphone, there is some initial bolus release of the drug, and the expected adverse effects of nausea, vomiting, and sedation do occur. These adverse effects are less obvious after the first hour of administration when the drug kinetics become closer to steady state. In a study to evaluate potential adverse effects on ventilation and oxygenation after DPPC-C hydromorphone administration, a serial blood gas analysis was performed in healthy dogs given placebo, DPPC-C hydromorphone, or standard hydromorphone (Wunsch et al., 2010). In that study, modest decreases were observed in PaO_2 after dogs were given

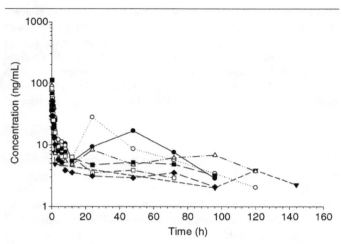

Figure 9.6. Plasma hydromorphone concentrations (ng/mL) in dogs after subcutaneous administration of 3.0 mg/kg of DPPC-C hydromorphone (From Smith, L.J., KuKanich, B., Hogan, B.K., Brown, C., Heath, T.D. & Krugner-Higby, L.A. (2008) Pharmacokinetics of a controlled-release liposome-encapsulated hydromorphone administered to healthy dogs. *Journal of Veterinary Pharmacology and Therapeutics*, 31(5), 415–422. With permission.)

either standard hydromorphone or DPPC-C hydromorphone, and similarly modest increases in $PaCO_2$ were observed in both groups (Wunsch et al., 2010). Changes in PaO_2 still remained within a range that would suggest close to 100% hemoglobin saturation, and $PaCO_2$ did not increase above 45 mm Hg in any dog (Wunsch et al., 2010).

Recently, the laboratory has synthesized and tested a formulation of liposome-encapsulated oxymorphone and/or hydromorphone made by an ammonium sulfate gradient loading (ASG) technique (Tu et al., 2010). A preliminary pharmacokinetic study in rhesus macaques suggested that ASG liposome-encapsulated oxymorphone, when administered subcutaneously, results in measureable serum concentrations of the drug for up to 21 days (Krugner-Higby et al., 2011). Analgesia in these studies was not assessed, as these were healthy, nonpainful primates. A pharmacokinetic study was recently completed to assess the theoretical duration of ASG liposome-encapsulated oxymorphone or hydromorphone in healthy dogs (Smith et al., 2013). Data suggested that serum hydromorphone concentrations greater than 1 ng/mL persisted for over 480 hours.

Systemic administration of liposome-encapsulated opioids has many theoretical advantages, including excellent bioavailability compared to extended-release oral formulations of opioids, particularly in veterinary patients. Other advantages include ease of administration, lack of necessary IV access or long-term catheter placement, established analgesic and safety profile of this class of drugs in veterinary medicine, and inability of the injected liposome-encapsulated drug to be accessed by children or diverted for abuse. A potential disadvantage is the long-acting nature of these formulations in the event that a patient has an adverse reaction to the drug. Additionally, the cost of manufacture, and existence of patents that use similar technology but with different classes of drugs may limit the commercialization of these drug delivery systems.

SUMMARY

Drug delivery technology is a huge area of future development in the analgesic world. Entire journals are devoted to this topic (Drug Delivery, Drug Delivery Technology, Journal of Drug Delivery). By the time this chapter is published, there will likely be new developments that have promise or application in the veterinary world. To date, some of the limitations in veterinary medicine to novel analgesic drug delivery systems have been due to lack of commercial availability, the need for patient-control for drug delivery, lack of bioavailability in veterinary patients, and cost. One can hope that, in the future, established analgesics or novel drugs will be incorporated into delivery systems that meet the needs of many veterinary patients. In the meantime, practitioners should use novel drug delivery systems or methods with the knowledge that many have not been tested or validated for analgesic efficacy in companion animals.

REFERENCES

Abbo, L.A., Ko, J.C., Maxwell, L.K., et al. (2008) Pharmacokinetics of buprenorphine following intravenous and oral transmucosal administration in dogs. *Veterinary Therapeutics*, 9(2), 83–93.

Anand, P. & Bley, K. (2011) Topical capsaicin for pain management: therapeutic potential and mechanism of action of the new high-concentration capsaicin 8% patch. *British Journal of Anaesthesia*, 107(4), 490–502.

Andaluz, A., Moll, X., Ventura, R., Abellán, R., Fresno, L., & García, F. (2009) Plasma buprenorphine concentrations after the application of a 70 µg/hour transdermal patch in dogs. Preliminary report. *Journal of Veterinary Pharmacology and Therapeutics*, 32(5), 503–505.

Anderson, D., Kollias-Baker, C., Colahan, P., Keene, R.O., Lynn, R.C., & Hepler, D.I. (2005) Urinary and serum concentrations of diclofenac after topical application to horses. *Veterinary Therapeutics*, 6(1), 57–66.

Aragon, C.L., Read, M.R., Gaynor, J.S., Barnhart, M.D., Wilson, D., & Papich, M.G. (2009) Pharmacokinetics of an immediate and extended release oral morphine formulation utilizing the spheroidal oral drug absorption system in dogs. *Journal of Veterinary Pharmacology and Therapeutics*, 32(2), 129–136.

Bidwell, L.A., Wilson, D.V., & Caron, J.P. (2007) Lack of systemic absorption of lidocaine from 5% patches placed on horses. *Veterinary Anesthesia and Analgesia*, 34(6), 443–446.

Broomhead, A., Kerr, R., Tester, W., et al. (1997) Comparison of a once-a-day sustained-release morphine formulation with standard oral morphine treatment for cancer pain. *Journal of Pain and Symptom Management*, 14(2), 63–73.

Brown, M.B., Martin, G.P., Jones, S.A., & Akomeah, F.K. (2006) Dermal and transdermal drug delivery systems: current and future prospects. *Drug Delivery*, 13(3), 175–187.

Caldwell, J.R. (2004) Avinza: 24-h sustained-release oral morphine therapy. *Expert Opinion on Pharmacotherapy*, 5(2), 469–472.

Caldwell, J.R., Rapoport, R.J., Davis, J.C., et al. (2002) Efficacy and safety of a once-daily morphine formulation in chronic, moderate-to-severe osteoarthritis pain: Results from a randomized, placebo-controlled, double-blind trial and an open label extension trial. *Journal of Pain and Symptom Management*, 23(4), 278–291.

Catbagan, D.L., Quimby, J.M., Mama, K.R., Rychel, J.K., & Mich, P.M. (2011) Comparison of the efficacy and adverse effects of sustained-release buprenorphine hydrochloride following subcutaneous administration and buprenorphine hydrochloride following oral transmucosal administration in cats undergoing ovariohysterectomy. *American Journal of Veterinary Research*, 72(4), 461–466.

Clark, M.D., Krugner-Higby, L., Smith, L.J., Heath, T.D., Clark, K.L., & Olson, D. (2004) Evaluation of liposome encapsulated (LE) oxymorphone hydrochloride in mice after splenectomy mice. *Comparative Medicine*, 54(5), 558–563.

Dohoo, S.E. & Tasker, R.E. (1997) Pharmacokinetics of oral morphine sulfate in dogs: A comparison of sustained release and conventional formulations. *Canadian Journal of Veterinary Research*, 61(4), 251–255.

Dunn, R.L., Yewey, G.L., Fugita, S.M., et al. (1996) Sustained release of cisplatin in dogs form an injectable implant delivery system. *Journal of Bioactive Compatible Polymers*, 11, 286–300.

Egger, C.M., Glerum, L.E., Allen, S.W., & Haag, M. (2003) Plasma fentanyl concentrations in awake cats and cats undergoing anesthesia and ovariohysterectomy using transdermal administration. *Veterinary Anesthesia and Analgesia*, 30(4), 229–236.

Egger, C.M., Glerum, L., Haag, M.K., & Rohrbach, B.W. (2007) Efficacy and cost-effectiveness of transdermal fentanyl patches for the relief of post-operative pain in dogs after anterior cruciate ligament and pelvic limb repair. *Veterinary Anesthesia and Analgesia*, 34(3), 200–208.

Ellison, N., Loprinzi, C.L., Kugler, J., et al. (1997) Phase III placebo-controlled trial of capsaicin cream in the management of surgical neuropathic pain in cancer patients. *Journal of Clinical Oncology*, 15(8), 2974–2980.

Ferreira, T.H., Rezende, M.L., Mama, K.R., Hudachek, S.F., & Aguiar, A.J. (2011) Plasma concentrations and behavioral, antinociceptive, and physiologic effects of methadone after intravenous or oral transmucosal administration in cats. *American Journal of Veterinary Research*, 72(6), 764–771.

Foley, P.L., Liang, H., & Crichlow, A.R. (2011) Evaluation of a sustained-release formulation of buprenorphine for analgesia in rats. *Journal of the American Association for Laboratory Animal Science*, 50(2), 198–204.

Frisbie, D.D., McIlwraith, C.W., Kawcak, C.E., Werpy, N.M., & Pearce, G.L. (2009) Evaluation of topically administered diclofenac liposomal cream for the treatment of horses with experimentally induced osteoarthritis. *American Journal of Veterinary Research*, 70(2), 210–215.

Galer, B.S., Jensen, M.P., Ma, T., Davies, P.S., & Rowbotham, M.C. (2002) The lidocaine patch 5% effectively treats all neuropathic pain qualities: results of a randomized, double-blind, vehicle-controlled, 3 week efficacy study with use of the neuropathic pain scale. *Clinical Journal of Pain*, 18(5), 297–301.

Gibbon, K.J., Cyborski, J.M., Guzinski, M.V., Viviano, K.R., & Trepanier, L.A. (2003) Evaluation of adverse effects of EMLA (lidocaine/prilocaine) cream for the placement of jugular catheters in healthy cats. *Journal of Veterinary Pharmacology and Therapeutics*, 26(6), 439–441.

Giordano, T., Steagall, P.V.M., Ferreira, T.H., et al. (2010) Postoperative analgesic effects of intravenous, intramuscular, subcutaneous, or oral transmucosal buprenorphine administered to cats undergoing ovariohysterectomy. *Veterinary Anesthesia and Analgesia*, 37(4), 357–366.

Hofmeister, E.H. & Egger, C.M. (2004) Transdermal fentanyl patches in small animals. *Journal of the American Animal Hospital Association*, 40(6), 468–478.

Kim, T., Kim, J., & Kim, S. (1993) Extended-release formulation of morphine for subcutaneous administration. *Cancer Chemotherapy and Pharmacology*, 33(3): 187–190.

Kim, T., Murande, S., Gruber, A., & Kim, S. (1996) Sustained-release morphine for epidural analgesia in rats. *Anesthesiology*, 85(2), 331–338.

Ko, J.C., Maxwell, L.K., Abbo, L.A., & Weil, A.B. (2008) Pharmacokinetics of lidocaine following the application of 5% lidocaine patches to cats. *Journal of Veterinary Pharmacology and Therapeutics*, 31(4), 359–367.

Ko, J., Weil, A., Maxwell, L., Kitao, T. & Haydon, T. (2007) Plasma concentrations of lidocaine in dogs following lidocaine patch application. *Journal of the American Animal Hospital Association*, 43(5), 280–283.

Krugner-Higby, L.A., KuKanich, B., Schmidt, B.K., Heath, T.D., & Brown, C. (2011) Pharmacokinetics and behavioral effects of liposomal hydromorphone suitable for perioperative use in rhesus macaques. *Psychopharmacology*, 330, 511–523

Krugner-Higby, L.A., Smith, L.J., Schmidt, B.K., et al. (2011) Experimental pharmacodynamics and analgesic efficacy of liposome-encapsulated hydromorphone in dogs. *Journal of the American Animal Hospital Association*, 47(3), 185–195.

Krugner-Higby, L., Smith, L.J., Clark, M., et al. (2003) Liposome-encapsulated oxymorphone hydrochloride provides prolonged relief of post-surgical visceral pain in rats. *Comparative Medicine*, 53(3), 270–279.

KuKanich, B., Hogan, B.K., Krugner-Higby, L.A., & Smith, L.J. (2008) Pharmacokinetics of hydromorphone hydrochloride in healthy dogs. *Veterinary Anesthesia and Analgesia*, 35(3), 256–264.

KuKanich, B., Lascelles, B.D.X., & Papich, M.G. (2005) Pharmacokinetics of morphine and plasma concentrations of morphine-6-glucuronide following morphine administration to dogs. *Journal of Veterinary Pharmacology and Therapeutics*, 28, 371–376.

Lee, D.D., Papich, M.G., & Hardie, E.M. (2000) Comparison of pharmacokinetics of fentanyl after intravenous and transdermal administration in cats. *American Journal of Veterinary Research*, 61(6), 672–677.

Lesser, G.J., Grossman, S.A., Leong, K.W., Lo, H., & Eller, S. (1996) In vitro and in vivo studies of subcutaneous hydromorphone implants designed for the treatment of cancer pain. *Pain*, 65(2–3), 265–272.

Levine, D.G., Epstein, K.L., Neelis, D.A., & Ross, M.W. (2009) Effect of topical application of 1% diclofenac sodium liposomal cream on inflammation in healthy horses undergoing intravenous regional limb perfusion with amikacin sulfate. *American Journal of Veterinary Research*, 70(11), 1323–1325.

Linton, D.D., Wilson, M.G., Newbound, G.C., et al. (2012) The effectiveness of a long-acting transdermal fentanyl solution compared to buprenorphine for the control of postoperative pain in dogs in a randomized, multicentered clinical study. *Journal of Veterinary Pharmacology and Therapeutics*, 35(S2), 53–64.

Lynn, R.C., Hepler, K.I., Kelch, W.J., Bertone, J.J., Smith, B.L., & Vatistas, N.J. (2004) Double-blinded placebo-controlled clinical field trial to evaluate the safety and efficacy of topically applied 1% diclofenac liposomal cream for the relief of lameness in horses. *Veterinary Therapeutics*, 5(2), 128–138.

Moore, R.A., Tramer, M.R., Carroll, D., Wiffen, P.J., & McQuay, H.J. (1998) Quantitative systematic review of topically applied non-steroidal anti-inflammatory drugs. *British Medical Journal*, 316(7128), 333–338.

Murrell, J.C., Robertson, S.A., Taylor, P.M., McCown, J.L., Bloomfield, M., & Sear, J.W. (2007) Use of a transdermal matrix patch of buprenorphine in cats: Preliminary pharmacokinetic and pharmacodynamic data. *Veterinary Record*, 160(17), 578–583.

Palazzo, E., Luongo, L., de Novellis, V., Berrino, L., Rossi, F., & Maione, S. (2010) Moving towards supraspinal TRPV1 receptors for chronic pain relief. *Molecular Pain*, 6, 66.

Portenoy, R.K., Southam, M.A., Gupta, S.K., et al. (1993) Transdermal fentanyl for cancer pain: repeated dose pharmacokinetics. *Anesthesiology*, 78(1), 36–43.

Posner, L.P., Pavuk, A.A., Rokshar, J.L., Carter, J.E., & Levine, J.F. (2010) Effects of opioids and anesthetic drugs on body temperature in cats. *Veterinary Anesthesia and Analgesia*, 37(1), 35–43.

Rains, C. & Bryson, H.M. (1995) Topical capsaicin. A review of its pharmacological properties and therapeutic potential in post-herpetic neuralgia, diabetic neuropathy and osteoarthritis. *Drugs & Aging*, 7(4), 317–328.

Robertson, S.A., Taylor, P.M., & Sear, J.W. (2003) Systemic uptake of buprenorphine by cats after oral transmucosal administration. *Veterinary Record*, 152(22), 675–678.

Roy, S.D. & Flynn, G.L. (1990) Transdermal delivery of narcotic analgesics: pH, anatomical, and subject influences on cutaneous permeability of fentanyl and sufentanil. *Pharmaceutical Research*, 7(8), 842–847.

Sathyan, G., Guo, C., Sivakumar, K., Gidwani, S., & Gupta, S. (2005) Evaluation of the bioequivalence of two transdermal fentanyl systems following single and repeat applications. *Current Medical Research and Opinion*, 21(12), 1961–1968.

Schmiedt, C.W. & Bjorling, D.E. (2007) Accidental prehension and suspected transmucosal or oral absorption of fentanyl from a transdermal patch in a dog. *Veterinary Anesthesia and Analgesia*, 34(1), 70–73.

Smith, L.J., KuKanich, B., Hogan, B.K., Brown, C., Heath, T.D. & Krugner-Higby, L.A. (2008) Pharmacokinetics of a controlled-release liposome-encapsulated hydromorphone administered to healthy dogs. *Journal of Veterinary Pharmacology and Therapeutics*, 31(5), 415–422.

Smith, L.J., Valenzuela, J.R., Krugner-Higby, L., Brown, C., & Heath, T.D. (2006) A single dose of liposome-encapsulated hydromorphone provides extended relief of hyperalgesia in a rodent model of neuropathic pain. *Comparative Medicine*, 56(6), 487–492.

Smith, L.J., KuKanich, B.K., Krugner-Higby, L.A., Schmidt, B.H., & Heath, T.D. (2013) Pharmacokinetics of ammonium sulfate gradient loaded liposme-encapsulated oxymorphone and hydromorphone in healthy dogs. *Veterinary Anaesthesia and Analgesia*, 40(5), 537–545.

Stanos, S. (2009) Overview of topical analgesics. *Pain Medicine News Special Edition*, 21–26.

Steagall, P.V.M., Taylor, P.M., Brondani, J.T., Luna, S.P., Dixon, M.J., & Ferreira, T.H. (2007) Effects of buprenorphine, carprofen, and saline on thermal and mechanical nociceptive thresholds in cats. *Veterinary Anesthesia and Analgesia*, 34(5), 344–350.

Taddio, A. (2001) Pain management for neonatal circumcision. *Paediatric Drugs*, 3(2), 101–111.

Taylor, A.L., Gostin, L.O., & Pagonis, K.A. (2008) Ensuring effective pain treatment: a national and global perspective. *Journal of the American Medical Association*, 299(1), 89–91.

The Capsaicin Study Group. (1991) Treatment of painful diabetic neuropathy with topical capsaicin. A multicenter, double-blind, vehicle controlled study. *Archives of Internal Medicine*, 151(11), 2225–2229.

Tu, S., McGinnis, T., Krugner-Higby, L., & Heath, T.D. (2010) A mathematical relationship for hydromorphone loading into liposomes with trans-membrane ammonium sulfate gradients. *Journal of Pharmaceutical Sciences*, 99(6), 2672–2680.

Turnbull, A. (1850) *Tincture of Capsicum as a Remedy for Chilblains and Toothache*, vol. 95, Dublin Medical Press, pp. 6–7.

Viscusi, E.R., Kopacz, D., Hartrick, C.T., Martin, G., & Manvelian, G. (2006) Single-dose extended-release epidural morphine for pain following hip arthroplasty. *American Journal of Therapeutics*, 13(5), 423–431.

Viscusi, E.R., Martin, G., Hartrick, C.T., Singla, N., Manvelian, G., & EREM Study Group. (2005) Forty-eight hours of postoperative pain relief after total hip arthroplasty with a novel, extended-release epidural morphine formulation. *Anesthesiology*, 102(5), 1014–1022.

Wagner, K.A., Gibbon, K.J., Strom, T.L., Kurian, J.R., & Trepanier, L.A. (2006) Adverse effects of EMLA (lidocaine/prilocaine) cream and efficacy for the placement of jugular catheters in hospitalized cats. *Journal of Feline Medicine and Surgery*, 8(2), 141–144.

Wunsch, L.A., Schmidt, B.K., Krugner-Higby, L.A., & Smith, L.J. (2010) A comparison of the effects of hydromorphone HCl and a novel extended release hydromorphone on arterial blood gas values in conscious healthy dogs. *Research in Veterinary Science*, 88(1), 154–158.

Yaksh, T.L., Provencher, J.C., Rathbun, M.L., & Kohn, F.R. (1999) Pharmacokinetics and efficacy of epidurally delivered sustained release encapsulated morphine in dogs. *Anesthesiology*, 90(5), 1402–1412.

Zempsky, W.T., Robbins, B., Richards, P.T., Leong, M.S., & Schechter, N.L. (2008) A novel needle-free powder lidocaine delivery system for rapid local analgesia. *The Journal of Pediatrics*, 152(3), 405–411.

Zhang, H., Zhang, J., & Streisand, J.B. (2002) Oral mucosal drug delivery: clinical pharmacokinetics and therapeutic applications. *Clinical Pharmacokinetics*, 41(9), 661–680.

10
Pharmacokinetic Principles for the Design of Intravenous Infusions

Bruno H. Pypendop

Intravenous infusions are being increasingly used to administer analgesic drugs such as opioids, lidocaine, ketamine, and α-2 agonists. The main advantage of intravenous infusions is that they allow the maintenance of constant plasma drug concentrations, which, in turn, may result in constant effect site concentrations and, therefore, a constant effect. Design of intravenous infusions can be either empirical or based on pharmacokinetics. The empirical approach relies on the selection of an initial dose and titration of subsequent doses based on the response of the patient, or on historical experience with the drug. The pharmacokinetic approach is based on the knowledge of the drug concentration that produces the desired effect (target concentration C_T) and the rate at which the drug concentration changes, therefore allowing calculation of the drug dose to be administered in order to maintain C_T. The optimal method involves both approaches, combining knowledge of drug pharmacokinetics and the ability to modify the administration scheme based on the patient's response. While knowledge of the concentration–effect relationship is essential to the use of pharmacokinetics for the design of dosing regimens, these relationships will not be discussed here.

Pharmacokinetics is the study of the time course of drug concentration in the body (Gabrielsson & Weiner, 2006). Pharmacokinetic analysis is a powerful tool in which mathematical equations are fitted to observations on the disposition of drugs; these equations can therefore be used to reconstruct the likely plasma drug concentration from any dose given to a patient, whether as a bolus or an infusion.

DEFINITIONS

Before discussing the pharmacokinetic principles governing the design of infusion schemes, it is useful to define a few terms to ensure that the correct terminology is used and understood.

Volume of Distribution
The volume of distribution (V) is the volume in which the drug *appears* to be diluted. In compartmental pharmacokinetic analysis,

one or several volumes of distribution are calculated, according to the number of compartments. The volume of distribution at steady state is the sum of the volumes of the different compartments. It is important to realize that these volumes are not the actual physical or physiological volumes. Compartment models are abstract constructs that allow the description of the changes in drug concentration, over time, in terms of the simplest possible mathematical equation, and do not attempt to accurately describe physiological events.

Clearance
Clearance is the body's ability to remove a drug from the blood or plasma. Clearance is the volume of plasma or blood from which the drug has been irreversibly removed per unit of time. This definition applies to "central" or "metabolic" clearance. Distribution clearance(s) is the transfer of drug from the central to the peripheral compartment(s) in multi-compartment models, for which the removal of the drug from the central compartment is reversible; that is, the drug moves back into the central compartment as plasma concentrations drop.

Half-life
The half-life is the time necessary for the plasma drug concentration to decrease by 50%. The concentration-time data of drugs that fit multi-compartment models show different phases with different slopes, and therefore different half-lives. The elimination (or terminal) half-life, most commonly quoted, refers to the final phase.

Zero-order Process
The zero-order process is a process occurring at a constant rate, for example, a constant rate infusion (CRI).

First-order Process
A first-order process is a process occurring at a rate proportional to the amount of drug present in the system. For example, most processes governing drug absorption, distribution, and elimination are first-order processes. With first-order processes, changes in plasma drug concentration over time are exponential functions.

Pain Management in Veterinary Practice, First Edition. Edited by Christine M. Egger, Lydia Love and Tom Doherty.
© 2014 John Wiley & Sons, Inc. Published 2014 by John Wiley & Sons, Inc.

DESIGN OF INFUSION SCHEMES

Constant Rate Infusion

The simplest form of infusion is a CRI. When using pharmacokinetics to establish an appropriate CRI, only two parameters are necessary: C_T and the (metabolic) clearance (Cl). The CRI can be calculated as (Shafer & Schwinn, 2005),

$$CRI = C_T \times Cl$$

We can see from this equation that such a CRI will replace the amount of drug irreversibly lost by the system through metabolic clearance (Figure 10.1). At steady state, this will result in a stable plasma concentration equal to C_T since the system is in equilibrium, and the only net movement of drug is through metabolic clearance. Before steady state, this method will result in plasma concentrations less than C_T, but exponentially approaching C_T. This is due to the fact that the calculation does not take into account the distribution from central to peripheral compartment(s), and that the input (infusion) is, in this case, a zero-order process, whereas the disposition (distribution and elimination) is a first-order process.

It is important to note that, for most drugs, steady state is slow to be reached. The rule of thumb is that steady state is reached after 4–5 terminal half-lives, thus it can take several hours for most drugs in clinical use to reach steady state. However, the desired concentration usually falls within a range. One method to reach the target concentration faster is to target the higher end of the desired concentration range. Another method is to target a concentration higher than the desired concentration, with the risk of reaching that high concentration, and the potential for associated adverse effects, depending upon the drug used.

Loading Dose

Another method to reach C_T faster with a CRI is by using a loading dose (Figure 10.2). A loading dose is typically given as an intravenous bolus, and will therefore be diluted in the volume of

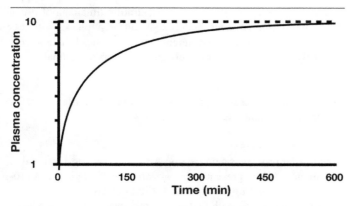

Figure 10.1. Changes in plasma concentration during administration of a constant rate infusion of two arbitrary units/min of a drug. Note that the concentrations are plotted on a logarithmic scale. Clearance of the drug is 0.2 L/min, and its terminal half-life is 120 minutes. The dashed line shows the C_T of 10 arbitrary units/L.

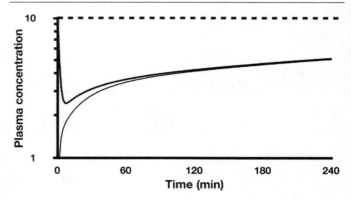

Figure 10.2. Changes in plasma concentration following the bolus administration of 100 arbitrary units of a drug as a loading dose calculated based on the volume of the central compartment, followed by a constant rate infusion (CRI) of 10 arbitrary units/min. Note that the concentrations are plotted on a logarithmic scale. The drug has a central volume of distribution of 10 L, and a clearance of 1 L/min. The thin line shows the changes in plasma concentration during the administration of the CRI without the loading dose. The dashed line shows the C_T of 10 arbitrary units/L, which is not achieved during the first 4 hours of infusion shown on the figure.

distribution of the drug. The loading dose D can therefore be calculated as (Shafer & Schwinn, 2005),

$$D = C_T \times V.$$

If a one-compartment model fits the concentration-time data, the situation is simple. When multi-compartment models fit the concentration-time data, there is an inherent problem in the selection of the appropriate volume of distribution. After intravenous bolus administration, the drug is, by definition, instantaneously diluted in the central compartment. If the volume of the central compartment is used in the above equation, C_T will be reached at time 0. However, the drug will immediately start distributing to the peripheral compartment(s) and also begin to undergo elimination, resulting in an immediate decrease below C_T. A CRI started at the same time as the bolus administration will only slowly return the plasma concentration toward C_T.

If the volume of distribution at steady state (V_{SS}) is used for the loading dose calculation instead of the volume of the central compartment, the initial plasma concentration will be much greater than C_T, because the drug is initially diluted in a volume much smaller than V_{SS}. A CRI will slowly return concentrations toward C_T (Figure 10.3).

This technique would only be safe for drugs with a very large therapeutic index, or if the difference between the volume of the central compartment and V_{SS} is small. Therefore, the volume of the central compartment is more commonly used. An alternative approach, using the volume of distribution at the time of the maximum effect, has been proposed. At that time, the volume of distribution will likely be intermediate between the volume of the central compartment and V_{SS}, resulting in concentrations transiently greater than C_T, but to a much lesser extent than if V_{SS} is used.

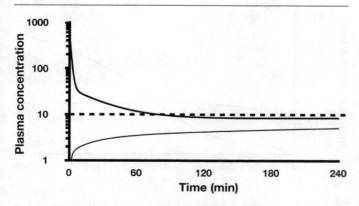

Figure 10.3. Changes in plasma concentration following the bolus administration of 5000 arbitrary units of a drug as a loading dose calculated based on the volume of distribution at steady state, followed by a constant rate infusion (CRI) of 10 arbitrary units/min. Note that the concentrations are plotted on a logarithmic scale. The drug has a volume of distribution at steady state of 500 L, and a clearance of 1 L/min. The thin line shows the changes in plasma concentration during the administration of the CRI without the loading dose. The dashed line shows the C_T of 10 arbitrary units/L, which is exceeded for the first hour of infusion in this example. In this example, the peak concentration is 50 times higher than C_T.

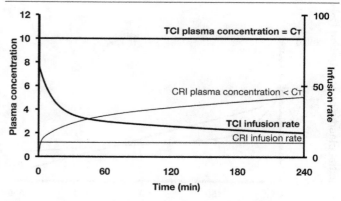

Figure 10.4. Changes in plasma drug concentrations and infusion rate over time for a target-controlled infusion (TCI, bold lines) and a constant rate infusion (CRI, thin lines). C_T is 10 arbitrary units/L. Note that the TCI produces a stable plasma concentration by using a variable infusion rate, while the CRI produces a variable plasma concentration (before steady state, not shown on this figure) by using a stable infusion rate.

Target-controlled Infusion

A better way to rapidly reach and maintain a target plasma concentration is to use a target-controlled infusion. With this approach, instead of using a zero-order input (a CRI) to match first-order processes (drug disposition), a first-order input is used. After delivering a loading dose calculated using the volume of the central compartment to reach C_T, C_T is maintained by administering an exponentially decreasing infusion rate. This allows the input to match the distribution and elimination kinetics (Figure 10.4).

As shown in this figure, a target-controlled infusion can achieve constant plasma concentrations by using a variable infusion rate, whereas, before steady state is reached, a CRI will result in variable plasma concentrations. Target-controlled infusions rely heavily on pharmacokinetic models, and have only been used for research in veterinary medicine.

Variable Infusion Rates

An intermediate solution between CRI and target-controlled infusion is the use of sequential CRIs. With this technique, a loading dose is administered, followed by a series of CRIs at decreasing rates, administered for fixed durations (Figure 10.5).

As illustrated in this figure, variable infusion rates allow rapid achievement and maintenance of plasma concentrations close to C_T. Simulations using known pharmacokinetic parameters can assist in the design of such infusion schemes.

DURATION OF EFFECT

Predicting the duration of effect of a drug after termination of an infusion is complex. It is commonly considered that the duration

of effect of a drug can be estimated from its terminal half-life, or that the duration of effect of different drugs can be compared by comparing their terminal half-lives. A drug with a short terminal half-life may be preferred when termination of effect shortly after discontinuing the drug is desirable. The use of half-lives to predict the time course of drug effect is problematic for several reasons (Shafer & Varvel, 1991):

1. The dose administered will affect the duration of effect independent of the terminal half-life. Only the half-lives of drugs administered at equipotent doses would be at all informative.

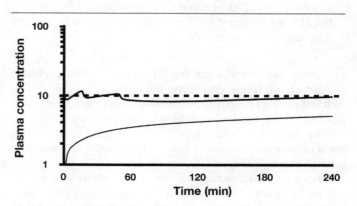

Figure 10.5. Changes in plasma drug concentration following administration of a loading dose followed by a "fast" constant rate infusion (CRI) for 15 minutes, then an "intermediate" CRI for 30 minutes and finally a "maintenance" CRI. Note that the concentrations are plotted on a logarithmic scale. The thin line shows the changes in plasma concentration during the administration of a CRI targeting 10 arbitrary units/L, calculated based on drug clearance. The dashed line shows C_T of 10 units/L.

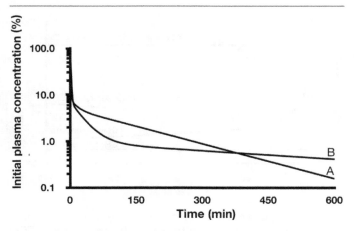

Figure 10.6. Changes in plasma concentration indexed to the initial concentration following a bolus of two drugs. Note that the concentrations are plotted on a logarithmic scale. The terminal half-lives of drugs A and B are 120 and 500 minutes, respectively.

2. If a CRI is used and discontinued before steady state is reached, the concentration reached will be difficult to predict (although less than C_T), and will differ among drugs. If a target-controlled infusion is used, the same principles apply, because even though the plasma concentration is known, the different compartments will contain different amounts of the drug depending on the duration of the infusion, which will influence the decrease in plasma concentration after the end of the infusion.

3. The effect may disappear at different fractions of the effective plasma concentration, depending on the drug, which complicates comparison. As an example, if the effect disappears when plasma concentration is 50% of the effective concentration for one drug but 25% for another drug, it will take one half-life for the first drug and two for the second.

In reality, duration of action depends on the interaction between volumes of distribution, clearances, and pharmacodynamic factors such as the ratio of effective concentration to concentration at which the effects disappear, hysteresis in the concentration – effect relationship, and so on. Therefore, predicting the time course of effect based on pharmacokinetics is more complicated than comparing terminal half-lives (Figure 10.6).

This figure illustrates that the relative concentration of drug B will be lower than that of drug A for more than 6 hours after bolus administration, despite the much shorter terminal half-life of drug A.

CONTEXT-SENSITIVE HALF-TIME

Using target-controlled infusion, it can be demonstrated that the duration of effect of a drug depends on the duration of infusion. This has led to the concept of "context-sensitive half-time," the

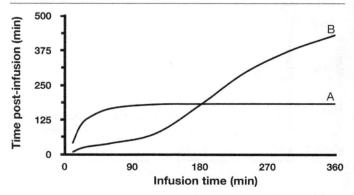

Figure 10.7. Time necessary to achieve a fixed decrease in plasma concentration (70% of the concentration at the time at which the infusion is stopped) as a function of the duration of infusion for two drugs.

context being the duration of the infusion (Hughes et al. 1992) (Figure 10.7).

This figure demonstrates that drug A has lower "context-sensitivity" than drug B. However, depending on the duration of infusion, drug B may produce faster recoveries: in this example, this would be the case for infusion times shorter than about 170 minutes.

If a CRI is used instead, the time needed to reach a given plasma concentration (e.g., concentration for the termination of the effect) before steady state is achieved will depend on the infusion time, because the plasma concentration at which the infusion is discontinued will depend on the infusion time (Figure 10.8).

This figure illustrates that if the effect disappears when plasma concentration is one arbitrary unit for both drugs, the effects of drug B would disappear faster than those of drug A when infusion time is 120 minutes despite the much shorter terminal half-life of drug A, but not if infusion time is 240 minutes.

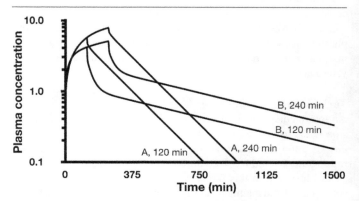

Figure 10.8. Changes in plasma concentration following a 120 and 240 minutes constant rate infusion targeting 10 arbitrary units/L for two drugs. Note that the concentrations are plotted on a logarithmic scale. The terminal half-lives of drugs A and B are 120 and 500 minutes, respectively.

SUMMARY

In conclusion, pharmacokinetics can be a useful tool for the design of intravenous infusions and the appropriate selection of drugs. However, it is important to remember that pharmacokinetic compartments do not necessarily correspond to physiological compartments, that predictions based on pharmacokinetic parameters can only be accurate if the model closely represents the drug disposition in the individual receiving the infusion, and that pharmacokinetics predict changes in plasma concentration, whereas the effect site for drugs used for analgesia is remote from the plasma. In veterinary medicine, the lack of models adequately describing drug disposition in a population and the common lack of knowledge of the drug concentration–effect relationship, limit the use of pharmacokinetics for designing intravenous infusion regimens.

REFERENCES

Gabrielsson, J. & Weiner, D. (2006). Pharmacokinetic concepts, in *Pharmacokinetic & Pharmacodynamic Data Analysis: Concepts and Applications*, 4th edn (eds J. Gabrielsson & D. Weiner), Swedish Pharmaceutical Press, Stockholm.

Hughes, M.A., Glass, P.S., & Jacobs, J.R. (1992). Context-sensitive half-time in multicompartment pharmacokinetic models for intravenous anesthetic drugs. *Anesthesiology*, 76(3), 334–341.

Shafer, S.L. & Schwinn, D.A. (2005). Basic principles of pharmacology related to anesthesia, in *Miller's Anesthesia*, 6th edn (ed. R.D. Miller), Elsevier Churchill Livingstone, Philadelphia.

Shafer, S.L. & Varvel, J.R. (1991). Pharmacokinetics, pharmacodynamics, and rational opioid selection. *Anesthesiology*, 74(1), 53–63.

Section 3
Nonpharmacological Pain Therapy

11
Canine Rehabilitation

Lowri Davies

The cornerstone of rehabilitation is the ability to simultaneously manage pain and restore function. A successful therapist will be an individual who is well-versed in acute and chronic pain management, has an understanding of the biomechanics of movement and how tissues respond to stress and strain patterns, is familiar with the principles of exercise physiology, and is able to apply these principles to the treatment of patients with neurological or musculoskeletal injuries.

A comprehensive approach requires a multidisciplinary team, as it is unlikely that one individual will possess all the skills required of a rehabilitation practitioner. Such a team may consist of a veterinary neurologist or orthopedic surgeon, a veterinarian skilled in rehabilitation, a certified physical therapist with further training in animal physical therapy, and appropriately trained technicians or assistants. Furthermore, a compliant owner and patient are fundamental to the success of the program.

The World Health Organization's (1992) definitions for impairment and disability are pertinent to veterinary patients. Impairment is defined as "Any loss or abnormality of psychological, physiological, or anatomic structure or function." Disability is defined as "Any restriction (resulting from impairment) of ability to perform an activity in the manner or within the range considered normal for the species." To restore function it is essential to understand the motor adaptations of the patient in response to pain. If altered function was merely a response to nociception then the administration of analgesics should resolve the problem. This is often not the case, however, and many aspects of motor adaptation persist despite resolution of pain (Hodges & Richardson, 1996).

This chapter outlines some of the adaptive changes in movement that arise as a consequence of pain and how these changes may provide treatment guidelines for the rehabilitation practitioner. It will consider clinical examination of the patient from a rehabilitation perspective and examine some of the most commonly used modalities in a rehabilitation program and how to develop a safe framework for their use. The reader is referred to texts on veterinary physical therapy for further information (McGowan et al., 2007).

UNDERSTANDING PAIN IN REHABILITATION PATIENTS

Musculoskeletal pain is a consequence of repetitive strain and overuse. These injuries include a variety of disorders that cause pain in bones, joints, muscle, or surrounding structures. Muscle pain may also be referred to other deep somatic and visceral structures.

The causes of musculoskeletal pain are not fully understood but likely involve inflammation, fibrosis, tissue degradation, and neurotransmitter and neurosensory disturbances, and may include central and peripheral hypersensitivity and impairment of descending inhibition of incoming nociceptive impulses (IASP, 2009).

Restoring or improving the neuromotor control of skeletal movement is fundamental for managing pain associated with the musculoskeletal system.

Why is Movement Different with Pain?
The fact that animals move differently when in pain cannot be disputed; however, the physiological basis for why this occurs is poorly understood. A recent theory (Hodges, 2011; Hodges & Tucker, 2011) (Figure 11.1) examines the concept that excitatory and inhibitory activity is redistributed in response to pain, and this modification of mechanical behavior is designed to protect tissues from injury. Hodges (2011) has concluded that muscle adaptation to pain involves redistribution of activity within and between muscles; modification of mechanical behavior, including decreased variability of movement and increased stiffness; and protection from further pain or injury through reduced voluntary activity, increased muscle splinting, and redistribution of load. These changes are mediated at multiple levels, centrally and peripherally, and while they provide short-term antinociception, they result in long-term negative consequences due to increased load, decreased movement, and decreased variability of movement.

Mounting evidence suggests that pain also affects postural function by altering balance (Mok et al., 2004) and causing changes in anticipatory and reactive postural mechanisms (MacDonald et al., 2009). Thus, the ability of the body to make subtle adjustments in posture and balance is hampered, and dynamic stability is lost (Hodges, 2011).

ASSESSMENT OF THE REHABILITATION PATIENT

Anamnesis
The reported history should identify the primary problem, for example, fracture, lameness, or poor performance. It should note

---

Pain Management in Veterinary Practice, First Edition. Edited by Christine M. Egger, Lydia Love and Tom Doherty.
© 2014 John Wiley & Sons, Inc. Published 2014 by John Wiley & Sons, Inc.

New theory for adaptation to pain

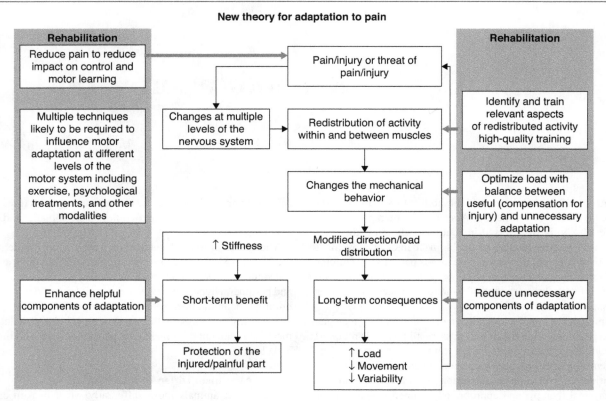

Figure 11.1. New theory of motor adaptation to pain and its implication for rehabilitation. The central column postulates that pain and injury or the potential threat of pain and injury lead to changes at multiple levels of the nervous system. The resultant changes lead to the redistribution of activity within and between muscle groups and altered mechanical behavior. Although an increase in stiffness can confer short-term benefit through the protection of the injured part, in the long term it leads to increased load on individual components of the musculoskeletal system, reduced movement, and loss of variability of movement. This model necessitates high quality rehabilitation through precise neuromotor training targeting multiple sites within the nervous system, e.g., cortical, spinal, and motor end plate. Reproduced with permission, Hodges, P.W. (2011) Pain and motor control: from the laboratory to rehabilitation. *Journal of electromyography and Kinesiology* 21, 220–228.

past surgical procedures, if any, and how satisfied the surgeon was with the result; that is, is the repair stable and have joint biomechanics been altered? Other factors to consider when evaluating a candidate for physical rehabilitation include the time post surgery or injury, tissues involved, duration of dysfunction, age, body condition, preinjury activity level of the patient, and desired outcome.

A detailed history should also include correct identification of the animal's degree of pain and disability. By identifying how the patient copes with the activities of daily living, a true picture of the animal's disability can be constructed. Information regarding the following should be gathered:

- Ability to ascend and descend stairs
- Ability to enter and exit vehicles
- Ability to cope with difficult surfaces such as wooden or tiled floors
- Ability to remain standing while eating
- Willingness to exercise and exercise tolerance
- Ability to remain squatting while defecating
- Ability to posture for urination
- Inappropriate elimination

- Willingness to play
- Change in demeanor
- Response to grooming
- Response or lack thereof to medication
- Effect of exercise on the lameness
- Effect of rest on the lameness
- Duration and intensity of the lameness
- Changes in sleep patterns

It is important to understand how pain developed in each patient and how the patient is coping. Some owners will report a gradual decline in their pet's mobility where the pet chooses to exercise less as pain progresses. Secondary issues, such as weight gain and mood changes, can develop. These patients often appear to have a depressed demeanor and are termed "passive" copers. "Active" copers are patients who bounce into the consulting room on three legs, dragging their owners behind them. These individuals are always keen to exercise, in spite of pain and lameness, and appear to be less susceptible to mood changes (Butler & Mosely, 2003). From a musculoskeletal perspective active copers can be challenging to treat as they often have weight shifting, compensatory movement, and novel neuromotor recruitment patterns that are well established in order to facilitate exercise. In contrast, chronic musculoskeletal and nervous system changes may not have occurred in passive copers, but they may have more immune and endocrine system dysfunction. They benefit from stress reduction, may require more coaxing through the therapeutic exercise regimen, and take longer to respond to treatment than would be expected in view of the degree of dysfunction observed. This is referred to as a disability-dysfunction mismatch (Butler & Mosely, 2003).

Questionnaires, such as the acute pain questionnaire (Thomas et al., 1996) or the Helsinki Chronic Pain Index (Eskelinen et al., 2012) (Chapter 22), can be given to owners to complete during anamnesis and at various points during treatment to help evaluate the patient's progress. Good communication will improve outcome, and recent studies have shown that the relationship between the clinician and the patient and owner is of primary importance in successful management of chronic pain (Jamison, 2011).

Assessment of the Patient for Pain

Diagnosis of altered pain states in animals can prove extremely challenging. Relying on lameness alone is inadequate, particularly after the acute period has passed, and signs may include tenderness, weakness, limited motion, and stiffness (IASP, 2009).

Identifying Movement Adaptations to Pain

Once discomfort has been identified, the next challenge in the design of a rehabilitation plan is to detect the movement adaptations that led to the changes in gait pattern and altered biomechanics of limb and trunk movement.

Much of conventional veterinary medicine emphasizes a reductionist approach, but a systems-based approach is required. The systems-based approach considers the joint to be an organ system in which all tissues comprising the joint work together, biomechanically and biologically, to maintain joint health and allow full, pain-free function. Thus, successful treatment should consider, for example, not only the cranial cruciate ligament but also the synovium, joint capsule, articular cartilage, menisci, and subchondral bone (Cook, 2010). Consideration should also be given to the neuromuscular consequences of injury, such as alterations in somatosensory and proprioceptive function (Ingersoll et al., 2008). Any rehabilitation program should consider how changes within the affected joint influence the system as a whole, including the back, trunk, and other limbs. For example, if the diagnosis is simply "torn cruciate ligament" and the treatment is simply "surgical correction of instability", it will be difficult to develop a safe and effective rehabilitation protocol. Instead, the diagnosis should be lameness, pain, and dysfunction due to inflammation, changes within the passive stabilizers of the joint, changes within the dynamic stabilizers of the joint, and altered neuromotor, somatosensory, and proprioceptive function. This provides a better understanding of the patient's impairment and dysfunction as well as the underlying causes, and can inform an effective rehabilitation plan (Panjabi, 1992).

Clinical Examination

STATIC ASSESSMENT

Static assessment includes assessment of muscle hypertrophy or atrophy, head and tail position, abdominal muscle tone, scarring or swelling, symmetry of the axial and appendicular skeleton, deviation in the sagittal plane of the thoracic and lumbar spine or lordosis or kyphosis, distribution of body weight among all four limbs, and any adduction or abduction of the limbs in the animal at rest. Note the limb alignment (including joint angles or goniometry), angular deformities (valgus and varus), and internal and external rotation of limbs. Determine if the deformity is bony in nature and thus, not correctable by rehabilitation alone, or whether it is functional in nature. If the deformity is functional, a neutral alignment is restored when the limb is elevated; thus, therapy is directed at maintaining this alignment during weight bearing.

DYNAMIC ASSESSMENT

Dynamic assessment involves moving the limbs and noting reactions and resistance in the muscles as joints are flexed and extended or limbs are advanced and retracted, observing the patient as it moves from standing to sitting and vice versa, and assessing quality and control of movement. Symmetry of the animal when sitting, and any tendency to lean or to brace with the forelimbs, is assessed. Observation should be made of the spinal column and of the interaction between the neck and back during flexion and extension.

GAIT ASSESSMENT

This portion of the assessment allows grading of the severity of the lameness, localization of the lameness, and description of the gait in terms of cranial and caudal phases, arc of flight, and linearity of the movement. Assess gait at the walk and trot, in a straight line and in a circle, on a flat, nonslippery surface, and then on a variety of surfaces. Observe the movement of the pelvis, lumbar, thoracic, and cervical spine, observing for bilateral symmetry. Observe how the patient positions the limbs and curves the trunk when walked or trotted in a right and left circle. Observe the animal on the left and right sides of body and note any differences. Observe the animal as it walks over low poles or up and down stairs.

NEUROLOGICAL EXAMINATION

A neurological examination should be part of the assessment to help differentiate poor balance due to stiffness and pain from ataxia due to a neurological lesion, as each has different rehabilitation requirements and prognosis.

PALPATION AND RANGE OF MOTION

Palpation and manipulation should occur with the patient during standing and in lateral recumbency. It is best to develop a systematic approach: palpate muscles for their overall symmetry, texture, and tone, presence of edema, trigger point formation, and the presence of lactic acid, which confers a feeling of crackling tissue paper within the muscle.

During palpation of joints, subtle effusion and temperature changes should be identified. Any remodeling in response to stress, for example, the formation of a medial stifle buttress in response to instability, should be noted. The stability of a joint should be determined through its full range of motion (ROM) while remembering that associated changes, such as muscle atrophy, may increase joint laxity without direct involvement of the joint. The quality of movement should be established as well as the total and pain-free ROM and the nature of the end stop (see below). Note pain on extension and flexion and internal and external rotation and assess medial and lateral instability of each joint.

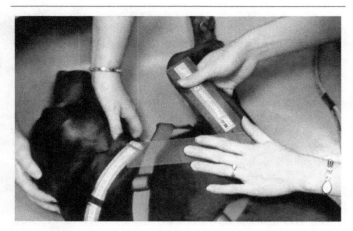

Figure 11.2. Using a hand-held goniometer to measure range of motion in the elbow joint.

The axial skeleton should be examined as a system and on an individual vertebral basis. Ventrodorsal and lateral motion should be evaluated and any restriction noted. Active and passive ROM should be established.

Range of Motion and End Stop Assessment of Joints
Range of motion within a joint is the degree of motion that joint is capable of undergoing from full flexion to full extension in the sagittal plane. It can also be used to describe the degree of abduction and adduction afforded to an individual joint.

A more useful measure to assess joint function may be the functional ROM. This is the degree of motion required within a joint to allow for normal motion to take place, that is, for an individual to move normally and comfortably. For many individuals, pain within the extreme ROM is not limiting to function; however, for the canine athlete, pain within the outer ranges of motion will become limiting to performance.

Range of motion is measured with a manual or laser goniometer (Figure 11.2). Studies with a group of Labrador Retrievers have demonstrated repeatable measures for the joints of the distal limbs (Jaegger et al., 2002). To increase accuracy, a mean of three measurements should be taken with the dog placed in lateral recumbency. The joint should be measured in both limbs, and it is often easier to start with the "normal" joint. Interbreed variation occurs and factors such as emaciation, obesity, and muscle atrophy may also affect values.

End stop, or feel, is a term used to describe the normal end point of motion within a joint, and each joint has a typical end stop. For example, the elbow joint will exhibit a soft end stop when flexed, as the biceps brachii limits further flexion. This type of end stop feels very different from the capsular or firm end stop felt in elbow extension. This stop has a firm feel but with a slight give to the end point, and it is abnormal if it occurs too early in the motion, as may occur in an osteoarthritic stifle joint. In a bony end stop, the stopping motion is abrupt and hard, and this may be observed in a joint affected by severe bony remodeling. A springy end stop is felt when the joint rebounds from the limit of motion, and it indicates the presence of a loose fragment within the joint. An empty end stop is one where no end point is reached, for example, with a fracture.

A painful end stop is one whereby the end point is never reached, as pain becomes a limiting factor to movement early on in flexion or extension.

Goniometry and measurement of a joint's ROM can be useful outcome measures when assessing the rehabilitation patient. Even small increases in joint motion, particularly within the functional range, can significantly improve mobility. End stop evaluation is important when assessing how much improvement in joint ROM is possible. A bony end stop is unlikely to change, and may contribute to a mechanical lameness that will be refractory to any rehabilitation technique. Such a gait may not necessarily be painful, provided the compensatory pattern adopted during motion is not too severe. On the other hand, an abnormal capsular, soft, or painful end stop to a joint's motion may well benefit significantly from rehabilitation.

For further information on detailed examination of the canine the reader is referred to McGowan et al., (2005).

TREATMENT OF MUSCULOSKELETAL PAIN

Many of the modalities used in rehabilitation medicine are appropriate for treating musculoskeletal pain (Table 11.1). The act of standing can be considered an exercise, and even 1 minute of standing in the correct position can be difficult for a dog that has been lying down for most of the day over a period of several months. The degree of pain and level of dysfunction are not necessarily linearly related, and an animal showing the greatest dysfunction is not necessarily in the most pain. Progression is essential and, once a baseline therapeutic exercise regimen is established, the aim should be to gradually increase the complexity and duration of the regimen over the subsequent weeks. This will vary from patient to patient, so each animal should be carefully assessed throughout therapy. A helpful strategy is to ask the owner to keep a diary of the pet's progress, and to repeat the pain questionnaire at regular intervals.

Movement and Exercise
Continued movement is beneficial as it improves joint nutrition and soft tissue function and facilitates fine motor control (Bennel et al., 2009). A challenge in treatment is establishing an appropriate level of exercise that does not further damage tissues. "No pain, no gain" is not a viable management strategy for the rehabilitation patient.

Table 11.1. Treatment options for musculoskeletal pain

Anti-inflammatory and centrally acting analgesics
Acupuncture
Transcutaneous electrical nerve stimulation
Improve biomechanics of movement and redistribute load
Therapeutic exercises
Massage
Hot and cold therapy
Therapeutic modalities—ultrasound, cold laser, neuromuscular
    electrostimulation
Osteopathy
Chiropractic
Environmental enrichment and play
Weight loss/dietary modification
Nutraceuticals/supplements

The aim should always be to reduce pain, although some discomfort may be required for the rehabilitation program to progress, particularly with therapeutic exercise. Pain management techniques, such as acupuncture and ice therapy and the judicious use of analgesics, may be required, especially early in the course of treatment.

Stress Distribution within the Joint
The load across a joint is not simply a reflection of the patient's body weight. Rather, it is a vector summation of body weight, the forces of acceleration and deceleration of the segment or moving part, and the muscular forces required to stabilize the joint and move the limb (Radin et al., 1979). Joints are configured to maximize the surface area for load distribution and, as the joint is loaded, cartilage and cancellous bone deform to further increase the surface area. Cartilage deforms under stress through the outflow of water and small solutes. Under a constant load this outflow occurs rapidly in the early stages, but as the material compresses it becomes more difficult for particles to escape; thus deformation is nonlinear. Another unique behavior of cartilage is that deformation is closely related to the rate at which external force is applied. The faster it is squeezed the harder it is for the particles to exit, and the harder it is for the cartilage to deform. This type of nonlinear deformation is termed viscoelastic, and has implications for the rehabilitation practitioner. By slowing or controlling joint motion there is both increased compliance of the cartilage, and reduced load across the joint. Exercises to improve neuromotor control of joint motion and enhance each joint's postural support will serve to reduce the load acting on a joint.

Mechanical Factors and Erosion of Articular Cartilage
Although the yield strength of articular cartilage is reduced by chemical, enzymatic, and metabolic factors, the actual wearing away of cartilage from weight-bearing surfaces requires mechanical forces. Cracks and tears beginning in the superficial tangential fiber layer are initiated by tensile stress—that is, the cartilage is pulled apart. If articular cartilage were compressed evenly across its entire surface, no tensile stresses would exist. In whole joints this is probably never the case, and only part of the joint is bearing the load at any given time. If one part of the cartilage surface is compressed and another is not, tensile stresses are created at the margins of loaded areas. Repetitive loading results in crack formation (Radin et al., 1979). Cartilage "wear" occurs when its ultimate tensile strength is exceeded. Failure to heal may be due to persistent high levels of stress in the joint. If these stresses can be decreased, a degree of functional healing of both bone and load-bearing surfaces can take place.

Stresses within a joint are reduced by increasing the surface area over which the load is distributed and reducing the overall load. By taking a broad view of the patient, it should be possible to determine what, if any, global changes in trunk and limb positioning have occurred to result in increased loading of an individual limb. Furthermore, load distribution within the limb should also be considered; that is, how the limb is positioned under the body will determine whether more weight is sent through the cranial or caudal, lateral or medial aspect of the joint, which again will lead to stress concentrations within the joint, and cause further remodeling in the diaphysis and associated connective tissue along the lines of stress. Thus, prior to carrying out even the simplest of weight-shifting exercises, the clinician must assess limb positioning and how this affects the distribution of load through its constituent parts. Repeating an exercise on a poorly positioned limb will only serve to accentuate the pain and dysfunction and serve no therapeutic purpose. In contrast, positioning the limb correctly and subsequently loading it should serve to stress the tissues in a functional manner and promote appropriate neuromotor adaptations.

Dynamic Stability
During rehabilitation, exercise regimens are often used to target specific areas of the body. In the face of a nociceptive stimulus the initial response is to attempt to reduce motion in the painful area through increased muscle activation and localized splinting and stiffening (Hodges, 2010). While decreasing localized motion is an effective short-term strategy, it becomes self-defeating in the long term and often results in a loss of dynamic stability, increasing movement on a global scale. Dynamic stability represents the ability to continue moving in the desired trajectory in the face of external forces, as it allows the patient to absorb these forces, remain stable, and not be thrown off course. However, as tissues stiffen, stability is reduced and the animal becomes incapable of absorbing external forces and, consequently, stumbles or alters the course of movement.

The concept of increasing muscle mass without any thought to how that muscle actually functions is not the aim of rehabilitation. Excessive muscle mass will increase static stability but impede performance through increasing stiffness, restricted ROM, and reduced dynamic stability, resulting in little predictability of movement. In contrast, a training regimen that develops strength without stiffness will achieve a high error tolerance and predictability during movement. The ultimate goal for any rehabilitation therapist should be to develop dynamic stability through improving muscle function and creating sufficient muscle mass to support the athletic requirements of that individual. Only in this way can controlled movement patterns that minimize the load placed on the musculoskeletal system during movement be generated.

Formulating a Treatment Plan and Ongoing Assessment
Treatment goals include correction of posture, movement, and muscle activation. When correcting posture, every attempt must be made to avoid reinforcing the maladaptive posture. Thus, when carrying out weight-shifting exercises not only must the limb be aligned squarely but also the whole body must be aligned squarely and maintained in such a position during the exercise. When correcting for movement, ensure that poor gait patterns are not reinforced. For example, during rehabilitation of the spinal patient a treadmill can be used to develop a functional neuromotor recruitment pattern by actively moving the patient's limbs (Figure 11.3). The animal should not be allowed to move freely at other times if this uncontrolled movement re-enforces poor or nonfunctional neuromotor recruitment patterns.

A rehabilitation program should aim to restore the injured tissue to preinjury levels of activity by promoting healing of the injured tissue and minimizing further tissue damage. As a result of the injury systemic changes in cardiovascular and neuromotor function will have occurred and the rehabilitation program must take this into account. The rehabilitation plan should also feature techniques to improve core stability, proprioception, muscle strength, muscle endurance, and cardiovascular function.

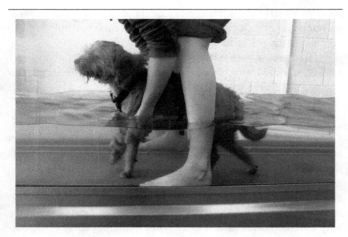

Figure 11.3. Gait training of a quadriplegic patient in the underwater treadmill.

Ongoing clinical reasoning allows the practitioner to evaluate the effect of each treatment, and determine whether the patient is improving or deteriorating. The animal cannot verbalize if it feels better, if the treatment was beneficial, or if it was very painful. The clinician has to rely on clinical reasoning to accurately read the patient's response. Detailed questioning of the owner on the patient's behalf can also assist with this process.

Muscle pain during and after exercise is common. During rehabilitation, it is essential to not only avoid potentiating inflammation at the site of injury but also to minimize muscle pain generated as a result of exercise. When assessing the patient it is also essential to differentiate between the two, so as to prevent over- or undertraining. Possible causes of muscle pain include ischemic muscle pain, pain caused by local areas of muscle contraction, muscle stiffness possibly as a result of muscle edema, and inflammation.

PRINCIPLES OF PROTOCOL DESIGN

Protocol design should take into account the unique solutions adopted by individual patients to manage their pain and disability. In general, rehabilitation patients may have reduced muscle function and strength, altered proprioception, muscle shortening and stiffness, joint effusion, scar tissue and adhesion formation, reduced range of motion, and pain inhibition of movement. By factoring in the nature of the injury and repair, the patient's age and body condition, and the preinjury level of activity, the practitioner can fine-tune the program. While therapies such as thermal modalities, therapeutic exercises, or hydrotherapy are likely to be used repeatedly, the frequency and intensity of application will vary from patient to patient. Each individual will vary in his or her need for pain relief and in response to treatment. It is this response, rather than a specific time frame, that will determine whether a regimen can be intensified.

It is outside the scope of this chapter to review protocol design for every common neurological and orthopedic condition; however, many common principles apply. The basic aim in each case is to promote healing and restore function without creating further tissue damage. Each protocol must address the neuromotor control of motion and the active (ligaments, tendons, muscles) and passive

(bony skeleton, joints, pelvis, spine) components of movement. The relative importance each component assumes will vary among individuals and also within an individual during the course of the rehabilitation program. Once a program has begun, the patient must be reevaluated at each visit to assess the benefits, if any, of therapy and the protocol should be adjusted accordingly.

It is also essential that the client's expectations be considered. For example, client expectation for treatment of a cranial cruciate injury in a 4-year-old working sheepdog competing in agility will be different from client expectations for treatment of a cruciate ligament rupture in an 8-year-old, overweight Labrador belonging to an elderly person who exercises the dog for 20 minutes twice daily. Though each case is equally challenging, a different management strategy will be required to achieve success. A plan that focuses clearly on each patient's needs and establishes short- and long-term goals should be drawn up for each patient.

Rehabilitation of the Orthopedic Patient
with Musculoskeletal Pain

Rehabilitation programs for orthopedic conditions have traditionally focused on restoration of muscle strength. However, dynamic stability depends upon the interaction of many passive soft tissues and active muscle forces, and is not dependent on muscle strength alone (Schipplein & Andriacchi, 1991). Equally, loss of muscle strength cannot be wholly attributable to a reduction in muscle cross-sectional area. Rather, recent studies have demonstrated poor or no correlation between cross-sectional area and quadriceps strength in human anterior cruciate ligament injury (Lysholm et al., 1998; Roberts et al., 1999; Herzog & Longino, 2007). Loss of strength is largely attributed to altered afferent feedback from mechanoreceptors in the torn ligament resulting in reduced activation of normal muscle fibers. Pain, effusion, anxiety, and aberrant joint mechanics will also contribute to loss of muscle strength. It is likely that much of what was traditionally thought to be due to loss of strength is in fact due to loss of function. Similarly, even though many therapeutic exercise regimens are nominally designed to improve muscle strength, it is likely that they also improve muscle function.

Choosing an exercise regimen that focuses primarily on stressing the muscle to facilitate strengthening in the early stages of recovery will drastically increase the load placed on joint surfaces, ligaments, tendons, and muscles, and can serve to potentiate pain, inflammation, and injury. Furthermore, without first correcting global posture and movement, it is likely that the forces of movement will not be transferred uniformly through a limb. This, in turn, leads to uneven load bearing at the joint surface, potentiating articular wear and tear.

Correction of posture and movement can only be achieved through the adoption of exercise regimens that promote correct muscle function and recruitment patterns. In conjunction with this, gait re-education or training may also be required. Exercises that facilitate neuromotor training are high in skill but low in strength requirements, and are generally safe to use. They require intense concentration on the animal's part, and if carried out correctly in the early stages, will lead to rapid fatigue. Once adequate motor control of movement has been achieved and a functional gait pattern developed, it is relatively easy to move on to improving muscle and cardiovascular endurance. Finally, during the last phase of rehabilitation exercises targeting muscle strengthening and discipline-specific exercises can be employed.

PHASES OF REHABILITATION FOR MUSCULOSKELETAL INJURY

For musculoskeletal cases the rehabilitation program can broadly be divided into four phases. Phase 1 is the immediate postinjury and acute inflammatory period. In phase 1, the primary focus is control of pain and minimization of inflammation. The focus of treatment and treatment options for phase 1 are listed in Table 11.2. Rapid application of these techniques within the first few hours of injury can help reduce recovery time. Although anecdotal evidence supports the use of techniques such as acupuncture, therapeutic ultrasound, and low-intensity laser, clinical evidence to support their efficacy is scant.

In most individuals, there is a shift toward tissue repair (Phase 2; subacute phase) after a few days. This transition is dependent on individual variation and on the degree of trauma. During phase 2 (Table 11.3), the focus changes to maintaining ROM with active ROM exercises and improving muscle function. It remains essential to control inflammation and minimize swelling. As a functional pattern of movement develops and the patient becomes more willing

Table 11.2. Focus and treatment options for musculoskeletal injury in phase 1 of the rehabilitation program

Focus	Treatment options
Pain control	Anti-inflammatory therapy
	Centrally acting analgesics
	Cryotherapy
	Immobilization-splinting, bandaging, cage rest
	Modification of environment
	Massage
	Acupuncture
Reduce inflammatory mediators	Cryotherapy
	Anti-inflammatory drugs
	Omega-3 fatty acid supplementation
Reduce tissue metabolic requirements and minimize cell death	Cryotherapy
Improve cell perfusion and minimize edema	Cryotherapy
	Massage
	Acupuncture
Promote functional neuromotor recruitment—prevent loss of muscle function and strength	Supported standing, gentle weight shifting exercises, neuromuscular stimulation when reflex arc is lost (i.e., lower motor neuron injury)
Maintain joint range of motion (ROM) (Figure 11.4)	Passive and active ROM exercises

Table 11.3. Focus and treatment options for musculoskeletal injury in phase 2 of the rehabilitation program

Focus	Treatment options
Ongoing management of pain and inflammation	As outlined in Table 11.2
Correct orientation of collagen fibers within healing tissue	Gentle loading normal weight distribution
Maintain ROM (Figure 11.4)	Regular passive and active ROM exercises
Maintain postural muscle function	Supported standing
Promote functional neuromotor recruitment	Gentle weight shifting with correct limb and trunk positioning
Proprioceptive enhancement	Weight shifting on different surfaces
	Proprioceptive road walking
Develop/maintain flexibility and work on core strength	Head turns with or without support
Gait training (Figure 11.3)	Aquatic treadmill
	Controlled lead walking

to load the injured limb, the duration of lead walks and aquatic treadmill work can be increased, provided pain and inflammation are not increased.

Phase 3 (Table 11.4) typically starts approximately 4–6 weeks postsurgery or injury. Tissue healing should now be well advanced, and the focus is on more complex neuromotor recruitment patterns and improving muscle endurance. Functional exercises targeting specific muscles and exercises to improve cardiovascular function can be added to the regimen at this time. During phase 4 of healing-specific exercises to match individual requirements should be introduced (Table 11.5).

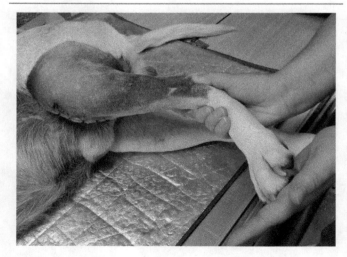

Figure 11.4. Using passive range of motion to assist with pain management in a postsurgical patient.

Table 11.4. Focus and treatment options for musculoskeletal injury in phase 3 of the rehabilitation program

Focus	Treatment option
Neuromotor training	Walking on challenging surfaces; e.g., gentle undulations, small steps, pebbles
	Figure of eight work
	Balancing on three or two legs
Advanced proprioceptive training (Figure 11.5)	Balance cushion or boards
	Blindfold work
Endurance training	Reduce frequency and increase length of walks as appropriate
	Increase duration of aquatic treadmill work
Cardiovascular training	Jogging on the lead
	Off-lead work
Maintain/improve joint ROM	Walking over poles (Figure 11.6)
	Stair climbing
	Sit to stand exercises
	Theraball work

Table 11.5. Focus and treatment options in phase 4

Focus	Treatment option
Muscle strengthening	Running, jumping, work on soft sand, high-resistance aquatic treadmill work, Therabands
Discipline-specific training	Focus on task specific work—agility, obedience, gun dogs, working sheepdogs, physical assistance, and rescue dogs

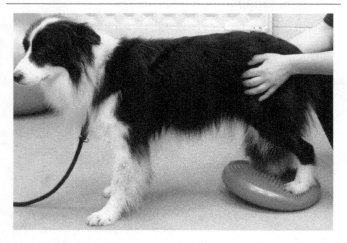

Figure 11.5. Improving core stability through exercising on the balance cushion.

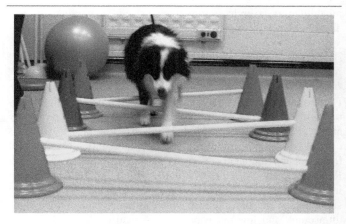

Figure 11.6. Walking over poles can improve joint range of motion.

COMMON PHYSICAL THERAPY MODALITIES

Aquatic Treadmill Therapy

It is necessary to understand the basic principles and properties of water including relative density, buoyancy, viscosity, resistance, hydrostatic pressure, and surface tension to appreciate the benefits of aquatic therapy. These are important components when planning an aquatic rehabilitation program. The higher the water level, the greater the buoyancy and the less a joint is compressed during movement. However, the higher the water level, the greater the resistance to movement and the more anaerobic the nature of the exercise. This will promote rapid fatigue and increase pain post exercise. Turbulent movement, such as occurs when motor control of movement is poor, also increases the demands of the exercise.

In order for aquatic treadmill therapy to assist with functional rehabilitation, it must promote functional neuromotor recruitment, enhance dynamic stability, and avoid overdevelopment of inappropriate musculature that only serves to stiffen the animal. The aim is always to enhance the patient's ability to walk on land. In the author's experience, this can only be achieved through the use of as low a water level as possible (Figure 11.7), provided the animal is ambulatory. High water levels (Figure 11.8), while reducing the load on the joint, reduce the need for the animal to control its own movement to any significant degree, and do not assist with developing functional stability. In nonambulatory cases, maximum buoyancy is initially desirable. As soon as the patient can move independently, however, an attempt should be made to reduce the water level, with extra support being provided by the therapist, with the lightest possible touch.

The demands of aquatic therapy should never be underestimated, and it has greater potential than any other exercise for increasing pain and contributing to tissue injury. For the purpose of rehabilitation and utilization of the plastic nature of the neuromotor system, all learning should be functional and precise aquatic treadmill therapy is the only appropriate form of hydrotherapy.

Superficial Thermal Modalities

Superficial heat and cold have been used for centuries to manage soft tissue and joint injuries. The aims of such treatment are to

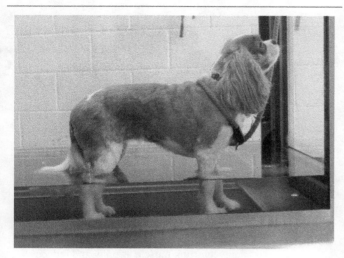

Figure 11.7. The aim of the aquatic treadmill exercise is to enhance the patient's ability to walk on land. This is best achieved through the use of as low a water level as possible, provided the animal is ambulatory.

reduce pain and inflammation, increase tissue plasticity, and facilitate healing and a return to function. Thermotherapy applications fall within the infrared portion of the electromagnetic spectrum just beyond the wavelength and frequency ranges for visible light, and the shorter the wavelength, the greater the frequency and depth of penetration. The estimated depth of penetration for most infrared thermal modalities (hot, cold, luminous infrared) is 1 cm. Cold will penetrate more deeply than superficial heating agents.

CRYOTHERAPY

Cryotherapy is applicable during the acute stage of tissue inflammation to assist with reducing the intensity of the inflammatory process (Heinrichs, 2004). It may also be used post exercise to control the secondary inflammatory effect of remobilization of tissues. Cryotherapy results in vasoconstriction and reduces tissue metabolism, oxygen requirements, sensory and motor nerve

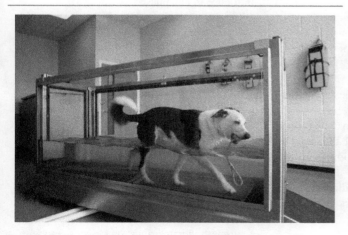

Figure 11.8. Increase resistance to movement by raising the water level of the aquatic treadmill.

conduction velocity, edema, and muscle spasm (possibly due to a change in the activity of the muscle spindle and the Golgi tendon organ).

Cold is most often applied with ice packs due to ease of application and cost. Ice packs should never be placed directly on the skin, and application at any one time should not exceed 10 minutes. Treatment should be repeated several times a day and continued throughout the acute stage of tissue inflammation. Certain precautions apply in the application of cold. Care should be taken to avoid frostbite through overvigorous application, and when placing the ice packs in the region of a peripheral nerve, as there have been reports of peripheral nerve palsy in humans (Knight, 1995).

HEAT

Heat treatment should be avoided in the acute stage of tissue injury, as it may exacerbate pain and swelling. The application of heat will result in local vasodilation due to histamine and bradykinin release in response to increased skin temperature. A reduction in local sympathetic activity, via the spinal dorsal root ganglia, reduces smooth muscle contraction and facilitates vasodilation. Heat will increase nerve conduction velocity (2 m/s for every 1°C rise). Muscle relaxation occurs as a result of reduced firing rate of the type II muscle spindle afferents and gamma efferents, increased firing rate of the type II fibers of the Golgi tendon organ, and decreased firing of the α motor neuron innervating extrafusal fibers (Ratanunga, 1981).

As with cold therapy, the pain threshold may be increased with local heat application. Stimulation of cutaneous thermal receptors has been postulated as a mechanism for inhibition of pain transmission at the level of the dorsal horn. Increased perfusion, with the subsequent resolution of local ischemia, and switching off of local pain receptors may also play a role in pain inhibition. Reduced muscle spasm also facilitates local perfusion. As heat increases, the rate of biochemical reactions will increase the rate of oxygen uptake and facilitate tissue healing; however, it may increase tissue catabolism through increased production of destructive enzymes such as collagenases.

Superficial heat application will only work to a depth of 1 cm. Deeper damage requires treatment from a modality with greater powers of penetration, such as ultrasound or laser. Heat will increase connective tissue extensibility, but only in the most superficial tissues. Heat may be applied through hot packs or warm baths. Treatment should last for 15–20 minutes, and be repeated as frequently as possible.

Stretching and Massage

Stretching is often best performed after warming. It can assist with increasing connective tissue extensibility and enhance joint ROM. Massage reduces muscle spasm and increases local blood flow. It can also promote vascular and lymphatic drainage. Techniques to release fascial planes can significantly enhance limb mobility and assist with pain management and restoration of motor function (Garfin et al., 1981).

Range of Motion Exercises

Range of motion exercises are important for maintaining or improving motion after injury or surgery, thereby reducing pain (Figure 11.4) (Salter et al., 1984). They also assist with recovery from neural injuries and promote motor learning (Udina et al., 2011). Passive ROM describes movement performed without active muscle

Table 11.6. Therapeutic exercises

Exercise	Target	Difficulty Level
Assisted standing Figure 11.9	Aid proprioception Improve circulation Neuromuscular re-education Muscle strength and endurance	Suitable for all nonambulatory patients
Standing weight shifting Figure 11.10	Enhance proprioception Enhance coordination Enhance muscle strength and endurance Improve joint nutrition	Safe exercise for early orthopedic rehabilitation and for neurological patients once they can stand unassisted Can be extremely difficult to carry out in a functional manner
Head turns	Enhance proprioception Enhance coordination Develop core muscles Improve flexibility	Safe exercise for early orthopedic rehabilitation Can also perform in the recumbent animal to prevent trunk muscle atrophy and reduce stiffness
Controlled lead walking	Enhance proprioception Gait training Improve muscle function and endurance Strengthen muscle	Safe exercise for early orthopedic rehabilitation Essential that the dog does not pull on the lead and that a non-functional gait pattern is not enhanced
Proprioceptive road walking Figure 11.11	Enhance proprioception Improve balance and coordination	Safe exercise for early orthopedic rehabilitation Must be done slowly and without pulling
Balance cushion work Figure 11.5	Enhance proprioception Enhance coordination and balance Develop core muscle function	More demanding exercise, likely to be suitable for Phase 2 onward Can be used under one or both fore or hind limbs
Figure of 8/weaves Figure 11.12	Promote side bending Enhance proprioception Strengthen limb adductors and abductors Introduce nonlinear motion and increase the load on individual joints	More demanding exercise, likely to be suitable for Phase 2 onward
Gradient walking	Walking up hill promotes loading of hind limbs, promotes knee and hip extension, improves ROM Walking down an incline increases difficulty level and promotes hock, stifle, and hip flexion	Introduce in late phase 2 or in phase 3 Difficulty can be varied by altering incline level
Pole or Cavaletti work Figure 11.6	Increase ROM Promote abdominal muscle recruitment Improve balance and coordination Improve proprioception and motor control	Introduce in late phase 2 or phase 3 Difficulty can be varied by altering pole height
Forelimb Lift Figure 11.13	Increase load on hind limbs Improve balance and coordination Improve back and abdominal muscle function	Introduce in late phase 2 or phase 3 Difficulty can be varied by lifting diagonal fore and hind limb pairs
Theraball work Figure 11.14	Develop core stability, increase load on fore or hind limbs depending on how ball is used Develop balance and proprioception	Introduce in phase 3
Stair climbing	Strengthen hind limbs Increase ROM and improve coordination	Introduce in phase 3
Sit to stand	Strengthen hip and stifle extensors Improve active ROM	Introduce in phase 3 Perform cautiously, as this requires reasonable strength in hamstrings, quadriceps, and gastrocnemius A "square" sit is essential

(continued)

Table 11.6. (*Continued*)

Exercise	Target	Difficulty Level
Balance board Figure 11.15	Enhance proprioception Enhance balance and coordination	Phase 3—increased level of challenge from balance cushion alone
Jogging	Improve muscle strength and endurance Improve cardiovascular fitness	Phase 3—Increase duration and frequency as program progresses
Dancing	Increase load on hind and fore limbs	Phase 3 and 4
Wheel-barrowing	Improve balance and coordination Improve proprioception	
Walking over difficult terrain—soft sand, pebbles, uneven ground	Improve muscle strength and endurance Improve cardiovascular fitness Improve coordination	Phase 3 and 4
Advanced Theraball work Figure 11.16	Enhance balance and coordination Increase core stability Advanced neuromotor skill training	Phase 4
Running	Increase muscle strength and endurance and Cardiovascular fitness	Phase 4
Blindfold work	Motor learning—enhance somatosensory feedback	Phase 4

contraction, whereas in active ROM a degree of active muscle contraction occurs as the therapist moves the limb or joint. Apart from patients with severe deficiencies, most movement is accompanied by a degree of muscle contraction. Passive ROM exercises are used to enhance pain management in inflamed joints, enhance neuromotor signaling, and to assist with tissue stretching in the subacute and chronic state where full range of motion has not been restored. Active range of motion exercises are required to prevent muscle atrophy, increase strength and endurance, and enhance circulation.

Therapeutic Exercises
Therapeutic exercises (Table 11.6), by their ability to influence motor plasticity and learning, are often the single most important component of any rehabilitation program. They include exercises to develop correct gait patterns, enhance proprioceptive function, improve coordination and balance, and increase pain-free joint ROM. They also function to improve muscle and cardiovascular endurance and increase muscle strength. Therapeutic exercises are fundamental to any rehabilitation program, but can also be integrated into all stages of life and activity from puppy growth and development to injury prevention in the sporting dog. They have the benefit of being relatively inexpensive, and allow the owner to be actively engaged in the pet's recovery.

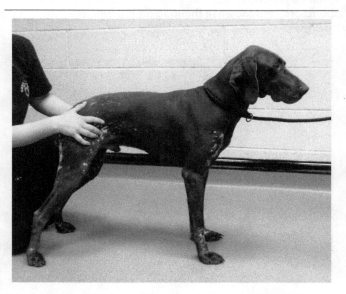

Figure 11.9. Supported standing on a peanut ball in a quadriplegic patient.

Figure 11.10. Gentle standing weight shifts used to enhance proprioception and prevent postural muscle atrophy.

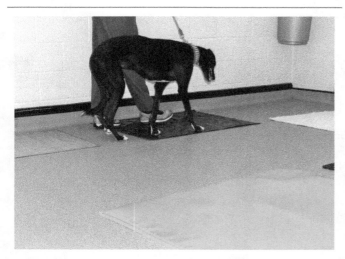

Figure 11.11. Walking along a proprioceptive road to enhance proprioception and promote neuromotor control.

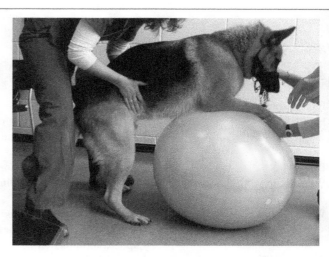

Figure 11.14. Working with a Theraball to increase the load on the hind limbs.

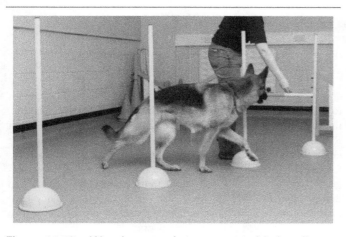

Figure 11.12. Weaving exercises promote side bending, enhance proprioception, strengthen limb adductors and abductors, and increase the load on individual joints.

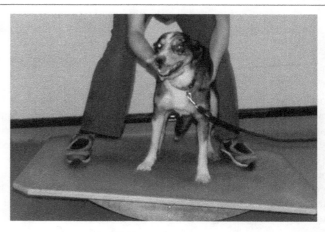

Figure 11.15. Balance board work enhances balance, coordination, and proprioception.

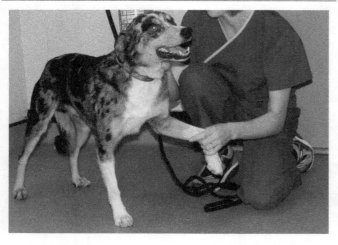

Figure 11.13. The forelimb lift will increase the load on the hind limbs, improve balance and coordination, and improve back and abdominal muscle function.

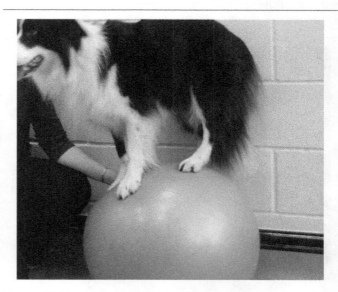

Figure 11.16. Advanced Theraball work to further enhance core stability.

Therapeutic exercises can be as simple as controlled lead walking for 1–2 minutes or as complex as balance and core recruitment exercises on a gym ball. Whatever the exercise, it is essential that it be carried out in a correct and functional manner, as training an inappropriate response is deleterious. Numerous studies highlight the fact that the ability of any intervention to change motor function depends on the quality of training; higher-quality training induces larger changes in temporal aspects of muscle activation (Tsao & Hodges, 2007).

The choice of exercises should meet the particular disabilities and requirements of the individual and, as with any exercise regimen, should be progressive in nature. Variation can be achieved through increasing the frequency and/or duration of an individual task. In general, it is best to introduce one new exercise at a time, and to increase the intensity of the exercise no more frequently than every other day. It is important to consider the effect of each exercise on the body as a whole. For example, it may be desirable to introduce pole work to increase hip or stifle flexion. However, if remodeling has occurred to such a degree that the joint's ROM will not allow for this, introducing such an exercise would merely accentuate compensatory movement patterns and increase the load on other structures.

Other Modalities

Acupuncture can assist with pain relief in many rehabilitation patients. Other useful techniques include therapeutic ultrasound therapy, neuromuscular stimulation, and transcutaneous electrical nerve stimulation (TENS).

Modification of Home Environment

Simple modifications, like keeping the patient warm through the use of coats and neck warmers, can significantly reduce musculoskeletal pain and stiffness. Similarly, providing a supportive bed can enhance comfort and promote sleep. Avoiding slippery surfaces and steps can also benefit many individuals, as can elevating the feeding bowl. Entry and exit from motor vehicles can be made easy through the use of a ramp, and all can be achieved at minimum cost to the owner.

SUMMARY

Successful rehabilitation requires a team approach to managing pain and restoring function. By adopting a global approach to diagnosis and management an individually tailored management protocol can be designed. Any attempt to make treatment prescriptive should be avoided and veterinary physical therapists must be innovative in their approaches. The ultimate aim should be to restore the patient to an active and pain free lifestyle, whether this is in the context of a slow leisurely walk or full athletic activity. When such an approach is adopted, the results can be spectacular and often life-changing for the patient.

REFERENCES

Bennel, K.L., Hunt, M.A., Wrigley, T.V., et al. (2009) Muscle and exercise in the prevention and management of knee osteoarthritis: an internal medicine specialist's guide. *Medical Clinics of North America*, 93(1), 161–177.

Butler, D. & Mosely, L. (2003) *Explain Pain*, NOI Group Publications, Adelaide, Australia.

Cook, J.L. (2010) Cranial cruciate ligament disease in dogs: biology versus biomechanics. *Veterinary Surgery*, 39(3), 270–277.

Eskelinen, E.V., Liska, W.D., Hyytiainen, H.K., & Hielm-Björkman, A. (2012) Canine total knee replacement performed due to osteoarthritis subsequent to distal femur fracture osteosynthesis: two-year objective outcome. *Veterinary Comparative Orthopedics and Traumatology*, 25(5), 427–432.

Fischer-Rasmussen, T. & Jensen, P. (2000) Proprioceptive sensitivity and performance in anterior cruciate ligament-deficient knee joints. *Scandinavian Journal of Medical Science Sports*, 10, 85–89.

Garfin, S.R. Tipton, C.M., Mubarak, S.J., Woo, S.L., Hargens, A.R., & Akeson, W.H. (1981) Role of fascia in maintenance of muscle tension and pressure. *Journal of Applied Physiology*, 51(2), 317–320.

Heinrichs, K. (2004) Superficial thermal modalities, in *Canine Rehabilitation and Physical Therapy* (eds D.L Millis, D. Levine, & R.A. Taylor), Saunders, St. Louis, MO, pp. 279–282

Herzog, W. & Longino, D. (2007) The role of muscles in joint degeneration and osteoarthritis. *Journal of Biomechanics*, 40, 54–63.

Hodges, P.W. & Richardson, C.A. (1996) Inefficient Muscular Stabilisation of the lumbar spine associated with low back pain: a motor control evaluation of transversus abdominis. *Spine*, 21(22), 2640–2650.

Hodges, P.W. (2010) Clinical update: emerging trends in exercise management of spinal pain. *Journal of the American Veterinary Medical Association*, 222(11), 552–558.

Hodges, P.W. (2011) Pain and motor control: from the laboratory to rehabilitation. *Journal of Electromyography and Kinesiology*, 21, 220–228.

Hodges, P.W. & Tucker, K. (2011) Moving differently in pain. *Pain*, 152, S90–S98.

IASP (2009) Exercise in the management of musculoskeletal pain. Arendt-Nielsen, L., Barbe, M.F., Bement, M.H., et al. IASP web resource. www.iasp-pain.org.

Ingersoll, C.D., Grindstaff, T.L., Pietrosimone, B.G., & Hart, J.M. (2008) Neuromuscular consequences of anterior cruciate ligament injury. *Clinics in Sport Medicine*, 27, 383–404.

Jaegger, G., Marcellin-Little, D.J., & Levine, D., 2002. Reliability of goniometry in Labrador retrievers. *American Journal of Veterinary Research*, 63(7), 979–986.

Jamison, R.N., 2011. Nonspecific treatment effects in pain medicine. *IASP Pain Clinical Updates*, XIX(2), 1–7.

Jeffery, N.D. & Blakemore, W.F. (1999) Spinal cord injury in small animals I. Mechanisms of spontaneous recovery. *Veterinary Record*, 144, 407–413.

Knight, K.L. (1995) Temperature changes resulting from cold application, in *Cryotherapy in Sports Injury Management*, Human Kinetics Publishers, Champaign, IL.

Lysholm, M., Ledin, T., Odkvist, L.M, & Good, L. (1998) Postural control – a comparison between patients with chronic anterior cruciate ligament insufficiency and healthy individuals. *Scandinavian Journal of Medical Science Sports*, 8, 432–438.

MacDonald, D., Mosely, G.L., & Hodges, P.W. (2009) Why do some patients keep hurting their back? Evidence of ongoing muscle dysfunction during remission from recurrent back pain. *Pain*, 142, 183–188.

McGowan, C., Goff, L., & Stubbs, N. (2005): *Animal physiotherapy: Assessment, Treatment and Rehabilitation of Animals*. Wiley-Blackwell.

McGowan, C., Goff, L., Stubbs, N. Eds. (2007) *Animal Physiotherapy: Assessment, Treatment and Rehabilitation of Animals*. Wiley-Blackwell, Ames, IA.

Mok, N., Brauer, S., & Hodges, P. (2004) Hip strategy for balance control in quiet standing is reduced in people with low back pain. *Spine*, 29, 107–112.

Panjabi, M. (1992) The stabilising system of the spine. Part I. Function, dysfunction, adaptation and enhancement. *Journal of Spinal Disorders*, 5(4), 383–389.

Radin, E.L., Simon, S.R., Rose, R.M., & Paul, I.L. (1979) Biomechanics of the spine, in *Practical Biomechanics for the Orthopedic Surgeon* (eds E.L. Radin, S.R. Simon, R.M. Rose, & I.L. Paul), John Wiley and Sons, New York, pp. 1–28.

Ratanunga, K.W. (1981) Influence of temperature on the velocity of shortening and rate of tension development in mammalian skeletal muscle. *Journal of Physiology*, 316, 35–36.

Roberts, D., Friden, T., Zatterstrom, R., Lindstrand, A., & Moritz, U. (1999) Proprioception in people with anterior cruciate ligament deficits: comparison of symptomatic and asymptomatic patients. *Journal of Orthopaedic Sports Physiotherapy*, 10, 587–594.

Salter, R.B., Hamilton, H.W., Wedge, J.H., et al. (1984) Clinical application of basic research on continuous passive motion for disorders and injuries of synovial joints: a preliminary report of a feasibility study. *Journal of Orthopaedic Research*, 1, 325–342.

Schipplein, O.D. & Andriacchi, T.P. (1991) Interaction between active and passive knee stabilizers during level walking. *Journal of Orthopaedic Research*, 9, 113–119.

Thomas, R.J., McEwen, J., & Asbury, A.J. (1996) The Glasgow Pain Questionnaire: a new generic measure of pain. *International Journal of Epidemiology*, 25(5), 1060–1067.

Tsao, H. & Hodges, P.W. (2007) Immediate changes in feedforward postural adjustments following voluntary motor training. *Experimental Brain Research*, 181(4), 537–546.

Udina, E., Puigdemasa, A., & Navarro, X. (2011) Passive and active exercise improve regeneration and muscle re-innervation after peripheral nerve injury in the rat. *Muscle and nerve*, 43(4), 500–509.

Minaire, P. (1992) Disease, illness and health: theoretical models of the disablement process. *WHO Bulletin OMS*, 70, 374.

12

Equine Rehabilitation

Lowri Davies

The equine rehabilitation therapist must consider numerous factors when designing a treatment plan. The majority of horses presented for rehabilitation are athletes of some type; thus, owner expectation for a full return of function is very high. Because of the close interaction between horse and rider, any attempt to rehabilitate the horse without paying attention to farriery, saddle fit, and the role of the rider in creating or amplifying the lameness may result in treatment failure. The rider may be required to undergo a personal rehabilitation regimen because it may be impossible to rehabilitate the horse in the face of ongoing issues with the rider's posture and balance.

Little formal research exists regarding the benefit of various therapeutic techniques and exercise regimens in horses. Accurate diagnosis remains essential, coupled with an understanding of associated tissue changes and appropriate choice of techniques for restoring function. Restoration of movement requires a combination of techniques, but the importance of restoring dynamic stability through enhanced neuroregulation cannot be overemphasized (see previous chapter). Veterinarian, physical therapist, master saddler, farrier, and owner will have to work as a team to achieve the desired goal.

RISK FACTORS FOR EQUINE LAMENESS

Risk factors that have been identified as predisposing to musculoskeletal injury include exercise frequency, stabling, body condition score, and breed, though controversy exists as to whether an individual's conformation has a significant role to play (Van Weeren et al., 2006).

Lameness from limb and back disorders accounts for a significant percentage of health problems in the domestic horse (Ross & Kaneene, 1996). The link between lameness and back pain is often ignored, even though problems within the axial skeleton will lead to asymmetrical limb loading and subsequent lameness in the distal limbs (Landmann et al., 2004).

Although it is well established in humans that movement assists healing and pain management (Salter, 1982; Jones & Amendola, 2007), equine athletes are frequently prescribed arbitrary periods of stall rest. The absence of loading within the musculoskeletal system may result in maladaptive responses within its components

(Enneking & Horowitz, 1972; Fitts & Brimmer, 1985; Appell, 1986). Postural feedback, proprioception, and overall tonus are inhibited by stall or stable rest, which has a significant impact on how a horse moves when it is finally led out of the box (McGreevy et al., 2011). Uncoordinated movements will increase the pressure or load on joints, tendons, and ligaments while muscle atrophy inhibits its inherent ability to absorb shock and protect these structures from the impact of movement. Care must be taken to restore neuromotor control prior to embarking on any form of strenuous activity.

In the wild, horses spend a significant proportion of time with the head and cervical spine lowered while grazing, a posture which may facilitate stretching of the soft tissues along the dorsum, including the longissimus dorsi and scalenus muscles (McGreevy et al., 2011). Flexion and lowering of the cervical spine also generates tension in the nuchal and supraspinous ligaments, elevating and separating the thoracolumbar spinous processes (Denoix & Pailloux, 2004). Stabled horses, particularly when fed from hayracks or nets, do not utilize this "natural" stretching action, and this may increase the risk of injury (Goodship & Birch, 2001).

Tack and Lameness

During motion, the saddle should support the rider's weight and distribute it evenly over as large an area as possible in order to reduce pressure. It should also facilitate normal spinal motion through flexion, extension, rotation, and lateroflexion. de Cocq et al. (2004) examined the effect of tack and weight on the equine back. They concluded that both caused overall extension of the thoracolumbar spine without any reduction in spinal range of motion (ROM). Limb kinematics was affected at the walk and trot due to increased limb retraction.

A poorly fitting saddle will cause pain and inhibit movement and lead to local (under the saddle) and general (distal limb) muscle atrophy and impairment of cybernetic muscle function. Cybernetic muscles are mainly composed of Type I muscle fibers, and their main function is to sense motion and produce adaptive postural responses. In contrast to gymnastic (i.e., movement-generating) muscles, cybernetic muscles are richly innervated, which allows for very precise control of movement (Denoix & Pailloux, 2004). They are present in the upper lip, around the eye, around the vertebral column, and next to joints. Cybernetic muscles are extremely

Pain Management in Veterinary Practice, First Edition. Edited by Christine M. Egger, Lydia Love and Tom Doherty.

important in controlling posture and fine tuning movement in response to the rider's commands. The function of these muscles may be impaired if the horse is stressed, in pain, or if movement is mechanically hampered, for example, by the saddle.

Devices that force a horse into an outline, such as draw reins and standing martingales, decrease the horse's ability to hold itself in position while inhibiting normal head and neck motion at the walk and canter. Such abnormal positioning has an adverse effect on balance and coordination and will alter locomotion and may result in pain (McGreevy et al., 2011).

Training and Exercise

Overexercising may predispose to back pain and injury when horses are poorly prepared for competition. Poor training, both in hand and under saddle, can result in distress and anxiety that, if prolonged, can lead to confusion, bad behavior, flight responses, and musculoskeletal degeneration. Overtraining can be a significant risk factor for the development of degenerative joint disease in elite athletes (Taylor et al., 2002), and may be associated with weight loss, reduced exercise tolerance, reduced red blood cell volume (PCV), altered immune function and an increase in muscle enzyme activity (McGowan & Whitworth, 2008).

PATIENT ASSESSMENT

The horse and the horse and rider unit should be assessed prior to embarking on a rehabilitation program. During anamnesis, an attempt should be made to establish the pattern of lameness and what, if any, activities provoke the lameness; for example, a horse with mild to moderate back pain can demonstrate normal or subtly altered behavior and gait patterns when ridden on the flat, but may demonstrate significant discomfort and move with a markedly altered gait when faced with a decline.

Pain Assessment

Behavioral changes that are associated with pain in the horse include kicking or biting when the tender area is touched, generalized restlessness, sweating, frequent movement of the painful limb, or continuous shifting of weight from one limb to another. Changes associated with back pain, such as poor performance, poor appetite, and slight changes in demeanor may be very subtle initially. These may progress to tail swishing or holding the tail to one side, bruxism, head shaking, resistance to saddling and grooming, loss of flexibility, stumbling, bucking, and rearing (Marks, 2000; Haussler & Paulekas, 2009). The horse may become withdrawn in nature, and tension in the abdominal muscles may lead to a "herring-gutted" or tucked appearance. Breed and an individual's temperament must be taken into consideration when trying to assess pain in horses.

Objective measurements of pain in the horse that may assist in diagnosing and treating pain include heart rate (not consistently increased in pain), pressure algometry, thermography (Figure 12.1), kinematic gait analysis, and response to analgesia (e.g., nerve blocks). Response to analgesic therapy is often quoted as an objective measure of pain. Frequently, however, only nonsteroidal anti-inflammatory drugs (NSAIDs) have been administered, and other classes of analgesics or multimodal pain management techniques have not been tried. The author has regularly

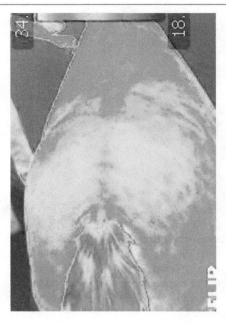

Figure 12.1. The use of thermal imagery to detect subtle alterations in regional blood flow, which determines tissue temperature.

encountered horses deemed to "not be in pain" when their behavior did not alter in response to an NSAID. Such horses are often subject to progressively harsher riding and controlling techniques in an attempt to counter what is deemed as bad behavior rather than a normal response to pain.

Assessment of Conformation, Muscle Tone, and Posture

A horse's posture should be assessed from both sides, cranial and caudal and from above. Limb alignment and weight distribution should be evaluated along with any irregularities in hoof or shoe wear and discrepancies in hoof size. Lordosis or kyphosis should be noted along with any conformational anomalies, as these often predispose to lameness (Kirkendall & Garrett, 1999).

Evaluation of muscle tone can give valuable information regarding an animal's psychological and physical well-being. Basic tonus is the light contractile tension in every skeletal muscle, which allows maintenance of posture at rest and changes in response to internal and external influences. External influences can increase (e.g., perceived threat) or decrease (e.g., calm and familiar environment) tonus. Internal influences, such as pain and anxiety, will generally increase tonus while fatigue will reduce it (Denoix & Pailloux, 2004). Although an increase in tonus through mild anxiety and stress may serve to enhance a horse's athletic ability, it can lead to muscle rigidity and poor performance if poorly managed.

Palpation

Systematic palpation of the whole body should be undertaken. This should serve to identify distention in the tendon sheaths and joint capsules, along with focal areas of pain and heat. Hoof testers should be used to assist with localizing pain in the foot.

An internal pelvic examination may be required to identify any pelvic and lumbosacral abnormalities as well as patency of the iliac arteries.

Manipulation of each joint should establish ROM and whether discomfort is associated with that movement (Chapter 11). These findings provide a benchmark against which to measure either improvement or exacerbation of clinical signs.

Gait Evaluation

Gait evaluation should identify the lame limb(s) as well as any subsequent compensatory changes. The horse should be observed at walk and trot on a straight line and on a left and right circle. The arc of flight should be noted along with limb placement (i.e., adducted or abducted). An attempt should also be made to identify any increase or decrease in an individual joint's ROM. The overall character of the movement should be evaluated for its fluidity and coordination, which may be affected by spinal stiffness or lordosis.

The horse should then be examined under tack and, finally, a ridden assessment should be carried out in order to evaluate how the gait is modified in response to external influences. Video assessment at each stage can be useful, both as an aid to diagnosis and as a way of monitoring progress.

Neurological Assessment

A neurological examination should be part of the assessment to help differentiate between neurological cases exhibiting gross central pathological change or vertebral malformation, and those that merely have impaired neuromotor control.

Neuromotor Control Assessment

Motor control relies on intact sensory and proprioceptive afferent input, well-developed central control of coordination and motor output, adequate motor neuron recruitment of muscle fibers, and

Table 12.1. Stages of tissue healing

Stage of tissue healing	Rehabilitation Objective	Techniques
Phase 1: Immediate postinjury period	Pain management Minimize tissue swelling and promote tissue perfusion Reduce movement at the trauma site	NSAID and centrally acting analgesics Cryotherapy, light compressive bandage Rest and external support if appropriate
Phase 2: Subacute phase	Ongoing pain management Minimize tissue swelling, promote tissue perfusion and healing Maintain range of motion (ROM) Promote functional neuromotor recruitment with controlled movement or loading Early reintroduction of exercise	NSAID & centrally acting analgesic, acupuncture Cryotherapy, massage, therapeutic ultrasound, low level laser therapy Gentle active and passive ROM exercises Regular short periods (5 minutes; 4–6 times daily) of in-hand walking to include proprioceptive stimulation such as proprioceptive track or weight shifting Aquatic treadmill therapy (Herzog & Longino, 2007)
Phase 3: Repair	Promote tissue healing Promote correct alignment of collagen fibers along the lines of stress and minimize adhesions Neuromotor recruitment Enhance proprioception Maintain joint ROM Develop core strength and improve posture Correct for compensatory changes; e.g., abnormal hoof wear, back and neck pain, contralateral limb loading	Acupuncture, ultrasound, massage, local heat, low-level laser therapy Controlled exercise gradually increasing in duration and intensity; e.g., introduce poles on proprioceptive track. Turn out in confined area. Gentle stretches 1–2 times daily. Cross-fiber massage over the scar. Therapeutic exercises Active ROM and stretching exercises Various therapeutic exercises Corrective farriery, physical therapy, acupuncture
Phase 4: Remodeling	Ongoing neuromotor training and proprioceptive enhancement Improve muscle strength and endurance Improve cardiovascular fitness Discipline-specific training	Stretching, increase in level of difficulty and duration of therapeutic exercises Introduction of short periods of fast work during the latter stages. Reintroduce specific tasks such as jumping or dressage

Table 12.2. Techniques to improve mobility and reduce pain in patients with osteoarthritis

Focus	Treatment option
Joint inflammation	Cryotherapy; low-grade joint mobilization; NSAIDs; chondroprotectants; nutraceuticals; weight management
Stiffness and pain: joint and associated soft tissue structures	Heat (infrared lamp, heat pack, rugs and wraps); therapeutic ultrasound; low-level laser therapy; massage, ROM, and stretching exercises; acupuncture
Muscle atrophy	Therapeutic exercises
Altered proprioception and neuromotor recruitment	Therapeutic exercises

the ability of the muscle fibers to respond to an electrical stimulus. Subsequent to injury, the sensory receptors within the joint capsule, ligaments, and tendons, as well as the muscle spindles, exhibit altered function. Inadequate proprioceptive input changes the frequency and rate of muscle fiber recruitment and adversely affects balance and coordination leading to clumsy, erratic movement that persists in the absence of nociceptive signals. Neuromotor control can be tested by watching a horse walk up and down slopes,

Table 12.3. Techniques to treat back pain in horses

Focus	Treatment option
Management	Increase time at pasture to encourage natural stretching of the longissimus dorsi; feed from the floor rather than hay nets
Reduce stress	Promote interaction with other horses; adopt a relaxed manner when handling and riding; increase time at pasture; acupuncture
Reduce pain	Analgesics; acupuncture; physical therapy; local heat; osteopathy; chiropractic; massage
Increase flexibility	Stretching exercises
Improve abdominal muscle tone	Therapeutic exercises
Improve iliopsoas function	Therapeutic exercises
Improve balance and proprioception	Therapeutic exercises
Improve core stability	Therapeutic exercises

turning tightly, or navigating obstacles. It can also be tested through assessing the horse's ability to maintain its trajectory in the face of external forces, such as tail pulling. Adequate time must be given during rehabilitation to allow for proprioceptive re-education and restoration of balanced, controlled movement.

Core Stability Assessment

When the abdominal muscles contract against the resistance of the diaphragm, hydrostatic pressure inside the abdominopelvic cavity increases and the pressure generated counters the pressure from the back, the rider, and gravity. In well-conditioned muscle with appropriate tonus, the abdominal muscles function as a system of stays supporting the intervertebral joints (Denoix & Pailloux, 2004). Reinforcement of this support is a critical part of any therapeutic exercise program. Assessment of abdominal muscle mass and tone should be an integral part of a lameness evaluation.

REHABILITATION FOR MUSCULOSKELETAL DISEASE AND INJURY

As outlined in the section on canine rehabilitation, the design of any treatment program should be influenced by the degree of inflammation and the rate of progress through the different stages of tissue healing. Table 12.1 describes the phases of healing, the rehabilitation goals, and techniques used to achieve them for acute injuries in horses.

Osteoarthritis and back pain are the most commonly encountered musculoskeletal diseases in horses. Frequently, the two are interlinked and should be addressed simultaneously. Osteoarthritis is not merely a problem of cartilage degradation within the joint; it is the end result of abnormal mechanical wear and tear. Local changes in muscle function may well be a precursor to its development (White et al., 2007). Joint instability due to ligament laxity and loss of functional control through altered proprioception and neuromotor function are also important predisposing factors. A multimodal approach to managing osteoarthritis in the equine is likely to have

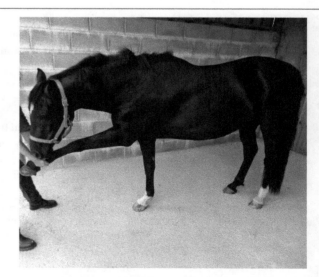

Figure 12.2. Stretching may provide pain relief through central mechanisms.

Table 12.4. Therapeutic exercises for horses

Exercise	Therapeutic effect
In-hand walking on a proprioceptive road (3–6 m lengths of alternating surfaces)	Proprioceptive re-education, rapid neuroreceptor adaptation
5 minutes sessions repeated twice daily	
Tail pulling—axial traction: Grasp the end of the tail and gently apply caudoventral traction in line with the sacrum	Reduces tension in the lumbar epaxial and gluteal musculature
Wait for the horse to pull against you and hold for 1 minute, repeat twice daily	
Lateral tail pulls:	Rhythmic movement stimulates activation of the spinal stabilizers (cybernetic muscles) and core musculature
Apply gentle tail traction on both the left and right sides	Activates joint mechanoreceptors and assists development of neuromuscular coupling at the lumbosacral junction
1 minute, repeat twice daily (Figure 12.5)	Improves balance and triggers a stabilizing response in the fore and hind limb muscle groups
Rocking:	As above
Stand parallel to the horse and place your hands over the withers or sacrum	
Rock the horse gently from side to side	
Move around to the other side and repeat	
1 minute twice daily	
Serpentine, figure of eight, and labyrinth work:	Promotes side bending, enhances proprioception, strengthens limb adductors and abductors
Start with large, wide turns and tighten them progressively to increase the level of difficulty	Introduces nonlinear motion and increases the load on individual joints
1 minute twice daily	Labyrinth work teaches the horse to step medially across the midline
(Figure 12.3)	Promotes concentration and requires the horse to drop his head
Ground pole work:	Increases ROM, promotes abdominal muscle recruitment, improves balance and coordination, improves proprioception and motor control
Place at intervals equal to the horse's stride length	
1 minute repeated twice daily; duration increased as horse progresses	Promotes limb flexion and pelvic limb protraction
(Figure 12.4)	
Walking over a low bridge	Novel proprioceptive and auditory stimulus
	Promotes cervical flexion
	Stimulates abdominal muscle contraction
Walking uphill:	Stimulates abdominal and iliopsoas muscle contraction and lifts the back
Use a short slope	Strengthens the gymnastic muscles of the pelvic limb
The severity of the incline can be increased as rehabilitation progresses	Increases flexion and protraction of the pelvic limb
Similarly, start with short sessions (2–3 minutes) and increase the duration (up to 10–15 minutes)	Improves shock absorbing capacity of pelvic limb
Walking uphill over poles:	Enhances concentration, coordination and proprioception
Increases the difficulty of the exercise	Encourages a caudal shift in the horse's center of gravity and increases the load on the hind limbs while reducing the load on the forelimbs
Walking downhill:	Eccentrically strengthens the pelvic limb as the limb is placed under the body in descent
Use a short slope; the severity of the decline can be increased as rehabilitation progresses	Improves abdominal muscle function
Similarly start with short sessions (2–3 minutes) and increase the duration (up to 10–15 minutes)	Improves balance and coordination
Walking downhill over poles	Enhances concentration, coordination, and proprioception
	Improves abdominal muscle function
	Improves balance

(continued)

Table 12.4. (*Continued*)

Exercise	Therapeutic effect
Backing uphill: Start with short sessions of 30–60 seconds repeated twice daily Trotting over ground poles and Cavaletti rails Start on the ground and progress to ridden work, 2–3 minutes repeated twice daily The height of the rail and duration of the exercise can be increased as the horse progresses	Enhanced proprioceptive stimulation Strengthens the pelvic limb Increase ROM Promote abdominal muscle recruitment Improve balance and inter limb coordination Improve proprioception and motor control Elevates the forehand Encourages poll flexion

the best outcome. Such an approach should include appropriate surgical intervention, pain management through traditional pharmacological means, acupuncture (Deyle et al., 2000), physical therapy (Frick, 2010), therapeutic exercises to enhance proprioception and neuromuscular activation, weight loss and nutritional management, and nutraceuticals and chondroprotectants. Techniques that can improve mobility and reduce pain in the osteoarthritic patient are listed in Table 12.2.

Back Pain

Any condition which induces a change in a horse's normal pattern of movement, whether through changes in management (enforced stabling), introduction of tack and rider, or disease and injury, may well predispose to back pain.

The longissimus dorsi muscle, under normal circumstances, should be able to control lateral and dorsoventral movements of the spine through sequential relaxation and contraction. However, if the muscle is permanently shortened or in a state of increased tonus, the horse will be unable to carry out these maneuvers or support the weight of the rider. Another contributing factor in the recovering athlete or in young horses is the lack of ability to contract the abdominal muscles, iliopsoas, or the cervical flexors. An inability to flex the spine results, and passive support mechanisms are altered. Factors that should be considered when designing a program to strengthen the back and reduce pain are listed in Table 12.3. Initially, therapeutic exercises should focus on groundwork, with ridden work only being reintroduced when the horse is capable of elevating the back and keeping the longissimus muscles relaxed.

Stretching

Some studies have demonstrated that stretching (Figure 12.2) assists with pain relief through centrally mediated effects (Frick, 2010). As stretch tolerance increases, the application of a constant force produces less pain, and it is hypothesized that this is due to an antinociceptive effect mediated by the stretch of the muscle (Shrier, 2002).

Stretching improves flexibility, which relieves pain, prevents injury, and enhances performance (Marko, 1979; Taylor et al., 1990; Thacker et al., 2004). These exercises also improve balance, body awareness, and proprioception. By increasing tissue compliance and reducing the viscoelasticity of resting muscle, stretching can enhance the ROM in a single joint or a system of joints. Compliance represents the ability of tissues to lengthen under minimal force, and poor compliance during active muscle contraction is a significant factor in tissue injury (Shrier, 2002; Krivikas, 2006).

Spinal reflexes mediated by motor muscle spindles and the Golgi tendon organs influence flexibility. The muscle spindle responds to an absolute change in length of muscle fibers and the rate of change in fiber length. When activated during rapid muscle contraction, the muscle spindle stimulates the primary afferent fibers and promotes muscle shortening and an increase in tension. The Golgi tendon organ, on the other hand, is located at the muscle–tendon interface and senses muscle tension. It relays information to the spinal cord that results in inhibition of the agonist muscle and contraction of the antagonist, thus enhancing the ability of the muscles to stretch. Thus, the aim of any stretching exercise should be to activate the Golgi tendon organ and inhibit the spindle reflex (Marko, 1979).

Other factors that influence flexibility include myofascial compliance, local skin elasticity, the presence of adhesions and scar tissue, hydration status, local joint and tissue temperature, and the type of joint.

Tissues should be warmed prior to stretching to minimize the risk of further injury. This can be achieved through the application of heat packs, the use of infrared radiation, massaging the tissues, or by gently walking the patient. Heat increases the firing rate of the Golgi tendon organ while inhibiting muscle spindle activity, and increases tissue elasticity. In general, it is recommended that stretching be carried out prior to exercise to improve flexibility and help prevent injury. It is also effective during the cooling down period, as it helps reduce postexercise muscle stiffness, fatigue, and shortening (Thacker et al., 2004).

Any performance horse will benefit from a regular stretching routine. This becomes particularly important in stabled horses that undergo very little "natural" stretching through grazing activity. Stretching should initially be introduced at a basic level, with the intensity or level of difficulty only being increased when the horse has demonstrated adequate improvement. It is essential that the horse is relaxed before starting, and has been adequately warmed up, as previously outlined. When teaching owners to perform a stretch, it is imperative that the purpose of the stretch be explained, and that clear written and pictorial instructions are issued for them to follow. The number and frequency of repetitions should be clarified as well as instructions on the duration of the stretch. Although some immediate improvement can be seen, it may take as long as 6 weeks for the full benefit to be witnessed. For more detailed information the reader is referred to the textbook entitled *Physical Therapy and Massage for the Horse* (Denoix & Pailloux, 2004).

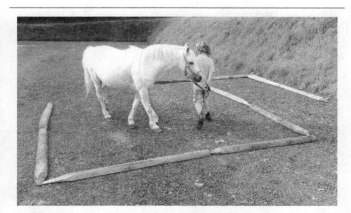

Figure 12.3. Movement through a labyrinth enhances neuromotor control, flexibility, and fore- and hind limb adductor function.

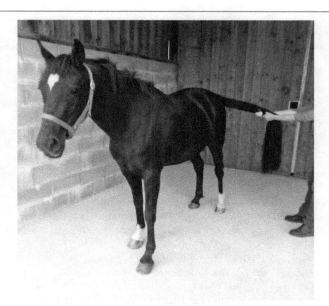

Figure 12.5. Lateral tail pull activates the spinal stabilizers and core musculature, enhances proprioception, and stabilizes responses in the fore and hind limbs.

Therapeutic Exercises

In the equine, a therapeutic exercise (Table 12.4) regimen serves to restore or develop balance and coordination, enhance proprioception, develop core strength, and improve gymnastic muscle function and cardiovascular endurance. Examples of therapeutic exercises for the equine include walking on a proprioceptive road, figure eights, or labyrinth work (Figure 12.3), ground pole work (Figure 12.4), walking up and down hills, and walking over poles and Cavaletti rails. For more detailed information the reader is referred to the textbook entitled *Physical Therapy and Massage for the Horse* (Denoix & Pailloux, 2004).

SUMMARY

Rehabilitation is an integral part of pain management in the equine athlete. When carried out correctly it will enhance tissue repair and increase the likelihood of an early return to athletic activity. Moreover it can help to minimize reinjury in the future. However, these goals can only be achieved through a holistic approach where retraining of the musculoskeletal system is accompanied by environmental modification, good podiatry, well-fitting tack, and an eye to the rider where appropriate.

REFERENCES

Appell, H.J. (1986) Skeletal muscle atrophy during immobilisation. *International Journal of Sports Medicine*, 7, 1–5.

de Cocq, P., van Weeren, P.R., & Back, W. (2004) Effects of girth, saddle and weight on movements of the horse. *Equine Veterinary Journal*, 36(8), 758–763.

Denoix, J.M. & Pailloux, J.P. (2004) *Physical Therapy and Massage for the Horse*, Manson Publishing, London.

Deyle, G.D., Henderson, N.E., Matekel, R.L., Ryder, M.G., Garber, M.B., & Allison, S.C. (2000) Effectiveness of manual physical therapy and exercise in osteoarthritis of the knee. A randomised, controlled trial. *Annals of Internal Medicine*, 132, 173–181.

Enneking, W.F. & Horowitz, M. (1972) The intra-articular effects of immobilisation on the human knee. *Journal of Bone and Joint Surgery*, 54, 973–985.

Fitts, R.H. & Brimmer, C.J. (1985) Recovery in skeletal muscle contractile function after prolonged hind limb immobilisation. *Journal of Applied Physiology*, 59, 916–923.

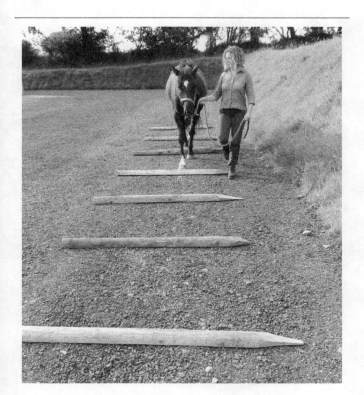

Figure 12.4. Ground pole work is used to improve ROM, activates the abdominal musculature, and enhances proprioception and motor control.

Frick, A. (2010) Stretching exercises for horses: Are they effective? *Journal of Equine Veterinary Science*, 30, 50–59.

Goodship, A.E. & Birch, H.L. (2001) Exercise effects on the skeletal tissues, in *Equine Locomotion* (eds W. Back & H.M. Clayton), W. B. Saunders, London, pp. 227–250.

Paulekas, R. & Haussler, K.K. (2009) Principles and practice of therapeutic exercises for horses. *Journal of Equine Veterinary Science*, 29, 870–893.

Herzog, W. & Longino, D. (2007) The role of muscles in joint degeneration and osteoarthritis. *Journal of Biomechanics*, 40, 54–63.

Jones, M.H. & Amendola, A.S. (2007) Acute treatment of inversion ankle sprains: Immobilisation versus functional treatment. *Clinical Orthopaedic Related Research*, 55, 169–172.

Kirkendall, D.T. & Garrett, W.E. (1999) Muscle strain injuries: research findings and clinical applicability. *Medscape General Medicine*, 1(2).

Krivikas, L.S (2006) Training flexibility, in *Exercise in Rehabilitation Medicine*, 2nd edn (ed. W.R. Frontera), Human Kinetics Publishers, Champaign, IL, pp. 33–43.

Landmann, M.A., de Blaauw, J.A., van Weeren, P.R., & Hofland, L.J. (2004) Field study of the prevalence of lameness in horses with back pain. *Veterinary Record*, 155, 165–168.

Marko, P.D. (1979) Ipsilateral and contralateral effect of proprioceptive neuromuscular facilitation techniques on hip motion and electromyographic activity. *Physical Therapy*, 59, 1366–1373.

Marks, D. (2000) Conformation and soundness. *American Association of Equine practitioners' proceedings*, 46, 39–45.

McGowan, C. & Whitworth, D.J. (2008) Overtraining syndrome in horses. *Comparative Exercise Physiology*, 5(2), 57–65.

McGreevy, P., McLean, A., Buckley, P., McConaghy, F., & McLean, C. (2011) How riding may affect welfare: what the equine veterinarian needs to know. *Equine veterinarian*, 10, 1–9.

Ross, W.A. & Kaneene, R.B. (1996) An individual animal level prospective study of risk factors associated with the occurrence of lameness in the Michigan USA equine population. *Preventative Veterinary Medicine*, 29, 59–75.

Salter, R.B. (1982) Motion versus rest: why immobilise joints? Presidential address. Canadian Orthopaedic Association. *Journal of Bone Joint Surgery*, 64, 62–65.

Shrier, I. (2002) Does stretching help prevent injuries? in *Evidence-based Sports Medicine* (eds D. MacAuley & T. Best), BMJ Publishing Group, Blackwell Publishing, Oxford, UK, pp. 36–38. .

Taylor, D.C., Dalton, J.D. Jr., Seaber, A.V., & Garrett, W.E. Jr. (1990) Viscoelastic properties of muscle-tendon units. The biomechanical effects of stretching. *American Journal of Sports Medicine*, 18, 300–309.

Taylor, P.M., Pascoe, P.J., & Mama, K.R. (2002) Diagnosing and treating pain in the horse. Where are we today? *Veterinary Clinical Equine Practice*, 18, 1–19.

Thacker, S.B., Gilchrist, J., Stroup, D.F., & Kimsey, C.D. Jr. (2004) The impact of stretching on sports injury risk: a systematic review of literature. *Medicine and Science in Sports and Exercise*, 36, 371–378.

Van Weeren, P.R. & Crevier-Denoix, N. (2006) Equine conformation: Clues to performance and soundness. *Equine Veterinary Journal*, 38, 591–596.

White, A., Foster, N.E., Cummings, M., & Barlas, P. (2007) Acupuncture treatment for chronic knee pain: A systematic review. *Rheumatology*, 46, 384–390.

13

Custom External Coaptation as a Pain Management Tool: Veterinary Orthotics and Prosthetics

Martin W. Kaufmann and Patrice M. Mich

The historical record of the field of human orthotics and prosthetics (H-OP) dates back to 2700 and 1500 BC, respectively (Seymour, 2002). Modern H-OP has been advanced by experiences gained from treating catastrophic wartime injury, sports injury, complications of diabetes, and congenital limb deformities.

Today the use of mechanical appliances to improve function and to manage pain associated with mobility is no longer solely the purview of human medicine. The techniques and materials used in H-OP are now being utilized in veterinary medicine. Veterinary-OP (V-OP) has made great strides in the past decade from the simple adaptation of PVC pipes, aluminum rods, thermoplastics, and fiberglass or plaster casting to the use of veterinary specific hinges, vacuum-molded composite high-temperature plastics, titanium, and carbon fiber, alongside a growing understanding of the intricacies of quadruped mobility and biomechanics (Adamson et al., 2005). The advantages afforded by custom orthoses and prostheses include prevention of cast-related wounds and resultant pain; management of primary pain generators associated with functional impairments; improvement of biomechanics, allowing for greater activity and a significant decrease in secondary pain; earlier return to active lifestyle, resulting in decreased obesity and associated comorbidities; improvement in quality of life and functional independence, possibly preventing a premature decision to euthanize; and the availability of treatment options where none existed before.

PRIMARY AND SECONDARY PAIN GENERATORS ASSOCIATED WITH LIMB DYSFUNCTION OR ABSENCE

Primary pain generators are those directly and specifically caused by an injury. For example, hyperextension injury of an osteoarthritic carpus during weight bearing produces pain stimuli above and beyond the pain associated with osteoarthritis in the resting state. The former, evoked pain, and the latter, spontaneous pain, can be significant sources of primary pain and subsequent loss of mobility. In both instances the peripheral nociceptors are activated, resulting in the perception of localized pain.

Secondary pain generators are those arising from compensation for pain or mechanical or functional impairment. Secondary pain compounds discomfort and can become a greater strain on the quality of life than the original injury. In the example above, decreased weight bearing through the affected carpus will result in a weight shift to the contralateral thoracic limb and potentially an increase in pelvic limb weight bearing. The contralateral triceps brachii, latissimus dorsi, and pectoral muscles will be excessively loaded and strained, resulting in myofascial trigger points within these muscle bellies. Additionally, the cervical, epaxial, and core muscles may be similarly affected due to a loss of homeostasis in structural supports. Lastly, increased weight bearing and compensatory gait shifting may exacerbate any concomitant ligament or joint pathology in the remaining limbs or trunk. The alert pain management clinician will carefully assess for gait and postural changes secondary to the presenting complaint. Common compensatory adjustments include ventral displacement of the head and neck, head bobbing, "hip hiking," pelvic tilt, spinal kyphosis or scoliosis, medially displaced limbs, and wide-based stance, among others (DeCamp, 1997; Renberg, 2001; Burton et al., 2008; Gomez Alvarez et al., 2008; Weishaupt, 2008).

THE ROLE OF CUSTOM EXTERNAL COAPTATION IN PAIN MANAGEMENT

Orthoses

Orthoses are any medical device attached to the body to support, align, position, immobilize, prevent or correct deformity, assist weak muscles, or improve function (Deshales, 2002) (Figure 13.1). Goals of orthotic use may include reduction of pain and/or swelling, prevention of contractures, or provision of joint stability (Melvin, 1989). Human medical conditions partly or wholly managed with orthoses include: rheumatoid arthritis (Egan et al., 2003), mild-to-moderate carpal tunnel syndrome (De Angelis et al., 2009); lateral epicondylitis (tennis elbow) (Jafarian et al., 2009); osteoarthritis of the digits (e.g., halicus limitus) and midfoot region (Kruizinga

Pain Management in Veterinary Practice, First Edition. Edited by Christine M. Egger, Lydia Love and Tom Doherty.
© 2014 John Wiley & Sons, Inc. Published 2014 by John Wiley & Sons, Inc.

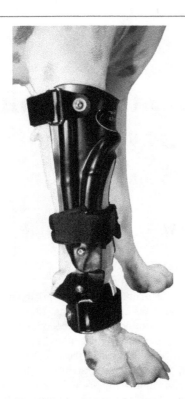

Figure 13.1. Articulating carpal device for carpal hyperextension injury; allows freedom of motion in flexion while providing hyperextension stop for "arthrodesis on demand."

et al., 2002; Rao et al., 2009; Ibuki et al., 2010); plantar fasciitis; mild-to-moderate lateral collateral ligament sprains of the ankle; mild-to-moderate Achilles tendon sprain (Petersen et al., 2007; Knobloch et al., 2008); and medial compartment syndrome of the osteoarthritic knee (Hewett et al., 1998; Barnes et al., 2002; Finger & Paulos, 2002; Pollo et al., 2002; Dennis et al., 2006; Ramsey et al., 2007). Patients with osteoarthritis may benefit from orthoses used to unload, support, or protect the joint (Seymour, 2002). Additionally, orthoses may be used preoperatively or as a protective supplement to surgical repair. These devices may also be used as an alternative to surgery or when no surgical option exists.

Surgical management of many orthopedic conditions in veterinary species remains the standard of care and the preferred therapeutic choice. Custom external coaptation can be used to provide security before and after the surgical repair and help prevent wounds or surgical failures caused by splinting, wet bandages, splint material fatigue/breakdown, and lack of patient tolerance of a support splint. The term coaptation refers to approximation and involves transmitting compressive or corrective forces through skin to the boney structures beneath. As a general rule, molded external coaptation devices are more efficient stabilizers of bones and joints than premade ones (Piermattei et al., 2006). The advantages of custom-fitted devices are that, in closely approximating the patient's individual topography and dispersing corrective forces over a larger surface area, fewer soft tissue problems arise and devices are better tolerated (Piermattei et al., 2006).

A good example is the surgical repair of an avulsed gastrocnemius tendon. Once repaired, rigid fixation of the tarsus in extension

greater than 165° is maintained for approximately 8 weeks, with transition to a gradual reloading of the tendon over an additional 4–8 weeks. Painful complications may arise when a traditional caudolateral or lateral rigid splint is used and followed by serial padded bandages including: maceration of skin and contamination of surgical incisions (Piermattei et al., 2006); moist dermatitis of the interdigital space; tape associated dermatitis; pressure wounds usually associated with the lateral metatarsal head (fifth metatarsal bone), the lateral malleolus, and/or the calcaneal tuberosity; pressure wounds from splint edges; and with an insufficiently rigid splint, flexion of the tarsus resulting in premature tendon loading at best, and surgical failure at worst. The use of a custom orthosis can obviate these complications because it can be altered from a rigid device, used during the initial tendon healing phase, to a dynamically articulating device which allows gradual controlled loading of the tendon as it heals (Figure 13.2). Ultimately, this device can be adapted to a sports brace as the patient resumes normal

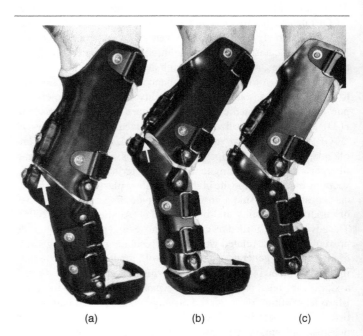

(a)   (b)   (c)

Figure 13.2. Progressively dynamic tarsus–paw orthosis for acute common calcaneal tendon injury used for postsurgical and nonsurgical support. (a) Articulating paw, nonarticulating tarsus configuration. Used during the healing phase. Large arrow indicates motion limiter in locked position; tarsus locked in extension 165–170°. (b) Articulating paw, progressively articulating tarsus configuration. Used during early loading phase of rehabilitation. The small arrow indicates adjustable motion limiter allowing variable flexion for controlled tendon loading as healing progresses. This device is set at 5° of freedom articulation. (c). Sports brace. Used after healing and rehabilitation are complete. Paw segment removed for increased freedom of motion. Fully articulating tarsus with controlled flexion stop to prevent end range flexion trauma during high intensity activity. (Mich, P.M., Fair, L., & Borghese, I. (2013) Assistive devices, orthotic, prosthetics, bandaging, in *Canine Sports Medicine and Rehabilitation* (eds M.C. Zink & J.B. VanDyke), Wiley-Blackwell.)

Table 13.1. Orthopedic conditions amenable to veterinary orthotic devices

Some common pathologies amenable to thoracic limb orthoses

Elbow instability (subluxation, osteoarthritis)
Carpal hyperextension
Carpus bi or triplanar instability
Carpal arthrodesis failure
Carpal support orthosis for contralateral thoracic limb amputation
Carpal instability secondary to contralateral amputation
Paw injuries including tendon laceration and digit amputation
Peripheral neuropathy
Brachial plexus distal neuropathy (carpus distad)

Some common pathologies amenable to pelvic limb orthoses

Cranial cruciate ligament rupture
Patellar luxation (grades 1 and 2)
Stifle collateral ligament injury
Tarsal hyperextension
Tarsal collateral ligament injury
Failed Achilles tendon repair
Achilles tendon rupture or avulsion
Achilles tendon sprain without rupture or avulsion
Sciatic neuropathy (tarsal collapse)
Paw injuries including tendon laceration and digit amputation
Peripheral neuropathy: degenerative myelopathy
Sciatic nerve trauma secondary to pelvic fracture or repair
IVDD, spinal canal stenosis, cervical spinal instability
Fibrocartilagenous embolus (FCE)

Special conditions

Hoppy vest/"monoski"/"Can-do" wheels for bilateral forelimb amputee
Toe-up sciatic sling for peripheral neuropathy of hindlimbs
Helmet as postcraniotomy protective device

activity. Although "off-the shelf" coaptation devices have been used in these cases, such devices cannot provide articulation or controlled, progressive reloading of tendon or bone; furthermore, the absence of customization often leads to soft tissue complications.

A number of patients are not surgical candidates for a variety of reasons including financial, personal preference, advanced patient age, perceived increased anesthetic risk, comorbidities, or circumstances requiring a delay of surgery. Until recently, veterinarians had no viable option for these patients. The development of V-OP has provided choices for applications using customized, articulated (as needed), external coaptation in the pre- or postoperative periods or in lieu of surgical intervention (Table 13.1).

Prosthetics

Biomechanical implications of agenesis of a limb segment ("congenital amputation" or amelia) or limb amputation include remaining limb breakdown and the development of secondary pain generators in myofascial tissue, joints, and spine by virtue of altered gait and structural support. Based on the significant consequences

of full limb amputation consideration of subtotal level amputation and application of prostheses becomes an attractive alternative. For perspective, consider human medical practice in which removal of normal proximal limb segments as a result of catastrophic injury to a distal limb segment is untenable.

The structural consequences of a missing or nonweight-bearing thoracic limb have not been fully elucidated, but conceivably are made more significant by virtue of the normal asymmetrical weight distribution of the quadruped. Normal weight distribution is approximately 60% to the thoracic limbs and 40% to the pelvic limbs. Importantly, body condition becomes a critical factor because obesity affects the thoracic limbs to a greater extent than the pelvic limbs. With the loss of a single thoracic limb or limb segment, the following compensatory adjustments can be seen during ambulation: ventral displacement of the head and neck during the weight-bearing phase of the gait; propulsion of the cranial half of the body during the swing phase, requiring an explosive thrust of the neck, trunk, and remaining thoracic limb; medially displaced remaining thoracic limb, which supports a disproportionate percentage of body mass (>30%) and absorbs the full concussive force of landing; and kyphosis of the lumbar spine with associated ventral rotation of the pelvis about the sacrum as body mass is distributed over the remaining three limbs (Figure 13.3). Clinical signs associated with these compensatory conformational changes may include: pectoral, rhomboideus, latissimus dorsi, triceps, and cervical, thoracic, and lumbar epaxial muscle tension and pain and myofascial trigger point development; shortening of the iliopsoas with reduced pelvic limb extension range; pain on palpation of the cervical and lumbar spine due to abnormally hyper- and hypomobile segments (Wada et al., 1992; Gómez Alvarez et al., 2007); frontal and sagittal plane collapse of the remaining carpus; and splayed thoracic limb digits due to collapse of the transverse paw arch.

The structural consequences of a missing or non-weight-bearing pelvic limb are similar, with some unique aspects. In this case, the propulsive thrust of the caudal half of the body is dependent on a single pelvic limb. This increases the requirement for spinal and core effort in driving the body forward. Balance is maintained by limiting the range of tail movement and ventral placement of the head. The resulting conformation bears some resemblance to that of a kangaroo in motion, with an even greater majority of body mass shifted onto the forelimbs (>60%). Additionally, in most cases the pelvis is tilted to the side of the missing limb with concomitant rotation of the lumbar spine (Figure 13.4). This asymmetrically alters lumbar epaxial muscle tension. Hypermobility of the lumbar spine in the sagittal, frontal, and transverse planes may increase the potential for altered kinematics and back pain (Wada et al., 1992; Landman et al., 2004; Gomez Alvarez et al., 2008).

Whenever possible, it is advantageous to re-establish a normal quadruped structure. Fortunately, veterinary patients are amenable to prosthetic limbs and adapt rapidly. This means that with distal limb injury or tumor, careful surgical planning for a subtotal limb amputation as opposed to the traditional complete limb amputation can enable the application of a custom prosthesis. The new paradigm is preservation of as much normal tissue as possible.

At the time of this writing, in order to suspend a prosthetic on the thoracic limb of a quadruped, preservation of 40% of the radius and ulna is required, and in the case of the pelvic limb, at minimum, 40% of the tibia and fibula is required (Syme's amputation (Shurr & Cook, 1990)). Technological advances, such as

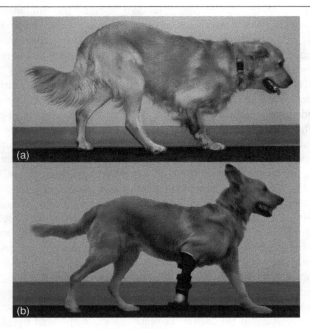

Figure 13.3. Thoracic limb prosthesis. (a) Impact of right thoracic limb loss on biomechanics. Because propulsion of the thoracic half of the body is driven from the left thoracic limb and cervical or thoracic spine, head and neck are shifted ventrally to move the center of mass cranially, absorb a portion of ground reaction force, improve balance, and most importantly, absorb and store energy to provide a means for forward propulsion; left thoracic limb absorbs greater than normal 30% of body mass; pelvic limbs shifted forward beneath the trunk to provide further balance and decrease impact to the left thoracic limb; subsequent kyphosis of the lumbar spine and ventral rotation of pelvis (transverse axis); pelvic limb stride length shortened in order to keep limbs beneath the trunk.
(b) Improved biomechanics with the addition of a right thoracic limb prosthesis. Propulsion of thoracic half of body no longer driven from left thoracic limb and cervical or thoracic spine alone; head and neck are properly elevated taking weight off of the left thoracic limb and decreasing repetitive strain on the cervical or thoracic spine; the back is more level from shoulders to pelvis; lumbar kyphosis and pelvic rotation (transverse axis) are reduced; pelvic limbs are shifted into more normal position centered beneath the pelvis allowing normalization of stride length. The end result is decreased myofascial and orthopedic biomechanical strain. (Mich, P.M., Fair, L., & Borghese, I. (2013) Assistive devices, orthotic, prosthetics, bandaging, in *Canine Sports Medicine and Rehabilitation* (eds M.C. Zink & J.B. VanDyke), Wiley-Blackwell.)

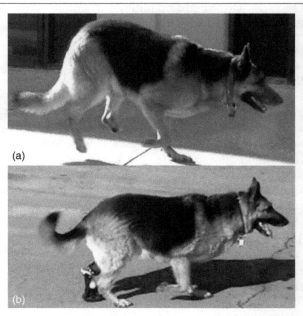

Figure 13.4. Pelvic limb prosthesis. (a) Impact of left pelvic limb loss on biomechanics. Because propulsion of the pelvic half of the body is driven from the right pelvic limb and lumbar spine, the head and neck are shifted ventrally for balance and the body mass is shifted cranially away from the pelvic limbs; the thoracic limbs are positioned caudally for balance and support; ventral rotation of the pelvis (transverse axis), kyphosis of the lumbar spine, and shortened right pelvic-limb stride length provide a means for energy storage for propulsion; the right pelvic limb is shifted medially beneath the trunk to provide balance and decrease impact to the left thoracic limb; subsequent rotation of pelvis (craniocaudal axis) alters spinal and limb biomechanics; the tail is low and shifted to the right for balance. (b) Improved biomechanics with the addition of a pelvic limb prosthetic. Propulsion of the pelvic half of the body is no longer driven by the right pelvic limb and lumbar spine alone. The head and neck are elevated as the body mass is shifted caudally to the pelvic limbs; the back is more level from the shoulders to the pelvis; lumbar kyphosis and pelvic rotation (craniocaudal and transverse axis) are reduced; the right pelvic limb is shifted laterally away from the midline as the prosthetic limb shares in weight bearing; the tail is elevated and in motion. The end result is decreased myofascial and orthopedic biomechanical strain. (Mich, P.M., Fair, L., & Borghese, I. (2013) Assistive devices, orthotic, prosthetics, bandaging, in *Canine Sports Medicine and Rehabilitation* (eds M.C. Zink & J.B. VanDyke), Wiley-Blackwell.)

osteointegration and implantable bone topographical segments, may alter these level limits in the near future. The tremendous variability in veterinary patients requires adaptability in socket design, componentry, and prosthetic limb mechanics to accommodate differences in the degree of injury, body type and condition, species, breed, size, lifestyle, sport or activity, and terrain (Table 13.2).

PATIENT EVALUATION FROM A V-OP PERSPECTIVE: DIAGNOSIS TO DEVICE

Patient evaluation for a V-OP device must be thorough and incorporate at least five separate examinations in order to fully define the presenting deficit, characterize biomechanical implications, identify comorbidities and potential complicators, and diagnose all

Table 13.2. Orthopedic conditions amenable to veterinary prosthetic devices

Thoracic limb prosthetics

Subtotal midshaft radius or ulna amputation (40% antebrachium retention required)

Subtotal radiocarpal disarticulation

Subtotal intercarpal disarticulation

Subtotal carpometacarpal disarticulation

Amelia

Congenital limb derangements

Traumatic limb amputation

Pelvic limb prosthetics

Subtotal midshaft tibia or fibula amputation (40% crus retention required)

Subtotal tarsocrural disarticulation

Subtotal level intertarsal disarticulation

Subtotal level tarsometatarsal disarticulation

Amelia

Congenital limb derangements

Traumatic limb amputation

primary and secondary pain generators. These examinations include a general wellness examination, an orthopedic (joint) examination, a myofascial (muscle) examination, a biomechanical (how joints and muscles work together) examination, and a neurological examination. The following issues must be identified and addressed: the type of injury or deficit and the functional and mechanical impairment resulting from it; comorbidities or complicators, lifestyle, environment, family dynamic, sport or activity; the goals and desired outcome of the client, the veterinarian, and the V-OP professional; and the alignment of goals with orthotic or prosthetic device functionality.

Because V-OP is a hands-on specialty, care must be taken to manage the case through a team approach. The ideal team includes the owner, the family veterinarian, a V-OP specialist, and a certified rehabilitation therapist.

Once case evaluation is complete and design of the device has been determined, custom fabrication and fitting of the device can proceed. The patient's primary and secondary pain generators must be re-evaluated in the device to assure that both functionality and quality of life goals have been addressed. Initiation of a professional rehabilitation and conditioning program is ideal when coupled with an appropriate device orientation program.

SUMMARY

Careful analysis of biomechanics challenges the long-held belief that quadrupeds are not adversely affected by a dysfunctional or missing limb. A new paradigm dictates that functional adaptability cannot be the only consideration. Custom orthoses provide a new alternative to static splinting and bandaging, minimizing associated wounds and improving long-term outcomes over these traditional techniques. Additionally, the use of veterinary prosthetics can significantly decrease chronic pain states and improve short and long-term quality of life in patients missing a limb or requiring amputation.

REFERENCES

Adamson, C., Kaufmann, M., Levine, D., Millis, D.L., & Marcellin-Little, D.J. (2005) Assistive devices, orthotics, and prosthetics. *Veterinary Clinics of North America:Small Animal Practice*, 35(6), 1441–1451.

Barnes, C.L., Cawley, P.W., & Hederman, B. (2002) Effect of Counterforce brace on symptomatic relief in a group of patients with symptomatic unicompartmental osteoarthritis: a prospective 2-year investigation. *American Journal of Orthopedics*, 31(7), 396–401.

Burton, N.J., Dobney, J.A., Owen, M.R., & Colborne, G.R. (2008) Joint angle, moment and power compensations in dogs with fragmented medial coronoid process. *Veterinary Comparative Orthopedic Traumatology*, 21(2), 110–118.

De Angelis, M.V., Pierfelice, F., Di Giovanni, P., Staniscia, T., & Uncini, A. (2009). Efficacy of a soft hand brace and a wrist splint for carpal tunnel syndrome: a randomized controlled study. *Acta Neurologica Scandinavia*, 119(1), 68–74.

DeCamp, C.E. (1997). Kinetic and kinematic gait analysis and the assessment of lameness in the dog. *Veterinary Clinics of North America: Small Animal Practice*, 27(4), 825–840.

Dennis, D.A., Komistek, R.D., Nadaud, M.C., & Mahfouz, M. (2006) Evaluation of off-loading braces for treatment of unicompartmental knee arthrosis. *Journal of Arthroplasty*, 21(4 Suppl 1), 2–8.

Deshales, L.D. (2002) Upper extremity orthoses, in *Occupational Therapy for Physical Dysfunction*, 5th edn (eds C.A. Trombly & M.V. Radomski), Lippincott, Williams & Wilkins, Baltimore, pp 313–349.

Egan, M., Brosseau, L., Farmer, M., et al. (2003) Splints and Orthosis for treating rheumatoid arthritis. *Cochrane database of systematic reviews*, (1):1469–1493.

Finger, S. & Paulos, L.E (2002) Clinical and biomechanical evaluation of the unloading brace. *Journal of Knee Surgery*, 15(3), 155–159.

Hewett, T.E., Noyes, F.R., Barber-Westin, S.D., & Heckmann, T.P. (1998) Decrease in knee joint pain and increase in function in patients with medial compartment arthrosis: a prospective analysis of valgus bracing. *Orthopedics*, 21(2), 131–138.

Gómez Alvarez, C.B., Wennerstrand, J., Bobbert, M.F., et al. (2007) The effect of induced forelimb lameness on thoracolumbar kinematics during treadmill locomotion. *Equine Veterinary Journal*, 39(3), 197–201.

Gomez Alvarez, C.B., Bobbert, M.F., Lamers, L., Johnston, C., Back, W., & van Weeren, P.R. (2008) The effect of induced hindlimb lameness on thoracolumbar kinematics during treadmill locomotion. *Equine Veterinary Journal*, 40(2), 147–152.

Ibuki, A., Cornoiu, A., Clarke, A., Unglik, R., & Beischer, A. (2010) The effect of orthotic treatment on midfoot osteoarthritis assessed using specifically designed patient evaluation questionnaires. *Prosthetics and orthotics international*, 34(4), 461–471.

Jafarian, F.S., Demneh, E.S, & Tyson, S.F. (2009) The immediate effect of orthotic management on grip strength of patients with lateral epicondylosis. *Journal of Orthopedics Sports and Physical Therapy*, 39(6), 484–489.

Knobloch, K., Schreibmueller, L., Longo, U.G., & Vogt, P.M. (2008) Eccentric exercises for the management of tendinopathy of the main body of the Achilles tendon with or without the AirHeel Brace. A randomized controlled trial. A: effects on pain and microcirculation. *Disability Rehabilitation*, 30(20–22), 1685–1691.

Kruizinga, C.P., Boonstra, A.M., Groothoff, J.W, Elzinga, A., & Göeken, L.N. (2002) Health complaints and disabilities in patients supplied with foot orthoses for degenerative foot disorders. *Prosthetics and Orthotics International*, 26(3), 235–242.

Landman, M.A., de Blaauw, J.A., van Weeren, P.R., & Hofland, L.J. (2004) Field study of the prevalence of lameness in horses with back problems. *Veterinary Record*, 155(6), 165–168.

Melvin, J.L. (1989) *Rheumatic Disease in the Adult and Child: Occupational Therapy and Rehabilitation*. 3rd edn, Davis Publications, Philadelphia.

Mich, P.M., Fair, L., & Borghese, I. (2013) Assistive devices, orthotic, prosthetics, bandaging, in *Canine Sports Medicine and Rehabilitation* (eds M.C. Zink & J.B. VanDyke), Wiley-Blackwell.

Piermattei, D.L., Flo, G.L., & DeCamp, C.E. (2006) Fractures: classification, diagnosis, and treatment, in *Handbook of Small Animal Orthopedics and Fracture Repair*, 4th edn Saunders-Elsevier, St. Louis, MO, pp. 25–159.

Petersen, W., Welp, R., & Rosenbaum, D. (2007) Chronic Achilles tendinopathy: a prospective randomized study comparing the therapeutic effect of eccentric training, the AirHeel brace, and a combination of both. *American Journal of Sports Medicine*, 35(10), 1659–1667.

Pollo, F.E., Otis, J.C., Backus, S.I., Warren, R.F., & Wickiewicz, T.L. (2002) Reduction of medial compartment loads with valgus bracing of the osteoarthritic knee. *American Journal of Sports Medicine*, 30(3), 414–421.

Ramsey, D.K., Briem, K., Axe, M.J., & Snyder-Mackler, L. (2007) A mechanical theory for the effectiveness of bracing for medial compartment osteoarthritis of the knee. *Journal of Bone and Joint Surgery*, 89(11), 2398–2407.

Rao, S., Baumhauer, J.F., Becica, L., & Nawoczenski, D.A. (2009) Shoe inserts alter plantar loading and function in patients with midfoot arthritis. *Journal of Orthopedics and Sports Physical Therapy*, 39(7), 522–531.

Renberg, W.C. (2001) Evaluation of the lame patient. *Veterinary Clinics of North America Small Animal Practice*, 31(1), 1–16.

Seymour, R. (2002). Introduction to prosthetics and orthotics, in *Prosthetics and Orthotics: Lower Limb and Spinal*, Lippincott Williams & Wilkins, Baltimore, pp. 3–35.

Shurr, D.G. & Cook, T.M. (1990) Below knee amputations and prosthetics, in *Prosthetics and Orthotics*, Appleton and Lange, Norwalk, CT, pp. 53–82.

Wada, E., Ebara, S., Saito, S., & Ono, K. (1992) Experimental spondylosis in the rabbit spine. Overuse could accelerate the spondylosis. *Spine*, 17(3 Suppl), S1–S6.

Weishaupt, M.A. (2008) Adaptation strategies of horses with lameness. *Veterinary Clinics of North America Equine Practice*, 24(1), 79–100.

14
Myofascial Pain Syndrome in Dogs

Rick Wall

Myofascial pain syndrome (MPS) in people is defined by Simons et al. (1999), as "...the sensory, motor, and autonomic symptoms caused by myofascial trigger points (MTrPs)." They further define an MTrP as "...a hyperirritable spot in skeletal muscle that is associated with a hypersensitive nodule in a taut band."

Rarely has MPS been discussed or recognized as a cause of pain in dogs, and few articles on the topic exist. Janssens (1991) discussed MTrPs in 48 dogs and in an additional article discussed therapy (Janssens, 1992). Simons and Stolov (1976), in attempting to establish an animal model for research, described palpable bands and contraction knots in the muscles of dogs. Nielsen and Pluhar (2005) briefly mention MTrPs in a review of pelvic limb lameness in dogs; however, they conclude that muscle strain was the cause of myalgia in the 22 patients discussed. To date, Wright (2010) has by far done the best job of describing MTrPs and their possible etiology in the veterinary patient. The relative absence of veterinary literature on the subject necessitates an understanding of myofascial pain and MTrPs in humans, combined with clinical observation and experience in dogs.

CHARACTERISTICS OF MYOFASCIAL TRIGGER POINTS

Myofascial trigger points have sensory, motor, and autonomic nervous system abnormalities. Muscle pain associated with MTrPs is described as diffuse and difficult to localize, and is accompanied by defined referred pain patterns and central and peripheral sensitization. However, when the MTrP is stimulated manually, localized pain is additionally appreciated. In humans and dogs, a sensory response referred to as a "jump sign" is observed during examination and manual stimulation of the MTrP. Referred pain probably exists in dogs with MTrPs; however, this remains difficult, if not impossible, to validate.

Features of the motor abnormality include the development of a taut band within the muscle, a local twitch response (LTR) when stimulated, muscle weakness without atrophy, and loss of reciprocal inhibition (Simons & Stoloff, 1976). Reciprocal inhibition is defined as the contraction of one muscle being inhibited by contraction of its antagonist muscle, and is reduced or absent when the contracted muscle contains an MTrP, potentially impairing fine motor control and coordination.

The taut band is a localized, usually linear, discrete band of hardened muscle that does not have the softer, homogeneous consistency of normal muscle. The taut band can be defined as a localized contracture within the muscle without nerve-initiated activation of the motor endplate or neuromuscular junction (Gerwin et al., 1997). In contrast, muscle spasm is the result of increased neuromuscular tone of the entire muscle, and is due to nerve-initiated contraction. The tender point within the taut band is what distinguishes the MTrP from other painful areas in muscle (Mense & Gerwin, 2010).

Another motor component recognized with MTrPs is the LTR. The LTR is local contraction of the taut band alone, elicited by manual strumming, palpation, or intramuscular stimulation with a needle. An intact spinal cord reflex arc must be present for an LTR to occur and severing the peripheral nerve abolishes the LTR. The LTR differs from the myotatic reflex in that the latter involves contraction of the entire muscle in response to stretch (Simons & Stolov, 1976). The LTR is not to be confused with patient reaction to palpation of an MTrP (the "Jump Sign").

In humans, described autonomic disturbances associated with trigger point activation include changes in skin temperature and color, piloerection, and lacrimation (Mense & Gerwin, 2010).

ETIOLOGY OF MYOFASCIAL TRIGGER POINTS

The mechanisms resulting in the formation of the taut band and MTrPs within the muscle remain unknown; however, ischemia appears to be the dominant factor in their development (Mense, 1997). Capillary compression resulting from forces generated within the taut band is thought to cause local ischemia. The release of vasodilating substances such as calcitonin gene-related peptide (CGRP) and substance P (SP) lead to local noninflammatory edema and further capillary compression and ischemia (Gerwin et al., 1997; Mense, 1997). Several theories exist to explain the etiology of MTrPs.

Integrated Trigger Point Hypothesis—"Energy Crisis"
Simons and Travell (1981) were the first to offer a scientific hypothesis to explain the formation of taut bands based on both electrophysiological and histopathological data. The *Integrated Trigger Point Hypothesis* postulates that muscle injury leads to increased calcium concentrations outside the sarcoplasmic reticulum, possibly due to mechanical rupture of the sarcoplasmic reticulum or

Pain Management in Veterinary Practice, First Edition. Edited by Christine M. Egger, Lydia Love and Tom Doherty.
© 2014 John Wiley & Sons, Inc. Published 2014 by John Wiley & Sons, Inc.

the sarcolemma. Increased calcium concentrations result in sustained muscle fiber contraction. This hypothesis was later refined to include a dysfunctional motor endplate occurring secondary to muscle injury, and resulting in excessive release of acetylcholine (ACh). Sustained maximal contraction of the muscle fibers in the vicinity of the dysfunctional endplate causes increased metabolic demand and decreased concentrations of adenosine triphosphate (ATP). The calcium pump that returns calcium to the sarcoplasmic reticulum is ATP dependent, as is the uncrosslinking of actin and myosin; thus, calcium concentrations and contractile activity remain increased.

Gerwin et al. (2004) further expanded the integrated hypothesis by stating that the most likely cause leading to development of the taut band is altered activity of the motor endplate or neuromuscular junction. Muscle injury alters the normal equilibrium between the release and breakdown of ACh and its removal by acetylcholinesterase from acetylcholine receptors in the postsynaptic membrane. Substances such as CGRP and SP, released during muscle injury, facilitate increased release of ACh, inhibition of breakdown, and upregulation of acetylcholine receptors. A persistent muscle fiber contraction develops leading to the development of the taut band and subsequent MTrP.

Central Modulation—A New Hypothesis

A new hypothesis, proposed by Hocking (2010), to explain the pathogenesis of MTrPs examines the role of the central nervous system and its modulatory mechanisms. Hocking, a practicing veterinarian in Australia, submits that most clinically relevant MTrPs in dogs (those that restrict stride and distort posture) are found in the flexor muscles, in contrast to Gerwin et al.'s (2004) conclusion that taut bands and subsequent MTrPs are the result of a dysfunctional motor endplate. Hocking proposes that their origin is rather a chronic expression of an intrinsic α-motoneuron property: the plateau potential or sustained partial depolarization. α-motoneurons are large lower motor neurons with cell bodies located in the brainstem and spinal cord and whose axons provide motor innervation of skeletal muscles.

Hocking identifies two classifications of MTrPs, "antecedent" MTrPs formed in nociceptive withdrawal reflex agonist muscles, and "consequent" MTrPs formed in nociceptive withdrawal reflex antagonist muscles, generally extensor muscles. Sustained stimulation of peripheral nociceptors and ensuing central sensitization result in persistent efferent α-motoneuron activation of agonist muscles and simultaneous inhibition of antagonist muscles. Facilitation of C fiber withdrawal reflexes, due to central sensitization, predisposes to antecedent MTrPs formation, while consequent MTrPs are proposed to be due to tonic reticulospinal or reticulotrigeminal facilitation or plateau potentials in the α-motoneurons innervating these muscles. Hocking submits that consequent MTrPs develop from changes in patient posture brought about by pain and/or impairment, counteraction of C fiber withdrawal reflex reciprocal inhibition of antagonist muscles, and counteraction of postural changes induced by antecedent MTrPs.

Muscle-related Mechanisms of MTrP Development

Low-level muscle contractions, uneven intramuscular pressure distribution, direct trauma, unaccustomed eccentric contractions, eccentric contraction in unconditioned muscle, and maximal or submaximal concentric contractions can lead to muscle injury and

subsequent development of MTrPs (Gerwin et al., 2004; Dommerholt & Huijbregts, 2011).

LOW-LEVEL MUSCLE CONTRACTIONS

Hagg (2003) postulated that myalgia was related to submaximal repetitive activity resulting in selective overloading of the earliest recruited and last derecruited motor units (Dommerholt & Huijbregts, 2011). This is referred to as the "Cinderella Hypothesis." Muscle forces generated at submaximal levels, also known as low-level muscle contractions, do not allow the recruited smaller type I fibers to rest and, thus, they become overworked. The result is metabolically overloaded muscle units with loss of cellular calcium homeostasis, subsequent activation of autogenic destructive processes, and myalgia. Hocking's (2010) hypothesis describes low-level muscle contractions as a response to C fiber nociceptor input.

UNEVEN INTRAMUSCULAR PRESSURE DISTRIBUTION

Otten (1988) confirmed, based on mathematical modeling applied to a frog gastrocnemius muscle, that during static low-level muscle contractions capillary pressures increase dramatically, especially near the muscle insertions. Increased intramuscular pressures lead to excessive capillary pressure, decreased circulation, ischemia, and hypoxia. The pathological changes brought about by increased pressure could lead to the formation of MTrPs and support Simon and Travell's *Integrated Trigger Point Hypothesis*.

DIRECT TRAUMA

Direct trauma to the muscle and muscle fibers may generate injury to the sarcoplasmic reticulum and/or the sarcolemma resulting in increased calcium concentrations, sustained contraction, and development of taut bands.

ECCENTRIC AND (SUB) MAXIMAL CONCENTRIC CONTRACTIONS

Eccentric muscle contraction is defined as muscle lengthening under tension. Eccentric muscle contraction is defined as muscle lengthening under tension, as opposed to concentric muscle contraction, during which the muscle shortens. Numerous studies in people indicate that mechanisms applicable to the development of MTrPs occur with muscle damage from eccentric exercise, exercise in unconditioned muscle, or maximal or submaximal concentric exercise (Gerwin et al., 2004; Dommerholt et al., 2006; Dommerholt & Huijbregts, 2011). Steiss and Levine (2005) suggests that eccentric contractions may be an explanation for muscle damage in the canine athlete. Muscle damage linked to these types of contractions is due to contraction-induced capillary constrictions, hypoperfusion, ischemia, and hypoxia. These changes result in a local acidic environment, release of protons (H^+), potassium ions (K^+), CGRP, bradykinin (BK), and SP, leading to activation of muscle nociceptors (Gerwin et al., 2004; Dommerholt & Huijbregts, 2011).

PAIN INITIATION IN MYOFASCIAL PAIN SYNDROME

The inflammatory model of muscle pain has been well studied, but no models of inflammation-induced MTrPs are known (Mense & Gerwin, 2010). Serum creatine phosphokinase (CPK) is not increased, thus global muscle inflammation does not appear to play a role in MTrP development. However, the ultrastructural muscle fiber derangements brought about by the aberrant muscle contractions result in profound biochemical changes localized at the trigger point zone including: decreased pH and increased concentrations of BK, CGRP, SP, tumor necrosis factor-α (TNF-α), interleukin-1β (IL-1β), serotonin, and norepinephrine (Shah et al., 2005). Substance P and CGRP are primarily produced in the dorsal root ganglion and transmitted antidromically down the neural process. The increased release of these substances results in prolonged nociceptive activation (Shah et al., 2008).

PERPETUATING FACTORS IN MYOFASCIAL PAIN

Gerwin states in the fourth chapter of *Travell and Simons' Myofascial Pain and Dysfunction*, "the clinical importance of factors that perpetuate myofascial trigger points is generally underestimated." The clinician must be acutely aware of perpetuating factors and how they affect the development of MTrPs. Gerwin also states "attention to perpetuating factors often spells the difference between successful and failed therapy."

Mechanical Stresses

Mechanical stresses are by far the most common perpetuating factors for MTrPs in dogs. Acute traumatic events may activate MTrPs, but are not responsible for perpetuating them. Sudden activation of MTrPs may occur after acute muscle strain, joint strain, fractures, direct muscle trauma, or excessive or unusual exercise. Such MTrPs are generally easy to treat once the soft tissue injury has healed. More commonly in dogs, MTrPs are both activated and perpetuated by chronic muscle overload. Postural changes in the dog resulting from orthopedic injury, postoperative surgical trauma and pain, neuropathy, joint dysfunction, and pain related to osteoarthritis create muscle overload. Many of the same muscle-related mechanisms that lead to the development of MTrPs also maintain them.

A canine patient with chronic osteoarthritis has compensatory postural changes that activate and perpetuate MTrPs in numerous muscles. Moderate to severe osteoarthritis of the coxofemoral joints activates and perpetuates MTrPs in the functional unit muscles of the coxofemoral joint, mainly flexors (including iliopsoas) and adductors. The cranial shift in weight overloads muscles in the thoracic limbs, namely the m. infraspinatus, m. deltoideus, and the long head of the m. triceps brachii. Repeated lateral flexion of the spine, which assists in ambulation by advancing the pelvis and pelvic limb while limiting coxofemoral flexion and extension, results in overloading of the miliocostalis lumborum. A dog with a non-weight-bearing pelvic limb adopts hopping actions during ambulation of the weight-bearing limb, and this results in unaccustomed eccentric contractions of the coxofemoral and stifle extensors in an attempt to limit flexion. Lumbar paraspinal muscles become overloaded, as they must now assist with ambulation in addition to spinal stabilization. The m. iliopsoas, which is actually two separate muscles, the m. psoas major and m. iliacus that join shortly before their insertion on the medial proximal femur, develops MTrPs, becomes shorter in length, and kyphosis can develop.

Nutritional Factors

In humans, deficiencies of vitamin B_{12} (cobalamin) and folic acid have been described as perpetuating factors for MPS (Simons et al., 1999; Mense & Gerwin, 2010; Dommerholt & Huijbregts, 2011). There are no references in the veterinary literature pertaining to

deficiencies of these substances causing pain of any type; however, cobalamin deficiency causes malaise and failure to thrive. Both substances currently have clinical application as markers for small bowel disease and the Gastrointestinal Laboratory at Texas A&M University offers assays for each. Cobalamin deficiency in the dog can occur with exocrine pancreatic insufficiency.

Iron insufficiency has been identified as a perpetuating factor for MTrPs in people; however, the relationship between the two is not clearly understood. In dogs, iron deficiency is recognized as a cause of anemia, and may be due to inadequate intake, malabsorption, and/or iron loss via chronic hemorrhage (Shell, 2006). The relationship of iron deficiency to MTrPs in animals is unknown.

Metabolic Factors

Hypothyroidism is the most common endocrine disorder in dogs, and is associated with a variety of clinical signs; however, the veterinary literature does not mention pain as a consequence of hypothyroidism. In humans, muscle pain, stiffness, weakness, and cramps and pain on exertion are reported with hypothyroidism (Simons et al., 1999).

Nerve Impingement

In people, peripheral nerve entrapments and radiculopathies can result in the development and perpetuation of MTrPs. Myofascial trigger points tend to be formed in the muscles of the extremities innervated by nerves arising at the same spinal cord segment as the entrapped nerve. This could be a potential cause of MTrPs in animals.

Visceral–somatic Pain Representations

Gerwin (2002) states that visceral pain can activate and perpetuate MTrPs in the area of referred pain. Neurons in the dorsal horn of the spinal cord receive input from the viscera and from receptors in the skin and deeper soft tissues. As a result of this overlap, visceral nociceptive activation of the dorsal horn neurons may result in muscle pain, and may be a cause of MTrPs in animals. Visceral disease should be ruled out when MTrPs are found.

DIAGNOSIS OF MTrPS

Manual Identification of MTrPs

Due to the lack of objective laboratory or diagnostic imaging techniques to confirm the existence of MTrPs, a diagnosis based upon palpation has been questioned frequently in the medical literature. However, Gerwin et al. (1997) and Bron et al. (2007) demonstrated good interindividual reliability of palpation skills for locating MTrPs. Currently, clinical examination with palpation is the only method of diagnosis in veterinary patients. Palpation skills require initial expert guidance and instruction followed by frequent clinical application.

An excellent knowledge of anatomy is required, as well as an understanding of the actions of each muscle to be examined. Clinical knowledge of "functional muscle units," defined as a unit of muscles that exercise action upon a given joint or joints, is critical. Muscle dysfunction leads to joint dysfunction and vice versa. When muscle dysfunction occurs MTrPs can develop (Dommerholt & Huijbregts, 2011).

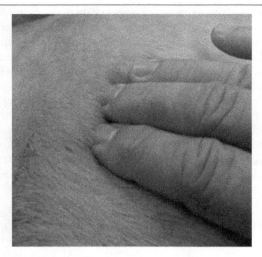

Figure 14.1. Flat palpation—examination with finger pressure across muscle fibers while compressing against firm underlying structure such as bone.

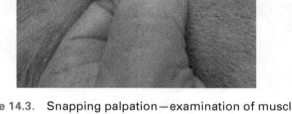

Figure 14.3. Snapping palpation—examination of muscle by pincer grasp while rapidly drawing back and rolling muscle fibers under fingers.

Clinical (Myofascial) Examination

There are three basic palpation techniques employed in a myofascial examination as defined by Simons and Travell (1999).

Flat Palpation: Examination by finger pressure that proceeds across the muscle fibers at a right angle to their length while compressing them against a firm underlying structure, such as a bone. This technique could be used for the m. infraspinatus (Figure 14.1).

Pincer Palpation: Examination of a part of a muscle by holding it in a pincer grasp between the thumb and fingers. Groups of muscle fibers are rolled between the tips of the digits to detect taut bands. This technique could be used for the m. triceps, m. sartorius, and m. tensor fascia latae (Figure 14.2).

Snapping Palpation: A fingertip is placed against the tense band of muscle at right angles to the direction of the band, and suddenly

pressed down while the examiner draws the finger back, rolling the underlying fibers under the finger. The motion is similar to that used to pluck a guitar string, except that the finger does not slide over the skin but moves the skin with it. To most effectively elicit an LTR, the taut band is palpated and snapped at the MTrP, with the muscle positioned to eliminate slack (Figure 14.3). Snapping palpation can be performed on the same muscles described for pincer palpation.

The patient can be examined in either the standing position or in lateral recumbency. However, taut bands are easier to appreciate in the recumbent patient with the muscle in a more relaxed state. In each position, an assistant is needed to provide gentle patient restraint, because examination can induce a jump sign. Education of the client prior to the myofascial examination is needed to avoid concern when pain is elicited.

Palpation of a muscle containing a taut band reveals a discrete hardness of the muscle in the area of the band. The taut band will parallel the direction of the muscle fibers and, when located, its length is examined to locate the hyperirritable MTrP. Patient response to palpation aids in localization of the MTrP rather than appreciation of a knot or swelling.

Simons et al. (1999) define the jump sign in people as "a general pain response of the patient who winces, may cry out, and may withdraw in response to pressure applied on the trigger point." This definition also applies to canine patients that show varying degrees of withdrawal or wincing but less commonly vocalize. Adequate digital pressure is needed to localize the taut band and MTrP; however, pressure must not be excessive in order to avoid generating significant patient reaction not due to localization of MTrPs. The jump sign is not to be confused with the LTR. In the canine patient, the LTR is rarely observed during examination as factors such as hair coat and muscle location limit observation.

In people, MTrPs are classified as either "active" or "latent." Active MTrPs produce pain spontaneously, whereas the latent MTrP produces pain only with stimulation. Other than the clinical presence of pain, the two types of MTrPs are similar in that they both cause muscle weakness and reduced range of motion. In the canine

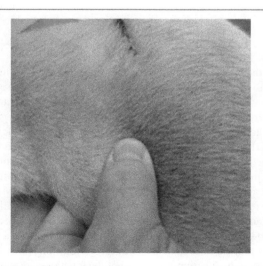

Figure 14.2. Pincer palpation—examination of muscle by holding it in a pincer grasp between thumb and fingers.

patient, it is impossible to determine which MTrPs are active or latent. Hocking (2010) states that in dogs, "all MTrPs feel similar, palpation elicits similar pain reactions, and appropriate stimulation induces a similar local twitch response."

Objective Criteria for Diagnosis of MTrPs

No objective criteria exist that can validate the clinical criteria used to diagnose MTrPs (Mense & Gerwin, 2010). However, recent advances in ultrasound and magnetic resonance imaging of MTrPs may have clinical application in human and veterinary patients (Sikdar et al., 2009; Chen et al., 2010).

TREATMENT OF MTrPS

Treatment of MTrPs in dogs consists of noninvasive and invasive therapies. Currently, there are no studies to validate the effectiveness of any therapy in dogs, and reported results remain strictly anecdotal. In people, numerous studies exist regarding noninvasive and invasive MTrP therapy; however, in many the diagnosis of MPS may lack validity. Tough et al. (2007), after an extensive literature review, reported variability in criteria used to diagnose MPS and MTrPs in people.

Noninvasive MTrP Therapy

THERAPEUTIC LASERS
Currently, lasers are a popular modality for the treatment of pain in the veterinary patient. Class IIIa (3a) lasers provide a maximum output power of 5 milliwatts (mW), Class IIIb lasers provide output power up to 500 mW, and Class IV lasers provide output power greater than 500 mW, and one currently marketed veterinary model claims a maximum output power of 15 W. The amount of laser energy delivered during a treatment session is reported in Joules (J), and one Joule is equal to 1 W/s. The dose is reported as the energy per session in Joules divided by the area (cm^2) where the energy is directed; therefore, the therapeutic laser dose is indicated in J/cm^2.

Studies regarding myofascial pain and MTrPs in people are limited to Class III lasers. This is due, in part, to the inability to calculate an accurate therapeutic dose when using a Class IV laser. Class IV lasers cannot be directly focused on a defined area due to the risk of thermal injury, and must be constantly moved over a region during treatment.

Treatment with Class IIIa and Class IIIb lasers is more commonly referred to in the literature as low-level laser therapy (LLT). LLT has been widely used in the treatment of MTrPs in people. Several double-blind placebo-controlled studies report positive effects of LLT on MTrPs (Hakguder et al., 2003; Gur et al., 2004; Ilbuldu et al., 2004). However, other studies report no therapeutic benefit (Altan et al., 2005; Dundar et al., 2007). Proper therapeutic dosages for treatment are not known, and conflicting information exists in humans and in animal models. Hakguder et al. (2003) suggested that inadequate dosage may be the cause of the unpredictability in the reported efficacy of laser therapy. However, Gur et al. (2004) reported efficacy with a lower dosage, and in a recently published paper using the rabbit as an animal model, Chen et al. (2010) reported better treatment outcomes with energy of 5.4 J per session versus 14.4 J per session.

ELECTROTHERAPIES
Several references exist that discuss the use of transcutaneous electrical nerve stimulation (TENS) in the management of pain in dogs; however, no specific mention of its use in myofascial pain was found (Steiss & Levine, 2005; Mlacnik et al., 2006; Canapp, 2007). Hou et al. (2002) reported that TENS combined with other physical modalities appeared to have an immediate effect with regard to decreasing myofascial pain in people. However, Dommerholt and Huijbregts (2011) concluded that insufficient evidence is available to determine the effectiveness of TENS in myofascial pain.

THERAPEUTIC ULTRASOUND
In a randomized controlled study, Aguilera et al. (2009) reported an immediate reduction in MTrP sensitivity with therapeutic ultrasound in humans. Draper et al (2010) used therapeutic ultrasound to decrease stiffness of latent MTrPs in the m. trapezius in humans. In that study, a 3 mHz therapeutic ultrasound was used at 1.4 W/cm^2 for 5 minutes in a circular motion on an area twice the size of the 7 cm^2 ultrasound head. In contrast, previous studies by Gam et al. (1998) and Lee et al. (1997) reported that therapeutic ultrasound was no more effective than placebo. Gam et al. (1998) surveyed patients up to 6 months after treatment by means of a patient questionnaire, and the studies reporting benefits from therapeutic ultrasound were based on immediate response only.

PHYSICAL/MANUAL THERAPIES
Mense and Gerwin (2010) concluded that data are either inadequate or conflicting regarding most manual therapies for treatment of MPS. Dommerholt and Huijbregts (2011), referring to physical and manual therapies, state that current evidence did not exceed the moderate level. They additionally assert that most trials examined multimodal treatment programs, so positive effects cannot exclusively be credited to a particular therapy.

Ischemic compression, also known as trigger point pressure release, is a commonly described manual therapy for the treatment of MTrPs in humans. Studies in humans show that ischemic compression may be of benefit in treatment of MTrPs associated with shoulder pain, neck pain, headaches, and carpal tunnel syndrome (Hou et al., 2002; Hains et al., 2010a, 2010b; Montanez-Aguilera et al., 2010). Numerous descriptions of the technique can be found in the academic medical literature as well as in the lay literature regarding massage therapy. Digital compression of the MTrP for 60–90 seconds with increasing pressure is the most commonly described method. In dogs the taut band is identified and examined for the exquisitely tender MTrP, then digital pressure is applied to the point of patient recognition. After 15–20 seconds, pressure may gradually be increased in most patients. Providing a gentle stretch to the muscle while applying pressure may assist in release of the MTrP.

Invasive MTrP Therapy
Several types of invasive MTrP therapy have been described in people, including trigger point dry needling with an acupuncture needle and MTrP injections with local anesthetics and other substances. In the author's experience, trigger point injection is not well accepted by many canine patients compared with dry needling. A hypodermic needle is much larger than an acupuncture needle, and the injection of lidocaine is painful, possibly explaining canine objection to this technique. Numerous substances have been used in trigger point

injections in people. Local anesthetics, corticosteroids, and vitamin B_{12} are most commonly described. Iwama and Akama (2000), in a randomized, double-blinded trial, reported a water-diluted 1% lidocaine mixture (1:3) resulted in better efficacy and less pain on injection. Iwama et al. (2001) later determined that water-diluted 0.25% lidocaine and water-diluted 0.25% mepivacaine were less painful on injection than saline-diluted 0.25% lidocaine and water-diluted 0.25% bupivacaine. The study additionally concluded that water-diluted (1:3) concentrations of 0.2–0.25% lidocaine or mepivacaine were the most effective dilutions for trigger point injections.

Confusion exists in the literature as to what constitutes myofascial trigger point dry needling. Myofascial trigger point dry needling is the insertion of an acupuncture needle into an MTrP within a taut band identified during clinical examination. It is not the insertion of a needle into a traditional acupuncture point, superficially over an MTrP, or into a prespecified location.

A systematic review of the literature by Furlan et al. (2005) suggested that myofascial trigger point dry needling appeared to be a useful adjunct to other therapies for lower back pain in humans. A more recent review and meta-analysis by Tough et al. (2009) concluded that there was at least limited evidence that supported the efficacy of myofascial trigger point dry needling in humans; however, the reviewers commented that additional studies are needed. In more recent studies in humans, Fernandez-Carnero et al. (2010) showed dry needling of MTrPs in the m. masseter to be effective in the treatment of myofascial temporomandibular disorders. Srbely et al. (2010) demonstrated short-term antinociceptive effects using dry needling of MTrPs. This effect was limited to muscles innervated by the same spinal cord segment. When an MTrP in the m. infraspinatus was needled, pain thresholds to pressure were increased in MTrPs in the m. supraspinatus (segments C5 and C6) while no change in pain threshold to pressure was found in MTrPs in the m. gluteus medius (segments L4, L5, and S1). Tsai et al. (2010) demonstrated that pressure point thresholds in active MTrPs located in the upper m. trapezius were increased with dry needling of MTrPs located in the m. extensor carpi radialis longus. Improvement in the range of motion of the neck was an additional finding. Osborne and Gatt (2010) were able to manage pain and improve the active joint range of motion (ROM) in acute shoulder injury during intense competition by performing dry needling of MTrPs in the scapulohumeral muscles of elite female athletes.

The clinician who undertakes invasive therapy for the treatment of MTrPs needs not only a thorough knowledge of anatomy, but also must develop the kinesthetic skills to accurately place the needle into the MTrP. Employing the examination techniques previously described, the taut band is identified and its length examined to localize the MTrP. The acupuncture needle (Seirin J Type No. 5 [0.25] with insertion tube) is rapidly inserted, with the aid of the insertion tube, into the superficial tissues and then directed into the deep tissues and muscle to the taut band (Figure 14.4). An appreciation of an increase in resistance as the needle enters the taut band develops with experience. If needle placement is accurate, a LTR may be appreciated in the taut band (Figure 14.5). The needle is moved in and out of the MTrP, slowly, until no further LTRs are appreciated. In dogs, the LTR confirms the presence of an MTrP, but does not distinguish between an active MTrP and a latent MTrP.

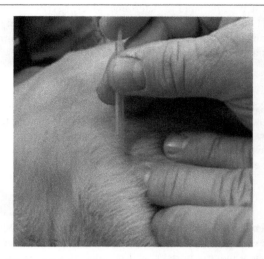

Figure 14.4. The taut band is identified and its length examined to localize the MTrP. The acupuncture needle (Seirin J Type No. 5 [0.25] with insertion tube) is rapidly inserted, with the aid of the insertion tube, into the superficial tissues and then directed into the deep tissues and muscle to the taut band.

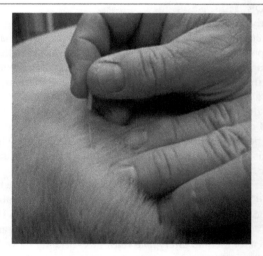

Figure 14.5. An increase in resistance, as the needle enters the taut band, is expected. If needle placement is accurate, an LTR may be appreciated in the taut band. The needle is moved in and out of the MTrP, slowly, until no further LTRs are appreciated.

Two landmark studies by Shah et al. (2005; 2008) have helped to validate invasive MTrP dry needling and the therapeutic importance of the LTR. After induction of the LTR by the needle entering the MTrP, local concentrations of biochemical mediators such as SP and CGRP decreased. This may explain the observed decrease in pain in people after release of the MTrP. In the later study, not only were there similarities in the biochemical milieu of the active MTrPs, but increased concentrations of analytes were found in remote muscle sites that did not contain MTrPs. Study participants with active MTrPs in the m. trapezius had increased concentrations of inflammatory mediators, neuropeptides, catecholamines, and cytokines in the m. gastrocnemius, which did not contain MTrPs. The cause of this is not completely understood, however, it could be related to central sensitization. There is also the possibility that widespread release of these analytes is a precursor to the development of MTrPs. Both studies offer explanations of the proposed therapeutic benefits of invasive therapeutic intervention and the secondary hyperalgesia that is often present in people with MPS.

TRIGGER POINT DRY NEEDLING VERSUS ACUPUNCTURE

In the small body of literature regarding MTrPs in veterinary medicine there has often been a flawed attempt to relate MTrPs to acupuncture points (Janssens, 1991; Janssens, 1992; Wright, 2010). Melzack et al. (1977) published a review examining the possible correspondence of acupuncture points and MTrPs for the treatment of pain. They concluded that there was a 71% correlation, and that MTrP and acupuncture points "represent the same phenomenon." Birch (2003), a well-known acupuncturist, conducted a thorough study of current literature and concluded that Melzack's study had had a profound impact, particularly on the further development of the theoretical knowledge regarding acupuncture for pain and treatment of MTrPs. Birch noted that 60% of the acupuncture points identified in Melzack's study are not routinely used for the treatment of pain, 47% of the points are not recommended for anything, 18% are commonly recommended for the treatment of pain, and 16% are recommended for any ailment. Melzack also made the flawed assumption that MTrPs had fixed anatomical locations, making comparisons to charts of classical acupuncture points reasonable. However, it should be understood that MTrPs could occur in any part of the muscle. Birch concluded that there may be some overlap in the location of acupuncture points and MTrPs, but it is likely to be coincidental, and such similarity of location does not imply a correlation. His findings suggested that if MTrPs had any correlation with acupuncture points it would be "Ah-Shi" points rather than the "channel/meridian" or "extra" points that Melzack studied. "Ah-Shi" points are defined as sensitive nonspecific acupuncture points.

INTRAMUSCULAR ELECTRICAL STIMULATION

Electrical stimulation is easily introduced into the MTrP through the acupuncture needle. In addition to the term intramuscular electrical stimulation (IES), several other descriptive names are used in the literature including percutaneous electrical nerve stimulation (PENS), percutaneous electrical muscle stimulation (PEMS), percutaneous neuromodulation therapy, and electroacupuncture (EA). The negative electrode is usually placed in the MTrP and the positive in the taut band outside of the MTrP (Dommerholt & Huijbregts, 2011). Frequencies between 2–4 Hz with high intensity are commonly used. Lee et al. (2008) demonstrated positive effects on MTrPs in people using a frequency of 2 Hz and an intensity that kept muscular contraction visible. Total application durations were 3 minutes for each MTrP. The induced muscle contraction may simulate the LTR.

A recent clinical study by Pérez-Palomares et al. (2010) compared MTrP dry needling to PEMS in 122 people suffering from nonspecific chronic lower back pain. The study results showed both techniques to be equally effective in the short term.

SUMMARY

This chapter included a brief review of the history of MTrP therapy, the characteristics of the MTrP, and current hypotheses explaining how the taut band and the MTrP develop. Examination techniques were described to assist clinicians in determining the causes of myalgia in their patients. The importance of perpetuating factors was stressed to aid clinicians in the treatment and prevention of myofascial pain. Exploration of the biochemical milieu of the MTrP, and the changes brought about by invasive therapy, verify the immediate benefits of MTrP needling.

Clinical studies in people are accumulating and they appear to validate the importance of myofascial pain in chronic pain syndromes. Information from these studies has application in veterinary medicine, and provides us with a foundation of knowledge to apply to the canine patient; however, clinical studies in dogs are needed to form evidence-based therapeutic recommendations.

REFERENCES

Aguilera, F.J., Martin, D.P., Masanet, R.A., Botella, A.C., Soler, L.B., & Morell, F.B. (2009) Immediate effect of ultrasound and ischemic compression techniques for the treatment of trapezius latent myofascial trigger points in healthy subjects: a randomized controlled study. *Journal of Manipulative Physiology and Therapy*, 32(7), 515–520.

Altan, L., Bingol, U., Aykac, M., & Yurtkuran, M. (2005) Investigation of the effect of GaAs laser therapy on cervical myofascial pain syndrome. *Rheumatology International*, 25(1), 23–27.

Birch, S. (2003) Trigger point-acupuncture point correlations revisited. *Journal of Alternative and Complementary Medicine*, 9(1), 91–103.

Bron, C., Franssen, J., Wensing, M., & Oostendorp, R.A. (2007) Interrater reliability of palpation of myofascial trigger points in three shoulder muscles. *Journal of Manual and Manipulative Therapy*, 15(4), 203–215.

Canapp, D.A. (2007) Select modalities. *Clinical Techniques in Small Animal Practice*, 22(4), 160–165.

Chen, K.H., Hong, C., Hsu, H., Shyi-Kuen, W., Fang-Chuan, K., & Yueh-Ling, H. (2010) Dose-dependent and ceiling effects of therapeutic laser on myofascial trigger spots in rabbit skeletal muscles. *Journal of Musculoskeletal Pain*, 18(3), 235–245.

Dommerholt, J., Bron, C., & Franssen, J. (2006) Myofascial trigger points: an evidence-informed review. *Journal of Manual and Manipulative Therapy*, 14(4), 203–221.

Dommerholt, J. & Huijbregts, P. (2011) *Myofascial Trigger Points—Pathophysiology and Evidence-Informed Diagnosis and Management*, Jones and Bartlett Publishers, Sudbury, MA.

Draper, D.O., Mahaffey, C., Kaiser, D., Eggett, D., & Jarmin, J. (2010) Thermal ultrasound decreases tissue stiffness of trigger points in upper trapezius muscles. *Physiotherapy Theory and Practice*, 26(3), 167–172.

Dundar, U., Eveik, D., Samili, F., Pusak, H., & Kavuncu, V. (2007) The effect of gallium arsenide aluminum laser therapy in the management of cervical myofascial pain syndrome: a double blind, placebo-controlled study. *Clinical Rheumatology*, 26(6), 930–934.

Fernandez-Carnero, J., La Touche, R., Ortega-Santiago, R, et al. (2010) Short-term effects of dry needling of active myofascial trigger points in the masseter muscle in patients with temporomandibular disorders. *Journal of Orofacial Pain*, 24(1), 106–112.

Furlan, A.D., van Tulder, M., Cherkin, D., et al. (2005) Acupuncture and dry needling for low back pain: an updated systemic review within the framework of the cochrane collaboration. *Spine*, 30(8), 944–963.

Gam, A.N., Warming, S., Larsen, L.E., et al. (1998) Treatment of myofascial trigger-points with ultrasound combined with massage and exercise—a randomized controlled trial. *Pain*, 77(1), 73–79.

Gerwin, R.D., Shannon, S., Hong, C.Z., Hubbard, D., & Gevirtz, R. (1997) Interrater reliability in myofascial trigger point examination. *Pain*, 69(1–2), 65–73.

Gerwin, R.D. (2002) Myofascial and visceral pain syndromes: visceral-somatic pain representations. *Journal of Musculoskeletal Pain*, 10(1–2), 165–175.

Gerwin, R.D., Dommerholt, J., & Shah, J.P. (2004) An expansion of Simons' integrated hypothesis of trigger point formation. *Current Pain and Headache Reports*, 8(6), 468–475.

Gur, A., Sarac, A.J., Cevik, R., Altindag, O., & Sarac, S. (2004) Efficacy of 904nm gallium arsenide low-level laser therapy in the management of pain in the neck: a double-blind and randomized-controlled trial. *Lasers in Surgery and Medicine*, 35(3), 229–235.

Hagg, G.M. (2003) The cinderella hypothesis, in *Chronic Work-Related Myalgia* (eds H. Johansson), Gavle University Press, Gavle, Sweden, pp. 127–132.

Hains, G., Descarreaux, M., & Hains, F. (2010a) Chronic Shoulder pain of myofascial origin: a randomized clinical trial using ischemic compression therapy. *Journal of Manipulative and Physiological Therapy*, 33(5), 362–369.

Hains, G., Descarreaux, M., Lamy, A.M., & Hains, F. (2010b) A randomized controlled (intervention) trial of ischemic compression therapy for chronic carpal tunnel syndrome. *Journal of the Canadian Chiropractic Association*, 54(3), 155–163.

Hakguder, A., Birtane, M., Gurcan, S., Kokino, S., & Turan, F.N. (2003) Efficacy of low level laser therapy in myofascial pain syndrome: an algometric and thermographic evaluation. *Lasers in Surgery and Medicine*, 33(5), 339–343.

Hocking, M. (2010) Trigger points and central modulation – A new hypothesis. *Journal of Musculoskeletal Pain*, 18(2), 186–203.

Hou, C.R., Tsai, L.C., Cheng, K.F., Chung, K.C., & Hong, C.Z. (2002) Immediate effects of various physical therapeutic modalities on cervical myofascial pain and trigger-point sensitivity. *Archives of Physical Medicine and Rehabilitation*, 83(10), 1406–1414.

Ilbuldu, E., Cakmak, A., Disci, R., & Aydin, R. (2004) Comparison of laser, dry needling, and placebo laser treatments in myofascial pain syndrome. *Photomedicine and Laser Surgery*, 22(4), 306–311.

Iwama, H. & Akama, Y. (2000) The superiority of water-diluted 0.25% to neat 1% lidocaine for trigger-point injections in myofascial pain syndrome: a prospective, randomized, double-blinded trial. *Anesthesia and Analgesia*, 91(2), 408–409.

Iwama, H., Ohmori, S., Kaneko, T., & Watanabe, K. (2001) Water-diluted local anesthetic for trigger-point injection in chronic myofascial pain syndrome: evaluation of types of local anesthetic and concentrations in water. *Regional Anesthesia and Pain Medicine*, 26(4), 333–336.

Janssens, L.A. (1991) Trigger points in 48 dogs with myofascial pain syndromes. *Veterinary Surgery*, 20(4), 274–278.

Janssens, L.A. (1992) Trigger point therapy. *Problems in Veterinary Medicine*, 4(1), 117–124.

Lee, J.C., Lin, D.T., & Hong, C. (1997) The effectiveness of simultaneous thermotherapy with ultrasound and electrotherapy with combined AC and DC current on the immediate pain relief of myofascial trigger points. *Journal of Musculoskeletal Pain*, 5(1), 81–90.

Lee, S.H., Chen, C.C., Lee, C.S., Lin, T.C., & Chan, R.C. (2008) Effects of needle electrical intramuscular stimulation on shoulder and cervical myofascial pain syndrome and microcirculation. *Journal of the Chinese Medical Association*, 7(4), 200–206.

Melzack, R., Stillwell, D.M., & Fox, E.J. (1977) Trigger points and acupuncture points for pain: correlations and implications. *Pain*, 3(1), 3–23.

Mense, S. (1997) Pathophysiologic basis of muscle pain syndromes, in *Myofascial Pain Update in Diagnosis and Treatment* (ed. A.A. Fischer), W.B. Saunders Company, Philadelphia, PA, pp. 23–53.

Mense, S. & Gerwin, R.D. (2010) *Muscle Pain: Diagnosis and Treatment*, Springer-Verlag, Berlin Heidelberg, Berlin, Germany.

Mlacnik, E., Bockstahler, B., Muller, M., Tetrick, M.A., Nap, R.C., & Zentek, J. (2006) Effect of caloric restriction and moderate or intense physiotherapy program for treatment of lameness in overweight dogs with osteoarthritis. *Journal of the American Veterinary Medical Association*, 229(11), 1756–1760.

Montanez-Aguilera, F.J., Valtuena-Gimeno, N., Pecos-Martin, D., Arnau-Masanet, R., Barrios-Pitarque, C., & Bosch-Morell, F. (2010) Changes in a patient with neck pain after application of ischemic compression as a trigger point therapy. *Journal of Back and Musculoskeletal Rehabilitation*, 23(2), 101–104.

Nielsen, C. & Pluhar, G.E. (2005) Diagnosis and treatment of hind limb muscle strain injuries in 22 dogs. *Veterinary Comparative Orthopedics and Traumatology*, 18(4), 247–253.

Osborne, N.J. & Gatt, I.T. (2010) Management of shoulder injuries using dry needling in elite volleyball players. *Acupuncture Medicine*, 28(1), 42–45.

Otten, E. (1988) Concepts and models of functional architecture in skeletal muscle. *Exercise and Sports Sciences Review*, 16, 89–137.

Pérez-Palomares, S., Oliván-Blázuez, B., Magallón-Botaya, R., et al. (2010) Percutaneous electrical nerve stimulation versus dry needling: effectiveness in the treatment of chronic low back pain. *Journal of Musculoskeletal Pain*, 18(1), 23–30.

Shah, J.P., Phillips, T.M., Danoff, J.V., & Gerber, L.H. (2005) An in vivo microanalytical technique for measuring the local biochemical milieu of human skeletal muscle. *Journal of Applied Physiology*, 99(5), 1977–1984.

Shah, J.P., Danoff, J.V., Desai, M.J., et al. (2008) Biochemicals associated with pain and inflammation are elevated in sites near to and remote from active myofascial trigger points. *Archives of Physical Medicine and Rehabilitation*, 89(1), 16–23.

Shell, L. (2006) *Iron Deficiency Anemia*. Veterinary Information Network.

Sikdar, S., Shah, J.P., Gebreab, T., et al. (2009) Novel applications of ultrasound technology to visualize and characterize myofascial trigger points and surrounding soft tissue. *Archives of Physical Medicine and Rehabilitation*, 90(11), 1829–1838.

Simons, D.G. & Stolov, W.C. (1976) Microscopic features and transient contraction of palpable bands in canine muscle. *American Journal of Physical Medicine*, 55(2), 65–88.

Simons, D.G. & Travell, J.G. (1981) Myofascial trigger points, a possible explanation. *Pain*, 10(1), 106–109.

Simons, D.G., Travell, J.G., & Simons, L.S. (1999) *Travell and Simons' Myofascial Pain and Dysfunction: The Trigger Point Manual. Volume 1: Upper Half of Body*, 2nd edn, Williams & Wilkins, Baltimore, MD.

Srbely, J.Z., Dickey, J.P., Lee, D., & Lowerison, M. (2010) Dry needle stimulation of myofascial trigger points evokes segmental antinociceptive effects. *Journal of Rehabilitation Medicine*, 42(5), 463–468.

Steiss, J.E. & Levine, D. (2005) Physical agent modalities. *Veterinary Clinics of North America: Small Animal Practice*, 35(6), 1317–1333.

Tough, E.A., White, A.R., Richards, S., & Campbell, J. (2007) Variability of criteria used to diagnose myofascial trigger point pain syndrome–evidence from a review of the literature. *Clinical Journal of Pain*, 23(3), 278–286.

Tough, E.A., White, A.R., Cummings, T.M., Richards, S.H., & Campbell, J.L. (2009) Acupuncture and dry needling in the management of myofascial trigger point pain: a systematic review and meta-analysis

of randomized controlled trials. *European Journal of Pain*, 13(1), 3–10.

Tsai, C.T., Hsieh, L.F., Kuan, T.S., Kao, M.J., Chou, L.W., & Hong, C.Z. (2010) Remote effects of dry needling on the irritability of the myofascial trigger point in the upper trapezius muscle. *American Journal of Physical Medicine and Rehabilitation*, 89(2), 133–140.

Wright, B. (2010) Management of chronic soft tissue pain. *Topics in Companion Animal Medicine*, 25(1), 26–31.

15
Traditional Chinese Herbal Medicine and Homeopathy in Pain Management

Lynelle Graham, Mona Boudreaux, and Steve Marsden

Complementary or alternative medicine pain management techniques, used alone or integrated into Western medicine-based protocols, include, but are not limited to acupuncture, herbal medicine, homeopathic remedies, chiropractic, and massage. Complementary methods may provide analgesia with fewer adverse effects, and may contribute to multimodal analgesia (Peilin, 2008). In fact, the integration of complementary therapies may allow for more comprehensive patient care and improved quality of life (Xie, 2005; Zareba, 2009).

The mechanisms underlying traditional Chinese medicine (TCM) methods, such as acupuncture and herbal medicine, can be approached from many angles. A biomedical approach stresses Westernized, scientific principles and evidence-based medicine. Others view the clinical application of these methods from a TCM perspective, which some regard as more holistic, because in addition to history, physical examination, and past responses to therapies, the patient's emotional state, home environment, diet, and other factors are considered. From a TCM perspective, the function of each organ is intimately related to the function of other organs; thus, the interaction of the organ systems is also considered when making a diagnosis and developing a treatment plan. Although older, the TCM approach is neither lost in antiquity or extraordinarily better. The biomedical and TCM approaches to integrative therapies are applicable to today's clinical practice and research (Huang, 2004).

CHINESE HERBAL MEDICINE AND ANALGESIA

Although the analgesic effect of acupuncture is more widely accepted in Western society, herbal therapy is the foundation of pain management within TCM (Peilin, 2008). The anti-inflammatory effects of Chinese herbal drugs have been a popular area of research worldwide (Li et al., 2009). Syndrome differentiation is the analysis of clinical information according to the paradigms of TCM, and in a clinical study comparing prescription of Chinese herbal medicine formulas based on syndrome differentiation, to Western therapeutics (e.g., NSAIDs, glucosamine, intra-articular steroid injections) for management of posttraumatic elbow pain, human patients were less painful when treated with Chinese herbal formulas. Pain assessment was based on total pain scores, joint pain scores, objective range of motion assessment, and patient self-assessment of daily activity (Min et al., 2010). The use of traditional Chinese herbal therapies in the management of cancer pain has been widely studied, and the data support the use of Chinese herbs for reducing cancer pain with fewer adverse effects compared to conventional analgesics (Xu et al., 2007).

Early herbal research focused on the isolation of active ingredients and individual compounds (Griffin, 1979); more recently, researchers are focusing on the action of single herbal ingredients and herbal formulas and on comparison of Western drugs and TCM formulas. A great need still exists for the evaluation of TCM formulas in veterinary clinical studies. This section provides an overview of current thinking regarding mechanisms and effectiveness of key individual herbs and classical Chinese herbal formulas. The reader is encouraged to explore other references for dosing parameters and more extensive information. Several veterinary-based texts provide this information (Wynn & Marsden, 2003; Marsden, 2006).

SINGLE HERBS WITH ANALGESIC PROPERTIES

Many individual herbs, often part of classical Chinese herbal formulas, including Yan Hu Suo (*Corydalis ambigua*), Bai Shao (white peony; *Paeoniae lactiflorae*), Bai Zhi (*Angelicae dahuricae*), Du Huo (*Angelica pubescens*), Mu Gua (Chinese quince; *Chaenomeles lagenaria* or *Chaenomeles sinensis*), Mo Yao (myrrh; *Commiphora myrrha*) and Ru Xiang (frankincense; *Boswellia carterii*), offer antinociceptive properties.

Yan Hu Suo, or *Corydalis*, is an herb commonly used for analgesia. Nicknamed "herbal morphine," Yan Hu Suo has approximately 40% of the efficacy of morphine (Bensky & Gamble, 1993). The corydalis alkaloids in the plant are thought to provide the antinociceptive properties, with dl-tetrahydropalmatine being the most important one (Yuan et al., 1996; Chen & Chen, 2004). The antinociceptive properties of dl-tetrahydropalmatine are thought to be related to agonist activity at supraspinal dopamine-2 receptors (Hu & Jin, 1999). Cannabinoid receptors are thought to impart the neuropathic antinociceptive properties of Yan Hu Suo (Huang et al, 2010).

Pain Management in Veterinary Practice, First Edition. Edited by Christine M. Egger, Lydia Love and Tom Doherty.

A number of studies have investigated the antinociceptive efficacy of Yan Hu Suo. Intraperitoneal injection of crude herbal extracts of Yan Hu Suo was evaluated in a model of chemically induced hyperalgesia in rats. Yan Hu Suo significantly increased the peak thermal threshold and reduced hyperalgesia compared to saline controls (Wei et al., 1999). A dose-related, clinical analgesic effect was noted with the administration of Yan Hu Suo to healthy humans subjected to mild-to-moderate noxious stimuli (Yuan et al., 2004). Other studies have shown a dose-related enhancement of the analgesic effects of Yan Hu Suo by adding other analgesic herbs such as *A. dahuricae* (Liao et al., 2010). In addition to analgesia, Yan Hu Suo inhibits neoplastic cell proliferation and metastasis (Gao et al., 2008; Xiao et al., 2008). Addition of the herb E Zhu (*Curcuma phaeocaulis*) enhanced the antineoplastic properties of Yan Hu Suo (Gao et al., 2009). Cancer-related pain can be debilitating, and slowing the cancer growth or the metastases can indirectly reduce pain.

Bai Zhi, or *A. dahuricae*, has analgesic activity sufficient for mild-to-moderate pain (Yuan et al., 2004). Bai Zhi decreases inducible nitric oxide synthase concentrations and the production of nitric oxide in experimental settings and inhibits cyclooxygenase and lipoxygenase (Kang et al., 2008; Moon et al., 2008). The analgesic actions of Bai Zhi are also partly due to central endogenous opioid mechanisms (Nie & Shen, 2002). Bai Zhi is an important analgesic component in the classical Chinese herbal formula Xian Fang Huo Ming Yin.

Another form of *Angelica*, Du Huo, or *A. pubescens*, affects the lipoxygenase and cyclooxygenase pathways (Liu et al., 1998). Intraperitoneal administration of Du Huo provided antinociception in inflammatory (Chen & Chen, 2004) and hyperalgesic pain models (Wei et al., 1999). Additionally, Du Huo appears to act synergistically with other herbs, such as Bai Shao (white peony), resulting in improved antinociception and decreased tissue swelling (Xu, 2007). Du Huo is an important part of analgesic formulas such as Du Huo Ji Sheng Tang and Yi Yi Ren Tang.

Bai Shao, known as *P. lactiflora* or white peony, contains paeoniflorin, which has analgesic properties via agonism of endogenous opioid receptors (Yu et al., 2007). Bai Shao is an important part of several analgesic herbal formulas, including Yi Yi Ren Tang and Gui Zhi Tang.

Mu Gua, known as *C. lagenaria* or Chinese quince, has been studied for its analgesic properties. Mu Gua reduced arthritic swelling in a mouse model (Bensky & Gamble, 1993). Glucosides of Mu Gua have demonstrated antinociception in a rat model of arthritis (Dai et al., 2003). A 10% ethanol fraction of *Chaenomeles*, containing the active component chlorogenic acid, provided antinociception in an inflammatory model in mice (Li et al., 2009). Mu Gua is an important part of Bu Gan Tang, a classical Chinese herbal formula used for treating pain due to muscle spasms.

Mo Yao, *C. myrrha* or myrrh, has anti-inflammatory constituents (Shen & Lou, 2008). Mo Yao is best known for its topical anti-inflammatory effects and improved wound healing (Haffor, 2010; Walsh et al., 2010). In addition, sesquiterpenes have been identified in myrrh and they mediate analgesia that is reversible with naloxone (Dolara et al., 1996).

Ru Xiang, *Boswellia* or frankincense, contains 17 different constituents with anti-inflammatory effects (Banno et al., 2006). The anti-inflammatory actions of boswellic acids are related to their anti-prostaglandin effects (Siemoneit et al., 2011). Ru Xiang extract has

beneficial effects in arthritis by decreasing inflammatory mediators (Sengupta et al., 2008), and the dried form of Ru Xiang has significant anti-inflammatory effects in rats (Fan et al., 2005) and humans (Kimmatkar et al., 2003). Despite extensive research, systematic reviews regarding the clinical analgesic efficacy of *Boswellia* extracts are equivocal (Ernst, 2008). Newer research, however, demonstrates the antineoplastic effects of *Boswellia* (Frank et al., 2009; Park et al., 2011). Chinese herbal formulas that contain both Mo Yao and Ru Xiang include Xiao Huo Luo Dan and Xian Fang Huo Ming Yin. Shen Tong Zhu Yu Tang contains Mo Yao only.

Numerous studies have reported that curcumin (Yu Jin), the main active compound of *Curcuma longa*, also known as turmeric, exhibits antinociceptive and anti-inflammatory properties. Curcumin appears to exhibit its antinociceptive effects through multiple mechanisms by affecting μ, δ, TRPV1, and 5-HT receptors, and ATP-sensitive potassium channels. Curcumin also inhibits release of tumor necrosis factor-alpha (TNF-α), interleukins, nitric oxide, and other key inflammatory mediators, and inhibits matrix metalloproteinase activity (Sharma et al., 2007; Yeon et al., 2010; Shen et al., 2012; Zhao et al., 2012).

HERBAL FORMULAS WITH ANALGESIC PROPERTIES

Unlike Western herbal analgesics, TCM herbs are rarely used individually. Instead, individual herbs might be included in or added to a classical formula in order to improve the analgesic effect (Zhu & Woerdenbag, 1995). Formulas that provide analgesia include: Du Huo Ji Sheng Tang, Xiao Huo Luo Dan, Yi Yi Ren Tang, Xian Fang Huo Ming Yin, Si Miao San, Xiao Chai Hu Tang, Bu Gan Tang, and Shen Tong Zhu Yu Tang.

Du Huo Ji Sheng Tang, or "Angelica and Lorthanus/Mulberry Mistletoe Combination," relieves pain, partly via anti-inflammatory mechanisms (Chen et al., 2011), and is suggested as an alternative to NSAIDs (Chen & Chen, 2009). Several studies, published in China, have evaluated the effectiveness of Du Huo Ji Sheng Tang for cervical pain, sciatica, osteoarthritis, spondylosis, and intervertebral disk herniation (Lin & Chen, 2007; Chen & Chen, 2009).

Xiao Huo Luo Dan, translated as "Minor Invigorate the Collaterals Pill" and also known as "Myrrh and Aconite Formula," is an effective analgesic formula for chronic musculoskeletal pain and joint pain (Allen & Boudreaux, 2009). Aconite is considered a warming herb in this formula. Interestingly, a blinded study demonstrated that oral ingestion of aconite results in increased body heat in dogs, as detected by infrared thermography, as soon as 30 minutes and for as long as 6 hours after ingestion (Chen et al., 2009). Aconite can be toxic, and its presence in Xiao Huo Luo Dan prevents the long-term use of this formula. The analgesic action of Xiao Huo Luo Dan may be related to nitric oxide synthase induction caused by aconite. An increased concentration of nitric oxide, allowing improved blood flow and resolution of clinical signs, has been observed in humans after aconite administration (Yamada et al., 2005).

Yi Yi Ren Tang, or "*Coix* Combination," is a commonly used formula for providing analgesia in lame large-breed dogs (Marsden, 2006); however, there are no scientific studies of the clinical use of Yi Yi Ren Tang.

Xian Fang Huo Ming Yin, translated as "The Sublime Formula for Surviving or Sustaining Life" and also known as "Angelica and

Mastic Combination," is a good analgesic for chronic arthritis in overweight dogs. Xian Fang Huo Ming Yin was originally used for infections and abscesses (Bensky & Barolet, 1990; Chen & Chen, 2009). This formula contains red peony or Chi Shao (related to Bai Shao, or white peony), Ru Xiang, and Mo Yao (Chen & Chen, 2009). The anti-inflammatory effects of Ru Xiang and Mo Yao makes Xian Fang Huo Ming Yin useful for arthritic dogs (Marsden, 2006).

Xian Fang Huo Ming Yin treats chronic inflammation, and Si Miao San, translated as "Four Marvels Powder," is better suited for treating acute inflammation. A modified version of Si Miao San had anti-inflammatory effects in hepatocytes *in vitro* (Liu et al., 2011). The inhibitory effect of Si Miao San on inflammatory mediators, such as TNF-α, interleukin-6, and nitric oxide, has been demonstrated (Fan et al., 2010). One of the key anti-inflammatory agents in Si Miao San is thought to be the Huang Bai (*Phellodendron amurense* or *Phellodendron chinense*), which contains high concentrations of berberine (Yang et al., 2010). Berberine inhibits the production of TNF-α, interleukin-6, and monocyte chemoattractant protein 1, resulting in the inhibition of prostaglandin E2 production. Berberine also downregulates the expression of COX-2 and matrix metalloproteinases through mitogen-activated protein kinase (MAPK) and NF–κB signaling pathways (Tillhon et al., 2012).

Xiao Chai Hu Tang, or "Minor Bupleurum Combination," contains Chai Hu (*Bupleurum chinensis*). The analgesic action of Chai Hu is thought to be due, in part, to increased plasma β-endorphin concentrations and decreased plasma epinephrine and dopamine concentrations (Chen et al., 2005). By adding Bai Shao or Gui Zi, this formula can be ideal for acute thoracolumbar disc disease, because the antispasmodic effects of Bai Shao decrease muscle spasms. Xiao Chai Hu Tang helped in the resolution of pancreatitis and gastric pain in people (Chen & Chen, 2009).

Bu Gan Tang is also known as "Tonify the Liver Decoction" or "Rehmannia and Peony Combination." Although research about Bu Gan Tang is lacking, the anti-inflammatory effects of two of the individual herbs, Bai Shao and Mu Gua, were discussed earlier.

The first four herbs comprising Bu Gan Tang actually make Si Wu Tang ("Four Materials Decoction"). Si Wu Tang has anti-inflammatory and antihistaminic effects, and Bai Shao is thought to play a key role (Dai et al., 2002), as the paeoniflorins in Bai Shao are some of the active constituents of Si Wu Tang (Wang et al., 2009). The action of the phthalides in Si Wu Tang in inhibiting uterine contraction was evaluated by in a randomized, double-blind, placebo-controlled, pilot clinical study (Tang et al., 2010). Additionally, the phthalides in Si Wu Tang are associated with uterine relaxation in mice (Tang et al., 2010). Si Wu Tang was not associated with any adverse reactions, and was also shown to provide perimenstrual analgesia to women (Yeh et al., 2007).

Shen Tong Zhu Yu Tang, translated as "Drive Stasis from a Painful Body Decoction" and also known as "Cnidium and Notopterygium Combination," is used for generalized muscle soreness (Chen & Chen, 2009). Two studies have evaluated the use of Shen Tong Zhu Yu Tang for pain in the lower back and legs in humans, and the majority of patients in both studies experienced either complete recovery or significant improvement (Chen and Chen, 2009). Du Huo Ji Sheng Tang and Shen Tong Zhu Yu Tang are formulas that promote blood circulation and relieve pain, in part, by anti-inflammatory mechanisms (Chen et al., 2011).

HOMEOPATHY FOR PAIN MANAGEMENT

Homeopathy is a type of medicine in which patients are treated with diluted preparations of the materials that cause the symptoms being treated. As a system of treatment, homeopathy was founded by Samuel C. Hahnemann in late eighteenth century Germany. Homeopathy is more culturally accepted in Europe, and many of the studies are published in German. Purists argue that homeopathy should be used to the exclusion of all other therapies. However, selected homeopathic formulations have been commonly suggested for relief of pain in veterinary patients, and may prove useful adjuncts for pain relief. Homeopathic remedies can be purchased over the counter in most health food stores, and should be given twice a day for chronic conditions, up to 3–4 times a day for subacute conditions, and even hourly for acute, severe conditions.

Although some plants, such as *Arnica* and *Symphytum*, can be toxic if ingested in their natural states, the dilution principles involved in making homeopathic agents eliminate toxicity. Therefore, oral forms of *Arnica* and *Symphytum* are only sold as homeopathic agents in the United States.

Homeopathic *Arnica*

Homeopathic *Arnica* (*A. montana*) is used to treat bruising and hemorrhage, especially when traumatic or surgical in origin. When given soon after the injury, arnica can reduce swelling and bruising, potentially lessening postoperative pain. Homeopathic *Arnica* has been investigated in blinded, placebo-controlled studies for its effect on postoperative swelling and pain associated with knee surgery in human patients, including arthroscopy, knee replacement, and cruciate ligament reconstruction. Patients treated with arnica had significantly less postoperative swelling after cruciate ligament reconstruction, and there was a trend towards less swelling following arthroscopy and knee replacement (Brinkhaus et al., 2006). In a randomized, double-blind, placebo controlled study of post-tonsillectomy adults, those receiving arnica had lower pain scores in the first 2 weeks postoperatively (Robertson et al., 2007). Clinical experience demonstrates that arnica is effective for acute and peracute injury.

Homeopathic *Symphytum*

Homeopathic *Symphytum* (*S. officinale*), also known as comfrey, is used to augment bone healing. In a placebo-controlled study of rats, treated with homeopathic *Symphytum* for up to 56 days after a titanium tibial implant placement, improved bone formation, based on radiographic and mechanical torque assessment, was confirmed (Spin-Neto et al., 2010). Additionally, nonhomeopathic, topical *Symphytum* demonstrated rapid and significant analgesic effects in a double-blind, placebo-controlled study of acute lower back pain in humans, using a visual analog scale and pressure algometry for pain assessment (Giannetti et al., 2010). In a blinded, placebo-controlled study, topical *Symphytum* reduced pain, decreased edema, and increased joint mobility after ankle sprains in humans (Koll et al., 2004). Although research in veterinary patients is lacking, *Symphytum* is often recommended for analgesia and to promote healing of fractures, especially with nonhealing bone injuries, and may aid in the management of subchondral bone defects, including osteochondritis dessicans and ununited anconeal processes.

Other Homeopathic Remedies

Based on clinical experience, other homeopathic remedies can be used for pain management in veterinary patients. *Ruta graveolens* is a common remedy for lameness, particularly for subacute or chronic ligamentous and tendonous injuries (e.g., anterior cruciate ligament tears). *R. graveolens* is considered useful for pain that is worse in cold, damp weather or pain that is worse with opposing extremes of physical activity, either after rest and/or with excessive exercise. *Rhus toxicodendron* is another lameness remedy used for more mild, subacute, or chronic soft tissue injury to muscles, joints, and ligaments. Often patients that benefit from this homeopathic remedy are worse upon initially rising or with early motion but improve with gentle continued motion and warmth. *Hypericum perfoliatum* is effective for neuropathic pain related to nerve trauma (nerve root injury, neuralgia, extensive dental work, declaw complications, and intervertebral disc disease). Although a literature search revealed no published studies on these remedies, clinical experience suggests that future research in the use of analgesic homeopathic agents may be beneficial.

SUMMARY

TCM and homeopathy offer veterinarians complementary or alternative options for managing pain in their patients. These tools may allow for better clinical control with fewer adverse effects than Western pharmaceuticals. As the use of these complementary methods grows among human patients, it is likely that there will be a greater demand for such therapies in veterinary patients.

REFERENCES

Allen, G. & Boudreaux, M. (2009) *Traditional Chinese Medicine: Desk Reference for Chinese Herbology*. Self-published.

Banno, N., Akihisa, T., Yasukawa, K., et al. (2006) Anti-inflammatory activities of the triterpene acids from the resin of *Boswellia carteri*. *Journal of Ethnopharmacology*, 107(2), 249–253.

Bensky, D. & Barolet, R. (1990) *Chinese Herbal Medicine: Formulas and Strategies*, Eastland Press, Seattle, WA.

Bensky, D. & Gamble, A. (1993) *Chinese Herbal Medicine: Materia Medica*, revised edition. Eastland Press, Seattle, WA.

Brinkhaus, B., Wilkens, J.M., Lüdtke, R., Hunger, J., Witt, C.M., & Willich, S.N. (2006) Homeopathic arnica therapy in patients receiving knee surgery: results of three randomised double-blind trials. *Complementary Therapies in Medicine*, 14(4), 237–246.

Chen, J. & Chen, T. (2004) *Chinese Medical Herbology and Pharmacology*, Art of Medicine Press, City of Industry, CA.

Chen, J. & Chen, T. (2009) *Chinese Herbal Formulas and Applications: Pharmacological Effects and Clinical Research*, Art of Medicine Press, City of Industry, CA.

Chen, J.X., Ji, B., Lu, Z.L., & Hu, L.S. (2005) Effects of chai hu (radix burpleuri) containing formulation on plasma beta-endorphin, epinephrine and dopamine on patients. *American Journal of Chinese Medicine*, 33(5), 737–745.

Chen, C.W., Sun, J., Li, Y.M., Shen, P.A., Chen, Y.Q. (2011) Action mechanisms of du-huo-ji-sheng-tang on cartilage degradation in a rabbit model of osteoarthritis. *Evidence Based Complementary and Alternative Medicine*, 2011, 7.

Chen, T.T., Qi, C., Guo, H., et al. (2009) The effects of Fu Zi on changes in the body heat of dogs. *Journal of Acupuncture and Meridian Studies*, 2(1), 71–74.

Dai, M., Wei, W., Shen, Y.X., & Zheng, Y.Q. (2003) Glucosides of Chaenomeles remit rat adjuvant arthritis by inhibiting synoviocyte activity. *Acta Pharmacologica*, 24, 1161–1166.

Dai, Y., But, P.P., Chan, Y.P., Matsuda, H., & Kubo, M. (2002) Antipruritic and anti-inflammatory effects of aqueous extract from Si-Wu-Tang. *Biological and Pharmaceutical Bulletin*, 25(9), 1175–1178.

Dolara, P., Luceri, C., Ghelardini, C., et al. (1996) Analgesic effects of myrrh. *Nature*, 379(29), 1038.

Ernst, E. (2008) Frankincense: systematic review. *British Medical Journal*, 17, 337.

Fan, A.Y., Lao, L., Zhang, R.X., et al. (2005) Effects of an acetone extract of *Boswellia carterii* Birdw. (Burseraceae) gum resin on adjuvant-induced arthritis in Lewis rats. *Journal of Ethnopharmacology*, 101(1–3), 104–109.

Fan, J., Liu, K., Zhang, Z., et al. (2010) Si-Miao-San extract inhibits the release of inflammatory mediators from lipopolysaccharide-stimulated mouse macrophages. *Journal of Ethnopharmacology*, 129(1), 5–9.

Frank, M.B., Yang, Q., Osban, J., et al. (2009) Frankincense oil derived from *Boswellia carteri* induces tumor cell specific cytotoxicity. *Biomedcentral Complementary and Alternative Medicine*, 9, 6.

Gao, J.L., He, T.C., Li, Y.B., & Wang, Y.T. (2009) A traditional Chinese medicine formulation consisting of Rhizoma Corydalis and Rhizoma Curcumae exerts synergistic anti-tumor activity. *Oncology Reports*, 22, 1077–1083.

Gao, J.L., Shi, J.M., He, K., et al. (2008) Yanhusuo extract inhibits metastasis of breast cancer cells by modulating mitogen-activated protein kinase (MAPK) signaling pathways. *Oncology Reports*, 20, 819–824.

Giannetti, B.M., Staiger, C., Bulitta, M., & Predel, H.G. (2010) Efficacy and safety of comfrey root extract ointment in the treatment of acute upper or lower back pain: results of a double-blind, randomised, placebo controlled, multicentre trial. *British Journal of Sports Medicine*, 44(9), 637–641.

Griffin, R.J. Jr. (1979) Herbal medicine revisited: science looks anew at ancient Chinese pharmacology. *American Pharmacologist*, 19(10), 16–22.

Haffor, A.S. (2010) Effect of myrrh (Commiphora molmol) on leukocyte levels before and during healing from gastric ulcer or skin injury. *Journal of Immunotoxicology*, 7(1), 68–75.

Hu, J.Y. & Jin, G.Z. (1999) Supraspinal D2 receptor involved in antinociception induced by l-tetrahydropalmatine. *Acta Pharmacologica Sinica*, 20, 715–719.

Huang, J.Y., Fang, M., Li, Y.J., Ma, Y.Q., & Cai, X.H. (2010) [Analgesic effect of Corydalis yanhusuo in a rat model of trigeminal neuropathic pain]. *Nan Fang Yi Ke Da Xue Xue Bao*, 30(9), 2161–2164.

Huang, Q.F. (2004) [Strategy and approaches of pathological and pathophysiological research in integrated traditional Chinese and western medicine]. *Zhong Xi Yi Jie He Xue Bao*, 2(4), 245–251.

Kang, O.H., Chae, H.S., Oh, Y.C., et al. (2008) Anti-nociceptive and anti-inflammatory effects of *Angelicae dahuricae* radix through inhibition of the expression of inducible nitric oxide synthase and NO production. *American Journal of Chinese Medicine*, 36(5), 913–928.

Kimmatkar, N., Thawani, V., Hingorani, L., & KhiyaniR. (2003) Efficacy and tolerability of *Boswellia serrata* extract in treatment of osteoarthritis of knee–a randomized double blind placebo controlled trial. *Phytomedicine*, 10(1), 3–7.

Koll, R., Buhr, M., Dieter, R., et al. (2004) Efficacy and tolerance of a comfrey root extract (Extr. Rad. Symphyti) in the treatment of ankle distortions: results of a multicenter, randomized, placebo-controlled, double-blind study. *Phytomedicine*, 11(6), 470–477.

Li, H.Y., Cui, L., & Cui, M. (2009) Hot topics in Chinese herbal drugs research documented in PubMed/MEDLINE by authors inside China and outside of China in the past 10 years: based on co-word cluster analysis. *Journal of Alternative and Complementary Medicine*, 15(7), 779–785.

Li, X., Yang, Y.B., Yang, Q., Sun, L.N., & Chen, W.S. (2009) Anti-inflammatory and analgesic activities of Chaenomeles speciosa fractions in laboratory animals. *Journal of Medicinal Food*, 12(5), 1016–1022.

Liao, Z.G., Liang, X.L., Zhu, J.Y., et al. (2010) Correlation between synergistic action of Radix Angelica dahurica extracts on analgesic effects of Corydalis alkaloid and plasma concentration of dl-THP. *Journal of Ethnopharmacology*, 129(1), 115–120.

Lin, X.J. & Chen, C.Y. (2007) [Advances in the study of treatment of lumbar disk herniation by Chinese medicinal herbs]. *Zhongguo Zhong Yao Za Zhi*, 32(3), 186–191.

Liu, J.H., Zschocke, S., Reininger, E., & Bauer, R. (1998) Inhibitory effects of *Angelica pubescens* f. biserrata on 5-lipoxygenase and cyclooxygenase. *Planta Medica*, 64(6), 525–529.

Liu, K., Luo, T., Zhang, Z., et al. (2011) Modified Si-Miao-San extract inhibits inflammatory response and modulates insulin sensitivity in hepatocytes through an IKKβ/IRS-1/Akt-dependent pathway. *Journal of Ethnopharmacology*, 136(3), 473–479.

Marsden, S. (2006) *Guide to Chinese Veterinary Herbal Medicine for Small Animals*. Self-published by Natural Path Herbal Company, Edmonton, AB.

Min, Z.H., Zhou, Y., & Zhang, H.M. (2010) Effect of treatment based on syndrome differentiation by Chinese medicine on post-traumatic elbow arthritis. *Chinese Journal of Integrative Medicine*, 16(3), 264–269.

Moon, T.C., Jin, M., Son, J.K., & Chang, H.W. (2008) The effects of isoimperatorin isolated from *Angelicae dahuricae* on cyclooxygenase-2 and 5-lipoxygenase in mouse bone marrow-derived mast cells. *Archives of Pharmacological Research*, 31(2), 210–215.

Nie, H. & Shen, Y.J. (2002) [Effect of essential oil of Radix *Angelicae dahuricae* on beta-endorphin, ACTH, NO and proopiomelanocortin of pain model rats]. *Zhongguo Zhong Yao Za Zhi*, 27(9), 690–693.

Park, B., Sung, B., Yadav, V.R., Cho, S.G., Liu, M., & Aggarwal, B.B. (2011) Acetyl-11-keto-β-boswellic acid suppresses invasion of pancreatic cancer cells through the downregulation of CXCR4 chemokine receptor expression. *International Journal of Cancer*, 129(1), 23–33.

Peilin, S. (2008) *The Treatment of Pain with Chinese Herbs and Acupuncture*, 2nd edn, Elsevier, St Louis, MO.

Robertson, A., Suryanarayanan, R., & Banerjee, A. (2007) Homeopathic *Arnica montana* for post-tonsillectomy analgesia: a randomised placebo control trial. *Homeopathy*, 96(1), 17–21.

Sengupta, K., Alluri, K.V., Satish, A.R., et al. (2008) A double blind, randomized, placebo controlled study of the efficacy and safety of 5-Loxin for treatment of osteoarthritis of the knee. *Arthritis Research and Therapy*, 10(4), R85.

Sharma, S., Chopra, K., & Kulkarni, S.K. (2007) Effect of insulin and its combination with resveratrol or curcumin in attenuation of diabetic neuropathic pain: participation of nitric oxide and TNF-alpha. *Phytotherapy Research*, 21, 278–283.

Shen, C.L., Smith, B.J., Lo, D.F., et al. (2012) Dietary polyphenols and mechanisms of osteoarthritis. *Journal of Nutritional Biochemistry*, 23(11), 1367–1377.

Shen, T. & Lou, H.X. (2008) Bioactive constituents of myrrh and frankincense, two simultaneously prescribed gum resins in Chinese traditional medicine. *Chemistry and Biodiversity*, 5(4), 540–553.

Siemoneit, U., Koeberle, A., Rossi, A., et al. (2011) Inhibition of microsomal prostaglandin E2 synthase-1 as a molecular basis for the anti-inflammatory actions of boswellic acids from frankincense. *British Journal of Pharmacology*, 162(1), 147–162.

Spin-Neto, R., Belluci, M.M., Sakakura, C.E., Scaf, G., Pepato, M.T., & Marcantonio, E. Jr. (2010) Homeopathic *Symphytum officinale* increases removal torque and radiographic bone density around titanium implants in rats. *Homeopathy*, 99(4), 249–254.

Tang, Y., Zhu, M., Yu, S., et al. (2010) Identification and comparative quantification of bioactive phthalides in essential oils from si-wu-tang, fo-shou-san, radix angelica and rhizoma chuanxiong. *Molecules*, 15(1), 341–351.

Tillhon, M., Guaman Ortiz, L.M., Lombardi, P., et al. (2012) Berberine: new perspectives for old remedies. *Biochemical Pharmacology*, 84(10), 1260–1267.

Walsh, M.E., Reis, D., & Jones, T. (2010) Integrating complementary and alternative medicine: use of myrrh in wound management. *Journal of Vascular Nursing*, 28(3), 102.

Wang, Z., Woa, S.K., Wang, L. et al. (2009) Simultaneous quantification of active components in the herbs and products of Si-Wu-Tang by high performance liquid chromatography–mass spectrometry. *Journal of Pharmaceutical and Biomedical Analysis*, 50, 232–244.

Wei, F., Zou, S., Young, B., et al. (1999) Effects of four herbal extracts on adjuvant-induced inflammation and hyperalgesia in rats. *The Journal of Alternative and Complementary Medicine*, 5(5), 429–436.

Wynn, S. & Marsden, S. (2003) *Manual of Natural Veterinary Medicine: Science and Tradition*. Mosby, St Louis, MO.

Xiao, Y., Yang, F.Q., Li, S.P., Hu, G., Lee, S.M., & Wang, Y.T. (2008) Essential oil of Curcuma wen yu jin induces apoptosis in human hepatoma cells. *World Journal of Gastroenterology*, 14, 4309–4318.

Xie, Z.F. (2005) [On the methodology for integration of traditional Chinese and Western medicine]. *Zhong Xi Yi Jie He Xue Bao*, 3(1), 3–5.

Xu, L., Lao, L.X., Ge, A., Yu, S., Li, J., & Mansky, P.J. (2007) Chinese herbal medicine for cancer pain. *Integrative Cancer Therapies*, 6(3), 208–234.

Yamada, K., Suzuki, E., Nakaki, T., Watanabe, S., & Kanba, S. (2005) Aconiti tuber increases plasma nitrite and nitrate levels in humans. *Journal of Ethnopharmacology*, 96(1–2), 165–169.

Yang, Q., Zhang, F., Gao, S.H., Sun, L.N., & Chen, W.S. (2010) Determination of bioactive compounds in Cortex Phellodendri by high-performance liquid chromatography. *Journal of AOAC International*, 93(3), 855–861.

Yeh, L.L., Liu, J.Y., Lin, K.S., et al. (2007) A randomised placebo-controlled trial of a traditional Chinese herbal formula in the treatment of primary dysmenorrhoea. *PLoS ONE*, 2(8), e719.

Yeon, K.Y., Kim, S.A., Kim, Y.H., et al. (2010) Curcumin produces an antihyperalgesic effect via antagonism of TRPV1. *Journal of Dental Research*, 89, 170–174.

Yu, H.Y., Liu, M.G., Liu, D.N., et al. (2007) Antinociceptive effects of systemic paeoniflorin on bee venom-induced various 'phenotypes' of nociception and hypersensitivity. *Pharmacology, Biochemistry, and Behavior*, 88, 131–140.

Yuan, C.S., Mehendale, S.R., Wang, C.Z., et al. (2004) Effects of Corydalis yanhusuo and *Angelicae dahuricae* on cold pressor-induced pain in humans: a controlled trial. *Journal of Clinical Pharmacology*, 44(11), 1323–1327.

Yuan, Y.F., Liu, Z.L., & Li, X.L. (1996) Use of silica gel with reversed-phase eluents for the separation and determination of alkaloids in Corydalis Yanhusuo and its preparations. *Biomedical Chromatography*, 10, 11–14.

Zareba, G. (2009) Phytotherapy for pain relief. *Drugs Today*, 45(6), 445–467.

Zhao, X., Xu, Y., Zhao, Q., Chen, C.R., Liu, A.M., & Huang, Z.L. (2012) Curcumin exerts antinociceptive effects in a mouse model of neuropathic pain: descending monoamine system and opioid receptors are differentially involved. *Neuropharmacology*, 62, 843–854.

Zhu, Y.P., & Woerdenbag, H.J. (1995) Traditional Chinese herbal medicine. *Pharmacy World and Sciences*, 17(4), 103–112.

16
Mechanisms of Acupuncture Analgesia

Shauna Cantwell

Acupuncture is a medical technique that has been practiced for over 3000 years. Although scientific efficacy has remained controversial, the US National Institutes of Health recently recognized acupuncture as a complementary medicine. The use of acupuncture is becoming more common in veterinary medicine, and it can play a role in the management of acute, inflammatory, and chronic pain. Western medical etiology, pathophysiology, diagnosis, and treatment should always be considered before applying acupuncture.

Acupuncture originated in China, and is part of traditional Chinese medicine (TCM) and traditional Chinese veterinary medicine (TCVM). This discipline of medicine uses a metaphoric language to describe the pathophysiology of disease and its treatment. The traditional concept surrounds *Qi* (pronounced "chee"), which is usually translated as energy or life force. The *Qi* circulates through all parts of the body via pathways called meridians. Up to 350 points along and around these meridians are thought to have increased bioactivity and are called acupuncture points.

Practitioners of TCVM use pattern differentiation to diagnose and treat patients, and to provide prognostic information. Diagnosis is attained through evaluation of multiple parameters including: history, physical examination, behavior, and environmental interaction. Point selection is individualized based on TCVM principles. Acupuncture can also be applied from a biomedical approach.

MECHANISMS OF ACUPUNCTURE ANALGESIA

The action of acupuncture is broad and varied depending on needle location, type of needle manipulation, and treatment duration. Generally, the effects of acupuncture are thought to be neurohormonal and immunomodulatory. Acupuncture inhibits nociceptive transmission (Leung et al., 2008), improves blood flow, inhibits inflammation, reduces muscle tension and spasm, resets proprioceptive mechanisms and posture, and affects the autonomic nervous system (Zhao, 2008; Leung, 2012).

Percutaneous needling stimulates A-β sensory fibers and causes reflex changes in motor neuron tone and vascular tone, and contributes to local spinal inhibition of nociception (see Chapter 2). A-δ and C nociceptive fibers are also stimulated by needle placement, but pain transmission is inhibited by spinal release of endogenous opioids and activation of inhibitory interneurons and descending inhibitory pathways (Leung, 2012).

The anti-inflammatory activity of acupuncture is due to both endogenous opioid and nonopioid factors. Electroacupuncture decreased both T- and B-cell activity in arthritic mice (Yim et al., 2007). Leukocyte migration and activity is also affected by acupuncture (Lee et al., 2004).

Some studies suggest that acupuncture significantly affects the autonomic nervous system (Kimura & Sato, 1997; Kimura & Hara, 2008). Sato's early work is instrumental in correlating somatic stimulation with visceral function through autonomic pathways. Adrenal gland activity and an intact sympathoadrenal medullary axis are necessary for electroacupuncture-induced anti-inflammatory effects and reduction in thermal hyperalgesia in patients with long-term neuropathic pain (Kim et al., 2008). Blockade of the peripheral sympathetic postganglionic neurons with propranolol blocks the anti-inflammatory effect of low-frequency electroacupuncture (Kim et al., 2008). The cholinergic anti-inflammatory pathway is also affected by acupuncture, as is demonstrated in the field of cancer research (Kavoussi & Ross, 2007). Vagal stimulation through acupuncture stimulates regulatory T cells that inhibit inflammation, and this approach is being investigated for the treatment of rheumatoid arthritis (Koopman et al., 2011).

The Acupuncture Point: Neural Stimulation Unit

Most acupuncture points are located in palpable depressions, and are classically defined by anatomical location. According to Zhang et al. (2012), points are defined by a combination of local tissue components called the "neural stimulation unit," which result in particular electrodermal properties of the points including higher conductance, lower impedance, and higher capacitance than adjacent tissues. Normalization of these properties is linked to therapeutic response.

Acupuncture points tend to occur at nerve bifurcations or where nerves penetrate tissue planes. Histologically, acupuncture points consist of free nerve endings, small arterioles, veins, lymphatics, and an increased concentration of mast cells (Egerbacher, 1971). They vary in the density of autonomic fibers. Points are in close proximity to somatic afferent terminals, suggesting the likelihood of interaction and modulation of afferent signals by needle placement.

Stimulation of a point results in tissue damage, activation of the inflammatory cascade, histamine and substance P (SP) release, and

Pain Management in Veterinary Practice, First Edition. Edited by Christine M. Egger, Lydia Love and Tom Doherty.
© 2014 John Wiley & Sons, Inc. Published 2014 by John Wiley & Sons, Inc.

neural excitation. Interestingly, mechanical displacement of connective tissue creates a shear wave, which is much greater when needles are placed in acupuncture points rather than in nearby sham (nonacupuncture) points. Calcium ion channels and adenosine are subsequently activated (Yang et al., 2011). Acupuncture points also contain sympathetically innervated small blood vessels, lymphatics, fibroblasts, lymphocytes, and platelets. These cells release neurotransmitters and inflammatory and immunomodulatory factors (Zhang et al., 2012). Factors that inhibit afferent fibers include: acetylcholine, norepinephrine, GABA, β-endorphin, SP, somatostatin, nitric oxide, ATP/cGMP, and adenosine. Stimulatory mediators released include: various cytokines, prostaglandins, bradykinin, glutamate, and many others. Serotonin and histamine can be either excitatory or inhibitory depending on which receptors they are acting upon. The predominant effect of acupuncture in pain conditions is to enhance the activity of inhibitory mediators (Hurt & Zylka, 2012).

Spinal and Supraspinal Mechanisms

Through the last decade, studies on neural mechanisms underlying acupuncture analgesia have focused on the cellular and molecular substrates involved. Diverse signaling molecules and receptors contribute to acupuncture analgesia, including opioid peptides (μ, δ, and κ receptors), glutamate (NMDA and AMPA/KA receptors), 5-hydroxytryptamine (serotonin), and cholecystokinin-8 (CCK-8). Whereas CCK-8 antagonizes acupuncture analgesia, opioid peptides and their receptors in the spinal dorsal horn play a pivotal role in mediating acupuncture analgesia. The release of opioid peptides evoked by electroacupuncture is frequency-dependent. Electroacupuncture at 2 Hz and 100 Hz cause the release of enkephalin and dynorphin in the spinal cord, respectively.

Evidence also exists for spinal microglial involvement in the antinociception of electroacupuncture (Zhao, 2008). Analgesic effects may be associated with inhibition of spinal glial activation, and thereby provide a potential strategy for the treatment of arthritis or other inflammatory conditions.

Several spinal and supraspinal areas are involved in acupuncture analgesia (Bowsher, 1998). The trigeminal, spinothalamic, and spinoreticular tracts receive afferent signals from their respective receptive fields and transmit the information to subcortical and cortical areas. The dorsal column may also have an important role in modulation of acupuncture effects, particularly in regulating visceral functions (Chen & Ma, 2003). Mechanoreceptor-activated signals are believed to be the dominant components of afferent impulses from the majority of points, and the dorsal column-medial lemniscus tract receives sensory information from multiple sources, including cutaneous pain and visceral sensations in addition to fine touch and proprioception.

Many brain regions are affected by acupuncture, and imaging studies demonstrate heterogeneity of response rather than a somatotopic representation of points. This widespread and diverse modulation of brain activity that occurs with acupuncture is most likely related to the multiple central pathways that are affected by point stimulation.

Multiple brain nuclei, composing a complicated network, are involved in processing of acupuncture stimulation, including the nucleus raphe magnus, periaqueductal gray area, locus coeruleus, arcuate nucleus, preoptic area, nucleus submedius, habenular nucleus, accumbens nucleus, caudate nucleus, septal area, and amygdala. Most of these nuclei are constituent parts of the endogenous descending inhibitory system, with serotonin and catecholamine-containing neurons projecting to the spinal cord (Li et al., 2007; Zhang et al., 2011; Zhang et al., 2012).

NEURAL NETWORKS

Neural networks, very similar to pattern generators, are groupings of facilitated pathways that need very little input or control after initiation to create a complex physiological or motor response. Acupuncture, and especially electroacupuncture, may have global central nervous system (CNS) impact by altering the neural networks. Functional MRI studies provide an integrated view of the specificity of dry needle acupuncture, with needle sensation and the subsequent neural cascade contributing to a reconfiguration of complex neural networks (Faingold 2008; Qin et al., 2011).

The neuronal network that serves acupuncture analgesia is thought to activate structures of the descending inhibitory pathways and deactivate limbic structures within the ascending nociceptive pathway (Campbell, 2006).

Acupuncture is a slow-acting modality, and changes in the neural connectivity continue to occur for a prolonged period after needles are applied. Liu et al. (2010) describe time-varied characteristics of acupuncture on distinct brain networks. This is consistent with the observation of a continuing effect over days, and even longer, after acupuncture.

MERIDIANS

Many of the bioactive acupuncture points are considered to lie along anatomically described lines. The points on a meridian have common functions and are thought to communicate. Observations supporting the existence of meridians include: changes of impedance, thermal and sense propagation, radioisotope uptake, and light and sound wave transmission (Yan et al., 1992). There is some thought that meridians follow lymphatic flow. It has also been suggested that electrical conductance follows Bonghan channels, which are threadlike tissues that have been found floating in blood and lymph vessels and covering organs. Their presence has been confirmed in lymph vessels with the use of magnetic nanoparticles (Johng et al., 2007). Others have suggested that the meridians might be a functional, rather than an anatomical, concept that includes the nervous, circulatory, endocrine, and immune systems (Zhao, 2008).

CLINICAL PRACTICE OF ACUPUNCTURE

In clinical practice, acupuncture treatment regimens generally use multiple points located in different parts of the body. Empirical and experimental evidence suggests that the combination of local and distant points produces greater treatment effects than the use of single points. Simultaneous stimulation of different points appears to elicit a more widespread and intense regional brain response (Zhang et al., 2012). Given that superior therapeutic response appears to be associated with synergistic or additive effects of point stimulation at local and distant sites, the clarification of this relationship will provide valuable information in the development of more efficient acupuncture treatment regimens.

Increasingly, clinical veterinary studies demonstrate the effectiveness of acupuncture. A return to function has been described in a cat with multifocal disc disease (Choi & Hill, 2009). Another study describes electroacupuncture as the sole analgesic required for bovine surgery (e.g., caesarian section, rumenotomy) (Kim et al., 2004). In a clinical study of dogs with intervertebral disc disease and long-standing severe neurological deficits, acupuncture treatment alone was reported to be superior to surgery alone (Joaquim et al., 2010). Acupuncture treatment combined with Western treatment in dogs with thoracolumbar disease and no deep pain was superior to Western treatment alone for return to ambulation (Hayashi et al., 2007). The return of deep pain was not significantly different between the two groups; however, three out of six dogs receiving acupuncture, and one out of eight dogs not receiving acupuncture, had an acceptable return to function. Laim et al. (2009) reported that electroacupuncture initially improved analgesia, though less so after the first 12 hours, when applied adjunctively post surgery to dogs undergoing hemilaminectomy. Shorter time to ambulation and deep pain perception occurred in dogs with thoracolumbar intervertebral disc disease when Western treatment was combined with electroacupuncture (Han et al., 2010). Gold bead acupuncture in dogs with hip dysplasia was reported to improve mobility and lessen pain scores for at least 2 years (Jaeger et al., 2006, 2007). Bilateral stimulation of acupuncture points induced a shorter latency period, greater intensity, and longer duration of analgesia in dogs subjected to thermal and mechanical nociceptive stimuli (Cassu et al., 2008). Preoperative electroacupuncture (EA) provided better post-ovariohysterectomy analgesia than did butorphanol in dogs (Groppetti et al., 2011), though not in horses with rectal distention (Skarda & Muir, 2003). Dogs treated with EA had a reduced need for postmastectomy rescue analgesics than did dogs treated with morphine (Gakiya et al., 2011). Peri-incisional treatment with transcutaneous electrical stimulation at acupuncture points, as opposed to nonacupuncture points, decreased the initial postovariohysterectomy pain scores, and decreased the dose of rescue analgesics needed in dogs (Cassu et al., 2012). Electroacupuncture improved lameness scores and increased serum β-endorphin concentrations in an experimental equine lameness model (Xie et al., 2001). Multiple sessions of EA was reported to be superior to phenylbutazone for treating horses with chronic back pain (Xie et al., 2005).

Modes of Therapy

Several methods of stimulation of acupuncture points can be employed, and traditionally each has a different purpose. A session typically lasts for 30 minutes, during which needles are intermittently rotated, electrically stimulated, or in some cases, heated. The needling sensation, known as *de-qi* (pronounced "day-chee"), is a predictor of acupuncture analgesia in human patients (Leung, 2012). It entails a sharp pricking sensation, but is also reported as a dullness, heaviness, deep ache, numbness, or flooding warmth. In animals, it is manifested by a strong response to the needle followed by a sudden relaxation.

Dry Needle

The most common veterinary application is to apply needles alone to acupuncture points. A subsequent *de-qi* response, such as a strong reaction, local hyperemia, or sudden sedation, signifies that the point has been located. The angle and depth of insertion vary with the anatomical location, age, size, and health of the patient. Moving the needles with a gentle thrust in a clockwise direction is tonifying (strengthening), and moving the needle with a forceful thrust and twisting counterclockwise is sedating, and is used to diminish an excessive physiological state. Duration of needle stimulation is commensurate with the needs of the animal.

Aqua Acupuncture

Fluid may be injected into acupuncture points to prolong the effect of point stimulation. Practitioners use various substances including saline, vitamin B12, and Adequan®. Bee venom injected at acupuncture point ST36 potentiated analgesia in neuropathic pain states in rodent models (Yoon et al., 2009), and is used in some TCVM practices. Autologous blood is used in acupuncture points for an anti-inflammatory effect. Injection into acupuncture points is quick, and can be used in animals that do not tolerate prolonged needling or EA.

Laser Acupuncture

Laser-emitting diode devices can be used to stimulate acupuncture points. Low-power (5–30 mW) energy of wavelengths 630–960 nm is common in veterinary medicine. Laser has been shown to be analgesic and anti-inflammatory (Lorenzini et al., 2010). Laser light refracts within 15 mm in tissue, so it is useful for shallow acupuncture points, or in areas of thin integument. More powerful lasers are being developed, and may become useful in veterinary acupuncture.

Material Implantation

Acupuncture points can be stimulated over a long period of time by inserting various materials including: surgical suture, skin staples, or gold beads or wire. The most common technique is to implant gold periarticularly in animals with hip dysplasia or degenerative joint disease. Gold bead implantation is reported to be associated with diminished pain and increased ambulation, but variable results have been reported (Jaeger et al., 2006, 2007).

Electroacupuncture

Applying electrical stimulus to peripheral nerves through percutaneously placed needles can produce prolonged analgesia lasting from hours to days or longer. This form of acupuncture is commonly applied to animals. Electric frequencies are usually set anywhere from 1 Hz to 200 Hz, and the millivoltage is set such that the animal barely notices it.

Electroacupuncture results in the release of endomorphin, dynorphin, enkephalin, and β-endorphin (Lin & Chen., 2008), and is an effective method shown to attenuate inflammatory, neuropathic, and cancer pain. Many neurochemicals, in particular endogenous opiate peptides, 5-HT, and catecholamines, exhibit a frequency-dependent release during EA. Though there is inconsistency in study results, different analgesic mechanisms have been demonstrated with high- and low-frequency stimulation. High-frequency (80–120 Hz) electrical stimulation at local points is recommended for segmental inhibition, and is associated with the release of dynorphins, serotonin, and GABA. Low-frequency (0.5–20 Hz) stimulation is more effective at remote sites for a more diffuse systemic effect, and is associated with the release of endorphins (Xing et al., 2007). Of note, alternating frequencies between 2 Hz and 100 Hz will cause a release of a full spectrum of endorphins (Wang et al., 2008).

In contrast to Xing et al. (2007), White et al. (2008) reported that high-intensity, but not low-intensity, EA applied unilaterally generates a significant and persistent bilateral hypoalgesic effect.

The underlying mechanism of long-term synaptic alterations is still unclear, but the NMDA receptor is involved. It seems that low-frequency stimulation (2 Hz) results in subsequent diminishment of neuropathic pain that relies on NMDA receptor stimulation to depress C-fiber evoked potentials in the dorsal horn (Xing et al., 2007). This is counter to the widely held belief that the NMDA receptor must be antagonized in the resolution of chronic pain. It is possible that the activity of this receptor plays a role in modulation of neurotransmission through depression as well as potentiation. Higher frequencies, such as 100 Hz, seem to be dependent on GABAergic and serotonergic inhibitory pathways, and seem to be less effective in diminishing neuropathic pain than the lower frequencies.

Hypothalamic neuroendocrine functions are also affected. Immediate and repeated electroacupuncture normalized behavioral and biochemical abnormalities in various models of animal stress, including immobilization, maternal separation, chronic mild stress, surgical trauma, chronic administration of corticosteroids, cold stimulation, tooth-pulp stimulation, and mechanical colon distention (Zhang et al., 2012).

CHRONIC PAIN

Although some acupuncture procedures are effective in acutely terminating signs, it is often necessary to use a repetitive protocol to achieve full therapeutic effect, particularly with chronic pain. This may be, in part, due to a cumulative effect needed to produce a persistent CNS change.

Treatment of chronic pain usually requires the use of local points, segmental points, and points with an autonomic effect; points related to tissue and structural compensation, such as trigger points, or myofascial origins or insertions often distant to the location in question. Table 16.1 briefly lists basic examples of points that can be added to an analgesic protocol.

Recent work has looked at the effect of acupuncture in hyperalgesic, allodynic, and neuropathic animals. Acupuncture can diminish the sensitization and CNS changes that are pivotal to the development of neuropathic pain. Acupuncture has been shown consistently to minimize or prevent neuropathic pain in animal models, and electroacupuncture as well as laser stimulation of points appears to be effective. In a study of irritable bowel syndrome in rats, a form of visceral neuropathic pain, treatment with ST 36 and ST 37, but not gall bladder (GB) points, was effective in diminishing pain and gut pathology (Tian et al., 2008). Electroacupuncture of low frequency at ST 2 has been shown to confer analgesia in a visceral pain model in rats, and in human patients with trigeminal neuralgia.

It is important to NOT needle the affected area when treating neuropathic pain if an autonomic component is suspected, because the needle stimulation can cause excruciating allodynic pain. Needling surrounding affected areas is helpful, as is treating the underlying pattern with TCVM principles. For specific local effect, treating the segmental paravertebral association and *Hua-tuo Jia Ji* points is beneficial. The literature suggests that for significant neuropathic pain reduction to occur, at least five biweekly sessions are necessary.

Trigger Points

Trigger points (also known in TCVM as *Ashi* points) commonly develop subsequent to postural changes occurring secondary to painful states, such as osteoarthritis. Trigger points, small firm painful foci within a muscle belly, are traditionally treated by a dispersing and sedating needle technique, moxibustion, deep acupressure massage (*tui na*), cupping (in humans) or rubbing. Needles can be inserted just until the "gummy" feeling is contacted. Sometimes a trigger point needs to be needled deeply, and with a pecking motion, to reflexively relieve the spasm. Needles are left in for varying periods, between a moment and 60 minutes. Dispersing and sedating techniques vary in the literature, but this author tends to use techniques of counterclockwise, and fast pecking insertion. Occasionally, simply placing the needle will be sufficient to cause relaxation of the trigger point and normalization of the area. Then the needle can be immediately removed. Once the trigger point is treated, systems become functional again: often lymphatic drainage, venous transport, arterial circulation, neural conduction, and regulatory and immune function can resume. See Chapter 14 for a more detailed discussion of trigger points.

Visceral Pain

Acupuncture can be useful in patients with functional GI disorders because of its effects on GI motility and visceral pain (Takahashi, 2011). Commonly, pain is referred to axial or extremity muscles, creating regional trigger points. Similar regional trigger points resulting from other causes can look identical to visceral pain-induced trigger points. Therefore, visceral disorders are part of the differential diagnosis of regional trigger points.

Cancer Pain

Acupuncture analgesia is an adjunctive treatment for patients with cancer pain. Control of pain and local swelling postoperatively, shortening the resolution of hematoma and tissue swelling, and minimizing use of medications and their attendant adverse effects, are reasons to utilize acupuncture for cancer management. In a Sloan–Kettering study of radiation mucositis, a neuropathic state following upper body radiation, 39% of 70 head and neck cancer patients demonstrated an improvement when treated with acupuncture compared to a 7% improvement of patients treated with physical therapy (Pfister et al., 2010). Zhang et al. (2012) demonstrated in rats that acupuncture can counteract the cancer-driven expression

Table 16.1. Common acupuncture points used for variable pain states and locations

Pain state and location	Common acupuncture points used
Inflammation	LI4, GV14, LI11
General pain	LIV3, GB34, BL60, GV20, SP6
Neuropathic pain	ST36, PC6, TH5
Bone and arthritic pain	BL23, KID1, KID3, BL11
Neck pain	*Jing Jia Ji*, SI3, BL23, BL24, BL25
Hip pain	GB27, GB28, BL54, *Jian-Jiao*
Elbow pain	SI8, PC3, HT1, LI11, LU5
Back pain	*Hua-tuo Jia Ji, Bai Hui, Shen Shu,* BL40

of the transient receptor potential vanilloid 1, thereby attenuating cancer pain.

Bone pain in cancer is a predominant issue. One study involving a rat model for bone cancer pain (Zhang et al., 2008), reported that electroacupuncture over the sciatic nerve (at acupuncture point GB 30 (Huantiao)) significantly attenuated cancer-related hyperalgesia and the expression of dynorphin and interleukin-1beta (IL-1β).

SUMMARY

Acupuncture is a complex intervention that has been used clinically for thousands of years to reduce pain in a variety of disease states. The physiological mechanisms underlying analgesia produced by acupuncture are being defined. In the meantime, practitioners of both traditional and Western forms of acupuncture can offer patients relief from suffering.

REFERENCES

Bowsher, D. (1998) Mechanisms of acupuncture, in *Medical Acupuncture: A Western Scientific Approach* (eds J. Filshie and A. White), Churchill Livingstone, Edinburgh, UK, pp. 69–82.

Campbell, A. (2006) Point specificity of acupuncture in the light of recent clinical and imaging studies. *Acupuncture Medicine*, 24(3), 118–122.

Cassu, R.N., Luna, S.P., Clark, R.M., & Kronka, S.N. (2008) Electroacupuncture analgesia in dogs: is there a difference between uni- and bi-lateral stimulation? *Veterinary Anaesthesia and Analgesia*, 35(1), 52–61.

Cassu, R.N., Silva, D.A., Genari, F.T., & Stevanin, H. (2012) Electroanalgesia for the postoperative control pain in dogs. *Acta Cirurgica Brasileira*, 27(1), 43–48.

Chen, S. & Ma, X. (2003) Nitric oxide in the gracile nucleus mediates depressor response to acupuncture (ST36). *Journal of Neurophysiology*, 90(2), 780–785.

Choi, K.H. & Hill, S.A. (2009) Acupuncture treatment for feline multifocal intervertebral disc disease. *Journal of Feline Medicine and Surgery*, 11(8), 706–710.

Egerbacher, M. (1971) Anatomische und histologische untersuchungen zur morphologic ausgewahlter akupunkturpunkte bei rind und hund, Doctoral dissertation. Vienna Veterinary Medicine University.

Faingold, C.L. (2008) Electrical stimulation therapies for CNS disorders and pain are mediated by competition between different neuronal networks in the brain. *Medical Hypotheses*, 71(5), 668–681.

Gakiya, H., Silva, D, Gomes, J., Stevanin, H., & Cassu, R.N. (2011) Electroacupuncture versus morphine for the postoperative control pain in dogs. *Acta Cirurgica Brasileira*, 26(5), 346–351.

Groppetti, D., Pecile, A.M., Sacerdote, P., Bronzo, V., & Ravasio, G. (2011) Effectiveness of electroacupuncture analgesia compared with opioid administration in a dog model: a pilot study. *British Journal of Anaesthesia*, 107(4), 612–618.

Han, H.J., Yoon, H.Y., Kim, J.Y., et al. (2010) Clinical effect of additional electroacupuncture on thoracolumbar intervertebral disc herniation in 80 paraplegic dogs. *American Journal of Chinese Medicine*, 38(6), 1015–1025.

Hayashi, A.M., Matera, J.M., & Fonseca Pinto, A.C. (2007) Evaluation of electroacupuncture treatment for thoracolumbar intervertebral disk disease in dogs. *Journal of the American Veterinary Medical Association*, 231(6), 913–918.

Hurt, J.K. & Zylka, M.J. (2012) PAPupuncture has localized and long-lasting antinociceptive effects in mouse models of acute and chronic pain. *Molecular Pain*, 8(1), 28.

Jaeger, G.T., Larsen, S., Søli, N., & Moe, L. (2006) Double-blind, placebo-controlled trial of the pain-relieving effects of the implantation of gold beads into dogs with hip dysplasia. *Veterinary Record*, 158(21), 722–726.

Jaeger, G.T., Larsen, S., Søli, N., & Moe, L. (2007) Two years follow-up study of the pain-relieving effect of gold bead implantation in dogs with hip-joint arthritis. *Acta Veterinaria Scandinavica*, 49, 9.

Joaquim, J.G., Luna, S.P., Brondani, J.T., Torelli, S.R., Rahal, S.C., & de Paula Freitas, F. (2010) Comparison of decompressive surgery, electroacupuncture, and decompressive surgery followed by electroacupuncture for the treatment of dogs with intervertebral disk disease with long-standing severe neurologic deficits. *Journal of the American Veterinary Medical Association*, 236(11), 1225–1229.

Johng, H.M., Yoo, J.S., Yoon, T.J., et al. (2007) Use of magnetic nanoparticles to visualize threadlike structures inside lymphatic vessels of rats. *Evidence Based Complementary and Alternative Medicine*, 4(1), 77–82.

Kavoussi, B. & Ross, B.E. (2007) Neuroimmune basis of anti-inflammatory acupuncture. *Integrative Cancer Therapy*, 6(3), 251–257.

Kim, D.H., Cho, S.H., Song, K.H., et al. (2004) Electroacupuncture analgesia for surgery in cattle. *American Journal of Chinese Medicine*, 32(1), 131–140.

Kim, H.W., Uh, D.K., Yoon, S.Y., et al. (2008) Low-frequency electroacupuncture suppresses carageenan-induced paw inflammation in mice via sympathetic post-ganglionic neurons, while high frequency EA suppression is mediated by the sympathoadrenal medullary axis. *Brain Research Bulletin*, 75, 689–705.

Kimura, A. & Sato, A. (1997) Somatic regulation of autonomic functions in anesthetized animals–neural mechanisms of physical therapy including acupuncture. *Japan Journal of Veterinary Research*, 45(3), 137–145.

Kimura, Y. & Hara, S. (2008) The effect of electro-acupuncture stimulation on rhythm of autonomic nervous system in dogs. *Journal of Veterinary Medical Science*, 70(4), 349–352.

Koopman, F., Stoof, S., Straub, R., et al. (2011) Restoring the balance of the autonomic nervous system as an innovative approach to the treatment of rheumatoid arthritis. *Molecular Medicine*, 17(9–10), 937–948.

Laim, A., Jaggy, A., Forterre, F., Doherr, M.G, Aeschbacher, & Glardon, O. (2009) Effects of adjunct electroacupuncture on severity of postoperative pain in dogs undergoing hemilaminectomy because of acute thoracolumbar intervertebral disk disease. *Journal of the American Veterinary Medical Association*, 234(9), 1141–1146.

Lee, H.G., Lee, B., Choi, S.H., et al. (2004) Electroacupuncture reduces stress-induced expression of c-fos in the brain of the rat. *American Journal of Chinese Medicine*, 32, 597–606.

Leung, A., Kim, S., Schulteis, G., & Yaksh, T. (2008) The effect of acupuncture duration on analgesia and peripheral sensory thresholds. *BMC Complementary Alternative Medicine*, 8, 18.

Leung, L. (2012) Neurophysiological basis of acupuncture induced analgesia—an updated review. *Journal of Acupuncture and Meridian Studies*, 5(6), 261–270.

Li, A., Wang, Y., Xin, G., et al. (2007) Electroacupuncture suppresses hyperalgesia and spinal Fos expression by activating the descending inhibitory system. *Brain Research*, 1186, 171–179.

Lin, J.G. & Chen, W.L. (2008) Acupuncture analgesia: a review of its mechanisms of action. *The American Journal of Chinese Medicine*, 36(4), 635–645.

Liu, J., Qin, W., Guo, Q., et al. (2010) Distinct brain networks for time-varied characteristics of acupuncture. *Neuroscience Letters*, 468, 353–358.

Lorenzini, L., Giuliani, A., Giardino, L., & Calzà, L. (2010) Laser acupuncture for acute inflammatory, visceral and neuropathic pain relief: an experimental study in the laboratory rat. *Research in Veterinary Science*, 88(1), 159–165.

Pfister, D.G., Cassileth, B.R., Deng, G.E., et al. (2010) Acupuncture for pain and dysfunction after neck dissection: results of a randomized controlled trial. *Journal of Clinical Oncology*, 28(15), 2565–2570.

Qin, W., Bai, L., Dai, J., et al. (2011) The temporal-spatial encoding of acupuncture effects in the brain. *Molecular Pain*, 7, 19.

Skarda, R.T. & Muir, W.W., 3rd. (2003) Comparison of electroacupuncture and butorphanol on respiratory and cardiovascular effects and rectal pain threshold after controlled rectal distention in mares. *American Journal of Veterinary Research*, 64(2), 137–144.

Takahashi, T. (2011) Mechanism of acupuncture on neuromodulation in the gut–a review. *Neuromodulation*, 14(1), 8–12.

Tian, S.L., Wang, X.Y., & Ding, G.H. (2008) Repeated electro-acupuncture attenuates chronic visceral hypersensitivity and spinal cord NMDA receptor phosphorylation in a rat irritable bowel syndrome model. *Life Science*, 83(9–10), 356–363.

Wang, S.M., Kain, Z.N., & White, P. (2008) Acupuncture analgesia: I. The scientific basis. *Anesthesia and Analgesia*, 106, 602–610.

White, A., Cummings, M., Barlas, P., et al. (2008) Defining an adequate dose of acupuncture using a neurophysiological approach–a narrative review of the literature. *Acupuncture Medicine*, 26(2), 111–120.

Xie, H., Colahan, P., & Ott, E.A. (2005) Evaluation of electroacupuncture treatment of horses with signs of chronic thoracolumbar pain. *Journal of the American Veterinary Medical Association*, 227(2), 281–286.

Xie, H., Ott, E.A., & Colahan, P. (2001) *Influence of Acupuncture on Experimental Lameness in Horses*. Proceedings of the American Association of Equine Practitioners, November 24–28, 2001, San Diego, CA.

Xing, G., Liu, F., & Qu, X. (2007) Long-term synaptic plasticity in the spinal dorsal horn and its modulation by electroacupuncture in rats with neuropathic pain. *Experimental Neurology*, 208, 323–332.

Yan, Z., Wang, P., Cheng, J., et al. (1992) Studies on the luminescence of channels in rats and its law of changes with "syndromes" and treatment of acupuncture and moxibustion. *Journal of Traditional Chinese Medicine*, 12(4), 283–287.

Yang, E., Li, P., Nilius, B., & LiG. (2011) Ancient Chinese medicine and mechanistic evidence of acupuncture physiology. *Pflugers Archives - European Journal of Physiology*, 462, 645–653.

Yim, Y.K., Lee, H., Hong, K.E., et al. (2007) Electroacupuncture at acupoint ST36 reduces inflammation and regulates immune activity in collagen-induced arthritic mice. *Evidence Based Complementary and Alternative Medicine*, 4, 51–57.

Yoon, S.Y., Roh, D.H., Kwon, Y.B., et al. (2009) Acupoint stimulation with diluted bee venom (apipuncture) potentiates the analgesic effect of intrathecal clonidine in the rodent formalin test and in a neuropathic pain model. *Journal of Pain*, 10(3), 253–263.

Zhang, J., Wang, X.M., & McAlonan, G. (2012) Neural acupuncture unit: a new concept for interpreting effects and mechanisms of acupuncture. *Evidence-Based Complementary and Alternative Medicine*.DOI: 10.1155/2012/429412.

Zhang, R.X., Li, A., Liu, B., et al. (2008) Electroacupuncture attenuates bone-cancer-induced hyperalgesia and inhibits spinal preprodynorphin expression in a rat model. *European Journal of Pain*, 12(7), 870–878.

Zhang, Y., Li, A., Xin, J., et al. (2011) Involvement of spinal serotonin receptors in electroacupuncture anti-hyperalgesia in an inflammatory pain rat model. *Neurochemical Research*, 36(10), 1785–1792.

Zhang, Y., Zhang, R.X., Zhang, M., et al. (2012) Electroacupuncture inhibition of hyperalgesia in an inflammatory pain rat model: involvement of distinct spinal serotonin and norepinephrine receptor subtypes. *British Journal of Anaesthesia*, 109(2), 245–252.

Zhang, Z., Wang, C., Gu, G., et al. (2012) The effects of electroacupuncture at the ST36 (Zusanli) acupoint on cancer pain and transient receptor potential vanilloid subfamily 1 expression in Walker 256 tumor-bearing rats. *Anesthesia and Analgesia*, 114(4), 879–885.

Zhao, Z. (2008) Neural mechanisms underlying acupuncture analgesia. *Progress in Neurobiology*, 85, 355–375.

17
Equine Acupuncture

Arthur I. Ortenburger

The use of acupuncture to reduce or eliminate pain can be an important option in many clinical situations. Acupuncture may be a useful adjunct to pharmaceutical analgesics, may be effective when other analgesics are not, can be used in cases where nonsteroidal anti-inflammatory drugs (NSAIDs) are contraindicated, is considered a very safe therapy, and can be less expensive for the treatment of chronic (lifetime) pain problems than pharmaceuticals. The practice of placing very fine gauge needles in specific places called acupuncture points is familiar to most people, but there are other means of stimulating these points, including heat, injection (both with drugs and inert fluids), microamperage electrical current, milliwatt laser light, and permanent implants of gold wire. Each method has its indications, and the fact that there is more than one way to stimulate an acupuncture point emphasizes its versatility and adaptability to unusual clinical problems and circumstances. The practice of acupuncture in horses is not difficult, and some of the more basic techniques may be used without training. Yet, there are a number of specifics unique to the discipline, and formal training to learn these will greatly increase opportunities to use this important therapeutic.

Effective use of the conventional, often pharmaceutical, analgesics for chronic pain conditions in horses is subject to a standard set of limitations well known in the healing arts. A high level of owner compliance is assumed, yet cannot always be obtained. The experienced clinician will instantly recognize that there are patients which refuse medication, which are NSAID-intolerant, which show confusing waxing and waning of the signs of pain over weeks and months, and which cannot undergo indicated surgical treatments for reasons of cost or other client concerns. The rules for horses in athletic competition may deny treatment with indicated analgesics, though the condition causing pain may not of itself prevent continued athletic use. Very often, these are the same patients for whom acupuncture may prove to be an important part of the integrated solution to their pain problem. While it can be effective for long-term analgesia, acupuncture avoids the risks of contributing to adverse drug events and of adverse drug–drug interactions related to polypharmacy.

The comparable virtues of the different schools of acupuncture thought, including traditional Chinese medicine (TCM), eight principles, empirical point selection, medical acupuncture, and French energetic, are less clear. These schools of acupuncture philosophy differ in their approach to identifying and resolving the essential *acupuncture lesion*—imbalance or obstruction of flow through acupuncture channels, also known as meridians. In fact, in some views there is no acupuncture lesion. Instead, the use of needles is seen as a peripheral manipulation of central somatic and autonomic pathways to achieve acupuncture analgesia. In application, however, it is often the case that for a given clinical problem, the same types of needles are inserted into the same acupuncture points to achieve the same therapeutic result, regardless of the philosophy employed to arrive at the solution. It has not been shown that the cognitive process of any particular acupuncture school is superior to another.

The use of acupuncture for acute pain may be appropriate in an outpatient or hospital setting, and includes pain of postoperative wounds, ileus, gastrointestinal ischemia, inflammation, abdominal distension, burns, ophthalmic inflammation, and orthopedic trauma.

ACUPUNCTURE TECHNIQUES AND PROCEDURES

Acupuncture points may be stimulated or treated by a variety of methods. For each, there are varying levels of research to document efficacy and clinical utility, though seldom for more than one animal species. This aspect of the discipline (i.e., which method of acupuncture point treatment is best for a given clinical problem) remains poorly understood and, for the moment, we must rely on clinical impressions and expert opinion to decide these matters. In this author's opinion, the routine use of acupuncture needles (sometimes referred to as "dry needles"), injection of acupuncture points, electroacupuncture, milliwatt diode laser light, gold implants, and moxibustion are all reasonable methods, and have sufficient clinical evidence of efficacy.

Acupuncture is most easily, if not quickly, performed in the unsedated horse handled by an experienced assistant. Very often, insertion of the needles is not perceived, and the usual methods of physical restraint are not needed. The routine use of guide tubes is recommended, with the caveat that these were designed for the thickness of human skin and are entirely too long for use where the skin is much thicker, especially over the dorsum. When guide tubes fail to send the needle through the entire thickness of the skin, a needle pinching technique is suggested (Figures 17.1a & 17.1b).

Pain Management in Veterinary Practice, First Edition. Edited by Christine M. Egger, Lydia Love and Tom Doherty.

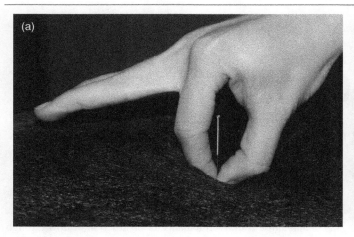
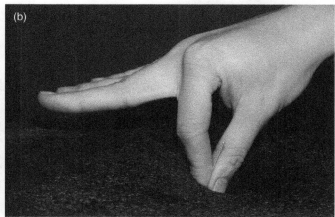

Figure 17.1. Needle placement through thick skin. (a) The thumb and forefinger are strongly flexed against each other while pinching the needle, and together press firmly into the skin over the acupuncture point. (b) Thumb and finger are suddenly extended, and the needle is sent through the horse's skin, which is stretched at the same time by the fingertips.

In the world of competitive athletes, it is quite common to encounter a horse experienced with many different kinds of needles, and which resists them all with vigor and determination. This behavior is usually known in advance of treatment, and appropriate sedation or physical restraint should be employed before acupuncture treatment even begins. Concerns that sedated animals do not respond to acupuncture normally or as well as unsedated animals have not been substantiated. Horses do display a unique seasonal response to the presence of acupuncture needles during a treatment session, with increased use of the panniculus "fly-shaking" reflex during the warmer months when biting arthropods are about; this response is reduced or absent during colder seasons. For horses which are doing a lot of fly-shaking in response to needle insertion, simply bending the needle handle flat to the skin and taping it down with Micropore® or other suitable tape will prevent dislodgement of the needle (Figure 17.2).

Electroacupuncture is preferred for the first two treatments to obtain the quickest possible treatment effect (Takeshige, 2001), followed by ordinary dry needle treatments for as long as needed. Conditions of acute pain (e.g., colic, ileus, orthopedic trauma) are treated daily for 3 days, then on alternate days. Chronic orthopedic pain (e.g., tarsal osteoarthritis, palmar heel pain) is treated at weekly intervals for 3–6 weeks, followed by maintenance therapy of one to four times each year.

Systemic, regional, and local points are generally needled, and a tonifying or sedating technique (Table 17.1) can be used. Local points are needled with a tonifying technique. Acupuncture points are found by anatomic location, as described in standard acupuncture texts. When treating any of the arthritides, it is prudent to locate and treat points proximal and distal to the plane of the joint, on dorsal, medial, and lateral surfaces of the limb. It may be difficult to perform electroacupuncture on the distal limbs due to lack of patient tolerance of the wires brushing against the skin of the limb, often eliciting stamping and tail wringing. Taping the wires to the skin may help reduce the horse's concern, as the sensation of needles and loose wires may be interpreted as the presence of flies.

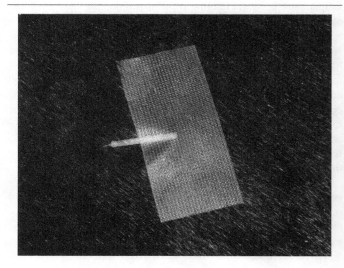

Figure 17.2. Securing needles in the summer. After placement of the acupuncture needle, the handle may be folded flat to the skin and covered with tape to prevent the panniculus reflex from shaking the needle out.

Acupuncture treatment of numerous disease problems, including pain, can be considered from two very different paths—use of a treatment formula or identification of the lesion. The understandable desire for a direct solution through treatment formulas (there is pain in the right forefoot, which acupuncture points will work?) is attractive and often effective (Table 17.2). However, there is much to recommend a more methodical and complete understanding of the problem, and from this, an effective and comprehensive treatment strategy will develop. In other words, acupuncture can be used to good effect even without an understanding of acupuncture science, but better results will be obtained when more specific treatment is developed in a context of the unique perspectives of what may be called "acupuncture medicine."

Table 17.1. Acupuncture point stimulation techniques and effects

Treatment variable	Tonification[a]	Sedation[a]
Needle manipulation	Gentle, brief	Vigorous, prolonged
Treatment duration	5–10 min	20–30 min
Electroacupuncture frequency	1–8 Hz	20–100 Hz
Laser dose	0.5–1.0 J	2–4 J
Injection volume (saline)	2–5 mL	10 mL

[a]The terms "tonify" and "sedate" are frequently used in acupuncture therapy to describe particular manipulations of the acupuncture point. These may be viewed as "strengthening" and "reducing," respectively, and are accomplished through particular movements of the needle, settings of frequency and signal strength in electrical stimulator equipment, and in different ways appropriate to other methods of acupuncture point stimulation.

ACUPUNCTURE FOR GENERALIZED, SYSTEMIC PAIN

There is growing recognition that a multimodal approach is the most effective, and probably the safest, method for many kinds of chronic pain (Lerche & Muir, 2009). Among the virtues of acupuncture in this role is the recognition that it elicits analgesia through unique neurological mechanisms, which do not duplicate or interfere with those produced by pharmaceutical, surgical, manipulative, bandaging, or behavioral methods of analgesia (Helms, 2012).

There is little published literature on the use of acupuncture in horses for systemic pain states, such as extensive burns or major trauma (collision with vehicles and other horses). Application of its principles with regard to selecting appropriate points to be needled should be straightforward, and the therapy might well be helpful when response to conventional pharmaceuticals is inadequate or

Table 17.2. Empirical acupuncture points for treatment of pain by location. Descriptive anatomical location of the named points will be found in any of the standard veterinary acupuncture texts. This table appears to suggest an empirical approach to acupuncture therapy. Instead, even a superficial understanding of the discipline will reveal that more appropriate combinations of points for a given patient are possible, requiring only a basic course in traditional Chinese medicine

Site of pain	Useful acupuncture points
Pain, not specific to a site	Bai hui, GV-20, BL-60, LI-4
Systemic (large-scale trauma, burns)	Bai hui, LI-4, 11, BL-60
Gastrointestinal	ST-2, BL-20, 21, ST-36
Temporomandibular joint	GB-2, 41, ST-7
Cervical spine	GB-39, BL-60, LU-7, Jiu-wei
Thoracolumbar spine	BL-40, Shu points three spinal segments cranial and caudal to the site of pain
Lumbosacral joints	Bai hui, BL-25
Pelvic region and sacroiliac joints	BL-25, 30, 35, 54
Hip joint	BL-54, GB-30
Stifle	GB-33, 34, ST-35
Hock	BL-37, 62, ST-42
Hind fetlock	BL-65, ST-43, LIV-2
Hind phalanx	KI-1, BL-66
Shoulder joint	GB-34, TH-14
Elbow joint	SI-9, HT-3, TH-10
Carpus	SI-9, TH-4
Fore tendinitis, suspensory desmitis	SI-9, GB-34, LU-10
Fore fetlock	TH-2, SI-3
Fore phalanx	PC-9, TH-1
Laminitis	SI-9, Ting points, LI-11
Palmar heel pain	SI-9, Qian ti men

their use contraindicated. The points Bai hui, BL-40, LI-4, LI-11, and SP-6 may be helpful in such cases, and may act to increase concentrations of central opioid neurotransmitters.

ACUPUNCTURE FOR LOCAL PAIN

Among the most frequent indications for acupuncture in equine practice is the control of chronic orthopedic pain (Fleming, 2001). Acupuncture is often effective, and may replace NSAIDs or allow smaller doses, thus reducing the potential for adverse effects. In the working athlete, acupuncture may also permit use of the horse in regulated competition without concern for a disqualifying blood or urine test detecting pharmaceuticals. Chronic orthopedic pain is most often localized in joints, and the common pathway leading to degenerative joint disease with concomitant pain may arise from excessive training, osteochondrosis, or the presence of osteochondral fracture fragments. Appropriate medical and surgical therapies must be considered and included in any discussion of acupuncture with the owner. It is often the case that there are other beneficial effects of acupuncture for athletes working at a high level of performance in their specialty, and at a comparable level of psychogenic stress, which might contribute to the onset of gastric ulcer syndrome, colic, and incidents and accidents which are always a concern in the confined, high-strung, and highly stressed animal (Xie, 2007a).

Palmar Heel Pain

In general, this author prefers to manage the lameness caused by any factor that results in palmar heel pain with conventional treatments. The analgesic benefits of corrective hoof trimming are considered essential to controlling pain as well as restoring a more physiological shape in horses with a variety of abnormalities of the hoof. However, there are individual animals that continue to demonstrate refractory chronic heel pain and which may benefit from acupuncture (Fleming, 2001). The usual systemic points have been of less value than the "extra" local points shown in Figure 17.3. Treatment is by tonification of the three points described, and will likely be needed at more frequent intervals than is usually the case for osteoarthritis or degenerative joint disease in more proximal joints. Given that the pain, manifested as lameness, usually seen with this syndrome waxes and wanes in the normal course of events, it can be particularly difficult to assess response to treatment in these cases.

Tendonitis and Desmitis

Acupuncture for therapy of tendonitis and desmitis is described, and is capable of reducing the pain that results (Xie & Preast, 2007). As of this writing, there is no research documenting improvement in quality or rate of healing of tendon injuries with acupuncture.

Sacroiliac Joint Pain

Accurate diagnosis of sacroiliac joint pain may be difficult, but often includes response to local treatment by intra-articular injection of anti-inflammatory medication. Acupuncture can be of value for this condition, especially in horses that will not allow treatment with drug injection, or if such treatment has been ineffective while there remains a strong likelihood that the diagnosis is correct. Although traditional principles suggest that a tonifying technique should be used with the needles placed in local points, tonification of local points will fail to obtain improvement in about 25%

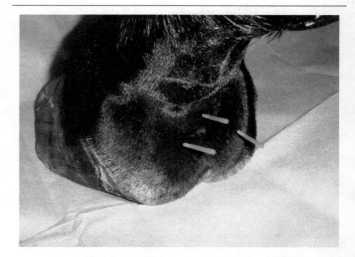

Figure 17.3. Palmar foot extra points. As part of the treatment for palmar heel pain, two extra points over the axial surface of both ungual cartilages are needled, as well as PC-9 (proximal center).

of cases. For those, sedation of these points succeeds in resolving pain. Electroacupuncture at 80 Hz and a relatively high current flow for a minimum of 10 minutes can result in marked improvement for a prolonged period (3–6 months). The points most often treated include Bai hui, GB-28, BL-25, 30, 35, and 54.

Chronic Cervical Pain

Osteoarthritis of the cervical zygapophyseal joints may be a significant cause of chronic pain in middle-aged athletes, and less often in younger flat racers (Dyson, 2003). Diagnosis is made by careful palpation and observation of restricted voluntary lateral flexion, and is confirmed by typical radiographic signs. The problem is most frequently seen in the caudal region of the neck, and may extend to the C7-T1 articulation. Treatment with systemic NSAIDs and local injection of glucocorticoids is effective, yet has an appreciable risk, including unintended subdural injection, laceration of the vertebral artery, infection, and those associated with prolonged use of NSAIDs. Chiropractic manipulation techniques should be considered for any signs of caudal neck pain in the horse. Acupuncture is usually very effective for alleviating pain and improving lateral bending of the neck. Transpositional acupuncture points are of less value for this condition, and the needed traditional Jiu-wei points (Figure 17.4) will be found in the classical texts (Westermayer, 1979). An extra point (Chingchung) is also of value, and located superficially to the dorsal tubercle of the transverse process of C-3.

Thoracolumbar Pain

The fact of back pain in horses of many different uses and breeds is well known to the observant practitioner, and has ample description in the veterinary literature (Denoix & Dyson, 2003). Yet, its diagnosis may be challenging, at least with respect to an accurate and specific anatomic location. It is helpful to understand that demonstration of pain in a somewhat general region of the back is a useful clinical accomplishment, and is quite adequate to allow institution of any of a number of treatments, of which acupuncture should

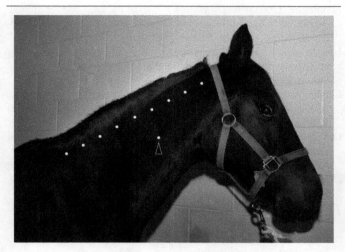

Figure 17.4. Traditional cervical points. The Jiu-wei point consists of nine sites, which may be needled on either side of the neck, appropriate to the location of cervical pain or disease. These sites are equidistant and divide a straight line between the center of the wing of the atlas and the craniodorsal angle of the scapula into 10 equal segments. An extra point is palpated over the dorsal tubercle of the transverse process of C-3 (arrowhead).

be one. Each type of equine athletic activity is prone to particular patterns of back pain, but for the clinician, the pain is where you find it, and local, physical methods of treatment will be far more effective than simply prescribing an NSAID. Most acupuncture treatments of back pain will include the use of bladder channel points which are in close proximity to the site of observed vertebral motion restrictions, epaxial muscle spasm, and trigger points. Conventional needling, electroacupuncture, and acupoint injection techniques are all effective; comparisons of the relative efficacy of these very different treatments in the horse remain indeterminate. When treating a long-established problem of back pain, it is common to find that each acupuncture treatment seems to result in movement of the pain from one region to another—from lumbosacral to mid-thoracic to thoracolumbar is one common pattern. In the author's experience, these cases simply require a few more treatments, and usually benefit from chiropractic therapy as well.

Lumbosacral Articulations

Pain originating from the intertransverse and lumbosacral joints is diagnosed by response to local motion palpation of these joints in a frontal plane (dorsal–ventral passive extension). The value of diagnostic imaging of these joints is unknown, and is likely to be misleading in revealing degenerative changes in the older animal that do not correlate to clinically relevant pain. For the present, we must evaluate abnormalities of gait and performance, restrictions to joint movement in this region, and signs of local pain by palpation to arrive at a diagnosis. The intertransverse joints in particular, seem to be very responsive to acupuncture, and a single treatment at BL-25 often has a long-lasting effect. The needle is inserted perpendicular to the skin with a tonifying technique.

Gastrointestinal Pain

Gastrointestinal pain in the horse is due to a wide range of pathophysiologies. In most cases, the available pharmaceuticals are safe, effective, and have rapid onset of analgesia. In circumstances where these analgesics are not ideal, for reasons related to owner preference, or as an adjunct to pharmaceutical treatment, acupuncture should be considered. Similar to allopathic medicine, the traditional Chinese view of colic recognizes numerous pathways for its development, and it is strongly advised that these be understood if the clinician will be using acupuncture to aid in the management of abdominal pain on a regular basis (Xie, 2007c). Otherwise, the empirical points ST-2, ST-25, Bl-20, Bl-21, and ST-36 may be of value in many cases, and will not interfere with conventional therapies. Whether acupuncture is capable of blocking pain to the extent that a surgical acute abdomen is not recognized is unknown at this time.

Ileus

Postoperative ileus is an occasional cause of pain that varies from slight to severe. Acupuncture can completely resolve such pain, but it must be said that the more severe cases may not respond adequately and will require the most potent pharmaceutical analgesics. Points used include BL-21, ST-36, and SP-6, all with a tonifying technique. These points are all associated in traditional Chinese medicine with function of the stomach, small intestine, and colon.

Laminar Degeneration (Laminitis)

In the author's experience, the use of acupuncture for acute laminitis pain has limited benefits, and is less effective than conventional analgesic methods. In the case of chronic laminitis pain, acupuncture has resulted in significant improvement of the lameness and affords substantial clinical benefit. The technique involves bleeding of the abnormal ting points (located along the coronary band on the front and hind hooves) in both forelimbs, accomplished with an 18-gauge hypodermic needle in the sedated horse (Fleming, 2001). A single full-thickness insertion and removal is quickly performed in each ting point, which is soft and "marshy" when palpated with a fingertip. The ting point of the pericardium channel is not treated.

USE OF ACUPUNCTURE IN COMPETITIVE ATHLETES

The question of fair and ethical treatment of athletes in competition with acupuncture has not been resolved. The definitive question may be phrased: "Should acupuncture treatment be provided to a competitive athlete when it is known or simply believed that such treatment will alter its performance?" The argument has any number of unique facets, which together do not lend themselves to resolving the question with a simple, blanket statement. As matters stand now, there are restrictions on the use of acupuncture in some European jurisdictions, but few in North America. The fact that acupuncture treatment cannot be physiologically detected by event stewards is entirely beside the point—the matter is an ethical and legal one, and the veterinarian can do nothing less than abide by the rules of the game. While acupuncture may be permitted in many venues, it is often a requirement that the treatment be reported to the show steward or veterinary authority.

ADVERSE EFFECTS

While the adverse effects of acupuncture are well documented in the human literature, there is little to be found related to animal acupuncture. One study reviewing the use of approximately 12,000 needles in 221 animals, including 74 horses, found a total of two major and two minor adverse events, of which one was a small area of local skin edema in the pastern of a horse treated for palmar heel pain (Ortenburger & Hopson, 2009).

SUMMARY

To practice acupuncture well requires an effort to learn this unique clinical discipline. It is not possible to convey the basic science knowledge and clinical skills necessary to practice acupuncture in this brief chapter. There are a number of educational courses available to learn this specialty, and such continuing education is recommended for veterinarians who have need for additional means to control pain in horses.

REFERENCES

Denoix, J-M. & Dyson, S. (2003) Thoracolumbar spine, in *Diagnosis and Management of Lameness in the Horse* (eds M.W. Ross & S.J. Dyson), Saunders, St. Louis, MO.

Dyson, S. (2003) The cervical spine and soft tissues of the neck, in *Diagnosis and Management of Lameness in the Horse* (eds M.W. Ross & S.J. Dyson), Saunders, St. Louis, MO.

Fleming, P. (2001) Acupuncture for musculoskeletal and neurologic conditions in horses, in *Veterinary Acupuncture Ancient Art to Modern Medicine* (ed. A.M. Schoen), Mosby Inc., St. Louis, MO.

Helms, J.M. (2012) *An Overview of Medical Acupuncture,* http://www.medicalacupuncture.org/acu_info/articles/helmsarticle.html (accessed January 10, 2012.

Lerche, P. & Muir, W. (2009) Pain management in horses and cattle, in *Handbook of Veterinary Pain Management* (eds J.S. Gaynor & W.W. Muir), Mosby Elsevier, St. Louis, MO.

Ortenburger, A. & Hopson, M. (2009) Adverse effects of animal acupuncture: review of 1,292 treatments. Proceedings of the 35th Annual International Congress on Veterinary Acupuncture, The International Veterinary Acupuncture Society, August 26–29, 2009, San Antonio, TX, pp. 57.

Takeshige, C. (2001) Mechanisms of acupuncture analgesia produced by low frequency electrical simulation of acupuncture points, in *Clinical Acupuncture Scientific Basis* (eds G. Stux & R. Hammerschlag), Springer-Verlag, Berlin.

Westermayer, E. (1979) *The Treatment of Horses by Acupuncture*, C.W. Daniel Company, Essex, UK.

Xie, H. (2007a) Acupuncture for acute and miscellaneous conditions, in *Xie's Veterinary Acupuncture*, (eds H. Xie, & V. Preast), Blackwell Publishing, Ames, IA.

Xie, H. & Preast, V. (2007b) Acupuncture for treatment of musculoskeletal and neurological disorders, in *Xie's Veterinary Acupuncture*, (eds H. Xie, & V. Preast), Blackwell Publishing, Ames, IA.

Xie, H. (2007c) Acupuncture for internal medicine, in *Xie's Veterinary Acupuncture*, (eds H. Xie, & V. Preast), Blackwell Publishing, Ames, IA.

18
Canine Chiropractic and Pain Management

Robin Downing

Chiropractic is a medical discipline based on spinal manipulation. The founder of chiropractic, D.D. Palmer, is recognized for stating a fundamental relationship between the skeleton and the nervous system. He did not view the spine or skeleton as isolated organs within the larger body, rather he viewed the spine as having a core role in the overall health. His primary contribution was to focus attention on the role of spinal movement in maintaining normal nerve function, and to develop a body of clinical knowledge and skills to address changes in spinal movement leading to nervous system dysfunction (Cleveland et al., 2001). Although D.D. Palmer is credited with discovering chiropractic, it was his son, B.J. Palmer, who developed chiropractic into a formal medical discipline.

Although pain is the leading reason human patients seek care from chiropractic practitioners (Leach, 1994a), and pain relief is central to the discipline of chiropractic (Bove & Swenson, 2001), the traditional paradigm of chiropractic medicine reflects the following core beliefs:

- The body is self-regulating and self-healing.
- The nervous system is the master system of the body.
- Alterations in spinal movement adversely affect the nervous system's ability to regulate function.
- Correcting, managing, or minimizing the vertebral subluxation complex (see Section The Vertebral Subluxation Complex) via chiropractic adjustment optimizes patient health (Cleveland et al., 2001).

Chiropractic is considered by practitioners (on human patients) to be a stand-alone system of health care, and the adaptation of chiropractic techniques for use in veterinary medicine is relatively recent (Pascoe, 2002). The American Veterinary Medical Association has published "Guidelines for Complementary and Alternative Veterinary Medicine" which contains the following description of chiropractic care: "... veterinary manual or manipulative therapy (similar to osteopathy, chiropractic, or physical medicine and therapy)..." (AVMA, 2001), thus placing chiropractic into the category of complementary care to be used (literally) to "complement" traditional allopathic veterinary medicine.

THE VERTEBRAL SUBLUXATION COMPLEX

A central tenet of chiropractic medicine is that pathology of the spine leads to nervous system dysfunction through the formation of a "vertebral subluxation complex (VSC)". Unlike an orthopedic luxation, where bones normally engaged in a structural relationship become disrupted or distracted (e.g., coxofemoral luxation), the VSC is a term that describes a functional rather than a structural abnormality. Segmental dysfunction is another term used to describe the VSC phenomenon (Leach, 1994b). The VSC describes a spinal segment that is restricted from moving throughout its normal range of motion (ROM). The complex describes this loss of movement within the context of one vertebra in relation to neighboring vertebrae. Vertebrae that do not function properly within the spinal framework generate mechanical stress and, thereby, accelerate the wear and tear on the surrounding spinal muscles, ligaments, discs, joints, and other spinal tissues. Pain, inflammation, tenderness to palpation, decreased mobility, and muscle spasm/tension result.

The American Chiropractic Association–endorsed definition of the VSC is a "...theoretical model of motion segment dysfunction which incorporates the complex interaction of pathological changes in nerve, muscle, ligamentous, vascular, and connective tissues" (Cleveland, 2001). Likewise, the Association of Chiropractic Colleges defines the VSC as "...a complex of functional, structural, and/or pathological articular changes that compromise neural integrity and may influence organ system function and general health" (Cleveland, 2001).

The commonality among all descriptions of the VSC is the loss of normal movement through the spinal segment. The VSC is thought to alter the normal neurophysiological balance found in a healthy individual. The restriction of movement at a spinal segment is theorized to lead to facilitation of nervous system activity that can, in turn, create pain and aberrations in homeostasis (Leach, 1994b). It is believed that once nerve functioning is compromised, nervous system communication within the body becomes less effective, jeopardizing the overall health and wellness of the individual. Persistent nociception and afferent bombardment result in facilitation and the subsequent decreased threshold for firing of neurons, leading to pain (Leach, 1994c).

Pain Management in Veterinary Practice, First Edition. Edited by Christine M. Egger, Lydia Love and Tom Doherty.
© 2014 John Wiley & Sons, Inc. Published 2014 by John Wiley & Sons, Inc.

The Lantz Model (Lantz, 1989; Cleveland, 2001) provides a very structured, nine-component description of the VSC, including a hierarchy of organization and a pattern of interrelation of its components. Movement (kinesiology) is represented at the apex of this model, thus emphasizing the importance of normal movement as well as describing the effect of loss of movement upon other components of the model. The nine interrelated components of the VSC according to Lantz are:

- Kinesiological (abnormal movement)
- Myological (muscle changes)
- Neurological (nerve roots, ganglia, and nociceptors affected by decreased motion)
- Vascular (local circulatory effects on the nervous system)
- Connective tissue (ligaments, tendons, intervertebral discs, and other supportive structures)
- Inflammatory response (initial cause of pain)
- Anatomical (alterations in tissue structure)
- Physiological (alterations in tissue function)
- Biochemical (closely related to the inflammatory response)

CHOOSING PATIENTS THAT WILL BENEFIT FROM CHIROPRACTIC TREATMENT

A primary care practitioner, by carefully palpating the patient for pain, can identify patients that would potentially benefit from chiropractic evaluation and adjustment. A systematic palpation will reveal areas of discomfort or altered sensation along the spine and over the pelvis. It is likely that the practitioner will also notice a relative lack of elasticity or tissue motion in these areas when compared to the surrounding tissues. The torso should be able to extend, flex, bend laterally, and rotate and it is critical to understand normal movement in order to recognize abnormal movement. A detailed description of a pain palpation in a dog is published elsewhere (Downing, 2011), but the key components include a systematic approach using pressure applied with the fleshy tissue over P3 of the first and second fingers. If back pain is noted or if areas along the back feel tense or less pliant than the surrounding areas, the patient may be a good candidate for chiropractic evaluation and adjustment.

In keeping with the AVMA Guidelines for Complementary and Alternative Veterinary Medicine, any canine patient receiving chiropractic care should also have a primary care provider. If the primary care veterinarian is appropriately trained, that individual may also serve in the capacity of providing chiropractic care. Should the primary care provider be other than the practitioner providing chiropractic care, the practitioner providing chiropractic care has an obligation to the patient and client to keep the primary care veterinarian informed of the patient's full complement of medical care. Before beginning any chiropractic treatment, informed consent should be obtained from the owner.

CHIROPRACTIC EVALUATION

Before any adjustments occur, the canine patient must be thoroughly evaluated to make as complete a diagnosis as possible. The examination should include, but may not be limited to, an evaluation of posture and gait, vertebral and extremity palpation, motion palpation, and an orthopedic and neurological evaluation.

When examining and treating the canine patient with chiropractic it is critical to keep the comfort of the patient, the comfort of the practitioner, and the safety of both parties in mind. Evaluation and adjustments should take place in an area large enough to accommodate the patient. A nonskid surface is necessary in order for the patient to be comfortable standing. It is also important to evaluate and adjust the patient in an area free of noise or distractions. An experienced assistant should gently restrain the dog during chiropractic diagnosis and treatment. The dog should be monitored carefully for signs of anxiety, agitation, or aggression, and if the dog cannot be calmed, the chiropractic session should be stopped until it can be resumed safely and comfortably. A painful dog is best adjusted after breaking the pain cycle pharmacologically.

Motion Palpation and the Chiropractic Listing

In order to know what to treat, the practitioner must perform a motion palpation to determine which spinal segment(s) are dysfunctional, and in which direction(s) motion is restricted. During a motion palpation to locate a VSC, the chiropractic practitioner evaluates the motion of each vertebral body as it interacts with the vertebral body immediately rostral to it. Motion palpation at each vertebra-to-vertebra connection should reveal dorsoventral movement as well as rotation to the right and left. Normal movement at each vertebral segment is subtle, and involves only millimeters of excursion in each direction. Likewise, palpation of the pelvis, including the sacroiliac joints and the lumbosacral junction, should demonstrate subtle movement. Restriction of movement in any direction at a vertebral segment defines the VSC that is subsequently adjusted. Often, there is apparent discomfort at these same segments. The dog may move away, may react negatively, or the soft tissues in the surrounding area may spasm under the practitioner's fingers.

The description of the VSC and its treatment are referred to as a "listing". The listing vernacular provides information about the location on the animal's body that will be contacted by the practitioner, the direction of reduced motion, as well as the direction in which the VSC will be adjusted or corrected. The listing vocabulary is taken from human chiropractic, specifically the Palmer Gonstead system (Scaringe & Cooperstein, 2001).

THE CHIROPRACTIC ADJUSTMENT

The adjustment is the core chiropractic interaction between the practitioner and the patient, and should only be performed by persons with chiropractic training. The chiropractic adjustment involves a specific, short-lever, high-velocity, controlled thrust to restore motion through a specific vector by forcing the facet joint surfaces to the anatomical limit of joint play (Leach, 1994d). It is the specificity of the adjustment in both the location and direction that differentiates the chiropractic adjustment from other less specific tissue manipulations. Sometimes during an adjustment a sound, called an "audible", will be caused by gas being liberated from synovial fluid (Leach, 1994d). Audibles do not occur as frequently in canine patients as in human patients.

The chiropractic adjustment is focused on the functional spinal unit comprised of two adjacent vertebrae, the joints that link them, the skeletal muscles that move the joints, and the supportive structures that span the distance between them. All chiropractic treatment occurs within the normal ROM of the specific functional spinal unit. The ROM of a spinal segment is comprised of several components. The active ROM is the extent of the motion in a specific direction the bones of a spinal segment can move via voluntary muscle contraction. The passive ROM is at the end of the active ROM and is initiated by an outside force. The end range of the passive ROM is called the elastic barrier and is determined by the ligaments in the spinal segments. Full ROM is defined by the anatomical barrier, which is the limit beyond which any additional motion would disrupt the anatomic structure of the spinal segment. Between the elastic barrier and the anatomical barrier is a theoretical space referred to as the "paraphysiological space", and it is within this space that the chiropractic adjustment occurs. This is an extremely small space, which means the adjusting thrust is a very low-amplitude movement (Scaringe & Cooperstein, 2001).

The adjustment is best accomplished by first taking the affected spinal segment to tension in the direction of the correction/adjustment. By taking up the "slack" in the tissue, the practitioner brings the segment to its elastic barrier at the end of the passive ROM, thus allowing the segment to be adjusted into the paraphysiological space. The timing of the thrust is crucial, as it is most effectively applied at the moment of greatest relaxation. Predicting or feeling for that moment takes practice, and involves palpating many patients in order to train the practitioner to most effectively diagnose and adjust VSCs (Options for Animals College of Animal Chiropractic, 2008).

Dogs are adjusted using a one-handed technique, allowing the practitioner to use the opposite hand and arm to stabilize the patient (Figure 18.1). Appropriate stabilization allows the practitioner to isolate the affected spinal segment for adjustment as well as to more easily take the segment to tension (to the elastic barrier). In addition, appropriate stabilization of the patient ensures that most of the force of the thrust employed during the adjustment will reach the intended tissues in the VSC (Options for Animals College of Animal Chiropractic, 2008). In the author's experience, appropriate stabilization without excessive restraint seems to reassure the patient, allowing it to relax into the adjustment and making the chiropractic treatment as effective as possible.

CONTRAINDICATIONS TO CHIROPRACTIC

Common sense dictates which patients or locations on the body should not be treated with chiropractic adjustment. Examples of conditions that should NOT be treated with chiropractic include (but are not limited to):

- Areas with active infection
- Fractures
- Acute prolapsed or ruptured intervertebral disc
- Areas of significant pain
- Joint luxation (e.g., traumatic coxofemoral luxation)
- Acute painful joint sprain or strain
- Meningitis/encephalitis

CHIROPRACTIC AND CATS

The same principles that apply to diagnosing and adjusting dogs apply to cats as well (Figure 18.2). This means decreasing significant pain before adjusting in order to provide the best outcome and experience for the patient. It also means appropriate gentle handling to keep the patient, assistants, and the practitioner safe. Cats may object more vigorously to restraint than the typical dog. Likewise, cats tend not to stand still for their assessments and adjustments,

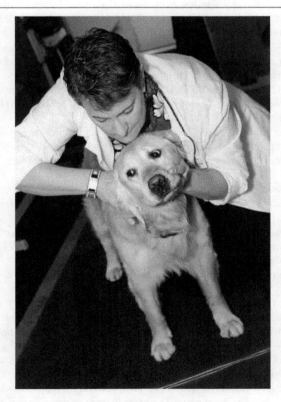

Figure 18.1. Cervical adjustment in a dog.

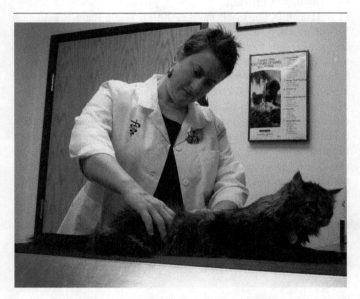

Figure 18.2. When adjusting cats, the exam table can be used to stabilize the patient.

and require flexibility on the part of the practitioner in order to accomplish appropriate chiropractic diagnosis and treatment.

TRAINING AND CERTIFICATION OPTIONS IN VETERINARY CHIROPRACTIC

Formal training in applying chiropractic techniques to animals began in 1988 through the American Veterinary Chiropractic Association (AVCA), thanks in large measure to the efforts of Dr. Sharon Willoughby. Dr. Willoughby was a veterinarian and a Doctor of Chiropractic (DC) who founded the AVCA in 1989. Animal chiropractic has evolved over time and continues to develop as a discipline, similar to the advances made in human chiropractic. As of this writing, training in veterinary chiropractic for certification includes a minimum of 210 contact hours of postgraduate education whether the student/candidate is a graduate veterinarian or a graduate chiropractor.

Training programs that prepare the student/candidate for credentialing examination with either the AVCA or the International Veterinary Chiropractic Association (IVCA) are found in the United States, Canada, Germany, Britain, and many other countries (see Section Resources).

Regardless of where training occurs, it is important for anyone pursuing animal chiropractic training to carefully review the relevant veterinary practice act and the chiropractic act in the appropriate geographic location in order to remain in compliance with applicable regional regulations.

THE FUTURE OF CANINE CHIROPRACTIC

Veterinarians and other conscientious health care providers have an obligation to practice evidence-based medicine (EBM). The gold standard for EBM is the randomized, double-blinded, placebo-controlled clinical study of patients with naturally occurring disease. One important challenge in establishing the efficacy of chiropractic adjustment for the treatment of pain or other conditions is the difficulty in providing a sham or placebo treatment or adjustment (Hawk et al., 1999; Pascoe, 2002). While there is evidence for the efficacy of chiropractic for pain relief via its effects on the spinal cord, there is some discordance in the results of meta-analyses. A 1992 meta-analysis reported that chiropractic outperformed the comparison treatments for pain relief (Anderson et al., 1992); however, a 2004 meta-analysis provided an equivocal conclusion (Assendelft et al., 2004). Chiropractic outperformed hospital outpatient management in patients with mild-to-moderate pain (Mead et al., 1995). In a 2004 review, spinal manipulative therapy for acute and chronic back pain compared favorably with placebo and other treatments (Bronfort et al., 2004). Finally, chiropractic has shown efficacy for treating migraine (Tuchin et al., 2000). While the author acknowledges that veterinarians must be cautious when extrapolating from human studies to animal patients, the human literature for chiropractic efficacy provides a starting place for understanding the role of chiropractic in pain management in quadrupeds.

SUMMARY

Although the need for animal patient chiropractic studies is clear, chiropractic care provides a reasonable strategy for enhancing the effects of pharmacological (and other) pain management strategies. The future position of chiropractic among accepted treatment modalities for pets will depend upon the results of rigorous clinical studies.

RESOURCES

Healing Oasis Wellness Center, Sturtevant, WI 53177, 262-878-9549, Fax 262-886-6460, www.thehealingoasis.com

Options for Animals, Wellsville, KS 66092, 309-658-2920, Fax: 309-658-2622, www.animalchiro.com

Parker College of Chiropractic, 2500 Walnut Hill Lane, Dallas, TX 75229, Post Graduate Department, Michelle Yungblut, 800-266-4723 or 214-902-2479, www.parker.edu/animal-chiropractic-program.aspx

Healing Oasis Wellness Centre of Canada, Brantford, Ontario, Canada, 519-448-1306, Fax 519-756-1597, www.veterinarychiropractic.ca.

BackBone Academy for Veterinary Chiropractic and Healing Arts, Kalbe, Germany, +49-4282-590688, Fax +49-721-151366446, www.backbone-academy.com

International Academy of Veterinary Chiropractic. Classes offered in Sittenson, Germany and Bournemouth, England www.i-a-v-c.com

REFERENCES

Anderson, R.A., Meeker, W.C., Wrick, B.E., et al. (1992) A meta-analysis of clinical trials of spinal manipulation. *Journal of Manipulative and Physiological Therapeutics*, 22, 181–194.

Assendelft, W.J., Morton, S.C., Yu, E.L., et al. (2004) Spinal manipulative therapy for low-back pain. *Cochrane Database of Systematic Reviews*, (1), Art. No.: CD000447. doi:10.1002/14651858.CD000447.pub3

AVMA. (2001) Guidelines for complementary and alternative veterinary medicine. *Journal of the American Veterinary Medical Association*, 218, 1731.

Bove, G. & Swenson, R. (2001) Nociceptors, pain, and chiropractic, in *Fundamentals of Chiropractic* (eds D. Redwood & C.S. Cleveland), Mosby, St. Louis, MO, pp. 187.

Bronfort, G., Haas, M., Evans, R.L., et al. (2004) Efficacy of spinal manipulation and mobilization for low back pain and neck pain: a systematic review and best evidence synthesis. *Spine Journal*, 4(3), 335–356.

Cleveland, A., Phillips, R., & Clum, G. (2001) The chiropractic paradigm, in *Fundamentals of Chiropractic* (eds D. Redwood & C.S. Cleveland), Mosby, St. Louis, MO, pp. 15–27.

Cleveland, C.S. (2001) Vertebral subluxation, in *Fundamentals of Chiropractic* (eds D. Redwood & C.S. Cleveland), Mosby, St. Louis, MO, pp. 129–153.

Downing, R. (2011) Managing chronic maladaptive pain. *NAVC Clinician's Brief*, 15–19.

Hawk, C., Azad, A., Phongphua, C., et al. (1999) Preliminary study of the effects of a placebo chiropractic treatment with sham adjustments. *Journal of Manipulative and Physiological Therapeutics*, 22, 436–443.

Lantz, C.A. (1989) The vertebral subluxation complex. *International Chiropractors Association Review*, 43, 37.

Leach, R.A. (1994a) Appendix B: integrated physiological model for VSC, in *The Chiropractic Theories: Principles and Clinical Applications*, 3rd edn, Williams & Wilkins, Baltimore, pp. 373–394.

Leach, R.A. (1994b) General introduction, in *The Chiropractic Theories: Principles and Clinical Applications*, 3rd edn, Williams & Wilkins, Baltimore, pp. 3–8.

Leach, R.A. (1994c) Facilitation hypothesis, in *The Chiropractic Theories: Principles and Clinical Applications*, 3rd edn, Williams & Wilkins, Baltimore, pp. 89–119.

Leach, R.A. (1994d) Manipulation terminology, in *The Chiropractic Theories: Principles and Clinical Applications*, 3rd edn, Williams & Wilkins, Baltimore, pp. 16–22.

Meade, T.W., Dyer, S., Brown, W., Frank, A.O. (1995) Randomised comparison of chiropractic and hospital outpatients management for low back pain: results from extended follow up. *British Medical Journal*, 311, 349–351.

Options for Animals College of Animal Chiropractic (2008), Basic animal chiropractic course notes, Options for Animals, Wellsville, KS.

Pascoe, P. (2002) Alternative methods for the control of pain. *Journal of the American Veterinary Medical Association*, 221(2), 222–229.

Scaringe, J.G. & Cooperstein, R. (2001) Chiropractic manual procedures, in *Fundamentals of Chiropractic* (eds D. Redwood & C.S. Cleveland), Mosby, St. Louis, MO, pp. 257–291.

Tuchin, P.J., Pollard, H., & Bonello, R. (2000) A randomized controlled trial of chiropractic spinal manipulative therapy for migraine. *Journal of Manipulative and Physiological Therapeutics*, 23, 91–95.

19
Equine Chiropractic

Henry S. Adair

Chiropractic (see also Chapter 18) is a form of manual therapy that uses controlled forces applied to specific articulations or anatomic regions to induce a therapeutic response via induced changes in joint structure, muscle function, and neurological reflexes (Haussler, 2000). It focuses on the relationship between structure (primarily the vertebral column) and function (as coordinated by the nervous system) (Haussler, 2000).

JOINT MOTION

Spinal joint motion can be categorized into three zones: physiological, paraphysiological, and pathological (Figure 19.1). The physiological zone of movement includes both active and passive ranges of motion (ROM). The elastic barrier is at the end of the passive ROM, which is determined by the ligaments in the spinal segment. The full ROM of the joint is limited by the anatomical barrier—the limit beyond which any additional motion would disrupt the anatomic structure and cause joint injury (the pathological zone). The paraphysiological zone exists between the elastic barrier and the anatomical barrier, and it is within this zone that the chiropractic adjustment is performed (Leach, 1994).

Vertebral Motion Segment and Vertebral Subluxation Complex

The vertebral motion segment includes two adjacent vertebrae, the facet joints, and the associated soft tissues that bind them together (Haussler, 2000). A vertebral subluxation complex (VSC) is a vertebral lesion characterized by joint asymmetry or loss of normal joint motion in one or more planes resulting in altered articular neurophysiology, biochemical alterations, joint capsule pathology, and articular degeneration (Leach, 1994; Haussler, 2000). These changes alter intervertebral disc and joint biomechanics and proprioception, and cause tenderness or diminished pain threshold to pressure in the adjacent paraspinal tissues or osseous structures, protective muscle guarding, abnormal paraspinal muscle tension, increased tension and stress on the joint capsules and adjacent ligaments, and visible or palpable signs of active inflammatory processes (e.g., edema, fibrosis, hyperemia, or altered temperature) (Leach, 1994; Haussler, 2000).

CHIROPRACTIC AND THE RELIEF OF PAIN

When spinal joints are restricted in their ROM low-grade inflammation occurs. Inflammation leads to radiculopathy and further fixation of the spinal segment. This can progress to spondylosis of one or more facet joints and changes in the disc, which result in further loss of normal joint movement within that motion segment (Ridgway, 2005). The inflammatory response and radiculopathy result in persistent afferent nociceptive bombardment, and appear to be the key components of facilitation and the subsequent decreased threshold to pain (Leach, 1994). There is poor transmission of the afferent signal, and the nature and appropriateness of the efferent signal is affected; muscles become shortened (i.e., hypertonic) and painful.

The goals of chiropractic treatment are to restore normal spinal joint motion, stimulate neurological reflexes, and reduce pain and muscle hypertonicity (Haussler, 2000). Chiropractic has been used extensively in the treatment of pain (Ridgway, 2005), and it is likely that manual therapies affect nociceptive processes at many levels (Haussler, 2010). The exact mechanisms by which manual therapies relieve pain are unknown, and may include local biochemical changes due to increased local blood flow, effects on primary afferent neurons from paraspinal tissues, reduction of central sensitization of segmental dorsal horn neurons by stretching of spinal mechanoreceptors, and activation of descending pain inhibitory systems projecting from the brain to the spinal cord, resulting in the release of endorphins and serotonin (Vernon et al., 1986; Haussler, 2010).

Spinal manipulation, as a short-lasting, dynamic, mechanical stimulus, may take advantage of two signaling characteristics of the nervous system: (1) inherent high-frequency signaling properties of dynamically sensitized primary afferent neurons and (2) response properties of postsynaptic neurons (Pickar & Bolton, 2012). Experimental studies reveal that spinal manipulation evokes a high-frequency discharge in some primary afferents. Spinal manipulation could affect the nervous system by activating paraspinal sensory

Pain Management in Veterinary Practice, First Edition. Edited by Christine M. Egger, Lydia Love and Tom Doherty.
© 2014 John Wiley & Sons, Inc. Published 2014 by John Wiley & Sons, Inc.

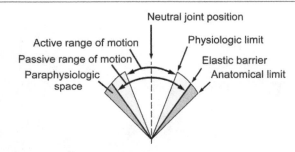

Figure 19.1. Joint mechanics as it relates to active and passive joint ranges of motion. The physiological limit demarcates active versus passive joint range of motion. The paraphysiological space is defined by the elastic barrier and the anatomic limit of the articulation. Inducing motion beyond the anatomic limit of the joint induces tissue damage and results in joint subluxation or luxation. From Haussler (2010), with permission.

neurons during the maneuver or by altering spinal biomechanics (Pickar & Bolton, 2012).

INDICATIONS FOR CHIROPRACTIC TREATMENT

Most of the current knowledge about equine manual therapies is based on human chiropractic (Haussler, 2010). Indications for spinal manipulation in horses include neck or back pain, localized or regional spinal joint stiffness, poor performance, and altered gait that is not associated with overt lameness (Haussler, 2010). Chiropractic treatment aims to resolve musculoskeletal disorders that are primarily induced by biomechanical factors, and a thorough diagnostic workup is required to identify soft tissue and osseous disorders, neurological disorders, or other lameness conditions that may not be responsive to manual therapy. Clinical signs indicating a primary spinal biomechanical disorder that may respond to chiropractic manipulation include: localized musculoskeletal pain, muscle hypertonicity, and abnormal spinal joint motion (i.e., hypermobility or hypomobility) (Haussler, 2010). If an area is found to be abnormal it should be further investigated prior to referral for chiropractic treatment. Additional diagnostic modalities include radiography, ultrasonography, scintigraphy, and, depending on the location of the abnormality (i.e., cranial cervical region), an MRI examination may be possible.

CONTRAINDICATIONS TO CHIROPRACTIC MANIPULATION

Chiropractic is not a panacea for all back problems, and is contraindicated for treatment of fractures, infections, neoplasia, metabolic disorders, nonmechanically related joint disorders, or neurological disease (Haussler, 2000). Acute episodes of sprains or strains, degenerative joint disease, or impinged spinous processes are also relative contraindications for chiropractic adjustments (Haussler, 2000). The above conditions should be ruled out by appropriate diagnostic modalities prior to institution of chiropractic manipulation.

CHIROPRACTIC MANIPULATION

Spinal manipulation should only be performed by persons trained in chiropractic. When VSCs occur, loss of ROM may occur along one or several vectors and, before attempting correction, a thorough and in-depth knowledge of anatomy and physiology is critical to correctly identify the vectors involved. A properly performed manipulation, typically a high-velocity, low-amplitude thrust of proper force along the determined line of correction, reestablishes full ROM. The properly performed chiropractic manipulation moves the involved joint or joints through both active and passive ranges of motion and into the paraphysiological space, and in the direction of the appropriate vectors. This must be accomplished without disturbing the anatomical barrier of the joint or joints.

This adjustment and manipulation, when performed correctly, is thought to enhance normal afferent signal transmission into the spinal cord, brainstem, or brain for interpretation. Correct interpretation allows an appropriate efferent response and restoration of normal segment movement (Haldeman, 2000). A correctly performed manipulation also decreases the hypertonic/hyperesthetic response of shortened muscle fibers and reduces muscle electroactivity (Shambaugh, 1987; Nansel et al., 1993). When the ROM is reestablished, the radiculopathy diminishes along with muscle shortening and the associated pain.

COMPLICATIONS

Adverse reactions to chiropractic manipulations are uncommon. Transient stiffness or temporary worsening of the condition are potential complications (Haussler, 2000). These usually will appear within the first 24 hours and resolve with conservative therapy, such as rest, gentle exercise, and analgesics, in 24–48 hours. Most complications occur from inexperienced or untrained individuals applying the manipulations or from a failure to perform adequate diagnostics.

CURRENT RESEARCH

The focus of equine chiropractic research has been assessment of the clinical effects of spinal manipulation on pain relief, flexibility, muscle hypertonicity, and spinal motion symmetry (Haussler, 2010). Randomized, controlled clinical trials, using pressure algometry to assess mechanical nociceptive thresholds in the thoracolumbar region of horses, indicate that manual and instrument-assisted spinal manipulation can increase mechanical nociceptive thresholds (Haussler & Erb, 2003; Haussler & Erb, 2006; Sullivan et al., 2008). The effect of manipulation on asymmetrical spinal movement patterns in horses with documented back pain suggests that chiropractic treatment elicits slight but significant changes in thoracolumbar and pelvic kinematics, and that some of these changes are likely to be beneficial (Haussler, 2010). Spinal manipulative therapy increases dorsoventral displacement of the trunk, producing increased passive spinal flexibility in actively ridden horses (Haussler et al., 2010). In horses with clinically diagnosed back problems, Alvarez et al. (2008) reported that the main overall effects of chiropractic manipulation included less extension of the thoracic back, a reduced inclination of the pelvis, and improved symmetry of the pelvic motion pattern.

SUMMARY

Spinal manipulation has been shown in several studies to be effective for reducing pain, improving flexibility, reducing abnormal muscle tone, and improving symmetry of spinal kinematics in horses (Cassidy et al., 1992; Nansel et al., 1993; Bronfort et al., 2004; Haussler, 2010). In order to utilize this therapeutic modality properly, a thorough knowledge of equine anatomy, biomechanics, and pathology is required to understand the principles and theories behind chiropractic manipulations. Chiropractic can provide additional diagnostic and therapeutic tools to assist the equine practitioner in identifying and treating the primary cause of equine lameness or poor performance (Wolf, 2002; Goff, 2009; Haussler, 2009; Haussler, 2010).

REFERENCES

Alvarez, C.B.G., L'Ami, J.J., Moffatt, D., et al. (2008) Effect of chiropractic manipulations on the kinematics of back and limbs in horses with clinically diagnosed back problems. *Equine Veterinary Journal*, 40(2), 153–159.

Bronfort, G., Haas, M., Evans, R.L., et al. (2004) Efficacy of spinal manipulation and mobilizationfor low back pain and neck pain: a systematic review and best evidence synthesis. *Spine Journal*, 4(3), 335–356.

Cassidy, J.D., Lopes, A.A., & Yong-Hing, K. (1992) The immediate effect of manipulation versus mobilization on pain and range of motion in the cervical spine: a randomized controlled trial. *Journal of Manipulative and Physiological Therapeutics*, 15(9), 570–575.

Goff, L.M. (2009) Manual therapy for the horse – A contemporary perspective. *Journal of Equine Veterinary Science*, 29(11), 799–808.

Haldeman, S. (2000) Neurologic effects of the adjustment. *Journal of Manipulative and Physiological Therapeutics*, 23(2), 112–114.

Haussler, K.K. (2000) Equine chiropractic: general principles and clinical applications, in *Proceedings of the American Association of Equine Practitioners*, pp. 84–93.

Haussler, K.K. (2009) Review of manual therapy techniques in equine practice. *Journal of Equine Veterinary Science*, 29(12), 849–869.

Haussler, K.K. (2010) The role of manual therapies in equine pain management. *Veterinary Clinics of North America: Equine Practice*, 26, 579–601.

Haussler, K.K. & Erb, H.N. (2003) Pressure algometry: objective assessment of back pain and effects of chiropractic treatment, in *Proceedings of the 49th Annual Convention of the American Association of Equine Practitioners,* The 49th Annual Convention of the American Association of Equine Practitioners, New Orleans, LA, pp. 66–70.

Haussler, K.K. & Erb, H.N. (2006) Pressure algometry for the detection of induced back pain in horses: a preliminary study. *Equine veterinary journal*, 38(1), 76–81.

Leach, R.A. (1994) *The Chiropractic Theories: Principles and Clinical Applications,* 3rd edn, Williams & Wilkins, Baltimore.

Lerche, P. & Muir, W.W. (2009) Perioperative pain management, *Equine Anesthesia* (eds W.W. Muir & J.A.E. Hubbell), Elsevier Inc., St. Louis, MO, pp. 369–380.

Nansel, D.D., Waldorf, T., & Cooperstein, R. (1993) Effect of cervical spinal adjustments on lumbar paraspinal muscle tone: evidence for facilitation of intersegmental tonic neck reflexes. *Journal of Manipulative and Physiological Therapeutics*, 16(2), 91–95.

Pickar, J.G. & Bolton, P.S. (2012) Spinal manipulative therapy and somatosensory activation. *Journal of Electromyography and Kinesiology*, 22(5), 785–794.

Ridgway, K.J. (2005) Diagnosis and treatment of equine musculoskeletal pain. The role of the complementary modalities: acupuncture and chiropractic, in *Proceedings of the 51st Annual Convention of the American Association of Equine Practitioners*, Seattle, WA, pp. 403–408.

Shambaugh, P. (1987) Changes in electrical activity in muscles resulting from chiropractic adjustment: a pilot study. *Journal of Manipulative and Physiological Therapeutics*, 10(6), 300–304.

Sullivan, K.A., Hill, A.E. & Haussler, K.K. (2008) The effects of chiropractic, massage and phenylbutazone on spinal mechanical nociceptive thresholds in horses without clinical signs. *Equine Veterinary Journal*, 40(1), 14–20.

Vernon, H.T., Dhami, M.S., Howley, T.P., et al. (1986) Spinal manipulation and beta-endorphin: a controlled study of the effect of a spinal manipulation on plasma beta-endorphin levels in normal males. *Journal of Manipulative and Physiological Therapeutics*, 9(2), 115–123.

Wolf, L. (2002) The role of complementary techniques in managing musculoskeletal pain in performance horses. *Veterinary Clinics of North America: Equine Practice*, 18(1), 107–115.

Section 4
Management of Pain in Veterinary Species

Pain Management in Veterinary Practice, First Edition. Edited by Christine M. Egger, Lydia Love and Tom Doherty.
© 2014 John Wiley & Sons, Inc. Published 2014 by John Wiley & Sons, Inc.

20

Recognition and Assessment of Acute Pain in the Dog

Kate L. White

The primary duty of veterinary health care professionals is relieving the suffering and pain in the animals under their care. Understanding of the mechanisms of pain has progressed at a far greater rate than the science of assessing pain in animals. Veterinarians are well trained in assessing and diagnosing complaints involving discrete body systems, but when it comes to pain, the assessment markers are not so obvious or universally applicable.

One might assume that pain assessment in humans would be easier because these patients can report, localize, describe, and demonstrate their pain; however, this ability to communicate can make the assessment of pain very subjective. In addition, pain assessment in humans and animals has to take into account other factors, such as psychological and situational influences, and concurrent disease that may be modifying the pain behaviors. It remains for the veterinary profession to develop a robust and validated pain assessment tool that is as objective as possible. Further studies are needed in this area, but the temptation to ignore pain, because of uncertainties and lack of consensus in the assessment of pain, must be avoided.

Attempts have been made to classify veterinarians' and animal health workers' ideas and views about pain in animals (Dohoo & Dohoo, 1998). From studies investigating analgesic use by veterinarians, it is possible to extrapolate the frequency and standard of pain assessment. Since the late 1980s, there has been a gradual and expansion of analgesic use in the veterinary industry driven by the increased awareness of pain behaviors, welfare concerns, and increased availability of a range of analgesics. A study conducted in the mid-1980s in the United States veterinary teaching hospitals revealed that only 40% of dogs and cats were given postoperative analgesics, even for relatively invasive surgery (Hansen & Hardie, 1993). The minimal use of analgesics may well be explained by the lack of discrete behaviors that traditionally encourage analgesic use, and the fact that the overt behaviors may disappear as animals become sicker. During the 1990s, studies of analgesic use after neutering showed minimal use of analgesics by veterinarians for these so-called "routine" procedures. Analgesics were administered to 10.5–12.6% of dogs undergoing neutering in a Canadian survey, (Dohoo & Dohoo, 1996), and 4–6% of animals in an Australian survey (Watson et al., 1996). A UK study conducted in 1996 reported that analgesics were administered to 32% of dogs for castration and 53% of bitches for ovariohysterectomy (Capner et al., 1999). In 2004, a study in France documented that analgesics were administered to 17.2% and 36.3% of dogs after castration and ovariohysterectomy, respectively (Hugonnard et al., 2004). In New Zealand, a study of analgesic use and attitudes to pain reported an increased use of analgesics for neutering and other procedures compared with the earlier studies (Williams et al., 2005). Veterinary school curricula have changed significantly in the last three decades, and now place great emphasis on analgesia, pain scoring, and a multimodal approach to patient comfort.

LIMITATIONS OF PAIN ASSESSMENT TOOLS

When embarking on pain assessment in dogs it is worth remembering the following points:

- Dogs manifest pain in differing ways.
- Some behaviors are strongly suggestive of pain.
- No behavior in isolation is pathognomonic for pain.
- Objective and subjective assessments can be used together to assess pain.
- The absence of certain behaviors does not mean the dog is not experiencing pain.
- Knowledge of the dog's normal behavior (either from the owner's reports or via observation prior to surgery) is useful when assessing the change in behavior in the face of pain.
- Pain behaviors can be modified by concurrent disease.
- Pain behaviors should be assessed during observation of the patient and during interaction with the patient
- Inter- and intra-assessor variability will occur, highlighting the subjective nature of pain assessment.
- Some "pain behaviors" can be associated with general ill health or other emotions such as fear, apprehension, and anxiety.
- Pain behaviors can be very subtle and can take a long time to recognize, so much so that clinicians or staff may miss these signs if enough time is not taken to assess the animal.

Pain Management in Veterinary Practice, First Edition. Edited by Christine M. Egger, Lydia Love and Tom Doherty.
© 2014 John Wiley & Sons, Inc. Published 2014 by John Wiley & Sons, Inc.

PAIN BEHAVIORS

Vocalization

Vocalization describes a number of behaviors including whining, whimpering, growling, howling, barking, screaming, crying, and groaning. Vocalization is, however, a nonspecific behavior and may be expressed in the absence of pain. Dogs may vocalize for other reasons, for example, anxiety, fear, dysphoria, hunger, or the need to urinate or defecate. It must also be remembered that some animals become very quiet when they are in pain, and this lack of vocalization can sometimes be misinterpreted as a sign of comfort.

Vocalization by a dog in response to movement, for example, getting up, lying down, or during wound palpation or dressing changes can be more suggestive of pain and can be a useful objective signal of the presence of pain. Determining whether vocalization during recovery from anesthesia is due to pain or the dysphoric effects of inhalational anesthetics or opioids is sometimes difficult. In these cases, additional analgesia is warranted to rule out pain, and if the vocalization persists in the face of analgesic administration, then an anxiolytic or sedative is administered. Vocalization during emergence from inhalational anesthesia is usually short-lived and often responds to sedation. Vocalization can also occur due to the dysphoric effects of the opioids, and this has been reported in studies evaluating pain behaviors following ovariohysterectomy in bitches (Fox et al., 2000).

Mobility and Posture

Abnormal movement and locomotion are obvious signs of musculoskeletal discomfort. The discomfort may be from the limbs, the pelvic girdle, the thorax, or spinal column. Although lameness can be mechanical in nature, it is more often the animal's protective response to guard the injured or painful area from weight bearing, which may exacerbate the injury or cause further pain. In order to properly assess musculoskeletal pain, dogs should be brought out of their cages and, if possible, walked on a lead to assess mobility. Signs such as a stilted gait or reluctance to start walking suggest pain. Often, when the dog starts to move it will vocalize or show other pain behaviors, reaffirming that the reluctance to move was due to pain. Some animals may show an abnormal loading of the thoracic limbs when there is pain associated with the hind limbs, and this is particularly obvious in dogs with acute pain of the hind legs or pelvis (e.g., post cruciate ligament repair) or with chronic osteoarthritic pain of the pelvic limbs and pelvis. Force plate analysis and thermographic imaging techniques can give further information about the gait changes and localization of the pathological changes that may be responsible for the pain.

Reluctance to move or change position once recumbent may also be indicative of pain. Conversely, some dogs in pain show restlessness and frequent changes of position. In these cases, it should be ascertained that the restlessness is not due to other reasons such as a need to urinate or defecate, and attention must be paid to providing appropriately padded bedding. Some dogs may be reluctant to lie down, this is often the case in dogs with abdominal discomfort or thoracic pain (Figure 20.1). These dogs will then become very tired if they cannot rest in a recumbent position, and this will lead to their eventual falling or slumping over and vocalizing in acute pain at that point. These dogs will often sit for long periods of time or adopt a "praying" position. Dogs with

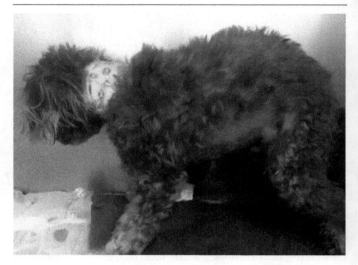

Figure 20.1. A dog showing typical signs of abdominal pain after exploratory laparotomy (abdominal splinting, reluctance to lie down, leaning against the side of the cage). (Courtesy of Gregory Hirshoren, University of Tennessee CVM)

abdominal pain may also show tenseness to their abdominal wall, also known as "splinting." Dogs in severe pain may thrash and roll about in the kennel becoming increasingly aggressive and difficult to manage.

Computer acquisition of behavioral data is available with automatic video tracking systems and software that can detect and analyze spatial behaviors. This offers a further tool for pain assessment, as this allows the capturing of the temporal changes in behavior that might be missed with the assessments at intervals. This technique is still in its infancy, but shows promise. Devices such as accelerometers are also being used in assessing the mobility and quality of life in chronic pain states (Hansen et al., 2007).

Interactive Behaviors and Attitude

It is useful to know about the dog's normal behavior, especially in terms of attitude and interaction with the humans. A dog may become aggressive when approached or manipulated and this may be a sign of acute pain, but aggression must be interpreted with careful consideration of the dog's normal behaviors. Some dogs will become submissive when they are in pain; others will become withdrawn and depressed and may constantly stare at the painful area or become oblivious to their surroundings. A subtle change in behavior, as reported by the owner, is often the first sign of pain and, in many cases, may cause the owner to seek veterinary attention despite the lack of other more obvious clinical signs. Some dogs that are in pain stop grooming and their coats look unkempt and take on a lackluster appearance.

Appetite, Urination, and Defecation

A change in appetite can occur for many reasons, but anorexia is common in painful animals. In all cases of anorexia, causes other than pain should be investigated. Dogs in pain may also show changes in urination and defecation, and may begin to soil in the house. The cause may be a reluctance to move and go outside or the painful condition may be altering sensation required for bowel and bladder control.

Physiological Signs Associated with Pain

Clinical signs such as heart rate, respiratory rate, and blood pressure can also be used to assess pain. These parameters are useful and easy to measure using noninvasive techniques, but are relatively nonspecific for pain. Holton et al. (1998a) reported that heart rate and respiratory rate in isolation were poor indicators of pain in hospitalized dogs, and that pupillary dilation was also limited in its value. Measurement of blood epinephrine, norepinephrine, and cortisol concentrations is questionable as concentrations can be altered by many factors. A study evaluating cortisol concentrations in dogs undergoing ovariohysterectomy reported that cortisol values increased from baseline even in the control groups, and this was attributable to handling of the dogs (Fox et al., 1994). These parameters may be of greater value when combined with other assessment methods.

PAIN SCALES AND PAIN ASSESSMENT

Quantifying the degree of pain that an animal is suffering from is challenging and highly subjective. Pain scales have been developed to try to standardize the assessment of pain and a few validated examples are currently used on a daily basis by practitioners, with varying degrees of success.

Simple Descriptive Scales

Prior to the 1990s there was little research into pain scales per se in animals, although different analgesics were often compared. Since then, there have been significant and exciting developments in pain assessment scales, and these scales are now in regular use in all manner of veterinary establishments and form an important part of analgesic studies. Initially, pain scales in animals were extrapolated from those used for children. The first types of pain scales that were used for animals were simple descriptive scales (SDS) with a 3- or 5-point scale with answers ranging from mild through moderate to severe. There was no further information on the scale as to what constituted mild, moderate, or severe pain, and it was up to the assessor to judge clinically the degree of pain being experienced by the animal. These ordinal verbal scales are very basic and not validated. The scales are also nonlinear, and the definitions of the descriptive words are open to different interpretations.

Numerical Rating Scales

Ordinal scales with numeric units offered an alternative method of assessment. With these scales, an assessor assigned arbitrary values to a linear scale in an effort to simplify and organize the assessment. These scales consisted of a 4-, 5- or 10-point scale of pain severity. The issue of nonlinearity in these scales is immediately obvious. A linear scale, such as a 10-point scale, would suggest that a dog with a score of four is in twice as much pain as a dog with a score of two, and a dog with a score of eight is in four times as much pain as a dog with a score of two. In practice, however, this degree of precision is not borne out.

Categorized Numerical Rating Scales

These numerical rating scales (NRS) can be expanded to have categories of behaviors, and within each category points are assigned for the different behaviors observed. These are known as categorized numerical rating scales. One example of a categorized NRS is the University of Melbourne Pain Scale (UMPS), which was designed based on specific physiological and behavioral indices to categorize the pain in dogs after surgery (Firth & Haldane, 1999). There are six categories, and within each category there are various behaviors or physiological parameters. This scale seems to have increased accuracy over the SDS and standard NRS, and has the added benefit of being able to rank the importance of certain behaviors, thereby increasing the specificity and sensitivity of the assessment scale. Similar scales, such as that used at Colorado State University (canine acute pain scale), have been developed for the use in clinical situations. This simple scale is intended for the assessment of dogs that may be experiencing pain after surgery or trauma. Three categories are assessed and assigned a score from 0 to 4; additionally, there is space for writing further comments and annotating a diagram to localize tension, pain, and heat. This scale is available to download at http://csuanimalcancercenter .org/assets/files/csu_acute_pain_scale_canine.pdf

Another example of a modified numerical rating score is the Canine Brief Pain Inventory (CBPI) (Figure 20.2), which is designed to record the owner's assessment of the severity of chronic pain. The CBPI has been modified to explore how the pain interferes with the animal's normal function. This scale has been used to measure pain in dogs with osteoarthritis and bone cancer (Brown et al., 2007, 2008, 2009) and is available to download at www.CanineBPI.com.

All scales have limitations, and the UMPS limitations are illustrated by an example of a severely injured dog that has undergone a limb amputation. The dog is depressed, anorexic, lying quietly, and unable to move. The UMPS does not capture all the details about this dog, and the dog scores four out of a possible total 27, suggestive of very mild pain (Hansen, 2003). It is important to stress that pain scales do not offer an alternative to good clinical judgment and thorough evaluation. Neither do scales offer a rigid system of when to start or stop administering analgesics.

Visual Analog Scale

A visual analog scale (VAS) was developed in an attempt to better capture subtleties and nuances of the pain experience. This is another semi-objective type of scale, which consists of a horizontal 10 cm (100 mm) line representing the pain experience. The left-hand end of the line is tethered at 0 and represents no pain, and the right-hand end is tethered at 10 and represents the worst possible pain for that condition. Using these descriptive terms at the ends of the line increased the scale's sensitivity (Holton et al., 1998a; Lascelles et al., 1998). The assessor draws a vertical line or cross on the scale that corresponds to the amount of pain he or she thinks is being experienced. These scales are used extensively in human pain assessment, somewhat modified to include descriptors at either end of "no relief at all from the pain," and "complete relief" to improve sensitivity. With the VAS there will again be significant variability among observers, and this type of scale is also prone to observer bias. The VAS is a very simple scale to use and can give information about trends of the pain experience. A modification of the VAS, using a 10-point ordinal scale has also been used with terms "no pain" and "pain could not be worse" at either end of the 10 cm line (Holton et al., 1998b).

Today's Date: ☐☐ / ☐☐ / ☐☐
　　　　　　　　Month　Day　Year

　　　　　　　　　　　　　　　　　　　　　　Patient/Study ID# _____

Canine Brief Pain Inventory (CBPI)

Description of Pain:

Rate your dog's pain.

1. Fill in the oval next to the <u>one number</u> that best describes the pain at its **worst** in the last 7 days.

　○0　○1　○2　○3　○4　○5　○6　○7　○8　○9　○10
　No Pain　　　　　　　　　　　　　　　　　　　Extreme Pain

2. Fill in the oval next to the <u>one number</u> that best describes the pain at its **least** in the last 7 days.

　○0　○1　○2　○3　○4　○5　○6　○7　○8　○9　○10
　No Pain　　　　　　　　　　　　　　　　　　　Extreme Pain

3. Fill in the oval next to the <u>one number</u> that best describes the pain at its **average** in the last 7 days.

　○0　○1　○2　○3　○4　○5　○6　○7　○8　○9　○10
　No Pain　　　　　　　　　　　　　　　　　　　Extreme Pain

4. Fill in the oval next to the <u>one number</u> that best describes the pain as it is **right now**.

　○0　○1　○2　○3　○4　○5　○6　○7　○8　○9　○10
　No Pain　　　　　　　　　　　　　　　　　　　Extreme Pain

Description of Function:

Fill in the oval next to the **one number** that describes how during the past 7 days **pain has interfered** with your dog's:

5. **General Activity**

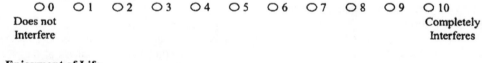

　○0　○1　○2　○3　○4　○5　○6　○7　○8　○9　○10
　Does not　　　　　　　　　　　　　　　　　　Completely
　Interfere　　　　　　　　　　　　　　　　　　Interferes

6. **Enjoyment of Life**

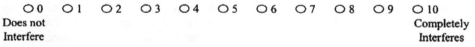

　○0　○1　○2　○3　○4　○5　○6　○7　○8　○9　○10
　Does not　　　　　　　　　　　　　　　　　　Completely
　Interfere　　　　　　　　　　　　　　　　　　Interferes

Figure 20.2. The Canine Brief Pain Inventory. This scale has been used to measure pain in dogs with osteoarthritis and bone cancer (Brown et al., 2007, 2008, 2009).

Dynamic Interactive Visual Analog Scale

A dynamic interactive form (DIVAS) is an expanded VAS that was developed to capture more information. This type of scale overcomes the limitation of scales that rely on observation alone, as these scales also assess interaction with the handler and wound palpation.

Pre-emptive Pain Scoring

Another method of assessing pain or attempting to quantify pain includes the pre-emptive scoring system that attempts to predict or anticipate the amount of pain that will be experienced based on the procedure. This approach has been adopted and summarized by several authors (Mathews, 2000; Mich & Hellyer, 2009).

SHORT FORM OF THE GLASGOW COMPOSITE PAIN SCALE

Dog's name _____

Hospital Number _____ **Date** / / **Time**

Surgery Yes/No (delete as appropriate)

Procedure or Condition _____

_____

In the sections below please circle the appropriate score in each list and sum these to give the total score.

A. Look at dog in Kennel

Is the dog?

(i)

Quiet	0
Crying or whimpering	1
Groaning	2
Screaming	3

(ii)

Ignoring any wound or painful area	0
Looking at wound or painful area	1
Licking wound or painful area	2
Rubbing wound or painful area	3
Chewing wound or painful area	4

> In the case of spinal, pelvic or multiple limb fractures, or where assistance is required to aid locomotion do not carry out section **B** and proceed to **C**
> *Please tick if this is the case* ☐ then proceed to C.

B. Put lead on dog and lead out of the kennel.

When the dog rises/walks is it?

(iii)

Normal	0
Lame	1
Slow or reluctant	2
Stiff	3
It refuses to move	4

C. If it has a wound or painful area including abdomen, apply gentle pressure 2 inches round the site.

Does it?

(iv)

Do nothing	0
Look round	1
Flinch	2
Growl or guard area	3
Snap	4
Cry	5

D. Overall

Is the dog?

(v)

Happy and content or happy and bouncy	0
Quiet	1
Indifferent or non-responsive to surroundings	2
Nervous or anxious or fearful	3
Depressed or non-responsive to stimulation	4

Is the dog?

(vi)

Comfortable	0
Unsettled	1
Restless	2
Hunched or tense	3
Rigid	4

© University of Glasgow

Total Score (i+ii+iii+iv+v+vi) = _____

Figure 20.3. The short form composite measure pain score (CMPS-SF) can be applied quickly and reliably in a clinical setting and has been designed as a clinical decision making tool which was developed for dogs in acute pain. It includes 30 descriptor options within six behavioral categories, including mobility. Within each category, the descriptors are ranked numerically according to their associated pain severity, and the person carrying out the assessment chooses the descriptor within each category that best fits the dog's behavior or condition. It is important to carry out the assessment procedure as described on the questionnaire, following the protocol closely. The pain score is the sum of the rank scores. The maximum score for the six categories is 24, or 20 if mobility is impossible to assess. The total CMPS-SF score has been shown to be a useful indicator of analgesic requirement and the recommended analgesic intervention level is 6/24 or 5/20 (Reid et al., 2007). Reprinted with permission.

Composite Scales

Researchers at Glasgow University Veterinary School have developed a scoring system for acute pain assessment in dogs (Holton et al., 2001). The Glasgow Composite Measure Pain Scale (CMPS) has been extensively validated and appears to produce reliable results. The questionnaire was developed in a similar manner to the method adopted by Melzack and Torgerson to design the McGill pain questionnaire (Melzack & Torgerson, 1971). The scale examines many behavioral traits and then derives a pain score from these. The prototype CMPS was developed into an interval scale for assessing acute pain in dogs by using the Thurstone scaling model to calculate the weights for each item (Thurstone, 1927). The scale then underwent validity testing and was proven in a clinical setting (Morton et al., 2005). Assessing dogs with this scoring system can be quite time consuming and would typically be too much to undertake on a regular basis, hence the development of a short form of the questionnaire (CMPS-SF) (Figure 20.3) that is more manageable (Reid et al., 2007). This compressed form of the questionnaire can be completed in less than 5 minutes.

The questionnaire is composed of six categories of 30 descriptors. The descriptors are ranked numerically within each category according to the severity of the pain. The pain score is the sum of the ranked scores with a maximum of 24, or 20 if mobility cannot be assessed. Intervention in the form of analgesic administration is suggested at 6/24 or 5/20. This type of assessment can be easily used on hospitalized patients and the author uses laminated forms of this scale attached to the dog kennels prompting regular assessment of the patients. A copy of the CMPS-SF and instructions for use can be downloaded at: http://www.gla.ac.uk/schools/vet/research/painandwelfare/downloadacutepainquestionnaire/

SUMMARY

Pain scales offer a useful tool in the assessment of pain but should not be used in isolation. Every dog should be assessed and have its analgesic regimen tailored to its requirements. A pain scale may assist the clinician in deciding when to taper the analgesics, and when intervention may be necessary, but should not replace sound clinical judgment. Pain scales are most useful in prompting the team to regularly reassess patients and are at best an adjunct to a comprehensive clinical assessment. Pain assessment should become a routine part of every animal's care and well-being. The entire veterinary team should be educated and supported in learning the skills necessary to undertake the assessment. Education of owners about pain behaviors is also an important part of the veterinarian's role to ensure that they can detect relevant behavioral changes and seek appropriate veterinary care.

REFERENCES

Brown, D.C., Boston, R., Coyne, J., & Farrar, J.T. (2007) The Canine Brief Pain Inventory (CBPI): Development and psychometric testing of an instrument designed to measure chronic pain in companion dogs with osteoarthritis. *American Journal Veterinary Research*, 68(6), 631–637.

Brown, D.C., Boston, R., Coyne, J., & Farrar, J.T. (2009) A novel approach to the use of animals in studies of pain: validation of the Canine Brief Pain Inventory in Canine Bone Cancer. *Pain Medicine*, 10(1), 133–142.

Brown, D.C., Boston, R., Coyne, J., et al. (2008) Ability of the Canine Brief Pain Inventory to detect response to treatment in dogs with osteoarthritis. *Journal of the American Veterinary Medical Association*, 233(8), 1278–1283.

Capner, C.A., Lascelles, B.D., & Waterman-Pearson, A.E. (1999) Current British veterinary attitudes to perioperative analgesia for dogs. *Veterinary Record*, 145(4), 95–99.

Dohoo, S.E., & Dohoo, I.R. (1996) Factors influencing the postoperative use of analgesics in dogs and cats by Canadian veterinarians. *The Canadian Veterinary Journal*, 37(9), 552–556.

Dohoo, S.E. & Dohoo, I.R. (1998) Attitudes and concerns of Canadian animal health technologists toward postoperative pain management in dogs and cats. *The Canadian Veterinary Journal*, 39(8), 491–496.

Firth, A.M. & Haldane, S.L. (1999) Development of a scale to evaluate postoperative pain in dogs. *Journal of the American Veterinary Medical Association*, 214(5), 651–659.

Fox, S.M., Mellor, D.J., Firth, E.C., Hodge, H., & Lawoko, C.R. (1994) Changes in plasma cortisol concentrations before, during and after analgesia, anaesthesia and anaesthesia plus ovariohysterectomy in bitches. *Research in Veterinary Science*, 57(1), 110–118.

Fox, S.M., Mellor, D.J., Stafford, K.J., Lowoko, C.R., & Hodge, H. (2000) The effects of ovariohysterectomy plus different combinations of halothane anaesthesia and butorphanol analgesia on behaviour in the bitch. *Research in Veterinary Science*, 68(3), 265–274.

Hansen, B.D. (2003) Assessment of pain in dogs: veterinary clinical studies. *Institute of Laboratory Animal Resources Journal*, 44(3), 197–205.

Hansen, B. & Hardie, E. (1993) Prescription and use of analgesics in dogs and cats in a veterinary teaching hospital: 258 cases (1983–1989). *Journal of the American Veterinary Medical Association*, 202(9), 1485–1494.

Hansen, B.D., Lascelles, B.D.X., Keene, B.W., Adams, A.K., & Thomson, A.E. (2007) Evaluation of an accelerometer for at-home monitoring of spontaneous activity in dogs. *American Journal Of Veterinary Research*, 68(5), 468–475.

Holton, L.L., Scott, E. M., Nolan, A. M., Reid, J., & Welsh, E. (1998a) Relationship between physiological factors and clinical pain in dogs scored using a numerical rating scale. *The Journal of Small Animal Practice*, 39(10), 469–474.

Holton, L.L., Scott, E.M., Nolan, A.M., Reid, J., Welsh, E., & Flaherty, D. (1998b) Comparison of three methods used for assessment of pain in dogs. *Journal of the American Veterinary Medical Association*, 212(1), 61–66.

Holton, L., Reid, J., Scott, E.M., Pawson, P., & Nolan, A. (2001) Development of a behaviour-based scale to measure acute pain in dogs. *Veterinary Record*, 148(17), 525–531.

Hugonnard, M., Leblond, A., Keroack, S., Cadoré, J.L., & Troncy, E. (2004) Attitudes and concerns of French veterinarians towards pain and analgesia in dogs and cats. *Veterinary Anaesthesia and Analgesia*, 31(3), 154–163.

Lascelles, B.D., Cripps, P.J., Jones, A., & Waterman-Pearson, A.E. (1998) Efficacy and kinetics of carprofen, administered preoperatively or postoperatively, for the prevention of pain in dogs undergoing ovariohysterectomy. *Veterinary Surgery*, 27(6), 568–582.

Mathews, K.A. (2000) Pain assessment and general approach to management. *Veterinary Clinics of North America Small Animal Practice*, 30(4), 729–755.

Melzack, R. & Torgerson, W. S. (1971) On the language of pain. *Anesthesiology*, 34(1), 50–59.

Mich, P.M. & Hellyer, P.W. (2009) Objective, categoric methods for assessing pain and analgesia, in *Handbook of Veterinary Pain*

Management, 2nd edn (eds Gaynor, J.S., Muir, W.W.), Mosby Elsevier, St Louis, MO, pp. 78–109

Morton, C.M., Reid, J., Scott, E.M., Holton, L.L., & Nolan, A.M. (2005) Application of a scaling model to establish and validate an interval level pain scale for assessment of acute pain in dogs. *American Journal of Veterinary Research*, 66(12), 2154–2166.

Reid, J., Nolan, A., Hughes, J., Lascelles, D., Pawson, P., & Scott, E.M. (2007) Development of the short-form Glasgow Composite Measure Pain Scale (CMPS-SF) and derivation of an analgesic intervention score. *Animal Welfare*, 16(Suppl. 1), 97–104.

Thurstone, L.L. (1927) A law of comparative judgment. *Psychological Review*, 34(4), 273–286.

Watson, A.D., Nicholson, A., Church, D.B., & Pearson, M.R. (1996) Use of anti-inflammatory and analgesic drugs in dogs and cats. *Australian Veterinary Journal*, 74(3), 203–210.

Williams, V.M., Lascelles, B.D. X., & Robson, M.C. (2005) Current attitudes to, and use of, peri-operative analgesia in dogs and cats by veterinarians in New Zealand. *New Zealand Veterinary Journal*, 53(3), 193–202.

21

Treatment of Acute Pain in the Dog

Kate L. White

Acute pain can follow surgery, diagnostic procedures, or trauma. In addition, there are many medical conditions that cause acute inflammatory pain (e.g., pancreatitis). Acute pain after surgery or a diagnostic intervention is preventable with the pre-emptive use of analgesics. The concept of pre-emptive analgesia is well recognized, and most practitioners provide analgesia in the form of an opioid and/or an NSAID in the premedication protocol. Acute pain from trauma cannot be pre-empted, and its treatment may require the use of combinations of drugs and larger dosages.

The drugs used to treat acute pain can be divided into five main classes: opioids, local anesthetics, NSAIDs, α-2 adrenoceptor agonists, and miscellaneous drugs or adjuncts.

An effective analgesic plan will, in many cases, involve a combination of drugs from different classes (i.e., multimodal or balanced analgesia).

OPIOIDS

Opioids (Table 21.1) (Chapter 4) are the most commonly used class of drugs for the treatment of acute pain in dogs. These drugs are subject to stringent regulatory control.

Adverse Effects of Opioids in Dogs

Although the opioids are primarily used for relieving pain they also produce a host of adverse effects. Opioids can produce sedation or arousal and excitement. This latter effect is not only species-dependent, but is also affected by the route, dose, and patient characteristics, such as presence of pain and the animal's temperament.

In humans, post-operative nausea and vomiting (PONV) is a multifactorial and unpleasant adverse effect of opioids and various strategies are employed to reduce its incidence. The true incidence of PONV in dogs is impossible to define because of the lack of ability to detect nausea other than by gross clinical signs, for example, licking of lips and salivation. Studies in dogs have identified individual drugs that are more likely to induce vomiting, morphine being the opioid most frequently cited. Opioid-induced vomiting occurs due to stimulation of the chemoreceptor trigger zone in the medulla, and seems to be less likely when opioids are given to dogs that are in pain (Lamont & Mathews, 2007). Other gastrointestinal effects associated with opioids in dogs include defecation, and ileus and constipation after repeated dosing (Papich, 2000).

Most opioids have minimal effects on the cardiovascular system and, consequently, are often used in protocols for dogs suffering from cardiovascular disease (Dyson, 2008). Some opioids can cause a vagally mediated bradycardia (e.g., fentanyl), and some may cause histamine release (e.g., morphine, meperidine/pethidine), especially if administered intravenously.

Adverse effects on the respiratory system are due to a μ-receptor-mediated, dose-dependent depression of ventilation, and are much less significant in dogs compared to humans.

Opioids can have a variable effect on urine production, some producing oliguria and some causing diuresis (Papich, 2000). Opioids given epidurally or spinally can induce urine retention, necessitating manual bladder emptying (Valverde, 2008). Other adverse effects of some of the opioids include suppression of the cough reflex, miosis or mydriasis, panting, and altered thermoregulation.

Full μ Agonists

FENTANYL

Fentanyl is a potent synthetic μ opioid agonist that is highly lipid soluble with a rapid onset of action (2–3 minutes) (Pascoe, 2000) and a short duration of action (20–30 minutes). The drug is reported to have a relative potency of 75–100 times that of morphine, and this may be attributable to its lipophilic nature and ability to cross the blood–brain barrier. After a single IV injection, fentanyl has a short distribution half-life (4.5 minutes ± 1.5 minutes) and an elimination half-life of 45.7 ± 8.6 minutes (Sano et al., 2006). Fentanyl can be administered IV or IM for acute pain, as a premedication, during anesthesia, or as a co-induction agent. When used as a CRI during anesthesia, the lower end of the dose range is used. Fentanyl has market authorization for dogs in Europe, and is indicated for intraoperative and postoperative analgesia as a CRI following an IV bolus.

Fentanyl has a relatively short context or elimination half-time, and a fentanyl CRI is often employed perioperatively or after trauma to maintain constant plasma concentrations after an IV loading dose (LD). A fentanyl CRI decreases minimum alveolar concentration (MAC) in a dose-dependent manner. Steagall et al. (2006) reported a 66% reduction in end-tidal isoflurane concentration after an LD of fentanyl (5 mcg/kg) and a fentanyl CRI of 0.5 mcg/kg/min in female dogs undergoing soft tissue procedures. During an infusion of fentanyl in humans, plasma concentrations gradually increase

Pain Management in Veterinary Practice, First Edition. Edited by Christine M. Egger, Lydia Love and Tom Doherty.
© 2014 John Wiley & Sons, Inc. Published 2014 by John Wiley & Sons, Inc.

Table 21.1. Opioids used for the treatment of acute pain in dogs

Drug	Indication	Dose	Comments	References
Buprenorphine	Mild-to-moderate pain	5–20 mcg/kg, IM, IV, q4-8h 20–120 mcg/kg OTM TD patch SR formulation available	Peak time to onset 45–60 minutes Bioavailability of OTM route ~30–50% TD patches available in various sizes, lag phase 12–36 hours before antinociceptive effects detectable. Anecdotal reports of depression and anorexia in dogs[a]	Slingsby et al., 2006; Slingsby et al., 2011; Krotscheck et al., 2008; Andaluz et al., 2009; Ko et al., 2011; Abbo et al., 2008; Pieper et al., 2011
Butorphanol	Mild-to-moderate pain	0.1–0.4 mg/kg SC, IM, IV, q2–3h 0.5–2 mg/kg PO 0.1–0.4 mg/kg/h CRI	Short duration of action up to 2 hours. Peak time to onset 15–30 minutes	Caulkett et al., 2003; Vettarato & Bacco, 2011
Codeine	Mild-to-moderate pain	0.5–2 mg/kg PO q6–12h	Onset of action approximately 30 minutes after dosing. Analgesic effects persist for 4–6 hours Also available in combination with acetaminophen, (give 1–2 mg/kg codeine)	Gaynor, 2008; KuKanich, 2010
Hydromorphone	Moderate-to-severe pain	0.08–0.3 mg/kg SC, IM, IV q2–6h	Onset of action 15–30 minutes depending on the route of administration	Guedes et al., 2008; Hansen, 2008; KuKanich et al., 2008; Smith et al., 2008
Fentanyl	Moderate-to-severe pain	1–10 mcg/kg IV bolus q20min or CRI 1–5 mcg/kg/h. Can increase dose during anesthesia to 10–45 mcg/kg/h for MAC reduction in severe pain	Short duration of effect 15–30 minutes. Onset of action 2–5 minutes after IV injection	Pascoe, 2000; Sano et al., 2006; Steagall et al., 2006
Fentanyl TD patch	Moderate-to-severe pain	2–4 mcg/kg/h	A patch lasts approx 3 days but there is significant interpatient variability	Egger et al., 1998; Hofmeister & Egger, 2004; Bellei et al., 2011
Fentanyl TD Recuvyra® "patchless"	Moderate-to-severe pain following procedures likely to require up to 4 days analgesia	2.6 mg/kg applied between the shoulder blades once to provide analgesia for up to 4 days	Dogs >30 kg to remain hospitalized for 48 hours following application of Recuvyra	EMA EPAR (2011b); KuKanich & Clark, 2012
Meperidine (pethidine)	Mild-to-moderate pain	3–10 mg/kg SC or IM q1–2h	Do not administer IV, due to risk of histamine release. Peak analgesic effects 30–60 minutes after IM injection	Vettarato & Bacco, 2011; Pascoe, 2000

(continued)

Table 21.1. (*Continued*)

Drug	Indication	Dose	Comments	References
Methadone	Moderate-to-severe pain	0.3–1 mg/kg SC, IM, IV (slowly) q1–4h	May cause less vomiting than morphine. Time to onset 10–60 minutes depending on route administered	Ingvast-Larsson et al., 2010; Murrell, 2011; KuKanich et al., 2008
Morphine	Moderate-to-severe pain	0.3–1 mg/kg SQ, IM, q1–4h For IV use inject slowly. CRI 0.1–0.4 mg/kg/h Epidural 0.1–0.2 mg/kg (PF) q12–24h	For severe pain administer high dose (1 mg/kg). Time to peak onset depends on route administered.	Barnhart et al., 2000 Dohoo et al., 1994 KuKanich et al., 2005 Valverde, 2008 Day et al., 1995
Morphine sustained release tablets and syrup	Moderate-to-severe pain	2–5 mg/kg PO q12h 0.5 mg/kg for syrup q4–6h	Bioavailability is poor (≈25%) Significant interpatient variability following the oral route	Dohoo et al., 1994
Oxymorphone	Moderate-to-severe pain	0.05–0.2 mg/kg SC, IM, IV q2–4h	Analgesic effects evident 3–5 minutes after IV injection	Smith et al., 2001
Remifentanil	Mild-to-moderate pain	4–10 mcg/kg/h, can increase to 20–60 mcg/kg/h for surgical analgesia	Rapid elimination	Anagnostou et al., 2011
Tramadol	Mild-to-moderate pain.	5–10 mg/kg PO q6–8h	Used in acute and chronic pain, maximum effects may take 14 days. Not licensed. Useful as an adjunct in multimodal therapy.	Mastrocinque & Fantoni, 2003; KuKanich & Papich, 2004; McMillan et al., 2008; Teresinha et al., 2010; Mastrocinque et al., 2012

[a]Personal communication Lydia Love, DVM, DACVAA 2012.

CRI, continuous rate infusion; IM, intramuscular; IV, intravenous; SQ, subcutaneously; OTM, oral transmucosal route; PF, preservative free; TD, transdermal.

and pharmacokinetic variables are dependent on the duration of the infusion. Furthermore, studies suggest that analgesia provided by fentanyl infusions may persist after the termination of the infusion, particularly when infusions in excess of 3–4 hours are used (Sano et al., 2006). Infusions of fentanyl may be of particular use in patients with cardiovascular compromise during anesthesia because of the MAC reduction.

Fentanyl is also available, in various sizes (12.5, 25, 50, 75, and 100 mcg/h), as a transdermal patch that is applied to a clipped area of skin prior to or immediately after surgery or trauma (Bellei et al., 2011). Plasma concentrations only reach steady state after 12–24 hours in dogs, thereby necessitating other analgesics in the interim period (Hofmeister & Egger, 2004). There seems to be significant individual variation in drug delivery (Kyles et al., 1996; Egger et al., 1998), and this is based on multiple factors. The advantages of fentanyl patches include ease of use, noninvasiveness,

continuous drug delivery over a period of time, and a perceived reduction in overall cost. Nevertheless, fentanyl patches were not superior to IM morphine in dogs undergoing cruciate ligament repair or pelvic limb surgery (Egger et al., 2007) nor did they offer any advantage when compared to epidural morphine in dogs undergoing ovariohysterectomy (Pekcan & Koc, 2010).

There is a novel 'patchless' topical preparation of fentanyl (Recuvyra®) for application between the shoulder blades of dogs 2–4 hours prior to surgery. It is claimed that one application of Recuvyra provides long-acting, continuous systemic delivery of fentanyl for up to 4 days. It is recommended that dogs greater than 30 kg in weight remain hospitalized for 48 hours post-administration to minimize the risk of a child coming into contact with fentanyl residues on the skin. In the limited number of clinical studies that have been performed, the formulation compared similarly to buprenorphine (Recuvyra, European Medicines Agency,

European Public Assessment Records (EMA EPAR) 2011b; Linton et al., 2012).

HYDROMORPHONE

Hydromorphone is a synthetic μ agonist opioid with efficacy and potency similar to oxymorphone. There are reports of hydromorphone causing more sedation than oxymorphone (Pascoe, 2000), and others consider it to be less sedating than oxymorphone or morphine (Wagner, 2009). It can induce histamine release but the effect is mild and unlikely to be clinically significant (Wagner, 2009). Hydromorphone often causes panting and vomiting in dogs that are not painful. Epidurally administered hydromorphone results in regional analgesia with a faster onset of action and a shorter duration (6–12 hours) when compared to morphine (Brose et al., 1991). Hydromorphone can also be administered as a CRI (Hansen, 2008). Currently, hydromorphone is a cheaper alternative to oxymorphone.

MORPHINE

Morphine is useful in the management of moderate-to-severe pain and provides profound analgesia in the dog. Its duration of action is 3–4 hours, but it can be given more frequently to dogs in severe pain or those exhibiting signs of breakthrough pain. There may be a degree of accumulation after several doses, and this may allow the dosing interval to be increased. Constant rate infusions (CRI) are frequently used after trauma and perioperatively, and infusions of morphine along with other drugs such as lidocaine and ketamine provide balanced analgesia. Variable rate infusions of morphine allow more precise dose titration, and compare favorably with intramuscular administration (Lucas et al., 2001). Morphine infusions can also be administered subcutaneously, and epidural morphine can be administered intermittently or as a CRI (Valverde, 2008). The discovery of opioid receptors elsewhere in the body has meant that other routes of administration, such as instillation into inflamed and painful joints (Day et al., 1995; Sammarco et al., 1996) and topical application to corneas to provide analgesia (Stiles et al., 2003), can be used in dogs.

Morphine may cause histamine release if given rapidly IV, resulting in vasodilation and hypotension (Robinson et al., 1988); thus, morphine is best diluted and given over 2–5 minutes. Morphine frequently causes vomiting, and should be avoided in dogs with increased intracranial or intraocular pressure, obstructive gastrointestinal lesions, or laryngeal paralysis.

Morphine is available in many different formulations and concentrations including injectable formulations (10, 15, 20, or 30 mg/mL), preservative-free formulations for epidural, spinal, or intra-articular use (1 and 10 mg/mL), oral tablets (10, 30, 60, or 100 mg tablets), suspensions and granules, and slow-release capsules and tablets. Rectal suppositories are also available.

The first pass effect is significant after oral administration of morphine, and this results in 25% or less bioavailability in the dog (Dohoo et al., 1994). The dose can be altered to take account of this and, in the author's experience, oral morphine therapy may provide a longer duration of action compared to the intravenous or intramuscular route.

Hepatic metabolism of morphine, specifically conjugation, results in the formation of morphine 6-glucuronide (M6G) and morphine 3-glucuronide (M3G). M6G has properties identical to morphine and M3G may contribute to excitation but has little activity at the opioid receptor. These metabolites are excreted in the urine and, in humans with renal dysfunction, there are reports of accumulation of the metabolites leading to a prolonged duration of action caused by the M6G metabolite (Milne et al., 1992), and implicating the M3G metabolites in neuroexcitatory effects such as allodynia, myoclonus, and seizures (Smith, 2009). There are no specific guidelines for administration of opioids to dogs with hepatic or renal disease, but their use should probably be similar to that adopted in humans – "start low and go slow" (Smith, 2009).

METHADONE

Methadone is a synthetic μ receptor agonist widely used as an analgesic in dogs. Methadone has marketing authorization in continental Europe and in the United Kingdom for use in dogs. It is available as a racemic mixture in a multidose bottle. Although methadone has affinity for the μ receptor, it also has activity at other receptor sites including the N-methyl-D-aspartate (NMDA) receptor and α-2 receptors (Codd et al., 1995). Activation of the NMDA receptor is recognized as a significant event in the generation of central sensitization and hyperalgesia. The use of NMDA antagonists can result in a reduction of central sensitization (Davis & Inturrisi, 1999). It is possible that the treatment or prevention of acute pain with methadone is superior to other opioids because of the additional action of the drug on the NMDA receptor, and potential reduction of central sensitization in the face of sustained nociceptive input (Murrell, 2011). The clinical significance of the drug's action on α-2 receptors has not been clarified. Furthermore, methadone reduces serotonin and noradrenergic uptake, and increased descending inhibition may contribute to the antinociceptive effect (Codd et al., 1995; Gorman et al., 1997).

Methadone is considered to have a half-life of 1.5–4 hours (KuKanich et al., 2005; Ingvast-Larsson et al., 2010), and can be administered via the subcutaneous, intramuscular or intravenous route. Analgesic efficacy is dose-dependent, and a dosing interval of 4 hours is suggested. In animals exhibiting signs of acute pain, methadone could be administered more frequently. One experimental study detected more whining in beagle dogs that had received methadone (Ingvast-Larsson et al., 2010). This study was performed in experimental dogs that were not subjected to a painful stimulus, and increased whining was not detected in the greyhounds studied. KuKanich et al. (2008) reported that greyhounds had a large volume of distribution compared to beagles and a greater clearance but similar elimination half-lives for methadone, leading to the suggestion that a greater dose of methadone would be necessary for greyhounds. Methadone does not induce vomiting, which may favor its use over morphine when vomiting is undesirable.

A few studies investigated the administration of methadone epidurally (Leibetseder et al., 2006; Campagnol et al., 2012). It had a longer duration of action when administered epidurally, and its isoflurane-sparing effects were significantly greater compared to the intravenous route (Leibetseder et al., 2006). However, this was not proven to be the case in a separate study (Campagnol et al., 2012). Further work is required to investigate the efficacy and duration of postoperative analgesia provided by epidural methadone.

OXYMORPHONE

Oxymorphone hydrochloride is a pure μ agonist considered to be 10 times more potent than morphine and comparable in terms of duration of effect and efficacy. Oxymorphone can be administered by SQ, IM, and IV routes and offers a degree of sedation without risk of histamine release (Smith et al., 2001). Oxymorphone is less likely to cause vomiting in dogs compared to morphine, but dogs are more likely to pant when given oxymorphone. In cases of severe pain, oxymorphone can be administered slowly IV, with peak effects in 6–8 minutes. Oxymorphone can be titrated to effect and continued as a CRI. Oxymorphone has been administered epidurally, but because it is more lipid soluble than morphine its duration of effect is shorter (Vesal et al., 1996; Torske et al., 1999).

Pethidine/Meperidine

Pethidine (meperidine) is a short-acting pure μ agonist used to treat dogs with mild-to-moderate pain. It has a similar efficacy profile but lower potency when compared to morphine. It has an onset of action of approximately 10–15 minutes after intramuscular administration, and its duration is between 30 and 120 minutes (Pascoe, 2000). A recent study demonstrated satisfactory analgesia and sedation for up to 4 hours after acepromazine and meperidine in dogs undergoing ovariectomy or ovariohysterectomy (Vettarato & Bacco, 2011). However, not all the dogs that received pethidine in that study were assessed for analgesia throughout the 4 hour period. The longer than expected duration of analgesia identified in that and in another study (Lascelles et al., 1997) may be explained by the pre-emptive administration of the drugs, which reduced noxious stimulation during surgery, thereby reducing the incidence of hypersensitivity. Lascelles et al. (1997) demonstrated the pre-emptive effect of meperidine in dogs undergoing ovariohysterectomy, and a significant difference in the duration of analgesia was provided by meperidine in dogs receiving the drug prior to surgery and in those receiving it post-operatively.

Interestingly, a third of the dogs that were given meperidine in one study (Vettarato & Bacco, 2011) vomited in the post-operative period, which contrasts to similar studies in which no vomiting was recorded after administration of meperidine (Grint et al., 2009). The causes of vomiting are multifactorial and may involve the type of procedure, the degree of pain, the combination of drugs used, patient gender and age, and individual variation.

Meperidine is likely to cause histamine release and should not be administered IV. Local urticarial reactions seen in one study following IM administration may also have been caused by histamine release, although there may be individual and breed variations, and this reaction may be more prevalent in dogs with atopy (Grint et al., 2009).

Remifentanil

Remifentanil is a structural analog of fentanyl, and is usually administered during anesthesia as an infusion in cases requiring intense analgesia or blunting of the sympathetic nervous system. The MAC-sparing effects of remifentanil infusions have been demonstrated (Hoke et al., 1997; Monteiro et al., 2010). The metabolism of remifentanil is different from other opioids as it is metabolized by nonspecific plasma esterases, making it useful in cases with liver or renal dysfunction (Hoke et al., 1997; Anagnostou et al., 2011). Remifentanil exhibits a relatively insensitive context half-time, meaning that the duration of the infusion has little impact on the time taken for plasma concentrations to decrease by 50% after stopping the infusion. A CRI is necessary for sustained analgesia because of the rapid clearance of remifentanil.

Partial Agonist and Agonist–Antagonist Opioids

These drugs occupy opioid receptors but do not elicit a maximal response. The concurrent administration of opioids with different receptor-binding profiles has revealed that the effects can be additive, synergistic, or antagonistic, hence the general advice not to mix the pure μ agonists with the partial agonists or agonist–antagonists.

Butorphanol

Butorphanol is a synthetic opioid that is an agonist at the κ receptor and an antagonist at the μ receptor. The clinical effect is dependent on dose, pain model, species, and route but, in general, butorphanol is considered to be useful for mild pain (Sawyer et al., 1991). Butorphanol has 7–10 times the receptor-binding potency as morphine but is not efficacious in moderate-to-severe pain (Pascoe, 2000). Butorphanol can be administered via the IM, SQ, and IV routes, and does not cause histamine release. It is also available as a tablet, and has antitussive effects.

Butorphanol alone produces mild sedation, but in combination with phenothiazines, α-2 agonists, or benzodiazepines provides sedation and analgesia for diagnostic and minimally invasive procedures. The duration of action of butorphanol is debatable, with some studies suggesting up to 2 hours and some significantly less. In general, its effects are quoted as being shorter lived than morphine, between 1 and 3 hours (Lamont & Mathews, 2007). A ceiling effect for provision of analgesia has been demonstrated in some studies (Sawyer et al., 1991). As with other drugs, there does seem to be a significant degree of individual variation in response. There is a general consensus that butorphanol may be more effective for treating visceral than somatic pain. Butorphanol CRIs can be efficacious for mild-to-moderate pain. A bolus dose of butorphanol is administered IV to achieve analgesia (e.g., 0.4 mg/kg) and is followed by a CRI. The infusion rate can be calculated by dividing the bolus dose that was effective in relieving the pain by 2 or 3 and administering this dose as the hourly CRI rate. However, butorphanol was less efficacious than meloxicam for post-operative analgesia in bitches undergoing ovariohysterectomy (Caulkett et al., 2003).

Butorphanol has minimal effects on the cardiovascular system, and is a suitable choice for compromised patients requiring analgesia and sedation. Butorphanol can also be used to partially antagonize the sedative or respiratory depressant effects of pure μ agonists without totally reversing the analgesia. This technique may be used in the recovery period to help restore laryngeal reflexes in preparation for extubation. A dose of 0.05–0.1 mg/kg of butorphanol, diluted and titrated to effect over 5 minutes, can be used.

Buprenorphine

Buprenorphine is an agonist–antagonist with strong affinity for the μ receptor and antagonist activity at the κ receptor. It is considered to be a partial agonist at the μ receptor, incapable of eliciting a full response (i.e., there is a ceiling effect). Interestingly, research in rats suggests that buprenorphine may not have a ceiling effect with respect to its antinociceptive effects, although it may for its respiratory depressant effects (Yassen et al., 2008).

The time to peak effect is 20–30 minutes after IV injection and 45–60 minutes after IM injection, thus another form of analgesia may be required in the interim. The long duration of effect (6–8 hours) makes this drug attractive to the practitioner. After 3 or 4 hours a further increment can be administered, if necessary, or the dose can be repeated after 5–6 hours have elapsed without untoward effects. Increasing the dose from 20 mcg/kg to 40 mcg/kg had no additional benefit for dogs undergoing ovariohysterectomy (Slingsby et al., 2011). It is advisable not to exceed recommended doses as the avid binding of the drug to the receptor makes reversal difficult if adverse effects occur. In practice, however, adverse effects such as respiratory depression are rarely seen with clinical doses. Buprenorphine is used regularly in the post-operative period, but is rarely sufficient when used alone to treat severe pain following thoracotomy or extensive orthopedic surgery. Buprenorphine has been evaluated transmucosally in dogs, and further studies are required to confirm reports of this route providing an alternative for post-operative analgesia in dogs undergoing ovariohysterectomy (Ko et al., 2011).

Buprenorphine is commonly administered for pre-emptive analgesia and is often combined with a sedative and an NSAID. Interestingly, despite the emphasis on multimodal analgesia, a recent study showed no superior analgesia when buprenorphine was combined with carprofen for dogs undergoing ovariohysterectomy (Shih et al., 2008). Despite widespread use, buprenorphine pharmacokinetics after IV administration at clinically relevant doses in dogs were only recently published (Krotscheck et al., 2008).

Other formulations of buprenorphine are available and are being tested in dogs. Buprenorphine transdermal delivery systems (TDS) have been developed for use in humans (Evans & Easthope, 2003; Griessinger et al., 2005). The patch is available in three sizes designed to release buprenorphine into the circulation at rates of 35, 52.5 or 70 mcg/h. The pharmacokinetics after application of a 70 mcg/h transdermal buprenorphine patch applied to four dogs have been described (Andaluz et al., 2009). Buprenorphine was detected in the plasma of all four dogs, but there was a variable time to peak plasma concentrations. The 70 mcg/h transdermal buprenorphine patches applied to dogs undergoing ovariohysterectomy provided analgesia comparable to 20 mcg/kg buprenorphine SQ given pre-emptively (Moll et al., 2011). An injectable sustained release formulation of buprenorphine has been developed and tested in rats (Foley et al., 2011) and cats (Catbagan et al., 2011), but currently there are limited data in dogs (Chapter 9).

TRAMADOL

Tramadol is a weak μ agonist and also provides analgesia through inhibition of neuronal uptake of norepinephrine and serotonin and modulation of serotonin release. Tramadol is often referred to as an "atypical opioid" and is not a controlled substance in the European Union and United Kingdom, although it is controlled in some states in the United States. Several studies investigated its use in acute and chronic pain in dogs. For acute surgical pain in dogs undergoing ovariohysterectomy it performed similarly to morphine (Mastrocinque & Fantoni, 2003). Tramadol is most commonly used in chronic pain states, such as osteoarthritis, often in conjunction with an NSAID. The use of such combinations has not yet been rigorously evaluated and, in all cases of "off label" use of drugs caution must be exercised. Additive effects of rofecoxib and tramadol were demonstrated in rats (Garcia-Hernandez et al., 2007). In human patients hospitalized for treatment of peptic ulcers, the use of tramadol was associated with a greater incidence of gastric ulceration and mortality compared to NSAID use alone (Tørring et al., 2008). That study suggests that the visceral analgesia provided by tramadol may have masked the pain associated with the

peptic ulcer, thereby delaying the patient seeking medical intervention. These studies serve to remind us to exercise caution and vigilance when administering unlicensed drugs and combinations of drugs.

NONSTEROIDAL ANTI-INFLAMMATORY DRUGS (NSAIDs)

NSAIDs (Table 21.2) (Chapter 5) offer an ever expanding choice of drugs for the treatment of acute and chronic pain. These drugs are licensed for soft tissue and orthopedic surgical pain and inflammatory conditions (i.e., osteoarthritis). Several NSAIDs are also licensed for administration prior to surgery in healthy animals.

The pharmacokinetic data of NSAIDs approved for dogs are available from the EMA EPARs and the Food and Drug Administration Freedom of Information sources (FDA FOIs). Excellent reviews are also available (Lees et al., 2004; KuKanich et al., 2012).

Adverse Effects of NSAIDs

The most common adverse effects reported are those associated with the gastrointestinal tract. Signs include vomiting, diarrhea, anorexia, bleeding, and in some cases death from gastrointestinal ulceration and perforation. These adverse effects can be caused directly by gastrointestinal mucosa irritation or indirectly through PGE_2 and PGI_2 inhibition (Wolfe et al., 1999). As yet, there is no extensive clinical trial comparing different NSAIDs, thus making direct comparisons about adverse effects difficult. It seems that the more recently approved NSAIDs may offer a lower incidence of gastrointestinal lesions compared to the older licensed NSAIDs (e.g., aspirin, ketoprofen, phenylbutazone, tolfenamic acid and flunixin), possibly attributable to their COX-1-sparing properties (KuKanich et al., 2012). It may not be as simple as that, because recent studies demonstrated that dogs with pre-existing gastric damage given the COX-2 selective NSAIDs had larger lesions at biopsy sites compared to dogs receiving placebo or the dual COX inhibitor tepoxalin. The conclusion from that study was that the COX-2 selective NSAIDs may decrease gastric healing (Goodman et al., 2009).

Adverse renal effects of NSAIDs are also well documented, and arise from the inhibition of prostaglandins that control blood vessel tone and salt and water balance in the kidney. Typically, NSAID-induced renal damage is associated with higher doses of NSAIDs and comorbidities and other factors such as dehydration and anesthesia. Studies in healthy dogs showed no indicators of renal damage in a 3-month period with carprofen, etodolac, ketoprofen, meloxicam, and flunixin (Luna et al., 2007). Guidelines for the use of NSAIDs advise against their use in dogs with renal compromise (Lascelles et al., 2005) but, interestingly, 2011 saw the European market authorization of cimicoxib (Cimalgex®, Vetoquinol®) for use in dogs. This NSAID has no contraindication for the use in dogs suffering from mild-to-moderate renal disease (IRIS stage 1 and 2), and is indicated for the treatment of soft tissue and orthopedic perioperative pain and osteoarthritis (Cimalgex EMA EPAR, 2011a).

There appears to be two types of hepatic injury induced by NSAIDs: idiosyncratic and intrinsic. The idiosyncratic adverse effects are dose-independent and the intrinsic injury is predictable and dose-dependent. MacPhail et al. (1998) suggested that the majority of hepatopathies associated with NSAID use occur within

Table 21.2. NSAIDs commonly used in dogs for treatment of acute pain due to inflammation, OA, trauma, and surgery

Drug	Subclass	Dose	Comments	References
Acetaminophen	Para-aminophenol derivative	10 mg/kg PO q12h, or 15 mg/kg q8h	Licensed formulation in UK (combined with codeine)	Mburu, 1991; Papich, 2008
Aspirin	Salicylic ester of acetic acid	10–25 mg/kg PO q12h	Not commonly employed in acute pain	Morton & Knottenbelt, 1989; Reimer et al., 1999
Carprofen	Propionic acid	2.2 mg/kg PO q12h, preop 4.4 mg/kg SQ	Licensed for perioperative use pre-emptively.	Leece et al., 2005; Shih et al., 2008
Cimicoxib	Coxib	2 mg/kg PO daily, can be given 2 hours prior to surgery and then for 3–7 days postop	No contraindication in mild-to-moderate renal dysfunction. Can be used in chronic pain.	Cimalgex® EMA EPAR, 2011a
Deracoxib	Coxib	1–2 mg/kg PO q24h postop 3–4 mg/kg PO q24h		Roberts et al., 2009
Etodolac	Pyrano-carboxylic acid	10–15 mg/kg PO q24h	Used for chronic pain more than acute pain	Borer et al., 2003; Budsberg et al., 1999
Firocoxib	Coxib	5 mg/kg PO q24h	Licensed for postoperative pain and inflammation associated with soft tissue, orthopedic and dental surgery and for chronic pain associated with osteoarthritis	Hanson et al., 2006; Kondo et al., 2012; Pollmeier et al., 2006
Flunixin	Nicotinic acid derivative	1 mg/kg IV, IM, SQ or PO q24h once	Licensed for surgical pain, safer NSAIDs are available	Mathews et al., 1996
Ketoprofen	Propionic acid derivative	2 mg/kg IV, SQ, IM, PO then 1 mg/kg q24h	For use postoperatively, can be used for chronic pain (short courses)	Martins et al., 2010
Ketorolac	Heterocyclic acetic acid derivative	0.3–0.5 mg/kg IV, IM q8-12h once or twice	Not licensed Also indicated for panosteitis, 5–10 mg/kg (depending on size) daily for 2–3 days	Mathews et al., 1996
Mavacoxib	Coxib	2 mg/kg PO Days 1, 14, 30 days, then once monthly	Do not exceed 6.5 dosing cycles, for use in chronic pain	Cox et al., 2011
Meclofenamic acid	Anthranilic derivative	1.1 mg/kg daily for 5–7 days		

(*continued*)

Table 21.2. *(Continued)*

Drug	Subclass	Dose	Comments	References
Meloxicam	Oxicam	0.2 mg/kg PO, IV, or SQ once then 0.1 mg/kg PO, IV, SQ q24h	Also available as an oromucosal "mist" in the UK	Lees et al., 2013 Aragon et al., 2007; Sanderson et al., 2009
Piroxicam	Oxicam	0.3 mg/kg PO q48h		Papich, 2008
Phenylbutazone	Pyrazolone	20 mg/kg daily in divided doses for 7 days, then 10 mg/kg daily in divided doses	Use gastroprotectants	
Robenacoxib	Coxib	2 mg/kg SQ once perioperatively 1 mg/kg PO once daily	Administer 30 minutes prior to surgery	Gruet et al., 2011; Schmid et al., 2010
Tepoxalin	Hydroxamic acid derivative	10 or 20 mg/kg PO once then 10 mg/kg PO q24h		Lamont & Mathews, 2007; Gilmour & Lehenbauer, 2009
Tolfenamic acid	Fenamate derivative	4 mg/kg PO SC	Licensed for acute and chronic pain, once daily for 3 days, then 4 days off	McKellar et al., 1994
Vedaprofen	Propionic acid derivative	0.5 mg/kg PO daily		Nell et al., 2002; Hoeijmakers et al., 2005

The general precautions for NSAIDs apply: do not use in patients with GI or renal disease (exception is cimicoxib, see EMA EPAR); discontinue use in case of vomiting or diarrhea; NSAIDs are not recommended in hypovolemic or hypotensive patients or those with bleeding disorders and not for concurrent use with other NSAIDs or corticosteroids.

the first 3 weeks of starting treatment, leading to the obvious conclusion that monitoring dogs early in their treatment plan is sensible, and baseline hepatic and renal panels are advisable (MacPhail et al., 1998). Although the incidence of hepatopathies is low, there is the consensus that they can occur with any of the NSAIDs, and no predisposing factors have been identified. There is a paucity of data describing the use of NSAIDs in dogs with pre-existing hepatic disease, and no proof, as yet, of an increased incidence of hepatic adverse effects in dogs with hepatic disease. However, it would be sensible to assume that hepatic disease could cause a reduction in the rate of NSAID metabolism and increase the risk of NSAID accumulation.

NSAIDs that inhibit COX-1 have the potential to affect coagulation, and concern has been expressed about the use of NSAIDs in the perioperative period or in animals with pre-existing clotting disorders. The magnitude of the disruption to the clotting profile depends on the NSAID administered. Aspirin irreversibly inhibits thromboxane synthesis in platelets and prolongs bleeding time; this effect lasts for the lifetime of the platelet and can therefore persist after treatment has ceased. A 5-day course of carprofen will decrease platelet aggregation in dogs, but this is not reflected in a change in the buccal mucosal bleeding time (Hickford et al., 2001). Longer courses of NSAIDs alter the coagulation profile to varying extents and, while "clinically unimportant" (Luna et al., 2007), the necessity to undertake periodic patient re-evaluation remains.

Interaction with Other Drugs

There is a significant rate of adverse events when one or more NSAIDs are co-administered or when corticosteroids are prescribed with NSAIDs, and these combinations should be avoided. In the face of an adverse event or a lack of efficacy, dogs are often prescribed an alternative NSAID. The question often arises concerning the period of washout between treatments when a different subclass of NSAID is chosen. Similarly, what are the consequences of using an injectable NSAID of one class perioperatively and then continuing with an oral course of another type of NSAID? Most experts recommend a washout period between NSAIDs when switching from one to another (Lascelles et al., 2005), and while this necessity of switching is more likely to occur in cases of chronic pain management it may also be necessary in acute pain management. An arbitrary period of 5–7 days is often suggested (Ryan et al., 2007), but there are no clinical studies to confirm these assumptions.

Contraindications to the Use of NSAIDs in Dogs

NSAIDs should only be administered in well-hydrated, normotensive dogs with no comorbidities such as renal or hemostatic dysfunction. Dogs should not be given an NSAID if they are receiving corticosteroids or another NSAID. Pre-emptive NSAID analgesia is encouraged, but if there is any doubt about the dog's hydration status the drug may be administered at the end of anesthesia or during recovery, with attention being paid to fluid therapy and blood pressure monitoring and support. If an NSAID is omitted, reliance on other drug categories will be necessary. Pain may be easier to manage postoperatively in the dogs that have received a pre-emptive NSAID (Lascelles et al., 1998).

Clinical NSAID Selection

When selecting an NSAID for treating acute pain in dogs there are many choices, but fundamental commonalities exist (Papich, 2008). The choice of which NSAID to use is often based on factors such as convenience for the pet owner rather than claims of efficacy, and the lack of clinical studies making direct comparisons among NSAIDs makes the decision more difficult.

ACETAMINOPHEN (PARACETAMOL)

Acetaminophen is an effective analgesic when administered to dogs, but at clinical doses offers minimal anti-inflammatory effects (Mburu, 1991). The target site for acetaminophen is contentious, with a new COX-3 isomer being proposed in the dog, although some investigators now consider COX-3 to be a CNS variant of COX-1 (Kis et al., 2005). There is also evidence that acetaminophen modulates serotonin, providing analgesia in a similar way to tramadol. Acetaminophen is not commonly prescribed to dogs in acute pain despite significant safety with its use, and is more frequently administered to dogs with chronic conditions with or without an opioid. It can be very useful when transitioning patients off of injectable opioids. Formulations combined with opioids are available and licensed in some countries.

ASPIRIN

The salicylic ester of acetic acid, aspirin (acetylsalicylic acid), is available in different pharmaceutical preparations including plain, buffered, and enteric-coated tablets as well as topical and rectal preparations. In veterinary medicine, aspirin is used primarily for the relief of mild-to-moderate pain associated with musculoskeletal inflammation or osteoarthritis. However, aspirin is not approved for use in dogs, and definitive efficacy studies have not been performed to establish effective dosages.

CARPROFEN

Carprofen can be used pre-emptively prior to orthopedic and soft tissue surgery and continued into the post-operative period. Carprofen is a propionic acid derivative available in tablet and injectable formulations.

CIMICOXIB

Cimicoxib is a coxib recently licensed in Europe for pain and inflammation associated with osteoarthritis, and the management of perioperative pain due to orthopedic or soft tissue surgery. The tablet can be administered prior to surgery and continued in the postoperative period. In clinical trials, cimicoxib was comparable to carprofen for post-surgical pain, and to firocoxib for pain associated with chronic osteoarthritis (Cimalgex EMA EPAR, 2011a). Cimicoxib has no contraindication or warning for mild-to-moderate renal disease (IRIS stage 1 and 2) in dogs.

DERACOXIB

Deracoxib was the first NSAID of the coxib class approved for use in dogs. It is available, in the USA, as a beef-flavored chewable tablet. Deracoxib is indicated for the control of post-operative pain and inflammation associated with orthopedic surgery for up to 7 days, and for the control of pain and inflammation associated with osteoarthritis.

ETODOLAC

Etodolac is indicated for managing pain and inflammation associated with canine osteoarthritis. It is not often used in acute pain management. It is considered to be a COX-2 preferential NSAID with adverse effects primarily associated with the GI tract, although keratoconjunctivitis sicca has been reported (Klauss et al., 2007).

FIROCOXIB

Firocoxib has been recently licensed in the United States and Europe for the control of pain and inflammation associated with osteoarthritis in dogs. It is available in a chewable tablet formulation. It compares well with carprofen, and there was lower incidence of diarrhea with firocoxib compared to carprofen and etodolac (Papich, 2008).

FLUNIXIN MEGLUMINE

Flunixin meglumine is reported to be an effective analgesic for acute surgical pain in dogs (Mathews et al., 1996). Chronic administration of flunixin meglumine to dogs results in severe GI ulceration and renal damage, and its use in this species is not recommended. There are safer NSAIDs now available for acute and chronic pain management.

KETOPROFEN

Ketoprofen is licensed (in Europe) for treating dogs with acute pain for up to 5 days. It is preferable to reserve ketoprofen for postoperative use to reduce the likelihood of hemorrhage, as it decreases anti-thromboxane activity. Several studies show that preoperative use of ketoprofen decreases platelet aggregation in healthy dogs but does not alter clotting times (Lemke et al., 2002). Nevertheless, Grisneaux et al. (1999) demonstrated increased bleeding in dogs undergoing orthopedic surgery.

KETOROLAC

Ketorolac is not approved for use in dogs, but several reports document its use in refractory panosteitis, and for post-operative pain where it was comparable to oxymorphone and ketoprofen (Mathews et al., 1996). A maximum of two doses should be administered, and it is prudent to give the drug with food or gastroprotectants.

MAVACOXIB

This coxib NSAID exhibits very slow clearance, and this is reflected in the dosing interval. The initial dose is followed 14 days later by a second dose, and, thereafter, one dose a month for a total of seven consecutive doses. While this may not be a popular choice for the dog in acute pain, it does offer the possibility of providing analgesia with less frequent dosing, which may suit some owners and pets.

MELOXICAM

Meloxicam has potent anti-inflammatory and analgesic properties. It is suitable for orthopedic and soft tissue inflammatory conditions and can be administered pre-emptively. It is available as an injectable formulation, syrup, tablets, and as a spray for oromucosal delivery, and the relatively long half-life allows for once daily dosing.

PHENYLBUTAZONE

Phenylbutazone does not represent a "first line" treatment in dogs suffering from acute pain in the United States and Europe. This is a drug more commonly used in chronic pain when other NSAIDs have failed in efficacy. It is licensed in the UK for the treatment of osteoarthritis, acute musculoskeletal trauma, spondylitis, bursitis and inflammation of ligaments, and rheumatoid and other arthritic diseases. There are few studies investigating the use of phenylbutazone for acute pain in dogs.

PIROXICAM

Piroxicam is an oxicam NSAID that is associated with a high incidence of adverse GI effects. It is often prescribed as an antineoplastic drug for the treatment of bladder transitional cell carcinoma and other cancers. It is also reported to be very efficacious in the treatment of pain associated with cystitis and urethritis. It is possible that the licensed oxicam, meloxicam, may offer similar properties with fewer adverse effects, but studies are required to prove this.

ROBENACOXIB

Robenacoxib is recommended for the treatment of pain and inflammation associated with chronic osteoarthritis in dogs. It is available in tablet form, and clinical trials demonstrated better efficacy of robenacoxib when administered without food or at least 30 minutes before or after a meal. It is also available in Europe in injectable form that is recommended for the treatment of pain and inflammation associated with orthopedic or soft tissue surgery in dogs. It should be administered subcutaneously approximately 30 minutes before the start of surgery.

TEPOXALIN

Tepoxalin is a dual COX inhibitor with an efficacy comparable to carprofen or meloxicam, which is licensed for the relief of inflammation and pain caused by acute and chronic musculoskeletal problems (Lamont & Mathews, 2007). The product is formulated as a lyophilized tablet that can be placed in the dog's food if direct oral administration is difficult.

TOLFENAMIC ACID

Tolfenamic acid has antipyretic and analgesic properties, and is licensed for inflammatory and painful post-operative syndromes. It is also used in some chronic pain scenarios, and is administered daily for 3 days followed by a 4-day interval without the drug. Tolfenamic acid has significant antithromboxane activity, so caution should be exercised in the post-surgical period (McKellar et al., 1994).

VEDAPROFEN

Vedaprofen is recommended for pain and inflammation associated with musculoskeletal disorders. It is available as an oral formulation for dogs, and has similar pharmacokinetic and pharmacodynamic properties to ketoprofen. It was as efficacious as meloxicam in dogs with acute and chronic osteoarthritic pain with a similar incidence of adverse effects (Nell et al., 2002).

LOCAL ANESTHETICS

Local anesthetics (Chapter 6) are useful for acute surgical, procedural, or traumatic pain. Local anesthetics can be administered epidurally and perineurally (Figure 21.1) to target specific nerves (Duke, 2000; Egger & Love 2009a, 2009b, 2009c, 2009d) or infiltrated into wounds (Figure 21.2) or fractures directly or via fenestrated

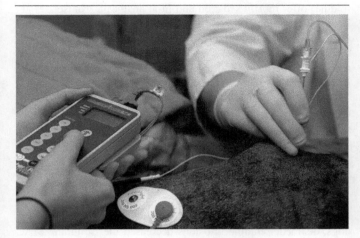

Figure 21.1. Use of a nerve locator to locate the sciatic nerve of a dog for blockade with a local anesthetic drug for pre-emptive, intra- and postoperative analgesia (Courtesy of Gregory Hirshoren, University of Tennessee CVM).

soaker catheters (Figure 21.3). Lidocaine can be administered as a constant rate intravenous infusion, and local anesthetic creams and gels can be applied topically.

Local anesthetics have a narrow therapeutic index. Doses should be based on lean body weight, and the total dose carefully calculated. Dogs with hepatic dysfunction should be given a reduced dose (approximately 50% less), as should pregnant bitches, neonates, and geriatric dogs. Intravenous administration of bupivacaine can be catastrophic, and aspirating prior to injecting the local anesthetic is imperative to prevent intravascular injection.

Lidocaine
Lidocaine can be administered into wounds and repeated at 2–3 hour intervals (2–4 mg/kg) or via fenestrated "soaker catheters".

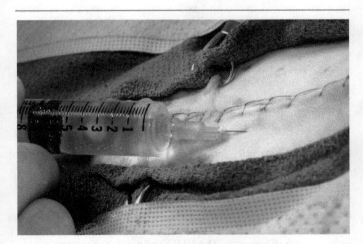

Figure 21.2. A local anesthetic incisional block can be administered before making the incision (providing pre-emptive analgesia), or prior to or after closure of the incision (Courtesy of Gregory Hirshoren, University of Tennessee CVM).

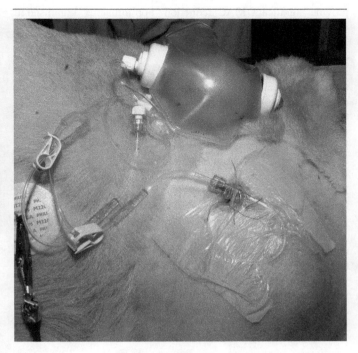

Figure 21.3. A soaker catheter can be placed in large wounds to provide continuous analgesia with local anesthetics (Courtesy of Gregory Hirshoren, University of Tennessee CVM).

Placement of these catheters is well covered elsewhere (Hansen, 2008; Egger & Love, 2009a). Boluses of local anesthetic can be administered via these catheters or CRI may be utilized; in the author's experience the latter has yielded less than optimal effects.

LIDOCAINE PATCHES
Lidocaine patches are efficacious for treating postherpetic neuralgia in humans, and have been investigated in dogs. There is some systemic absorption of lidocaine when these patches are applied, but plasma concentrations are less than those achieved via CRI. The role of lidocaine patches in acute pain management in dogs remains uncertain (Ko et al., 2007).

EMLA® CREAM
Eutectic mixture of local anesthetic (EMLA®) cream is a nonsterile mixture of lidocaine and prilocaine dosed in a similar way to the injectable formulations. A 2% gel contains 2 g/100 mL of local anesthetic, and it should be applied to the skin 45–60 minutes prior to IV catheter placement to provide anesthesia of the area. Sterile gels of lidocaine are also available, and these may facilitate urinary catheter placement.

SYSTEMIC CONSTANT RATE INFUSIONS (CRI) OF LIDOCAINE
Systemic lidocaine infusions have been used in dogs and provide anesthetic-sparing effects and analgesia with minimal cardiovascular effects; lidocaine CRIs are also used for their antiarrhythmic effects. After an LD (1–2 mg/kg) administered over 5–10 minutes, the CRI can be administered to achieve the desired effect. Doses of 1–3 mg/kg/h provide analgesia, but doses of 6–12 mg/kg/h also

provide significant MAC reduction. For infusions administered during anesthesia, it is recommended to reduce the CRI dose to 2–5 mg/kg/h after an hour to minimize the risk of toxic plasma concentrations.

Lidocaine may also be useful in managing head trauma patients, as it may reduce intracranial pressure (Dyson, 2008). Head trauma patients given opioids as analgesics may experience excessive sedation and respiratory depression, potentially resulting in increased risk of increased intracranial pressure and tentorial herniation. A lidocaine CRI can reduce the opioid dose required, thereby reducing complications associated with opioid use.

LIDOCAINE COMBINATION CRIs

Multi-drug infusions can be used in the perioperative period as part of a multimodal regimen to treat acute pain. Combinations of lidocaine (L) and morphine (M) and ketamine (K) have been investigated. One paper documenting effects of an MLK cocktail reported an isoflurane MAC reduction of 45% (Muir et al., 2003). Infusions of lidocaine and fentanyl are also frequently utilized and provide analgesia and MAC reduction. Separate infusions of these drugs will allow the clinician to tailor each infusion to each individual patient.

Bupivacaine

Bupivacaine has a longer onset of action (15–20 minutes) and a longer duration of action (4–6 hours) than lidocaine, and the dose should not exceed 2 mg/kg. Bupivacaine can be used perineurally or via soaker catheter with the total daily dose via this route not exceeding 12 mg/kg. Combining bupivacaine and lidocaine gives a faster onset but a shorter duration of action than bupivacaine alone. The total dose should not exceed 2 mg/kg (1 mg/kg of each local anesthetic). Bupivacaine should never be injected intravenously.

α-2 AGONISTS

Veterinarians commonly use α-2 agonists (Chapter 7) for sedative and analgesic effects, and those used in dogs include xylazine, dexmedetomidine, and medetomidine. Currently, the cardiovascular effects of α-2 agonists limit their widespread use in pain protocols, and they are usually used as adjuncts to the other classes of analgesics. These drugs should only be administered to clinically healthy dogs.

α-2 agonists exert their effect on α-2 receptors in the dorsal horn of the spinal cord, the brain stem, and in the periphery. α-2 agonists are reported to provide excellent visceral analgesia, and their duration of action is between 1 and 2 hours (Lemke, 2007). Data from the EMA EPAR supports the view that analgesia is not always optimal with medetomidine or dexmedetomidine, with one study rating analgesia scores as good or excellent in 50% of dogs receiving dexmedetomidine IV compared to 55% receiving medetomidine IV. The analgesia scores were good or excellent in 40% of dogs receiving IM dexmedetomidine compared with 65% of dogs receiving IM medetomidine. However, it is often difficult to assess analgesia and sedation separately because sedation affects the behavioral evaluation of analgesia, especially with supraspinally organized pain-related behaviors.

Recommended doses of α-2 agonists for analgesia vary, and, although some suggest that low doses (e.g., 1–2 mcg/kg/h medeto-

midine) offer mostly sedation and little analgesia (Kuusela et al., 2000), these microdose infusions may offer a more constant and titratable level of analgesia (Murrell & Hellebrekers, 2005; Valtolina et al., 2009). Studies in humans have shown that postoperative analgesic dose requirements are reduced after perioperative infusions of dexmedetomidine (Unlugenc et al., 2005).

Even at low infusion rates (1–3 mcg/kg/h), significant hemodynamic changes can occur with medetomidine infusions in dogs (Carter et al., 2010). In that study, cardiac output was reduced by 50–70% and this must be carefully considered when medetomidine and dexmedetomidine are used. The author typically uses an LD of 0.5 mcg/kg dexmedetomidine IV followed by a CRI of the drug (0.5–1 mcg/kg/h).

When using CRIs of α-2 agonists in anesthetized dogs one must be cognizant of the MAC-reducing properties of these drugs. In dogs, dexmedetomidine infusions decreased the isoflurane MAC by up to 59% at 3 mcg/kg/h (Pascoe et al., 2006), but lower doses (0.1 mcg/kg/h) did not have a significant effect on the MAC of isoflurane.

α-2 agonists demonstrate synergism with opioids, supporting their use as a part of a multimodal regimen (Ossipov et al., 1990). Their effects, including analgesia, can be completely reversed using atipamezole or yohimbine.

α-2 agonists can also be used in the recovery period in the face of dysphoria and anxiety (0.5–1 mcg/kg IV), and while perhaps offering little in the way of analgesia at these doses, can be very useful to sedate hemodynamically stable patients.

Locoregional Use of α-2 Agonists

Some studies have investigated the use of epidural medetomidine in dogs, and while it may offer an additive or synergistic effect when combined with opioids or local anesthetics its regional analgesic effects are relatively short-lived due to its lipophilicity and systemic absorption. Epidural dexmedetomidine reduces the MAC of isoflurane in dogs, and has a potent antinociceptive effect via this route (Campagnol et al., 2007).

Several studies in humans and dogs (Lamont & Lemke, 2008) have investigated the use of α-2 agonists perineurally or intra-articularly. These routes would seem sensible in the face of discovery of α-2 adrenoceptors on the terminals of primary afferent nociceptive fibers. There are many studies investigating the use of clonidine perineurally in humans (and also intrathecally, intravenously, and epidurally) but few studies looking at dexmedetomidine. It is likely that the mechanism by which they act spinally and supraspinally is different from the perineural mechanism (Brummett et al., 2010).

KETAMINE

In cases of acute pain, opioids are often the first choice with the addition of NSAIDs and local anesthetics as indicated. α-2 agonists may be included but their negative cardiovascular and sedative effects limit their use. Ketamine has recently gained popularity as an analgesic adjunct (Chapter 8). The NMDA glutamate receptor has long been recognized as contributing to central sensitization and hyperalgesia, and therapies directed at this receptor have been sought to minimize "wind up" and modify the plasticity of the nervous system (Chapter 2). In humans, ketamine is used primarily for neuropathic pain but also in acute post-operative and post-traumatic pain, with some limited evidence of a pre-emptive benefit (Galinski et al., 2007). In dogs, the use of low-dose ketamine in the perioperative period has become more popular, and the anesthetic-sparing properties of ketamine in dogs have been demonstrated (Pypendop et al., 2007; Wilson et al., 2008; Love et al., 2011). The analgesic effects of low-dose ketamine are more difficult to prove, and studies conducted in dogs did not demonstrate any reduction in post-operative opioid requirements, in contrast with studies in humans (Wagner et al., 2002; Bell et al., 2006; Sarrau et al., 2007). Rates of infusions of ketamine between 0.1 and 0.5 mg/kg/h following a 0.5 mg/kg LD may offer a useful analgesic adjunct in dogs (Lamont & Mathews, 2007).

PHYSICAL MODALITIES

Physical therapy techniques including passive range of motion, massage, ultrasound, low-level laser, and acupuncture can be useful adjuncts to pharmaceutical treatment of acute pain in dogs (Chapter 11 and Chapter 16).

NURSING STRATEGIES

There are a number of nonpharmacological techniques that can be used to relieve anxiety and consequently improve pain control. Physical and psychological factors have been shown to have an impact on how humans cope with pain, and it is appropriate to consider these in animals as well.

Consideration should be given to the ambient temperature of the room, the noise levels, and lighting. Nervous animals may fare better in a calmer environment rather than in a noisy ward of barking dogs. Conversely, some dogs may respond better in a busy area, benefitting from constant words of encouragement and occasional stroking by the team of nurses, technicians, and clinicians working there. Attention to nutrition is also of great importance during recuperation. Dogs need to be offered appropriate varieties of food and some may require hand feeding. The nares should be cleaned so that the animals can smell and detect the food. Increased coping ability, as a result of improved feeding and comfort is not well understood, but it would seem sensible to adopt the approach of "the animal will feel better when it eats" rather than "the animal will eat when it feels better".

An unfamiliar environment may cause the animal anxiety and stress. "White coat" syndrome is well recognized in humans, resulting in increased blood pressure readings in patients visiting the hospital, and may be present in a significant number of our patients. Therefore, sedation and tranquilization can also benefit the animal in some cases.

When a dog is presented in acute pain it is usually accompanied by owners that may be experiencing an emotional crisis because of the suffering of their pet and their helplessness in being unable to alleviate the perceived pain. Consideration needs to be given to the owner–animal bond and support of the owner and their family.

SUMMARY

The treatment of acute pain in the dog is a daily challenge for most veterinarians. The ever-expanding range of drugs allows us to adopt a multimodal approach to acute pain treatment. Large prospective multicenter trials are necessary to provide the evidence that underpins our clinical decision-making to ensure we can prevent and treat acute pain in our canine patients.

REFERENCES

Abbo, L.A., Ko, J.C., Maxwell, L.K., et al. (2008) Pharmacokinetics of buprenorphine following intravenous and oral transmucosal administration in dogs. *Veterinary Therapeutics*, 9(2), 83–93.

Anagnostou, T.L., Kazakos, G.M., Savvas, I., Papazoglou, L.G., Rallis, T.S., & Raptopoulos, D. (2011) Remifentanil/isoflurane anesthesia in five dogs with liver disease undergoing liver biopsy. *Journal of the American Animal Hospital Association*, 47(6), 103–109.

Andaluz, A., Moll, X., Abellán, R., et al. (2009) Pharmacokinetics of buprenorphine after intravenous administration of clinical doses to dogs. *The Veterinary Journal*, 181(3), 299–304.

Andaluz, A., Moll, X., Ventura, R., Abellán, R., Fresno, L., & García, F. (2009) Plasma buprenorphine concentrations after the administration of a 70 mcg/h transdermal patch in dogs. Preliminary report. *Journal of Veterinary Pharmacology and Therapeutics*, 32(5), 503–505.

Aragon, C.L., Hofmeister, E.H., & Budsberg, S.C. (2007) Systematic review of clinical trials of treatments for osteoarthritis in dogs. *Journal of American Veterinary Medical Association*, 230(4), 514–521.

Barnhart, M.D., Hubbell, J.A., Muir, W.W., Sams, R.A., & Bednarski, R.M. (2000) Pharmacokinetics, pharmacodynamics, and analgesic effects of morphine after rectal, intramuscular, and intravenous administration in dogs. *American Journal of Veterinary Research*, 61, 24–28.

Bell, R.F., Dahl, J.B., Moore, R.A., et al. (2006) Perioperative ketamine for acute postoperative pain. *Cochrane Database Systemic review*, 1, CD004603.

Bellei, E., Roncada, P., Pisoni, L., Joechler, M., & Zaghini, A. (2011) The use of fentanyl patches in dogs undergoing spinal surgery: plasma concentrations and analgesic efficacy. *Journal of Veterinary Pharmacology and Therapeutics*, 34, 437–441.

Borer, L.R., Peel, J.E., Seewald, W., Schawalder, P., & Spreng, D.E. (2003) Effect of carprofen, etodolac, meloxicam, or butorphanol in dogs with induced acute synovitis. *American Journal of Veterinary Research*, 64(11), 1429–1437.

Brose, W.G., Tanelian, D.L., Brodsky, J.B., Mark, J.B., & Cousins, M.J. (1991) CSF and blood pharmacokinetics of hydromorphone and morphine following lumbar epidural administration. *Pain*, 45, 11–15.

Brummett, C.M., Amodeo, F.S., Janda, A.M., Padda, A.K., & Lydic, R. (2010) Perineural dexmedetomidine provides an increased duration of analgesia to a thermal stimulus when compared with a systemic control in a rat sciatic nerve block. *Regional Anesthesia and Pain Medicine*, 35(5), 427–431.

Budsberg, S.C., Johnston, S.A., Schwarz, P.D., DeCamp, C.E., & Claxton, R. (1999) Efficacy of etodolac for the treatment of osteoarthritis of the hip joints in dogs. *Journal of American Veterinary Medical Association*, 214, 206–210.

Campagnol, D., Teixeira-Neto, F.J., Giordano, T., Ferreira, T.H., & Monteiro, E.R. (2007) Effects of epidural administration of dexmedetomidine on the minimum alveolar concentration of isoflurane in dogs. *American Journal of Veterinary Research*, 68(12), 1308–1318.

Campagnol, D., Teixeira-Neto, F.J., & Peccinini, R.G. (2012) Comparison of the effects of epidural or intravenous methadone on the minimum alveolar concentration of isoflurane in dogs. *Veterinary Journal*, 192(3), 311–315.

Carter, J.E., Cambell, N.B., Posner, L.P., & Swanson, C. (2010) The hemodynamic effects of medetomidine continuous rate infusion in the dog. *Veterinary Anaesthesia and Analgesia*, 37(3), 197–206.

Catbagan, D.L., Quimby, J.M., Mama, K.R., et al. (2011) Comparison of the efficacy and adverse effects of sustained-release buprenorphine hydrochloride following subcutaneous administration and buprenorphine hydrochloride following oral transmucosal administration in cats undergoing ovariohysterectomy. *American Journal of Veterinary Research*, 272(4), 461–466.

Caulkett, N., Read, M., Fowler, D., & Waldner, C. (2003) A comparison of the analgesic effects of butorphanol with those of meloxicam after elective ovariohysterectomy in dogs. *Canadian Veterinary Journal*, 44(7), 565–570.

Codd, E., Shank, R.P., Schupsky, J.J., & Raffa, R.B. (1995) Serotonin and norepinephrine uptake inhibiting activity of centrally acting analgesics: Structural determinants and role in antinociception. *The Journal of Pharmacology and Experimental Therapeutics*, 274(3), 1263–1270.

Cox, S.R., Liao, S., Payne-Johnson, M., Zielinski, R.J., & Stegemann, M.R. (2011) Population pharmacokinetics of mavacoxib in osteoarthritic dogs. *Journal of Veterinary Pharmacology and Therapeutics*, 34(1), 1–11.

Davis, A.M. & Inturrisi, C.E. (1999) d-Methadone blocks morphine tolerance and N-Methyl-D-Aspartate-induced hyperalgesia. *The Journal of Pharmacology and Experimental Therapeutics*, 289(2), 1048–1053.

Day, T.K., Pepper, W.T., Tobias, T.A., Flynn, M.F., & Clarke, K.M. (1995) Comparison of intra-articular and epidural morphine for analgesia following stifle arthrotomy in dogs. *Veterinary Surgery*, 24(6), 522–530.

Dohoo, S., Tasker, R.A., & Donald, A. (1994) Pharmacokinetics of parenteral and oral sustained-release morphine sulphate in dogs. *Journal of Veterinary Pharmacology and Therapeutics*, 17, 426–433.

Duke, T. (2000) Local and regional anesthetic and analgesic techniques in the dog and cat: Part I, Pharmacology of local anesthetics and topical anesthesia. *The Canadian Veterinary Journal*, 41(11), 883–884.

Dyson, D.H. (2008) Analgesia and chemical restraint for the emergent veterinary patient. *Veterinary Clinics of North America Food Small Animal Practice*, 38, 1329–1352.

Egger, C.M., Duke, T., Archer, J., et al. (1998) Comparison of plasma fentanyl concentrations by using three transdermal fentanyl patch sizes in dogs. *Veterinary Surgery*, 21, 159–166.

Egger, C.M., Glerum, L., Haag, K.M., et al. (2007) Efficacy and cost-effectiveness of transdermal fentanyl patches for the relief of postoperative pain in dogs after anterior cruciate ligament and pelvic limb repair. *Veterinary Anaesthesia and Analgesia*, 34(3), 200–208.

Egger, C. & Love, L. (2009a) Local and regional anesthesia techniques, Part 1: Overview and five simple techniques. *Veterinary Medicine*, Advanstar Communications. http://veterinarymedicine.dvm360.com/vetmed/Anesthesia/Local-and-regional-anesthesia-techniques/ArticleStandard/Article/detail/575560

Egger, C. & Love, L. (2009b) Local and regional anesthesia techniques, Part 2: Stifle, intercostal, intrapleural, and forelimb techniques. *Veterinary Medicine*, Advanstar Communications. http://veterinary medicine.dvm360.com/vetmed/Medicine/Local-and-regional-anesthesia-techniques-Part-2-St/ArticleStandard/Article/detail/585255.

Egger, C. & Love, L. (2009c) Local and regional anesthesia techniques, Part 3: Blocking the maxillary and mandibular nerves. *Veterinary Medicine*, Advanstar Communications. http://veterinarymedicine.dvm360.com/vetmed/Medicine/Local-and-regional-anesthesia-techniques-Part-3-Bl/ArticleStandard/Article/detail/601619.

Egger, C. & Love, L. (2009d) Local and regional anesthesia techniques, Part 4: Epidural anesthesia and analgesia. *Veterinary Medicine*, Advanstar Communications. http://veterinarymedicine.dvm360.com/vetmed/Medicine/Local-and-regional-anesthesia-techniques-Part-4-Ep/ArticleStandard/Article/detail/632170.

EMA EPAR (2011a) Cimalgex. European Public Assessment Report. London, UK.

EMA EPAR (2011b) Recuvyra. European Public Assessment Report. London, UK.

Evans, H.C. & Easthope, S.E. (2003) Transdermal buprenorphine. *Drugs*, 63, 1999–2010.

Foley, P.L., Liang, H., & Crichlow, A.R. (2011) Evaluation of a sustained-release formulation of buprenorphine for analgesia in rats. *Journal of the American Association of Laboratory Animal Science*, 50(2), 198–204.

Galinski, M., Dolveck, F., Combes, X., et al. (2007) Management of severe acute pain in emergency settings; ketamine reduces morphine consumption. *American Journal of Emergency Medicine*, 25, 385–390.

Garcia-Hernandez, L., Deciga-Campos, M. Guervara-Lopez, U., López-Muñoz, F.J. (2007) Co-administration of rofecoxib and tramadol results in additive or sub-additive interaction during arthritic nociception in rat. *Pharmacology Biochemistry and Behaviour*, 87, 331–340.

Gaynor, J.S. (2008) Control of cancer pain in veterinary patients. *Veterinary Clinics of North America Small Animal Practice*, 38, 1429–1448.

Gilmour, M.A. & Lehenbauer, T.W. (2009) Comparison of tepoxalin, carprofen, and meloxicam for reducing intraocular inflammation in dogs. *American Journal of Veterinary Research*, 70(7), 902–907.

Goodman, L., Torres, B., Punke, J., et al. (2009) Effects of firocoxib and tepoxalin on healing in a canine gastric mucosal injury model. *Journal of Veterinary Internal Medicine*, 23, 56–62.

Gorman, A.L., Elliott, K.J., & Inturrisi, C.E. (1997) The d- and l-isomers of methadone bind to the non-competitive site on the N-methyl-D-aspartate (NMDA) receptor in rat forebrain and spinal cord. *Neuroscience Letters*, 223, 5–8.

Griessinger, N., Sittl, R., & Likar, R. (2005) Transdermal buprenorphine in clinical practice – a post-marketing surveillance study in 13,179 patients. *Current Medical Research and Opinion*, 21, 1147–1156.

Grint, N.J., Burford, J., & Dugdale, A.H. (2009) Does pethidine affect the cardiovascular and sedative effects of dexmedetomidine in dogs? *The Journal of Small Animal Practice*, 50(2), 62–66.

Grisneaux, E., Pibarot, P., Dupuis, J., & Blais, D. (1999) Comparison of ketoprofen and carprofen administered prior to orthopedic surgery for control of postoperative pain in dogs. *Journal of the American Veterinary Medical Association*, 15, 215(8), 1105–1110.

Gruet, P., Seewald, W., & King, J.N. (2011) Evaluation of subcutaneous and oral administration of robenacoxib and meloxicam for the treatment of acute pain and inflammation associated with orthopedic surgery in dogs. *American Journal of Veterinary Research*, 72(2), 184–193.

Guedes, A.G., Papich, M.G., Rude, E.P., & Rider, M.A. (2008) Pharmacokinetics and physiological effects of intravenous hydromorphone in conscious dogs. *Journal of Veterinary Pharmacology and Therapeutics*, 31(4), 334–343.

Hansen, B. (2008) Analgesia for the critically ill dog or cat: An update. *Veterinary Clinics of North America Small Animal Practice*, 38, 1353–1363.

Hanson, P.D., Brooks, K.C., Case, J. et al. (2006) Efficacy and safety of firocoxib in the management of canine osteoarthritis under field conditions. *Veterinary Therapeutics*, 7, 127–140.

Hickford, F.H., Barr, S.C., & Erb, H.N. (2001) Effect of carprofen on hemostatic variables in dogs. *American Journal of Veterinary Research*, 62(10), 1642–1646.

Hoeijmakers, M., Coert, A., Helden, H., & Horspool, L.J. (2005) The pharmacokinetics of vedaprofen and its enantiomers in dogs after single and multiple dosing. *Journal of Veterinary Pharmacology and Therapeutics*, 28(3), 305–312.

Hofmeister, E.H. & Egger, C.M. (2004) Transdermal fentanyl patches in small animals. *Journal of the American Animal Hospital Association*, 40(6), 468–478.

Hoke, J.F., Cunningham, F., James, M.K., Muir, K.T., & Hoffman, W.E. (1997) Comparative pharmacokinetics and pharmacodynamics of remifentanil, its principle metabolite (GR90291) and alfentanil in dogs. *Journal of Pharmacology and Experimental Therapeutics*, 281, 226–232.

Ingvast-Larsson, C., Holgersson, A., Bondesson, U., Lagerstedt, A.S., Olsson, K. (2010) Clinical pharmacology of methadone in dogs. *Veterinary Anaesthesia and Analgesia*, 37(1), 48–56.

Kis, B., Snipes, J.A., & Busija, D.W. (2005) Acetaminophen and the cyclooxygenase-3 puzzle: sorting out the facts, fiction, and uncertainties. *Journal of Pharmacology and Experimental Therapeutics*, 315(1), 1–7.

Klauss, G., Giuliano, E.A., Moore, C.P., et al. (2007) Keratoconjunctivitis sicca associated with administration of etodolac in dogs: 211 cases (1992–2002). *Journal of the American Veterinary Medical Association*, 230(4), 541–547.

Ko, J., Weil, A., Maxwell, L., Kitao, T., & Haydon, T. (2007) Plasma concentrations of lidocaine in dogs following lidocaine patch application. *Journal of the American Animal Hospital Association*, 43(5), 280–283.

Ko, J.C., Freeman, L.J., Barletta, M., et al. (2011) Efficacy of oral transmucosal and intravenous administration of buprenorphine before surgery for postoperative analgesia in dogs undergoing ovariohysterectomy. *Journal of the American Veterinary Medical Association*, 238(3), 318–328.

Kondo, Y., Takashima, K., Matsumoto, S., et al. (2012) Efficacy and safety of firocoxib for the treatment of pain associated with soft tissue surgery in dogs under field conditions in Japan. *Journal of Veterinary Medical Science*, 74(10), 1283–1289.

Krotscheck, U., Boothe, D.M., & Little, A.A. (2008) Pharmacokinetics of buprenorphine following intravenous administration in dogs. *American Journal of Veterinary Research*, 69(6), 722–727.

KuKanich, B. (2010) Pharmacokinetics of acetaminophen, codeine, and the codeine metabolites morphine and codeine-6-glucuronide in healthy Greyhound dogs. *Journal of Veterinary Pharmacology and Therapeutics*, 33(1), 15–21.

KuKanich, B., Bidgood, T., & Knesl, O. (2012) Clinical pharmacology of nonsteroidal anti-inflammatory drugs in dogs. *Veterinary Anaesthesia and Analgesia*, 39, 69–90.

KuKanich, B. & Borum, S.L. (2008) The disposition and behavioural effects of methadone in Greyhounds. *Veterinary Anaesthesia and Analgesia*, 35, 242–248.

KuKanich, B., & Clark, T.P. (2012) The history and pharmacology of fentanyl: relevance to a novel, long-acting transdermal fentanyl solution newly approved for use in dogs. *Journal of Veterinary Pharmacology and Therapeutics*, 35(suppl 2), 3–19.

KuKanich, B., Hogan, B.K., Krugner-Higby, L.A., & Smith, L.J. (2008) Pharmacokinetics of hydromorphone hydrochloride in healthy dogs. *Veterinary Anaesthesia and Analgesia*, 35, 256–264.

KuKanich, B., Lascelles, B.D., Aman, A.M., Mealey, K.L., & Papich, M.G. (2005) The effects of inhibiting cytochrome P450 3A, p-glycoprotein, and gastric acid secretion on the oral bioavailability of methadone in dogs. *Journal of Veterinary Pharmacology and Therapeutics*, 28, 461–466.

KuKanich, B., Lascelles, B.D., & Papich, M.G. (2005) Pharmacokinetics of morphine and plasma concentrations of morphine-6-glucuronide following morphine administration to dogs. *Journal of Veterinary Pharmacology and Therapeutics*, 28(4), 371–376.

KuKanich, B. & Papich, M.G. (2004) Pharmacokinetics of tramadol and the metabolite O-desmethyltramadol in dogs. *Journal of Veterinary Pharmacology and Therapeutics*, 27, 239–246.

Kuusela, E., Raekallio, M., Antilla, M., Falck, I., Mölsä, S., & Vainio, O. (2000) Clinical effects and pharmacokinetics of medetomidine and its enantiomers in dogs. *Journal of Veterinary Pharmacology and Therapeutics*, 23, 15–20.

Kyles, A.E., Papich, M., & Hardie, E.M. (1996) Disposition of transdermally administered fentanyl in dogs. *American Journal of Veterinary Research*, 57, 715–719.

Lamont, L.A. & Lemke, K.A. (2008) The effects of medetomidine on radial nerve blockade with mepivacaine in dogs. *Veterinary Anaesthesia and Analgesia*, 35(1), 62–68.

Lascelles, B.D., Cripps, P., Jones, A., & Waterman, A.E. (1997) Postoperative central hypersensitivity and pain: the pre-emptive value of pethidine for ovariohysterectomy. *Pain*, 73(3), 461–471.

Lascelles, B.D., Cripps, P.J., & Jones, A., (1998) Efficacy and kinetics of carprofen, administered preoperatively or postoperatively, for the prevention of pain in dogs undergoing ovariohysterectomy. *Veterinary Surgery*, 27, 568–582.

Lamont, L.A. & Mathews, K.A. (2007) Opioids, nonsteroidal anti-inflammatories and analgesic adjuncts, in *Lumb and Jones' Veterinary Anesthesia*, 4th edn (eds W.J. Tranquilli, J.C. Thurmon, & K.A. Grimm), Williams and Wilkins, Baltimore, MD, pp. 241–271.

Lascelles, B.D., McFarland, J.M., & Swann, H. (2005) Guidelines for safe and effective use of NSAIDs in dogs. *Veterinary Therapeutics*, 6, 237–251.

Leece, E.A., Brearley, J.C., & Harding, E.F. (2005) Comparison of carprofen and meloxicam for 72 hours following ovariohysterectomy in dogs. *Veterinary Anaesthesia and Analgesia*, 32(4), 184–192.

Lees, P., Cheng, Z., Keefe, T.J., et al. (2013) Bioequivalence in dogs of a meloxicam formulation administered as a transmucosal oral mist with an orally administered pioneer suspension product. *Journal of Veterinary Pharmacology and Therapeutics*, 36(1), 78–84.

Lees, P., Landoni, M.F., Giraudel, J., & Toutain, P.L. (2004) Pharmacodynamics and pharmacokinetics of nonsteroidal anti-inflammatory drugs in species of veterinary interest. *Journal of Veterinary Pharmacology and Therapeutics*, 27, 479–490.

Leibetseder, E.N., Mosing, M., & Jones, R.S. (2006) A comparison of extradural and intravenous methadone on intraoperative isoflurane and postoperative analgesia requirements in dogs. *Veterinary Anaesthesia and Analgesia*, 33, 128–136.

Lemke, K.A. (2007) Anticholinergics and sedatives, in *Lumb and Jones' Veterinary Anesthesia*, 4th edn (eds W.J. Tranquilli, J.C. Thurmon, & K.A. Grimm), Williams and Wilkins, Baltimore, MD, pp. 203–239.

Lemke, K.A., Runyon, C.L., & Horney, B.S. (2002) Effects of preoperative administration of ketoprofen on whole blood platelet aggregation, buccal mucosal bleeding time, and hematologic indices in dogs undergoing elective ovariohysterectomy. *Journal of the American Veterinary Medical Association*, 220(12), 1818–1822.

Linton, D.D., Wilson, M.G., Newbound, G.C., Freise, K.J., & Clark, T.P. (2012) The effectiveness of a long-acting transdermal fentanyl solution compared to buprenorphine for the control of postoperative pain in dogs in a randomized, multicentered clinical study. *Journal of Veterinary Pharmacology and Therapeutics*, 35(S2), 53–64.

Love, L., Egger, C., Rohrbach, B., Cox, S., Hobbs, M., & Doherty, T. (2011) The effect of ketamine on the MACBAR of sevoflurane in dogs. *Veterinary Anaesthesia and Analgesia*, 38(4):292–300.

Lucas, A.N., Firth, A.M., Anderson, G.A., Vine, J.H., & Edwards, G.A. (2001) Comparison of the effects of morphine administered by constant-rate intravenous infusion or intermittent intramuscular injection in dogs. *Journal of American Veterinary Medical Association*, 218(6), 884–891.

Luna, S.P., Basílio, A.C., Steagall, P.V., et al. (2007) Evaluation of adverse effects of long-term oral administration of carprofen, etodolac, Flunixin meglumine, ketoprofen, and meloxicam in dogs. *American Journal of Veterinary Research*, 68(3), 258–264.

MacPhail, C.M., Lappin, M.R., Meyer, D.J., et al. (1998) Hepatocellular toxicosis associated with administration of carprofen in 21 dogs. *Journal of American Veterinary Medical Association*, 212(15), 1895–1901.

Martins, T.L., Kahvegian, M.A., Noel-Morgan, J., Leon-Román, M.A, Otsuki, D.A., & Fantoni, D.T. (2010) Comparison of the effects of tramadol, codeine, and ketoprofen alone or in combination on postoperative pain and on concentrations of blood glucose, serum cortisol, and serum interleukin-6 in dogs undergoing maxillectomy or mandibulectomy. *American Journal of Veterinary Research*, 71(9), 1019–1026.

Mastrocinque, S., Almeida, T.F., Tatarunas, A.C., et al. (2012) Comparison of epidural and systemic tramadol for analgesia following ovariohysterectomy. *Journal of the American Animal Hospital Association*, 48(5), 310–319.

Mastrocinque, S. & Fantoni, D.T. (2003) A comparison of preoperative tramadol and morphine for the control of early postoperative pain in canine ovariohysterectomy. *Veterinary Anaesthesia and Analgesia*, 30, 220–228.

Mathews, K.A., Paley, D.M., Foster, R.A., Valliant, A.E., & Young, S.S. (1996). A comparison of ketorolac with flunixin, butorphanol and oxymorphone in controlling postoperative pain in dogs. *Canadian Veterinary Journal*, 37, 557–567.

Mburu, D.N. (1991) Evaluation of the anti-inflammatory effects of a low dose of acetaminophen following surgery in dogs. *Journal of Veterinary Pharmacology and Therapeutics*, 14, 109–111.

McKellar, Q.A., Lees, P., & Gettingby, G. (1994) Pharmacodynamics of tolfenamic acid in dogs: Evaluation of dose response relationships. *European Journal of Pharmacology*, 253, 191–200.

McMillan, C.J., Livingston, A., Clark, C.R., et al. (2008) Pharmacokinetics of intravenous tramadol in dogs. *The Canadian Journal of Veterinary Research*, 72(4), 325–331.

Milne, R.W., Nation, R.L., Somogyi, A.A., Bochner, F., Griggs, W.M. (1992) The influence of renal function on the renal clearance of morphine and its glucuronide metabolites in intensive-care patients. *British Journal of Clinical Pharmacology*, 34, 53–59.

Moll, X., Fresno, L., García, F., Prandi, D., Andaluz, A. (2011) Comparison of subcutaneous and transdermal administration of buprenorphine for pre-emptive analgesia in dogs undergoing elective ovariohysterectomy. *The Veterinary Journal*, 187, 124–128.

Monteiro, E.R., Neto, F.J.T., Campagnol, D., Garofalo, N.A., & Alvaides, R.K. (2010) Hemodynamic effects in dogs anesthetized with isoflurane and remifentanil-isoflurane. *American Journal of Veterinary Research*, 71, 1133–1141.

Morton, D.J. & Knottenbelt, D.C. (1989) Pharmacokinetics of aspirin and its application in canine veterinary medicine. *Journal of South African Veterinary Association*, 60(4), 191–194.

Muir, W.W., Wiese, A.J., & March, P.A. (2003) Effects of morphine, lidocaine, ketamine, and morphine-lidocaine-ketamine drug combination on minimum alveolar concentration in dogs anesthetized with isoflurane. *American Journal of Veterinary Research*, 64(9), 1155–1160.

Murrell, J. (2011) Clinical use of methadone in dogs and cats. *UK Vet Companion Animal*, 16, 56–61.

Murrell, J.C. & Hellebrekers, L.J. (2005) Medetomidine and dexmedetomidine: a review of cardiovascular effects and antinociceptive properties in the dog. *Veterinary Anaesthesia and Analgesia*, 32, 117–127.

Nell, T., Bergman, J., Hoeijmakers, M., Van Laar, P., & Horspool, L.J. (2002) Comparison of vedaprofen and meloxicam in dogs with musculoskeletal pain and inflammation. *Journal of Small Animal Practice*, 43(5), 208–212.

Ossipov, M., Harris, S., Lloyd, P., Messineo, E., Lin, B.S., Bagley, J. (1990) Antinociceptive interaction between opioids and medetomidine: systemic additivity and spinal synergy. *Anaesthesiology*, 73, 1227–1235.

Papich, M.G. (2000) Pharmacologic considerations for opiate analgesic and nonsteroidal anti-inflammatory drugs. *Veterinary Clinics of North America Small Animal Practice*, 30, 815–837.

Papich, M.G. (2008) An update on nonsteroidal antiinflammatory drugs in small animals. *Veterinary Clinics of North America Small Animal Practice*, 38, 1243–1266.

Pascoe, P.J. (2000). Opioid analgesics. *Veterinary Clinics of North America Small Animal Practice*, 30, 757–772.

Pascoe, P.J., Raekallio, M., & Kuusela, E. (2006) Changes in the minimum alveolar concentration of isoflurane and some cardiopulmonary measurements during three continuous infusion rates of dexmedetomidine in dogs. *Veterinary Anaesthesia and Analgesia*, 33, 97–103.

Pekcan, Z. & Koc, B. (2010) The post-operative analgesic effects of epidurally administered morphine and transdermal fentanyl patch after ovariohysterectomy in dogs. *Veterinary Anaesthesia and Analgesia*, 37(6), 557–565.

Pieper, K., Schuster, T., Levionnois, O., Matis, U., Bergadano, A. (2011) Antinociceptive efficacy and plasma concentrations of transdermal buprenorphine in dogs. *The Veterinary Journal*, 187(3), 335–341.

Pollmeier, M., Toulemonde, C., Fleishman, C., & Hanson, P.D. (2006) Clinical evaluation of firocoxib and carprofen for the treatment of dogs with osteoarthritis. *The Veterinary Record*, 159, 547–551.

Pypendop, B.H., Solano, A., Boscan, P., & Ilkiw, J.E. (2007) Characteristics of the relationship between plasma ketamine concentration and its effect on the minimum alveolar concentration of isoflurane in dogs. *Veterinary Anaesthesia and Analgesia*, 34(3), 209–212.

Reimer, M.E., Johnston, S.A., Leib, M.S., et al. (1999) The gastroduodenal effects of buffered aspirin, carprofen, and etodolac in healthy dogs. *Journal of Veterinary Internal Medicine*, 13, 472–477.

Roberts, E.S., Van Lare, K.A., Marable, B.R., & Salminen, W.F. (2009) Safety and tolerability of 3-week and 6-month dosing of Deramaxx (deracoxib) chewable tablets in dogs. *Journal of Veterinary Pharmacology and Therapeutics*, 32, 329–337.

Robinson, E.P., Faggella, A.M., Henry, D.P., & Russell, W.L. (1988) Comparison of histamine release induced by morphine and oxymorphone administration in dogs. *American Journal of Veterinary Research*, 49, 1699–1701.

Ryan, W.G., Moldave, K., & Carithers, D. (2007) Switching NSAIDs in practice: insights from the Previcox (firocoxib) Experience Trial. *Veterinary Therapeutics*, 8(4), 263–271.

Sammarco, J.L., Conzemius, M.G., Perkowski, S.Z., et al. (1996) Postoperative analgesia for stifle surgery: a comparison of intra-articular bupivacaine, morphine, or saline. *Veterinary Surgery*, 25(1), 59–69.

Sanderson, R.O., Beata, C., Flipo, R.M., et al. (2009) Systematic review of the management of canine osteoarthritis. *The Veterinary Record*, 164(14), 418–424.

Sano, T., Nishimura, R., Kanazawa, H., et al. (2006) Pharmacokinetics of fentanyl after single intravenous injection and constant rate infusion in dogs. *Veterinary Anaesthesia and Analgesia*, 33, 266–273.

Sarrau, S., Jourdan, J., Dupuis-Soyris, F., & Verwaerde, P. (2007) Effects of postoperative ketamine infusion on pain control and feeding behaviour in bitches undergoing mastectomy. *Journal of Small Animal Practice*, 48(12), 670–676.

Sawyer, D.C., Rech, R.H., Durham, R.A., Adams, T., Richter, M.A., & Striler, E.L. (1991) Dose response to butorphanol administered subcutaneously to increase visceral nociceptive threshold in dogs. *American Journal of Veterinary Research*, 52, 1826–1830.

Schmid, V.B., Seewald, W., Lees, P., & King, J.N. (2010) In vitro and ex vivo inhibition of COX isoforms by robenacoxib in the cat: a comparative study. *Journal of Veterinary Pharmacology and Therapeutics*, 33(5), 444–452.

Schmid, V.B., Spreng, D.E., Seewald, W., Jung, M., Lees, P., & King, J.N. (2010) Analgesic and anti-inflammatory actions of robenacoxib in acute joint inflammation in dog. *Journal of Veterinary Pharmacology and Therapeutics*, 33(2), 118–131.

Shih, A.C., Robertson, S., Isaza, N., Pablo, L., & Davies, W. (2008) Comparison between analgesic effects of buprenorphine, carprofen, and buprenorphine with carprofen for canine ovariohysterectomy. *Veterinary Anaesthesia and Analgesia*, 35(1), 69–79.

Slingsby, L.S., Taylor, P.M., & Murrell, J.C. (2011) A study to evaluate buprenorphine at 40 mcg/kg compared to 20 mcg/kg as a postoperative analgesic in the dog. *Veterinary Anaesthesia and Analgesia*, 38(6), 584–593.

Slingsby, L.S., Taylor, P.M., & Waterman-Pearson, A.E. (2006) Effects of two doses of buprenorphine four or six hours apart on nociceptive thresholds, pain and sedation in dogs after castration. *The Veterinary Record*, 159(21), 705–711.

Smith, H.S. (2009) Opioid metabolism. *Mayo Clinic Proceedings*, 84(7), 613–624.

Smith, L.J., KuKanich, B., Hogan, B.K., Brown, C., Heath, T.D., & Krugner-Higby, L.A. (2008) Pharmacokinetics of a controlled-release liposome-encapsulated hydromorphone administered to healthy dogs. *Journal of Veterinary Pharmacology and Therapeutics*, 31(5), 415–422.

Smith, L.J., Yu, J.K., Bjorling, D.E., et al. (2001) Effects of hydromorphone or oxymorphone, with or without acepromazine, on preanesthetic sedation, physiologic values, and histamine release in dogs. *Journal of the American Veterinary Medical Association*, 218(7), 1101–1105.

Steagall, P.V., Teixeira-Neto, F.J., Minto, B.W., Campagnol, D.,& Corrêa, M.A. (2006) Evaluation of the isoflurane-sparing effects of lidocaine and fentanyl during surgery in dogs. *Journal of the American Veterinary Medical Association*, 229(4), 522–527.

Stiles, J., Honda, C.N., Krohne, S.G., Kazacos, E.A. (2003) Effect of topical administration of 1% morphine sulfate solution on signs of pain and corneal wound healing in dogs. *American Journal of Veterinary Research*, 64(7), 813–818.

Teresinha, L., Martins, M.A.P., Noel-Morgan, J., et al. (2010) Comparison of the effects of tramadol, codeine, and ketoprofen alone or in combination on postoperative pain and on concentrations of blood glucose, serum cortisol, and serum interleukin-6 in dogs undergoing maxillectomy or mandibulectomy. *American Journal of Veterinary Research*, 71(9), 1019–1026.

Tørring, M.L., Riis, A., Christensen, S., et al (2008) Perforated peptic ulcer and short-term mortality among tramadol users. *British Journal of Clinical Pharmacology*, 65, 565–572.

Torske, E.K., Dyson, D.H., & Conlon, P.D. (1999). Cardiovascular effects of epidurally administered oxymorphone and an oxymorphone-bupivacaine combination in halothane-anesthetized dogs. *American Journal of Veterinary Research*, 60(2), 194–200.

Unlugenc, H., Gunduz, M., Guler, T., Yagmur, O., & Isik, G. (2005) The effect of pre-anaesthetic administration of intravenous dexmedetomidine on postoperative pain in patients receiving patient-controlled morphine. *European Journal of Anesthesiology*, 22(5), 386–391.

Valtolina, C., Robben, J.H., Uilenreef, J., et al. (2009) Clinical evaluation of the efficacy and safety of a constant rate infusion of dexmedetomidine for postoperative pain management in dogs. *Veterinary Anaesthesia and Analgesia*, 36(4), 369–383.

Valverde, A. (2008) Epidural analgesia and anesthesia in dogs and cats. *Veterinary Clinics of North America Small Animal Practice*, 38, 1205–1230.

Vesal, N., Cribb, P.H., & Frketic, M. (1996) Postoperative and cardiopulmonary effects in dogs of oxymorphone administered epidurally and intramuscularly, and medetomidine administered epidurally: a comparative clinical study. *Veterinary Surgery*, 25, 361–369.

Vettarato, E. & Bacco, S. (2011) A comparison of the sedative and analgesic properties of pethidine (meperidine) and butorphanol in dogs. *The Journal of Small Animal Practice*, 52(8), 426–432.

Wagner, A. (2009) Opioids, in *Handbook of Veterinary Pain Management*, 2nd edn. (eds J.S. Gaynor & W.W. Muir), Mosby Elsevier, St Louis, MO, pp. 163–182.

Wagner, A.E., Walton, J.A., Hellyer, P.W., Gaynor, J.S., & Mama, K.R. (2002) Use of low dose ketamine administered by constant rate infusion as an adjunct for postoperative analgesia in dogs. *Journal of the American Veterinary Medical Association*, 221, 72–75.

Wilson, J., Doherty, T.J., Egger, C.M., Fidler, A., Cox, S., & Rohrbach, B. (2008) Effects of intravenous lidocaine, ketamine, and the combination on the minimum alveolar concentration of sevoflurane in dogs. *Veterinary Anaesthesia and Analgesia*, 35(4), 289–296.

Wolfe, M.M., Lichtenstein, D.R., & Singh, G. (1999) Gastrointestinal toxicity of nonsteroidal antiinflammatory drugs. *New England Journal of Medicine*, 340, 1888–1899.

Yassen, A., Olofsen, E, Kan, J., Dahan, A., & Danhof, M. (2008) Pharmacokinetic-pharmacokynamic modelling of the effectiveness and safety of buprenorphine and fentanyl in rats. *Pharmaceutical Research*, 25(1), 183–193.

22
Recognition and Assessment of Chronic Pain in Dogs

Anna Hielm-Björkman

Since the first guidelines for recognition of animal pain were published (Morton & Griffiths, 1985; Sanford et al., 1986), the general understanding that the animal experience of pain is similar to that of humans has grown (ACVA, 1998; Lascelles & Main, 2002; Robertson, 2002; Rutherford, 2002). However, veterinarians and pet owners continue to use analgesics quite sparingly (Lascelles et al., 2000; Raekallio et al., 2003; Hugonnard et al., 2004; Murrell & Johnson, 2006). This may be due to lack of recognition of pain, concerns about adverse effects and human abuse potential, and concerns about drug dependency and withdrawal. An understanding of how to recognize and assess chronic pain in dogs, the pathophysiology of chronic pain, and the pharmacology of analgesic drugs will greatly improve pain management in dogs with chronic pain.

RECOGNIZING CHRONIC PAIN IN DOGS

In human medicine, it has been suggested that pain be the fifth vital sign and should be assessed at every visit along with temperature, pulse, respiration, and blood pressure (Phillips, 2000). This should also be true in veterinary medicine, and it requires asking owners very specific questions, and training them to recognize the signs of chronic pain in their animals. Recognizing chronic pain in canine patients can be challenging. For example, a stoic dog in an unsecure environment may not demonstrate overt signs of pain. Behavioral changes that happen slowly are difficult for owners to detect and very often, the owner interprets signs of chronic pain as normal old age changes.

There is a need for scoring systems that can be used clinically and in studies investigating chronic pain (Schulz et al., 2006; Cook, 2007; Kapatkin, 2007). Pain indices and scoring systems should be validated and tested for reliability. Reliability refers to the extent to which the measure yields the same score each time it is administered, all other things being equal, or that the score will change because of an intervention. Validity is the ability to measure what is supposed to be measured; thus, a chronic pain instrument would measure chronic pain. Validity has four components. Face validity is the extent to which the scale or index is subjectively viewed by knowledgeable individuals as measuring what it is reported to measure. Content validity is related to whether the scale or the index is sufficiently comprehensive to cover all of the generally accepted variables of, for example, chronic pain, that is, does it ask about mood, posture, and movement? Criterion validity is used when describing the correlation between a scale and another already validated external measurement of the same phenomenon. This correlation can be measured using statistical correlation methods. Finally, construct validity is the ability of the scale or the index to measure other phenomena related to the phenomenon that the scale purports to measure. For a chronic pain index, this might be that the scale can be used to evaluate lameness.

Some reliable and validated chronic pain assessment tools have emerged to aid in the assessment of pain in dogs and the response to treatment. The need for even more outcome assessment tools likely reflects the fact that there is more than one type of "chronic pain" in dogs, and it is unlikely that a single assessment tool will suffice. Chronic cancer pain, chronic osteoarthritis (OA) pain, chronic neuropathic pain, chronic trigger point pain, chronic dental pain, and chronic visceral pain may require different pain assessment tools.

Canine Pain Behavior
Wiseman et al. (2001) were the first to report a preliminary study of unstructured interviews with 13 owners of dogs with chronic pain. All owners reported some changes in their dogs' behavior, and most reported some change in demeanor. Six veterinarians were also questioned about how they assessed chronic pain and they reported clinical signs similar to those reported by owners.

Canine pain behavior can be divided into different types. The first type consists of genetically determined pain responses common to all dogs and most mammals, is usually associated with acute pain, and includes avoidance responses, physiological responses (pupillary dilation, increased heart and respiratory rate), and vocalization (Morton & Griffiths, 1985; Sanford et al., 1986; ACVA, 1998). There are, however, marked differences in pain behavior among and within species (Sanford, 1992; Dobromylskyj et al., 2000). Genetic manipulation of dogs has resulted in a variety of dog breeds with very different appearances and behavioral characteristics. Some breeds have a reputation for being stoic while others are less so (Dobromylskyj et al., 2000). To complicate matters further, distinct individual differences exist (Dobromylskyj et al., 2000).

Pain Management in Veterinary Practice, First Edition. Edited by Christine M. Egger, Lydia Love and Tom Doherty.
© 2014 John Wiley & Sons, Inc. Published 2014 by John Wiley & Sons, Inc.

The second type of pain behavior is that which is socially acquired. Just as humans learn some of their pain behavior from their parents at a very early age (Sargent & Liebman, 1985), dogs may learn their pain behavior from their dog pack or even from their owners (Dobromylskyj et al., 2000); some owners encourage their dogs to show pain while others do not.

Dogs can override genetically determined autonomic responses and muscle reactions (Wall, 1992), and appear more or less painful depending on the situation. All dogs can become "very lame" if they learn that they will gain more attention and perhaps treats from the family. On the other hand, a dog excited about a race, a hunt, or a trip to the veterinary office may be unlikely to show overt signs of pain (Dobromylskyj et al., 2000; Flecknell, 2000). Wall (1992) also points out the necessity of understanding a particular animal's relationship with its environment during assessment. The presence or absence of the owner, novel smells, and the sounds of other animals may influence how or if an animal shows signs of pain (Dobromylskyj et al., 2000). Because of this, the owner's observations should always be considered in the pain assessment (ACVA, 1998; Hardie, 2000; Wiseman et al., 2001). When asked specific questions, the owner is most likely to detect subtle changes in the dog's mood and behavior in its usual environment. However, one recent study clearly showed that although owners can score movement, demeanor, and behavior, they do not realize that these variables are indicators of pain (Hielm-Bjorkman et al., 2011). Thus, the use of a validated questionnaire containing specific questions about movement and behavior is critical in helping the veterinarian to determine if a dog is in pain, but the owner should be trained to recognize behaviors characteristic of a dog in pain (Hielm-Bjorkman et al., 2011). Typical behaviors and signs of chronic pain in dogs are listed in Table 22.1. It is important to note that many of these may also be typical behaviors of a normal dog, a dog with acute pain, or a dog with some other disease. A dog with chronic pain may show none, few, or many of these signs.

PAIN ASSESSMENT SCALES

A number of observational scales are used to assess chronic pain in dogs including: a visual analog scale (VAS), a numerical/numeric rating scale (NRS), a simple descriptive scale (SDS), a Likert scale, a comparative scale, or a combination of these.

Observational Scales

The observational pain VAS is a 10 cm (100 mm) line with the left endpoint (0) signifying "no pain" and the right endpoint (10 or 100) signifying the "worst possible pain." The observer places a mark on the line corresponding to the patient's perceived pain intensity. The VAS pain score is the distance, to the nearest millimeter, between the mark and the left end of the scale (Revill et al., 1976; Varni et al., 1987). In a human study, the VAS for constant or chronic pain was reproducible, had good correlation between repeated ratings of a recalled pain distant in time, and changes in ratings were likely to be real changes of opinion (Revill et al., 1976). The VAS method has been used by veterinarians and researchers to rate acute, postoperative, and chronic pain, and it can also be used to rate pain-related activities such as lameness (Conzemius et al., 1997; Innes & Barr, 1998; Holton et al., 1998; Hudson et al., 2004; Hielm-Bjorkman et al., 2011). It is reported that the canine observational pain VAS had no face validity, meaning that owners could not use

Table 22.1.   Signs of chronic pain in dogs

Positive behaviors reduced with chronic pain
Decreased socialization/play with human family
Decreased socialization/play with other dogs
Decreased movement (quality and quantity)
Decreased interest in hygiene/grooming
Decreased tail wagging
Hypo- or anorexic
Decreased curiosity

Negative behaviors more frequent with chronic pain
Aggression toward humans and/or toward other dogs
More dependent on owner, jealous, "clingy"
Sleeping more
Does not come up to greet owner
Fearful
Guarding behavior, guards body parts
Biting painful areas
Licking painful areas or dorsal aspects of front limbs
Sudden, excessive scratching
Sudden, excessive negative reaction (compulsive behavior)
Under or overactive

Abnormal posture or movement seen with chronic pain
Reluctance to move (walk, trot, gallop, jump . . .)
Inability to turn in one or both directions
Hind legs tucked under abdomen
Tail between hind legs
Ears back
Restlessness, wandering, circling
Rigid posture and gait
Sitting or laying down in the middle of walks
Head hanging; will not lift or turn head (neck pain)
Praying position (abdominal pain)
Decreased weight bearing (limb pain)
Sitting abnormally (e.g., knee out in stifle pain)
Trembling or shaking

Mental and physiological behavior
Depressed, sad, and/or anxious demeanor
Visible white sclera around the iris (not always pain; some breeds show this all the time)
Panting or tachypnea or tachycardia without exercise

Other
No change in behavior
Decreased vocalization and/or quiet whining or whimpering
Increased vocalization including screaming or howling with breakthrough pain or manipulation of painful area
Allodynia
Hyperesthesia or hyperalgesia

Source: Modified from Wiseman et al., 2001, Hielm-Bjorkman et al., 2003.

it for evaluating pain as they did not recognize the signs of pain in their dogs. It was also not valid for rating the response to treatment. It was reliable in that owners misinterpreted the pain each time in the same way (Hielm-Bjorkman et al., 2011). Nonetheless, the VAS is a useful observational report measure because of its ease of use, its reliability and validity for rating things other than pain, and its low cost (Varni et al., 1987; Huijer Abu-Saad & Uiterwijk, 1995). The VAS format may also be used to assess other factors such as quality of life (QOL) or specific abilities such as pacing, jumping, or trotting (Canapp et al., 1999; Hudson et al., 2004).

The NRS is used in the same way as the VAS. Instead of a line, it has 10 or 11 numbers (usually 0 or 1–10) written successively from left to right, and the assessor circles the number that corresponds best to their evaluation (Conzemius et al., 1997; Holton et al., 1998; Wiseman-Orr et al., 2006; Brown et al., 2007). A pain study in sheep confirmed that the VAS and NRS have good agreement, but that the VAS is more sensitive (Welsh et al., 1993). Quinn et al. (2007) found that the VAS and the NRS were interpreted differently by two out of three observers, that changes in the NRS did not result in proportional changes in the VAS, and that both scales correlate poorly with force plate data. This would indicate that the two scales are not interchangeable.

The SDS provides several (usually three to five) written answers, often corresponding to degree of severity (Holton et al., 1998; Hielm-Bjorkman et al., 2003). For example, when asked a question regarding the ease with which the dog rises, the possible answers include: with great ease, with ease, neither with ease nor with difficulty, with difficulty, or with great difficulty.

Likert-type scales have responses that are framed on an agree–disagree continuum from strongly disagree to strongly agree (Wiseman-Orr et al., 2006), and a comparative scale would ask questions that compare some variable now to some other time, usually a baseline or time before treatment, with the answers indicating better, worse, or unchanged.

Multifactorial Descriptive Scales

As chronic pain is multifactorial (i.e., includes changes in different domains such as mood, posture, movement), chronic pain scales will usually be made up of questions from several of these domains. Depending on how they are structured, these scales have different names including variable rating scale (VRS) (Hardie, 2000), multifactorial pain scale (MFPS) (Firth & Haldane, 1999; Dobromylskyj et al., 2000), and multifocus/multifactorial descriptive scale (MDS) (Hardie, 2000; Hielm-Bjorkman et al., 2003; Brown et al., 2007; Hielm-Bjorkman et al., 2009; Hercock et al., 2009). The questions and answers can be structured in the form of a VAS, NRS, SDS, Likert scale, or comparative scale. The questions can either be real time, in which the owners are asked to assess how their dog has been that day, week, or month, or comparative, in which questions are posed to compare a variable now to some other time, usually a baseline or time before treatment (Gibson et al., 1980; Bollinger et al., 2002; Vaisanen et al., 2004; Wiseman-Orr et al., 2006; Pollard et al., 2006; Jaeger et al., 2007). The different variables may be weighted differently, depending on how important the question is in relation to assessing pain (Hardie, 2000).

Validated Pain Indices

Several chronic pain indices have been developed and validated, based on answers to specific questions relating to movement, behav-

ior, and demeanor, for owners of dogs suffering from different types of chronic pain. Indices validated for the chronic pain of OA in various joints include: the SDS-based 11-question Helsinki Chronic Pain Index (HCPI) (Figure 22.1) (Hielm-Bjorkman et al., 2003, 2009, 2011; Wernham et al., 2011), the VAS-based 11-question lameness and pain questionnaire (Hudson et al., 2004), the Glasgow University Veterinary School Questionnaire (GUVQuest) (Wiseman-Orr et al., 2004, 2006), the NRS-based 11-question Canine Brief Pain Inventory (CBPI) (Brown et al., 2007; 2008; Imhoff et al., 2011; Walton, 2011; Wernham et al., 2011) (Chapter 20), and the Liverpool OsteoArthritis in Dogs (elbow) score (LOAD-e) (Hercock et al., 2009; Walton, 2011). They have all been tested and found to be useful for diagnosing chronic pain in dogs suffering from OA, and the CBPI was also tested and found to be useful in dogs with bone cancer pain (Brown et al., 2009). The HCPI is undergoing validation in Swedish, Norwegian, Estonian, German, French, Dutch, Greek, and Portuguese, and the English version has been updated in a new translation that better reflects the initial Finnish HCPI (the HCPI-E2). Both the old and the new English translation of the validated index can be downloaded at http://www.vetmed.helsinki.fi/english/animalpain/hcpi. The CBPI has been validated for OA and bone cancer pain, is presently only available in English, and can be downloaded at www.CanineBPI.com (Brown et al., 2007, 2008). A scale developed by Yazbek & Fantoni (2005) has been validated for chronic cancer pain.

Development of an instrument that may aid in the differentiation of a patient with chronic pain from otherwise depressed or lethargic patients is also underway (Wiseman, 2011). This 60-item structured questionnaire measures health-related QOL, and it showed promising initial results in differentiating dogs suffering from chronic pain due to OA from healthy dogs and dogs suffering from lymphoma. It includes five main domains: vitality, emotional well-being, anxiety, pain, and fear of pain (Wiseman, 2011). Another group of researchers have also introduced QOL questionnaires (Wojciechowska et al., 2005a, 2005b).

End of Trial/Treatment Questions

Questions regarding owner satisfaction or trial outcome can also be used to assess chronic pain and the response to treatment. These can include questions regarding the owners' willingness to continue their animal's treatment, use the same treatment again in a similar situation but in another dog, or recommend this treatment to a friend (Jaeger et al., 2007; Eskelinen et al., 2012). The questions can also be posed as a scale of satisfaction statements indicating whether the owner is very content, content, indifferent, discontent, or very discontent with the effect of a treatment on chronic pain. Special care must be taken when posing the questions, as the owner may be content with the treatment (e.g., because it helped the dog's atopy) but not feel that it helped relieve pain. In clinical research situations one can ask owners retrospectively to guess what group their dog was assigned (Kapatkin et al., 2006; Hielm-Bjorkman et al., 2007).

CLINICAL EVALUATION OF CHRONIC PAIN

For an evaluative instrument to be useful it has to be validated, reliable, and preferably tested for response to analgesic treatment. A number of different methods are used by veterinarians to evaluate chronic pain due to OA. Lameness scores from 0 or 1 to 4 or 5, and

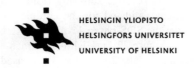

HELSINGIN YLIOPISTO
HELSINGFORS UNIVERSITET
UNIVERSITY OF HELSINKI

OWNER QUESTIONNAIRE: HCPI-E2

Date _____   Questionnaire no. 1   2   3   4   5   6   7   8   9   Pre ☐   Post ☐
(remember to mark date and if it is pre- or post treatment!)

Name of Dog _____   Diagnosis_____

Owner _____   Owner signature:_____
(is important so we know that the same owner completes the form every time!)

Points	0	1	2	3	4

Tick only one answer – the one that best describes your dog during the preceding week

1. The dog's mood is:

Very alert	alert	neither alert, nor indifferent	indifferent	very indifferent
☐	☐	☐	☐	☐

2. The dog plays:

Very willingly	willingly	reluctantly	very reluctantly	does not play at all
☐	☐	☐	☐	☐

3. Rate how often your dog vocalizes pain (audible complaining, whining, crying out etc.):

Never	hardly ever	sometimes	often	very often
☐	☐	☐	☐	☐

4. The dog walks:

With great ease	with ease	neither with ease, nor with difficulty	with difficulty	with great difficulty
☐	☐	☐	☐	☐

5. The dog trots (moving diagonal limbs at the same time; "jogging"):

With great ease	with ease	with some difficulty	with great difficulty	does not trot at all
☐	☐	☐	☐	☐

6. The dog gallops (high-speed running):

With great ease	with ease	with some difficulty	with great difficulty	does not gallop at all
☐	☐	☐	☐	☐

Kliinisen hevos- ja pieneläinlääketieteen laitos   PL 57 (Viikintie 49), 00014 Helsingin yliopisto
Eläinlääketieteellinen tiedekunta   Puhelin (09) 1911 (vaihde), faksi (09) 191 57298, www.vetmed.helsinki.fi

Institutionen för klinisk häst- och smådjursmedicin   PB 57 (Viksvägen 49), FIN-00014 Helsingfors universitet
Veterinärmedicinska fakulteten   Telefon +358 9 1911 (växel), fax +358 9 191 57298, www.vetmed.helsinki.fi/svenska/

Department of Equine and Small Animal Medicine   P.O. Box 57 (Viikintie 49), FIN-00014 University of Helsinki
Faculty of Veterinary Medicine   Telephone +358 9 1911, fax +358 9 191 57298, www.vetmed.helsinki.fi/english/

Figure 22.1.   The Helsinki chronic pain index (for veterinary use).

2(2)

7. The dog jumps (e.g., into car, onto sofa…):

With great ease	with ease	with some difficulty	with great difficulty	does not jump at all
☐	☐	☐	☐	☐

8. The dog lies down:

With great ease	with ease	neither with ease, nor with difficulty	with difficulty	with great difficulty
☐	☐	☐	☐	☐

9. The dog rises from a lying position:

With great ease	with ease	neither with ease, nor with difficulty	with difficulty	with great difficulty
☐	☐	☐	☐	☐

10. The dog moves after a long rest:

With great ease	with ease	neither with ease, nor with difficulty	with difficulty	with great difficulty
☐	☐	☐	☐	☐

11. The dog moves after major activity or heavy exercise:

With great ease	with ease	neither with ease, nor with difficulty	with difficulty	with great difficulty
☐	☐	☐	☐	☐

Points	*0*	*1*	*2*	*3*	*4*

Total up the answers to all 11 questions. Total chronic pain index score: _____
(The points and how to calculate the score should not be shown to the owners)

Thank You for your help!

Veterinarian's note:

_____

_____

_____

This Helsinki Chronic Pain Index has been developed at the University of Helsinki, Finland and is available in many languages.

For information about the HCPI, please contact Anna Hielm-Björkman, DVM, PhD
at   anna.hielm-bjorkman@helsinki.fi

Figure 22.1.   (*Continued*)

weight bearing measurements are commonly used (Holtsinger et al., 1992; Vasseur et al., 1995; Borer et al., 2003; Peterson & Keefe, 2004). Lameness has also been evaluated using a 10 cm VAS scale (Canapp et al., 1999). Other abnormalities of the locomotor system can also be scored including: limb circumference as a measure of atrophy (Dobromylskyj et al., 2000; Millis, 2004), limb range of motion (ROM) when extending or flexing joints (Holtsinger et al., 1992; Vasseur et al., 1995; Millis, 2004), swelling (Borer et al., 2003), crepitus (Holtsinger et al., 1992), pain from palpation (Holtsinger et al., 1992; Vasseur et al., 1995; Borer et al., 2003), or willingness to hold up a contralateral limb (Vasseur et al., 1995). Unfortunately, none of these techniques have been scientifically validated or shown to be reliable. On the contrary, subjective evaluation of lameness varied greatly among observers (three surgeons and three veterinary students) and agreed poorly with ground reaction forces (GRFs) from force plate analysis. Reliability of evaluation was not aided by having multiple observers (Waxman et al., 2008).

Hormonal Changes with Chronic Pain

Concentrations of various hormones have been used to assess stress and pain in animals (ACVA, 1998). Plasma epinephrine (adrenaline), norepinephrine (noradrenaline), β-endorphin, cortisol, and vasopressin concentrations are known to increase in stressful situations such as trauma and surgery (Desborough, 2000). In one study, epinephrine, cortisol, and vasopressin increased significantly, whereas β-endorphin decreased significantly (Hielm-Bjorkman et al., 2003). There is also considerable individual variation, and hormonal changes alone should not be used to identify chronic pain.

Diagnostic Imaging

Abnormalities found on radiographs, ultrasound, MRI, and CT that correspond with changes in locomotion resulting from chronic musculoskeletal pain are well documented in dogs (Smith, 1997; Slocum & Slocum, 1998; Levitski et al., 1999; Gordon et al., 2003; Akerblom & Sjoström, 2007). Although it is generally accepted that the degree of discomfort cannot be predicted from the pathological changes seen on radiographs (Dobromylskyj et al., 2000; Hielm-Bjorkman et al., 2003; Gordon et al., 2003) or CT (Jones & Inzana, 2000; Mayhew et al., 2002), abnormalities detected during imaging can be useful to help diagnose a source of chronic pain.

Thermography

There are no scientific publications on the use of thermographic cameras to locate the areas of chronic pain in dogs. A few studies demonstrate that myofascial trigger points can be diagnosed in humans using thermography (Diakow, 1988, 1992), and one study that shows changes in thermographic patterns associated with analgesic therapy in chronically painful horses (von Schweinitz, 1998).

Force Platform Analysis as a Measure of Chronic Pain

The most objective pain assessment method currently available for dogs with chronic limb pain is measurement of GRFs using force platform analyses. A normal healthy dog puts ~60% of its weight on the forelimbs and ~40% on the hind limbs. Force platform analysis is based on the assumption that a dog will put less weight on a limb if it is painful (Anderson & Mann, 1994; Wiseman et al., 2001; Hudson et al., 2004).

Force platform analysis (Figure 22.2) is considered to be the gold standard for evaluation of canine lameness (Quinn et al., 2007), and

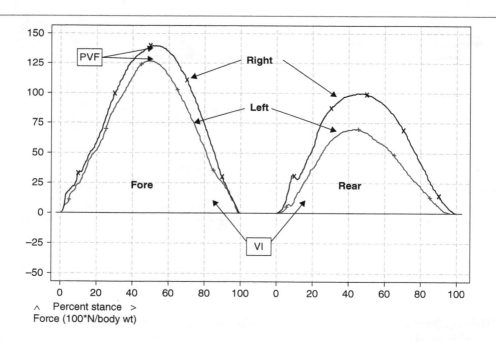

Figure 22.2. Force platform analysis is considered to be the gold standard for evaluation of canine lameness. It has been used to evaluate ground reaction forces (GRFs) in dogs with lameness due to pain. The two vertical GRFs most commonly used are the peak vertical force (PVF), or the highest force value recorded, and the vertical impulse (VI), or the force generated over time (Veterinary Surgery 36:293–301, 2007).

has been used to evaluate GRF in dogs with lameness due to pain. The two vertical GRFs most commonly used are the peak vertical force (PVF), or the highest force value recorded, and the vertical impulse (VI), or the force generated over time. These values are usually measured as a percentage of body weight (BW). The GRFs are evaluated one side at a time (either both right legs or both left legs). Dogs exhibit significantly reduced vertical forces in the painful limb, and stride length is increased. However, there was no difference in velocity, maximal foot velocity, stance duration, stride frequency, and impulse area, between dogs that are painful due to hip dysplasia and clinically normal dogs (Bennett et al., 1996).

Force platform analysis has been used to evaluate treatment of chronically painful OA of the hip (Vasseur et al., 1995; Budsberg et al., 1996, 1999; Budsberg, 2001; Moreau et al., 2003), the elbow joint (Bouck et al., 1995; Vasseur et al., 1995; Theyse et al., 2000; Moreau et al., 2003), and many other orthopedic conditions. Vertical impulse was found to be a better indicator of improvement than the PVF in the canine hip, and is frequently selected as the primary response variable (Budsberg et al., 1996, 1999; Budsberg, 2001). Because speed has an impact on the measured forces, it is important that speed and acceleration are kept constant. Trotting velocities of 0.8 to 2 or 3 m/s (Allen et al., 1994; Bennett et al., 1996; Budsberg et al., 1996; Jevens et al., 1996; Trumble et al., 2004, 2005; Kapatkin et al., 2007) and acceleration variation of $\pm$ 0.5 m/s^2 (Budsberg et al., 1996, 1999; Kapatkin et al., 2007) have been used. The mean of three to six runs is typically used, as variation among runs can be very large (Jevens et al., 1996; Tano et al., 1998; Budsberg et al., 1999).

Although force plate analysis is considered the "gold standard" in lameness research, this really applies only when all dogs are of the same breed or at least of the same weight and conformation, and only when a single joint in one leg is painful (Conzemius, 2010). This limits its use in clinical research where many joints may be involved and there is no breed standardization. Despite this, the new chronic pain scales have recently been validated against force plate analysis.

The LOAD-e owner questionnaire (Hercock et al., 2009) was the first one to be validated against force plate analysis. Correlation of LOAD-e with PVF was poor and not statistically significant. Further studies have failed to correlate force plate data with LOAD-e, the HPCI, and the VBPI (Fachon & Grandjean, 2007; Walton, 2011). However, LOAD-e, HPCI, and VBPI correlated significantly with each other, indicating construct validity and that they measure the same thing or are influenced by the same factors. This lack of correlation with force plate analysis indicates that these chronic pain scales have poor criterion validity, implying that the lameness that the force plate measures is not equal to the overall chronic pain that the indices measure. Quinn et al. (2007) evaluated two lameness scales in the form of a VAS and an NRS and also failed to find an association with the PVF using the same dogs. This group did find an association between the VAS lameness score and the force plate VI value, indicating that the human eye can perceive lameness that includes a time component (as in VI), but cannot perceive lameness during weight bearing (as in PVF) (Quinn et al., 2007). When experienced surgeons and first year students were asked to score a lameness using a VAS and then predict corresponding force plate GRF values, the agreement was low for all (Waxman et al., 2008). Increased sensory sensitivity was evaluated in dogs with chronic pain due to cruciate ligament disease (Brydges et al., 2012). In that study, vertical pressure and impulse were different compared to control dogs, though the difference was not significant, indicating that GRFs may not measure pain sensory sensitivity adequately. Further work is needed to elucidate the relationships between the pain scales and GRFs.

Weight-assessing Walkways and Carpets

A disadvantage of using the force plate is that it only evaluates one pair of ipsilateral legs per run across the platform. A weight-assessing carpet, consisting of a number of pressure sensors, can evaluate each footfall (Lascelles et al., 2006; Viguier et al., 2007; Collard et al., 2010; Light et al., 2010). Presently, there are at least two carpets that offer canine software; the longer GAITFour® and the shorter Tecscan.

Static Weight Bearing

Static weight bearing has also been used as a method of comparing a painful leg to a nonpainful contralateral one, and can be used as an easy in-practice evaluation tool. Each time the dog comes in to the practice, the painful leg and its contralateral pair are placed on two bathroom scales and if the difference in static weight bearing between the two limbs is more than 6%, it might be indicative of pain (Hyytiainen et al., 2012). Static weight bearing can also be measured using a pressure carpet or a plate (Lascelles et al., 2006; Brydges et al., 2012).

Activity Monitors

Some studies suggest that an activity monitor attached to the dog's collar may be a valid outcome assessment tool for documenting improved activity associated with treatment and decreased pain in dogs with OA (Hansen et al., 2007; Wernham et al., 2011).

Other Methods

As chronic pain is such a common diagnosis, new methods to validate pain are continuously emerging. Methods that have been used in human or rodent preclinical trials are now being evaluated for dogs. For example, the von Frey filament and sensitivity to cold thermal stimuli have been evaluated in dogs (KuKanich et al., 2005; Brydges et al., 2012).

Analgesic Drug Trial Period and Analgesic Withdrawal

Administration of an analgesic for a trial period, with the owner monitoring the change in behavior and demeanor, can be helpful. However, a study (Hielm-Bjorkman et al., 2011) found that owners did not perceive changes in their pets' mobility or behavior after starting an NSAID or after 2 or 4 weeks on an NSAID. It was only after the analgesic was withdrawn that owners perceived that their pets had improved on the analgesic. In practice, this may mean administering an analgesic for 2 weeks, having the owner evaluate changes, and then discontinuing the analgesic for a week, again with the owner evaluating changes. Validated pain questionnaires should be given to the owner before treatment and at regular intervals during treatment. If an analgesic drug appears to be a failure, other analgesics from the same or a different drug category should be administered, and the results reassessed until an effective treatment is found. Focused analgesic therapies based on assessment of the underlying pathophysiology are likely to be most effective.

SUMMARY

Pain scoring should become part of everyday clinical practice, and pain scoring systems must be validated to be helpful in the assessment of treatment results. As pain is considered the "fifth vital sign" all patients should have their pain assessed at each clinic visit and after any change in treatment. Owners, technicians, and veterinarians should become familiar with the signs of chronic pain in dogs and the use of chronic pain assessment tools. Periodic pain and QOL scoring will provide the veterinarian with baseline information that can be assessed over the lifetime of the dog, allowing earlier intervention and improved outcomes.

REFERENCES

American College of Veterinary Anaesthesiologists (ACVA) (1998) American College of Veterinary Anaesthesiologists' position paper on the treatment of pain in animals. *Journal of the American Veterinary Medical Association*, 213, 628–630.

Akerblom, S. & Sjoström, L. (2007) Evaluation of clinical, radiological and cytological findings compared to arthroscopic findings in shoulder joint lameness in the dog. *Veterinary and Comparative Orthopaedics and Traumatology*, 20, 136–141.

Allen, K., DeCamp, C.E., Braden, T.D., & Bahns, M. (1994) Kinematic gait analysis of the trot in healthy mixed breed dogs. *Veterinary and Comparative Orthopaedics and Traumatology*, 7, 148–153.

Anderson, M.A. & Mann, F.A. (1994) Force plate analysis: A non-invasive tool for gait evaluation. *The Compendium on Continuing Education for the Practicing Veterinarian*, 16, 857–867.

Bennett, R.L., DeCamp, C.E., Flo, G.L., Hauptman, J.G., & Stajich, M. (1996) Kinematic gait analysis in dogs with hip dysplasia. *American Journal of Veterinary Research*, 57, 966–971.

Bollinger, C., DeCamp, C.E., Stajich, M., et al. (2002) Gait analysis of dogs with hip dysplasia treated with gold bead implantation acupuncture. *Veterinary and Comparative Orthopaedics and Traumatology*, 2, 116–122.

Borer, L.R., Peel, J.E., Seewald, W., Schawalder, P., & Spreng, D.E. (2003) Effect of carprofen, etodolac, meloxicam, or butorphanol in dogs with induced acute synovitis. *American Journal of Veterinary Research*, 64, 1429–1437.

Bouck, G.R., Miller, C.W., & Taves, C.L. (1995) A comparison of surgical and medical treatment of fragmented coronoid process and osteochondritis dissecans of the canine elbow. *Veterinary and Comparative Orthopaedics and Traumatology*, 8, 177–183.

Brown, D.C., Boston, R.C., Coyne, J.C., & Farrar, J.T. (2007) Development and psychometric testing of an instrument to measure chronic pain in dogs with osteoarthritis. *American Journal of Veterinary Research*, 68, 631–637.

Brown, D.C., Boston, R.C., Coyne, J.C., & Farrar, J.T. (2008) Ability of the canine brief pain inventory to detect response to treatment in dogs with osteoarthritis. *Journal of the American Veterinary Medical Association*, 233, 1278–1283.

Brown, D.C., Boston, R., Coyne, J.C., & Farrar, J.T. (2009) A novel approach to the use of animals in studies of pain: validation of the canine brief pain inventory in canine bone cancer. *Pain Medicine*, 10(1), 133–142.

Brydges, N.M., Argyle, D.J., Mosley, J.R., Duncan, J.C., Fleetwood-Walker, S., & Clements, D.N. (2012) Clinical assessments of increased sensory sensitivity in dogs with cranial cruciate ligament rupture. *The Veterinary Journal*, 193(2), 545–550.

Budsberg, S.C. (2001) Long-term temporal evaluation of ground reaction forces during development of experimentally induced osteoarthritis in dogs. *American Journal of Veterinary Research*, 62, 1207–1211.

Budsberg, S.C., Chambers, J.N., Van Lue, S.L., Foutz, T.L., & Reece, L. (1996) Prospective evaluation of ground reaction forces in dogs undergoing unilateral total hip replacement. *American Journal of Veterinary Research*, 57, 1781–1785.

Budsberg, S.C., Johnston, S.A., Schwarz, P.D., DeCamp, C.E., & Claxton, R. (1999) Efficacy of etodolac for the treatment of osteoarthritis of the hip joints in dogs. *Journal of the American Veterinary Medical Association*, 214, 206–210.

Canapp, S.O., Jr., McLaughlin, R.M., Jr., Hoskinson, J.J., Roush, J.K., & Butine, M.D. (1999) Scintigraphic evaluation of dogs with acute synovitis after treatment with glucosamine hydrochloride and chondroitin sulfate. *American Journal of Veterinary Research*, 60, 1552–1557.

Collard, F., Maitre, P., Le Quang, T. et al. (2010) Canine hip denervation: comparison between clinical outcome and gait analysis. *Revue Médicine Vétrinaire*, 161, 277–282.

Conzemius, M. (2010) *Limitations of Force Platform Gait Analysis*, Proceedings of the 3rd World Veterinary Orthopaedic Congress, ESVOT-VOS 15th ESVOT Congress, Bologna, Italy, pp. 87–88.

Conzemius, M.G., Hill, C.M., Sammarco, J.L., & Perkowski, S.Z. (1997) Correlation between subjective and objective measures used to determine severity of postoperative pain in dogs. *Journal of the American Veterinary Medical Association*, 210, 1619–1622.

Cook, J.L. (2007) Outcomes-based patient care in veterinary surgery: What is an outcome measure? *Veterinary Surgery*, 36, 187–189.

Desborough, J.P. (2000) The stress response to trauma and surgery. *British Journal of Anaesthesia'*, 85, 109–117.

Diakow, P.R. (1988) Thermographic imaging of myofascial trigger points. *Journal of manipulative physiological therapeutics*, 11(2), 114–117.

Diakow, P.R. (1992) Differentiation of active and latent trigger points by thermography. *Journal of manipulative physiological therapeutics*, 15(7), 439–441.

Dobromylskyj, P., Flecknell, P.A., Lascelles, B.D., Livingston, A., & Taylor, P. (2000) Pain assessment, in *Pain Management in Animals* (eds P.A. Flecknell & A. Waterman-Pearson), W. B. Saunders, London, pp. 53–79.

Eskelinen, E.V., Liska, W.D., Hyytiäinen, H.K., & Hielm-Björkman, A. (2012) Canine total knee replacement performed due to osteoarthritis subsequent to distal femur fracture osteosynthesis: two-year objective outcome. *Veterinary and Comparative Orthopaedics and Traumatology*, 25(5), 427–432.

Fachon, L. & Grandjean, D. (2007) Accuracy of asymmetry indices of ground reaction forces for diagnosis of hind limb lameness in dogs. *American Journal of Veterinary Research*, 68, 1089–1094.

Firth, A.M. & Haldane, S.L. (1999) Development of a scale to evaluate postoperative pain in dogs. *Journal of the American Veterinary Medical Association*, 214, 651–659.

Flecknell, P.A. (2000) Animal pain - an introduction, in *Pain Management in Animals* (ed. A. Waterman-Pearson), W.B. Saunders, London, pp. 1–7, 53–79.

Gibson, R.G., Gibson, S.L.M., Conway, V., & Chappell, D. (1980) *Perna Canaliculus* in the treatment of arthritis. *The Practitioner*, 224, 955–960.

Gordon, W.J., Conzemius, M.G., Riedesel, E., et al. (2003) The relationship between limb function and radiographic osteoarthrosis in dogs with stifle osteoarthrosis. *Veterinary Surgery*, 32, 451–454.

Hansen, B.D., Lascelles, B.D., Keene, B.W., Adams, A.K, & Thomson, A.E. (2007) Evaluation of an accelerometer for at-home monitoring of spontaneous activity in dogs. *American Journal of Veterinary Research*, 68, 468–475.

Hardie, E.M. (2000) Recognition of pain behaviour in animals, in *Animal pain* (ed. L.J. Hellebrekers), Van der Wees, Utrecht, The Netherlands, pp. 51–69.

Hercock, C.A., Pinchbeck, G., Giejda, A., Clegg, P.D., & Innes, J.F. (2009) Validation of a client-based clinical metrology instrument for the evaluation of canine elbow osteoarthritis. *Journal of Small Animal Practice*, 50, 266–271.

Hielm-Bjorkman, A., Kuusela, E., Liman, A., et al. (2003) Evaluation of methods for assessment of pain associated with chronic osteoarthritis in dogs. *Journal of the American Veterinary Medical Association*, 222, 1552–1558.

Hielm-Bjorkman, A., Reunanen, V., Meri, P., & Tulamo, R.M. (2007) Panax Ginseng in combination with Brewers' Yeast as a stimulant for geriatric dogs: a controlled randomized blinded study. *Journal of Veterinary Pharmacology and Therapeutics*, 30, 295–304.

Hielm-Bjorkman, A., Rita, H., & Tulamo, R-M. (2009) Psychometric testing of the Helsinki chronic pain index by completion of a questionnaire in Finnish by owners of dogs with chronic signs of pain caused by osteoarthritis. *American Journal of Veterinary Research*, 70, 727–734.

Hielm-Bjorkman, A.K., Kapatkin, A.S., & Rita, H.J. (2011) Reliability and validity for use of a visual analogue scale by owners to measure chronic pain attributable to osteoarthritis in their dogs. *American Journal of Veterinary Research*, 72, 601–607.

Holton, L., Scott, E.M., Nolan, A.M., Reid, J., Welsh, E., & Flaherty, D. (1998) Comparison of three methods used for assessment of pain in dogs. *Journal of the American Veterinary Medical Association*, 212, 61–66.

Holtsinger, R.H., Parker, R.B., Beale, B.S., & Friedman, R.L. (1992) The therapeutic efficacy of carprofen (Rimadyl-V™) in 209 clinical cases of canine degenerative joint disease. *Veterinary and Comparative Orthopaedics and Traumatology*, 5, 140–144.

Hudson, J.T., Slater, M.R., Taylor, L., Scott, H.M., & Kerwin, S.C. (2004) Assessing repeatability and validity of a visual analogue scale questionnaire for use in assessing pain and lameness in dogs. *American Journal of Veterinary Research*, 65, 1634–1643.

Hugonnard, M., Leblond, A., Keroack, S., Cadoré, J.L., & Troncy, E. (2004) Attitudes and concerns of French veterinarians towards pain and analgesia in dogs and cats. *Veterinary Anaesthesia and Analgesia*, 31, 154–163.

Huijer Abu-Saad, H.H. & Uiterwijk, M. (1995) Pain in children with juvenile rheumatoid arthritis: a descriptive study. *Pediatric Research*, 38, 194–197.

Hyytiainen, H., Molsä, S., Junnila, J., Laitinen-Vapaavuori, O.M., & Hielm-Björkman, A.K. (2012) Use of bathroom scales in measuring asymmetry of hind limb static weight bearing in dogs with osteoarthritis. *Veterinary and Comparative Orthopaedics and Traumatology*, 25(5), 390–396.

Imhoff, D.J., Gordon-Evans, W.J., Evans, R.B., Johnson, A.L., Griffon, D.J., & Swanson, K.S. (2011) Evaluation of S-adenosyl l-methionine in a double-blinded, randomized, placebo-controlled, clinical trial for treatment of presumptive osteoarthritis in the dog. *Veterinary Surgery*, 40(2), 228–232.

Innes, J.F. & Barr, A.R. (1998) Can owners assess outcome following treatment of canine cruciate ligament deficiency? *Journal of Small Animal Practice*, 39, 373–378.

Jaeger, G.T., Larsen, S., Soli, N., & Moe, L. (2007) Two years follow-up study of the pain relieving effect of gold bead implantation in dogs with hip-joint arthritis. *Acta Veterinaria Scandinavica*, 49, 9.

Jevens, D.J., DeCamp, C.E., Hauptman, J., Braden, T.D., Richter, M., & Robinson, R. (1996) Use of force-plate analysis of gait to compare two surgical techniques for treatment of cranial cruciate ligament rupture in dogs. *American Journal of Veterinary Research*, 57, 389–393.

Jones, J.C. & Inzana, K.D. (2000) Subclinical CT abnormalities in the lumbosacral spine of older large-breed dogs. *Veterinary Radiology & Ultrasound*, 41, 19–26.

Kapatkin, A.S. (2007) Outcome-based medicine and its applications in clinical surgical practice. *Veterinary Surgery*, 36, 515–518.

Kapatkin, A.S., Arbittier, G., Kass, P.H., Gilley, R.S., & Smith, G.K. (2007) Kinetic gait analysis of healthy dogs on two different surfaces. *Veterinary Surgery*, 36, 605–608.

Kapatkin, A.S., Tomasic, M., et al. (2006) Effects of electrostimulated acupuncture on ground reaction forces and pain scores in dogs with chronic elbow joint arthritis. *Journal of the American Veterinary Medical Association*, 228, 1350–1354.

KuKanich, B., Lascelles, B.D., & Papich, M.G. (2005) Use of a von Frey device for evaluation of pharmacokinetics and pharmacodynamics of morphine after intravenous administration as an infusion or multiple doses in dogs. *American Journal of Veterinary Research*, 66, 1968–1974.

Lascelles, B.D.X. & Main, D.C.J. (2002) Surgical trauma and chronically painful conditions – within our comfort level but beyond theirs? *Journal of the American Veterinary Medical Association*, 221, 215–222.

Lascelles, B.D.X., Parry, A.T., Stidworthy, M.F., Dobson, J.M., & White, R.A. (2000) Squamous cell carcinoma of the nasal planum in 17 dogs. *Veterinary Record*, 147, 473–476.

Lascelles, B.D.X., Roe, S.C, Smith, E. et al. (2006) Evaluation of a pressure walkway system for measurement of vertical limb forces in clinically normal dogs. *American Journal of Veterinary Research*, 67, 277–282.

Levitski, R.E., Lipsitz, D., & Chauvet, A.E. (1999) Magnetic resonance imaging of the cervical spine in 27 dogs. *Veterinary Radiology & Ultrasound*, 40, 332–341.

Light, V.A., Steiss, J.E., Montgomery, R.D., Rumph, P.F., & Wright, J.C. (2010) Temporal-spatial gait analysis by use of a portable walkway system in healthy Labrador Retrievers at a walk. *American Journal of Veterinary Research*, 71, 997–1002.

Mayhew, P.D., Kapatkin, A.S., Wortman, J.A., & Vite, C.H. (2002) Association of cauda equina compression on magnetic resonance images and clinical signs in dogs with degenerative lumbosacral stenosis. *Journal of the American Animal Hospital Association*, 38, 555–562.

Millis, D.L. (2004) Assessing and measuring outcomes, in *Canine Rehabilitation & Physical Therapy* (eds D. Levine & R.A. Taylor), Saunders, Missouri, pp. 211–227.

Moreau, M., Dupuis, J., Bonneau, N.H., & Desnoyers, M. (2003) Clinical evaluation of a neutraceutical, carprofen and meloxicam for the treatment of dogs with osteoarthritis. *Veterinary Record*, 152, 323–329.

Morton, D.B. & Griffiths, P.H.M. (1985) Guidelines on the recognition of pain, distress and discomfort in experimental animals and a hypothesis for assessment. *Veterinary Record*, 116, 431–436.

Murrell, J.C. & Johnson, C.B. (2006) Neurophysiological techniques to assess pain in animals. *Journal of Veterinary Pharmacology and Therapeutics*, 29, 325–335.

Peterson, K.D. & Keefe, T.J. (2004) Effects of meloxicam on severity of lameness and other clinical signs of osteoarthritis in dogs. *Journal of the American Veterinary Medical Association*, 225, 1056–1060.

Phillips, D.M. (2000) JCAHO pain management standards are unveiled. Joint Commission on Accreditation of Healthcare Organizations. *Journal of the American Medical Association*, 284, 428–429.

Pollard, B., Guilford, W.G., Ankenbauer-Perkins, K.L., & Hedderley, D. (2006) Clinical efficacy and tolerance of an extract of green lipped mussel (Perna canaliculus) in dogs presumptively diagnosed with degenerative joint disease. *New Zealand Veterinary Journal*, 54, 114–118.

Quinn, M.M., Keuler, N.S., Lu, Y., Faria, M.L., Muir, P., & Markel, M.D. (2007) Evaluation of agreement between numerical rating scales, visual analogue scoring scales, and force plate gait analysis in dogs. *Veterinary Surgery*, 36, 360–367.

Raekallio, M., Heinonen, K.M., Kuussaari, J., & Vainio, O. (2003) Pain alleviation in animals: attitudes and practices of Finnish veterinarians. *The Veterinary Journal*, 165, 131–135.

Revill, S.I., Robinson, J.O., Rosen, M., & Hogg, M.I. (1976) The reliability of a linear analogue for evaluating pain. *Anaesthesia*, 31, 1191–1198.

Robertson, S.A. (2002) What is pain? *Journal of the American Veterinary Medical Association*, 221, 202–205.

Rutherford, K.M.D. (2002) Assessing pain in animals. *Animal Welfare*, 11, 31–53.

Sanford, J. (1992) Guidelines for detection and assessment of pain and distress in experimental animals, in *Animal Pain* (eds C.E. Short & A. Van Poznac), Churchill Livingstone, New York, pp. 515–524.

Sanford, J., Ewbank, R., Molony, V., et al. (1986) Working party of the Association of Veterinary Teachers and Research Workers: guidelines for the recognition and assessment of pain in animals. *Veterinary Record*, 118, 334–338.

Sargent, J. & Liebman, R. (1985) Childhood chronic illness: issues for psychotherapists. *Community Mental Health Journal*, 21(4), 294–311.

Schulz, K.S., Cook, J.L., Kapatkin, A.S., & Brown, D.C. (2006) Evidence-Based surgery: time for change. *Veterinary Surgery*, 35, 697–699.

Slocum, B. & Slocum, D.S. (1998) Hip - diagnostic tests, in *Current Techniques in Small Animal Surgery* (ed. M.J. Bojrab), Williams & Wilkins, Baltimore, MD, pp. 1127–1145.

Smith, G.K. (1997) Advances in diagnosing canine hip dysplasia. *Journal of the American Veterinary Medical Association*, 210(10), 1451–1457.

Tano, C.A., Cockshutt, J.R., Dobson, H., Miller, C.W., Holmberg, D.L., & Taves, C.L. (1998) Force plate analysis of dogs with bilateral hip dysplasia treated with a unilateral triple pelvic osteotomy: a long-term review of cases. *Veterinary and Comparative Orthopaedics and Traumatology*, 11, 85–93.

Theyse, L.F.H., Hazewinkel, H.A., & Van Den Brom, W.E. (2000) Force plate analyses before and after surgical treatment of unilateral fragmented coronoid process. *Veterinary and Comparative Orthopaedics and Traumatology*, 13, 135–140.

Trumble, T.N., Billinghurst, R.C., & McIlwraith, C.W. (2004) Correlation of prostaglandin E2 concentrations in synovial fluid with ground reaction forces and clinical variables for pain or inflammation in dogs with osteoarthritis induced by transaction of the cranial cruciate ligament. *American Journal of Veterinary Research*, 65, 1269–1275.

Trumble, T.N., Billinghurst, R.C., Bendele, A.M., & McIlwraith, C.W. (2005) Evaluation of changes in vertical ground reaction forces as indicators of meniscal damage after transaction of the cranial cruciate ligament in dogs. *American Journal of Veterinary Research*, 66, 156–163.

Vaisanen, M., Oksanen, H., & Vainio, O. (2004) Postoperative signs in 96 dogs undergoing soft tissue surgery. *Veterinary Record*, 155, 729–733.

Varni, J.W., Thompson, K.L., & Hanson, V. (1987) The Varni/Thompson pediatric pain questionnaire: I. Chronic musculoskeletal pain in juvenile rheumatoid arthritis. *Pain*, 28, 27–38.

Vasseur, P.B., Johnson, A.L., Budsberg, S.C., et al. (1995) Randomized, controlled trial of the efficacy of carprofen, a nonsteroidal anti-inflammatory drug, in the treatment of osteoarthritis in dogs. *Journal of the American Veterinary Medical Association*, 206, 807–811.

Viguier, E., Le Quang, T., Maitre, P. Gaudin, A., Rowling, M., & Haas, D. (2007) The validity and reliability of the GAITRite® system's measurement of the walking dog. *Computer Methods in Biomechanics and Biomedical Engineering*, 10(Suppl. 1), 113–114.

von Schweinitz, D.G. (1998) Thermographic evidence for the effectiveness of acupuncture in equine neuromuscular disease. *Acupuncture in Medicine*, 16(1), 14–17.

Wall, P.D. (1992) Defining "pain in animals", in *Animal Pain* (eds C.E. Short & A. Van Poznac), Churchill Livingstone, New York, pp. 63–79.

Walton, B. (2011) *Owner Based Metrology Instruments for Conditions of Canine Chronic Mobility Impairment: Construct and Criterion Validity of LOAD, HCPI and CBPI*. Scientific Proceedings of the BSAVA Congress 2011, British Small Animal Veterinary Association, Gloucester, p. 427.

Waxman, A.S., Robinson, D.A., Evans, R.B., Hulse, D.A., Innes, J.F., & Conzemius, M.G. (2008) Relationship between objective and subjective assessment of limb function in normal dogs with an experimentally induced lameness. *Veterinary Surgery*, 37(3), 241–246.

Welsh, E.M., Gettinby, G., & Nolan, A.M. (1993) Comparison of a visual analogue scale and a numerical rating scale for assessment of lameness, using sheep as the model. *American Journal of Veterinary Research*, 54, 976–984.

Wernham, B.G.J., Trumpatori, B., Hash, J., et al. (2011) Dose reduction of meloxicam in dogs with osteoarthritis-associated pain and impaired mobility. *Journal of Veterinary Internal Medicine*, 25, 1298–1305.

Wiseman, L. (2011) *Development of a 60-item structured questionnaire instrument to measure health-related quality of life (HRQL) in healthy dogs, dogs with degenerative joint disease and dogs with lymphoma*. Scientific Proceedings of the BSAVA Congress 2011, British Small Animal Veterinary Association, Gloucester, p. 486.

Wiseman, M.L., Nolan, A.M., Reid, J., & Scott, E.M., (2001) Preliminary study on owner-reported behavior changes associated with chronic pain in dogs. *Veterinary Record*, 149, 423–424.

Wiseman-Orr, M.L., Nolan, A.M., Reid, J., & Scott, E.M. (2004) Development of a questionnaire to measure the effects of chronic pain on health-related quality of life. *American Journal of Veterinary Research*, 65, 1077–1084.

Wiseman-Orr, M.L., Scott, E.M., Reid, J., & Nolan, A.M. (2006) Validation of a structured questionnaire to measure chronic in dogs on the basis of effects on health-related quality of life. *American Journal of Veterinary Research*, 67, 1826–1836.

Wojciechowska, J.I., Hewson, C.J., Stryhn, H., Guy, N.C., Patronek, G.J., & TimmonsV. (2005a) Development of a discriminative questionnaire to assess nonphysical aspects of quality of life in dogs. *American Journal of Veterinary Research*, 66, 1453–1460.

Wojciechowska, J.I., Hewson, C.J., Stryhn, H., Guy, N.C., Patronek, G.J., & Timmons, V. (2005b) Evaluation of a questionnaire regarding nonphysical aspects of quality of life in sick and healthy dogs. *American Journal of Veterinary Research*, 66, 1461–1467.

Yazbek, K.V. & Fantoni, D.T. (2005) Validity of a health-related quality-of-life scale for dogs with signs of pain secondary to cancer. *Journal of the American Veterinary Medical Association*, 226, 1354–1358.

23
Treatment of Chronic Pain in Dogs

Anna Hielm-Björkman

The International Association for the Study of Pain (IASP) has defined chronic pain as "pain without apparent biological value which has persisted beyond normal tissue healing time" (Merskey et al., 1994). Normal nociceptive or protective pain would have been alleviated with tissue healing. According to a new British survey, small animal veterinarians see pets with chronic pain, poor mobility, and orthopedic or neurological disease on a weekly basis (Yeates & Main, 2011), yet chronic pain is underdiagnosed and undertreated in dogs (Raekallio et al., 2003). There are many challenges to the treatment of canine chronic pain including: recognizing the signs of chronic pain (Chapter 22); determining if the pain is inflammatory, neuropathic, visceral, or somatic; lack of knowledge of appropriate use of analgesics, including fear of adverse effects; and management of treatment failures and breakthrough pain (BTP).

Chronic pain has many etiologies, and treatment of the cause rather than the signs should occur whenever possible (Wall & Melzack, 2003). The causes of chronic pain in a patient might be quite obvious, for example, a fracture callus causing nerve compression and neuropathic pain. At other times, the pain seems disproportionate to the initiating stimulus, and there are instances when the cause of chronic pain cannot be identified, even by using advanced diagnostic techniques (e.g., phantom limb pain or neuropathic pain). In these cases, the signs have become the disease, and must be treated as such.

Chronic pain can include inflammatory somatic pain, visceral pain, neuropathic pain, and breakthrough episodes of acute pain associated with a chronic pain syndrome. There may be inflammatory and/or autonomic signs including temperature and color changes and swelling. An osteoarthritic joint or an inflamed tooth result in inflammatory pain initially but, as the disease becomes chronic, primary nociceptive afferents become sensitized and inflammatory and neuropathic pain with peripheral and central sensitization may be present (Shenker et al., 2004). These more complex chronic pain syndromes have components of several types of pain. For example, a fast growing osteosarcoma may have components of somatic, visceral, and neuropathic pain mechanisms. Cancer pain is reviewed in two other chapters (Chapters 3 and 27), thus it will not be discussed in this chapter. In the following discussion we will review the main types of chronic pain.

TYPES OF CHRONIC PAIN

Chronic Canine Inflammatory Pain (Somatic)

Inflammatory pain can be somatic or visceral, but the neuroanatomy and physiology of visceral pain are very different from that of somatic inflammatory pain and are discussed below. Chronic inflammatory pain can be recognized in any somatic tissue (e.g., dermal, articular, and musculoskeletal tissues), and is a result of an abundance of inflammatory mediators. Osteoarthritis (OA) is a prime example of a canine chronic inflammatory pain syndrome, but inflammatory pain can also result from a variety of insults, including burns, trauma, surgery, or a chronic infection such as Lyme disease.

The typical signs of inflammation, including signs of redness, warmth, swelling, and pain, may or may not be present externally. Even when present, they may not be obvious because of the site, depth, and duration of the inflammatory process, and may be obscured by the hair coat. Generally, the dog is reluctant to move or to have the site manipulated. If the pain is very chronic, many secondary musculoskeletal signs will also be present, such as lameness, altered gait or standing position, muscle cramps, and trigger points. Inflammatory somatic pain in humans is described as throbbing or aching: a "dull" kind of pain that may be very localized.

Early inflammatory pain is best treated with nonsteroidal anti-inflammator drugs (NSAIDs), but is sometimes treated with corticosteroids. Other therapies have also been used, although many of them only have anecdotal evidence of success and randomized clinical trials are lacking. Persistent inflammatory pain will eventually lead to other types of pain, most often neuropathic pain. Even in these late-stage inflammatory pain syndromes, the inflammatory process is still a part of the disease, and NSAIDs are frequently combined with adjuvant analgesics and/or other pain treatments.

Chronic Canine Visceral Pain

Visceral pain is often a mixture of inflammatory and neuropathic pain, and may have an element of referred pain. The ratio of $A\delta$:C-fibers in somatic structures is 1:2, whereas the ratio is 1:10 in viscera. Visceral afferent fibers travel in parasympathetic nerves, such as the vagus nerve, and have large overlapping receptor fields

Pain Management in Veterinary Practice, First Edition. Edited by Christine M. Egger, Lydia Love and Tom Doherty.

(McMahon, 1997), making visceral pain more difficult to localize. Etiologies include peritonitis, gastric ulceration, irritable bowel syndrome, food hypersensitivities, malabsorption syndromes, constipation, colic, reflux disorders, chronic pancreatitis, cancer, and renal calculi.

As visceral neuroanatomy is different from that of the soma, the signs and treatments of visceral pain will also be very different from those of somatic inflammatory pain, despite the inflammatory element. Visceral pain results from smooth muscle spasm, mesenteric stretching, distension of hollow structures, ischemia, mechanical obstruction, or nerve damage; whereas normal surgical procedures, such as cutting or clamping, do not cause visceral pain. Humans describe visceral pain as deep, squeezing, gnawing, cramping, aching, and poorly localized. Associated symptoms in humans include nausea, perhaps something to consider when treating dogs with visceral pain.

Visceral pain is not easy to diagnose. The painful area is usually in the thorax or abdomen, but there might be sensitive sites of referred pain elsewhere on the body. There might also be autonomic signs (heat, swelling), but these may be hard to recognize in canine patients. The visceral signs may wax and wane, and may get better or worse with eating, drinking, urinating, or defecating. As in somatic inflammatory chronic pain, there may be secondary musculoskeletal pain as well.

Visceral pain is best treated by treating the inciting cause, whenever possible. If diagnostic work up is normal, a dietary change, for example, to a balanced, low carbohydrate, high protein, high fat diet supplemented with B-vitamins, minerals, pro- and prebiotics and omega-3 fatty acids has provided relief in some patients in the author's experience. Relief of gastrointestinal pain using antispasmodic agents may also be helpful. Visceral pain *per se* is usually hard to treat, but treatment with opioid agonist-antagonists or partial agonists, NSAIDs, metamizole sodium (dipyrone where available), tricyclic antidepressants (TCAs), serotonin reuptake inhibitors, and anticonvulsants can be tried.

Chronic canine neuropathic pain

Neuropathic pain is defined by the IASP (2007) as "pain initiated or caused by a primary lesion or dysfunction in the nervous system." Neuropathic pain can occur because of peripheral or central dysfunction or disease of the nervous system (Saarto & Wiffen, 2005) (Chapter 2).

As there are many underlying mechanisms contributing to neuropathic pain, including peripheral and central sensitization, central disinhibition, and phenotypic changes in neurons (Wolfe & Poma, 2010), the clinical signs of neuropathic pain will vary. Humans describe neuropathic pain as burning or shooting and it can be associated with motor, sensory, or autonomic deficits.

Diagnosing neuropathic pain is challenging in animals. In humans, diagnosis relies upon a thorough evaluation of the patient's medical history, asking specific questions about the symptoms of pain, ruling out inflammatory pain with an NSAID treatment trial, and formulating a placebo-controlled adjuvant drug trial. Questions to pose to the dog owner relate to the quantitative, qualitative, and time-related aspects of the pain signs, recollection of pain- or stress-related events in the dog's life, and successful and unsuccessful treatment trials. Because neuropathic pain may be associated with spontaneous and stimulated paresthesia, questions related to the dog's quality of life should be asked, including questions about quality and quantity of sleep, attention span, demeanor (nervousness, aggression, depression, anxiety), social withdrawal, resistance to stroking or palpation, pruritus or scratching or licking episodes, and tendency to clumsiness, resulting in wounds or other trauma. If the pain is very chronic, many secondary musculoskeletal signs will be present including lameness, altered gait or standing position, muscle cramps, and trigger points. A recent study described ways to assess altered sensitivity due to chronic neuropathic pain. Inter-digital von Frey filament application, thermal (cold) sensitivity, static weight bearing, and gait parameters were different in dogs with chronic neuropathic pain due to cruciate disease compared with healthy control dogs, although static weight bearing and gait parameters did not reach significance (Brydges et al., 2012).

Chronic neuropathic pain treatment protocols generally start with an NSAID trial. If pain is not controlled with an NSAID, analgesic adjuvants, such as TCAs, serotonin–norepinephrine reuptake inhibitors (SNRIs), anticonvulsants, or tramadol, can be added (Cashmore et al., 2009; Finnerup et al., 2009). If pain is still uncontrolled, an opioid should be considered. Each drug should be trialed for 2–4 weeks, because many require titration to achieve the desired effects.

In the past, opioids were considered to be ineffective in the treatment of chronic neuropathic pain; however, there is now evidence suggesting that some human individuals and some chronic neuropathic pain syndromes respond well to opioid therapy (Pergolizzi et al., 2008). Combination therapies have been shown to be more effective than using individual drug therapy in humans and dogs (Lascelles et al., 2008; Selph et al., 2011).

Breakthrough Pain

Breakthrough pain (also referred to as flares or flare-ups) occurs when a patient with chronic pain experiences transient flares of severe or excruciating pain, although the chronic pain is controlled. If a pain flare occurs regularly at the end of the medication period, just before the next dose is due, it is probably not BTP but a sign that the dosing interval needs to be altered.

The episodes of BTP can be a few seconds in duration, or may continue for minutes to hours, vary in frequency, and the onset can be sudden or gradual (Portenoy & Hagen, 1990). The pain may be so intense that the animal may scream or be unable to move, and they may also bite themselves or others. To treat episodes of BTP, the owner should have a "rescue" medicine, such as an opioid or tramadol, available. Opioid patches can be used for longer episodes of BTP (e.g., fentanyl or buprenorphine patches), though time to effective drug concentrations should be considered and a faster onset drug, such as tramadol, should be administered in the interim.

Trigger Point Pain

Another type of chronic pain that should be considered in chronic pain syndromes is the chronic referred pain that comes from myofascial trigger points (MTrPs) (Chapter 14). Trigger points are small nodules or taut bands in muscle tissue and are usually present in approximately the same areas in all individuals (Figure 23.1) (Janssens, 1991). These MTrPs are called "active" when they elicit pain spontaneously or with movement, or "passive"/"latent" when they elicit pain only on manipulation (Simons et al., 1999).

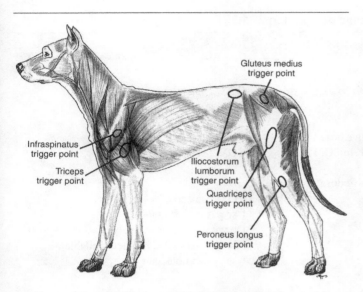

Figure 23.1. Common sites of myofascial trigger points in dogs (Janssens, 1991; Reprinted with permission).

MANAGEMENT OF CHRONIC PAIN

The goal when treating chronic pain is to provide effective analgesia with the fewest possible side effects. The goals of the owners, and the ability of the owner to assist with and pay for treatment must also be considered when formulating treatment plans. Realistic goals should be established with the input of the owner. It is important for the owners to know whether their pet will have to be treated for the next 3 months or the next 10 years. For example, OA will never be cured, and it generally deteriorates with time. In contrast, back pain due to spondylosis will nearly always get better when the bone bridge is stable, especially if there is no pressure on nerves. Because the expected duration varies, the importance of monitoring the treatment effect must be stressed. It is not ethical to continue medication if there is no treatment effect or if pain has resolved.

Multimodal Analgesia

Multimodal analgesia involves using drugs and modalities of various types to target different parts of the pain pathway, and is often referred to as balanced analgesia. When choosing a treatment protocol for a patient with chronic pain one must consider the type of pain (inflammatory, visceral, neuropathic, breakthrough, or some combination), the efficacy and duration of the proposed treatment versus its safety profile, and how the treatment response will be monitored. To minimize adverse effects, practitioners should combine as many low-risk drugs/modalities as possible with as few high-risk drugs/modalities as possible to achieve analgesia.

When treating chronic pain there are numerous modalities available, including surgery, analgesic drugs (e.g., NSAIDs, opioids, local anesthetics, anticonvulsants, antidepressants), physical modalities (e.g., TENS, acupuncture, physical therapy, laser therapy), dietary intervention (diet, nutraceuticals, supplements), and a number of old and new "alternative" treatments (e.g., magnetic field therapy, stem cell therapy, manipulation therapies). Making an evidence-based decision on what treatment to use may not be simple, as many of these therapies lack rigorous scientific evaluation, although many are supported by long-standing practice (Lamont, 2008a; 2008b; Greene, 2010; Grubb, 2010a, 2010b, 2010c; Rychel, 2010). There is strong evidence to support the use of some of the most commonly used NSAIDs, and some other therapies have moderate or weak evidence (Aragon et al., 2007; Mathews, 2008;, Sanderson et al., 2009).

PHARMACOLOGICAL CONTROL OF CHRONIC PAIN IN DOGS

Many different classes of analgesics can be used to treat canine patients suffering from chronic pain. Most of the pharmacological treatments described here are presented in Tables 23.1 and 23.2.

Nonsteroidal Anti-inflammatory Drugs

At the time of writing there are seven FDA approved NSAIDs (Table 23.1) (Chapter 5) on the US market for treatment of dogs with chronic pain, with a few more licensed in Canada, Europe, Australia, South America, and Asia. All have proven to be effective for the inflammatory component of chronic pain, and none appears to be more effective or safer (Gibofsky et al., 2003).

If there are no contraindications, NSAIDs are often the first choice in a patient suffering from chronic pain, with other analgesics and treatments added as needed. There are individual differences in patient responses to NSAIDs, so it may be necessary to try a few different NSAIDs in order to find the one that is best tolerated and most effective (Papich, 2008). If no improvement in chronic pain is seen after 10 days of treatment, the current NSAID administration should be stopped. A new NSAID can be tried after a 5–7-day washout period (Lascelles et al., 2005a, 2005b). If NSAIDs do not improve pain behaviors, it should be suspected that an inflammatory pain component is lacking and other analgesics should be tried. If the NSAID provided some relief, other classes of analgesics may be added.

All the currently FDA approved NSAIDs for dogs are COX-1 sparing/COX-2 selective. Nevertheless, all NSAIDs, regardless of COX-1/COX-2 specificity, are capable of producing vomiting, diarrhea, decreased appetite, gastrointestinal lesions and ulcers, and hepatic and renal injuries (Papich, 2008). Before starting any patient on an NSAID, it is advisable to evaluate renal and hepatic functions. A thorough history is also required to ensure that the dog is not taking any other steroidal or nonsteroidal drugs, including herbal formulations (e.g., pine bark or grape seed extracts, *Boswellia serrata*) or nephro- or hepatotoxic medicines (e.g., aminoglycosides). Gastroprotectants (e.g., omeprazole, famotidine, or misoprostol) should be considered when NSAIDs are used for more than a week. If mild gastrointestinal signs develop and persist for more than 1-2 days the NSAID should be discontinued. Another NSAID can be tried after a 5–7-day washout period (Lascelles et al., 2005a, 2005b), but pain will need to be treated during the washout period with other classes of analgesics and/or physical modalities. The ideal washout period is not known and the current recommendations are based on the elimination half-lives of NSAIDs. Most adverse effects of NSAIDs are dose dependent, so using the lowest effective dose is important (Papich, 2008).

There are some NSAIDs that are thought to work via COX-3 inhibition, and, therefore, cause fewer adverse effects. Metamizole (dipyrone), a potent analgesic frequently used in human patients

Table 23.1. Anti-inflammatory drugs used in treating chronic pain in dogs

Drug	Dose and duration of use	Comments
COX-1 and COX-2 inhibitor NSAIDs		
Meloxicam	Start 0.2 mg/kg, follow with 0.1 mg/kg q24h; PO, SC, IV Long-term use ≤ 0.1 mg/kg Use long term at lowest effective dose	COX-2 selective
Carprofen	4.4 mg/kg q24h; 2.2 mg/kg q12h; PO, IV, SC Use long term at lowest effective dose	COX-2 selective
Nimesulide	5 mg/kg q24h 3–5d PO	COX-2 selective
Aspirin	10–20 mg/kg q12h PO	Use gastroprotectant Do not use perioperatively Not recommended if other available
Ketoprofen	0.25 mg/kg q24h PO up to 30d 1–2 mg/kg q24h PO max 4–5d; 2 mg/kg q24h SC, IM, IV max 3d	Use gastroprotectant
Etodolac	10–15 mg/kg q24h PO	COX-1 selective Use gastroprotectant Can cause keratoconjunctivitis sicca
Tolfenamic acid	4 mg/kg q24h IM, SC max 2d 4 mg/kg q24h PO max 4d Can dose 3–4 days on and 3–4 days off for several weeks	
Coxibs		
Firocoxib	5 mg/kg q24h PO	COX-2 selective Liver disease potentially leads to overdosing with prolonged use
Deracoxib	High dose 3–4 mg/kg q24h PO 7 d max Long-term 1–2 mg/kg q24h PO Avoid long-term use of high dose	COX-2 selective
Robenacoxib	1–2 mg/kg q24h PO; 2 mg/kg q24h SC max 2 doses	COX-2 selective Do not administer together with food
Mavacoxib	2 mg/kg start q14d PO then q1month, max 7 doses First treatment provides 14 days of analgesia; thereafter each treatment gives 30 days of analgesia. Do not administer more than 6 months in a row. Can be re-started after a 1-month break	COX-2 selective Do not administer to animals under 5 kg or under 1 year of age, or to pregnant animals Always give with main meal If serious adverse effects occur, they may be long-acting and cannot be reversed
Dual inhibitors		
Tepoxalin	Start at 10–20 mg/kg q24h then 10 mg/kg q24h PO	COX/LOX dual inhibitor Give with food
COX-3 inhibitor		
Metamizole (dipyrone)	25(–100) mg/kg q8h PO, IV slowly Avoid IM and SC Sold as a singular or in Buscopan Compositum (butylscopolamine 4 mg/mL and metamizole 500 mg/mL)	Do not combine with chlorpromazine or barbiturates For spastic somatic and visceral chronic pain Injection site reactions Few GI or hepatic adverse effects Agranulocytosis in humans (very rare)

(continued)

Table 23.1. (*Continued*)

Drug	Dose and duration of use	Comments
Acetaminophen (Paracetamol)	10–15 mg/kg q8h–q12h PO q12h IV Long-term ≤10 mg/kg q12h Short-term 5 days Long-term months	Weak anti-inflammatory effects Toxic over 100 mg/kg. NEVER USE IN CATS! Possible serotonin syndrome candidate Few GI or hepatic adverse effects Can be used in patients with GI and renal problems and thrombocytopenia Can be used with other NSAIDs Synergism with opioids
Diclofenac	Topical cream over joint q12h and ≤10 days Treat only one joint at a time	Use rubber gloves when applying cream
SAIDs/Corticosteroids		
Dexamethasone	0.01–0.15 mg/kg q24h PO, SC, IM, IV 3–5 days max	Risk of GI ulceration if used with NSAIDs
Prednisolone	1.0–2.2 mg/kg q12–24h PO taper down to 0.25 mg/kg q48h, ≤7 days	Risk of GI ulceration if used with NSAIDs
Prednisone	1.0–2.2 mg/kg q12–24h PO taper down to 0.25 mg/kg q48h, 0.5 mg/kg q12–24h PO together with gabapentin or pregabalin for syringomyelia	Risk of GI ulceration if used with NSAIDs
Trimacinolone	10–20 mg/joint IA in severe OA Do not inject same joint more than 3 times	Risk of GI ulceration if used with NSAIDs
Methyl-prednisolone	10–20 mg/joint IA in severe OA Do not inject same joint more than three times	Risk of GI ulceration if used with NSAIDs

All drugs listed above are not available in all countries and some are not approved for the use in dogs. Some have been approved and tested for efficacy in canine inflammatory pain or osteoarthritis but are also used in other types of chronic pain. The doses listed come from the product leaflets, from the author's experience as well as from other people working with chronic pain, from references cited in the text and from books on pain management (adapted from Flecknell & Waterman-Pearson, 2000; Tranquilli et al., 2007; Gaynor & Muir III, 2009; Ramsey, 2011). Dosages should be taken as general guidelines as individual variations exist. Clinical judgment should always determine the final dose used. To avoid typical NSAID adverse effects, doctors should strive to find the smallest clinically effective dose and use multimodal analgesia (e.g., combined with nutraceuticals, acupuncture, TENS, laser, etc.).

COX, cyclooxygenase; COX/LOX, cyclooxygenase/lipoxygenase; GI, gastrointestinal; IA, intra-articular; IM, intramuscular; IV, intravenous; NSAID, nonsteroidal anti-inflammatory drug; OA, osteoarthritis; PO, per os (oral); SAID, steroidal anti-inflammatory drug; SC, subcutaneous.

in some countries, was banned in other countries because it was reported to be associated with severe adverse effects in some older studies. More recent studies have questioned those results and appropriate dosages have recently been tested in dogs (Imagawa et al., 2011).

Because of the potential adverse effects, there is a constant debate as to the duration of NSAID treatment for the chronically painful patient. A systematic review ($n = 1575$) suggested that there is clinical benefit of longer-term (≥4 weeks) NSAID use in dogs suffering from osteoarthritic pain (Innes et al., 2010), although careful monitoring is critical. In a study of outpatients with pain ($n = 1153$), 89% of dogs with chronic pain received NSAIDs, and only 63% of owners of these dogs considered the treatment to be effective (Muir et al., 2004). A similar study of nonsurgically treated dogs with hip dysplasia and chronic pain due to OA showed that at least 40.5% of the dogs were on an NSAID (duration ranging from 1 month to 12 years with a median duration 2 years and 7 months), with 70% of those dogs requiring daily dosing. However, 35.7% of the owners of the dogs receiving NSAIDs reported that the medication had no or little effect (Farrell et al., 2007). Although these results may partly be due to the fact that owners cannot assess pain, they do emphasize the need for continuous monitoring of chronic pain patients for adverse effects and efficacy. Habituation to NSAIDs has never been reported in humans or animals; thus,

Table 23.2. Adjuvants used in canine chronic pain

Drug	Canine dosing schedule (mg/kg)	Indications	Care/Contraindications	Possible adverse effects
Antidepressants				
Amitriptyline	1–2 mg/kg q12–24h PO Onset 10—14 days Trial at least 4 weeks Duration of treatment indefinite	Adjunctive analgesic in chronic pain such as OA and neoplasia, neuropathic pain. Especially good if anxiety, depression present	Can contribute to serotonin syndrome Caution with glaucoma, epilepsy, urinary retention, cardiac and renal patients	Sedation, excitability, dry mouth, vomiting, hypotension, syncope, weight gain reported in humans
Imipramine	0.5–1 mg/kg q8h; 1–2 mg/kg q12h; 2–4 mg/kg q24h PO	As above	As above	As above but less sedating
Clomipramine	1–2 mg/kg q12h PO The only TCA authorized for canine use Duration of treatment usually 8–12 weeks, even longer	Indicated only for separation anxiety but can be tried for chronic pain such as OA and neoplasia pain Neuropathic pain	As above Not recommended for male breeding dogs (testicular hypoplasia) May also potentiate quinidine, coumarin, sympathomimetics	Very seldom any adverse effects but can cause GI upset or lethargy
Anticonvulsants				
Gabapentin	10–60 mg/kg q8–24h PO (start with 5–10 mg/kg q12h) If patient also taking antacid, give Gabapentin 2 hours after Trial at least 4 weeks Duration of treatment indefinite Many patients require TID dosing	Neuropathic pain, allodynia, hyperalgesia. Adjunctive analgesic in chronic pain such as OA, amputees, syringomyelia, large areas of tissue damage, chronic wounds	Care with patients with renal or hepatic disease	Mild but in 25% of patients: drowsiness, ataxia Rare GI signs: nausea, anorexia, vomiting With time, adverse effects usually disappear.
Pregabalin	3–4 mg/kg q8–12h PO (start with 2 mg/kg q12h) Trial at least 4 weeks Duration of treatment indefinite	Neuropathic pain, allodynia, hyperalgesia. Adjunctive analgesic in chronic pain such as OA, amputees, syringomyelia/chiari, large areas of tissue damage	Do not use in pregnant animals	Many dogs develop drowsiness, sedation, ataxia. With time, adverse effects usually disappear. Hepatic enzymes might rise with long-term dosing.

NMDA antagonists

Drug	Dose	Indication	Cautions	Adverse effects
Amantadine	3–5 mg/kg q24h PO Onset of effect in 7–14 days Combine with an NSAID ± opioid Duration of treatment weeks to years Pulse therapy of 1–2 weeks as needed	Adjunctive analgesic in chronic pain Neuropathic pain, wind-up, opioid tolerant patients	Not known May induce serotonin syndrome	Rare, can include agitation, GI upset or diarrhea during first few days
Orphenadrine + Acetaminophen (paracetamol)	Dose according to acetaminophen 10–15 mg/kg q8–12h PO 1–3 days Can be given longer No research on long-term use	Spinal pain due to muscle spasm	Caution with dosing to avoid overdosage of either drug	Orphenadrine can lead to cardiac and respiratory arrest. See also Table 23.2 for acetaminophen.

α-2 adrenoreceptor agonists

Drug	Dose	Indication	Cautions	Adverse effects
Dexmedetomidine	IV bolus 0.0005–0.001 mg/kg CRI 0.0005–0.001 mg/kg/h; 3–5 µg/kg IM, SC, IV in combination with opioid	In hospital, breakthrough pain management, adjunct to opioid	Care with geriatrics, diabetes and cardiac patients Use in normovolemic patients	Sedation, muscle relaxation Vomiting common
Medetomidine	0.001 mg/kg IV; 0.002–0.015 mg/kg IM; CRI 0.0005–0.001 mg/kg/h 10–20 µg/kg in combination with an opioid IM, SC, IV	In hospital, breakthrough pain management, adjunct to opioid	As above	As above
Tizanidine	3 mg/d PO; 125 µg/h IT Start with low dose and titrate to effect	PO for muscle spasms, degenerative disc disease BTP: IT	Adverse effects decline with use	In humans: drowsiness, sedation

Sodium channel blockers

Drug	Dose	Indication	Cautions	Adverse effects
Lidocaine	4 mg/kg IM; 1–2 mg/kg IA; ED 2–8 mg/kg IV in 2 mg/kg boluses followed by a CRI of 0.025–0.1 mg/kg/min, T, I, NB, ED, S, TDP 5% Max total dose 7–8 mg/kg of 2% lidocaine, 2 mg/kg q4–6h PO in esophagitis	Local, regional and systemic analgesia, e.g., chronic nerve root or facet joint pain. Also together with corticosteroids As TDP in chronic pain. BTP: CRI, ED	Do not overdose. Care with lidocaine preparations that include epinephrine Concurrent cimetidine and propranolol may prolong lidocaine clearance.	CNS toxicity, seizures, depression, muscle trembling Cardiovascular depression
Mepivacaine	0.25–5 mL/ joint, depending on joint size Duration 2–4 h	Local, perineural, IA Less irritating and less vasodilatory effects than Lidocaine	Max total not known Do not use IV	As above

(continued)

Table 23.2. (Continued)

Drug	Canine dosing schedule (mg/kg)	Indications	Care/Contraindications	Possible adverse effects
Bupivacaine	1–2 mg/kg; ED SC, IP, NB, I, 1–2.3 mg/kg S, max 2 mg/kg IA. Duration 4–8 h Perineural 1–2 mL of 0.5% solution	For chronic nerve pain; nerve impingement, facet joint pain Also together with corticosteroids BTP: ED	Max total dose 2 mg/kg of 0.5% bupivacaine Do not use IV	
TRPV1 agonists				
Capsaicin	Transdermal as 0.025 or 0.075% cream, q6h Treat for a minimum of 4 weeks	Chronic muscle or joint pain, in animals that do not tolerate NSAIDs or opioids	Do not allow dog to lick the area. Owner should use gloves.	Can irritate skin
Resiniferatoxin	1 μg/kg IT over 10 min, followed by 0.2 mL sterile saline (under general anesthesia) Treatment effect 2–3 months	For unrelieved chronic pain in drug tolerant patients		
Muscle relaxants/Tranquilizers				
Diazepam	For skeletal muscle relaxation: 2–10 mg/kg PO q8h; 0.5–1 mg/kg IV slowly Do not dilute or mix	Especially spinal pain due to muscle cramps Can help visceral pain Alone or together with NSAID or TCA Tolerance may develop in long-term use	Not recommended with hepatic disease, CNS or respiratory depression, severe muscle weakness Interacts with opioids, antihistamines and digoxin	In humans sedation, muscle weakness, ataxia Interferes with memory

The table list adjuvants and other analgesics used in hospital settings in cases of breakthrough pain episodes as well as drugs that can be sent home with the patient. Dosages should be taken as general guidelines as individual variations exist. Clinical judgment should always determine the final dose used. All drugs listed are not available in all countries and most of the drugs above are not approved for use in dogs. Local and national laws may also restrict the use of some combination analgesics that include opioids, for dogs. Some of the drugs above have been approved and tested for efficacy in some specific canine conditions but are also used in other chronic pain conditions using extrapolated doses. The doses listed come from the author's experience as well as from other people working with chronic pain, from references cited in the text and from books of pain management (Flecknell & Waterman-Pearson, 2000; Tranquilli et al., 2007; Gaynor & Muir III, 2009; Ramsey, 2011).

BTP, breakthrough pain; CRI, constant rate infusion; ED, epidural; GI, gastrointestinal; I, infiltration; IC, intercostal; IM, intramuscular; IP, intrapleural; IT, intrathecal; IV, intravenous; NB, nerve block; OA, osteoarthritis; PO, per os (oral); S, spinal; SC, subcutaneous; T, topical; TCA, tricyclic antidepressants; TDP, transdermal patch; OTM, oral transmucosal.

if an NSAID stops working it is more probable that it is the type of chronic pain that has changed, and the pain is no longer primarily inflammatory in nature.

Information on dosing, indications, and adverse effects of the NSAIDs recommended for chronic pain can be found in Table 23.1.

CARPROFEN

Carprofen is a COX-2 selective NSAID available as a tablet and an injectable formulation and approved for chronic pain management and orthopedic and soft tissue surgery in Australia, Europe, and North America. It can be given to dogs as young as 6 weeks of age.

Two meta-analyses have evaluated the evidence of effect of carprofen and found it to be strong for treatment of dogs with OA (Aragon et al., 2007; Sanderson et al., 2009). Successful treatment effects were seen in about 65% of patients after 2 weeks and in 74% at 12 weeks, the rest reported no change or worsening pain (Mansa et al., 2007). The response seemed to be better in less severe cases, when the main type of pain was likely to be inflammatory in nature. The response was significantly poorer in dogs with lameness of 6-month duration or longer compared with those with lameness of 6-month duration or less (Mansa et al., 2007).

Carprofen is associated with the typical NSAID adverse effects, and gastrointestinal toxicity and idiopathic hepatotoxicity have been reported (MacPhail et al., 1998; Moreau et al., 2003). A combined adverse effect incidence of 3–6% has been suggested (Moreau et al., 2003; Raekallio et al., 2006; Mansa et al., 2007). In one study, mild adverse effects (including adipsia, polydipsia, anorexia, anxiety, constipation, diarrhea, and emesis) were reported in 34% of the trial dogs (Pollmeier et al., 2006). Carprofen has some limited positive effects on the synthesis of aggrecan in an *in vitro* model (Benton et al., 1997). Pelletier et al. (2000) reported a delay in the development of abnormal subchondral osteoblasts, although the significance of this is unclear.

MELOXICAM

Meloxicam is COX-2 selective NSAID approved for canine OA in the United States, and for acute and chronic canine musculoskeletal pain and inflammation in Europe. It is available as an oral liquid or an injectable formulation, and can be given to dogs over 6 weeks of age, except in the United States where dogs must be older than 6 months. Two systematic reviews evaluated 5 and 7 clinical trials on meloxicam for OA in dogs. Evidence exists for the efficacy of meloxicam, supporting a strong relationship between its use and decrease in OA pain (Aragon et al., 2007; Sanderson et al., 2009). The adverse effects may be less severe for meloxicam than for some other NSAIDs (Mathews et al., 1999; Poulsen Nautrep & Justus, 1999; Boston et al., 2003; Moreau et al., 2003; Brainard et al., 2007), although one study found carprofen to have fewer adverse effects (Luna et al., 2007). Dose reduction resulted in less effective pain control (Wernham et al., 2011).

ETODOLAC

Etodolac is mostly COX-1 selective, and is available in tablet form. It is approved for chronic pain associated with OA, for dogs 12 months or older in the United States. Etodolac has been shown to be effective as an analgesic for chronic pain due to OA in dogs in several studies (Budsberg et al., 1999; Hanson et al., 2006), and was moderately effective in two reviews (Aragon et al., 2007; Sanderson et al., 2009).

Aside from the expected adverse events associated with NSAIDs, keratoconjunctivitis sicca (KCS) has been reported when using etodolac in dogs (Klauss et al., 2007). The incidence of diarrhea in two clinical trials was 2.6% (Budsberg et al., 1999) and 8.3% (Hanson et al., 2006), respectively.

FIROCOXIB

Firocoxib is a COX-2 specific inhibitor that is only available as a chewable tablet form. It is approved for the treatment of chronic pain associated with OA, and for 3 days after soft tissue surgery. It can be administered to dogs 7 months of age or older. Firocoxib is associated with the same adverse effects as other NSAIDs. It was considered effective for canine OA pain in a recent systematic review (Sanderson et al., 2009). In two studies where firocoxib was compared to carprofen ($n = 218$) or etodolac ($n = 249$), firocoxib was associated with 14% and 19% fewer health problems, respectively, although none of the treatments were associated with clinically significant adverse effects (Hanson et al., 2004; Pollmeier et al., 2006). Firocoxib also had a significantly better treatment effect than carprofen after 30 days (Pollmeier et al., 2006). When administered to geriatric dogs with OA ($n = 54$) there were few adverse effects (diarrhea, vomiting, dark feces, and anorexia) after 3 months of treatment, and the treatment effect was positively time dependent. In a recent long-term efficacy study of 39 dogs, 5.1% were withdrawn because of adverse GI effects, 82% showed improvement by day 15, and 96% of the 25 dogs that remained in the study had improved by day 360 (Autefage et al., 2011).

DERACOXIB

Deracoxib, a COX-2 specific NSAID, is available as a chewable tablet, and is approved for OA and orthopedic surgery in North America and Europe for dogs as young as 4 months of age. In a 6-week long study it was found to be better than placebo for chronic pain due to canine OA.

Although Deracoxib is COX-1 sparing (McCann et al., 2004), a case series reported 29 cases of gastrointestinal tract perforations in a 2-year study period (Lascelles et al., 2005a). Most cases were associated with either concurrent steroid or NSAID use, or use of the larger, postoperative dose (3–4 mg/kg). Another case series reported that three dogs developed duodenal perforation, and two of these had received the approved dosage (Case et al., 2010). In a 28-day randomized controlled trial of eight dogs administered 1.5 mg/kg Deracoxib q12h, only one dog had severe diarrhea in the treatment group, and no other adverse effects were noted (Sennello & Leib, 2006). Interestingly, Deracoxib (2 mg/kg q24h) increased coagulability in dogs with OA (Brainard et al., 2007).

ROBENACOXIB

Robenacoxib, a COX-2 specific inhibitor, is available as a chewable tablet, and is approved for OA and orthopedic surgery in North America and Europe for dogs as young as 3 months of age. It should not be given to dogs less than 2.5 kg of body weight and should not be given with food. As it is quite new, it has not yet been evaluated in any of the recent NSAID reviews.

MAVACOXIB

Mavacoxib is the newest of the coxib NSAIDs and has a unique dosing schedule due to its long duration of action. The second dose is given 2 weeks after the first dose, and subsequent doses are given every 4 weeks. Its half-life in the dog is as long as 80 days, thus, one should be absolutely certain that there are no contraindications to the use of NSAIDs prior to administering mavacoxib. As a precaution, it is recommended that serum chemistry and urinalysis be repeated prior to administering the third tablet. It should not be given to dogs less than 1 year of age or less than 5 kg body weight, nor to dogs that are known to be allergic to sulfonamides. It should be given with food.

As it is quite new, it has not yet been evaluated in any of the recent NSAID reviews.

TEPOXALIN

Tepoxalin inhibits COX-1, COX-2, and lipoxygenase (Agnello et al., 2005), and is approved for treatment of dogs with OA that are older than 6 months of age. In an *in vitro* study, tepoxalin significantly reduced cartilage loss (Macrory et al., 2009). There are no studies evaluating the efficacy of this drug in chronic canine pain. Tepoxalin causes few adverse effects (Knight et al., 1996; Kay-Mugford et al., 2004; Punke et al., 2008).

TOLFENAMIC ACID

Tolfenamic acid is not approved for use in dogs in the United States, but it is approved for OA and chronic pain in Canada and some European countries. It is available as a tablet form and as an injectable solution for subcutaneous administration. It is approved for dogs over 6 weeks of age. It has an unusual dosing schedule of 3–4 days on and 3–4 days off. No studies evaluating its treatment effect in chronic canine pain are available. Adverse effects associated with its use include diarrhea and occasional vomiting.

KETOPROFEN AND VEDAPROFEN

Ketoprofen and vedaprofen are COX-1 and COX-2 inhibitors and come in tablet form only. Neither of them is approved for use in dogs in the United States. Both are approved in Canada and in some European countries for OA pain, and for 3 days after soft tissue surgery in dogs over 6 months of age. Neither is recommended for chronic use.

ACETAMINOPHEN (PARACETAMOL)

Acetaminophen (paracetamol) is not approved for dogs anywhere in the world, though oral formulations also containing codeine are approved in some countries. When appropriately dosed acetaminophen has a good safety record and can be efficacious in the treatment of chronic pain in dogs, particularly dogs that do not tolerate NSAIDs. It is thought to be COX-3 (a COX-1 variant) selective and lacks anti-inflammatory effects at recommended doses. In a Cochrane meta-analysis, it was concluded that traditional NSAIDs are superior to acetaminophen for OA pain in humans (Towheed et al., 2006). However, with chronic visceral pain, especially where there is need for a gastrointestinal sparing drug, acetaminophen can be useful. It is often coadministered with opioids, and is found in proprietary combination formulas with orphenadrine, codeine, or oxycodone, although the bioavailability of oral opioids in dogs is low. Adverse events, although uncommon, are mostly associated with the gastrointestinal system (Manley, 1995). Acetaminophen can be administered to patients with gastric ulcers (Ramsey, 2011). Renal toxicity is also uncommon, but hepatic damage can occur in dogs (Lascelles & Gaynor, 2007; Ramsey, 2011). Toxicity has not been reported in dogs until the dosage exceeds 100 mg/kg (Mburu et al., 1988).

In humans, the EULAR hip OA guidelines recommend acetaminophen as the oral analgesic of first choice for mild to moderate pain and, if successful, as the preferred long-term oral analgesic because of its efficacy and safety (Zhang et al., 2005). There are, however, no studies of the chronic use of acetaminophen in dogs.

Corticosteroids

Corticosteroids are available as injectable and tablet formulations, and are approved for OA and orthopedic surgery in North America and Europe in dogs at least 5 months of age. Due to adverse effects, corticosteroids are seldom used for the treatment of dogs with chronic pain. Short-term (1–3 weeks) relief of chronic knee pain was reported after intra-articular injection of corticosteroids in human patients (Bellamy et al., 2006). However, impaired chondrocyte function and prolonged proteoglycan and collagen inhibition have also been reported (Chunekamrrai et al., 1989). Triamcinolone hexacetonide is superior to betamethasone for analgesia and few adverse effects were reported (Bellamy et al., 2006). Corticosteroids have also been used in combination with local anesthetics in intra-articular injections and peripheral nerve blocks in humans (Kinzel et al., 2003).

In a recent study, intrathecal administration of methylprednisolone acetate, a treatment used in humans for chronic pain syndromes, caused meningeal inflammation and is no longer recommended (Rijsdijk et al., 2012). Some of the adverse effects of corticosteroids are similar to those of NSAIDs, and therefore, they should not be administered concurrently. Due to a relatively short duration of effect and potential adverse effects, the intra-articular injection of corticosteroids is controversial.

Local and Regional Anesthetic Techniques

Local anesthesia techniques are often used to provide perioperative analgesia, but are less commonly used to treat chronic pain syndromes. Local anesthetic blocks can assist in diagnosis and treatment of chronic pain, such as that due to facet joint OA and nerve root compression. In humans, articular facet joint arthrosis and nerve root compression affect 79% of patients with lower back or neck pain (Halla & Hardin, 1987). A study of nine dogs reported the results of infiltrating facet joints with uni- or bilateral arthroses with a combination of trimacinolone (10 mg per facet joint) and lidocaine hydrochloride (20 mg per facet joint) (Kinzel et al., 2003). Seven out of the nine dogs were pain free 4 months after a single injection. Thus, the modality warrants further study.

Analgesic Adjuvants

Often, chronic pain cannot be managed with NSAIDs alone and adjunctive analgesics (Table 23.2) are needed.

ANTIDEPRESSANT DRUGS

There are four main groups of antidepressants that have been used in chronic pain in dogs: TCAs, selective serotonin reuptake inhibitors (SSRIs), SNRIs, and monoamine oxidase inhibitors (MAOIs) (Chapter 8). Although antidepressants are often the drug of choice for neuropathic pain, there are potential problems with their use, including serotonin syndrome (Chapter 8) and withdrawal symptoms. Serotonin syndrome results from an excess of serotonin,

Table 23.3. Drugs implicated in development of serotonin syndrome

Drug class	Drug and herbs
MAO inhibitors	Selegiline
Antiparasitics/Antibacterials	Amitraz, furazolidone (used off label for giardiosis)
Tricyclic antidepressants	Amitriptyline, clomipramine, imipramine
Tetracyclic antidepressants	Mirtazapine
SSRI, SNRI	Fluoxetine, sertraline, duloxetine, tramadol
NMDA antagonists	Dextromethorphan, amantadine
Opioids	Tramadol, fentanyl, buprenorphine, oxycodone, pethidine, methadone
Serotonin agonists	Tryptans
Certain herbs	St. John's Wort (*Hypericum perforatum*), Panax ginseng, nutmeg
Certain foods	Foods containing tryptophan (serotonin precursor)
Other	Metoclopramide, L-Dopa

MAO, monoamine oxidase; NMDA, N-methyl-D-aspartate; SSRI, selective serotonin reuptake inhibitor; SNRI, serotonin–norepinephrine reuptake inhibitor.

and is usually a consequence of administering more than one drug that affects serotonin reuptake and/or breakdown. The TCAs are highly metabolized by the cytochrome P450 hepatic enzymes and toxicity may be seen with concurrent administration of other drugs that inhibit cytochrome P450 (such as cimetidine and calcium channel blockers). Drugs that one should avoid using together are listed in Table 23.3. It is still unclear if giving these medications with foods that contain large amounts of L-tryptophan, the precursor of serotonin, is contraindicated. Although there are no reports of serotonin syndrome in dogs given recommended doses of antidepressants, it has been reported in dogs after accidental ingestion (Johnson, 1990).

Patients should be slowly tapered off TCAs, SSRIs, SNRIs, and MAOIs to avoid withdrawal syndrome. Symptoms of withdrawal in humans include paresthesia, dizziness, tremors, insomnia, irritability, nightmares, movement disorders, and nausea. The dose should be tapered over a period of 2 weeks to several months, depending on the duration of administration. A total washout period of several weeks is also recommended before a new drug of the same category is administered.

The antidepressant drugs that have been used most frequently in chronic canine pain include amitriptyline, venlafaxine, imipramide, and clomipramine. Amitriptyline is used most frequently in dogs and clomipramine is the only one licensed for use in dogs, though not for chronic pain. Selegiline, an MAOI registered for cognitive dysfunction in dogs, will sometimes be efficacious for chronic pain when other drugs have not been (personal observation and anecdotal evidence).

Amitriptyline

Amitriptyline is frequently used off-label for chronic pain in dogs, especially when the pain has a neuropathic component. It is most often combined with other analgesics, as it is seldom efficacious when used alone. It is recommended that a low starting dose is used, and that the dose be slowly (every 3–7 days) titrated to effect. There are no randomized clinical trials of these drugs in dogs, but some case reports have been published (Cashmore et al., 2009). Mild adverse events include drowsiness, dizziness, excitement, and agitation (Grubb, 2010a), which may be more severe in patients receiving more than one drug of the same class.

ANTICONVULSANT DRUGS

Gabapentin and Pregabalin

Gabapentin and pregabalin are the anticonvulsant drugs that have been used most frequently for treating dogs with chronic pain (Chapter 8). Animal studies report that although gabapentin does not affect the nociceptive threshold, it is effective in reducing both allodynia and hyperalgesia, suggesting that it has a selective effect on the nociceptive process involved in central sensitization (Nicholson, 2000). Pregabalin has similar effects in dogs, but no studies have been published, and anecdotal evidence is sparse.

No randomized clinical trials have been published to date, but Wolfe and Poma (2010) reported a significant reduction in cervical hyperesthesia in two chronically painful dogs with syringomyelia, each receiving gabapentin and prednisone (at anti-inflammatory doses). The dogs were eventually tapered off prednisone but remained on gabapentin. In another case, neuropathic pain due to a suspected nerve root avulsion was successfully treated with gabapentin (Cashmore et al., 2009). Combining NSAIDs, opioids, and low-dose gabapentin with low-dose imipramine gave effective aid in human neuropathic cancer pain patients (Arai et al., 2010).

During the first weeks of administration gabapentin may cause sedation, nausea, and vomiting (Greene, 2010). To minimize sedation, gabapentin should be administered at low doses initially, slowly increasing the dose until effective analgesia is achieved. Most patients are dosed every 8 hours, but patients with compromised liver or renal function may only require twice daily dosing or less (Vollmer et al., 1986; Radulovic et al., 1995).

N-METHYL-D-ASPARTATE (NMDA) RECEPTOR ANTAGONISTS

Activation of the NMDA receptor is responsible for the development of central sensitization, hyperalgesia, and allodynia, and NMDA receptor antagonists are known to be antihyperalgesic; thus, they may be useful for treating patients with chronic pain. NMDA receptor antagonists also increase opioid receptor sensitivity, reduce opioid tolerance, and minimize opioid rebound hyperalgesia. Intravenous infusions of ketamine in humans have resulted in short- to long-term improvements in neuropathic pain (Kapural et al., 2009).

Amantadine

Amantadine is the most commonly used NMDA receptor antagonist for chronic pain conditions in dogs. It was developed as an antiviral drug in humans. Because it is antihyperalgesic it may be helpful in patients with long-lasting, poorly managed chronic pain, and is especially efficacious in preventing dorsal horn "wind-up." It can be used alone or with NSAIDs. A small study in dogs demonstrated high bioavailability of orally administered amantadine and a half-life of 8 hours (Bleidner et al., 1965). In one clinical study in dogs, amantadine was used with NSAIDs for chronic pain, and had a synergistic effect with NSAIDs (Lascelles et al., 2008).

α-2 Agonists

Tizanidine hydrochloride and clonidine hydrochloride have both been used in dogs for the treatment of painful muscle spasms, and tizanidine had fewer adverse effects (Kroin et al., 2003).

Opioids

Opioids (Table 23.4) are not practical for long-term use in chronic pain, as they have adverse effects and tolerance may develop over time. The pure μ agonists are the most efficacious and are indicated for severe BTP in patients with chronic pain conditions such as OA or back pain (Pergolizzi et al., 2008). However, a recent Cochrane study evaluated randomized controlled trials ($n = 2268$) of oral and transdermal opioids (excluding tramadol) for human hip or knee OA. The small to moderate beneficial effects of opioids were outweighed by large increases in the risk of adverse events. It was concluded that opioids should not be routinely used, even if OA pain is severe (Nuesch et al., 2010).

Recently, some studies on the use of opioids to treat neuropathic pain have been published (Simpson et al., 2007). A meta-analysis ($n = 6019$) of human patients, 80% with inflammatory pain and 12% with neuropathic pain, concluded that potent opioids, such as morphine and oxycodone, were significantly more efficacious than naproxen and amitriptyline for pain relief. Although constipation and nausea were the only clinically and statistically significant adverse effects, 33% of patients abandoned the trials (Furlan et al., 2006).

In humans, nausea and vomiting are common when beginning administration, but tolerance develops, usually in 1–2 weeks. Constipation, on the other hand, rarely disappears, so laxatives or high fiber foods should be administered when using opioids. Other potential adverse effects include excitement, respiratory depression, panting, cough suppression, bradycardia, histamine release, defecation, constipation, and urinary retention (Pettifer & Dyson, 2000).

Morphine withdrawal has been studied in the dog, as a model for human withdrawal syndrome. The clinical signs include hyperactivity, biting, digging, tremors, nausea, hyperthermia, increased wakefulness, and tachycardia and hypertension (Yoshimura et al., 1993). In addition, there was EEG evidence of activation in the amygdala and hippocampus, followed by dissociation of the EEG in the cortex (fast wave) from that in the limbic (slow wave) system (Yoshimura et al., 1993). These clinical signs can be misdiagnosed as pain when tapering a patient off opioids. Adequate analgesia, using drugs from other classes or other analgesic modalities, must be provided when weaning a dog off opioids.

Morphine and Oxycodone

Morphine is formulated in tablets (providing 2–4 hours of analgesia), oral liquids, and injectable solutions. Sustained release tablets provide up to 12 hours of analgesia and may be suitable for treatment of chronic pain, especiallyBTP, at home. Morphine and oxycodone have been recommended for oral administration (Gaynor, 2008), but conflicting data indicate that these drugs are less effective in dogs due to poor oral bioavailability and lack of active metabolites (Weinstein & Gaylord, 1979; Yoshimura et al., 1993; KuKanich et al., 2005). Other formulations can be used for severe BTP episodes in hospital settings.

No randomized clinical trials are available regarding the treatment of chronic pain in dogs with morphine or its synthetic derivatives. One study reported that intravenous oxymorphone and hydromorphone could be used, with similar effect, for treating dogs in pain. Hydromorphone, although cheaper, causes a greater incidence of vomiting in dogs (Pettifer & Dyson, 2000; Bateman et al., 2008).

Oral Codeine

Codeine has been recommended as an orally administered analgesic for dogs (Gaynor, 2008). Although codeine and the combination of codeine and acetaminophen are used in dogs suffering from chronic pain, the evidence for its efficacy is primarily anecdotal (KuKanich, 2010). Adverse effects are typical of those of opioids, and in the combination drug, acetaminophen-related adverse effects appear to be infrequent but hepatic damage, anemia, and methemoglobinemia have been reported (Grubb, 2010a).

Transdermal Fentanyl

The major advantage of a transdermal patch (Chapter 9) is that the dog can be cared for at home; disadvantages include the unpredictable plasma concentrations achieved and the cost (Hofmeister & Egger, 2004). The patches come in sizes ranging from 12.5 to 100 μg/h). It requires about 24 hours to achieve plasma fentanyl concentrations that are analgesic for dogs, and the patch provides analgesia for about 72 hours; if a longer period of analgesia is required the patch should be changed every 3 days (Egger et al., 1998).

Studies are published on the use of the fentanyl patch in dogs in the intra- or postoperative periods (Kyles et al., 1998; Robinson et al., 1999), but no clinical trials on use of the patch with chronic pain flare-ups are available. Most information comes from early pharmacological trials (Bailey et al., 1987; Schultheiss et al., 1995; Kyles et al., 1996; Egger et al., 1998; Kyles et al., 1998; Robinson et al., 1999; Pascoe, 2000; Welch et al., 2002), reviews (Hofmeister & Egger, 2004), or anecdotal use. There are some randomized clinical trials on the use of fentanyl patches for human chronic, noncancer pain (Dellemijn, 1998; Allan et al., 2001; Ringe et al., 2002; Jamison et al., 2003; Katz et al., 2003a, 2003b; Ackerman et al., 2004; Clark et al., 2004), but no trials of continuous use have been reported in dogs.

Anorexia, hyperthermia, sedation, and dysphoria were the most reported adverse events in early canine studies (Hofmeister & Egger, 2004). The patch should be removed if it causes skin irritation or other adverse reactions. An ingested patch can cause a lethal overdose, so dogs should wear an Elizabethan collar (Schmidt & Bjorling, 2007). As fentanyl is a pure μ agonist, its adverse effects can be reversed with naloxone, naltrexone, or nalorphine. The reversal agent may need to be administered several times to combat the adverse effects because the fentanyl plasma concentrations will decrease slowly after ingestion of a patch.

Transdermal Buprenorphine
Buprenorphine is available as a transdermal gel and patch (Chapter 9) and is adequate for mild to moderate pain. The buprenorphine patch is effective for 7 days in humans. In a canine trial there were no adverse effects and the dogs' appetite, weight, urination, and defecation remained normal (Pieper et al., 2011). In humans, buprenorphine seems to be the most efficacious opioid for the treatment of neuropathic pain (Pergolizzi et al., 2008).

Oral Tramadol
Tramadol (Chapter 4) is a centrally acting synthetic opiate that also acts through serotonergic and adrenergic pathways. Apart from its analgesic effects, it has mild antianxiety effects in humans and is efficacious for BTP with chronic pain syndromes. The pharmacokinetics of tramadol in the dog (McMillan et al., 2008) indicate a short half-life, thus, it should be dosed every 4–8 hours for adequate pain control. It is available as a tablet, an oral liquid, and an injectable formulation (in some countries).

No randomized clinical trials of tramadol use in chronic canine pain have been published, but there is a lot of anecdotal evidence that it is effective in dogs. Tramadol is usually well tolerated, but adverse effects, such as gastrointestinal upset, dysphoria, sedation, and aggression, have been observed. Large doses of tramadol may cause convulsions in dogs (Greene, 2010). However, in a study of healthy dogs ($n = 8$) premedicated with tramadol or morphine, tramadol produced no visible sedation and no vomiting (Guedes et al., 2005). In a pharmacokinetic study, 1, 2, and 3 mg/kg of tramadol was given to dogs IV. The dogs showed mild dose-related sedation but only one dog appeared to be nauseated (McMillan et al., 2008). Tramadol can cause serotonin syndrome in patients also receiving SSRI/SNRI drugs or MOA inhibitors. It is not advisable to combine these drugs. Tramadol is safe to use in patients with renal failure, but not in patients with liver failure, as it is metabolized by the liver.

Surgical Intervention
Surgery has the potential to relieve acute pain, such as in the case of nerve entrapment or intervertebral disc disease, and may be curative. In contrast, surgery for chronic pain is less likely to be completely successful as there are often secondary problems, such as an altered anatomy, altered neurophysiology and/or neuroendocrinology (e.g., disuse atrophy of nerve and muscle). Total joint replacements may be an exception.

Due to the availability of advanced imaging techniques such as computed tomography and magnetic resonance imaging that allow visualization of intervertebral disc degeneration, lumbosacral stenosis, cauda equina compression, and nerve root entrapment, diagnosis of the cause of chronic pain is often possible and individualized treatments can be planned. Current surgical therapies for chronic back pain include decompressive surgery and fixation and/or fusion techniques.

Improvement of degenerative lumbosacral stenosis pain treated by dorsal laminectomy ($n = 156$) occurred in 83 of 105 (79%) of dogs with follow-up data. Of the 38 owners that responded to questionnaires up to 5 years (median 2.1 years) after surgery, 76%

still perceived an improvement (Suwankong et al., 2008). In acute canine disc disease, surgical results are usually excellent: 96% of nonambulatory dogs with intact pain sensation and a Hansen type-1 disk extrusion in the thoracolumbar spine had successful decompressive surgery (Davis & Brown, 2002). In contrast, surgical decompression of long-standing, severe intervertebral disk disease (IVDD) has a success rate of only 40% (Joaquim et al., 2010). Combining decompressive surgery with electrical stimulation at acupuncture points increased the success rate to 74%, and, in dogs treated with acupuncture alone, the success rate was even greater (79%) (Joaquim et al., 2010). Cervical spondylomyelopathy (Wobblers syndrome) is a common and complex disease of the cervical spine of large and giant breed dogs. It has been referred to by 14 different names and 21 surgical techniques have been proposed to treat it, demonstrating the difficulty of treating this chronically painful disease (da Costa, 2010).

Eighty one percent of canine syringomyelia patients who underwent foramen magnum decompression surgery had improvement or resolution of chronic pain signs initially, but the signs recurred in 25% of cases, presumably because of new scar tissue in the area (Dewey et al., 2005). In humans, rehabilitation as an individualized exercise program is suggested to accompany spinal root compression surgery (Long, 2003).

For OA patients various surgical techniques are available. A human Cochrane meta-analysis of joint lavage ($n = 567$) showed no benefit for either pain or improved function (Reichenbach et al., 2010). No comparable reports exist in veterinary medicine. Total joint replacement techniques and femoral head and neck excision (FHNE) may be indicated for treatment of chronic OA, but there are no meta-analyses of the efficacy of these surgeries in dogs. One report suggested that total hip replacement may be associated with a greater degree of function in treated limbs, whereas FHNE may be associated with fewer and less severe complications; however, owner satisfaction rates were similar between the two surgical approaches (Franklin & Cook, 2011). In another study 96% of owners were satisfied with the results after FHNE, although 42% of dogs had poor functional results (Off & Matis, 2010). Multiple recent clinical trials suggest that cemented and cementless, and nano, micro, or routine hip arthroplasties provide effective relief of chronic OA pain when evaluated by lameness evaluations, owner questionnaires, gait analysis, or weight bearing (Marker et al., 2009; Lascelles et al., 2010; Liska, 2010; Gemmill et al., 2011; Drüen et al., 2012; Fitzpatrick et al., 2012; Forster et al., 2012; Ireifej et al., 2012; Marino et al., 2012; Seibert et al., 2012). Other reports indicate that other joint replacements, for example, of the stifle, are equally useful in treating other chronically painful canine joints (Eskelinen et al., 2012). In other joints arthrodesis has shown to be effective for chronic pain (Pucheu & Duhautois, 2008; Diaz-Bertrana et al., 2009).

Risks of surgery include further nerve injury, surgically induced instability and/or luxation, infection, and excessive scar or adhesion formation. Failure to correct the underlying pathology and failure to diagnose concurrent disease will also affect outcome (Long, 2003). In general, very chronic pain is associated with an altered pain physiology and surgical intervention is unlikely to be curative (Long, 2003). It is wise, therefore, to remember the dictum, "above all else, do no harm." It might be advisable to try less invasive techniques before considering an uncertain surgical procedure.

Myofascial Trigger Point Therapy

MTrPs (Chapter 14) may be one of the most under diagnosed conditions in humans (Cummings, 2007) and animals, likely because of a lack of validated diagnostic criteria (Lucas et al., 2009). The points are identified by manual palpation: a taut band, a "snapping" reaction, and a very painful point can be found repeatedly in the same position. In dogs, they vary from 3 mm in a 1 kg Yorkshire terrier to 8 cm in a large dog, and can even be located when the dog is deeply sedated. When practicing this diagnostic technique, it is helpful to start with sedated animals, as palpation is usually painful. Janssens (1991, 2001) has identified the most common anatomical sites for trigger points in the dog (Figure 23.1). There are a number of treatments for the deactivation of MTrPs, including muscle stretch techniques (Hong, 1994; Mense et al., 2001), MTrP injection techniques (e.g., lidocaine) (Alvarez & Rockwell, 2002), "dry" needling with acupuncture needles (Kalichman & Vulfsons, 2010; Ay et al., 2010), and therapeutic ultrasound (Srbely & Dickey, 2007; Srbely et al., 2008). In addition, correction of the factors that promoted MTrP formation (e.g., avoidance of a repetitive movement) is required. More information on MTrPs can be found in Chapter 14.

Environmental Modifications

Modification of the environment including placing carpets on slippery floors, installing ramps for stairs or for getting into the car, placing comfortable dog beds at floor level, or letting an outdoor dog move into the house during colder weather are all helpful. If the animal is being treated with corticosteroids or is otherwise polyuric, installing a litter box or incontinence pads nearby or opening up a doggy-door to the balcony, yard, or bathroom for urination can improve the quality of life.

Hygiene

Chronically painful dogs often take less interest in their hygiene or may simply be too painful to groom. The owner must be reminded to groom the animal regularly and guard against urine or fecal scalding.

NUTRITION

Chronically painful dogs should be fed a high-quality food that contains the nutrients required for normal physiology and tissue repair, and has anti-inflammatory and analgesic properties. Such diets can be obtained commercially or prepared at home. Some food items may be pronociceptive or proinflammatory, while others may be antinociceptive or anti-inflammatory. For example, fatty fish and flax contain anti-inflammatory omega-3 fatty acids and reduce pain in dogs (see under Nutritional Supplements). Many pet food companies have started adding cartilage "building blocks" and anti-inflammatory ingredients, such as omega-3 oils, to canine diets.

Another important aspect of diet is quantity. In humans, a relationship between obesity and chronic pain (Ray et al., 2011), and loss of body fat and improvement in symptoms of knee OA has been established repeatedly (Toda et al., 1998; Riecke et al., 2010). A lifetime study of Labrador retrievers demonstrated that limited food consumption reduced the incidence and severity of OA, and significantly increased the median age of onset of OA (12 years in the food restricted group compared to 6 years in the control group) (Kealy et al., 2000; Smith et al., 2006). Severity of shoulder OA was also significantly less at 6 and 8 years of age in the food restricted group (Runge et al., 2008). A clear correlation between losing weight and diminishing chronic pain in dogs with OA has been reported (Impellizeri et al., 2000; Mlacnik et al., 2006).

Providing a diet that aids in preventing adverse effects of the analgesic drug therapies in use is also important. If the patient is receiving opioids, the addition of fiber or stool softeners (e.g., high fiber cereals, berries, fruits, vegetables, canned pumpkin, psyllium seed husks, water) can help prevent constipation (August, 1983; Rouse et al., 1991; Ashraf et al., 1995). If a patient has visceral pain, all gas-producing foods should be avoided. Consideration should also be given to whether analgesics should be administered with or without food, and if there are dietary interactions affecting a drug's absorption or function.

Oral Nutritional Supplements

Nutritional supplements include both macro and micro minerals, vitamins, amino acids, fatty acids, and numerous other supplements of herbal, animal, or mineral origin. Supplements may be used as components in the formation of new tissues (e.g., cartilage), because of their analgesic or anti-inflammatory properties (omega-3 fatty acids), or because they improve normal physiological function (e.g., minerals and vitamins). Supplements are chosen based upon the underlying cause of the chronic pain.

Subchondral bone, cartilage, synovia, the joint capsule, synovial fluid, and intra-articular ligaments are all part of the OA process and all can contribute to pain with the exception of synovial fluid and cartilage (Little, 2009). Inflammation is the underlying pathology and there is evidence of chondritis, synovitis, and osteitis in OA (Dougados, 2006). This type of patient may benefit from a number of nutritional supplements, some of which have been proven scientifically to be beneficial. Doses, dosing intervals, indications, and adverse effects of some supplements are provided in Table 23.5.

OMEGA-3 FATTY ACIDS

The omega-3 fatty acids have an NSAID sparing anti-inflammatory effect in humans with chronic inflammatory pain (Goldberg & Katz, 2007; Galarraga et al., 2008). Omega-3 fatty acids exert their beneficial effect by substituting cell membrane lipids: the pro-inflammatory precursor arachidonic acid (AA) is substituted with the anti-inflammatory precursors eicosapentaenoic (EPA) or docosahexaenoic acid (DHA). This results in the production of more anti-inflammatory and fewer pro-inflammatory prostaglandins and leukotrienes and, hence, less pain (Siess et al., 1980; Goodnight et al., 1982; Hall et al., 2005; Smith, 2005). Omega-3 fatty acids from fish oils have been clinically tested in several canine studies, and a positive, albeit weak, effect was found (Roush et al., 2010a, 2010b; Fritsch et al., 2010a, 2010b; Hielm-Bjorkman, 2012). Dietary omega-3 fatty acid was the only nutraceutical that showed a high level of evidence for treatment effect in dogs in a recent review (Vandeweerd et al., 2012).

The optimal dose and optimal duration of treatment are not established, but some guidelines are given in Table 23.5 (Hansen et al., 2008; PARNUT, 2010).

GREEN LIPPED MUSSEL

Green lipped mussel (GLM) extract comes from a New Zealand offshore mussel species, *Perna canaliculus*. The active ingredients of the GLM are not known, but it contains small amounts of the omega-3 fatty acids eicosatetraenoic acid (ETA), EPA,

Table 23.4. Opioids used in canine chronic pain management

Opioid	Dosing Instructions	Indications	Precautions and Contraindications	Possible Adverse Effects
Morphine	Morphine sulfate 0.2–1 mg/kg PO q4–6h; Morphine sulfate sustained release 2–5 mg/kg PO q12h; 0.25–1 mg/kg IM q4–6h; 0.05–0.1 mg/kg IV q1–2h; epidural 0.1 mg/kg diluted with 0.26 mL/kg of sterile saline, max total volume 6 mL in all dogs, q8–12h (onset 30–60 min, treatment effect 18–24 h) CRI 0.15–0.2 mg/kg/h; 0.1 mg/kg IA	BTP management in hospital Outpatient PO dosing	Oral morphine has lower bioavailability and is less effective in dogs than in humans.	Defecation after administration Constipation Urinary retention Bradycardia Dysphoria Histamine release when given rapidly IV
Hydromorphone	0.05–0.2 mg/kg IM, SC; CRI 0.05–0.1 mg/kg/h; 0.05–0.1 mg/kg IV q2–6h	BTP management in hospital		
Oxycodone	0.1–0.3 mg/kg PO q8–12h	BTP management Outpatient PO dosing		
Oxycodone + acetaminophen (paracetamol)	Dose according to acetaminophen: 10–15 mg/kg PO q8–12h, long-term ≤10 mg/kg q12h	Broad spectrum analgesia in chronic inflammatory pain		
Oxymorphone	0.03–0.05 mg/kg IV; 0.05–0.2 mg/kg IM, SC q2–4h	BTP management in hospital		Fewer adverse effects but more panting than morphine
Fentanyl	Transdermal patch 2–5 μg/kg/h (e.g., a 100 μg/h depot patch for a 25 kg dog) Change skin area every time a new patch placed In hospital: 2–5 μg/kg IV CRI: 2–10 μg/kg/h slowly	BTP management Patient can go home Maintains mobility and facilitates physical therapy CRI: BTP management in hospital	Do not heat area with patch Avoid contact with children or other animals Wash hands after handling	Skin irritation Nausea and vomiting Constipation, urine retention, sedation, excitement, panting, dysphoria (especially northern breed dogs) Bradycardia and respiratory depression using IV, CRI, or rapid bolus of higher doses
Buprenorphine	0.005–0.03 mg/kg SC, IM, IV, OTM q4–8h; Onset slow: IV 5–15 min, IM 60 min but give 6–12h treatment effect One transdermal depot patch provides 7 days of analgesia in humans	BTP management Patient can go home with patch	Difficult to antagonize IM injection may be painful Do not combine with full μ agonist	Slight sedation potentiated when concomitant use with CYP P450 3A4 inhibitors (e.g., ketoconazole)

(continued)

Table 23.4. (*Continued*)

Opioid	Dosing Instructions	Indications	Precautions and Contraindications	Possible Adverse Effects
Butorphanol	0.2–2 mg/kg PO q6–8h, 0.2–1.2 mg/kg IM q2–6h, 0.1–0.8 mg/kg IV q0.5–2h Usually used together with NSAIDs	Mild and moderate pain, visceral pain Short duration of analgesia	Antitussive Do not combine with full μ agonist—can reverse affect	Sedation Rarely anorexia and diarrhea
Codeine	0.5–1 mg/kg PO q4–6h No research on long-term use	Outpatient PO dosing	Antitussive	
Codeine + acetaminophen (paracetamol)	Dose according to acetaminophen 10–15 mg/kg PO q8–12h and according to codeine 2 mg/kg q8–12h (eg. Acetaminophen 300 mg + codeine 30–60mg for a 20–30 kg dog) No research on long-term use	Outpatient PO dosing	Antitussive	Sedation
Tramadol	2–5 mg/kg PO q6–12h; 2 mg/kg IV No research on long-term use Usually used together with NSAIDs, adjuvants, and /or opioids	BTP management at home Adjunctive analgesic in chronic pain such as OA and neoplasia Neuropathic pain	Can contribute to serotonin syndrome Caution with hepatic disease	Sedation at high doses but otherwise less respiratory depression, sedation, and GI side effects than μ agonist opioids

The table list opioids used in hospital settings in cases of breakthrough pain episodes as well as opioids that can be sent home with the patient. Dosages should be taken as general guidelines as individual variations exist. Clinical judgment should always determine the final dose used. All drugs listed are not available in all countries and most are not approved for the use in dogs. Local and national laws may also restrict the use of opioids for dogs. Some opioids may have been tested for efficacy in some specific canine conditions but may also be used in other types of chronic pain using extrapolated doses. The doses listed come from the author's experience as well as from other people working with chronic pain, from references cited in the text and from books of pain management (Flecknell & Waterman-Pearson, 2000; Tranquilli et al., 2007; Gaynor & Muir III, 2009; Ramsey, 2011).

BTP, breakthrough pain; CRI, constant rate infusion; ED, epidural; IA, intraarticular; IM, intramuscular; IT, intrathecal; IV, intravenous; NSAID, nonsteroidal anti-inflammatory drug; OTM, oral transmucosal; PO, per os (oral); S, spinal; SC, subcutaneous; TDP, transdermal patch.

DHA, chondroitin and keratan sulfates, and other nutrients they obtain from their diet. These lipids have anti-inflammatory properties and could, thereby, be useful for chronic inflammatory pain, although the amount of omega-3 oils in GLM is minimal (Macrides et al., 1997; Whitehouse et al., 1997). The GLM also contains sulfates that may act as building blocks in cartilage regeneration.

At least four randomized clinical trials have demonstrated mild to moderate beneficial effects of GLM on chronic pain variables in dogs suffering from OA (Dobenacker et al., 2002; Bierer & Bui, 2002; Bui & Bierer, 2003; Hielm-Björkman et al., 2009). One clinical trial (with a placebo group receiving fish cartilage and brewer's yeast) found no difference between placebo and GLM in dogs with degenerative joint disease (Pollard et al., 2006). There

may be a dose–response relationship because trials using bigger daily doses have demonstrated more positive results (Bierer & Bui, 2002; Hielm-Björkman et al., 2009. In a recent review (four studies, $n = 266$), GLM treatment was considered promising but, because of inconsistencies among studies, its use was not recommended (Vandeweerd et al., 2012).

GLUCOSAMINE AND CHONDROITIN SULFATE
Repeating disaccharide units of glucosamine (GS) and galactosamine in cartilage make up chondroitin sulfate (CS). GS supplements are formulated as GS hydrochloride or GS sulfate, and are usually made from animal cartilage sources or from shellfish.

Table 23.5. Nutraceuticals, acupuncture, and electro-treatments used in treating a variety of chronic pain conditions in dogs

Treatment	Dose and frequency / Duration of onset and effect	Indications	Cautions/Contra-indications	Possible adverse effects
Nutraceuticals				
Omega-3 fatty acids	90 mg/kg/day PO of EPA and 4–5 mg/kg/day of DHA, EPA content in feed: 0.38% — At least 3 months to see effects — Administer for at least 6 months	Inflammatory pain	Caution in patients with bleeding disorders — Can be combined with NSAIDs or corticosteroids	Very rare — "Fishy" odor — Gastrointestinal upset reported
Green Lipped Mussel (GLM)	10–40 mg/kg/day PO—double dose the first 10 days — At least 3 months to see effects — Administer for at least 6 months — Effects may persist for 2 months after discontinuation	Inflammatory pain	None identified — Can be combined with NSAIDs or corticosteroids	None reported
Glucosamine (GS)	50 mg/kg PO Double dose the first 10 days — At least 3 months to see effects — Can be administered continuously	Chronic pain due to OA	None identified — Can be combined with NSAIDs or corticosteroids	None reported
Chondroitin sulfate (CS)	38 mg/kg/day PO Double dose the first 10 days — At least 3 months to see effects — Can be administered continuously	Chronic pain due to OA	None identified — Can be combined with NSAIDs or corticosteroids	None reported
Avocado + soybean unsaponifiables (ASU)	10 mg/kg/day PO — At least 2 months to see effects — Effects may persist for 2 months after discontinuation	Inflammatory pain	None identified — Can be combined with NSAIDs or corticosteroids	None reported
Injected supplements				
PPS	3 mg/kg, SC, IM four times, 1 week apart. — Effects may last 3–12 months	OA changes in joints		Side effects very rare — Prolonged coagulation time
PSGAG	5 mg/kg IM as twice weekly injections for 3–6 weeks — Effects may last 3–12 months	OA changes in joints		Side effects very rare — Dose-dependent prolonged coagulation time

(continued)

Table 23.5. (Continued)

Treatment	Dose and frequency Duration of onset and effect	Indications	Cautions/Contra-indications	Possible adverse effects
Hyaluronic acid	Dosage varies depending on molecular size, e.g., 1500 kD; 10 mg/0.67 mL of saline solution Give 3–5 injections IA, 1–3 weeks apart	OA changes in joints	None identified Use aseptic technique	None reported
Electrotherapies				
TENS	Depending on TENS unit. Continuous or pulse, variable amplitude, intensity, Hz (1–200). Several times a week to begin then less frequently as improvement occurs	All types of pain	Do not use over suspected carcinoma or over uterus during pregnancy. Analgesia might mask fractures and other severe pain pathology.	None reported
Therapeutic ultrasound	Typically 1–3 W/cm^2 several times a week to begin then less frequently as improvement occurs	All types of pain	Same as above	Exacerbation of pain if too high intensity or too long duration used
Therapeutic laser/Low-level laser (LLL)	Usually dosed as joules per area: 1–4 J/cm^2	All types of pain Can be used locally over painful areas or instead of needles on acupuncture points	Same as above	Pigmented skin requires less energy. Caution in rooms with mirrors or reflecting metal surfaces. Always use safety glasses.
Electroacupuncture (EA)	Low Hz and high intensity stimulates opioid analgesia, high Hz and low intensity stimulates GABA mediated analgesia Several times a week to begin then less frequently as improvement occurs	All types of pain Especially good for myofascial trigger points	Same as above	Adverse effects very rare Needle retention in muscle can occur.

The table list supplements that can be used in canine chronic pain at home and treatments performed by veterinarians, physiotherapists or rehabilitation specialists. Dosages should be taken as general guidelines as individual variations exist but none of the supplements listed have any known adverse reactions. The doses listed come from the author's experience as well as from other people working with chronic pain, from references cited in the text and from books of pain management (Flecknell & Waterman-Pearson, 2000; Tranquilli et al., 2007; Gaynor & Muir III, 2009).

EPA, eicosapentaenoic; DHA, docosahexaenoic; IA, intraarticular; IM, intramuscular; NSAID, nonsteroidal anti-inflammatory drug; OA, osteoarthritis; PO, per os (oral); PPS, pentosan polysulfate; PSGAG, polysulfated glycosaminoglycan; SC, subcutaneous; TENS, transcutaneous electric nerve stimulation.

Oral bioavailability of GS and CS in the dog is 87% and 70%, respectively (Setnikar et al., 1986).

Based on *in vitro* observations, there are several theories of how GS and CS work. They provide exogenous supplies for synthesis of proteoglycans and cartilage matrix by increasing aggrecan synthesis and gene expression of type II collagen (Lippiello et al., 2000; Henrotin et al., 2003; Kawcak et al. 2007; Chan et al., 2007). They have mild anti-inflammatory properties and decrease the synthesis of inflammatory mediators such as nitric oxide and prostaglandin E_2 (Setnikar et al., 1991; Henrotin et al., 1998; Meininger et al., 2000; Byron et al., 2003; Chan et al., 2005b; 2006). GS and CS also exhibit an antioxidant action (Valvason et al., 2008), and decrease the synthesis and activity of certain metalloproteinases, that is, enzymes that decrease cartilage metabolism (Henrotin et al., 1998; Kut-Lasserre et al., 2001; Nakamura et al., 2004; Chan et al., 2005a; 2006). They lack the adverse effects of NSAIDs, and it has also been proposed that their properties are not associated with inhibition of prostaglandin synthesis (Setnikar et al., 1991; Müller-Fassbender et al., 1994).

There are no canine clinical trials of GS alone or CS alone, but GS together with CS ($n = 35$) had a significant positive treatment effect for OA, starting from day 70 of supplementation (McCarthy et al., 2007). In the same study, the NSAID was significantly better than the GS + CS in all variables except pain. However, GS, CS, and manganese ascorbate together ($n = 71$) resulted in no effect when evaluated at day 60 (Moreau et al., 2003). As the effect was evident in the first study only at day 70, it might be that the second study ended too soon. When GS was given before an induced synovitis it had a protective effect against synovitis and bone remodeling and lameness was reduced (Canapp et al., 1999). In an equine study ($n = 25$), there was a 36% reduction in pain after 60 days of treatment and a 68% reduction after 150 days of treatment (Gupta et al., 2009).

Several human randomized clinical trials have demonstrated significant positive results for GS use compared to placebo (Crolle & DiEste, 1980; Pujalte et al., 1980; Drovanti et al., 1980; D'Ambrosio et al., 1981; Vaz, 1982; Tapadinhas et al., 1982), and for CS use compared to placebo (Uebelhart et al., 1998; Mazieres et al., 2001). In a recent human study of nearly 1600 patients suffering from pain due to knee OA, the response to GS and CS together was only significantly greater than in the placebo group in a subgroup of 354 patients that had moderate to severe pain. When all patients were included, there was no significant difference between treatment and placebo group (Clegg et al., 2006). Also, there was no positive effect reported in two recent human reviews; one of CS alone (Raichenbach et al., 2007) and the other of GS and CS combined ($n = 3803$) (Wandel et al., 2010).

Although several animal studies have reported a positive treatment effect with GS and CS, a final recommendation cannot be given. Lag time to appreciable effect is 2–3 months, and the effect appears to be weaker than that of an NSAID. In patients that cannot take NSAIDs, and as a part of a multimodal treatment, use of these supplements may be warranted. Ulbricht & Basch (2005) graded the evidence level as strong, for GS and as conflicting or unclear for CS.

Avocado and Soybean Unsaponifiables

Avocado-soybean unsaponifiables (ASU) are made from the unsaponifiable fractions of one-third avocado oil and two-thirds soybean oil. There are no published clinical trials investigating the usefulness of these compounds for naturally occurring OA in dogs. A randomized clinical trial with induced OA in canine stifles reported that ASU could inhibit early cartilage and bone lesions (Boileau et al., 2009). A meta-analysis concluded that there is good evidence that they help pain due to OA in humans and that there are no adverse effects (Ameye & Chee, 2006), whereas a small, randomized clinical trial ($n = 16$) reported no reduction of pain signs in horses, but did show disease-modifying effects in the treated group compared to placebo (Kawcak et al., 2007).

Injectable Nutritional and Autologous Treatments

Pentosan Polysulfates (PPS)

Early studies reported that intramuscular PPS (e.g., Cartrophen®) significantly decreased articular damage in dogs with OA (Rogachefsky et al., 1993, 1994). At least three randomized clinical trials found significantly positive clinical treatment outcomes after PPS administration (Bouck et al., 1995; Read et al., 1996; Budsberg et al., 2007). One study found no difference in functional outcome between oral calcium PPS and placebo, after surgical cruciate repair (Innes et al., 2000). In human studies, chronic pain significantly decreased in the PPS group compared to the control group (Ghosh et al., 2005).

Polysulfated Glycosaminoglycans (PSGAG)

Polysulfated glycosaminoglycans (PSGAG) (e.g., Adequan®, Arteparon®) are injectable chondroprotective agents used to treat OA pain, and their mode of action has been studied extensively (Mikulikova & Trnavsky, 1982; Nishikawa et al., 1985; Burkhard & Ghosh, 1987; Ghosh et al., 1987). Dogs with OA receiving IM injections of PSGAG had significant improvement in cartilage repair in several studies (Altman et al., 1989a; 1989b). De Haan (1994) found no significant difference between treatment and placebo groups of adult dogs suffering from OA. A study of younger dogs with hip dysplasia demonstrated less radiographical evidence of subluxation in the PSGAG group compared to the placebo (Lust et al., 1992), and another study showed some protection of cartilage after meniscectomy (Hannan et al., 1987).

Hyaluronic Acid

Intra-articular (IA) viscosupplementation includes natural hyaluronic acid (HA, hyaluronan) and synthetic hylan derivatives (e.g., Hylartin®, Legend®, Synacid®). There are varying opinions about the efficacy of this treatment in dogs (Hellström et al., 2003; Brandt et al., 2004; Smith et al., 2005), but its use seems to be more accepted in horses. A human Cochrane review of 76 trials, following patients for 5–13 weeks after injection, reported an improvement from baseline of 28–54% for pain and 9–32% for function. In general, efficacy was comparable to NSAIDs, and longer-term benefits were observed compared to intra-articular corticosteroids. Few adverse events were reported (Bellamy et al., 2006). A 40-month randomized clinical trial assessed repeated intra-articular injections of HA in human knee OA patients and reported improvement, and a marked carry-over effect of at least 1 year (Navarro-Sarabia et al., 2011). As study results are conflicting, more research is warranted.

Intra-articular Stem-cell, Autologous Conditioned Serum (ACS), Bioskaffold Therapy, and Other Similar Techniques

The use of autologous tissues to treat pain from chronic OA, lumbar stenosis, disc prolapse, and muscle and tendon injuries is gaining in popularity. The autologous conditioned serums, Orthokine®, tested in humans ($n = 84$ and 376), and IRAP® tested in horses ($n = 16$ and 262), have shown promising results with negligible adverse effects (Frisbie et al., 2007; Wehling et al., 2007; Jarloev & Weinberger, 2008).

Two studies investigated treatment of chronic canine elbow and hip OA with adipose-derived mesenchymal stem cells (Black et al., 2007; 2008). The hip study was a randomized clinical trial that reported significant improvement in the stem cell group for pain, lameness, and range of motion, compared to the placebo group. The primary objective of the elbow study was to evaluate the effectiveness of this therapy in 14 dogs with chronic OA of the humeroradial joint and to determine the duration of effect. Veterinarians assessed each dog for lameness, pain on manipulation, range of motion, and functional disability using a numeric rating scale at baseline and at intervals up to 180 days after treatment. Statistically significant improvement in outcome measures was demonstrated. A more recent study demonstrated that injection of adipose-derived mesenchymal stem cells improved chronic OA of the elbow joints in dogs (Guercio et al., 2012).

A significant improvement in pain and other pain-related outcome measures was associated with injectable bioscaffold (porcine urinary bladder) for canine hip OA in a 6-month randomized clinical trial (Rose et al., 2009). The effect was still evident 6 months after the injection.

Exercise

Exercise reduced chronic pain in human studies (Ettinger et al., 1997; van Baar et al., 1998; Hurley & Scott, 1998), and this is likely also the case for dogs. An exercise regimen for a dog with chronic pain due to OA might include walks and trotting on soft surfaces and on hilly terrain, underwater treadmill or swimming, or retrieving (Edge-Hughes, 2007). However, too much exercise may cause the pain to worsen (Mansa et al., 2007).

Manipulative Therapies

Manipulative therapies consist of those practices, such as chiropractic, osteopathy, and naprapathy, which incorporate handling and adjustment of the vertebrae. Subluxations in the spinal facet joints are thought to be the common inciting factor leading to arthritic hypertrophy, synovial cysts, and eroded cartilage and end plates. Techniques such as osteopathy also include "indirect techniques" that do not include any functional manipulation *per se*, but work more on myofascial tissue release. See discussion of canine chiropractic in Chapter 18.

There are no randomized clinical trials reporting successful treatment of dogs suffering from chronic pain, but anecdotal evidence abounds. Some meta-analyses in humans suggest that spinal manipulation is beneficial for patients suffering from chronic pain. There are few adverse effects from spinal manipulative therapies, provided they are performed by educated, experienced, and knowledgeable therapists. Research on all these modalities in dogs would be very welcome.

Physical Therapy

There are many physical therapy modalities that can be used to treat dogs with chronic pain. Massage, stretching, active and passive activation, transcutaneous electric nerve stimulation (TENS), therapeutic laser, ultrasound, magnetic therapy, microcurrent nerve stimulation, and the application of heat and cold can be helpful (McGowan et al., 2007). See chapter 11 for a detailed discussion of physical therapy.

THERAPEUTIC ULTRASOUND

No studies on the use of therapeutic ultrasound for canine chronic pain are available, although a case report of two dogs with acute muscle avulsion injuries described a positive treatment effect (Mueller et al., 2009). A Cochrane meta-analysis ($n = 341$) of therapeutic ultrasound for human OA of the knee and hip suggest that it might be beneficial for pain and improvement of function; however, due to some low-quality evidence the magnitude of the effect is still unclear (Rutjes et al., 2010).

Low-level or Therapeutic Lasers

Although there are no clinical studies reporting the use of low-level laser (LLL) for chronic pain in dogs, there are many studies describing its use for conditions such as OA, back pain, dental pain, fascial pain, neuropathic pain, and phantom pain in humans. However, the studies are not consistent in the wavelengths, wattage, or frequencies used. For painful joints, LLL provided superior pain relief compared to NSAIDs (Antipa et al., 1995; $n > 900$, Glazewski, 1996; $n = 224$), to LLL and NSAIDs combined (Haimovici et al., 1988, Nakaji et al., 2005), and to NSAIDs and massage/physiotherapy (Soriano et al., 1995; $n = 938$). Patients with OA in the upper extremities (Simunovic & Trobonjaca, 2000) and knee (Basirnia et al., 2002; Hegedus et al., 2009) had a 70% reduction in pain after LLL. Eighty one percent of patients with occipital neuralgia, 79% of patients with arm/shoulder/neck pain, and 50% of patients with back pain had good to excellent results with LLL (Mizokami et al., 1990). Toya et al. (1994) conducted a multicenter double-blinded randomized controlled trial and reported that 82% of patients with extremity joint, cervical, or lumbar spine pain had effective pain relief, compared to 42% in the placebo group. In another study, the risk ratio for chronic neck pain improvement after LLL was shown to be 4.05 (2.74–5.98), and the treatment effect lasted for up to 22 weeks (Chow et al., 2009). In double-blinded, cross-over studies of patients suffering from stage III–IV ankylosing spondyloarthritis pain, morning stiffness and waking during sleep were all significantly reduced after LLL, whereas range of motion and laboratory parameters did not change significantly (Gärtner, 1989, 1992). One single application of LLL relieved pain for up to 3 days in 83.5% of the patients. Application of LLL to the stellate ganglion provided pain relief in a double-blinded controlled study (Hashimoto et al., 1997).

In a double-blinded randomized controlled trial, treating myofascial pain syndrome with LLL resulted in significant amelioration of pain at rest and at movement, a reduction in the number of trigger points, and improvement in the Neck Pain and Disability Visual Analog Scale (NPAD), Beck depression inventory, and the Nottingham Health Profile, compared to placebo. The score for self-assessed improvement of pain was significantly different between the active and placebo laser groups (63% vs. 19%) (Gur et al., 2004). In a double-blinded randomized controlled trial of chronic neck pain ($n = 90$), the self-reported improvement was 48.5% in the LLL group compared to 3.99% in the placebo group, but other variables failed to show significant differences between groups (Chow et al., 2006).

Treatment of phantom pain has also been reported to improve with LLL (Taguchi, 1998). After LLL therapy for atypical facial pain, 76% of patients were pain-free and 44% remained pain-free 1 year later (Eckerdal et al., 1994). Painful oral conditions were improved in 60 of 100 cases (Bradley & Reynolds, 1994). However, in patients ($n = 40$) with chronic orofacial pain resistant to other treatments, there was no effect of LLL treatment (Hansen & Thoröe, 1990). Treatment effect with LLL may be dose dependent. In a meta-analysis of OA studies, there was a significant difference in outcome depending upon the dose range used (Bjordal et al., 2003).

No adverse effects of LLL have been described, and studies have concluded that there is no risk of tissue damage even after massive irradiation (Sasaki et al., 1992), although dark skin may be more sensitive to treatment (Shah & Alster, 2010). Patients may be more painful the day after treatment, as a chronic disease process is made more acute with the laser (Tunér & Hode, 2010).

ELECTROMAGNETIC FIELDS

So far, not many studies have employed either static (SMF) or pulsed electromagnetic fields (PEMF) as pain treatment in dogs, horses, or humans. In humans, there is an obvious problem with blinding the procedure, due to the magnetism. Anecdotal use and an abstract on canine use, indicate a potential benefit (Pinna et al., 2010).

Acupuncture

Acupuncture can be a helpful treatment for canine chronic pain conditions, and it has been used to treat pain in dogs since the early 1970s (Janssens, 1976; Schoen, 2001). Scientific literature supporting its efficacy is just starting to accumulate, but the results are conflicting and controversial. The use of appropriate sham procedures and controls for acupuncture studies is a source of controversy, and makes comparison of studies more difficult (ter Riet et al., 1990; Pomeranz, 1996; White & Ernst, 1999; Paterson & Dieppe, 2005). A recognized problem with placebo treatment is that needling a nonacupuncture point seems to provide the same kind of responses as needling a true acupuncture point (Debreceni, 1993). In functional MRI studies, sham acupuncture of nonacupuncture points led to analgesia or an increase in functional MRI activation in the same pain-related brain areas that are affected by needling a meridian acupuncture point (Cho et al., 2002a, 2002b). A recent systematic review that re-evaluated 13 randomized controlled studies of different human pain conditions ($n = 3025$) demonstrated a difference between real and sham acupuncture, and between sham and no acupuncture (Madsen et al., 2009). Thus, sham needling is not considered a placebo treatment as it has similar, though much weaker effects than acupuncture point needling.

There are only a few randomized controlled studies of acupuncture in dogs suffering from chronic pain. One study reported the results of treatment of nine dogs with forelimb lameness due to elbow OA that were treated weekly three times with acupuncture, sham, or nothing in a crossover design (Kapatkin et al., 2006). Although lameness, measured as ground reaction forces, was not different between treatments, changes in the VAS scoring by owners approached significance ($p < 0.08$) and eight of the nine owners

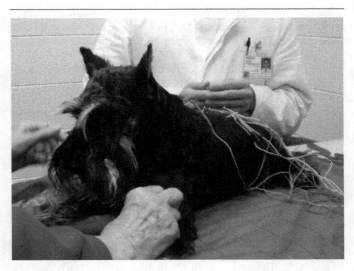

Figure 23.2. A dog receiving electroacupuncture for pain due to intervertebral disc disease (Courtesy of Gregory Hirshoren, University of Tennessee CVM).

recognized when their dogs had received acupuncture rather than sham ($p = 0.04$) (Kapatkin et al., 2006).

Some studies have evaluated electroacupuncture (Figure 23.2) in dogs suffering from IVDD. Electroacupuncture combined with standard "western" medical treatment was significantly more successful (88.5% vs. 58.3%) and resulted in significantly shorter recovery of ambulation and deep pain perception than did western treatment alone (Hayashi et al., 2007). Joaquim et al. (2010) reported that electroacupuncture was superior to decompressive surgery alone or surgery and electroacupuncture combined (clinical success rates of 79%, 40%, and 73% respectively) for treating chronic IVDD.

SUMMARY

Treating chronic pain in the dog requires a multimodal approach, including pharmacological and nonpharmacological modalities. Large randomized controlled clinical trials are not always available for veterinary species and a combination of clinical experience and extrapolation from research on human and laboratory animals may be necessary. The treatment of chronic pain requires dedication on the part of the owner and the veterinarian but can reduce suffering and improve the quality of life of dogs with chronic pain syndromes.

REFERENCES

Ackerman, S.J., Knight, T., Schein, J., et al. (2004) Risk of constipation in patients prescribed fentanyl transdermal system or oxycodone hydrochloride controlled-release in a California Medicaid population. *The Consultant Pharmacist*, 19, 118–132.

Agnello, K.A., Reynolds, L.R., & Budsberg, S.C. (2005) *In vivo* effects of tepoxalin, an inhibitor of cyclooxygenase and lipoxygenase, on prostanoid and leukotriene production in dogs with chronic osteoarthritis. *American Journal of Veterinary Research*, 66, 966–972.

Allan, L., Hays, H., Jensen, N.H., et al. (2001) Randomized crossover trial of transdermal fentanyl and sustained release oral morphine for treating chronic non-cancer pain. *British Medical Journal*, 322, 1154–1158.

Altman, R.D., Dean, D., Muniz, O., et al. (1989a) Prophylactic treatment of canine osteoarthritis with glycosaminoglycan polysulfuric acid ester. *Arthritis & Rheumatism*, 32(10), 759–766.

Altman, R.D., Dean, D., Muniz, O., et al. (1989b) Therapeutic treatment of canine osteoarthritis with glycosaminoglycan polysulfuric acid ester. *Arthritis & Rheumatism*, 32(10), 1300–1307.

Alvarez, D.J. & Rockwell, P.G. (2002) Trigger points: diagnosis and management. *American Family Physician*, 65, 653–660.

Ameye, L.G., & Chee, W.S.S. (2006) Osteoarthritis and nutrition. From neutroceuticals to functional foods: a systematic review of the scientific evidence. *Arthritis Research and Therapy*, 8, R127.

Antipa, C. et al. (1995) Low-energy laser treatment of rheumatic diseases: a long-term study, in *Proceedings of SPIE*, 2391, 658–662. (Laser-tissue interaction VI)

Aragon, C.L., Hofmeister, E.H., & Budsberg, S.C. (2007) Systematic review of clinical trials of treatments for osteoarthritis in dogs. *Journal of the American Veterinary Medical Association*, 230, 514–521.

Arai, Y.C.P, Matsubara, T., Shimo, K., et al. (2010) Low-dose gabapentin as useful adjuvant to opioids for neuropathic cancer pain when combined with low-dose imipramine. *Journal of Anesthesia*, 24, 407–410.

Ashraf, W., Park, F., Lof, J., et al. (1995) Effects of psyllium therapy on stool characteristics, colon transit and anorectal function in chronic idiopathic constipation. *Alimentary Pharmacology and Therapeutics*, 9, 639–647.

August, J.R. (1983) Gastrointestinal disorders of the cat. *Veterinary Clinics of North America: Small Animal Practice*, 13(3), 585–597.

Autefage, A., Palissier, F.M., Asimus, E., et al. (2011) Long-term efficacy and safety of firocoxib in the treatment of dogs with osteoarthritis. *The Veterinary Record*, 168(23), 617.

Ay, S., Evcik, D., & Tur, B.S. (2010) Comparison of injection methods in myofascial pain syndrome: a randomized controlled trial. *Clinical Rheumatology*, 29, 19–23.

Bailey, P.L., Port, J.D., McJames, S., et al. (1987) Is fentanyl an anesthetic in the dog? *Anesthesia & Analgesia*, 66, 542–548.

Basirnia, A., Sadeghipoor, G., Djavid, E.G., et al. (2002) The effect of low power laser therapy on osteoarthritis of the knee. *Laser in Medical Science*, 17(4), *Proc. 14th Annual Meeting of Deutsche Gesellschaft für Lazermedicin*, Munich, Germany, 2003.

Bateman, S.W., Haldane, S., & Stephens, J.A. (2008) Comparison of the analgesic efficacy of hydromorphone and oxymorphone in dogs and cats: a randomized blinded study. *Veterinary Anesthesia and Analgesia*, 35(4), 341–347.

Bellamy, N., Campbell, J., Robinson, V., et al. (2006) Intaarticular corticosteroid for treatment of osteoarthritis of the knee. *Cochrane Database of Systematic Reviews*. [Abstract]

Benton, H.P., Vasseur, P.B., BrodericVilla, G.A., et al. (1997) Effect of carprofen on sulfated glycosaminoglycan metabolism, protein synthesis, and prostaglandin release by cultured osteoarthritic canine chondrocytes. *American Journal of Veterinary Research*, 58, 286–292.

Bierer, T.L. & Bui, L.M. (2002) Improvement of arthritic signs in dogs fed green-lipped mussel (*Perna canaliculus*). *Journal of Nutrition*, 132, S1634–S1636.

Bjordal, J.M., Couppè, C., Chow, R.T., et al. (2003) A systematic review of low level laser therapy with location-specific doses for pain from chronic joint disorders. *Australian Journal of Physiotherapy*, 49, 107–116.

Black, L.L., Gaynor, J., Adams, C., et al. (2008) Effect of intraarticular injection of autologous adipose-derived mesenchymal stem and regenerative cells on clinical signs of chronic osteoarthritis of the elbow joint in dogs. *Veterinary Therapeutics*, 9, 192–200.

Black, L.L., Gaynor, J., Gahring, D., et al. (2007) Effect of adipose-derived mesenchymal stem and regenerative cells on lameness in dogs with chronic osteoarthritis of the coxofemoral joints: a randomized, double-blinded, multicenter, controlled trial. *Veterinary Therapeutics*, 8, 272–284.

Bleidner, W.E., Harmon, J.B., Hewes, W.E., et al. (1965) Absorption, distribution and excretion of amantadine hydrochloride. *Journal of Pharmacology and Experimental Therapeutics*, 150(3), 484–490.

Boileau, C., Martel-Pelletier, J., Caron, J., et al. (2009) Protective effects of total fraction of avocado/soybean unsaponifiables on the structural changes in experimental dog osteoarthritis: Inhibition of inducible nitric oxide synthase and matrix metalloproteinase-13. *Arthritis Research & Therapy*, 11, R41.

Boston, S.E., Moens, N.M., Kruth, S.A., et al. (2003) Endoscopic evaluation of the gastroduodenal mucosa to determine the safety of short-term concurrent administration of meloxicam and dexa-methasone in healthy dogs. *American Journal of Veterinary Research*, 64, 1369–1375.

Bouck, G.R., Miller, C.W., & Taves, C.L. (1995) A comparison of surgical and medical treatment of fragmented coronoid process and osteochondritis dissecans of the canine elbow. *Veterinary and Comparative Orthopaedics and Traumatology*, 8, 177–183.

Bradley, F.G. & Reynolds, P.A. (1994) Low reactive level laser therapy in Oral and Maxillofacial Surgery. Review of 100 cases. [Abstract]. *Laser Therapy*, 6, 67.

Brainard, B.M., Meredith, C.P., Callan, M.B., et al. (2007) Changes in platelet function, hemostasis, and prostaglandin expression after treatment with nonsteroidal anti-inflammatory drugs with various cyclooxygenase selectivities in dogs. *American Journal of Veterinary Research*, 68(3), 251–257.

Brandt, K.D., Smith, G.N., & Myers, S.L. (2004) Hyaluronan injection affects neither osteoarthritis progression nor loading of the OA knee in dogs. *Biorheology*, 41(3–4), 493–502.

Brydges, N.M., Argyle, D.J., Mosley, J.R., et al. (2012) Clinical assessments of increased sensory sensitivity in dogs with cranial cruciate ligament rupture. *Veterinary Journal*, 193(2), 545–50.

Budsberg, S.C., Johnston, S.A., Schwartz, P.D., et al. (1999) Efficacy of etodolac for the treatment of osteoarthritis of the hip joints in dogs. *Journal of the American Veterinary Medical Association*, 214, 206–210.

Budsberg, S.C., Bergh, M.S., Reynolds, L.R., et al. (2007) Evaluation of pentosan polysulfate sodium in the postoperative recovery from cranial cruciate injury in dogs: a randomized, placebo-controlled clinical trial. *Veterinary Surgery*, 36, 234–244.

Bui, L.M. & Bierer, T.L. (2003) Influence of green-lipped mussels (*Perna canaliculus*) in alleviating signs of arthritis in dogs. *Veterinary Therapeutics*, 4, 397–407.

Byron, C.R., Orth, M.W., Venta, P.J., et al. (2003) Influence of glucosamine on matrix metalloproteinase expression and activity in lipopolysaccharide-stimulated equine chondrocythes. *American Journal of Veterinary Research*, 64, 666–671.

Canapp, S.O., Jr., McLaughlin, R.M., Jr., Hoskinson, J.J., et al. (1999) Scintigraphic evaluation of dogs with acute synovitis after treatment with glucosamine hydrochloride and chondroitin sulfate. *American Journal of Veterinary Research*, 60, 1552–1557.

Case, J.B., Fick, J.L., & Rooney, M.B. (2010) Proximal duodenal perforation in three dogs following deracoxib administration. *Journal of the American Animal Hospital Association*, 46, 255–258.

Cashmore, R.G., Harcourt-Brown, T.R., Freeman, P.M., et al. (2009) Clinical diagnosis and treatment of suspected neuropathic pain in three dogs. *Australian Veterinary Journal*, 87, 45–50.

Chan, P.S., Caron, J.P., & Orth, M.W. (2005a) Effect of glucosamine and chondroitin sulfate on regulation of gene expression of proteolytic enzymes and their inhibitors in interleukin-1-challenged bovine articular cartilage explants. *American Journal of Veterinary Research*, 66, 1870–1876.

Chan, P.S., Caron, J.P., Rosa, G.J., et al. (2005b) Glucosamine and chondroitin sulfate regulate gene expressions and synthesis of nitric oxide and prostaglandin E(2) in articular cartilage explants. *Osteoarthritis and Cartilage*, 13, 387–394.

Chan, P.S., Caron, J.P., & Orth, M.W. (2006) Short-term gene expression changes in cartilage explants stimulated with interleukin 1beta plus glucosamine and chondroitin sulfate. *Journal of Rheumatology*, 33, 1329–1340.

Chan, P.S., Caron, J.P., & Orth, M.W. (2007) The effects of glucosamine and chondroitin sulfate on cartilage explants cultured for 2 weeks. *American Journal of Veterinary Research*, 68, 709–715.

Cho, Z.H., Oleson, T.D., Alimi, D., et al. (2002a) Acupuncture: the search for biologic evidence with functional magnetic resonance imaging and positron emission tomography techniques. *Journal of Alternative and Complementary Medicine*, 8, 399–401.

Cho, Z.H., Son, Y.D., Han, J.Y., et al. (2002b) fMRI neurophysiological evidence of acupuncture mechanisms. *Acupuncture in Medicine*, 14, 16–22.

Chow, R.T., Heller, G.Z., & Barnsley, L. (2006) The effect of 300mW, 830 nm laser on chronic neck pain: A double blind, randomized, placebo-controlled study. *Pain*, 124, 201–210.

Chow, R.T., Johnson, M.I., Lopes-Martins, R.A., et al. (2009) Efficacy of low-level laser therapy in the management of neck pain: a systematic review and meta-analysis of randomised placebo or active-treatment controlled trials. *Lancet*, 374, 1897–1908.

Chunekamrrai, S., Krook, L.P., Lust, G., et al. (1989) Changes in articular cartilage after intraarticular injections of methylprednisolone acetate in horses. *American Journal of Veterinary Research*, 50, 1733–1741.

Clark, A.J., Ahmedzai, S.H., Allan, L.G., et al. (2004) Efficacy and safety of transdermal fentanyl and sustained-release oral morphine in patients with cancer and chronic non-cancer pain. *Current Medical Research Opinion*, 20, 1419–1428.

Clegg, D.O., Reda, D.J., Harris, C.L., et al. (2006) Glucosamine, chondroitin sulfate, and the two in combination for painful knee osteoarthritis. *The New England Journal of Medicine*, 354, 795–808.

Crolle, G. & DiEste, E. (1980) Glucosamine sulphate for the management of arthrosis. *Current Therapeutic Research*, 7, 104–109.

Cummings, M. (2007) Regional myofascial pain: diagnosis and management. *Best Practice and Research Clinical Rheumatology*, 21, 367–387.

D'Ambrosio, E., Casa, B., Bompani, G., et al. (1981) Glucosamine sulfate: a controlled clinical investigation in arthrosis. *Pharmatherapeutica*, 2, 504–508.

da Costa, R.C. (2010) Cervical spondylomyelopathy (wobbler syndrome) in dogs. *Veterinary Clinics of North America: Small Animal Practice*, 40(5), 881–913.

Davis, G.J. & Brown, D.C. (2002) Prognostic indicators for time to ambulation after surgical decompression in non-ambulatory dogs with acute thoracolumbar disk extrusions: 112 cases. *Veterinary Surgery*, 31, 513–518.

Debreceni, L. (1993) Chemical releases associated with acupuncture and electric stimulation. *Critical Reviews in Physical and Rehabilitation Medicine*, 5, 247–275.

De Haan, J.J., Goring, R.L., & Beale, B.S. (1994) Evaluation of polysulfated glycosaminoglycan for the treatment of hip dysplasia in dogs. *Veterinary Surgery*, 23, 177–181.

Dellemijn, P.L., van Dujin, H., & Vanneste, J.A. (1998) Prolonged treatment with transdermal fentanyl in neuropathic pain. *Journal of Pain and Symptom Management*, 16, 220–229.

Dewey, C., Berg, J., Barone, G., et al. (2005) Foramen magnum decompression for treatment of caudal occipital malformation syndrome in dogs. *Journal of the American Veterinary Medical Association*, 227, 1270–1275.

Diaz-Bertrana, C., Darnaculleta, F., Durall, I., et al. (2009) The stepped hybrid plate for carpal panarthrodesis - Part II: a multicentre study of 52 arthrodeses. *Veterinary and Comparative Orthopaedics and Traumatology*, 22(5), 389–397.

Dougados, M. (2006) Symptomatic slow-acting drugs for osteoarthritis: what are the facts? *Joint Bone Spine*, 73, 606–609.

Drovanti, A., Bignamini, A.A., and Rovati, A.L. (1980) Therapeutic activity of oral glucosamine sulfate in osteoarthritis: a placebo controlled double blind investigation. *Clinical Therapeutics*, 3, 260–272.

Drüen, S., Böddeker, J., Meyer-Lindenberg, A., et al. (2012) Computer-based gait analysis of dogs: evaluation of kinetic and kinematic parameters after cemented and cementless total hip replacement. *Veterinary and Comparative Orthopaedics and Traumatology*, 25(5), 375–384.

Eckerdal, A. (1994) Kliniske erfaringer fra et 5-års icke-kontrolert studie af low power laser-behandling af periorale neuropatier. [Clinical experiences from a 5 year non-controlled study of low power laser treatment of periodal neuropatias]. (in Danish) *Tandlaegebladet*, 98, 526–529.

Edge-Huges, L. (2007) Osteoarthritis, in *Animal Physiotherapy – Assessment, Treatment and Rehabilitation of Animals* (eds C.M. McGowan, L. Goff, & N. Stubbs), pp. 213–215. Blackwell Publishing, Oxford, UK.

Egger, C.M., Duke, T., Archer, J., et al. (1998) Comparison of plasma fentanyl concentrations by using three transdermal fentanyl patch sizes in dogs. *Veterinary Surgery*, 27, 156–166.

Eskelinen, E.V., Liska, W.D., Hyytiäinen, H.K., et al. (2012) Canine total knee replacement performed due to osteoarthritis subsequent to distal femur fracture osteosynthesis and a two-year objective outcome. *Veterinary and Comparative Orthopaedics and Traumatology*, 25(5), 427–432.

Ettinger, W.H., Jr., Burns, R., Messier, S.P., et al. (1997) A randomized trial comparing aerobic exercise and resistance exercise with a health education program in older adults with knee osteoarthritis: the fitness arthritis and seniors trial (FAST). *Journal of the American Medical Association*, 277, 25–31.

Farrell, M., Clements, D.N., Mellor, D., et al. (2007) Retrospective evaluation of the long-term outcome of non-surgical management of 74 dogs with clinical hip dysplasia. *The Veterinary Record*, 160, 506–511.

Finnerup, N.B., Baastrup, C., & Jensen, T.S. (2009) Neuropathic pain following spinal cord injury pain: mechanisms and treatment. *Scandinavian Journal of Pain*, 1, 1, 3–11.

Fitzpatrick, N., Pratola, L., Yeadon, R., et al. (2012) Total hip replacement after failed femoral head and neck excision in two dogs and two cats. *Veterinary Surgery*, 41(1), 136–142.

Flecknell, P. & Waterman-Pearson, A. (2000) *Pain management in animals*. W.B. Saunders, London, UK.

Forster, K.E., Wills, A., Torrington, A.M., et al. (2012) Complications and owner assessment of canine total hip replacement: a multicenter internet based survey. *Veterinary Surgery*, 41(5), 545–550.

Franklin, S.P. & Cook, J.L. (2011) What is the evidence? Surgical treatment of large dogs with hip joint osteoarthritis. *Journal of the American Veterinary Medical Association*, 238(4), 440–442.

Frisbie, D.D., Kawcak, C.E., Werpy, N.M., et al. (2007) Clinical, biochemical, and histologic effects of intra-articular administration of autologous conditioned serum in horses with experimentally induced osteoarthritis. *American Journal of Veterinary Research*, 68, 290–296.

Fritsch, D., Allen, T.A., Dodd, C.E., et al. (2010a) Dose-titration effects of fish oil in osteoarthritic dogs. *Journal of Veterinary Internal Medicine*, 24(5), 1020–1026.

Fritsch, D.A., Allen, T.A., Dodd, C.E., et al. (2010b) A multicenter study of the effect of dietary supplementation with fish oil omega-3 fatty acids on carprofen dosage in dogs with osteoarthritis. *Journal of the American Veterinary Medical Association*, 236(5), 535–539.

Furlan, A.D., Sandoval, J.A., Mailis-Gagnon, A., et al. (2006) Opioids for chronic noncancer pain: a meta-analysis of effectiveness and side effects. *Canadian Medical Association Journal*, 174, 1589–1594.

Gakiya, H.H., Silva, D.A., Gomes, J., et al. (2011) Electroacupuncture versus morphine for the postoperative control of pain in dogs. *Acta Cirurgica Brasiliera*, 26(5), 346–351.

Galarraga, B., Ho, M., Youssef, H.M., et al. (2008) Cod liver oil (n-3 fatty acids) as a non-steroidal anti-inflammatory drug sparing agent in rheumatoid arthritis. *Rheumatology*, 47, 665–669.

Garcia Rodriguez, L.A. & Hernandez-Diaz, S. (2001) The relative risk of upper gastrointestinal complications among users of acetaminophen and non-steroidal anti-inflammatory drugs. *Epidemiology*, 12, 570–576.

Gaynor, J. (2008) Control of cancer pain in veterinary patients. *Veterinary Clinics of North America: Small Animal Practice*, 38, 1429–1448.

Gaynor, J. & Muir, III (2009) *Handbook of Veterinary pain management*, 2nd edn, Elsevier Mosby, St. Louis, Missouri, USA.

Gemmill, T.J., Pink, J., Renwick, A., et al. (2011) Hybrid cemented/cementless total hip replacement in dogs: seventy-eight consecutive joint replacements. *Veterinary Surgery*, 40(5), 621–630.

Ghosh, P., Collier, S., and Andrews, J. (1987) Synovial membrane-cartilage interactions: The role of serine proteinase inhibitors in interleukin-1 mediated degradation of articular cartilage. *Journal of Rheumatology*, 14, 122–124.

Ghosh, P., Edelman, J., March, L., et al. (2005) Effects of pentosan polysulfate in osteoarthritis of the knee: a randomized, double blind, placebo-controlled pilot study. *Current Therapeutic Research*, 66, 552–571.

Gibofsky, A., Williams, G.W., McKenna, F., et al. (2003) Comparing the efficacy of cyclooxygenase 2-specific inhibitors in treating osteoarthritis: appropriate trial design considerations and results of a randomized, placebo-controlled trial. *Arthritis & Rheumatism*, 48, 3102–3111.

Glazewski, J.B. (1996) Application of low-intensity lasers in rheumatology. The results of four-year observation in 224 patients, in *Proceedings of SPIE*, 2929, 80–91.

Goldberg, R.J. & Katz, J. (2007) A meta-analysis of the analgesic effects of omega-3 polyunsaturated fatty acid supplementation for inflammatory joint pain. *Pain*, 129, 210–223.

Goodnight, S.H., Jr., Harris, W.S., Connor, W.E., et al. (1982) Polyunsaturated fatty acids, hyperlipidemia, and thrombosis. *Arteriosclerosis*, 2, 87–113.

Greene, S. (2010) Chronic pain: Pathophysiology and treatment implications. *Topics in Companion Animal Medicine*, 25, 5–9.

Grubb, T. (2010a) What do we really know about the drugs we use to treat chronic pain? *Topics in Companion Animal Medicine*, 25, 10–19.

Grubb, T. (2010b) Chronic neuropathic pain in veterinary patients. *Topics in Companion Animal Medicine*, 25, 45–52.

Grubb, T. (2010c) Where do we go from here? Future treatment strategies for chronic pain. *Topics in Companion Animal Medicine*, 25, 59–63.

Guedes, A.G.P., Natalini, C.C., Rude, E.P., et al. (2005) Comparison of tramadol and morphine for pre-medication of dogs undergoing general anesthesia for orthopedic surgery. *Veterinary Anesthesia and Analgesia*, 32, 1–19.

Guercio, A., Di Marco, P., Casella, S., et al. (2012) Production of canine mesenchymal stem cells from adipose tissue and their application in dogs with chronic osteoarthritis of the humeroradial joints. *Cell Biology International*, 36(2), 189–194.

Gupta, R.C., Canerdy, T.D., Skaggs, P., et al. (2009) Therapeutic efficacy of undenatured type II collagen (UC-II) in comparison to glucosamine and chondroitin in arthritic horses. *Journal of Veterinary Pharmacology and Therapy*, 32(6), 577–584.

Gur, A., Sarac, A.J., Cevik, R., et al. (2004) Efficacy of 904 nm gallium arsenide low level laser therapy in the management of chronic myofascial pain in the neck: a double-blind and randomize-controlled trial. *Lasers in Surgery and Medicine*, 35, 229–235.

Hadley, H.S., Wheeler, J.L., & Petersen, S.W. (2010) Effects of intra-articular botulinum toxin a (botox) in dogs with chronic osteoarthritis: a pilot study. *Veterinary and Comparative Orthopaedics and Traumatology*, 23, 254–258.

Haimovici, N. (1988) Clinical use of anti-inflammatory action of the laser in activated osteoarthritis of small peripheral joints. LASER. *Journal of the European Medical Laser Association*, 1, 4–11.

Hall, J.A., Henry, L.R., Jha, S., et al. (2005) Dietary (n-3) fatty acids alter plasma fatty acids and leukotriene B synthesis by stimulated neutrophils from healthy geriatric Beagles. *Prostaglandins, Leukotrienes and Essential Fatty Acids*, 73, 335–341.

Halla, J.T. & Hardin, J.G., jr. (1987) Atlantoaxial (C1-C2) facet joint osteoarthritis: a distinctive clinical syndrome. *Arthritis and Rheumatism*, 30, 577–582.

Han, H.J., Yoon, H.Y., Kim, J.Y., et al. (2010) Clinical effect of additional electroacupuncture on thoracolumbar intervertebral disc herniation in 80 paraplegic dogs. *American Journal of Chinese Medicine*, 38(6), 1015–1025.

Hannan, N., Ghosh, P., Bellenger, C., et al. (1987) Systemic administration of glycosaminoglycan polysulfate (arteparon) provides partial protection of articular cartilage from damage produced by meniscectomy in the canine. *Journal of Orthopaedic Research*, 5, 47–59.

Hansen, H., & Thoroe, U. (1990) Low power laser biostimulation of chronic orofacial pain. A double-blind placebo controlled crossover study in 40 patients. *Pain*, 43, 169–179.

Hansen, R.A., Harris, M.A., Pluhar, G.E., et al. (2008) Fish oil decreases matrix metalloproteinases in knee synovia of dogs with inflammatory joint disease. *Journal of Nutritional Biochemistry*, 19, 101–108.

Hanson, P.D., Drag, M., Alva, L., et al. (2004) Safety of firocoxib for the treatment of osteoarthritis in dogs in United States field studies, in *Proceedings of ACVS congress*, Denver, USA, p. E9.

Hanson, P.D., Brooks, K.C., Case, J., et al. (2006) Efficacy and safety of firocoxib in the management of canine osteoarthritis under field conditions. *Veterinary Therapeutics*, 7, 127–140.

Hashimoto, T., Kemmutso, O., Otsuka, H., et al. (1997) Efficacy of laser irradiation on the area near the stellate ganglion is dose-dependent: a double-blind crossover placebo-controlled study. *Laser Therapy*, 9, 7–12.

Hayashi, A.M., Matera, J.M., & Fonseca Pinto, A.C. (2007) Evaluation of electroacupuncture treatment for thoracolumbar intervertebral disk disease in dogs. *Journal of the American Veterinary Medical Association*, 231(6), 913–918.

Hegedus, B., Viharos, L., Gervain, M., et al. (2009) The effect of low-level laser in knee osteoarthritis: a double blind, randomized, placebo-controlled trial. *Photomedicine and Laser Surgery*, 27(4), 577–584.

Henrotin, Y.E., Labasse, A.H., Jaspar, J.M., et al. (1998) Effects of three avocado/soybean unsaponifiable articular chondrocytes. *Clinical Rheumatology*, 17, 31–39.

Henrotin, Y.E., Sanchez, C., Deberg, M.A., et al. (2003) Avocado/soybean unsaponifiables increase aggrecan synthesis and reduce catabolic and pro-inflammatory mediator production by human osteoarthritic chondrocytes. *Journal of Rheumatology*, 30, 1825–1834.

Hielm-Björkman, A., Tulamo, R-M., Salonen, H., et al. (2009) Evaluating a complementary therapy for moderate to severe canine osteoarthritis. Part I: Green Lipped Mussel (Perna *Canaliculus*). *Evidence Based Complementary and Alternative Medicine*, 6, 365–373.

Hielm-Björkman, A., Roine, J., Elo, K., et al. (2012) An uncommissioned randomized, placebo-controlled double-blind study to test the effect of deep sea fish oil as a pain reliever for dogs suffering from canine OA. *BMC Veterinary Research*, 8, 157. doi:10.1186/1746-6148-8-157

Hofmeister, E.H. and Egger, C.M. (2004) Transdermal fentanyl patches in small animals. *Journal of the American Animal Hospital Association*, 40, 468–478.

Hong, C.Z. (1994) Lidocaine injection versus dry needling to myofascial trigger point. The importance of the local twitch response. *American Journal of Physical Medicine & Rehabilitation*, 73(4), 256–263.

Hurley, M.V. & Scott, D.L. (1998) Improvements in quadriceps sensorimotor function and disability of patients with knee osteoarthritis following a clinically practicable exercise regime. *British Journal of Rheumatology*, 37, 1181–1187.

IASP-International Association for the Study of Pain (2007) IASP Pain Terminology (accessed June 25, 2007).

Imagawa, V.H., Fantoni, D.T., Tatarunas, A.C. et al. (2011) The use of different doses of metamizole for post-operative analgesia in dogs. *Veterinary Anaesthesia and Analgesia*. 38(4), 385–393.

Impellizeri, J.A., Tetrick, M.A., & Muir, P. (2000) Effect of weight reduction on clinical signs of lameness in dogs with hip osteoarthritis. *Journal of the American Veterinary Medical Association*, 216, 1089–1091.

Innes, J.F., Barr, R.S., & Sharif, B.M. (2000) Efficacy of oral calcium pentosan polysulfate for the treatment of osteoarthritis of the canine stifle joint secondary to cranial cruciate ligament deficiency. *The Veterinary Record*, 146, 433–437.

Innes, J.F., Clayton, J., & Lascelles, B.D.X. (2010) Review of the safety and efficacy of long-term NSAID use in the treatment of canine osteoarthritis. *The Veterinary Record*, 166, 226–230.

Ireifej, S., Marino, D., & Loughin, C. (2012) Nano total hip replacement in 12 dogs. *Veterinary Surgery*, 41(1), 130–135.

Jamison, R.N., Schein, J.R. Vallow, S., et al. (2003) Neuropsychological effects of long-term opioid use in chronic pain patients. *Journal of Pain and Symptom Management*, 26, 913–921.

Janssens, L.A.A. (1976) Acupuncture therapy for the treatment of chronic osteoarthritis in dogs: a review of 61 cases. *Veterinary Medicine Small Animal Clinician*, 71, 465–468.

Janssens, L.A.A. (1991) Trigger points in 48 dogs with myofascial pain syndrome. *Veterinary Surgery*, 20, 274–278.

Janssens, L.A.A. (2001) Trigger point therapy, in *Veterinary Acupuncture-Ancient Art to Modern Medicine*, 2nd edn (ed. A.M. Schoen), Mosby, St Louis, USA, pp. 199–203.

Jarloev, N. & Weinberger, T. (2008) IRAP-Clinical experiences with autologous interleukin-1-receptor-antagonist (IL-1Ra) enriched protein solution (autologous conditioned serum) in equine joints. Part 2, in *Proceedings of the European Equine Meeting of the year 2008, XIV SIVE, FEEVA Congress*, Venice, Italy.

Joaquim, J., Luna, S., Brondani, J., et al. (2010) Comparison of decompressive surgery, electroacupuncture, and decompressive surgery followed by electroacupuncture for the treatment of dogs with intervertebral disk disease with long-standing severe neurologic deficits. *Journal of the American Veterinary Medical Association*, 236, 1225–1229.

Johnson, L.R. (1990) Tricyclic antidepressant toxicosis. *Veterinary Clinics of North America: Small Animal Practice*, 20, 393–403.

Kalichman, L. & Vulfsons, S. (2010) Dry needling in the management of musculoskeletal pain. *Journal of the American Board of Family Medicine*, 23, 19–23.

Kapatkin, A.S., Tomasic, M., & Beech, J. (2006) Effects of electrostimulated acupuncture on ground reaction forces and pain scores in dogs with chronic elbow joint arthritis. *Journal of the American Veterinary Medical Association*, 228, 1350–1354.

Kapural, L., Sessler, D.I., Kapural, M., et al. (2009) Opioid-sparing effect of intravenous, outpatient ketamine infusions may be short-lasting in chronic pain patients with opioid requirements. [Abstract]. in *ASA Annual Meeting 2009*.

Katz, N., Schein, J., & Kosinski, M. (2003a) HRQoL changes in chronic low back pain patients recieving either fentanyl transdermal system or oxycodone with acetaminophen. (Poster). in *American Pain Society*, Chicago, USA.

Katz, N., Schein, J., & Kosinski, M. (2003b) Sleep and somnolence changes in chronic lower back pain patients receiving opioid therapy. (Poster). in *American Pain Society*, Chicago, USA.

Kawaguchi, H., Pilbeam, C.C., Harrison, J.R., et al. (1995) The role of prostaglandins in the regulation of bone metabolism. *Clinical Orthopaedics and Related Research*, 313, 36–46.

Kawcak, C.E., Frisbie, D.D., McIlwraith, C.W., et al. (2007) Evaluation of avocado and soybean unsaponifiable extracts for treatment of horses with experimentally induced osteoarthritis. *American Journal of Veterinary Research*, 68, 598–604.

Kay-Mugford, P.A., Grimm, K.A., Weingarten, A.J., et al. (2004) Effect of preoperative administration of tepoxalin on hemostasis and hepatic and renal function in dogs. *Veterinary Therapeutics*, 5, 120–127.

Kealy, R.D., Lawler, D.F, Ballam, J.M., et al. (2000) Evaluation of the effect of limited food consumption on radiographic evidence of osteoarthritis in dogs. *Journal of the American Veterinary Association*, 217, 1678–1680.

Kinzel, S., Hein, S., Buecker, A., et al. (2003) Diagnosis and treatment of arthrosis of cervical articular facet joints in Scottish Deerhounds: 9 cases (1998–2002). *Journal of the American Veterinary Medical Association*, 223, 1311–1315.

Klauss, G., Giuliano, E.A., Moore, C.P., et al. (2007) Keratoconjunctivitis sicca associated with administration of etodolac in dogs: 211 cases (1992-2002). *Journal of the American Veterinary Medical Association*, 230, 541–547.

Knight, E.V., Kimball, C.M., Keenan, I.L., et al. (1996) Preclinical toxicity evaluation of tepoxalin, a dual inhibitor of cyclooxygenase and 5-lipoxygenase, in sprague-dawley rats and beagle dogs. *Fundamental and Applied Toxicology*, 33, 38–48.

Kroin, J.S., McCarthy, R.J., Penn, R.D., et al. (2003) Continuous intrathecal clonidine and tizanidine in conscious dogs: analgesic and hemodynamic effects. *Anesthesia & Analgesia*, 96(3), 776–782.

KuKanich, B., Lascelles, B.D., & Papich, M.G. (2005) Pharmacokinetics of morphine and plasma concentrations of morphine-6-glucuronide following morphine administration to dogs. *Journal of Veterinary Pharmacology and Therapeutics*, 28, 371–376.

KuKanich, B. (2010) Pharmacokinetics of acetaminophen, codeine, and the codeine metabolites morphine and codeine-6-glucuronide in healthy Greyhound dogs. *The Journal of Veterinary Pharmacology and Therapeutics*, 33(1), 15–21.

Kut-Lasserre, C., Miller, C.C., Ejeil, A.L., et al. (2001) Effect of avocado and soybean unsaponifiables on gelatinase A (MMP-2), stromelycin 1 (MMP-3), and tissue inhibitors of matrix metalloproteinase (TIMP-1 and TIMP-2) secretion by human fibroblast in culture. *Journal of Periodontology*, 72, 1685–1694.

Kyles, A.E., Hardie, E.M., Hansen, B.D., et al. (1998) Comparison of transdermal fentanyl and intramuscular oxymorphone on post-operative behavior after ovariohysterectomy in dogs. *Research in Veterinary Science*, 65, 245–251.

Kyles, A.E., Papich, M., & Hardie, E.M. (1996) Disposition of transdermally administered fentanyl in dogs. *American Journal of Veterinary Science*, 57, 715–719.

Lamont, L.A. (2008a) Multimodal pain management in veterinary medicine: The physiologic basis of pharmacologic therapies. *Veterinary Clinics of North America: Small Animal Practice*, 38, 1173–1186.

Lamont, L.A. (2008b) Adjunctive analgesic therapy in veterinary medicine. *Veterinary Clinics of North America: Small Animal Practice*, 38, 1187–1203.

Lascelles, B.D.X., Blikslager, A.T., Fox, S.M., et al. (2005a) Gastrointestinal tract perforation in dogs treated with a selective cyclooxygenase-2 inhibitor: 29 cases (2002-2003). *Journal of the American Veterinary Medical Association*, 227, 1112–1117.

Lascelles, B.D.X., McFarland, J.M., & Swann, H. (2005b) Guidelines for safe and effective use of NSAIDs in dogs. *Veterinary Therapeutics*, 6, 237–250.

Lascelles, D.X. & Gaynor, J.S. (2007) Cancer patients, in *Lumb & Jones' Veterinary Anesthesia and Analgesia*, 4th edn (eds W.J. Tranquilli, J.C. Thurmon, K.A. Grimm), Blackwell publishing, Oxford, UK, p. 1001.

Lascelles, B.D.X., Gaynor, J.S., Smith, E.S., et al. (2008) Amantadine in a multimodal analgesic regimen for alleviation of refractory osteoarthritis pain in dogs. *Journal of Veterinary Internal Medicine*, 22, 53–59.

Lascelles, B.D., Freire, M., Roe, S.C., et al. (2010) Evaluation of functional outcome after BFX total hip replacement using a pressure sensitive walkway. *Veterinary Surgery*, 39(1), 71–77.

Lippiello, L., Woodward, J., Karpman, R., et al. (2000) In vivo chondroprotection and metabolic synergy of glucosamine and chondroitin sulfate. *Clinical Orthopaedics and Related Research*, 381, 229–240.

Liska, W.D. (2010) Micro total hip replacement for dogs and cats: surgical technique and outcomes. *Veterinary Surgery*, 39(7), 797–810.

Little, C. (2009) Update on matrix degradation: role of matrix degradation in OA. *Osteoarthritis & Cartilage*, 17(Suppl 1), S6.

Long, D.M. (2003) Chronic back pain, in *Handbook of Pain Management,* (eds R. Melzack & P.D. Wall), Churchill Livingstone, Elsevier Limited, Edinburgh, UK, pp. 67–76.

Lucas, N., Macaskill, P., Irwing, L., et al. (2009) Reliability of physical examination for diagnosis of myofascial trigger points: a systematic review of the literature. *Clinical Journal of Pain*, 25, 80–89.

Luna, S.P.L., Basilio, A.C., Steagall, P.V.M., et al. (2007) Evaluation of adverse effects of long-term oral administration of carprofen, etodolac, flunixin meglumine, ketoprofen, and meloxicam in dogs. *American Journal of Veterinary Research*, 68, 258–264.

Lust, G., Williams, A.J., Burton-Wurster, N., et al. (1992) Effects of intramuscular administration of glycosaminoglycan polysulfates on signs of incipient hip dysplasia in growing pups. *American Journal of Veterinary Research*, 53, 1836–1843.

Macrides, T.A., Treschow, A.P., Kalafatis, N., et al. (1997) The anti-inflammatory effects of Omega-3 Tetraenoic fatty acids isolated from a lipid extract from the New Zealand Green-Lipped Mussel, in *Proceedings of the 88th American Oil Chemists Society Annual Meeting*, Seattle, USA.

MacPhail, C.M., Lappin, M.R., Meyer, D.J., et al. (1998) Hepatocellular toxicosis associated with administration of carprofen in 21 dogs. *Journal of the American Veterinary Medical Association*, 212, 1895–1901.

Macrory, L., Vaughan-Thomas, A., Clegg, P.D., et al. (2009) An exploration of the ability of tepoxalin to ameliorate the degradation of articular cartilage in a canine *in vitro* model. *BMC Veterinary Research*, 5, 25.

Madsen, M.V., Gøtzsche, P.C., & Hróbjartsson, A. (2009) Acupuncture treatment for pain: systematic review of randomised clinical trials with acupuncture, placebo acupuncture, and no acupuncture groups. *British Medical Journal*, 338, a3115.

Manley, P.A. (1995) Treatment of degenerative joint disease, in *Kirk's Current Therapy XII. Small Animal Practice* (eds J.D. Bonagura & R.W. Kirk), WB Saunders Co, Philadelphia, USA, pp. 1196–1199.

Mansa, S., Palmer, E., Grondahl, C., et al. (2007) Long-term treatment with carprofen of 805 dogs with osteoarthritis. *Veterinary Research*, 160, 427–430.

Marino, D.J., Ireifej, S.J., and Loughin, C.A. (2012) Micro total hip replacement in dogs and cats. *Veterinary Surgery*, 41(1), 121–129.

Marker, D.R., Strimbu, K., McGrath, M.S., et al. (2009) Resurfacing versus conventional total hip arthroplasty - review of comparative clinical and basic science studies. *Bulletin of the NYU Hospital for Joint Diseases*, 67(2), 120–127.

Mathews, K.A., Pettifer, G., & Foster, R.F. (1999) A comparison of the safety and efficacy of meloxicam to ketoprofen and butorphanol for control of post-operative pain associated with soft tissue surgery in dogs, in *Proceedings of the symposium on recent advances in non-steroidal anti-inflammatory therapy in small animals*, Paris, France, p. 67.

Mathews, K.A. (2008) Neuropathic pain in dogs and cats: if only they could tell us if they hurt. *Veterinary Clinics of North America: Small Animal Practice*, 38, 1365–1413.

Mazieres, B., Combe, B., Phan Van, A., et al. (2001) Chondroitin sulfate in osteoarthritis of the knee: a prospective, double blind, placebo controlled multicenter clinical study. *Journal of Rheumatology*, 28, 173–181.

Mburu, D.N., Mbugua, S.W., Skoglund, L.A., et al. (1988) Effects of paracetamol and acetylsalicylic acid on the post-operative course after experimental orthopaedic surgery in dogs. *Journal of Veterinary Pharmacology and Therapeutics*, 11, 163–171.

McCann, M.E., Anderson, D.R., Zhang, D., et al. (2004) In vitro effects and in vivo efficacy of a novel cyclooxygenase-2 inhibitor in dogs with experimentally induced synovitis. *American Journal of Veterinary Research*, 65, 503–512.

McCarthy, G., O'Donavan, J., Jones, B., et al. (2007) Randomized double blind, positive-controlled trial to assess the efficacy of glucosamine/chondroitin sulfate for the treatment of dogs with osteoarthritis. *Veterinary Journal*, 174, 54–61.

McGowan, C., Goff, L., & Stubbs, N. (2007) *Animal Physiotherapy - Assessment, Treatment and Rehabilitation of Animals*. Blackwell Publishing, Oxford, UK.

McMahon, S.B. (1997) Are there fundamental differences in the peripheral mechanism of visceral and somatic pain? *Behavioral and Brain Sciences*, 20, 381–391.

McMillan, C.J., Livingston, A., Clark, C.R., et al. (2008) Pharmacokinetics of intravenous tramadol in dogs. *The Canadian Journal of Veterinary Research*, 72, 325–331.

Meininger, C.J., Kelly, K.A., Li, H., et al. (2000) Glucosamine inhibits inducible nitric oxide synthesis. *Biochemical and Biophysical Research Communications*, 279, 234–239.

Mense, S., Simons, D.G., & Russell, I.J. (2001) *Muscle Pain. Understanding its Nature, Diagnosis, and Treatment*, Lippincott Williams & Wilkins, Philadelphia, USA, p. 385.

Merskey, H. & Bogduk, N. (1994) *Classification of Chronic Pain: Descriptions of Chronic Pain Syndromes and Definitions of Pain Terms*, IASP press, Seattle.

Mikulikova, D. & Trnavsky, K. (1982) Influence of glycosaminoglycan polysulfate (arteparon) on lysosomal enzyme release from human polymorphonuclear leukocytes. *Rheumatology International*, 41, 50–53.

Mizokami, T., et al. (1990) Effect of diode laser for pain: A clinical study on different pain types. *Laser Therapy*, 2, 35–40.

Mlacnik, E., Bockstahler, B.A., Müller, M., et al. (2006) Effects of caloric restriction and a moderate or intense physiotherapy program for treatment of lameness in overweight dogs with osteoarthritis. *Journal of the American Veterinary Medical Association*, 229(11), 1756–1760.

Moreau, M., Depuis, J., Bonneau, N.H., et al. (2003) Clinical evaluation of a nutraceutical, carprofen and meloxicam for the treatment of dogs with osteoarthritis. *The Veterinary Record*, 152, 323–329.

Mueller, M.C., Gradner, G., Hittmair, K.M., et al. (2009) Conservative treatment of partial gastrocnemius muscle avulsions in dogs using therapeutic ultrasound - A force plate study. *Veterinary and Comparative Orthopaedics and Traumatology*, 22(3), 243–248.

Muir, W.W.III., Wiese, A.J., & Wittum, T.E. (2004) Prevalence and characteristics of pain in dogs and cats examined as outpatients at a veterinary teaching hospital. *Journal of the American Veterinary Medical Association*, 9, 1459–1463.

Mukai, A. & Kancherla, V. (2011) Interventional procedures for cervical pain. *Physical Medicine and Rehabilitation Clinics of North America*, 22(3), 539–549.

Murnaghan, M., Li, G., & Marsh, D.R. (2006) Nonsteroidal anti-inflammatory drug-induced fracture non-union: an inhibition of angiogenesis? *Journal of Bone and Joint Surgery*, 88A3, 140–147.

Nakaji, S., Shiroto, C., Yodono, M., et al. (2005) Retrospective study of adjunctive diode laser therapy for pain attenuation in 662 patients: detailed analysis by questionnaire. *Photomedicine and Laser Surgery*, 23, 60–65.

Nakamura, H., Shibakawa, A., Tanaka, M., et al. (2004) Effects of glucosamine hydrochloride on the production of prostaglandin E2, nitric oxide and metalloproteases by chondrocytes and synoviocytes in osteoarthritis. *Clinical and Experimental Rheumatology*, 22, 293–299.

Navarro-Sarabia, F., Coronel, P., Collantes, E., et al. (2011) A 40-month multicentre, randomized placebo-controlled study to assess the efficacy and carry-over effect of repeated intra-articular injections of hyaluronic acid in knee osteoarthritis: the AMELIA project. *Annals of the Rheumatic Diseases*, 70, 1957–1962.

Nicholson, B. (2000) Gabapentin use in neuropathic pain syndromes. *Acta Neurologica Scandinavica*, 101, 359–371.

Nishikawa, H., Mori, I., & Umemoto, J. (1985) Influences of sulfated glycosaminoglycans on biosynthesis of hyaluronic acid in rabbit knee synovium. *Archives of Biochemistry and Biophysics*, 240, 146–153.

Nuesch, E., Rutjes, A.W.S., Husni, E., et al. (2010) Oral or transdermal opioids for osteoarthritis of the knee or hip (Review). *Cochrane Database of Systematic Reviews*, (4), CD003115.

Ochi, H., Hara, Y., Asou, Y., et al. (2011) Effects of long-term administration of carprofen on healing of tibial osteotomy in dogs. *American Journal of Veterinary Research*, 72, 634–641.

Off, W. & Matis, U. (2010) Excision arthroplasty of the hip joint in dogs and cats. Clinical, radiographic, and gait analysis findings from the Department of Surgery, Veterinary Faculty of the Ludwig-Maximilians-University of Munich, Germany. 1997. *Veterinary and Comparative Orthopedics and Traumatology*, 23(5), 297–305.

Papich, M.G. (2008) An update on non-steroidal anti-inflammatory drugs (NSAIDs) in small animals. *Veterinary Clinics of North America: Small Animal Practice*, 38, 1243–1266.

PARNUT: European Union Article 10, commission regulation No 767/2009 about feed regulation, new amendment 1070/2010. www address: http://eur-lex.europa.eu/LexUriServ/LexUriServ.do?uri=OJ:L:2010:306:0042:0043:EN:PDF (accessed May 2012).

Pascoe, P.J. (2000) Opioid analgesics. *Veterinary Clinics of North America: Small Animal Practice*, 30, 757–772.

Paterson, C. & Dieppe, P. (2005) Characteristic and incidental (placebo) effects in complex interventions such as acupuncture. *British Medical Journal*, 330, 1202–1205.

Pelletier, J.P. & Martel-Pelletier, J. (1993) Effects of minesulfide and naproxen on the degradation and metalloprotease synthesis of human osteoarthritic cartilage. *Drugs*, 46, 34–39.

Pelletier, J.P., DiBattista, J.A., Raynauld, J.P., et al. (1995) The in vivo effects of intraarticular corticosteroid injections on cartilage lesions, stromelysin, interleukin-1, and oncogene protein synthesis in experimental osteoarthritis. *Laboratory Investigation*, 72(5), 578–586.

Pelletier, J.P., Mineau, F., Fernandes, J., et al. (1997) Two NSAIDs, minesulide and naproxen, can reduce the synthesis of urokinase and IL-6 while increasing PAI-1 in human OA synovial fibroblasts. *Clinical and Experimental Rheumatology*, 15, 393–398.

Pelletier, J.-P., Lajeunesse, D., Jovanovic, D.V., et al. (2000) Carprofen simultaneously reduces progression of morphological changes in cartilage and subchondral bone in experimental dog osteoarthritis. *Journal of Rheumatology*, 27, 2893–2902.

Pergolizzi, J., Boger, R.H., Budd, K., et al. (2008) Opioids and the management of chronic severe pain in the elderly: Consensus statement of an international expert panel with focus on the six clinically most often used World Health Organisation step III opioids (buprenorphine, fentanyl, hydromorphone, methadone, morphine, oxycodone). *Pain Practice*, 8, 287–313.

Persillin, R.H. & Ziff, M. (1966) The effect of gold salt on lysosomal enzymes of the peritoneal macrophage. *Arthritis & Rheumatism*, 9, 57–65.

Pettifer, G. and Dyson, D. (2000) Hydromorphone: A cost-effective alternative to the use of oxymorphone. *Canadian Veterinary Journal*, 41, 135–137.

Pieper, K., Schuster, T., Levinnois, O., et al. (2011) Antinociceptive efficacy and plasma concentrations of transdermal buprenorphine in dogs. *The Veterinary Journal*, 187, 335–341.

Pinna, S., Tribuiani, A.M., Pizzuti, E., et al. (2010) PEMF therapy in the treatment of canine osteoarthritis: preliminary results, in *Proceedings of the World Veterinary Orthopaedic Congress*, Bologna, Italy.

Pollard, B., Guilford, W.G., Ankenbauer-Perkins, K.L., et al. (2006) Clinical efficacy and tolerance of an extract of green-lipped mussel *(Perna canaliculus)* in dogs presumptively diagnosed with degenerative joint disease. *New Zeeland Veterinary Journal*, 54, 114–118.

Pollmeier, M., Toulemonde, C., Fleishman, C., et al. (2006) Clinical evaluation of firocoxib and carprofen for the treatment of dogs with osteoarthritis. *The Veterinary Record*, 159, 547–551.

Pomeranz, B. (1996) Scientific research into acupuncture for the relief of pain. *Journal of Complementary Medicine*, 2(1), 53–60, 73–75.

Portenoy, R.K. & Hagen, N.A. (1990) Breakthrough pain: definition, prevalence and characteristics. *Pain*, 41, 273–281.

Poulsen Nautrep, B. & Justus, C. (1999) Effects of some veterinary NSAIDs on ex vivo thromboxane production and in vivo urine output in the dog. In: *Proceedings of the symposium on recent advances in non-steroidal anti-inflammatory therapy in small animals*, Paris, France, p.25.

Pucheu, B. and Duhautois, B. (2008) Surgical treatment of shoulder instability. A retrospective study on 76 cases (1993–2007). *Veterinary and Comparative Orthopaedics and Traumatology*, 21(4), 368–374.

Pujalte, J.M., Llavore, E.P., & Ylescupidez, F.R. (1980) Double blind clinical evaluation of oral glucosamine sulfate in the basic treatment of osteoarthritis. *Current Medical Research & Opinion*, 7, 110–114.

Punke, J.P., Speas, A.L., Reynolds, L.R., et al. (2008) Effects of firocoxib, meloxicam, and tepoxalin on prostanoid and leukotriene production by duodenal mucosa and other tissues of osteoarthritic dogs. *American Journal of Veterinary Research*, 69, 1203–1209.

Radulovic, L.L., Türck, D., von Hodenberg, A., et al. (1995) Disposition of gabapentin (neurontin) in mice, rats, dogs, and monkeys. *Drug Metabolism and Disposition*, 23, 441–448.

Raekallio, M., Heinonen, K.M., Kuussaari, J., et al. (2003) Pain alleviation in animals: attitudes and practices of Finnish veterinarians. *The Veterinary Journal*, 165, 131–135.

Raekallio, M., Hielm-Bjorkman, A., Kejonen, J., et al. (2006) Evaluation of adverse effects of long-term orally administered carprofen in dogs. *Journal of the American Veterinary Medical Association*, 228, 876–880.

Raisz, L.G. (1999) Prostaglandins and bone: physiology and pathophysiology. *Osteoarthritis Cartilage*, 7, 419–421.

Raisz, L.G. & Lorenzo, J.A. (2006) Prostaglandins and proinflammatory cytokines, in *Dynamics of Bone and Cartilage Metabolism: Principles and Clinical Applications*, 2nd edn (eds. M.J. Seibel, S.P. Robins, J.P Bilezikian), Academic Press Inc., New York, USA, pp. 115–128.

Ramsey, I. (2011) *BSAVA Small Animal Formulary*, 7th edn (ed. I. Ramsey), British Small Animal Veterinary Association, Gloucester, England.

Rashad, S., Revel, P., Hemingway, A., et al. (1989) Effect of non-steroidal anti-inflammatory drugs on the course of osteoarthritis. *Lancet*, 334(8662), 519–522.

Ray, L., Lipton, R.B., Zimmerman, M.E., et al. (2011) Mechanisms of association between obesity and chronic pain in the elderly. *Pain*, 152, 53–59.

Read, R.A., Cullis-Hill, D., & Jones, M.P. (1996) Systemic use of pentosan polysulfate in the treatment of osteoarthritis. *Veterinary Clinics of North America: Small Animal Practice*, 37, 108–114.

Reichenbach, S., Rutjes, A.W., Nuesch, E., et al. (2010) Joint lavage for osteoarthritis of the knee. *Cochrane Database Systematic Review*, 12(5), CD007320.

Reichenbach, S., Sterchi, R., Scherer, M., et al. (2007) Meta-analysis: chondroitin for osteoarthritis of the knee or hip. *Annals of Internal Medicine*, 146(8), 580–590.

Reymond, N., Speranza, C., Gruet, P., et al. (2012) Robenacoxib vs. carprofen for the treatment of canine osteoarthritis; a randomized, noninferiority clinical trial. *Journal of Veterinary Pharmacology and Therapeutics*, 35(2), 175–183.

Riecke, B.F., Christensen, R., Christensen, P., et al. (2010) Comparing two low-energy diets for the treatment of knee symptoms in obese patients: a pragmatic randomized clinical trial. *Osteoarthritis & Cartilage*, 18, 746–754.

Rijsdijk, M., van Wijck, A.J.M., Kalkman, C.J., et al. (2012) Safety assessment and pharmacokinetics of intrathecal methylprednisolone acetate in dogs. *Anesthesiology*, 116, 170–181.

Ringe, J.D., Faber, H. Bock, O., et al. (2002) Transdermal fentanyl for the treatment of back pain caused by vertebral osteoporosis. *Rheumatology International*, 22, 199–203.

Robinson, T.M., Kruse-Elliott, K.T., Markel, M.D., et al. (1999) A comparison of transdermal fentanyl versus epidural morphine for analgesia in dogs undergoing major orthopedic surgery. *Journal of the American Animal Hospital Association*, 35, 95–100.

Rogachefsky, R.A., Dean, D.D., Howell, D.S., et al. (1993) Treatment of canine osteoarthritis with insulin-like growth factor-1 (IGF-1) and sodium pentosan polysulfate. *Osteoarthritis Cartilage*, 1, 105–114.

Rogachefsky, R.A., Dean, D.D., Howell, D.S., et al. (1994) Treatment of canine osteoarthritis with sodium pentosan polysulfate and insulin-like growth factor-1. *Annals of the New York Academy of Sciences*, 6, 392–394.

Rose, W., Wood, J.D., Simmons-Byrd, A., et al. (2009) Effect of a xenogeneic urinary bladder injectible bioscaffold on lameness in dogs with osteoarthritis of the coxofemoral joint (hip): A randomized, double-blinded controlled trial. *International Journal of Applied Research in Veterinary Medicine*, 7, 13–22.

Rouse, M., Chapman, N., Mahapatra, M., et al. (1991) An open, randomised, parallel group study of lactulose versus ispaghula in the treatment of chronic constipation in adults. *The British Journal of Clinical Practice*, 45, 28–30.

Roush, J.K., Cross, A.R., Renberg, W.C., et al. (2010b) Evaluation of the effects of dietary supplementation with fish oil omega-3 fatty acids on weight bearing in dogs with osteoarthritis. *Journal of the American Veterinary Medical Association*, 236(1), 67–73.

Roush, J.K., Dodd, C.E., Fritsch, D.A., et al. (2010a) Multicenter veterinary practice assessment of the effects of omega-3 fatty acids on osteoarthritis in dogs. *Journal of the American Veterinary Medical Association*, 236(1), 59–66.

Runge, J.J., Biery, D.N., Lawler, D.F., et al. (2008) The effects of lifetime food restriction on the development of osteoarthritis in the canine shoulder. *Veterinary Surgery*, 37, 102–107.

Rutjes, A.W., Nuesch, E., Sterchi, R., et al. (2010) Therapeutic ultrasound for osteoarthritis of the knee or hip. *Cochrane Database Systematic Review*, p. 20, CD003132. [Abstract]

Rychel, J.K. (2010) Diagnosis and treatment of osteoarthritis. *Topics in Companion Animal Medicine*, 25(1), 20–25.

Saarto, E. & Wiffen, P.J. (2005) Antidepressants for neuropathic pain [Systematic Review]. *Cochrane Database of Systematic Reviews*, 4, 4.

Sanderson, R.O., Beata, C., Filipo, R.M., et al. (2009) Systematic review of the management of canine osteoarthritis. *The Veterinary Record*, 164, 418–424.

Sasaki, K., Calderhead, R.G., Chin, I., et al. (1992) To examine the adverse photothermal effects of extended dosage laser therapy in vivo on the skin and subcutaneous tissue in the rat model. *Laser Therapy*, 4, 69–74.

Schoen, A. (2001) Acupuncture for musculoskeletal disorders, in *Veterinary Acupuncture- Ancient art to modern mystery*, 2nd edn (ed. A. Schoen), Mosby Inc., Missouri, USA.

Schultheiss, P.J., Morse, B.C., & Baker, W.H. (1995) Evaluation of a transdermal fentanyl system in the dog. *Contemporary Topics in Laboratory Animal Science*, 54, 75–81.

Seibert, R., Marcellin-Little, D.J., Roe, S.C., et al. (2012) Comparison of body weight distribution, peak vertical force, and vertical impulse as measures of hip joint pain and efficacy of total hip replacement. *Veterinary Surgery*, 41(4), 443–447.

Selph, S., Carson, S., Fu, R., et al. (2011) *Drug Class Review: Neuropathic Pain: Final Update 1 Report [Internet]*. Oregon Health & Science University, Portland, Oregon.

Sennello, K.A. & Leib, M.S. (2006) Effects of deracoxib or buffered aspirin on the gastric mucosa of healthy dogs. *Journal of Veterinary Internal Medicine*, 20, 1291–1296.

Setnikar, I., Giacetti, C., & Zanolo, G. (1986) Pharmacokinetics of glucosamine in the dog and man. *Arzneimittelforschung*, 36, 792–835.

Setnikar, I., Cereda, R., Pacini, M.A., et al. (1991) Anti-reactive properties of glucosamine sulfate. *Arzneimittelforschung*, 41, 157–161.

Sewell, R.D., Gonzalez, J.P., & Pugh, J. (1984) Comparison of the relative effects of aspirin, mefenamic acid, dihydrocodeine, dextropropoxyphene and paracetamol on visceral pain, respiratory rate and prostaglandin biosynthesis. *Archives Internationales de Pharmacodynamie et de Therapie*, 268(2), 325–334.

Shah, S. & Alster, T.S. (2010) Laser treatment of dark skin: an updated review. *American Journal of Clinical Dermatology*, 11, 389–397.

Shenker, N.G., Blake, D.R., McCabe, C.S., et al. (2004) Symmetry, T cells and neurogenic arthritis, in *Osteoarthritic Joint Pain*, (eds D.J. Chadwick & J. Goode), John Wiley & Sons Ltd., Chichester, pp. 241–251.

Siess, W., Roth, P., Scherer, B., et al. (1980) Platelet-membrane fatty acids, platelet aggregation, and thromboxane formation during a mackerel diet. *Lancet*, 1, 441–444.

Simons, D.G., Travell, J.G., & Simons, L.S. (1999) *Travell & Simons' myofascial pain and dysfunction: the trigger point manual,* Williams & Wilkins, Baltimore, pp. 1–10.

Simpson, D.M., Messina, J., Xie, F., et al. (2007) Fentanyl buccal tablet for the relief of breakthrough pain in opioid-tolerant adult patients with chronic neuropathic pain: a multicenter, randomized, double blind, placebo-controlled study. *Clinical Therapeutics*, 29, 588–601.

Simunovic, Z. & Trobonjaca, T. (2000) Low-level laser therapy in the treatment of osteoarthrosis of joints of the upper extremity: a multicenter, double blind, placebo controlled clinical study of 154 patients. *Laser in Surgery and Medicine*, (Suppl. 12), 7.

Smith, G., Jr., Myers, S.L., Brandt, K.D., et al. (2005) Effect of intraarticular hyaluronan injection on vertical ground reaction force and progression of osteoarthritis after anterior cruciate ligament transaction. *Journal of Rheumatology*, 32, 325–334.

Smith, G.K., Paster, E.R., Powers, M.Y., et al. (2006) Lifelong diet restriction and radiographic evidence of osteoarthritis of the hip joint in dogs. *Journal of the American Veterinary Medical Association*, 229, 690–693.

Smith, W.L. (2005) Cyclooxygenases, peroxide tone and the allure of fish oil. *Current Opinion in Cell Biology*, 17, 174–182.

Soriano, F. et al. (1995) The analgesic effect of 902 nm gallium arsenide semiconductor low level laser therapy (laser therapy) on osteoarticular pain: a report on 938 irradiated patients. *Laser Therapy*, 7(2), 75–80.

Srbely, J.Z. & Dickey, J. (2007) Randomized control study of the antinociceptive effect of ultrasound on trigger point sensitivity: novel applications in myofascial therapy? *Clinical Rehabilitation*, 21, 411–417.

Srbely, J.Z., Dickey, J., Lowerison, M., et al. (2008) Stimulation of myofascial trigger points with ultrasound induces segmental antinociceptive effects: a randomized controlled study. *Pain*, 139, 260–266.

Suwankong, N., Meij, B.P., Voorhout, G., et al. (2008) Review and retrospective analysis of degenerative lumbosacral stenosis in 156 dogs treated by dorsal laminectomy. *Veterinary and Comparative Orthopaedics and Traumatology*, 21, 285–93.

Taguchi, Y. (1998) Clinical experiences of laser applications in physical therapy, in *Proceedings of 2nd Congress World Association for Laser Therapy*, Kansas City, USA, p. 106.

Tapadinhas, M.J., Rivera, I.C., & Bignamini, A.A. (1982) Oral glucosamine sulfate in the management of arthritis: report on a multicentre open investigation in Portugal. *Pharmatherapeutica*, 3, 157–168.

ter Riet, G., Kleijnen, J., Knipschild, P. (1999) Acupuncture and chronic pain: a criteria-based meta-analysis. *Journal of Clinical Epidemiology*, 43(11), 1191–1199.

Toda, Y., Toda, T., Takemura, S., et al. (1998) Change in body fat, but not body weight or metabolic correlates of obesity, is related to symptomatic relief of obese patients with knee osteoarthritis after a weight control program. *Journal of Rheumatology*, 25, 2081–2086.

Towheed, T.E., Maxwell, L., & Judd, M.G. (2006) Acetaminophen for osteoarthritis. *Cochrane Database Systematic Reviews*, 1, CD004257.

Toya, S., Motegi, M., Inomata, K., et al. (1994) Report on a computer-randomized double blind clinical trial to determine the effectiveness of the GaAlAs (830nm) diode laser for pain attenuation in selected pain. *Laser Therapy*, 6, 143–148.

Tranquilli, W.J., Thurmon, J.C., Grimm, K.A. (2007) *Lumb & Jones' Veterinary Anesthesia and Analgesia*, 4th edn,. Blackwell publishing, Ames, Iowa, USA.

Tunér, J. & Hode, L. (2010) Low-level laser therapy for hand arthritis-fact or fiction? *Clinical Rheumatology*, 30, 147–148.

Uebelhart, D., Thonar, E.J., Delmas, P.D., et al. (1998) Effects of oral chondroitin sulfate on the progression of knee osteoarthritis: a pilot study. *Osteoarthritis Cartilage*, 6, 39–46.

Ulbricht, C.E. & Basch, E.M. (2005) *Natural Standard – Herb & Supplement Reference,* Elsevier Mosby, St. Louis, USA, pp. 790–1000.

Valvason, C., Musacchio, E., & Pozzuoli, A. (2008) Influence of glucosamine sulfate on oxidative stress in human osteoarthritic chondrocytes: effects on HO-1, p22Phox and iNOS expression. *Rheumatology*, 47(1), 31–35.

van Baar, M.E., Dekker, J., Oostendorp, R.A.B., et al. (1998) The effectiveness of exercise therapy in patients with osteoarthritis of the hip or knee: a randomized clinical trial. *Journal of Rheumatology*, 25, 2432–2439.

Vandeweerd, J.M., Coisnon, C., Clegg, P., et al. (2012) Systematic review of efficacy of nutraceuticals to alleviate clinical signs of osteoarthritis. *Journal of Veterinary Internal Medicine*, 26(3), 448–456.

Vaz, A.L. (1982) Double blind clinical evaluation of the relative efficiency of ibuprofen and glucosamine sulfate in the management of osteoarthritis of the knee in outpatients. *Current Medical Research & Opinion*, 8, 145–149.

Vollmer, K.O., von Hodenberg, A., & Kolle, E.U. (1986) Pharmacokinetics and metabolism of gabapentin in rat, dog and man. *Arzneimittelforschung*, 36, 830–839.

Wall, P.D. & Melzack, R. (2003) *Handbook of Pain Management*, Churchill Livingstone, Edinburgh.

Wandel, S., Jüni, P., Tendal, B., et al. (2010) Effects of glucosamine, chondroitin, or placebo in patients with osteoarthritis of hip or knee: network meta-analysis. *British Medical Journal*, 341, c4675.

Wehling, P., Moser, C., Frisbie, D., et al. (2007) Autologous conditioned serum in the treatment of orthopaedic diseases. *Biodrugs*, 21, 323–332.

Welch, J.A., Wohl, J.S., & Wright, J.C. (2002) Evaluation of postoperative respiratory function by serial blood gas analysis in dogs treated with transdermal fentanyl. *Journal of Veterinary Emergency and critical care*, 12, 81–87.

Wernham, B.G., Trumpatori, B., Hash, J., et al. (2011) Dose reduction of meloxicam in dogs with osteoarthritis-associated pain and impaired mobility. *Journal of Veterinary Internal Medicine*, 25(6), 1298–1305.

White, A.R. & Earnst, E. (1999) A systematic review of randomized controlled trials of acupuncture for neck pain. *The Journal of Rheumatology*, 38, 143–147.

Whitehouse, M.W., Macrides, T.A., Kalafatis, N., et al. (1997) The anti-inflammatory activity of a lipid fraction from the New Zealand green lipped mussel. *Inflammopharmacology*, 5, 237–246.

Wolfe, K. & Poma, R. (2010) Syringomyelia in the Cavalier King Charles spaniel (CKCS) dog. *The Canadian Veterinary Journal*, 51, 95–102.

Yeates, J.W. & Main, D.C.J. (2011) Veterinary surgeons' opinions on dog welfare issues. *Journal of Small Animal Practice*, 52, 464–468.

Yoshikawa, T., Tanaka, H., & Kondo, M. (1983) Effect of vitamin E on adjuvant arthritis in rats. *Biochemical Medicine*, 29, 227–234.

Yoshimura, K., Horiuchi, M., Konishi, M., et al. (1993) Physical dependence on morphine induced in dogs via the use of miniosmotic pumps. *Journal of Pharmacological and Toxicological Methods*, 30(2), 85–95.

Zhang, W., Doherty, M., Arden, N., et al. (2005) EULAR evidence based recommendations for the management of hip osteoarthritis: report of a task force of the EULAR Standing Committee for International Clinical Studies Including Therapeutics (ESCISIT). *Annals of the Rheumatic Diseases*, 64(5), 669–681.

24

The Recognition and Assessment of Pain in Cats

Kersti Seksel

Pain is defined as "An unpleasant sensory and emotional experience associated with actual or potential tissue damage" (IASP, 1994). Thus, pain is characterized by physical discomfort, and typically leads to evasive action and acute mental or emotional distress or suffering. Although animal welfare was once heavily weighted in terms of the physical health of the animal and its environment (e.g., provision of shelter and food), the psychological well-being of nonhuman animals is now included in the assessment of welfare (e.g., the OIE Terrestrial Animal Health Code, 2012). Pain negatively affects quality of life, induces behavioral changes, and causes unnecessary fear, anxiety, and stress. The recent AAHA and AAFP pain management guidelines were developed to help practitioners identify situations in which pain management may be required, and to provide resources to help improve their analgesic practice in cats (Hellyer et al., 2007)

SOURCES OF PAIN IN CATS

Pain may be classified as acute or chronic, localized or generalized, and adaptive (inflammatory or nociceptive) or maladaptive (neuropathic or functional), and an individual may experience several types of pain concurrently. Common sources of mild to moderate pain in cats include, but are not limited to, castration, mild gingivitis, cystitis, otitis, dermatitis, mild osteoarthritis, and soft tissue injury (including bite wounds, lacerations, contusions). Sources of moderate to severe pain in cats include osteoarthritis, enucleation of the eye, dental extractions, severe gingivitis, pancreatitis, neoplasia, abdominal procedures (exploratory laparotomy), and orthopedic procedures (Hellyer et al., 2007; Robertson, 2008).

PAIN AND BEHAVIOR

One of the most commonly recognized signs of pain in animals is a change in their behavior, and this may be the first indication that an animal is unwell (Seksel, 2008; McKune & Robertson, 2012). A behavioral response involves not only what an animal does but also when, how, where, and why it exhibits the behavior. Behavior should never be considered in isolation, but always in the context in which it occurs.

The behavioral signs of pain may be overt or covert and vary with the type of pain, species (Overall, 1997; Dobromylskyj et al., 2000), gender and hormonal status (Unruh, 1996; Cook, 1997; Page, 1999; Craft, 2003; Craft et al., 2004; Fillingim & Gear, 2004), and age (Sternberg et al., 2004). Previous exposure to noxious or stressful stimuli, and the outcome of that experience, will affect the behavior exhibited (Overall, 1997). Moreover, the environment or situation in which the animal is assessed for pain may affect how a behavior is expressed. For example, the presence or absence of others (conspecifics as well as members of other species), familiar or unfamiliar surroundings, and novel stimuli (e.g., weather) play a part in determining what behaviors are expressed, and the duration and frequency of the behavior (Flecknell, 2000).

ASSESSMENT OF PAIN

Typically, pain has been assessed by three approaches:

- Measurement of general body functions and homeostasis (e.g., food intake, weight gain, or reproductive success).
- Measurement of physiological responses (e.g., plasma cortisol concentrations, blood pressure, heart rate).
- Measurement of behavioral responses, such as vocalization and changes in body language and facial expression.

Assessment of pain by observing an animal's behavior is subjective, but, because it is generally noninvasive, there are considerable benefits from observing behavior. Signs of pain may include loss of normal behaviors as well as the expression of abnormal behaviors; furthermore, because pain alters motivation, avoidance or defensive behaviors are more likely to be exhibited. Three main techniques have been used to assess pain behaviors (Weary et al., 2006):

- Identification of pain-specific behaviors (e.g., increased vocalization).
- Observation of changes in normal behavior (e.g., decreased locomotor activity or appetite).
- Observation of preference or avoidance behaviors.

Pain is also assessed by response to therapy with analgesics. The signs of pain in cats are subtle, and likely vary with environment,

Pain Management in Veterinary Practice, First Edition. Edited by Christine M. Egger, Lydia Love and Tom Doherty.
© 2014 John Wiley & Sons, Inc. Published 2014 by John Wiley & Sons, Inc.

type of procedure, pre-existing conditions, and the individual. In addition, because they are not always compliant for palpation and manipulation, it can be challenging to perform orthopedic and neurological examinations on cats (Vainionpaa et al., 2012). To effectively assess if a cat is experiencing pain, it is essential to be familiar with the normal behavior of the cat. This involves not only being familiar with the species but also with the individual. Pet owners, for instance, are very astute at recognizing even minor changes in their pets' behavior.

Behavioral Signs of Fear, Anxiety, and Learned Helplessness in Cats

A painful experience may evoke fear and anxiety. Behavioral signs of fear are very similar to and many overlap with the signs of pain. Nevertheless, it is important to differentiate between fear and pain because the management and treatment regimens instigated in response to these behaviors will differ, and long-term problems, such as anxiety and panic, could result from inappropriate treatment (Overall, 1997).

Although the terms anxiety and fear are often used interchangeably, they are not the same. Fear is related to the specific behaviors of escape and avoidance, whereas anxiety is the result of threats that are perceived to be uncontrollable or unavoidable. Fear should be distinguished from anxiety, which typically occurs without any external threat. Fear is usually of acute onset and is transient, whereas anxiety, the anticipation of future danger or misfortune, is a more chronic state of nonspecific apprehension.

The emotion of fear induces the physiological effects of the sympathetic nervous system—the flight, fight, or freeze response. An increase in muscle tone is needed for physical movement and increased blood flow to those muscles is necessary to increase oxygen delivery. The physiological response also includes increased heart rate and respiratory rate (panting), sweating, trembling, pacing, and possibly urination and defecation (Notari, 2009).

Cats exhibit changes in body posture and activity when afraid, and may engage in avoidance responses such as fleeing or hiding. A fearful cat may assume body postures that are protective, such as lowering of the body and head, placing the ears closer to the head, and the tail tucked under the body. If the cat perceives a threat, the response can also include elements of defensive aggression (Notari, 2009). Displacement behaviors can also occur and, while they are normal behaviors, they are not normal in the context in which they are displayed. Displacement behaviors include lip licking, yawning, grooming, and sniffing.

Another complicating factor in identifying behavioral signs of pain is learned helplessness. If an animal cannot escape the source of pain, learned helplessness may result. The animal literally appears to "give up" and will not respond or react at all to manipulation or palpation of painful areas. This may give the false impression that the animal is not in pain.

Behavioral Signs of Pain in Cats

The most common behavioral indicators of pain in cats are listed in Table 24.1. Many of these clinical signs are used as indicators of pain because they are overt and easily recognized and measured. Covert signs of pain are more difficult, if not impossible, to detect in any species, and may manifest as sleeping or hiding. Thus, it should not be assumed that a sleeping or hiding cat is comfortable. It is critical to have knowledge of normal behavior for the cat being

Table 24.1.　Common clinical signs of pain in cats

Clinical Signs
Avoidance or flight response
Aggression or fight response: Pain may lower the threshold for aggression and lower tolerance to handling.
Restlessness or agitation
Depression and reluctance to move
Hunched posture with head held low
Squinting of the eyes
Vocalization (including purring)
Increased responsiveness when site of pain is manipulated
Gait changes (e.g., limping or other adaptations of gait in arthritic cats—these may persist after the pain has decreased)
Changes in locomotion (increase or decreased movement)
Changes in respiration rate and heart rate
Decreased appetite
Increased or decreased grooming
Decreased interactions with people or animals
Tail flicking
Changes in facial expression

evaluated; thus, owners and caregivers should be included in the evaluation process. Deviations from normal behavior suggest pain, anxiety, fear, or some combination of stressors (Robertson, 2008).

Cats do not always vocalize when in pain; however, if painful they may hiss, spit, and growl when approached or handled (Seksel, 2008; Notari, 2009). Several studies have shown that veterinarians are most likely to treat "painful" animals that vocalize. This means that animals that do not vocalize are less likely to be treated or that the treatment is inadequate.

PAIN ASSESSMENT IN CATS

Currently, there is no gold standard for assessing pain in animals, and there are no validated scales to assess pain or the efficacy of analgesic treatment in cats. Commonly used systems for assessing pain include simple descriptive scales, numeric rating scales, and visual analog scales (VAS).

A simple scale, intended for pain assessment of cats after surgery or trauma, has been developed at Colorado State University (feline acute pain scale) for use in clinical situations. This scale is available to download at http://csuanimalcancercenter.org/assets/files/csu_acute_pain_scale_feline.pdf.

Assessment of Acute Pain

Scoring systems that include observation and interaction with the animal are thought to be most reliable (Cambridge et al., 2000, Robertson, 2008; McKune & Robertson, 2012). Wound sensitivity correlated well with visual analog pain scores in cats with acute pain (Slingsby et al., 2001). In a study of cats undergoing tenectomy, onychectomy, or anesthesia alone, physiological parameters (heart rate, respiratory rate, rectal temperature) and plasma cortisol and β-endorphin concentrations did not differ among groups. However, there were significant differences among groups for response to handling and palpation of the forelimb (simple descriptive score), and the observational and interactive VAS. The authors concluded that determination of the presence of pain in cats could be made on the basis of observation and interaction by a trained observer (Cambridge et al., 2000).

Other studies have also failed to find reliable correlations between physiological variables, such as respiratory rate, heart rate, blood pressure, or plasma cortisol or β-endorphin concentrations, and pain scores in cats, and many factors other than pain can influence these variables (Smith et al., 1996; Smith et al., 1999; Cambridge et al., 2000).

An ethogram was used to identify pre- and postoperative behaviors in cats undergoing ovariohysterectomy (Waran et al., 2007). The study compared cats not given analgesics, cats given preoperative analgesics, and cats given pre- and postoperative analgesics. Cats not given postoperative analgesics more frequently assumed a "half-tucked up" posture and demonstrated a greater incidence of crouching behavior and attention to the surgical site (turning toward incision or physically touching it). These behaviors were thought to be indicative of pain because they were not seen prior to surgery, they occurred in the greatest frequency in the first hour post surgery, they had the greatest occurrence in the group not given postoperative analgesics, and there was a decrease in these behaviors after analgesics were administered. Vaisanen et al. (2007) asked owners to complete a questionnaire on their cats' behavior during the 3 days after ovariohysterectomy or castration, and to indicate their perceptions of the severity of postoperative pain using a 100 mm VAS. Owners consistently indicated that they observed changes in their cats' behavior including a decrease in overall activity level, an increase in time spent sleeping, a decrease in playfulness, and an altered way of movement. Pain was thought to be more severe in female cats, with an average VAS of 25 mm compared to 15 mm in male cats. Other behaviors reported included decreases in vocalization, increase in desire for human companionship, and hiding and attention seeking behaviors.

Variations of the VAS (Carroll et al., 2008; 2011) and the NRS (Ingwersen et al., 2012) have been used to assess acute pain and response to treatment in cats in the research setting. A multidimensional composite measure scale has been developed for cats and is currently undergoing further validation (Brondani et al., 2009; Brondani et al., 2011).

Assessment of Chronic Pain
In the assessment of chronic pain, a questionnaire using owner observation to evaluate quality of life has been validated in dogs (Wiseman–Orr, 2006), and several questionnaires have been developed to identify pain behaviors and assess response to treatment in cats, but all currently lack validation. Lascelles et al. (2007) compared a client-specific outcome measures questionnaire with an activity monitor for ability to characterize impairment in 13 cats. The cats were 10 years of age or older (mean age 14 years), and had painful arthritic joints, radiographic evidence of OA, and owner-assessed decreases in activity. In addition to the questionnaire, the owners were also asked to complete a simple global quality of life assessment. The cats' behavior was evaluated initially without medication, and again after treatment with placebo or meloxicam. Activity counts for the week when cats were administered meloxicam were significantly greater than baseline, but placebo treatment did not affect activity counts. The client questionnaire data showed that owners also considered their cats to be more active on meloxi-

cam compared with baseline and placebo, although some placebo effect was seen. Assessment of global quality of life improved significantly with meloxicam treatment.

The effects of meloxicam treatment on owner-observed behavioral and lifestyle changes were evaluated in 28 cats with clinical and radiographic evidence of osteoarthritis. The study evaluated lameness, general demeanor, activity levels, food and water intake, aggression, grooming, ability to jump, and elimination habits before treatment and after 28 days of treatment with meloxicam (Clarke & Bennett, 2006). The most obvious change after meloxicam treatment was an improvement in ability and willingness to jump, and overall activity levels.

Another study used a client questionnaire to evaluate the observed behavioral and lifestyle changes in cats with known musculoskeletal disease, before and after treatment with meloxicam. The questionnaire grouped behaviors into 4 domains: mobility, activity, grooming, and temperament, and was completed by the owner prior to treatment and again after 28 days of treatment. There was a significant improvement in behaviors within the four domains after treatment, and the authors concluded that owners' assessment of changes in their cats' behavior is an important method of identifying chronic pain in cats (Bennett and Morton, 2009).

Another study in cats with radiographic evidence of degenerative joint disease and clinical signs of musculoskeletal pain, found that behaviors relating to activity levels were very different between healthy cats and cats with DJD-associated pain. The authors were able to identify 15 potentially useful parameters that will be used to construct an owner-answered questionnaire, which the authors will attempt to validate to assess degenerative joint disease associated pain in cats (Zamprogno et al., 2010).

Slingerland et al. (2011) studied 100 cats and used a questionnaire to identify behavioral and lifestyle changes with OA in cats. They reported decreased mobility (less jumping, decreased height of jump, stiffness and problems walking up and down the stairs, and less grooming as being associated with OA, but these features also strongly correlated with increasing age. Increased elimination over the edge of the litter box was also associated with OA.

Interestingly, lameness does not appear to be a consistent finding in cats with musculoskeletal pain, and the prevalence of radiographic evidence of degenerative joint disease and osteoarthritis is greater than the prevalence of lameness (Hardie et al., 2002; Godfrey, 2005; Clarke et al., 2005; Bennett et al., 2012).

Complicating the identification and assessment of pain in cats are the recent findings of a study comparing thermographic imaging with physical examination and a client questionnaire and owner's estimation of whether the cat was in pain. The agreement between the owners estimation of pain and the questionnaire and the physical examination and thermographic imaging findings was low, and the agreement between the physical examination findings and thermography was moderate, perhaps suggesting that owners cannot reliably identify painful behaviors in their cats (Vainionpaa et al., 2012).

SUMMARY
Recognition of pain in cats is complex. It involves learning to recognize covert as well as overt signs of pain. Humans show large individual variation in responses to pain and its treatment and the same is probably true for cats. Thus, it is important to assess each

cat as an individual. Further research and training, including client education, in the recognition of pain in cats is required.

REFERENCES

Bennett, D. & Morton, C.A. (2009) A study of owner observed behavioural and lifestyle changes in cats with musculoskeletal disease before and after analgesic therapy. *Journal of Feline Medicine and Surgery*, 11, 997–1004

Bennett, D., Zainal Ariffin, S.M., & Johnston, P. (2012) Osteoarthritis in the cat 1. How common is it and how easy to recognise? *Journal of Feline Medicine and Surgery*, 14, 65–75.

Brondani, J.T., Luna, S.P.L., & Padovani, C.R. (2011) Refinement and initial validation of a multidimensional composite scale for use in assessing acute postoperative pain in cats. *American Journal of Veterinary Research*, 72, 174–183.

Brondani, J.T., Luna, S.P.L., Beier, S.L., et al. (2009) Analgesic efficacy of perioperative use of vedaprofen, tramadol or their combination in cats undergoing ovariohysterectomy. *Journal of Feline Medicine and Surgery*, 11, 420–429.

Cambridge, A., Tobias, K., Newberry, R., et al. (2000) Subjective and objective measurements of postoperative pain in cats. *Journal of the American Veterinary Medical Association*, 217(5), 685–690.

Carroll, G.L., Narbe, R., Peterson, K., et al. (2008) A pilot study: sodium urate synovitis as an acute model of inflammatory response using objective and subjective criteria to evaluate arthritis pain in cats. *Journal of Veterinary Pharmacology and Therapeutics*, 31, 456–465.

Carroll, G.L., Narbe, R., Kerwin, S.C., et al. (2011) Dose range finding study for the efficacy of meloxicam administered prior to sodium urate-induced synovitis in cats. *Veterinary Anaesthesia and Analgesia*, 38(4), 394–406.

Clarke, S.P. & Bennett, D. (2006) Feline osteoarthritis: a prospective study of 28 cases. *Journal of Small Animal Practice*, 47, 439–445.

Clarke, S.P., Mellor, D., Clements, D.N., et al. (2005) Radiographic prevalence of degenerative joint disease in a hospital population of cats. *The Veterinary Record*, 157, 793e9.

Cook, C.J. (1997) Sex related differences in analgesia in sheep (*Ovis ovis*). *New Zealand Veterinary Journal*, 45(4), 169–170.

Craft, R.M. (2003) Sex differences in opioid analgesia: "from mouse to man." *Clinical Journal of Pain*, 19(3), 175–176.

Craft, R.M., Mogil, J.S., & Aloisi, A.M. (2004) Sex differences in pain and analgesia: the role of gonadal hormones. *European Journal of Pain*, 8(5), 397–411.

Dobromylskyj, P., Flecknell, P.A., Lascelles, P.D., et al. (2000) Pain assessment, in *Pain management in Animals* (eds P. Flecknell & A. Waterman-Pearson), WB Saunders, London, pp. 53–79.

Fillingim, R.B. & Gear, R.W. (2004) Sex differences in opioid analgesia: clinical and experimental findings. *European Journal of Pain*, 8(5), 413–425.

Flecknell, P.A. (2000) Animal pain an introduction, in *Pain management in Animals* (eds P. Flecknell & A. Waterman-Pearson), WB Saunders, London, pp. 1–7.

Godfrey, D.R. (2005) Osteoarthritis in cats: a retrospective radiological study. *Journal of Small Animal Practice*, 46, 425–429.

Hardie, E.M., Roe, S.C., & Martin, F.R. (2002) Radiographic evidence of degenerative joint disease in geriatric cats: 100 cases (1994–1997). *Journal of the American Veterinary Medical Association*, 220, 628–632.

Hellyer, P., Rodan, I., Brunt, J., et al. (2007) AAHA/AAFP pain management guidelines for dogs and cats. *Journal of Feline Medicine and Surgery*, 9, 466–480.

IASP Task Force on Taxonomy (1994) Pain terms, a current list with definitions and notes on usage, in *Classification of Chronic Pain*, 2nd edn (eds H. Merskey & N. Bogduk), IASP Press, Seattle.

Ingwersen, W., Fox, R., Cunningham, G., et al. (2012) Efficacy and safety of 3 versus 5 days of meloxicam as an analgesic for feline onychectomy and sterilization. *The Canadian Veterinary Journal*, 53(3), 257–264.

Lascelles, B.D.X., Bernie, H.D., Roe, S., et al. (2007) Evaluation of client-specific outcome measures and activity monitoring to measure pain relief in cats with osteoarthritis. *Journal of Veterinary Internal Medicine*, 21, 410–416.

McKune, C. & Robertson, S. (2012) Analgesia, in *The Cat Clinical Medicine and Management* (ed. S. Little) Elsevier, St Louis, Missouri, pp. 90–111.

Notari, L. (2009) Stress in veterinary behavioural medicine, in *BSAVA Manual of Canine and Feline Behavioural Medicine*, 2nd edn (eds D.F. Horwitz & D.S. Mills), BSAVA, Gloucester, pp. 136–145.

OIE Terrestrial Animal Health Code (2012) www.oie.int/international-standard-setting/terrestrial-code.

Overall, K.L. (ed.) (1997) *Clinical Behavioral Medicine for Small Animals*. 1st edn, Mosby. St. Louis, Missouri.

Page, G.G. (1999) The multi-issue nature of sex differences in opioid analgesia. *Pain Forum*, 8(1), 45–47.

Robertson, S. A. (2005) Assessment and management of acute pain in cats. *Journal of Veterinary Emergency and Critical Care*, 15(4), 261–272.

Robertson, S.A. (2008) Managing pain in feline patients. *Veterinary Clinics of North America Small Animal Practice*, 38(6), 1267–1290.

Seksel, K. (2008) How pain affects animals, in *Animal Pain* (ed. D. Mellor), OIE publication.

Slingerland, L.I., Hazewinkel, H.A.W., Meij, B.P., et al. (2011) Cross-sectional study of the prevalence and clinical features of osteoarthritis in 100 cats. *Veterinary Journal*, 187, 304–309.

Slingsby, L., Jones, A., & Waterman-Pearson, A.E. (2001) Use of a new finger-mounted device to compare mechanical nociceptive thresholds in cats given pethidine or no medication after castration. *Research in Veterinary Science*, 70(3), 243–246.

Smith, J., Allen, S., & Quandt, J. (1999) Changes in cortisol concentration in response to stress and postoperative pain in client-owned cats and correlation with objective clinical variables. *American Journal of Veterinary Research*, 60(4), 432–436.

Smith, J., Allen, S., Quandt, J., et al. (1996) Indicators of postoperative pain in cats and correlation with clinical criteria. *American Journal of Veterinary Research*, 57(11), 1674–1678.

Sternberg, W.F., Ritchie, J., & Mogil, J.S. (2004) Qualitative sex differences in kappa-opioid analgesia in mice are dependent on age. *Neuroscience Letters*, 363(2), 178–181.

Unruh, A.M. (1996) Gender variations in clinical pain research. *Pain*, 65(2–3), 123–167.

Vainionpaa, M.H., Raekallio, M.R., Junnila, J.J.T., et al. (2012) A comparison of thermographic imaging, physical examination and modified questionnaire as an instrument to assess painful conditions in cats. *Journal of Feline Medicine and Surgery*, 0(0), 1–8.

Vaisanen, M.A.M., Tuomikoski, S.K., & Vainio, O.M. (2007) Behavioral alterations and severity of pain in cats recovering at home following elective ovariohysterectomy or castration.

Journal of the American Veterinary Medical Association, 231, 236–242.

Waran, N., Best, L., Williams, V., Salinsky, J., Clarke, N. (2007) A preliminary study of behaviour-based indicators of pain in cats. *Animal Welfare*, 16(Suppl 1),105–108.

Weary, D.M., Niel, L., Flower, F.C., et al. (2006) Identifying and preventing pain in animals. *Applied Animal Behavior Science*, 100(1–2), 64–76.

Wiseman–Orr, M.L., Scott, E.M., Reid, J., et al. (2006) Validation of a structured questionnaire as an instrument to measure chronic pain in dogs on the basis of effects on health related quality of life. *American Journal of Veterinary Research*, 67, 1826–1836.

Zamprogno, H., Hansen, B.D., Bondell, H.D., et al. (2010) Item generation and design testing of a questionnaire to assess degenerative joint disease-associated pain in cats. *American Journal of Veterinary Research*, 71(12), 1417–1424.

25
Treatment of Acute Pain in Cats

Jacob A. Johnson

Pain has been recognized in felines since at least the 1950s, when cats were used as research models for discovery of pain mechanisms in humans (Kennard, 1953; Kennard, 1954). However, the recognition that pain should be treated in cats did not come until much later (Davis & Donnelly, 1968), as is evidenced by painful studies performed on awake cats that were afforded no analgesia (Straw & Mitchell, 1964). The treatment of acute pain is important for medical and ethical reasons, and control of pain promotes healing, decreases morbidity, and reduces complications (Davis et al., 2007b). Veterinarians entering the profession swear an oath to relieve animal suffering, and professional organizations, such as the American Animal Hospital Association (AAHA) and the American Association of Feline Practitioners (AAFP), require assessment of pain and the use of analgesics for all surgical patients (Hellyer et al., 2007).

Data collected in a teaching hospital between 1983 and 1989 showed that only one in 15 cats undergoing major operations were administered analgesics in the postoperative period (Hansen & Hardie, 1993). This statistic appears to have improved by 1996, when 94% of feline orthopedic patients were reported to have been given analgesics, yet only 26% of ovariohysterectomy patients were given analgesics (Lascelles et al., 1999). A 2006 study reported that the percentage of cats being given analgesics post ovariohysterectomy had increased to 87.2% (Hewson et al., 2006).

There are four primary reasons cited as to why the treatment of acute pain in feline patients has been neglected (Lascelles & Waterman, 1997):

1. The difficulty of assessing pain in the feline patient.

2. Misconceptions about analgesic drugs, especially opioids, in felines.

3. The lack of products licensed for pain management in felines.

4. Reservations about the adverse effects of analgesics.

Fortunately, all these limitations have been addressed in recent years, and practitioners now have the resources necessary to address acute pain in feline patients.

CONSEQUENCES OF ACUTE PAIN

Acute pain is pain associated with an acute injury or event where the signs of chronic pain are absent. In human patients, chronic pain is defined as pain that persists past the normal time of healing (Merskey & Bogduk, 1994). Acute pain is most often experienced in the perioperative period, but other causes of acute pain include trauma, inflammation and/or infection, and illnesses, such as pancreatitis.

Prolonged, untreated acute pain has numerous negative physiological effects including activation of the sympathetic nervous system, increasing myocardial work and oxygen consumption; activation of the renin–angiotensin–aldosterone system (RAAS), causing fluid and sodium retention; and impaired wound healing and increased incidence of bacterial infections secondary to sympathetically induced vasoconstriction limiting blood flow to the periphery (Gaynor & Muir, 2009). Prolonged acute pain can lead to chronic pain and decreased quality of life (Carr & Goudas, 1999).

GOALS OF TREATMENT OF ACUTE PAIN IN CATS

Acute pain in the feline patient is best managed in a goal-directed manner. The four main goals to consider are patient comfort, preventing the development of chronic pain, avoidance of adverse effects, and optimization of physiological homeostasis.

Patient Comfort

In the ideal situation, a practitioner would be able to provide complete analgesia. Although analgesia means absence of pain, the term is a misnomer, as frequently the goal is to reduce the pain to a level that is tolerable for the patient. If pain is reduced to a tolerable level there is a reduction in sympathetic stimulation, thus avoiding many of the deleterious effects of the pain. Reducing pain to a tolerable level allows the patient to recover from surgery without undue suffering, thus speeding the time to discharge. Some techniques, such as local and regional blocks, do allow for the complete cessation of painful stimulus.

Pain Management in Veterinary Practice, First Edition. Edited by Christine M. Egger, Lydia Love and Tom Doherty.
© 2014 John Wiley & Sons, Inc. Published 2014 by John Wiley & Sons, Inc.

Preventing the Development of Chronic Pain

Persistent, uncontrolled noxious input can cause a maladaptive process referred to as neuropathic pain, a common type of chronic pain (Chapter 2). In human medicine, the transition from acute to chronic pain is assumed to occur at 3–6 months after acute injury or surgery (Merskey & Bogduk, 1994). A continued barrage of afferent input from a painful process causes physiological changes in the peripheral nerves and dorsal horn of the spinal cord, resulting in hyperalgesia, allodynia, and central sensitization. These pathological conditions can persist even after the initial insult has resolved. The role of acute pain in the establishment of chronic pain states continues to be a source of investigation (Andreae et al., 2008), but use of multimodal analgesia for acute pain has demonstrated benefit in reducing chronic pain (Clarke et al., 2012).

Prevention of Adverse Effects

No pharmacological intervention is without some unwanted effect. Historically, one of the reasons cited for practitioners' reluctance to administer analgesics to feline patients has been the potential for adverse effects (Lascelles et al., 1999). This is especially true of opioids, where the fear of excitement or "morphine mania" has caused practitioners to avoid their use in felines. Based on clinical experience, concerns about opioids in cats seem to be unfounded (Taylor & Robertson, 2004). Nevertheless, a balance must be struck between desired effects (i.e., adequate analgesia) and adverse effects, such as agitation, excess sedation, hypothermia, ileus, or cardiovascular depression.

Optimization of Physiological Homeostasis

This final goal requires balancing the effects of analgesics and other interventions to return the patient's internal physiological environment to the state it was prior to acute injury, illness, or surgery. Analgesia is critical in removing the excessive stress response and surge of endogenous catecholamines. At the same time, inappropriate use of analgesics may cause a decrease in body temperature, ventilation, or cardiac output.

TREATMENT STRATEGIES

Preventive Analgesia

An important strategy in developing an acute pain management plan is to employ preventive analgesia. The value of preemptive analgesia, that is, administering analgesics prior to the induction of pain, has been scrutinized, and numerous large studies have failed to demonstrate a benefit of this strategy (Campiglia et al., 2010). Part of the issue may be in the limited scope of the definition; that is, it may not be adequate to simply administer analgesics prior to nociceptive input to control pain. Kissin (2000) was the first to suggest a broader definition of preemptive analgesia that has now been further defined as preventive analgesia (Dahl & Kehlet, 2011). To be preventive, an analgesic treatment must be:

- Administered prior to the induction of nociceptive input.
- Of sufficient efficacy to control intense, acute nociceptive input.
- Of sufficient duration to last until nociceptive input has subsided.
- Capable of combating incisional/physiological pain and inflammatory pain.

Recent studies that incorporate these tenets have demonstrated the benefit of preventive analgesia (Ong et al., 2005; Hebl et al., 2008).

Unfortunately, the nociceptive process has already been initiated in patients that have experienced trauma or are suffering from systemic illness and, therefore, can be more difficult to control. Luckily, the most common cause of acute pain is surgery and, frequently, the nociceptive process is not induced until the initiation of the procedure. These patients benefit the most from preventive analgesic strategies. For those patients that are already sensitized to pain, additional treatment with drugs specifically targeted at neuroplastic changes (Chapter 8), such as N-methyl-D-aspartate (NMDA) receptor antagonists, selective calcium channel blockers (gabapentin) and/or sodium channel blockers (lidocaine) may be required to provide effective analgesia.

Locoregional Anesthesia

In addition to preventive analgesia, another beneficial concept to employ is management of pain at the lowest level on the nociceptive pathway. Local anesthesia provides several distinct advantages when applied appropriately for pain management: complete abolition of nociceptive input, decreased risk of maladaptive pain processes, and decreased risk of adverse effects. If nociceptive input can be eliminated peripherally by applying local anesthetics (Chapter 6), then there is no risk of peripheral sensitization, central sensitization, or perception of pain by the patient. Moreover, there is a reduced risk of adverse effects because of the smaller doses of drugs needed to provide analgesia.

Local anesthetics can be the sole analgesic provided for simple surgical procedures performed on sedated patients or can be incorporated into a multimodal approach to acute pain management, and can be beneficial even when the patient is under general anesthesia.

LOCAL ANESTHETIC DRUGS

Commonly used local anesthetics include lidocaine, bupivacaine, mepivacaine, and ropivacaine (Chapter 6). Ropivacaine is a newer local anesthetic with a lower potential for adverse cardiovascular effects. The agents vary in their onset and duration of action based on their physical properties, and can be selected based on the specific needs of a patient (Table 25.1). The goal is to use the largest volume and concentration possible while avoiding adverse effects resulting from absorption. This will speed onset, prolong the duration of action, and increase the likelihood of a successful block (Scott et al., 1980).

The toxic doses of local anesthetics used epidurally or subcutaneously for local anesthesia in cats have not been established. An injection of 3 mg/kg of lidocaine for intravenous regional anesthesia had no detrimental effects (Kushner et al., 2002). Intravenous infusion of lidocaine at a rate of 16 mg/kg/min produced the initial signs of neurotoxicity (first occurrence of EEG spike wave activity) after 0.8 minutes, and infusion of bupivacaine at 4 mg/kg/min caused similar signs at 1.1 minutes (Chadwick, 1985). A 20 mg dose of bupivacaine administered intratracheally induced a greater than 20% decrease in heart rate and blood pressure, and caused apnea (Ford et al., 1984). When used epidurally, it is recommended not to exceed 4 mg/kg of lidocaine or 1 mg/kg of bupivacaine (Robertson & Taylor, 2004). Intravenous constant rate infusion of lidocaine is discussed later in the chapter.

Table 25.1. Local Anesthetics for acute pain in cats

Drug	Dose	Concentration (%)	Onset (min)	Duration (h)	Indications	Cautions/ contraindications	Reference
Epidural							
Lidocaine	0.2 mL/kg	2	<10	1.5	Perineal, hindlimb, caudal abdominal analgesia	Clotting disorders, infection at administration site, uncorrected hypotension	Valverde, 2008
Bupivacaine	0.2 mL/kg	0.5	<15	2–4	As above	As above	As above
Ropivacaine	0.2 mL/kg	0.5	<15	2–4	As above	As above	As above
Local/Regional							
Lidocaine	0.1–0.5 mL/ site	1–2	Fast	1–2	Analgesia of limbs, oral cavity, globe, chest wall, local lesions	Avoid inadvertent vascular injection Avoid exceeding 4 mg/kg total dose	Skarda & Tranquilli, 2007
Bupivacaine	0.1–0.5 mL/ site	0.25–0.5	Intermediate	3–8	As above	Avoid inadvertent vascular injection Avoid exceeding 2 mg/kg total dose	As above
Ropivacaine	0.1–0.5 mL/ site	0.2–0.5	Intermediate	3–8	As above	Avoid inadvertent vascular injection	As above
Mepivacaine	0.1–0.5 mL/ site	1–2	Fast	1.5–3	As above	Avoid inadvertent vascular injection	As above
Wound Diffusion Catheter							
Bupivacaine	0.5–1 mg/kg q6h	0.125–0.25	N/A	6	Amputation, large mass removal, thoracotomy, sterile wound closure	Limit dose to 4 mg/kg/day	Davis et al., 2007a

No information is available on the toxicity of ropivacaine or mepivacaine in cats. In dogs, ropivacaine is very similar to bupivacaine in its neurotoxicity, but is less toxic to the cardiovascular system (Feldman et al., 1989).

In human medicine, the addition of α-2 agonists to local anesthetics for regional anesthesia shows some benefit, including increased duration of action (McCartney et al., 2007; Popping et al., 2009). In cats, no appreciable benefit has been demonstrated (Lawal & Adetunji, 2009). Limited information is available on the benefit of adding opioids to local anesthetics for epidural analgesia in cats (Troncy et al., 2002).

SELECTED LOCAL ANESTHETIC TECHNIQUES IN CATS

Topical Anesthesia
Certain formulations of local anesthetics (Chapter 9) applied topically will provide a limited degree of analgesia. Eutectic Mixture of Local Anesthetics (EMLA) cream is a prescription mixture of lidocaine and prilocaine formulated to permeate the epidermis. This product is applied over the area to be anesthetized, and covered with an occlusive bandage for 60 minutes. A similar product, liposome-encapsulated 4% lidocaine, is available over-the-counter. In human patients, this product, without the use of an occlusive dressing, is as effective as EMLA cream, and needs only a 30-minute application time (Eichenfield et al., 2002). These creams can provide effective analgesia for minor procedures, such as blood collections and catheter insertion, especially in fractious or hyperalgesic patients. Systemic absorption of the local anesthetic using this application results in nontoxic blood concentrations (Fransson et al., 2002; Wagner et al., 2006).

Local Infiltrative Anesthesia
Local anesthesia can be used as part of a multimodal approach to surgical analgesia. Local anesthesia is an excellent choice for removal of small skin lesions and repair of superficial lacerations under sedation. To anesthetize a localized area, local anesthetic is injected in and around the immediate area of injury or surgery. A series of injections of 0.1–0.3 mL of local anesthetic into the intradermal and/or subcutaneous tissue using a 25-gauge needle is sufficient to provide complete anesthesia of the subcutaneous tissue and skin. If the wound involves deeper layers of tissue, such as muscle, local anesthetic is injected into the deeper layers of tissue once the subcutaneous tissue and the skin have been blocked. To minimize pain on injection of the local anesthetic, the needle should be advanced through areas already anesthetized.

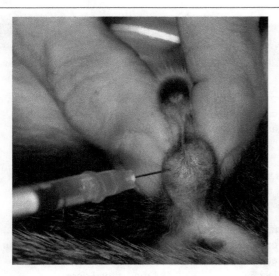

Figure 25.1. Intratesticular block is performed prior to castration (see text for description) (courtesy of Gregory Hirshoren, University of Tennessee CVM).

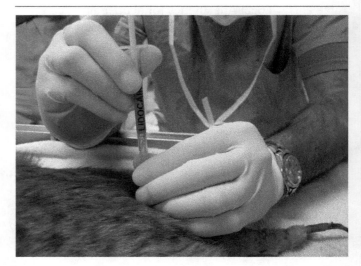

Figure 25.2. Placement of a coccygeal epidural block to provide intra- and postoperative analgesia in a patient undergoing tail amputation following a degloving injury (courtesy of Darci Palmer).

Intratesticular Local Anesthesia

Injection of lidocaine into the testicle prior to castration has proven efficacious in other species (Haga et al., 2006), and is recommended for felines (Figure 25.1). Lidocaine injected into the testicle rapidly distributes through the spermatic cord (Ranheim et al., 2005) so tissues external to the cord, such as the ligamentous attachments of the cord, may not be desensitized by this technique. To perform this block, 0.25–1 mL of 2% lidocaine (not to exceed 4 mg/kg total dose) or 0.25% or 0.5% bupivacaine (not to exceed 2 mg/kg total dose) is injected into the body of each testicle, through the scrotum, during final surgical preparation of the incision site. The suggested volumes vary, but a volume that results in the testicle feeling turgid, while not exceeding the maximum dose, is most commonly used.

Wound or Soaker Catheters

A drawback of local anesthetics is that onetime applications have a finite duration of action. In certain circumstances this can be overcome by providing intermittent boluses or constant rate infusions through wound diffusion or "soaker catheters." These catheters have been used for large invasive surgical procedures, such as removal of a fibrosarcoma or limb amputation (Davis et al., 2007a; Abelson et al., 2009). Soaker catheters are available from manufacturers (MILA International, Inc., http://milainternational.com) or can be assembled from raw materials in practice (Davis et al., 2007a; Egger & Love, 2009a). These finely fenestrated catheters are placed into a surgical incision prior to closing. If nerves were transected during the surgery, such as with an amputation, the catheter is placed in close proximity to the nerves. Once the wound is closed, bupivacaine is injected at a dose of 1–1.5 mg/kg every 6 hours (Abelson et al., 2009). Dilution of the bupivacaine to 0.125% allows for increased volume for each injection, thus a greater area of distribution within the wound.

Regional Anesthesia Techniques

If nociceptive input cannot be controlled at the local level, pain originating from particular segments of the body can be blocked regionally by applying drugs to afferent nerves. Although the nociceptors can be sensitized, and the portion of the nerve distal to the block can undergo neuroplasticity causing increased sensitivity to ongoing afferent input, nociceptive input is prevented from reaching the dorsal horn of the spinal cord. Regional anesthesia has the advantage of limiting adverse systemic effects and providing complete blockade of nociceptive input to the central nervous system. Local anesthetics, opioids, and α-2 agonists are used for regional anesthesia. Most of the blocks performed in dogs can be performed using similar techniques in cats including brachial plexus block, paravertebral block, intercostal block, intrapleural block, maxillary and mandibular blocks, retrobulbar blocks, epidural blocks (Figures 25.2 and 25.3), and spinal blocks. The reader is referred to several resources for specific information on how to perform locoregional blocks in dogs and cats (Lemke, 2007; Skarda & Tranquilli, 2007; Egger & Love, 2009a, 2009b, 2009c, 2009d).

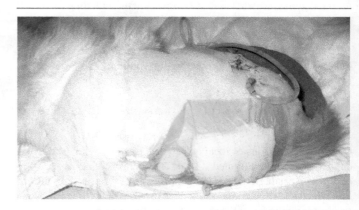

Figure 25.3. Epidural catheter in a patient being treated for severe pain due to bacterial cellulitis following a dog bite injury.

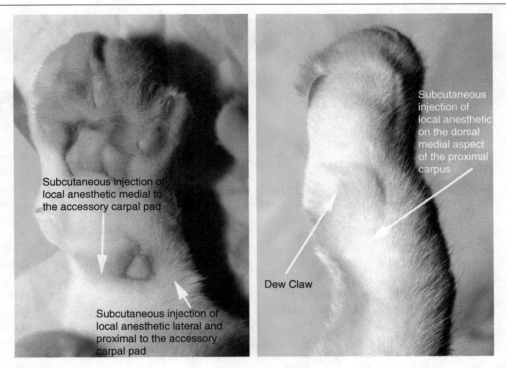

Subcutaneous injection of local anesthetic medial to the accessory carpal pad

Subcutaneous injection of local anesthetic lateral and proximal to the accessory carpal pad

Subcutaneous injection of local anesthetic on the dorsal medial aspect of the proximal carpus

Dew Claw

Figure 25.4. (a) and (b) Declaw or onychectomy block (see text for description) (courtesy of Gregory Hirshoren, University of Tennessee CVM).

Forefoot Block This nerve block is very useful for forelimb phalangeal amputation (declaw or onychectomy) (Figure 25.4). When properly applied using a long-acting anesthetic, such as bupivacaine, it provides complete anesthesia for the procedure and provides analgesia well into the postoperative period. Inject 0.2–0.3 mg/kg of bupivicaine subcutaneously at three sites on each forelimb: lateral and proximal to the accessory carpal pad to block the dorsal branch of the ulnar nerve, medial to the accessory carpal pad to block the median nerve and palmar branch of the ulnar nerve, and at the dorsal–medial aspect of the proximal carpus to block the superficial branches of the radial nerve.

Systemic Analgesia

If pain cannot be managed at the local or regional level, the next intervention point in the pain pathway is by inhibition of nociceptive input at the dorsal horn of the spinal cord and brain. Hypersensitization of the peripheral nociceptors and peripheral nerves is still possible, but the effect is dampened during processing in the dorsal horn and in the brain by the administration of systemically administered analgesics.

OPIOIDS

Clinically, the opioids (Table 25.2) (Chapter 4) are grouped according to the opioid receptor with which they interact. The primary opioid receptors involved in analgesia are μ and κ, and opioids can be agonists, partial agonists, or antagonists at these receptors. Patient specific responses to different classes of opioids appear to exist, and may be based on genetic profiles. In one study, some cats showed superior analgesia from a κ agonist, others showed superior analgesia from a μ agonist, and others did not appear to

benefit from either drug (Johnson et al., 2007). This is important to keep in mind clinically, and individuals should be monitored for efficacy of treatment. If a particular opioid does not produce the desired analgesic effect another opioid or class of opioid should be administered.

κ agonists, such as butorphanol, provide analgesia that is appropriate for minimally invasive procedures (Hellyer et al., 2007). For many years, butorphanol was the most commonly used opioid in feline patients. Although still popular, it is being replaced with more efficacious and longer-acting agents. Butorphanol has a short duration of action in other species, but feline studies show wide patient variability in the duration of action, from 0 minutes to 6 hours (Sawyer & Rech, 1987). Its efficacy demonstrates a ceiling effect, whereby increasing amounts do not provide any additional analgesia. Nalbuphine, another κ agonist, has a pharmacodynamic profile similar to butorphanol (Murphy & Hug, 1982). Overall, the κ agonists tend to exhibit fewer adverse effects and more profound sedation when compared to μ agonists. Respiratory depression and vomiting are minimal after administration of κ agonists.

Mu agonists are the primary analgesics used to combat moderate to severe pain arising from deep somatic and visceral input. Fears of excitation traditionally limited their use in feline patients, but experience has shown that they are efficacious in clinically relevant doses, and the adverse behavioral effects are minimal (Robertson & Taylor, 2004).

Adverse Effects of Opioids in Cats

Adverse and desired effects can occur with any of the full μ agonists and tend to do so in a dose-dependent manner. Dysphoria is more common at supratherapeutic doses, while euphoria, a desirable effect, is more common at clinical doses (Robertson & Taylor,

Table 25.2.   Opioids for acute pain in cats

Drug	Dose	Route	Onset (min)	Duration (h)	Cautions/ Contraindications	Reference
Butorphanol	0.1–0.8 mg/kg	IV, IM, SC	<5	0–8	Not suitable alone for moderate to severe pain	Robertson et al., 2003; Lascelles & Robertson, 2004a; Johnson et al., 2007
Nalbuphine	0.75–3 mg/kg	IV	<15	2.5–3		Sawyer & Rech, 1987
Morphine	0.1–0.2 mg/kg	IV (slow), IM, SQ	5–45 (depends on route)	6	Rapid IV injection may cause histamine release	Lascelles & Waterman, 1997; Taylor et al., 2001; Steagall et al., 2006
Hydromorphone/ oxymorphone	0.1 mg/kg	IM, IV	<15	7.5		Wegner et al., 2004
Meperidine	3–10 mg/kg	IM, SQ	Rapid	1	IV injection causes histamine release	Robertson, 2008
Methadone	0.1–0.6 mg/kg	IM, IV, OTM	<10	1.5–6.5		Ferreira et al., 2011
Fentanyl	1–5 μg/kg	IV, IM	Rapid	0.5	Apnea	Lamont, 2002
Buprenorphine	5–100 μg/kg	IV, IM, SQ, OTM	15	4–8	Ceiling effect	Dyson, 2008; Steagall et al., 2009
Opioid Continuous Rate Infusions						
Butorphanol	0.05–0.2 mg/ kg/h	IV			Dysphoria at higher doses	
Hydromorphone	5–10 μg/kg/h	IV			Titrate to effect Monitor for hyperthermia	Dyson, 2008
Fentanyl	2–4 μg/kg/h	IV, TD			Titrate to effect	Hansen, 2008
Remifentanil	15–60 μg/kg/h	IV			Dysphoria at higher doses	Brosnan, 2009
Buprenorphine	2–4 μg/kg/h	IV				Hansen, 2008

IM, intramuscular; IV, intravenous; OTM, oral transmucosal; PO, per os; SC, subcutaneously, TD, transdermal.

2004). Vomiting occurs more frequently in nonpainful patients and varies by route of administration (Bateman et al., 2008; Robertson et al., 2009). Administration may initially stimulate and then suppress bowel motility. Feline patients have a decrease in minute ventilation, which is primarily a function of decreased respiratory rate, but apnea is uncommon (Florez et al., 1968). Bradycardia can occur at very high doses, but does not compromise blood pressure or cardiac output (Grimm et al., 2005).

Hyperthermia may occur when opioids are administered to healthy patients. This has been historically associated with hydromorphone (Niedfeldt & Robertson, 2006), but can occur with any opioid (Posner et al., 2007). Although temperatures have been shown to increase to 105.3°F, no long-term deleterious effects have been documented. The temperature returns to normal within 5 hours without any intervention. The occurrence of hyperthermia should not dissuade the use of μ agonists in feline patients.

Morphine
Morphine is the basis of comparison for all the μ agonists and it exhibits a linear dose–response curve, meaning that increasing the drug dose increases the degree of analgesia. Some of the analgesic effects of morphine are exerted by an active metabolite, morphine 6-glucuronide. Although cats produce minimal amounts of this metabolite (Taylor et al., 2001), research supports the supposition that morphine produces an analgesic effect in cats (Steagall et al., 2006; Pypendop et al., 2008). Morphine causes histamine release when given intravenously, causing vasodilation and compensatory tachycardia, and thus should be administered IM or subcutaneously or slowly IV.

Hydromorphone and Oxymorphone
Hydromorphone and oxymorphone are synthetic μ agonists that are more lipid soluble than morphine; thus, their onset is more rapid and their duration of action is shorter. These products are active without metabolism, so they provide a more consistent response when compared to morphine in feline patients. Using a thermal nociceptive model, hydromorphone had a maximum antinociceptive response for at least 3 hours, with a significant antinociceptive response lasting for 7 hours (Wegner et al., 2004). When oxymorphone and hydromorphone were compared in a clinical study, the only difference noted was an increased incidence of nausea and vomiting with hydromorphone (Bateman et al., 2008).

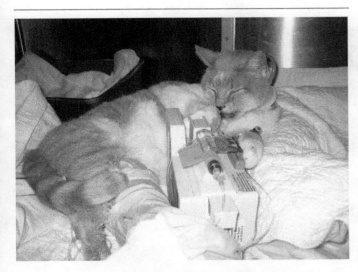

Figure 25.5. Patient on a fentanyl constant rate infusion to provide postoperative analgesia after surgery to correct multiple injuries sustained from being hit by a car.

Meperidine

Meperidine is a μ agonist that is similar to morphine. Its duration of action is about 2 hours; thus, it requires frequent administration for continued analgesia. Like morphine, meperidine causes histamine release when given intravenously.

Methadone

Methadone is a synthetic μ agonist with a similar potency to morphine. It may also provide analgesia through its actions as an NMDA receptor antagonist and through uptake inhibition of serotonin and norepinephrine. Methadone did not induce vomiting or signs of dysphoria when given to healthy cats (Ferreira et al., 2011).

Fentanyl

Fentanyl is a highly lipid-soluble synthetic μ agonist which has a faster onset than hydromorphone and a rapid elimination (Lee et al., 2000). These properties make it a reasonable choice for short procedures when ongoing analgesia is not required. Longer analgesia with fentanyl can be provided via a continuous rate infusion (Figure 25.5) or transdermal application (see below).

Remifentanil

Remifentanil, an analog of fentanyl, is the most recent addition to the μ agonist class of opioids. Remifentanil has some unique characteristics that provide advantages for the feline patient. It is ultra short acting (Pypendop et al., 2008), so it is almost exclusively administered by constant rate infusion. It is eliminated by tissue esterases; thus, it does not rely on liver metabolism or renal elimination for termination of effect (Glass et al., 1999).

Buprenorphine

Buprenorphine is a unique μ agonist, classified as a partial agonist. It binds tightly to the μ receptor, but does not activate it to the same degree as a pure μ agonist; thus it exhibits a ceiling effect on the dose–response curve and causes fewer adverse effects. Buprenorphine has a long onset of action after any route of administration, but also has the longest duration of action (Slingsby et al., 2010). It is useful for moderate pain, and it eliminates frequent redosing. However, because buprenorphine binds to μ receptors very tightly, it can prevent the binding of more efficacious pure mu agonists to the receptor if administered concurrently. Thus, if buprenorphine is not providing adequate analgesia, a more efficacious opioid, given concurrently, may not be effective. Oral transmucosal administration of buprenorphine to cats results in bioavailability and analgesic effects similar to intravenous administration (Robertson et al., 2005a).

Continuous Rate Infusions of Opioids in Cats

All opioids have a finite duration of action, and will not provide extended analgesia without repeated injections or constant rate infusions. Pure μ agonists (morphine, hydromorphone, oxymorphone, fentanyl, remifentanil) are suitable for application as a constant rate infusion for long-term analgesia of the hospitalized patient. Agent selection is dependent on several factors, including onset of action, duration of action, and cost. If a patient's pain is well controlled at a set rate, then the longer-acting agents such as morphine and hydromorphone provide a more affordable option. If a patient's pain is unregulated, and frequent adjustments in the amount of medication are needed, then the shorter-acting agents (fentanyl and remifentanil) with a rapid onset of action are more appropriate, although more expensive.

Extended Release Application of Opioids in Cats

Transdermal applications (Chapter 9) are available, but have limitations. A commercially available fentanyl transdermal patch has the ability to provide therapeutic plasma concentrations for up to 100 hours after one application. A high interpatient variability in absorption rates appears to exist, and constant plasma concentrations do not occur until 12–18 hours after application (Lee et al., 2000). Transdermal creams containing any one of a variety of opioids can be formulated by compounding pharmacies, but studies have shown disappointing results (Robertson et al., 2005b). Extended release formulations of injectable opioids show promise for providing consistent results (Krugner-Higby et al., 2011), but further studies are needed in felines. The reader is referred to Chapter 9 for a detailed discussion of transdermal and injectable extended release formulations.

α-2 AGONISTS

α-2 agonists (Table 25.3) represent an underutilized systemic analgesic for felines. This class of drugs (Chapter 7) provides profound analgesia but also has significant sedative properties, which may be a desired or undesired effect. Their application, especially in regard to perioperative pain management, has been limited due to the profound cardiovascular changes. However, they are a safe class of agents to use when properly applied to appropriate patients.

The pharmacodynamic properties of the various agents can be loosely categorized by their specificity for the α-2 versus the α-1 adrenergic receptor (Virtanen, 1989). Greater specificity for the α-2 receptor leads to increased potency, increased duration of action, more profound analgesia and sedation, and a decrease in adverse cardiovascular effects (Selmi et al., 2005).

Xylazine and dexmedetomidine are approved, in the United States, for use in feline patients. Other α-2 agonists, such as

Table 25.3. α-2 agonists for acute pain in cats

Drug	Dose	Route	Onset (min)	Duration (h)	Indications	Cautions/ Contraindications	Reference
Xylazine	0.25–1 mg/kg	IV, IM	<5	0.25–0.5	Acute analgesia/sedation	Cardiovascular depression, emesis	Selmi et al., 2004
Romifidine	0.1–0.4 mg/kg	IM	5–30	0.5–1	As above	As above	Selmi et al., 2004
Detomidine	0.5 mg/kg	PO	20	>1	Intractable patient	Very limited information available on use in felines	Grove & Ramsay, 2000
Dexmedetomidine	2–40 μg/kg	IM	15	2	Acute analgesia/sedation; synergistic analgesia with opioids	Cardiovascular depression, emesis	Slingsby & Taylor, 2008

IM, intramuscular; IV, intravenous; PO, per os.

detomidine and romifidine, have similar clinical effects in felines, but have no advantages over the approved products.

Xylazine

Xylazine has a low selectivity for the α-2 receptor, with a ratio of 160:1 (Virtanen et al., 1988), and therefore demonstrates more significant risks (Clarke & Hall, 1990) and less profound desired effects when compared to more selective α-2 agonists (Selmi et al., 2005). Due to its low cost, it has an application in shelter medicine where an affordable, injectable analgesic is needed (Williams et al., 2002), even though concern exists about its increased association with perianesthetic mortality (Clark & Hall, 1990).

Dexmedetomidine

Dexmedetomidine is the newest α-2 agonist in the veterinary market, and is much more selective for the α-2 receptor than xylazine. It is a purified form of medetomidine, containing only the dextrorotary enantiomer. The levorotary form has no analgesic or sedative properties, but does contribute to some of the negative cardiovascular effects (Kuusela et al., 2001). Dexmedetomidine produces reliable analgesia in feline patients, producing significant effects for 120 minutes (Granholm et al., 2007). It can be used as a constant rate infusion in hospitalized patients. It is valuable as a synergist for opioids, and can be used to provide consistent analgesia in patients that are refractory to opioids (Slingsby et al., 2010).

Reluctance to administer α-2 agonists to feline patients is primarily due to concern about the adverse cardiovascular effects. Stimulation of the peripheral α-2 receptors and α-1 receptors causes vasoconstriction, increasing blood pressure and causing a reflex bradycardia. In feline patients, this effect is less pronounced with dexmedetomidine than with other α-2 agonists. Based on studies in the dog, cardiac output is decreased by up to 57% but blood flow to the core organs is preserved at acceptable values (Lawrence et al., 1996). The author has used dexmedetomidine as the sole perioperative analgesic in feline neonates (3–4 weeks old) in a research environment with reliable results. Sedation could be considered an adverse effect if analgesia is the sole desired effect, but typically the degree of sedation is acceptable or even desirable. Temperature, pulse, respiration, mucous membrane color, degree of sedation, and adequacy of analgesia should be closely monitored, particularly with prolonged dosing.

Mechanisms to eliminate the adverse cardiovascular effects of the α-2 agonists while preserving the desired effects of sedation and analgesia are being investigated. One promising technique is the simultaneous administration of an antagonist that does not cross into the central nervous system (Honkavaara et al., 2012).

Nonsteroidal Anti-Inflammatory Drugs

Nonsteroidal anti-inflammatory drugs (NSAIDs) (Table 25.4) (Chapter 5) act at multiple sites along the nociceptive pathway, and are used as part of a preventive approach to analgesia. NSAIDs reduce the peripheral inflammation that sensitizes the peripheral nociceptor, thus decreasing nociceptive input. They also act at the dorsal horn of the spinal cord, inhibiting nociceptive input through modulation. NSAIDs are the longest-acting class of analgesic agents, with a duration of action in feline patients of at least 24 hours. NSAIDs have a good safety profile when applied appropriately, and are a valuable addition to a multimodal analgesic plan where inflammatory pain will be involved.

Meloxicam

Meloxicam is labeled for single-dose administration for acute pain for cats in the United States. While other NSAIDs are eliminated through glucuronidation, a process felines are deficient in, meloxicam is eliminated either unchanged in the feces or through oxidation (Grude et al., 2010). Administration should be discontinued as soon as inflammatory pain has resolved, as there is risk of renal damage with repeated use. In the United States, labeled use of meloxicam is limited to a single perioperative injectable dose of 0.3 mg/mL. A US Food and Drug Administration (FDA) black box warning exists against the continued administration of injectable or oral meloxicam after one-time perioperative use, although longer-term dosing is approved for cats in Europe and Australia.

Table 25.4. Nonsteroidal anti-inflammatory drugs (NSAIDs) for acute pain in cats

Drug	Dose (mg/kg)	Route	Onset (min)	Duration (h)	Indications	Cautions/ Contraindications	Reference
Meloxicam	0.05-0.3[a]	PO, SQ, IV	60–120	>24	Acute inflammatory pain	Clotting disorders, volume depletion, gastric mucosal compromise; monitor closely for adverse effects if exceeding one dose	Lascelles, et al. 2007
Robenacoxib	1–2.4	PO	As above	As above	As above	Clotting disorders, volume depletion, gastric mucosal compromise	Giraudel, et al. 2010
Ketoprofen	1–2	PO, IV, SC	As above	As above	As above	As above	Lascelles, et al. 2007
Carprofen	1–2	IV, SC	As above	As above	As above	As above	Lascelles, et al. 2007

[a]For one-time dosing only in the United States.

IM, intramuscular; IV, intravenous; PO, per os; SC, subcutaneously.

Robenacoxib
Robenacoxib is the most recent NSAID approved for cats. Its effects are equivalent to ketoprofen (Giraudel et al., 2010) but superior to meloxicam (Kamata et al., 2012). Although it is only labeled for 3 days of administration, a safety study suggests that in healthy cats, administration for longer periods of time is feasible (King et al., 2012).

Ketoprofen
Ketoprofen is not approved for feline use in the United States, but is in other countries. It is equivalent to carprofen and meloxicam in its ability to control postoperative pain (Slingsby & Waterman-Pearson, 2000). Ketoprofen undergoes glucuronidation, but there appears to be alternate elimination pathways, potentially thioesterification, that prevent toxic accumulation after repeated dosing (Castro et al., 2000).

Carprofen
Carprofen is approved for cats as a single injection in Europe and Australia. Its analgesic effects are comparable to ketoprofen and meloxicam (Slingsby & Waterman-Pearson, 2000). Because of the wide interpatient variability in elimination (Parton et al., 2000), it is only recommended for use as a single dose (Lascelles et al., 2007).

TRAMADOL
Tramadol (Table 25.5) (Chapter 4) is a unique analgesic as it has actions at multiple receptors and is, therefore, difficult to classify. Structurally, tramadol is a synthetic analogue of the opioid codeine, but it has very weak affinity for the opioid receptor. Tramadol inhibits uptake of norepinephrine and serotonin, which may contribute to its clinically observed effects either as an analgesic or behavior altering drug. Tramadol is beneficial in the control of acute, moderate pain associated with surgery, especially when combined with an NSAID (Clarke et al., 2012). It had efficacy in a thermal acute pain model (Pypendop et al., 2009). It was not as efficacious as morphine, but can be considered a suitable alternative to injectable opioids when a parenteral route of administration is not available (Castro et al., 2009). The commercially available tablet has been reported to be unpalatable to cats, so reformulation into a gelatin capsule or oral suspension may be required for patient acceptance (Ko et al., 2008).

ADJUVANT ANALGESICS
This includes drugs indicated for other medical conditions, but which are also beneficial in the treatment of pain (Table 25.5) (Chapter 8). Most often, they are used in conjunction with traditional systemic analgesics. They are most commonly used in the treatment of chronic pain, but are efficacious in the treatment of acute pain and in limiting the conversion of acute pain to a chronic pain state.

NMDA Antagonists
Ketamine In subanesthetic doses, ketamine (Chapter 8) acts on the NMDA receptors in the spinal cord to decrease windup. Ketamine is most effective when it is administered prior to nociceptive input and continued through the duration of input (Nagasaka et al., 2000). Ketamine does not block acute nociceptive input, but inhibits the wide dynamic range (WDR) neurons associated with central sensitization. Ketamine, either as a bolus or constant rate infusion, provides analgesia in the postoperative period and, at subanesthetic doses, is devoid of adverse effects (Bell et al., 2006). An initial dose of 0.1–1 mg/kg IV, followed by an IV infusion of 2–5 µg/kg/min is recommended for the treatment of acute surgical pain. Doses greater than 20 µg/kg/min increase sympathetic stimulation in the awake patient and cause changes in mentation (Pascoe et al., 2007).

Table 25.5. Other/adjuvant analgesics for acute pain in cats

Drug	Dose	Route	Onset (min)	Duration (h)	Indications	Cautions/ Contraindications	Reference
Tramadol	2–4 mg/kg	PO	60	6	Acute, moderate pain	Avoid in patients on SSRI agents	Pypendop et al., 2009
Ketamine	0.1–1 mg/kg Constant rate infusion: 2–5 µg/kg/min	IV	Delayed	N/A	Prevention and treatment of central sensitization	Avoid in patients with severe renal impairment	Pascoe et al., 2007
Amantadine	3 mg/kg	PO	Delayed	24	Oral treatment of central sensitization		Gaynor, 2008
Gabapentin	10 mg/kg	PO	Unknown	8	Neuropathic pain	Sedation	Vettorato & Corletto, 2011

IV, intravenous; PO, per os; SSRI, selective serotonin reuptake inhibitor.

Amantadine Amantadine (Chapter 8) is unique among the NMDA receptor antagonists because it stabilizes the closed state of the channel, rather than blocking transmission of the open channel. Thus, it may have a greater role in the prevention of chronic pain than in the treatment of acute pain. Amantadine did not augment opioid analgesia in a feline thermal nociception model (Siao et al., 2012), but clinical trials in humans show promising results (Bujak-Gizycka et al., 2012). The bioavailability of amantadine exceeds 100% (Siao et al., 2011), indicating that this drug would be suitable for oral administration. The recommended dose is 3 mg/kg once a day (Gaynor, 2008).

Sodium Channel Blockers
Lidocaine Although lidocaine is known as an effective local anesthetic, there is interest in its analgesic properties when administered as a constant rate infusion intravenously. Intravenous lidocaine has proven to be beneficial in patients undergoing abdominal procedures when used in conjunction with traditional forms of analgesia (McCarthy et al., 2010). Intravenous lidocaine decreased the minimum alveolar concentration of isoflurane in cats (Pypendop & Ilkiw, 2005b), but was not beneficial in a model of acute pain (Pypendop et al., 2006). Constant rate infusions of lidocaine that reduce inhalational anesthetic requirements cause significant reductions in cardiac output and an increase in systemic vascular resistance, so lidocaine is not recommended for routine use in felines (Pypendop & Ilkiw, 2005a).

Calcium Channel Blockers
Gabapentin Gabapentin (Chapter 8) is an anticonvulsant that binds to the α2δ subunit of voltage-gated calcium channels, and likely mediates analgesia by reducing excitatory neurotransmitter release. In limited cases, it had a beneficial response in treating acute traumatic pain when combined with other analgesics (Vettorato & Corletto, 2011). It appears to have no effect on acute physiological pain, so its benefit may be in the treatment or prevention of neuropathic pain (Pypendop et al., 2010).

Nursing Care
Although this chapter has focused on the medical management of acute pain, it is vital not to neglect the impact that proper nursing

care can have on minimizing acute pain. Any stress placed on the feline patient from the environment and interaction with the veterinary team has the potential to exacerbate painful stimuli. Proper wound management and bandaging are vital to reduce pain from contact with surgical wounds. In the hospitalized patient, providing a warm and secluded area with minimum noise will reduce stress. The goal of the veterinary team should be to minimize restraint and adverse manipulation of the feline patient. A more thorough description of ways to implement feline nursing care can be found elsewhere (Carney et al., 2012).

SUMMARY

Historically, the treatment of acute pain in feline patients has been neglected. However, practitioners now appreciate the importance of recognizing and treating pain in cats and have the resources available to properly address it. By implementing goal-directed therapy, practitioners can focus on the overall benefit to the patient and implement effective treatment strategies. Many different classes of drugs are effective in managing acute pain and can be applied simultaneously in a multimodal fashion to ultimately reduce pain to an acceptable level for the feline patient.

REFERENCES

Abelson, A.L., Mccobb, E.C., Shaw, S., et al. (2009). Use of wound soaker catheters for the administration of local anesthetic for postoperative analgesia: 56 cases. *Veterinary Anaesthesia and Analgesia*, 36, 597–602.

Bateman, S.W., Haldane, S., & Stephens, J.A. (2008). Comparison of the analgesic efficacy of hydromorphone and oxymorphone in dogs and cats: a randomized blinded study. *Veterinary Anaesthesia and Analgesia*, 35, 341–347.

Bell, R.F., Dahl, J.B., Moore, R.A., & Kalso, E.A. (2006). Perioperative ketamine for acute postoperative pain. *Cochrane Database of Systematic Reviews*, CD004603.

Brosnan, R.J., Pypendop, B.H., Siao, K.T., & Stanley, S.D. (2009) Effects of reminfentanil on measures of anesthetic immobility and analgesia in cats. *American Journal of Veterinary Research*, 70(9), 1065–1071.

Bujak-Gizycka, B., Kacka, K., Suski, M., et al. (2012). Beneficial effect of amantadine on postoperative pain reduction and consumption of morphine in patients subjected to elective spine surgery. *Pain Medicine*, 13, 459–465.

Campiglia, L., Consales, G., & De Gaudio, A.R. (2010). Pre-emptive analgesia for postoperative pain control: a review. *Clinical Drug Investigation*, 30, 15–26.

Carney, H.C., Little, S., Brownlee-Tomasso, D., et al. (2012). AAFP and ISFM feline-friendly nursing care guidelines. *Journal of Feline Medicine and Surgery*, 14, 337–349.

Carr, D.B. & Goudas, L.C. (1999). Acute pain. *Lancet*, 353, 2051–2058.

Castro, D.S., Silva, M.F., Shih, A.C., Motta, P.P., Pires, M.V., & Scherer, P.O. (2009). Comparison between the analgesic effects of morphine and tramadol delivered epidurally in cats receiving a standardized noxious stimulation. *Journal of Feline Medicine and Surgery*, 11, 948–953.

Castro, E., Soraci, A., Fogel, F., & Tapia, O. (2000). Chiral inversion of R(-) fenoprofen and ketoprofen enantiomers in cats. *Journal of Veterinary Pharmacology and Therapeutics*, 23, 265–271.

Chadwick, H.S. (1985). Toxicity and resuscitation in lidocaine-infused or bupivacaine-infused cats. *Anesthesiology*, 63, 385–390.

Clarke, H., Bonin, R.P., Orser, B.A., Englesakis, M., Wijeysundera, D.N., & Katz, J. (2012). The prevention of chronic postsurgical pain using gabapentin and pregabalin: a combined systematic review and meta-analysis. *Anesthesia and Analgesia*, 115, 428–442.

Clarke, K.W. & Hall, L.W. (1990). A survey of anaesthesia in small animal practice: AVA/BSAVA report. *Journal of the Association of Veterinary Anaesthetists of Great Britain and Ireland*, 17, 4–10.

Dahl, J.B. & Kehlet, H. (2011). Preventive analgesia. *Current Opinions in Anaesthesiology*, 24, 331–338.

Davis, K.M., Hardie, E.M., Lascelles, B.D., & Hansen, B. (2007a). Feline fibrosarcoma: perioperative management. *Compendium on Continuing Education for the Practicing Veterinarian*, 29, 712–714, 716–720, 722–729 passim.

Davis, K.M., Hardie, E.M., Martin, F.R., Zhu, J., & Brownie, C. (2007b). Correlation between perioperative factors and successful outcome in fibrosarcoma resection in cats. *The Veterinary Record*, 161, 199–200.

Davis, L.E. & Donnelly, E.J. (1968). Analgesic drugs in the cat. *Journal of the American Veterinary Medical Association*, 153, 1161–1167.

Dyson, D.H. (2008) Perioperative pain management in veterinary patients. *Veterinary Clinics of North America Small Animal Practice*, 38-(6), 1309–1327.

Egger, C. & Love, L. (2009a) Local and regional anesthesia techniques, Part 1: Overview and five simple techniques. *Veterinary Medicine*, http://veterinarymedicine.dvm360.com/vetmed/Anesthesia/Local-and-regional-anesthesia-techniques/ArticleStandard/Article/detail/575560 (accessed July 7, 2013).

Egger, C. & Love, L. (2009b) Local and regional anesthesia techniques, Part 2: Stifle, intercostal, intrapleural, and forelimb techniques. *Veterinary Medicine*, http://veterinarymedicine.dvm360.com/vetmed/Medicine/Local-and-regional-anesthesia-techniques-Part-2-St/ArticleStandard/Article/detail/585255 (accessed July 7, 2013).

Egger, C. & Love, L. (2009c) Local and regional anesthesia techniques, Part 3: Blocking the maxillary and mandibular nerves. *Veterinary Medicine*, http://veterinarymedicine.dvm360.com/vetmed/Medicine/Local-and-regional-anesthesia-techniques-Part-3-Bl/ArticleStandard/Article/detail/601619 (accessed July 7, 2013).

Egger, C. & Love, L. (2009d) Local and regional anesthesia techniques, Part 4: Epidural anesthesia and analgesia. *Veterinary Medicine*, http://veterinarymedicine.dvm360.com/vetmed/Medicine/Local-and-regional-anesthesia-techniques-Part-4-Ep/ArticleStandard/Article/detail/632170 (accessed July 7, 2013).

Eichenfield, L.F., Funk, A., Fallon-Friedlander, S., & Cunningham, B.B. (2002) A clinical study to evaluate the efficacy of ELA-Max (4% liposomal lidocaine) as compared with eutectic mixture of local anesthetics cream for pain reduction of venipuncture in children. *Pediatrics*, 109, 1093–1099.

Feldman, H.S., Arthur, G.R., & Covino, B.G. (1989). Comparative systemic toxicity of convulsant and supraconvulsant doses of intravenous ropivacaine, bupivacaine, and lidocaine in the conscious dog. *Anesthesia & Analgesia*, 69, 794–801.

Ferriera, T.H., Rezende, M.L., Mama, K.R., Hudachek, S.F., & Aguiar, A.J. (2011). Plasma concentrations and behavorial, antinociceptive, and physiologic effects of methadone after intravenous and oral transmucosal administration in cats. *American Journal of Veterinary Research*, 72, 764–771.

Florez, J., McCarthy, L.E., & Borison, H.L. (1968). A comparative study in the cat of the respiratory effects of morphine injected intravenously and into the cerebrospinal fluid. *The Journal of Pharmacology and Experimental Therapeutics*, 163, 448–455.

Ford, D.J., Singh, P., Watters, C., & Raj, P.P. (1984). Duration and toxicity of bupivacaine for topical anesthesia of the airway in the cat. *Anesthesia & Analgesia*, 63, 1001–1004.

Fransson, B.A., Peck, K.E., Smith, J.K., Anthony, J.A., & Mealey, K.L. (2002). Transdermal absorption of a liposome-encapsulated formulation of lidocaine following topical administration in cats. *American Journal of Veterinary Research*, 63, 1309–1312.

Gaynor, J.S. (2008). Control of cancer pain in veterinary patients. *Veterinary Clinics of North America Small Animal Practice*, 38, 1429–1448.

Gaynor, J.S. & Muir, W. (2009). *Handbook of Veterinary Pain Management*, Mosby/Elsevier, St. Louis, MO.

Giraudel, J.M., Gruet, P., Alexander, D.G., Seewald, W., & King, J.N. (2010). Evaluation of orally administered robenacoxib versus ketoprofen for treatment of acute pain and inflammation associated with musculoskeletal disorders in cats. *American Journal of Veterinary Research*, 71, 710–719.

Glass, P.S., Gan, T.J., & Howell, S. (1999). A review of the pharmacokinetics and pharmacodynamics of remifentanil. *Anesthesia & Analgesia*, 89, S7–S14.

Granholm, M., McKusick, B.C., Westerholm, F.C., & Aspegrén, J.C. (2007). Evaluation of the clinical efficacy and safety of intramuscular and intravenous doses of dexmedetomidine and medetomidine in dogs and their reversal with atipamezole. *The Veterinary Record*, 160, 891–897.

Grimm, K.A., Tranquilli, W.J., Gross, D.R., et al. (2005). Cardiopulmonary effects of fentanyl in conscious dogs and dogs sedated with a continuous rate infusion of medetomidine. *American Journal of Veterinary Research*, 66, 1222–1226.

Grove, D.M. & Ramsay, E.C. (2000) Sedative and physiologic effects of orally administered alpha 2-adrenoceptor agonists and ketamine in cats. *Journal of the American Veterinary Medical Association*, 216(12), 1929–1932.

Grude, P., Guittard, J., Garcia, C., Daoulas, I., Thoulon, F., & Ebner, T. (2010). Excretion mass balance evaluation, metabolite profile analysis and metabolite identification in plasma and excreta after oral administration of [14C]-meloxicam to the male cat: preliminary study. *Journal of Veterinary Pharmacology and Therapeutics*, 33, 396–407.

Haga, H.A., Lykkjen, S., Revold, T., & Ranheim, B. (2006). Effect of intratesticular injection of lidocaine on cardiovascular responses to castration in isoflurane-anesthetized stallions. *American Journal of Veterinary Research*, 67, 403–408.

Hansen, B. (2008) Analgesia for the critically ill dog or cat: an update. *Veterinary Clinics of North America Small Animal Practice*, 38(6), 1353–1363.

Hansen, B. & Hardie, E. (1993). Prescription and use of analgesics in dogs and cats in a veterinary teaching hospital: 258 cases (1983-1989). *Journal of the American Veterinary Medical Association*, 202, 1485–1494.

Hebl, J.R., Dilger, J.A., Byer, D.E., et al. (2008). A pre-emptive multi-modal pathway featuring peripheral nerve block improves perioperative outcomes after major orthopedic surgery. *Regional Anesthesia in Pain Medicine*, 33, 510–517.

Hellyer, P., Rodan, I., Brunt, J., Downing, R., Hagedorn, J.E., & Robertson, S.A. (2007). AAHA/AAFP pain management guidelines or dogs and cats. *Journal of Feline Medicine and Surgery*, 9, 466–480.

Hewson, C.J., Dohoo, I.R., & Lemke, K.A. (2006). Perioperative use of analgesics in dogs and cats by Canadian veterinarians in 2001. *The Canadian Veterinary Journal*, 47, 352–359.

Honkavaara, J., Restitutti, F., Raekallio, M., et al. (2012). Influence of MK-467, a peripherally acting alpha2-adrenoceptor antagonist on the disposition of intravenous dexmedetomidine in dogs. *Drug Metabolism and Disposition*, 40, 445–449.

Johnson, J.A., Robertson, S.A., & Pypendop, B.H. (2007). Antinociceptive effects of butorphanol, buprenorphine, or both, administered intramuscularly in cats. *American Journal of Veterinary Research*, 68, 699–703.

Kamata, M., King, J.N., Seewald, W., Sakakibara, N., Yamashita, K., & Nishimura, R. (2012). Comparison of injectable robenacoxib versus meloxicam for peri-operative use in cats: Results of a randomised clinical trial. *The Veterinary Journal*, 193, 114–118.

Kennard, M.A. (1953). Sensitization of the spinal cord of the cat to pain-inducing stimuli. *Journal of Neurosurgery*, 10, 169–177.

Kennard, M.A. (1954). The course of ascending fibers in the spinal cord of the cat essential to the recognition of painful stimuli. *The Journal of Comparative Neurology*, 100, 511–524.

King, J.N., Hotz, R., Reagan, E.L., Roth, D.R., Seewald, W., & Lees, P. (2012). Safety of oral robenacoxib in the cat. *Journal of Veterinary Pharmacology and Therapeutics*, 35, 290–300.

Kissin, I. (2000). Preemptive analgesia. *Anesthesiology*, 93, 1138–1143.

Ko, J.C.H., Abbo, L.A., Weil, A.B., Johnson, B.M., Inoue, T., & Payton, M.E. (2008). Effect of orally administered tramadol alone or with an intravenously administered opioid on minimum alveolar concentration of sevoflurane in cats. *Journal of the American Veterinary Medical Association*, 12, 1834–1840.

Krugner-Higby, L., Smith, L., Schmidt, B., et al. (2011). Experimental pharmacodynamics and analgesic efficacy of liposome-encapsulated hydromorphone in dogs. *Journal of the American Animal Hospital Association*, 47, 185–195.

Kushner, L.I., Fan, B., & Shofer, F.S. (2002). Intravenous regional anesthesia in isoflurane anesthetized cats: lidocaine plasma concentrations and cardiovascular effects. *Veterinary Anaesthesia and Analgesia*, 29, 140–149.

Kuusela, E., Vainio, O., Kaistinen, A., Kobylin, S., Raekallio, M. (2001). Sedative, analgesic, and cardiovascular effects of lev-omedetomidine alone and in combination with dexmedetomidine in dogs. *American Journal of Veterinary Research*, 62, 616–621.

Lamont, L.A. (2002) Feline perioperative pain management. *Veterinary Clinics of North America Small Animal Practice*, 32(4), 747–763.

Lascelles, B., Capner, C., & Waterman-Pearson, A. (1999). Current British veterinary attitudes to perioperative analgesia for cats and small mammals. *The Veterinary Record*, 145, 601–604.

Lascelles, B.D., Court, M.H., Hardie, E.M., & Robertson, S.A. (2007). Nonsteroidal anti-inflammatory drugs in cats: a review. *Veterinary Anaesthesia and Analgesia*, 34, 228–250.

Lascelles, B.D. & Robertson, S.A. (2004a) Use of thermal threshold response to evaluate the antinociceptive effects of butorphanol in cats. *American Journal of Veterinary Research*, 65(8), 1085–1090.

Lascelles, B.D. & Robertson, S.A. (2004b) Antinociceptive effects of hydromorphone, butorphanol, or the combination in cats. *Journal of Veterinary Internal Medicine*, 18(2), 190–195.

Lascelles, D. & Waterman, A. (1997). Analgesia in cats. *In Practice*, 19, 203–213.

Lawal, F.M. & Adetunji, A. (2009). Evaluation of epidural anaesthesia with lignocaine - xylazine mixture in ketamine - sedated cats. *Israel Journal of Veterinary Medicine*, 64, 47–51.

Lawrence, C.J., Prinzen, F.W., & De Lange, S. (1996). The effect of dexmedetomidine on nutrient organ blood flow. *Anesthesia & Analgesia*, 83, 1160–1165.

Lee, D.D., Papich, M.G., & Hardie, E.M. (2000). Comparison of pharmacokinetics of fentanyl after intravenous and transdermal administration in cats. *American Journal of Veterinary Research*, 61, 672–627.

Lemke, KA. (2007) Pain management II: local and regional anaesthetic techniques. In: *BSAVA manual of canine and feline anaesthesia and analgesia* (eds C. Seymour & T. Duke-Novakovski) 2nd edn. British Small Animal Veterinary Association, Gloucester, UK, 104–114.

McCarthy, G.C., Megalla, S.A., & Habib, A.S. (2010). Impact of intravenous lidocaine infusion on postoperative analgesia and recovery from surgery: a systematic review of randomized controlled trials. *Drugs*, 70, 1149–1163.

McCartney, C.J., Duggan, E., & Apatu, E. (2007). Should we add clonidine to local anesthetic for peripheral nerve blockade? A qualitative systematic review of the literature. *Regional Anesthesia in Pain Medicine*, 32, 330–338.

Merskey, H. & Bogduk, N. (1994) *Classification of Chronic Pain: Descriptions of Chronic Pain Syndromes and Definitions of Pain Terms*, 2nd edn. IASP Press, Seattle, WA.

Murphy, M.R. & Hug, C.C. (1982). The enflurane sparing effect of morphine, butorphanol, and nalbuphine. *Anesthesiology*, 57, 489–492.

Nagasaka, H., Nakamura, S., Mizumoto, Y., & Sato, I. (2000). Effects of ketamine on formalin-induced activity in the spinal dorsal horn of spinal cord-transected cats: differences in response to intravenous ketamine administered before and after formalin. *Acta Anaesthesiologica Scandinavica*, 44, 953–958.

Niedfeldt, R.L. & Robertson, S.A. (2006). Postanesthetic hyperthermia in cats: a retrospective comparison between hydromorphone and buprenorphine. *Veterinary Anaesthesia and Analgesia*, 33, 381–389.

Ong, C.K., Lirk, P., Seymour, R.A., & Jenkins, B.J. (2005). The efficacy of preemptive analgesia for acute postoperative pain management: a meta-analysis. *Anesthesia & Analgesia*, 100, 757–773.

Parton, K., Balmer, T.V., Boyle, J., Whittem, T., & MacHon, R. (2000). The pharmacokinetics and effects of intravenously administered carprofen and salicylate on gastrointestinal mucosa and selected biochemical measurements in healthy cats. *Journal of Veterinary Pharmacology and Therapeutics*, 23, 73–79.

Pascoe, P.J., Ilkiw, J.E., Craig, C., & Kollias-Baker, C. (2007). The effects of ketamine on the minimum alveolar concentration of isoflurane in cats. *Veterinary Anaesthesia and Analgesia*, 34, 31–39.

Popping, D.M., Elia, N., Marret, E., Wenk, M., & Tramèr, M.R. (2009). Clonidine as an adjuvant to local anesthetics for peripheral nerve and plexus blocks: a meta-analysis of randomized trials. *Anesthesiology*, 111, 406–415.

Posner, L.P., Gleed, R.D., Erb, H.N., & Ludders, J.W. (2007). Post-anesthetic hyperthermia in cats. *Veterinary Anaesthesia and Analgesia*, 34, 40–47.

Pypendop, B.H., Brosnan, R.J., Siao, K.T., & Stanley, S.D. (2008). Pharmacokinetics of remifentanil in conscious cats and cats anesthetized with isoflurane. *American Journal of Veterinary Research*, 69, 531–536.

Pypendop, B.H. & Ilkiw, J.E. (2005a). Assessment of the hemodynamic effects of lidocaine administered IV in isoflurane-anesthetized cats. *American Journal of Veterinary Research*, 66, 661–668.

Pypendop, B.H. & Ilkiw, J.E. (2005b). The effects of intravenous lidocaine administration on the minimum alveolar concentration of isoflurane in cats. *Anesthesia & Analgesia*, 100, 97–101.

Pypendop, B.H., Ilkiw, J.E., & Robertson, S.A. (2006). Effects of intravenous administration of lidocaine on the thermal threshold in cats. *American Journal of Veterinary Research*, 67, 16–20.

Pypendop, B.H., Siao, K.T., & Ilkiw, J.E. (2009). Effects of tramadol hydrochloride on the thermal threshold in cats. *American Journal of Veterinary Research*, 70, 1465–1470.

Pypendop, B.H., Siao, K.T., & Ilkiw, J.E. (2010). Thermal antinociceptive effect of orally administered gabapentin in healthy cats. *American Journal of Veterinary Research*, 71, 1027–1032.

Pypendop, B.H., Siao, K.T., Pascoe, P.J., & Ilkiw, J.E. (2008b). Effects of epidurally administered morphine or buprenorphine on the thermal threshold in cats. *American Journal of Veterinary Research*, 69, 983–987.

Ranheim, B., Haga, H.A., & Ingebrigtsen, K. (2005). Distribution of radioactive lidocaine injected into the testes in piglets. *Journal of Veterinary Pharmacology and Therapeutics*, 28, 481–483.

Robertson, S.A. (2008) Managing pain in feline patients. *Veterinary Clinics of North America Small Animal Practice*, 38(6), 1267–1290.

Robertson, S.A., Lascelles, B.D., Taylor, P.M., & Sear, J.W. (2005a) PK-PD modeling of buprenorphine in cats: intravenous and oral transmucosal administration. *Journal of Veterinary Pharmacology and Therapeutics*, 28, 453–460.

Robertson, S.A. & Taylor, P.M. (2004). Pain management in cats–past, present and future. Part 2. treatment of pain–clinical pharmacology. *Journal of Feline Medicine and Surgery*, 6, 321–333.

Robertson, S.A., Taylor, P.M., Lascelles, B.D., & Dixon, M.J. (2003) Changes in thermal threshold response in eight cats after administration of buprenorphine, butorphanol and morphine. *Veterinary Record*, 153(15), 462–465.

Robertson, S.A., Taylor, P.M., Sear, J.W., & Keuhnel, G. (2005b). Relationship between plasma concentrations and analgesia after intravenous fentanyl and disposition after other routes of administration in cats. *Journal of Veterinary Pharmacology and Therapeutics*, 28, 87–93.

Robertson, S.A., Wegner, K., & Lascelles, B.D. (2009). Antinociceptive and side-effects of hydromorphone after subcutaneous administration in cats. *Journal of Feline Medicine and Surgery*, 11, 76–81.

Sawyer, D.C. & Rech, R.H. (1987). Analgesia and behavioral-effects of butorphanol, nalbuphine, and pentazocine in the cat. *Journal of the American Animal Hospital Association*, 23, 438–446.

Scott, D.B., McClure, J.H., Giasi, R.M., Seo, J., & Covino, B.G. (1980). Effects of concentration of local anaesthetic drugs in extradural block. *British Journal of Anaesthesia*, 52, 1033–1037.

Selmi, A.L., Barbudo-Selmi, G.R., Mendes, G.M., Figueiredo, J.P., & Lins, B.T. (2000) Sedative, analgesic and cardiorespiratory effects of romifidine in cats. *Veterinary Anaesthesia and Analgesia*, 31(3), 195–206.

Selmi, A.L., Mendes, G.M., Lins, B.T., Figueiredo, J.P., & Barbudo-Selmi, G.R. (2005). Comparison of xylazine and medetomidine as premedicants for cats being anaesthetised with propofol-sevoflurane. *The Veterinary Record*, 157, 139–143.

Siao, K.T., Pypendop, B.H., Escobar, A., Stanley, S.D., & Ilkiw, J.E. (2012). Effect of amantadine on oxymorphone-induced thermal antinociception in cats. *Journal of Veterinary Pharmacology and Therapeutics*, 35, 169–174.

Siao, K.T., Pypendop, B.H., Stanley, S.D., & Ilkiw, J.E. (2011). Pharmacokinetics of amantadine in cats. *Journal of Veterinary Pharmacology and Therapeutics*, 34, 599–604.

Skarda, R.T. & Tranquilli, W.J. (2007) Local and regional anesthetics; Local and regional anesthetic techniques: dogs; Local and regional anesthetic techniques: cats. In: *Lumb and Jones' Veterinary Anesthesia and Analgesia*, (eds W.J. Tranquilli, J.C. Thurmon, & K.A. Grimm), 4th edn. pp. 395–418, 561–604. Blackwell Publishing, Ames, IA.

Slingsby, L.S. & Taylor, P.M. (2008) Thermal antinociception after dexmedetomidine administration in cats: a dose-finding study. *Journal of Veterinary Pharmacology and Therapeutics*, 31(2), 135–142.

Slingsby, L.S. & Waterman-Pearson, A.E. (2000). Postoperative analgesia in the cat after ovariohysterectomy by use of carprofen, ketoprofen, meloxicam or tolfenamic acid. *Journal of Small Animal Practice*, 41, 447–450.

Slingsby, L.S., Murrell, J.C., & Taylor, P.M. (2010). Combination of dexmedetomidine with buprenorphine enhances the antinociceptive effect to a thermal stimulus in the cat compared with either agent alone. *Veterinary Anaesthesia and Analgesia*, 37, 162–170.

Steagall, P.V.M., Carnicelli, P., Taylor, P.M., Luna, S.P., Dixon, M., & Ferreira, T.H. (2006). Effects of subcutaneous methadone, morphine, buprenorphine or saline on thermal and pressure thresholds in cats. *Journal of Veterinary Pharmacology and Therapeutics*, 29, 531–537.

Steagall, P.V., Mantovani, F.B., Taylor, P.M., Dixon, M.J., & Luna, S.P. (2009), Dose-related antinociceptive effects of intravenous buprenorphine in cats. *The Veterinary Journal*, 182(2), 203–209.

Straw, R.N. & Mitchell, C.L. (1964). The effects of morphine, pentobarbital, pentazocine and nalorphine on bioelectrical potentials evoked in the brain stem of the cat by electrical stimulation of the tooth pulp. *The Journal of Pharmacology and Experimental Therapeutics*, 146, 7–15.

Taylor, P.M. & Robertson, S.A. (2004). Pain management in cats–past, present and future. Part 1. The cat is unique. *Journal of Feline Medicine and Surgery*, 6, 313–320.

Taylor, P.M., Robertson, S.A., Dixon, M.J., et al. (2001). Morphine, pethidine and buprenorphine disposition in the cat. *Journal of Veterinary Pharmacology and Therapeutics*, 24, 391–398.

Troncy, E., Junot, S., Keroack, S., et al. (2002). Results of pre-emptive epidural administration of morphine with or without bupivacaine in dogs and cats undergoing surgery: 265 cases (1997-1999). *Journal of the American Veterinary Medical Association*, 221, 666–672.

Valverde, A. (2008) Epidural analgesia and anesthesia in dogs and cats. *Veterinary Clinics of North America Small Animal Clinics*, 38, 1205–1230.

Vettorato, E. & Corletto, F. (2011). Gabapentin as part of multi-modal analgesia in two cats suffering multiple injuries. *Veterinary Anaesthesia and Analgesia*, 38, 518–520.

Virtanen, R. (1989). Pharmacological profiles of medetomidine and its antagonist, atipamezole. *Acta Veterinaria Scandanavia Supplement*, 85, 29–37.

Virtanen, R., Savola, J.M., Saano, V., & Nyman, L. (1988). Characterization of the selectivity, specificity and potency of medetomidine as an alpha 2-adrenoceptor agonist. *European Journal of Pharmacology*, 150, 9–14.

Wagner, K.A., Gibbon, K.J., Strom, T.L., Kurian, J.R., & Trepanier, L.A. (2006). Adverse effects of EMLA (lidocaine/prilocaine) cream and efficacy for the placement of jugular catheters in hospitalized cats. *Journal of Feline Medicine and Surgery*, 8, 141–144.

Wegner, K., Robertson, S.A., Kollias-Baker, C., Sams, R.A., & Muir, W.W. 3rd. (2004). Pharmacokinetic and pharmacodynamic evaluation of intravenous hydromorphone in cats. *Journal of Veterinary Pharmacology and Therapeutics*, 27, 329–336.

Williams, L.S., Levy, J.K., Robertson, S.A., Cistola, A.M., & Centonze, L.A. (2002). Use of the anesthetic combination of tiletamine, zolazepam, ketamine, and xylazine for neutering feral cats. *Journal of the American Veterinary Medical Association*, 220, 1491–1495.

26
Treatment and Assessment of Chronic Pain in Cats

Bonnie Wright and Jessica K. Rychel

Chronic pain may be defined as any ongoing discomfort that no longer serves a useful purpose for the patient. Regardless of the inciting etiology, chronic pain may lead to temporary or permanent adverse changes in homeostasis. Associated soft tissues and the surrounding cytokine milieu may be altered, and modifications in the processing of pain signals in the peripheral and central nervous system may occur.

BARRIERS TO TREATMENT OF CHRONIC PAIN IN CATS

One barrier to the effective treatment of chronic pain in cats is the implicit difficulty of assessing chronic pain in this species. Although progress has been made toward validated pain assessment and quality of life (QOL) questionnaires in dogs (Wiseman-Orr et al., 2004), chronic pain assessment in cats remains elusive. Despite a series of well-designed studies to define aspects of feline pain behavior, the repeatability remains questionable on an individual cat basis (Bennett & Morton, 2009).

Other factors that interfere with effective treatment of cats in pain include a reticence by cat owners to seek veterinary care, and a perception by veterinarians that treatment of cats is difficult due to the unique pharmacodynamic challenges posed by this species (Rodan et al., 2011). In addition, there is a large gap in the literature regarding analgesic treatment of cats as opposed to dogs, horses, and humans—although there are recent contributions to the literature regarding the detection and treatment of acute and chronic pain in cats (Zamprogno et al., 2010; Brondani et al., 2011). Data exists, based on research performed by pet food companies, regarding the use of dietary modification in cats with osteoarthritis (OA) (Yamka et al., 2006); however, all of these studies are weakened due to the lack of a validated, standardized chronic pain scoring system for cats.

Finally, chronic pain is frequently treated with a variety of physical medicine modalities such as physical therapy, acupuncture, exercise, and massage, which lack efficacy studies in cats. Clearly, this has dramatically delayed the scientific community's acceptance of these modalities. The challenge for this monograph is not only to present what is known, but also what is commonly thought or experienced, but which is mainly anecdotal in nature.

ASSESSMENT OF CHRONIC PAIN IN CATS

To date, the bulk of feline chronic pain assessment has focused on OA pain. A client-based QOL assessment that is effective at separating behaviors in cats with OA from cats without OA has been developed (Lascelles et al., 2007a; Zamprogno et al., 2010). However, when these questionnaires were applied to a series of cats being fed a potentially therapeutic diet for OA pain, the results were inconsistent, highly variable, and of little help in differentiating between the groups (Lascelles et al., 2010). While it is possible that the therapeutic diet did not resolve pain significantly enough to be measured, and that the null hypothesis was true, a similar study narrowly indicated that a nonsteroidal anti-inflammatory drug (NSAID) improved analgesia in painful cats with OA (Lascelles et al., 2001). These studies suggest that the difficulty in assessing chronic pain in cats interferes with the ability to test the efficacy of analgesic therapies. The same group of researchers did find some promise in using measures of movement and activity to assess chronic pain in cats. The assumption was that cats decrease their activity in response to chronic pain, and this appeared to be an accurate prediction in early studies (Lascelles et al., 2008). Cats treated with analgesics had an increased frequency of movement and spent less time sleeping. In the study evaluating dietary modification for treating OA pain in cats, the accelerometry data showed that cats fed the test diet were likely to be more active than the control group in the afternoon and evening, but no significant differences were found over a 24 hour time frame. Thus, although accelerometry appears promising as a tool for pain assessment in cats, interpretations are complex and appear to be dependent on specific time periods of the day when cats may be normally more active (Lascelles et al., 2010).

Ground reaction forces (Lascelles et al., 2007b), kinematics (Suter et al., 1998), and serum markers for OA pain have been investigated in cats. Each of these methods of pain assessment has limitations. For example, cats undergoing surgical transection of the cruciate ligament had a return to normal kinematics within 6 months, which they maintained for 5 years posttransection, despite extensive radiographic evidence of OA (Suter et al., 1998; Hasler et al., 1998).

INCIDENCE OF CHRONIC PAIN IN CATS

A rough estimate of the ratio of feline to canine patients that present to a typical chronic pain and physical rehabilitation practice is 1:50. However, recent studies investigating the prevalence of radiographic evidence of OA and the incidence of chronic pain in cats, indicate that this disparity cannot be attributed to an absence of painful conditions in cats as they age. Clarke et al. (2005) examined the radiographs and case records of 218 cats (median age: 10.2 years, range: 0.6–16.4 years) and reported a prevalence of 33.9% for degenerative joint disease (DJD) overall, and 16.5% for appendicular OA. Interestingly, only 16.7% of these cats were lame. Godfrey (2005) examined the radiographs of 292 cats with an average age of 9.5 years. He found a 22% prevalence of DJD in the appendicular skeleton with lameness in 17.5% of these cats. In a cohort of cats over 6 years of age, not showing overt signs of pain or thought to be suffering from pain, the incidence of OA considered severe enough to cause pain was greater than 61% (Slingerland et al., 2011). These studies simply looked for radiographic findings of OA as a potential source of pain and, therefore, would have missed any soft-tissue pain arising from the bladder, pancreas, nerve injury or compression, or myofascial pain. On the other hand, it is recognized that radiographic changes often fail to correlate with the level of pain experienced when evaluating OA (Wenham & Conaghan, 2009; Freire et al., 2011). Therefore, an objective knowledge of the incidence of chronic pain in cats is lacking, but it is evident that it is far greater than the incidence of painful cats being presented for assessment and treatment.

SOURCES OF CHRONIC PAIN IN CATS

A wide variety of underlying injuries and illnesses can lead to chronic pain, including: OA, dental pain, gingival disease, neurological pain (especially lumbosacral spondylopathy), cystitis, chronic pancreatitis, and ongoing pain from previous surgical procedures, especially declaw or tail injury and amputation. The incidence of ongoing pain after surgical procedures is reported to range from 10% to 70% in the human population (Kehlet et al., 2006). Furthermore, orthopedic conditions that result in altered kinesthetics may also result in secondary soft-tissue pain (Solomonow, 2006).

DIAGNOSIS OF PAIN IN CATS

Anamnesis and Quality of Life Assessment
In addition to obtaining a compete history, owners can be given QOL scales to aid in assessment of the cat at home (Bennett & Morton, 2009) (Tables 26.1 and 26.2). In general, home assessment is a key feature of identifying pain-associated behaviors such as decreased grooming, changes in activity level, reduction in mobility and jumping, and development of inappropriate elimination. The owner can complete these scales periodically to monitor efficacy of treatment and disease progression.

Table 26.1. Owner assessment of cat

1. Mobility level	*Normal/abnormal*	*Severity (1–10)*
2. Activity level	*Normal/abnormal*	*Severity (1–10)*
3. Grooming habits	*Normal/abnormal*	*Severity (1–10)*
4. Temperament	*Normal/abnormal*	*Severity (1–10)*
5. Overall severity of problem from 1 (mild) to 10 (severe)	*Normal/abnormal*	*Severity (1–10)*

Key signs of chronic musculoskeletal disease (see Table 26.2). If behavior is abnormal, please rate severity of problem from 1 to 10, where 1 is minor change and 10 is severe. (Bennett & Morton, 2009; with permission).

Response to treatment can be used as a diagnostic indicator, but it may be complicated by the fact that among individuals and types of pain conditions the response to treatment may vary widely. In humans, even intra-articular problems, such as meniscal injuries, may not present with typical joint pain, and may not respond well to OA treatments (Conaghan & Felson, 2004; Conaghan et al., 2006).

Physical Examination
In addition to a history and a standardized QOL questionnaire, the practitioner's most valuable tool is the physical examination (Hielm-Bjorkman et al., 2009). The physical examination should include general, neurological, and orthopedic examinations, as well as myofascial palpation to help elucidate painful conditions that would otherwise be missed. Low-stress physical examination in cats is particularly important to be able to elicit and evaluate painful conditions. Excessive restraint will elicit fear and stress, and the subsequent release of catecholamines and cortisol makes it unlikely that a feline patient will demonstrate behavioral indicators of pain. Minimal restraint, a comfortable location, and appropriate handling techniques will ensure patient comfort and minimize stress. A location where the cat can move about on a soft surface, without escaping to a hiding place, is the ideal place to start the evaluation. It often takes significant time and a willingness to take "breaks" in order to get a thorough evaluation of a cat with a painful condition. Similar conditions may cause vastly different levels of pain in different individuals, and a gentle, inquisitive examination will help to discern the regions and degree of pain and help direct the application of treatment. A gentle examination will go a long way in the veterinarian's relationship with the cat and client. Most forms of chronic pain will never completely resolve, and this is likely to be a long-term relationship; thus, a solid foundation of trust is essential.

The Myofascial Examination
The myofascial palpation examination (Chapter 14) takes advantage of the fact that muscle and fascia are closely associated with the patient's neurological framework, which governs both acute and chronic pain transduction, transmission, and perception. Pain, regardless of the underlying etiology, creates adverse activity within the nervous system and patterns of muscular compensation that can lead to soft-tissue discomfort. With excessive neuronal activity,

Table 26.2.   Examples of feline behaviors to consider for evaluation of pain states

Owner behavior watch:

Mobility	Jumping up or down	Refusing or hesitating to jump up or down
		Less agile on stairs
		No longer attempting to reach high spots
	Size/height of jump, up or down	Makes smaller jumps, e.g., takes several steps to reach high spots
		Frequency of jumps, e.g., jumps onto high surfaces less than before
	Gracefulness	Movement less graceful than before
		Becoming stiff and creaky
	Changes in toileting	Changes in location, e.g., reluctant/refusing to go outside or reluctant/refusing to use litter tray
		Difficulties in using litter tray, e.g., missing tray sometimes/often
Activity levels	Sleeping habits	Sleeping or resting more
		Lying in the same spot for long time, not moving location often
		Changes in resting place
	Playing	Playing less
		No longer instigating play
		More difficult to tempt to play
	Hunting	Hunting less than before
Grooming habits	Coat condition	Coat matted or scruffy, generally or in one particular place
		Observed grooming behavior less frequent or of shorter duration
	Scratching	Sharpens claws less frequently
		Change of location/height where scratching occurs
		Claws overgrown or catching on carpets or clicking on hard floors
Temperament (demeanor)	Tolerance to owner or other animals	Less keen to interact
		Grumpy with other cats
		Grumpy on contact with other animals and/or owner
	General attitude	Quieter
		Spending more time alone
		Not seeking/avoiding contact with other cats or other animals
		Not seeking/avoiding contact with owner

Think about how your cat used to be and compare this with how he/she is now, using the type of activities listed above as a guide. (Bennett & Morton, 2009; with permission).

associated muscles tighten, then spasm, causing them to enter an "energy crisis" (Wright, 2010). Myofascial trigger points (MTrPs) are thought to form for a variety of reasons, including simple strain, prolonged spasm due to compensatory kinesthetics from OA or pain, or the body's attempt to stabilize joint laxity. Once formed, MTrPs tend to become self-perpetuating, and adversely impact mobility.

MTrPs can be palpated as knotted regions within discrete bands of tightened muscle. When these regions are strummed in a cross-fiber fashion, reflex fasciculation within the affected or surrounding musculature can occur. In addition, these MTrPs are frequently painful, and close attention to the patient's demeanor, expression, breathing pattern, and posture can aid in the interpretation.

In addition to being painful in their own right, MTrPs contribute to changes in patient mobility and muscle strength and function, and put additional strain on joints and/or spinal segments served by the contracted muscle bellies. Over time, this myofascial restriction helps to create comorbid conditions that accumulate into a multifaceted pain experience.

Execution of the myofascial palpation examination requires a systematic approach, with gentle cross-fiber palpation of muscle

bellies, working down the muscles of the skull and neck, paraspinal muscles, pelvic muscles, and finally muscles of the limbs. An extremely painful patient may not allow a full myofascial examination, and should be treated appropriately with pain medication prior to complete examination. Intensity of discomfort, but not myofascial dysfunction, will lessen with administration of analgesic medication. The pattern of myofascial discomfort can help to localize the source of pain, give clues about underlying etiology, and guide patient treatment.

TREATMENT OF CHRONIC PAIN IN CATS

After combining information from the physical examination, history, QOL score, and relevant diagnostics (radiographs, CT, MRI, biochemical data, CBC), a treatment plan can be developed. Some painful conditions are treatable to resolution, as when an underlying etiology is identified and quickly resolved, and analgesia is required only during the resolution phase. Unfortunately, the vast majority of chronic pain conditions are not curable, and will require ongoing treatment. Pain evaluation should be repeated, and the therapeutic approach reevaluated at each visit to look for improvement or worsening of discomfort with treatment.

Pharmacological Approaches to Treatment of Chronic Pain in the Cat

Pharmacological treatments for chronic pain in cats include opioids, serotonin-specific and dual (serotonin and norepinephrine) reuptake inhibitors (SNRIs), antiepileptics, N-methyl D-Aspartate (NMDA) receptor modifying drugs, NSAIDs, and sodium channel blockers. When choosing analgesic strategies, it is important to consider evidence-based pharmaceutical choices and minimize adverse effects, based on relevant medical history and concurrent diseases. In cats, pharmaceutical data are limited primarily to opioids for acute, adaptive pain, and NSAIDs for acute, but also potentially for chronic pain conditions.

OPIOIDS

Opioid medications are the cornerstone of acute pain treatment in most veterinary species, and the use of opioids for acute pain in cats is discussed in Chapter 25. Opioids work via the endogenous enkephalin, endorphin, and dynorphin receptor systems, and have effects at peripheral, spinal, and brain sites. An extensive review of receptor subtypes, binding potential, efficacy, and potency may be found in Chapter 4, and reviews are available in the literature (Inturrisi, 2002). There is tremendous variability in the efficacy of opioids among individuals (Moore et al., 2011). A body of knowledge is building in humans documenting pharmacogenetic differences behind this observation, and feline patients likely show the same genetic variability (Somogyi et al., 2007).

There are limitations to long-term opioid use in cats, including a lack of efficacy data and knowledge of the required frequency of administration; adverse effects, such as mydriasis, inappetance, ileus, dysphoria, and euphoria; issues of tolerance (extrapolated from other species); and the possibility of enhanced pain response from direct activation of the glia (opioid-induced hyperalgesia (OIH)) (Mao & Mayer, 2001; Lee et al., 2011; Lesniak & Lipkowski, 2011). Some opioids for long-term use in cats include fentanyl patches, buprenorphine, and tramadol.

Fentanyl Patches

Fentanyl patches are frequently utilized in the perioperative period or for acute traumatic pain in cats, but they can be useful to control breakthrough pain and to provide palliative analgesic therapy. Fentanyl patches most commonly used in cats are 12.5 μg/h (cats <3 kg) and 25 μg/h (cats >4 kg), and a new patch should be placed in a new location every 72 hours when used for long-term pain relief. Fentanyl patches are discussed in greater detail in Chapter 9. Plasma concentrations of fentanyl after standardized placement of fentanyl patches were extremely variable (some cats having no measureable plasma concentrations at any point), so use of these patches on cats must be governed by close observation of pain behaviors.

Buprenorphine

The high bioavailability and ease of administration of sublingual buprenorphine make it ideal for long-term use in cats (Robertson et al., 2005). Although this is an expensive long-term treatment option, buprenorphine may be associated with fewer adverse effects compared to other opioids (Silverman, 2009) (Chapter 4). Furthermore, a long-acting buprenorphine formulation for subcutaneous administration has been developed that may provide analgesia for up to 72 hours in cats (Catbagan et al., 2011) (Chapter 9). As a partial agonist with strong affinity for the μ receptor, buprenorphine provides analgesia for mild to moderate pain. A concern surrounding long-acting buprenorphine use is that if inadequate analgesia is provided, other opioids are unlikely to be effective until the end of the sustained release period (up to 72 hours). A human-labeled buprenorphine patch is available, but as is commonly found with dermal delivery systems, the uptake is highly variable, and thought to be insufficient in cats (Murrell et al., 2007).

Tramadol

Tramadol is a weak μ agonist that also activates the serotonin/norepinephrine descending inhibitory systems (Chapter 4). As an opioid, tramadol has about one-tenth the potency of morphine, and has less affinity for the μ receptor. Tramadol is rapidly transformed into a variety of metabolites. In humans, the major metabolite, M1 (*O*-Desmethyltramadol), plays a significant role in its analgesic efficacy. At the μ receptor, M1 has greater affinity and a more marked analgesic effect. Cats produce an M1 metabolite as a result of phase 1 metabolism (demethylation), but it is not yet known how important different metabolites are in providing analgesia for cats (Pypendop & Ilkiw, 2008).

Data are available regarding the clinical analgesic efficacy of tramadol in cats. Several recent studies indicate that a 2–4 mg/kg dose increases the thermal nociceptive threshold (Pypendop et al., 2009), and may be efficacious as a perioperative analgesic (Brondani et al., 2009; Cagnardi et al., 2011). There is also evidence for the efficacy of epidural tramadol in cats (Castro et al., 2009). A study by Ko et al. (2008a) found that orally administered tramadol resulted in signficant sevoflurane minimum alveolar concentration (MAC) reduction that was reversible with naloxone. Chronic use of tramadol in cats has been associated with inappetance, poor palatability (the drug is very bitter), and undesirable behavioral changes, such as agitation or dysphoria.

NONSTEROIDAL ANTI-INFLAMMATORY DRUGS

NSAIDs (Chapters 5 and 25) are important cornerstones of pharmacological treatment of chronic pain in many species, but a combination of concerns limits the long-term use of NSAIDs in cats. An extensive review of NSAIDs and current knowledge about their use in cats is available (Lascelles et al., 2007c). Drugs that require glucuronidation often have prolonged elimination times in cats due to their well-recognized deficiency in this enzyme system. Drugs that require glucuronidation include aspirin, carprofen, and acetaminophen, and this is a contraindication for their long-term use; although all use of acetaminophen is contraindicated in cats. Other NSAIDS, such as meloxicam, piroxicam, and robenacoxib are cleared primarily by oxidative enzymes, and may have a more rapid or predictable elimination time in cats. Data are lacking regarding the precise elimination mechanism for a number of NSAIDs in cats, including flunixin, ketoprofen, and coxib classes (Lascelles et al., 2007c).

A widely held impression regarding the chronic use of NSAIDs is that cats may be more sensitive than other species to organ damage secondary to prostaglandin inhibition, particularly renal damage. For this reason, meloxicam, which is approved for use in feline chronic pain in the United Kingdom, now has a black box warning in the United States against repeated dosing in cats. This warning came after a large number of adverse event reports of cats becoming ill with renal failure and dying after repeat use of meloxicam, according to an October 2010 US Food and Drug Administration (FDA) report. Though most adverse events occurred as the result of inappropriately large doses, incorrect dosing frequency, or combinations of NSAIDs with medications that are more likely to cause an adverse event, it is important to remember that adverse effects can occur with any NSAID. Although meloxicam can still be prescribed for chronic use off label in the United States, the lowest effective dose given with the least possible frequency should be used, and owners must be aware of the risk–benefit ratio of administration of this medication.

A coxib class NSAID, robenacoxib, is available for chronic OA pain in cats in Europe, with a label-dosing interval of approximately 1 week, and has recently received approval for treatment of cats with acute perioperative pain in cats in the United States.

ADDITIONAL ANALGESICS

There are additional medications that can be used for chronic pain in cats, though species-specific information is limited for these medications. Antecdotally, many of them are used successfully in clinical cases, and are worthy of mention here. The medications include SNRIs, tricyclic antidepressants (TCAs), monoamine oxidase inhibitors (MAOIs), gabapentin, NMDA receptor antagonists, and sodium channel blockers (Table 26.3) (See Chapter 8 for more detailed discussion of these drugs).

Antidepressants

SNRIs, TCAs, and MAOIs work by increasing the concentration of either or both serotonin and norepinephrine in the spinal cord and brain by decreasing their uptake or metabolism. Serotonin and norepinephrine are central (along with enkephalins) to generation of descending pain inhibition from the brainstem.

Drugs in this class that have been studied in cats include fluoxetine (Pryor et al., 2001), amitriptyline (Chew et al., 1998), and clomipramine (Lainesse et al., 2006). These drugs are most commonly used for behavioral issues, such as urine spraying. The only analgesia study of these compounds investigated the efficacy of amitryptiline for chronic pain associated with interstitial cystitis, and it appeared to be effective, although it may not impact the disease process itself (Kraijer et al., 2003). For the most part, use of these drugs for painful conditions in cats is extrapolated from their use in the treatment of chronic pain and depression in humans.

Due to variable efficacy, use of these drugs is often based on clinical response, though long-term use (3–4 weeks) may be required before a beneficial response is seen.

Gabapentin

Gabapentin is an antiepileptic drug that is a GABA analog, but does not exert influence on the GABAergic system. Gabapentin appears to interact with a very specific part of the neuronal calcium channel complex, specifically the $\alpha2\delta$ subunit. This subunit appears more frequently with heavy neuronal firing, such as occurs with epilepsy or chronic pain. Gabapentin decreases expression of this subunit, restoring slower, or more normal firing via the calcium channels (Mich & Horne, 2008). Gabapentin is most effective during amplified pain facilitation in the spinal cord, and is likely of greatest benefit in chronic pain conditions, though clinical effect may take several days to weeks to become noticeable.

Enough information has been published on gabapentin pharmacokinetics in cats to allow for its clinical use (Siao et al., 2010). Two pharmacodynamic studies have failed to demonstrate reduction of MAC or thermal threshold in cats administered gabapentin (Pypendop et al., 2010; Reid et al., 2010), though this is not surprising given the specific mechanism of action of gabapentin, as neither group of cats in these studies had chronic pain. Therefore, data supporting analgesic efficacy of gabapentin for chronic pain in cats are lacking, but the potential for efficacy is good, and is supported by clinical evidence (Vettorato & Corletto, 2011).

Gabapentin may require compounding for use in the cat because the liquid formulation contains xylitol. Some practitioners use a relatively high starting dose, rather than having the drug compounded. Most cats tolerate the drug very well, and side effects, which are uncommon, are usually self-limiting and include sedation or mild gastrointestinal upset. Pregabalin, though currently expensive and lacking feline pharmacological data, may find use in treatment of chronic pain in cats.

NMDA Receptor Antagonists

Amantadine is a noncompetitive NMDA receptor antagonist that prevents NMDA receptors from being activated in the spinal cord, even in an environment of increasing glutamate neurotransmitter concentration, thus preventing windup. As an oral analog of ketamine, many of the suspected effects of amantadine are based on ketamine data. Much like gabapentin, NMDA antagonists are likely most effective in chronic or progressivly worsening pain

Table 26.3.   Adjunctive drugs used for chronic pain in cats

Drug class	Drug name	Common dose	Comment
SSRI	Fluoxetine	0.5–1.5 mg/kg PO q24h	Behavior changes possible
TCA	Amitriptyline	2.5–12.5 mg/cat PO q24h	Variable efficacy—may take up to 2 weeks to see improvement
	Imipramine	2.5–5 mg/cat PO q24h	See above
	Clomipramine	0.3–1.0 mg/kg PO q24h	See above
Antiepileptic	Gabapentin	10 mg/kg PO BID–TID	Do not use products containing xylitol!
NMDA antagonist	Amantadine	3–5 mg/kg PO q24h	Extrapolated from dogs
Sodium channel Blocker	Lidocaine CRI	10–20 µg/kg/min IV CRI	Caution with use in cats

conditions. Gabapentin and amantadine can be considered to be primarily antihyperalgesic drugs, rather than true analgesic drugs.

The pharmacokinetics of amantadine have recently been described in cats, but a specific dose and dosing intervals have not yet been established (Siao et al., 2011). The dose range being used in practice (2–5 mg/kg orally every 24 hours) has been extrapolated from other species, and is without any specific rationale for use in cats. A single study evaluated thermal threshold reduction in cats (Siao et al., 2012) and as expected, there was no statistical reduction in thermal threshold with the addition of amantadine to this population of cats, but the cats studied did not have chronic pain. Clinical use of amantadine has been growing, and the drug has been associated with minimal adverse effects, but it can cause occasional gastrointestinal upset or central nervous system agitation. An overdose of $10\times$ or greater may cause seizures.

Sodium Channel Blockers

Sodium channel blockers have long been established as effective for nerve blockade, though the short-acting nature of nerve blockade makes them a less logical choice for treating chronic pain. Intravenous administration of sodium channel blockers, however, has been shown to help reset hyperalgesia in humans with neuropathic pain (Finnerup et al., 2005). There are concerns associated with applying this information to cats due to the cardiovascular depression associated with intravenous use of lidocaine (Pypendop & Ilkiw, 2005). At plasma concentrations of lidocaine that cause cardiovascular depression in cats, thermal threshold nociception was not altered (Pypendop et al., 2006). However, thermal threshold testing is more appropriate for analgesic drug testing, rather than antihyperalgesic drug testing. Clinical use of intravenous lidocaine has appeared to help reset pain states in chronically painful cats, but caution should be exercised with use of intravenous lidocaine due to cardiovascular effects and the lack of efficacy data. Intravenous doses of lidocaine, usually 10–20 µ/kg/min, need to be carefully calculated to avoid toxicity, which can include seizures and cardiac arrest.

Lidocaine Transdermal Patches   Alternative formulations have allowed the possibility of prolonged administration of local anesthetics at sites of superficial discomfort. In particular, the availability of lidocaine in a transdermal patch can provide relief for a local or regional area of pain. Although efficacy data are not available for lidocaine patches in cats, safety data are available, and plasma concentrations of lidocaine remained low (Ko et al., 2008b). These patches can be cut to an appropriate size and shape for the region being treated, but do not adhere well to feline skin. Some adjustments, such as clipping surrounding fur, thorough cleaning of the skin, and use of bandage material (e.g., Elastikon @) have been employed to improve adhesion, but these measures can cause skin irritation with repeated application.

Nutrition and Supplements for Feline Pain Management

Dietary treatments to modulate chronic pain states primarily focus on treatment of inflammation and restoring joint health. Cartilage, menisci, joint capsules, and synovia are the major soft-tissue components within the joint that contribute to pain signaling. Dietary supplements that may impact joint health include green-lipped mussels, avocado soybean unsaponifiables, glucosamine, chondroitin, and omega-3 fatty acids (specifically eicosapentaenoic acid

(EPA) and docosahexaenoic acid (DHA)). Feline dietary manipulation (addition of omega-3 fatty acids, green-lipped mussels, glucosamine, and chondroitin) demonstrated equivocal results in QOL and pain evaluation; but there was some indication of improved overall comfort, as activity levels for these cats, as measured by accelerometry, were increased during the afternoon and evening time periods (Lascelles et al., 2010). Other oral supplements that are frequently discussed in chat groups and marketed for cats include Vitamins A, E, and C; *Boswellia*; yucca; microlactin; and elk-antler velvet. Clinical and research data for safety and efficacy of these supplements in cats are lacking. There are no studies showing optimal dosing for any of the dietary supplements.

Injectable alternatives for protection and healing of osteoarthritic joints are becoming increasingly appealing due to improved bioavailability to joints (less gastrointestinal degradation) and ease of administration (some cats tolerate injection more readily than oral medications). These options include injection of polysulfated glycosaminoglycans, hyaluronic acid, stem cells, and interleukin receptor antagonists. Despite a lack of labeling for cats, the company marketing the polysulfonated glycosaminoglycan product, Adequan®, has documented the deposition of the compound in the joints of cats. This treatment has, anecdotally, been reported to be efficacious in clinical practice. Cats have a tendency to develop injection-associated sarcomas, and this is an important consideration before suggesting repeated injections of any compound in cats.

PHYSICAL MEDICINE

Physical medicine modalities are defined herein as modalities that cause mechanical tissue deformation and induce healing. Cats are amenable to many physical medicine treatments, including acupuncture, stretching, therapeutic exercise, massage, joint mobilization, therapeutic ultrasound, therapeutic laser, extracorporeal shockwave therapy (ESWT), and environmental enrichment. Weight loss is an important consideration for treatment of pain associated with OA and, although a direct association has not been proven, studies have shown an increased incidence of OA pain in cats with higher body condition scores (Lascelles et al., 2010).

Much of physical medicine is based on an understanding of the physiological mechanisms for healing, rather than on objective data from placebo-controlled trials. Some of this departure is due to the fact that complex interventions are very poorly represented by placebo-controlled studies (Kaptchuk et al., 2009). Even with a simple intervention (such as swapping a sugar pill for an active drug) the medical ritual surrounding research trials has been shown to alter perceptions in both the "placebo" group and the treatment group (Hrobjartsson & Gotzsche, 2001). This impact is massively heightened when complex interventions such as acupuncture, touch, exercise, diet, and lifestyle are part of the treatment, as is the case with physical medicine. Unfortunately, data regarding cats will lag far behind that of humans, dogs, and horses, requiring that the clinician work from a physiological explanation of the tools of physical medicine rather than validated clinical trials.

The Benefits of Physical Medicine in Feline Patients

Because physical medicine bypasses drug safety and administration issues, and can help address underlying causes for chronic pain, it is an invaluable tool for successful pain management in feline patients.

Furthermore, these modalities are often dramatically effective at reducing behaviors thought to be associated with pain, and can improve activity level and family interaction in a painful patient. A true multimodal approach is usually best, employing a combination of diet, physical medicine, and pharmacology to achieve the best result of comfort and mobility.

A basic understanding of the physiology behind acupuncture, exercise, and other forms of tissue deformation is necessary because these are critical components of effective pain management in cats. Physical medicine interacts with the endogenous analgesic system, attempting to activate and maximize the patient's comfort with endogenous mechanisms. This interaction occurs along the entire pain sensing system from skin to brain, involving muscle, tendon, fascia, periosteum, and so on. More data are available regarding the efficacy of acupuncture than many of the other modalities, and there are a number of excellent reviews describing the current understanding of acupuncture mechanisms (Wang et al., 2008a, Wang et al., 2008b). Chapter 16 discusses the mechanisms of acupuncture-induced analgesia in more detail, and Chapter 11 discusses rehabilitation modalities and the underlying physiological mechanisms.

Acupuncture in Cats

Acupuncture is surprisingly well tolerated in feline patients, and can be a very valuable tool for treatment of an assortment of chronic pain conditions. The mechanism for acupuncture-induced analgesia is complex, but involves reduced transmission and amplification of pain signaling in the dorsal horn; release of endogenous analgesic neurotransmitters, including enkephalins and endorphins; and modification of inhibitory neurotransmitters and receptors (Wang et al., 2008a, 2008b). By providing a safe and effective alternative or addition to pharmaceutical intervention, acupuncture provides a way to achieve long-term comfort while minimizing the adverse effects and inconvenience of medications. Importantly, cats undergoing acupuncture treatment must be handled gently, to maximize their participation in this treatment. Providing a quiet, comfortable, and protected space for them to have their treatment is essential. Some cats may become too stressed by a trip to a veterinary hospital, and in-home treatment may be better for those patients.

Though clinial data on acupuncture in client-owned cats are limited, cats have been studied, using acupuncture, as models for certain human conditions (Wang et al. 2007). Extrapolation from these studies, in addition to clinical experience, can provide information on conditions in cats that may respond positively to acupuncture. Because acupuncture is safe, and usually well tolerated, a trial period of three to five sessions can usually be used to determine whether the patient will be amenable and responsive to acupuncture. Cats with orthopedic pain conditions, OA, neurological injuries, back and lumbosacral pain, and a variety of medical issues, are good candidates for an acupuncture trial.

Medical conditions that cause chronic pain and may respond to acupuncture can include gastrointestinal inflammation, constipation, and other motility issues; sterile cystitis; pancreatitis; and chronic respiratory conditions such as asthma or upper respiratory infection (Wang et al., 2007; Capodice et al., 2007; Carneiro et al., 2010). Treatment of these internal conditions can be achieved because of viscerosomatic neurological overlap within spinal cord segments (Cabioglu & Arslan, 2008), and the systemic effects of acupuncture, including effects on gastrointestinal motility, inflam-

mation, and immunomodulation, all of which can significantly impact painful conditions.

Musculoskeletal conditions can be successfully treated with acupuncture, but if a patient is initially too uncomfortable to tolerate acupuncture, pharmaceutical intervention may be required prior to treatment. The primary goals of acupuncture for these patients include alteration of the local cellular cytokine milieu to become anti-inflammatory, treatment of muscle tension and MTrPs, and provision of analgesia. The treatment of MTrPs in chronic pain patients is particularly important in breaking the cycle of ongoing pain.

MTrPs can be treated rapidly with acupuncture. Though MTrP acupuncture treatment can be very rewarding, it can create some discomfort during treatment, so it should be performed with caution in cats new to acupuncture. An acupuncture needle is inserted directly into an MTrP, at which time a characteristic twitch and muscle release can be noted. A limited number of MTrPs should be addressed in feline acupuncture sessions, as treating too many may be irritating and uncomfortable for the patient. Combining acupuncture with massage and stretching can lead to a more permanent solution to reducing MTrP dysfunction and pain (Trampas et al., 2010).

Physical Rehabilitation Techniques and Massage

Much of the focus of physical rehabilitation and massage techniques are directed at reducing pain, strengthening, and stretching of pathologically shortened muscles and their antagonistic muscle groups, and proprioceptive retraining of the neuromuscular system (see Chapter 11 for further discussion on rehabilitation techniques). Though the use of rehabilitation techniques has become common in other species, a barrier remains to the use of these techniques in cats. Often it is assumed that cats will not tolerate rehabilitation due to temperament, lifestyle, or age. In fact, cats respond well to rehabilitation techniques, and often enjoy the mental stimulation of therapeutic exercise, stretching, and massage in the hospital and at home.

Cryotherapy can be applied to regions of inflammation, particularly with an acute exacerbation of a chronic injury, to reduce hyperalgesia and slow local metabolism (Sluka et al. 1999). Heat therapy is also valuable, and often appreciated by feline patients. Application of a superficial hot pack over a tense muscle or region of chronic discomfort can help ease muscle spasm, improve blood flow, and reduce pain-associated behaviors (Sluka et al., 1999; Lane & Latham, 2009).

Therapeutic laser is a good option for feline patients, because in addition to providing analgesia, it can improve neurological function, blood flow, and regional healing (Hashmi et al., 2010). This technique is quick and nonpainful, so is often very well tolerated by feline patients, even those that do not allow other modalities.

Extracorporeal shock wave therapy (ESWT) is a technique novel to small animal veterinary medicine, but one that has been used with increasing success in human, equine, and research medical settings. This technique is being explored for its value in chronic pain conditions such as OA and lumbosacral instability and pain, very common findings in middle-aged to geriatric cats. Like other physical medicine modalities, ESWT likely works through bioneuromodulation as a result of mechanical deformation of tissues, resulting in a reduction in chronic inflammation (Yoo et al., 2012), altered neurotransmitters (Hausdorf et al., 2008), and improved joint health

(Wang et al., 2010). ESWT is uncomfortable and noisy, and because sedation or general anesthesia of the patient is usually necessary, ESWT may not be desirable for all patients. Typically, two to three treatments are performed, and the benefits may last for months.

The use of joint manipulation, joint mobilization, and stretching can also be beneficial for specific feline patients. In the hands of a skilled practitioner, these techniques can improve synovial fluid production, reduce edema, increase comfort, improve lymphatic and venous drainage, and improve the range of motion and flexibility.

It is noteworthy that the facet joints in the spinal column undergo similar changes to other joints, and respond to similar treatments. As with elsewhere in the body, when any structure becomes involved in pathology or pain, all of the associated structures are susceptible. Spinal arthritis implicates the paraspinal muscles and nerves. Back pain is a common condition in feline patients, and one that has been traditionally overlooked. The use of stretching, strengthening, and neuromuscular retraining can help a patient regain spinal comfort and mobility, though, as with most other chronic pain conditions, a multimodal approach is often required.

SUMMARY

As the literature concerning pain in cats trickles into the databases, an increasing number of tools will be available to identify and treat cats suffering from pain. In the meantime, the tools to diagnose pain, as well as a large number of effective treatments, lie, quite literally, in the hands of the practitioner. An inquisitive, gentle touch often helps locate the specific source of discomfort, perhaps with greater clarity than the classic reliance on radiographic evidence of arthritis, as it is so poorly correlated with clinical pain. While the body seems to have many ways of amplifying pain in multiple tissue types and regions, it also holds the keys to homeostasis. A skilled practitioner can often gently coax the body back into a place of balance with a combination of physical medicine modalities, pharmacological manipulations, and investment by the owner in exercise, diet, environmental enrichment, and weight loss.

REFERENCES

Bennett, D. & Morton, C. (2009) A study of owner observed behavioural and lifestyle changes in cats with musculoskeletal disease before and after analgesic therapy. *Journal of Feline Medicine and Surgery*, 11(12), 997–1004.

Brondani, J.T., Loureiro Luna, S.P., Beier, S.L., Minto, B.W., & Padovani, C.R. (2009) Analgesic efficacy of perioperative use of vedaprofen, tramadol or their combination in cats undergoing ovariohysterectomy. *Journal of Feline Medicine & Surgery*, 11(6), 420–429.

Brondani, J.T., Luna, S.P., & Padovani, C.R. (2011) Refinement and initial validation of a multidimensional composite scale for use in assessing acute postoperative pain in cats. *American Journal of Veterinary Research*, 72(2), 174–183.

Cabioglu, M.T. & Arslan, G. (2008) Neurophysiologic basis of backshu and huatuo-jiaji points. *The American Journal of Chinese Medicine*, 36(3), 473–479.

Cagnardi, P., Villa, R., Zonca, A., et al. (2011) Pharmacokinetics, intraoperative effect and postoperative analgesia of tramadol in cats. *Research in Veterinary Science*, 90(3), 503–509.

Capodice, J.L., Jin, Z., Bemis, D.L., et al. (2007) A pilot study on acupuncture for lower urinary tract symptoms related to chronic prostatitis/chronic pelvic pain. *Chinese Medicine*, 2, 1–7.

Carneiro, E.R., Xavier, R.A.N., Pedreira De Castro, M.A., Do Nascimento, C.M., & Silveira, V.L. (2010) Electroacupuncture promotes a decrease in inflammatory response associated with Th1/Th2 cytokines, nitric oxide and leukotriene B4 modulation in experimental asthma. *Cytokine*, 50, 335–340.

Castro, D.S., Silva, M.F., Shih, A.C., Motta, P.P., Pires, M.V., & Scherer, P.O. (2009) Comparison between the analgesic effects of morphine and tramadol delivered epidurally in cats receiving a standard noxious stimulation. *Journal of Feline Medicine & Surgery*, 11(12), 948–953.

Catbagan, D.L., Quimby, J.M., Mama, K.R., Rychel, J.K., & Mich, P.M. (2011) Comparison of the efficacy and adverse effects of sustained-release buprenorphine hydrochloride following subcutaneous administration and buprenorhpine hydrochloride following oral transmucosal administration in cats undergoing ovariohysterectomy. *American Journal of Veterinary Research*, 72(4), 461–466.

Chew, D.J., Buffington, C.A., Kendall, M.S., DiBartola, S.P., & Woodworth, B.E. (1998) Amitriptyline treatment for severe recurrent idiopathic cystitis in cats. *Journal of the American Veterinary Medical Association*, 213, 1282–1286.

Clarke, S.P., Mellor, D., Clements, D.N., et al. (2005) Prevalence of radiographic signs of degenerative joint disease in a hospital population of cats. *The Veterinary Record*, 157(25), 793–799.

Conaghan, P.G. & Felson, D.T. (2004) Structural associations of osteoarthritis pain: lessons from magnetic resonance imaging. *Novartis Foundation Symposium*, 260, 191–201.

Conaghan, P.G., Felson, D., Gold, G., Lohmander, S., Totterman, S., & Altman, R. (2006) MRI and non-cartilaginous structures in knee osteoarthritis. *Osteoarthritis and Cartilage*, 14, A87–A94.

Finnerup, N.B., Biering-Sorensen, F., Johannesen, I.L., et al. (2005). Intravenous lidocaine relieves spinal cord injury pain: a randomized controlled trial. *Anesthesiology*, 102(5), 1023–1030.

Freire, M., Robertson, I., Bondell, H.D., et al. (2011) Radiographic evaluation of feline appendicular degenerative joint disease versus macroscopic appearance of articular cartilage. *Veterinary Radiology & Ultrasound*, 52(3), 239–247.

Godfrey, D.R. (2005) Osteoarthritis in cats: a retrospective radiological study. *Journal of Small Animal Practice*, 46(9), 425–429.

Hashmi, J.T., Huang, Y.Y., Osmani, B.Z., Sharma, S.K., Naeser, M.A., & Hamblin, M.R. (2010) Role of Low-Level Laser Therapy in Neurorehabilitation. *Physical Medicine & Rehabilitation*, 12(S2), S292–S305.

Hasler, E.M., Herzog, W., Leonard, T.R., Stano, A., & Nguyen, H. (1998) In vivo knee joint loading and kinematics before and after ACL transection in an animal model. *Journal of Biomechanics*, 31, 253–262.

Hausdorf, J., Lemmens, M.A.M, Kaplan, S., et al. (2008) Extracorporeal shockwave application to the distal femur of rabbits diminishes the number of neurons immunoreactive for substance P in dorsal root ganglia L5. *Brain Research*, 1207, 96–101.

Hielm-Bjorkman, A.K., Rita, H., & Tulamo, R.M. (2009) Psychometric testing of the Helsinki chronic pain index by completion of a questionnaire in Finnish by owners of dogs with chronic signs of pain caused by osteoarthritis. *American Journal of Veterinary Research*, 70(6), 727–734.

Hrobjartsson, A. & Gotzsche, P.C. (2001). Is the placebo worthless? An analysis of clinical trials comparing placebo with no treatment. *New England Journal of Medicine*, 344(21), 1594–1602.

Inturrisi, C.E. (2002) Clinical pharmacology of opioids for pain. *The Clinical Journal of Pain*, 18(4 Suppl), S3–S13.

Kaptchuk, T.J., Shaw, J., Kerr, K.E. et al. (2009) "Maybe I made up the whole thing": placebos and patient's experiences in a randomized controlled trial. *Culture, Medicine and Psychiatry*, 33, 382–411.

Kehlet, H., Jensen, T.S., & Woolf, C.J. (2006) Persistent postsurgical pain: risk factors and prevention. *Lancet*, 367(9522), 1618–1625.

Ko, J.C., Abbo, L.A., Weil, A.B., Johnson, B.M., Inoue, T., & Payton, M.E. (2008a) Effect of orally administered tramadol alone or with an intravenously administered opioid on minimum alveolar concentration of sevoflurane in cats. *Journal of the American Veterinary Medical Association*, 232(12), 1834–1840.

Ko, J.C., Maxwell, L.K., Abbo, L.A., & Weil, A.B. (2008b) Pharmacokinetics of lidocaine following the application of 5% lidocaine patches to cats. *Journal of Veterinary Pharmacology & Therapeutics*, 31, 359–367.

Kraijer, M., Fink-Gremmels, J., Nickel, R.F. (2003) The short-term clinical efficacy of amitriptyline in the management of idiopathic feline lower urinary tract disease: a controlled clinical study. *Journal of Feline Medicine and Surgery*, 5(3), 191–196.

Lainesse, C., Frank, D., Meucci, V., Intorre, L., Soldani, G., & Doucet, M. (2006) Pharmacokinetics of clomipramine and desmethyl-clomipramine after single-dose intravenous and oral administrations in cats. *Journal of Veterinary Pharmacology & Therapeutics*, 29, 271–278.

Lane, E. & Latham, T. (2009) Managing pain using heat and cold therapy. *Pediatric Nursing*, 21(6), 14–18.

Lascelles, B.D., Henderson, A.J., & Hackett, I.J. (2001) Evaluation of the clinical efficacy of meloxicam in cats with painful locomotor disorders. *Journal of Small Animal Practice*, 42(12), 587–593.

Lascelles, B.D.X., Hansen, B.D., Roe, S., et al. (2007a) Evaluation of client specific outcome measures and activity monitoring to measure pain relief in cats with osteo-arthritis. *Journal of Veterinary Internal Medicine*, 21(3), 410–416.

Lascelles, B.D., Findley, K., Correa, M., Marcellin-Little, D., & Roe, S. (2007b) Kinetic evaluation of normal walking and jumping in cats, using a pressure sensitive walkway. *The Veterinary Record*, 160, 512–516.

Lascelles, B.D., Court, M.H., Hardie, E.M., & Robertson, S.A. (2007c) Nonsteroidal anti-inflammatory drugs in cats: a review. *Veterinary Anesthesia & Analgesia*, 34(4), 228–250.

Lascelles, B.D., Hansen, B.D., Thomson, A., Pierce, C.C., Boland, E., & Smith, E.S. (2008) Evaluation of a digitally integrated accelerometer-based activity monitor for the measurement of activity in cats. *Veterinary Anesthesia & Analgesia*, 35(2), 173–183.

Lascelles, B.D., Depuy, V., Thompson, A., et al. (2010) Evaluation of a therapeutic diet for feline degenerative joint disease. *Journal of Veterinary Internal Medicine*, 24(3), 487–495.

Lee, M., Silverman, S., Hansen, H., Patel, V.B., & Manchikanti, L. (2011) A comprehensive review of opioid-induced hyperalgesia. *Pain Physician*, 14, 145–161.

Lesniak, A. & Lipkowski, A.W. (2011) Opioid peptides in peripheral pain control. *Acta Neurobiologiae Experimentalis*, 71, 129–138.

Mao, J. & Mayer, D.J. (2001) Spinal Cord neuroplasticity following repeated opioid exposure and its relation to pathological pain. *Annals of the New York Academy of Sciences*, 933, 175–184.

Mich, P.M. & Horne, W.A. (2008) Alternative splicing of the Ca^{2+} channel $\beta 4$ subunit confers specificity for gabapentin inhibition for Ca2.1 trafficking. *Molecular Pharmacology*, 74(3), 904–912.

Moore, R.A., Derry, S., McQuay, H.J., & Wiffen, P.J. (2011) Single dose oral analgesics for acute postoperative pain in adults. *Cochrane Database of Systematic Reviews*, 7(9), CD008659.

Murrell, J.C., Robertson, S.A., & Taylor, P.M. (2007) Use of a transdermal matrix patch of buprenorphine in cats: preliminary pharmacokinetic and pharmacodynamic data. *The Veterinary Record*, 160(17), 578–583.

Pryor, P.A., Hart, B.L., Cliff, K.D., & Bain, M.J. (2001) Effects of a selective serotonin reuptake inhibitor on urine spraying behavior in cats. *Journal of the American Veterinary Medical Association*, 219(11), 1557–1561.

Pypendop, B.H. & Ilkiw, J.E. (2005) Assessment of the hemodynamic effects of lidocaine administered IV in isoflurane-anesthetized cats. *American Journal of Veterinary Research*, 66, 661–668.

Pypendop, B.H., Ilkiw, J.E., & Robertson, S.A. (2006) Effects of intravenous administration of lidocaine on the thermal threshold in cats. *American Journal of Veterinary Research*, 67, 16–20.

Pypendop, B.H. & Ilkiw, J.E. (2008) Pharmacokinetics of tramadol, and its metabolite O-desmethyl-tramadol, in cats. *Journal of Veterinary Pharmacology & Therapeutics*, 31(1), 52–59.

Pypendop, B.H., Siao, K.T., & Ilkiw, J.E. (2009) Effects of Tramadol hydrochloride on the thermal threshold in cats. *American Journal of Veterinary Research*, 70(12), 1465–1470.

Pypendop, B.H., Siao, K.T., & Ikliw, J.E. (2010) Thermal antinociceptive effect of orally administered gabapentin in healthy cats. *American Journal of Veterinary Research*, 71(9), 1027–1032.

Reid, P., Pypendop, B.H., & Ilkiw, J.E. (2010) The effects of intravenous gabapentin administration on the minimum alveolar concentration of isoflurane in cats. *Anesthesia & Analgesia*, 111(3), 633–637.

Robertson, S.A., Lascelles, B.D., Taylor, P.M., & Sear, J.W. (2005) PK-PD modeling of buprenorphine in cats: intravenous and oral transmucosal administration. *Journal of Veterinary Pharmacology & Therapeutics*, 28(5), 453–460.

Rodan, I., Sundahl, E., Carney, H., et al. (2011) AAFP and ISFM feline friendly-handling guidelines. *Journal of Feline Medicine & Surgery*, 13(5), 364–375.

Siao, K.T., Pypendop, B.H., & Ilkiw, J.E. (2010) Pharmacokinetics of Gabapentin in cats. *American Journal of Veterinary Research*, 71(7), 817–821.

Siao, K.T., Pypendop, B.H., Stanley, S.D., & Ilkiw, J.E. (2011) Pharmacokinetics of amantadine in cats. *Journal of Veterinary Pharmacology & Therapeutics*, 34(6), 599–604.

Siao, K.T., Pypendop, B.H., Escobar, A., Stanley, S.D., & Ilkiw, J.E. (2012) Effect of amantadine on oxymorphone-induced thermal antinociception in cats. *Journal of Veterinary Pharmacology & Therapeutics*, 35(2), 169–174.

Silverman, S.M. (2009) Opioid induced hyperalgesia: clinical implications for the pain practitioner. *Pain Physician*, 12(3), 679–684.

Slingerland, L.I., Hazewinkel, H.A., Meij, B.P., Picavet, P., & Voorhout, G. (2011) Cross-sectional study of the prevalence and clinical features of osteoarthritis in 100 cats. *The Veterinary Journal*, 187(3), 304–309.

Sluka, K.A., Christy, M.R., Peterson, W.L., Rudd, S.L., & Troy, S.M. (1999) Reduction of pain-related behaviors with either cold or heat treatment in an animal model of acute arthritis. *Archives of Physical Medicine and Rehabilitation*, 80(3), 313–317.

Solomonow, M. (2006) Sensory-motor control of ligaments and associated neuromuscular disorders. *Journal of Electromyography & Kinesiology*, 16(6), 549–567.

Somogyi, A.A., Barratt, D.T., & Coller, J.K. (2007) Pharmacogenetics of opioids. *Clinical Pharmacology & Therapeutics*, 81(3), 429–444.

Suter, E., Herzog, W., Leonard, T.R., & Nguyen, H. (1998) One-year changes in hind limb kinematics, ground reaction forces and knee stability in an experimental model of osteoarthritis. *Journal of Biomechanics*, 31, 511–517.

Trampas, A., Kitsios, A., Sykaras, E., Symeonidis, S., & Lazarou, L. (2010) Clinical massage and modified proprioceptive neuromuscular facilitation stretching in males with latent myofascial trigger points. *Physical Therapy in Sport*, 11, 91–98.

Vettorato, E. & Corletto, F. (2011) Gabapentin as part of multi-modal analgesia in two cats suffering multiple injuries. *Veterinary Anaesthesia & Analgesia*, 38(5), 518–520.

Wang, C., Zhou, D.F., Shuai, X.W., Liu, J.X., & Xie, P.Y. (2007) Effects and mechanisms of electroacupuncture at PC6 on frequency of transient lower esophageal sphincter relaxation in cats. *World Journal of Gastroenterology*, 13(36), 4873–4880.

Wang, C.J., Weng, L.H., Ko, J.Y., et al. (2010) Extracorporeal shockwave shows regression of osteoarthritis of the knee in rats. *Journal of Surgical Research*, 171(2), 601–608.

Wang, S.M., Kain, Z.N., & White, P. (2008a) Acupuncture analgesia: I. The scientific basis. *Anesthesia & Analgesia*, 106(2), 602–610.

Wang, S.M., Kain, Z.N., & White, P.F. (2008b) Acupuncture analgesia: II. Clinical considerations. *Anesthesia & Analgesia*, 106(2), 611–621.

Wenham, C.Y. & Conaghan, P.G. (2009) Imaging the painful osteoarthritic knee joint: what have we learned? *Nature Clinical Practice Rheumatology*, 5(3), 149–158.

Wiseman-Orr, M.L., Nolan, A.M., Reid, J., & Scott, E.M. (2004) Development of a questionnaire to measure the effects of chronic pain on health-related quality of life in dogs. *American Journal of Veterinary Research*, 65(8),1077–1084.

Wright, B. (2010) Management of chronic soft tissue pain. *Topics in Companion Animal Medicine*, 25(1), 26–31.

Yamka, R.M., Friesen, K.G., Lowry, S.R., & Coffman, L. (2006) Measurement of arthritic and bone serum metabolites in arthritis, nonarthritic, and geriatric cats fed wellness foods. *The International Journal of Applied Research in Veterinary Medicine*, 4, 265–273.

Yoo, S.D., Choi, S., Lee, G.J., et al. (2012) Effects of extracorporeal shockwave therapy on nanostructural and biomechanical responses in the collagenase-induced Achilles tendinitis animal model. *Lasers in Medical Science*, 27(6):1195–1204.

Zamprogno, H., Hansen, B.D., Bondell, H.D., et al. (2010) Development of a questionnaire to assess degenerative joint disease-associated pain in cats: item generation and questionnaire format. *American Journal of Veterinary Research*, 71(12), 1417–1424.

27
Cancer-associated Pain and its Management

Lydia Love and Lisa DiBernardi

Cancer is a group of diseases that are defined by the uninhibited replication of cells. Most cancers arise from a single cell that has suffered a disruption of the mechanisms regulating proliferation and self-elimination. Malignant tumors may damage normal organ architecture and function, invade adjacent tissues, and metastasize to distant sites in the body. Unrestrained growth of cells creates pain via several mechanisms: directly through destruction of soft or bony tissues and indirectly via secondary infection, inflammation, edema, visceral distention or obstruction, or paraneoplastic syndromes. In addition, therapeutic interventions may also cause pain in patients with cancer, including acute perioperative pain, and chemotherapy- and radiation-induced adverse effects.

Identification of the underlying mechanisms of pain helps to delineate management strategies. Addressing cancer-associated pain (Chapter 3) can be difficult because of the potential coexistence of both adaptive and maladaptive pain states. Adaptive pain is acute in nature, includes nociceptive and inflammatory pain, and occurs in the presence of an intact nervous system. Nociceptive pain is transitory and results in the development of a protective reflex in order to avoid further damage to the organism. Inflammatory pain is associated with tissue damage and leads to changes in peripheral and central processing of noxious stimuli. Maladaptive pain refers to several different mechanisms of pain that do not specifically promote healing and essentially are, in and of themselves, disease processes. Examples of maladaptive pain include ongoing inflammatory pain; neuropathic pain consisting of anatomical or physiological dysfunction of the nervous system; and sympathetically maintained pain syndromes (Dickinson et al., 2010; Voscopoulos & Lema, 2010).

To complicate matters, cancer-associated pain can be somatic or visceral in origin. Somatic pain is typically easily localized, whereas visceral pain is more diffuse in nature and may manifest as referred pain (Robinson & Gebhart, 2008). Most research into the mechanisms and treatment of pain has focused on somatic pain sensation. Visceral and somatic afferents differ in density, morphology, and nociceptor characteristics as well as in central distribution and processing. Development of management strategies for visceral pain lags well behind that of somatic pain.

The prevalence of cancer-associated pain in veterinary species is unknown. A meta-analysis of studies published from 1966 to 2005 indicates that the prevalence of pain in human cancer patients is 59%, whereas in those with terminal disease, the prevalence is 64%. Even in states of remission, cancer-associated pain was determined to have a prevalence of 33% (van den Beuken-van Everdingen et al., 2007). It is probable that the prevalence of cancer-associated pain is similar in veterinary species, and 20–30% of deaths in dogs over 2 years of age are due to neoplasia (Fleming et al., 2011). It is essential that veterinarians are attentive to the potential existence of pain and resulting disturbances in quality of life (QOL) in patients with cancer, and are vigilant in their attempts to relieve such pain.

ASSESSING THE CANCER PATIENT

Evaluation of the cancer patient must be integrative in nature, with attention to a wide variety of factors that affect the QOL of the patient. Pain certainly will affect QOL, but other issues, including organ function and appetite, can have profound consequences on behavior and activity. Detailed questioning of the human caretakers regarding activity level, grooming behaviors, interest in play, perceived comfort and mobility, interaction with household members, behavioral responses, and digestive function, including bowel movements and appetite, should occur at every clinical evaluation. This information is central to a comprehensive analysis of the daily life of the patient (Yazbek & Fantoni, 2005; Wiseman-Orr et al., 2006; Lynch et al., 2011). Coexisting diseases such as osteoarthritis, cardiac insufficiency, and dental disease should be assessed and managed because these conditions can profoundly affect QOL. Development of a questionnaire that is repeatedly administered over time can help veterinarians and owners gain an objective view of the patient's condition and lifestyle. Several examples have been validated in dogs and are available in the veterinary literature (Yazbek & Fantoni, 2005; Wiseman-Orr et al., 2006; Lynch et al., 2011).

A complete catalog of the prescription medications and herbal, nutritional, and nutraceutical supplements that are being administered to the patient should be included in the anamnesis. Cancer patients may have multiple providers involved in their care, and careful inventory of medications and treatments is essential to avoid unnecessary polypharmacy or drug interactions. Attention should be paid to any drugs that: may cause painful conditions and affect QOL; may be addressing pain states; or may interact with analgesic therapies. For example, administration of prednisone may cause gastrointestinal ulceration or muscle wasting and associated weakness; vinca alkaloids may cause ileus or peripheral neuropathies; and platinum drugs may affect renal function or cause gastrointestinal distress.

The physical examination is an essential portion of the cancer patient evaluation and should include all major organ systems. Specifically regarding pain states, attention should be paid to the demeanor and behavioral responses of the patient, location of primary and metastatic neoplastic disease, site of surgical interventions, musculoskeletal conditions, mobility, neurological function, and dermatological conditions such as radiation-induced erythema and desquamation. Secondary conditions, such as edema due to lymphatic blockage, or pathological fractures (which typically manifest as an acute decline in function and comfort), should also be carefully investigated.

ANALGESIC STRATEGIES

The management strategy of cancer-related pain should be multifaceted in nature, including: modification or removal of the source of pain via surgical resection and/or curative intent radiation therapy (CRT); pharmacological manipulation of the pain pathway; adjunctive therapies such as acupuncture and physical rehabilitation modalities; interventional analgesic techniques; and palliative care, including reduced fraction radiation therapy.

Restorative Techniques

Restorative techniques are those treatments that are intended to induce remission of the cancer state, and can include surgical removal and radiation therapy, with the objective of long-term tumor control.

SURGICAL RESECTION

The primary goal in the treatment of cancer is to rid the body of neoplastic disease. Surgical intervention in the treatment of cancer may be definitive or palliative. Although definitive therapy will accomplish tumor control and result in alleviation or elimination of pain, palliative surgical therapy is an important tool for control of oncological pain. The benefits of a limb amputation in a dog with osteosarcoma are obvious: a limping Rottweiler with a destructive lesion of the proximal humerus is in pain, and this pain can be alleviated by removal of the forelimb. However, visceral oncological pain, resulting from an expansile mass and associated inflammation and edema, and the relief that may be provided by surgical resection, may be overlooked in veterinary species. For example, resection of a hepatocellular carcinoma in a cat may be beneficial in controlling visceral pain in the short-term; but the invasive nature of the surgical procedure must be judged in light of the benefit to the patient and the owner's goals. Surgical interventions will create acute nociceptive and inflammatory pain in the short-term that should be anticipated and addressed.

Interestingly, perioperative anesthetic and analgesic practices, including administration of opioid analgesics and nonsteroidal anti-inflammatory drugs (NSAIDs), use of local anesthetic techniques, precipitation of the neuroendocrine stress response, temperature regulation, and transfusion of blood products may influence long-term outcomes such as recurrence and metastasis (Gottschalk et al., 2010; Afsharimani et al., 2011).

CURATIVE INTENT RADIATION THERAPY

CRT delivers a measured dose of ionizing radiation to a predefined tumor volume with the goal of eradicating the tumor. In addition, the radiation specialist strives to preserve healthy tissue, maximize QOL, and prolong survival. With these goals in mind, CRT is delivered in small, defined doses called fractions. This differs from palliative intent radiation therapy in which larger doses of radiation are delivered in smaller fractions over a shorter time period.

The most common form of radiation-induced cell death is caused by injury to DNA, leading to the loss of reproductive integrity. Apoptosis, or programmed cell death, is the less common mechanism by which radiation can reduce cell populations, and is characteristic of hemopoietic and lymphoid cells.

A gratifying consequence of solid tumor remission can be a reduction of pain through the elimination of neoplastic invasion into normal tissues, alleviation of pressure on neural structures, or reduction of associated organ expansion and inflammation. Unfortunately, adverse effects of CRT can occur and may cause temporary discomfort (Carsten et al., 2008). Anticipated adverse effects are largely dependent on the normal tissues within the irradiated field as well as the inherent tumor features and calculated parameters of radiation delivery. Cellular effects of radiation ensue within minutes through a series of cytoplasmic signaling and transduction pathways; however, these changes may take weeks to years to become clinically detectable and relevant. Early effects (days to weeks) involve rapidly proliferating tissues, and are often self-limiting. Late effects (months to years) involve slowly proliferating tissues, such as bone, lung, kidney, and spinal cord. These late effects may be more difficult to manage, and may result in fibrosis, necrosis, and loss of function or even death.

The advent of intensity modulated radiation therapy (IMRT) has provided the opportunity to reduce the number and severity of adverse effects. IMRT uses 3D computed tomography images of a patient to aid in computerized treatment planning. The total treatment dose is divided through 5–9 beams, and within a single-beam radiation, beam-shaping devices, called collimators, create beamlets, which allow the intensity of the radiation beam to vary during treatment sessions. This dose modulation permits different areas of a tumor or nearby normal tissues to receive drastically different doses of radiation. When compared with conventional radiation techniques, IMRT has proven effective in the reduction of both acute and delayed toxicities including hematological, gastrointestinal, and dermatological complications, while decreasing the occurrence of xerostomia and osteoradionecrosis, in a variety of malignancies (Veldeman et al., 2008; Ahmed et al., 2009; Pepek et al., 2010). IMRT resulted in improved ocular sparing and reduced the frequency and severity of acute and late ocular toxicity compared to conventionally delivered RT in dogs with sinonasal tumors (Lawrence et al., 2010). As the use of IMRT expands, substantiation of reduced normal tissue toxicity for other organ systems will likely emerge, with a consequential improvement in tumor control and QOL.

A radiation-induced adverse effect scoring system has been published by the Veterinary Radiation Therapy Oncology Group, and was adapted for veterinary patients from scoring systems published by the Radiation Therapy Oncology Group and the European Organization for Research and Treatment of Cancer (LaDue & Klein, 2001).

Because the most common tumors treated in veterinary medicine are of the skin and subcutis (soft tissue sarcoma and mast cell tumor), commonly recognized radiation-induced adverse effects are epilation, inflammation, erythema, and desquamation in the tissues within and surrounding the targeted treatment field (Collen & Mayer, 2006). Moist desquamation is usually accompanied by pruritus and often takes 2–4 weeks to resolve. Topical treatments for radiation-induced dermatitis include silver sulfadiazine ointments, aloe vera gel, commercial wound dressings, and topical corticosteroids (Collen & Mayer, 2006). Petroleum-based products should be avoided, and a porous biological dressing designed to mimic skin should be applied. Currently, there are no prospective, controlled clinical studies evaluating the commonly used products for treating radiation-induced adverse effects. Washing the affected area with water or water with a mild soap has been thought to alleviate pruritus; however, a randomized study involving 99 women who received breast irradiation failed to identify statistical evidence in support of this claim (Roy et al., 2001). Because veterinary patients do not participate in a daily hygiene regimen, washing with a mild soap solution and gently patting dry is recommended. It is also best to plan ahead to prevent self-trauma such as licking, rubbing, or scratching that may exacerbate discomfort and delay healing. Elizabethan collars, padded bandages on paws to prevent scratching, or cotton clothing to prevent access to pruritic areas may be beneficial.

Pharmacological Management

Pharmacological manipulation of the pain pathway is the foundation of analgesic management in a variety of pain states. When prescribing analgesic agents, it is important to perform a full assessment of the current therapeutic and palliative treatment strategies in order to avoid unnecessary polypharmacy and to gauge the caretaker's emotional and financial resources.

NONSTEROIDAL ANTI-INFLAMMATORY DRUGS

NSAIDs (Chapter 5) are the mainstay of treatment for mild to moderate pain caused by inflammatory mechanisms. Many neoplastic processes involve inflammatory cascades that lead to pain and discomfort. These effects can be ameliorated by the use of NSAIDs. NSAIDs affect both peripheral and central cyclooxygenase (COX) enzymes (Yaksh et al., 2001). In addition to analgesic effects, inhibition of COX enzymes may interfere with tumor promoting mechanisms such as angiogenesis and metastasis (Ghosh et al., 2010). For well over a decade, piroxicam (0.3 mg/kg q24h) has been used as a palliative treatment for transitional cell carcinoma (TCC) of the bladder. In the original study of 34 dogs, the nonselective COX inhibitor piroxicam achieved a median survival time of 181 days, and owners described an improved QOL (Knapp et al., 1994). More recently, COX-2 inhibition has been investigated in cancer prevention and therapy (Moreira et al., 2010; Khan et al., 2011). The COX-2 selective NSAID, deracoxib, has an antitumor profile in dogs with TCC similar to that of piroxicam (McMillan et al., 2011). The use of piroxicam or carprofen increased the median survival time of dogs affected with prostatic carcinoma from 0.7 months in untreated dogs to 6.9 months (Sorenmo et al., 2004). In canine osteosarcoma, three of four dogs that experienced spontaneous regression were receiving carprofen (Mehl et al., 2001).

Chronic use of NSAIDs can induce gastrointestinal complications and renal damage, and discontinuation of the NSAID is

the foundation of treatment. Careful monitoring of gastrointestinal signs is warranted, as slightly fewer than 20% of dogs receiving piroxicam or deracoxib will experience effects related to gastrointestinal ulceration (Knapp et al., 1994; McMillan et al., 2011). In humans, proton pump inhibitors, H_2 receptor blockers, and the prostaglandin analog, misoprostol, decrease the incidence of gastric and duodenal ulceration. Only misoprostol has been shown to reduce the risk of serious complications, such as GI perforation, in human patients taking NSAIDs (Rostom et al., 2002).

ACETAMINOPHEN

Although acetaminophen has been utilized for more than half a century, the mechanisms by which it produces analgesia are still largely unknown. Because of pharmacological similarities to NSAIDs, inhibition of COX enzymes has received the most attention and, like NSAIDs, acetaminophen is an efficacious analgesic and antipyretic; however, its anti-inflammatory effects are weak (Ouellet & Percival, 2001). It has been hypothesized that acetaminophen cannot inhibit COX enzymes in highly oxidative environments, such as that created by inflammation, and so is limited to COX inhibition in the central nervous system (Mattia & Coluzzi, 2009). Interestingly, serotonergic, endocannabinoid, and TRPV1 receptor mechanisms have also been implicated in the analgesic mechanisms of acetaminophen (Mallet et al., 2008; Mallet et al., 2010). Acetaminophen is toxic to cats at doses of approximately 60 mg/kg, and primarily results in methemoglobinemia, cyanosis, and death (Savides et al., 1984). Due to decreased feline hepatic glucuronyltransferase activity, reactive metabolic intermediates accumulate and cause oxidative damage to hemoglobin (Shrestha et al., 2011). Acetaminophen should not be used in cats at any dose. In dogs, acute toxicity occurs at approximately 200 mg/kg, and the target organ is the liver (Savides et al., 1984). Human data indicate that the combination of acetaminophen with an NSAID can be advantageous and safe (de Vries et al., 2010; Mehlisch et al., 2010). Acetaminophen can be used carefully in dogs with normal hepatic function, either instead of NSAIDS or in combination with them, though long-term safety data are not available.

TRAMADOL AND TAPENTADOL

Tramadol, a centrally acting analgesic with weak μ-opioid receptor agonist activity, is commonly used in dogs and is currently not controlled at the federal level in the United States. The primary metabolite, O-desmethyltramadol or M1, has a much stronger affinity for the μ receptor, and is responsible for the naloxone-reversible analgesia (Ide et al., 2006). Dogs do not appear to be very efficient producers of this metabolite (KuKanich & Papich, 2011), whereas cats rapidly produce M1 (Pypendop & Ilkiw, 2008). Tramadol also activates descending inhibitory spinal pathways originating in the periaqueductal grey matter and rostral ventral medulla via modification of serotonergic and noradrenergic release and reuptake (Bamigbade et al., 1997). Tramadol demonstrates antinociceptive effects in a variety of species and pain states (Mastrocinque & Fantoni, 2003; Pypendop et al., 2009; Norrbrink & Lundeberg, 2009). Adverse effects include a lowered seizure threshold, dysphoria, constipation, and serotonin syndrome. In particular, serotonin syndrome can be serious and potentially fatal; care should be taken with coadministration of drugs that affect the serotonin system, such as selegiline, serotonin reuptake inhibitors, and tricyclic antidepressants.

Tapentadol is also a centrally acting analgesic that is an agonist of the μ-opioid receptor as well as an inhibitor of norepinephrine reuptake. Unlike tramadol, the parent compound is the effector at the μ-opioid receptor, avoiding the need for metabolic activation of the drug and, thereby, decreasing individual differences in response due to variable cytochrome p450 enzyme activity. In addition, tapentadol does not affect serotonergic pathways and, therefore, bears no risk of precipitating serotonin syndrome (Tzschentke et al., 2007). Analgesic effects are evident in acute and chronic pain states in both laboratory (Schröder et al., 2011) and human clinical settings (Hartrick & Rozek, 2011). Serious adverse effects can occur, including respiratory depression and seizures. Tapentadol is a federally controlled schedule II drug, and pharmacokinetic data indicate that bioavailability in dogs is low (Giorgi et al., 2012). Pharmacodynamic data have not been published. The multimodal analgesic profile makes tapentadol a promising drug in the treatment of cancer pain, though specific recommendations for its use cannot be made until more research in veterinary species is conducted.

Gabapentin and Pregabalin

Gabapentin and pregabalin (Chapter 8) decrease neuronal excitability by interacting with a subunit of voltage-gated Ca^{2+} channels. By decreasing intracellular Ca^{2+} concentrations these antiepileptic drugs decrease release of the excitatory neurotransmitter glutamate (Quintero et al., 2011). Gabapentin, in particular, has a long history of use in neuropathic pain states in people, and its use has been reported in several veterinary species (Davis et al., 2007; Cashmore et al., 2009; Shaver et al., 2009). The pharmacokinetics of pregabalin are favorable in dogs (Salazar et al., 2009), and though it is relatively expensive and federally controlled, pregabalin may be an excellent addition to the armamentarium against neuropathic pain states.

Tricyclic Antidepressants and Serotonin– Norepinephrine Reuptake Inhibitors

Antidepressant agents of various types, most notably the tricyclic antidepressants (TCAs) and serotonin–norepinephrine reuptake inhibitors (SNRIs) are effective in the management of neuropathic pain states (Chapter 8). In fact, TCAs are standard in the treatment of neuropathic pain in humans and have been used since the middle of the twentieth century (Dharmshaktu et al., 2012). Although there are many cellular mechanisms that may contribute to the analgesic and antihyperalgesic effects of antidepressant drugs, efficacy is most likely determined by augmented activity of descending modulatory pathways through increased serotonin and norepinephrine concentrations at spinal and supraspinal sites. Though some reports exist (Chew et al., 1998; Cashmore et al., 2009), use of antidepressant agents for pain management has not been researched extensively in veterinary species, and support for efficacy is mostly anecdotal in nature.

NMDA Antagonists

Sustained or intense nociceptive input allows activation of NMDA receptors on the postsynaptic membrane, augmenting rostral projection and reinforcing peripheral nociceptive signals. Antagonism of NMDA receptors decreases windup and central sensitization at the level of the dorsal horn of the spinal cord. Unfortunately, contradictory evidence for the efficacy of NMDA antagonists in chronic neuropathic pain states exists in human pain literature (Collins et al., 2010), and this is likely due to the wide variation in underlying pathophysiology, as well as differences in receptor distribution and composition. The oral NMDA antagonist, amantadine (Chapter 8), is most commonly used in veterinary species, and one clinical study has demonstrated improvement in activity levels in dogs with chronic noncancer pain (Lascelles et al., 2008).

Opioids

The foundation of analgesic therapy for centuries, opioids (Chapter 4) are effective in a variety of acute pain states. As such, they are an integral part of the management of cancer pain in veterinary patients. Unfortunately, outpatient use of opioids is somewhat hampered in companion animal species due to poor oral absorption of most formulations, and concerns about the use of controlled drugs in veterinary species.

Oral bioavailability of immediate release oral morphine was about 5% and somewhat erratic in a laboratory-based study in beagles (KuKanich et al., 2005a), and a formulation of oral morphine containing both immediate- and sustained-release components also resulted in relatively low plasma concentrations and high variability (Aragon et al., 2009). Oral preparations of methadone and codeine with acetaminophen have yielded similar results, displaying low but variable oral absorption and fast elimination times (KuKanich et al., 2005b). Inhibition of a specific cytochrome p450 enzyme, p-glycoprotein activity, or gastric acid secretion did not increase blood methadone concentrations in dogs (KuKanich, 2010). Although experimental pharmacokinetic studies are less than promising, it may be reasonable to use oral opioids in some dogs for breakthrough pain due to the high variability in absorption. Owners should be warned that the clinical effect is somewhat unpredictable and that adverse effects, such as constipation and respiratory depression, may occur.

Transmucosal administration of the partial μ-agonist buprenorphine is an option in cats (Robertson et al., 2003) and dogs (Abbo et al., 2008). It is important that the drug is not swallowed due to high first-pass hepatic extraction; rather, it should be administered onto the buccal mucosa or underneath the tongue. Oral transmucosal administration of buprenorphine is probably most easily employed in cats and small dogs due to both the volume that must be administered and the expense. Recently, a sustained-release (SR) injectable formulation of buprenorphine has become available (Chapter 9). Though not FDA approved, limited investigations have demonstrated efficacy in acute pain settings in cats (Catbagan et al., 2011) and rats (Foley et al., 2011). Anecdotally, buprenorphine SR has been successfully used in cats to treat oncological pain. No published pharmacokinetic data are currently available; however, one injection appears to be effective for three days. Collective experience suggests that dogs tend to become depressed and anorexic with the use of buprenorphine SR, even at low doses.

Fentanyl patches are marketed for the treatment of chronic pain in human patients but are used in an off-label manner in veterinary species for acute and chronic pain. Effective plasma fentanyl concentrations may not be reached for 6–8 hours in cats and up to 24 hours in dogs; in addition, individual variation can occur. There are no published data regarding length of efficacy of fentanyl patches in dogs or cats. Plasma concentrations thought to be consistent with analgesia are documented for 72 hours in dogs (Egger et al., 1998) and cats (Egger et al., 2003); however, interindividual variation is marked. If multiple patches are used in succession, it is probably best to rotate patch site placement so that buildup of adhesive does not occur. The chosen site should be clipped gently so as not to abrade the skin, and the patch should be held in place for 60 seconds to ensure good adhesion. Care should be taken to make certain that the pet or children in the household do not ingest the patch.

Interesting variations on conventional opioid receptor targeting are currently being investigated, and may become useful for veterinary cancer pain patients. μ- and δ-opioid receptors form heterogeneous complexes that modulate physiological responses to exogenous opioid administration (Ananthan, 2006). Leveraging the resulting pharmacological characteristics may allow for increased opioid efficacy with concurrent reduction in adverse effects. Other research has focused on decreasing the adverse effects of long-term opioid use, such as constipation, by coadministration of an opioid antagonist that is restricted from the central nervous system. The peripheral opioid antagonists, alvimopan and methylnaltrexone are currently available for use in humans, and may prove useful in veterinary species as palliative oncological care develops.

AMINOBISPHOSPHONATES

Primary bone tumors and bony metastases can be associated with debilitating pain, and may result in pathological fractures. Restorative techniques for primary bone tumors, such as amputation, stereotactic radiosurgery, or CRT, are effective in the treatment of bone pain of neoplastic origin. Limb-sparing procedures can offer long-term local tumor control and improvement in limb function (Farese et al., 2004). However, provision of palliative care may be necessary with metastatic bone tumors or even with primary tumors in certain situations. Palliative care in dogs with analgesics alone offers an expected survival time of 1–3 months. Palliative care management options are discussed below and in Chapter 40.

Nitrogen-containing bisphosphonates prevent resorption of bone by localizing to areas of active osteolysis, disrupting intracellular signaling pathways, and interfering with production of regulatory proteins, thereby inducing apoptosis of osteoclasts (Roelofs et al., 2006).

Pain associated with bone metastasis and skeletal-related morbidity, such as pathological fractures, are common features of advanced neoplastic disease in humans. Aminobisphosphonates decrease skeletal complications and metastatic bony pain in humans with osteolytic neoplasias (Wong & Wiffen, 2002; Cameron et al., 2006). Pamidronate is used most commonly in veterinary medicine to assist in the palliative management of osteosarcoma. Intravenous administration of pamidronate to dogs with neoplasia was considered safe, and resulted in reduction in subjective assessment of pain in 4 of 10 dogs with osteosarcoma. In addition, markers of bone metabolism were reduced (Fan et al., 2005). In a prospective study of dogs with appendicular osteosarcoma, pamidronate infusion resulted in alleviation of pain for more than 4 months in 28% of patients, as well as decreases in bone biologic activity (Fan et al., 2007). Similarly, zoledronate also reduced markers of bone resorption and reduced pain in a subset of dogs with malignant osteolysis (Fan et al., 2008). A small prospective clinical trial to evaluate pain control was initiated in osteosarcoma-bearing dogs perceived to be poor surgical candidates. This protocol combined intravenous zoledronate (0.1 mg/kg on day 2, then every 28 days), oral analgesics (continuous combination of NSAIDs, tramadol, and gabapentin), and accelerated palliative radiation therapy (PRT) (10 Gray (Gy) administered on days 1 and 2). Pain relief was evaluated utilizing a client pain score system and biomechanical limb function tests (computerized gait analysis and videotape assessment). Median time to response data was not available; nonetheless, the findings suggest that this combination protocol provided durable pain alleviation. Dogs achieving pain control for more than 3 months had the additional benefit of positive bone biological and biomechanical effects (Garrett et. al., 2011). However, in dogs undergoing a course of palliative radiation for appendicular osteosarcoma, addition of pamidronate did not enhance pain alleviation (Fan et al., 2009). Oral aminobisphosphonates, such as alendronate (Fosamax®) are available, but oral absorption in dogs is quite poor (Lin et al., 1991). Because generic alendronate is inexpensive, its use may be considered if administration of injectable aminobisphosphonates is prohibitively expensive.

For the management of pain associated with neoplasia of bone, 1–2 mg/kg of pamidronate is diluted into 250 mL of 0.9% saline and administered over 2–4 hours. Administration can be repeated every 3–4 weeks, but renal function and electrolyte concentrations should be monitored closely.

In people receiving bisphosphonate therapy, osteonecrosis of the jaw may develop. Bisphosphonate-related osteonecrosis of the jaw (BRONJ) is defined as exposed, necrotic bone in the maxillofacial region that has persisted for more than 8 weeks in a patient who has received bisphosphonate treatment and has no history of radiation therapy (AAOMS, 2009). Although no clinical veterinary reports of BRONJ exist, histopathological remodeling and necrosis of the mandible have been precipitated by long-term bisphosphonate therapy in dogs in experimental settings (Burr & Allen, 2009). Development of BRONJ appears to be related to the bisphosphonate potency and length of treatment, and caution should be taken when considering long-term bisphosphonate therapy. In particular, excellent oral care should be maintained as inflammatory oral disease and dentoalveolar surgery increase the risk of BRONJ (AAOMS, 2009).

Adjunctive Techniques

Many nonpharmacological modalities may lessen pain and improve strength and overall QOL in cancer patients. Complementary techniques, including acupuncture, massage, and herbal remedies, are used by more than 50% of cancer patients participating in FDA clinical trials, and almost a quarter of those patients reported that they did not fully disclose this information to their physician (Naing et al., 2011). It is probable that similar circumstances occur in the course of veterinary cancer treatment, and specific inquiry into the use of complementary techniques and pharmacological agents is part of a thorough anamnesis.

ACUPUNCTURE

Acupuncture is a complex intervention that encompasses a wide range of theoretical and clinical practices. Mechanistic theory ranges from the traditional Chinese medicinal approach of balancing Qi to the more recent Western attempt to explain the effects through manipulation of neurophysiological pathways. The actual practice of acupuncture incorporates many forms, including dry needling, laser acupuncture, and electroacupuncture, and possibly acupressure or herbal medicine. Available evidence is promising though somewhat difficult to interpret; many studies demonstrate efficacy, but conclusions may be limited by methodological issues

(Paley et al., 2011). Acupuncture is reviewed elsewhere in this book (Chapter 16). Specific considerations for acupuncture in the presence of cancer include avoidance of insertion of needles into or near tumors and attention to the risk of infection in immunocompromised patients.

PHYSICAL REHABILITATION

Physical rehabilitation therapy (Chapter 11) may be helpful in the management of cancer pain, as well as comorbidities such as lymphedema, restricted mobility, or muscle wasting. Techniques include passive range of motion, massage therapy, cryotherapy, heat therapy, transcutaneous electrostimulation, low-level laser therapy, and aquatic treadmill work. These techniques may help improve pain management and overall QOL. Specific examples from the human literature include the use of therapeutic laser for the prevention and treatment of radiation-induced oral mucositis (Bjordal et al., 2011) and postmastectomy lymphedema (Carati et al., 2003), and the use of massage therapy in improving sleep, mood disturbances, and overall QOL (Listing et al., 2009; Sturgeon et al., 2009). Application of any external heating modality such as low-level laser or therapeutic ultrasound should be used cautiously, if at all, in the presence of cancer, and application directly over the neoplastic cells should be avoided (Frigo et al., 2009).

Interventional Analgesic Techniques

Interventional analgesic techniques are those procedures that invasively attempt to modify the pain pathway without addressing the underlying disease process. Examples include epidural and intrathecal injections or catheter placement, specific peripheral nerve blocks, ganglion blocks or neurolysis, spinal cord stimulation, and percutaneous vertebroplasty. Various interventional techniques are considered in human palliative care settings when standard oral and injectable protocols have failed. In veterinary practice, the assorted interventional techniques are uncommonly employed in cancer pain management due to invasiveness, expense, lack of training, and the option of euthanasia. Of these modalities, epidural placement of analgesic drugs is most familiar to veterinarians, and is often used in perioperative period to control acute pain (Valverde, 2008). Many drugs can be placed into the epidural and subarachnoid spaces to provide pain relief, including opioids, ketamine, α-2 agonists, and corticosteroids, and these routes of administration may be considered for management of severe cancer pain in companion animal species. In-patient care is recommended for patients that require such interventions, and QOL, goals, and prognosis should be considered.

PALLIATIVE THERAPY

The experience of pain in cancer is widely accepted as a major threat to QOL. Pain may be associated with disease, as well as the treatments to mitigate disease (Eguchi, 2010). The concept of palliative therapy has several goals: to provide relief from pain and other distressing effects; to neither hasten nor postpone death; to offer a support mechanism to help the family cope during illness (pre-emptive bereavement and bereavement), to permit pets to live with their companions as actively as possible until death, and to enhance QOL. Palliative care may also positively influence the course of disease, though it is not specifically designed to do so (Eguchi, 2010).

The American Cancer Society projected the number of newly diagnosed human cancer cases to be 1,596,670 in 2011 and, currently, one in four deaths are due to cancer (Siegel et al., 2011). With these staggering statistics it is rare to find a person who has not been witness to cancer-related therapies. Of 106 persons responding to a recent survey, slightly more than 50% were aware of veterinary oncology as a specialty (Harland et al., 2011). Palliative therapies are frequently employed in veterinary medicine because veterinary patients often present with advanced disease, and owners may be unable to emotionally or financially support curative intent treatment.

Palliative Radiation Therapy

The goals of PRT are to relieve clinical signs, prevent imminent complications, improve QOL, and possibly extend survival duration. PRT is instituted for relief in companion animals with discomfort or dysfunction and limited expected survival. The prescribed radiation dose can be quantitated in fraction (treatment dose) or cumulative treatment dose, and is expressed as tissue absorbed dose in the unit of gray (Gy). PRT is the administration of hypofractionated radiation. Hypofractionation refers to the delivery of a radiotherapy dose in a smaller number of treatments than would be used to deliver a standard, curative intent dosing scheme. In PRT, the daily fraction size is larger than with CRT and larger fraction sizes may result in greater damage to late responding tissues. Most pets will not survive to face the increased risk of long-term effects associated with PRT. In addition to alleviation of bone pain, external beam irradiation generates reossification and healing in 65–85% of nonfractured lytic bone lesions (Ratanatharathorn et al., 2004). For fractured long bones, rigid immobilization with internal fixation is required for healing.

The mechanism of radiation-induced pain amelioration is currently undefined. Mechanisms that may initiate and sustain bone cancer pain (Chapter 3) include osteolysis through production of mediators such as endothelin A and nerve growth factor, tumor-mediated nerve injury, direct stimulation of nociceptors, periosteal stretching, microfractures within the bone, reactive muscle spasms, or nerve root infiltration (Vakaet & Boterberg, 2004; Goblirsch et al., 2006). Reorganization of the dorsal horn of the spinal cord occurs and expression of glial fibrillary acidic protein, a marker of astrocyte hypertrophy, increases markedly in association with bone cancer pain (Goblirsch et al., 2006). Pain may also ensue from the dysregulation of cytokine homeostatic balance favoring inflammation. The microenvironment of tumors is complex and includes several classes of cytokines that promote tumor cell survival. Reduction of inflammatory cells through irradiation inhibits the release of chemical pain mediators and is probably responsible for the rapid reduction in pain in some patients (Mercadante, 1997). Decreased activity of osteoclasts in the bone microenvironment reduces bone destruction and predicts the relief of pain through irradiation (Hoskin et al., 2000). Alternatively, reduction of tumor burden has been suggested as the sole mechanism of radiation-induced analgesia (Goblirsch et al., 2005). The absence of a dose–response relationship suggests that tumor shrinkage may not be that important. In addition, a relationship between the radiosensitivity of the tumor and amelioration of pain is lacking (Vakaet & Boterberg, 2004).

Regardless of the mechanism, the degree and onset of pain relief provided by irradiation varies. Pain relief may range from none to complete, and may occur in as short as hours to weeks after the delivery of radiation. Within the context of alleviating pain, minimizing cost, inconvenience, and risk of adverse effects, many palliative protocols have been formulated. The application of PRT varies widely amongst radiation oncologists, and may be altered for client convenience and cost. Currently, the majority of veterinary radiation facilities are using megavoltage radiation therapy that can deliver electron or photon beam energy greater than 1000 kVp. This creates a tissue dose profile that targets the maximum dose at some distance beneath the skin surface, reducing skin toxicity.

In a survey of radiation oncologists, a dose of 8 Gy given on days 0, 7, and 21 or 4 weekly fractions was reported as the most commonly employed palliative protocol. Other common protocols consist of 4 Gy delivered in 5 fractions and 6 Gy in 6 fractions, delivered in a weekly or biweekly fashion (Prescott, 2010; Farrelly et al., 2004). An abbreviated protocol has been devised to provide comfort for pets with appendicular bone tumors while affording convenience for owners lacking nearby access to a radiation therapy facility. The protocol consists of 8 Gy delivered in daily fractions on 2 consecutive days. Pain relief occurred in 91% of dogs within 2 days with a median duration of relief of 67 days (Knapp-Hoch et al., 2009). There are a number of other protocols reported in the veterinary literature for canine osteosarcoma, and response rates vary from 50% to 93% with duration of response 53–130 days, and a median onset of response of 2–21 days (McEntee et al., 1993; Thrall & LaRue, 1995; Ramirez et al., 1999; Green et al., 2002; Coomer et al., 2009; Knapp-Hoch et al., 2009). One study verified improved limb function through the use of force plate analysis measurement (Weinstein et al., 2009). The comparison of these protocols is complicated by the low power of some of the studies, varied stage and extent of local disease, as well as use and timing of adjunctive treatments such as bisphosphonates, chemotherapy, and analgesics.

Aside from the successful alleviation of discomfort in bone tumors, PRT may offer relief for a variety of tumor types. In situations where surgical excision of canine oral melanoma would lead to unacceptable aesthetics or result in poor function, use of RT has been described. In dogs irradiated on days 0, 7, and 21 with a dose of 8 Gy, more than 50% of dogs experienced complete remission usually by 5 weeks from the start of treatment, and 30% of dogs achieved a partial remission. Because melanoma is highly metastatic, patients treated with local radiation therapy had a limited mean survival of 7.9 months (Bateman et al., 1994). Unfortunately, a small group of cats treated with the same protocol did not fare as well as their canine counterparts. While three of the five cats evaluated, responded, the duration of response was short and median survival was 4.8 months (Farrely et al., 2004). Although these studies did not specifically evaluate pain, remission of disease can be associated with a reduction in discomfort.

Most patients treated with PRT will not be afforded long-term survival. The common early adverse effects associated with RT are often acceptable whereas late reactions can be undesirable and life threatening. Tumor reirradiation is possible, provided the owners are aware that continued treatment will eventually produce late onset adverse effects.

The appeal of PRT lies not only in improved QOL through relief of clinical signs, but compared to CRT, the cost incurred is minimal. Prior to referral for either CRT or PRT, consideration should be given to the pet's cardiac and pulmonary functions because the patient will require anesthesia for irradiation. Depending on the tumor location, advanced imaging may also be advantageous to avoid critical normal structures.

RADIOPHARMACEUTICALS

Radioisotopes are unstable forms of chemical elements that transition to more stable forms with the release of radioactivity. Systemic administration of radioactive isotopes with an affinity for active bone pathology ameliorates bone pain in humans with primary or metastatic bone neoplasias (Morris et al., 2009). Several radionuclides have been assessed for efficacy in the primary treatment of bone tumors and for provision of analgesia. The radioisotopes Strontium-89, Samarium-153, Rhenium-186, and Phosphorus-32 provide a significant though small benefit in patients experiencing pain at the start of treatment (Roqué et al., 2011). Sixty to eighty percent of patients receiving Samarium-153 experience a decrease in pain scores that is often accompanied by a decreased requirement for other analgesic agents (Ripamonti et al., 2007; Sartor et al., 2007). Samarium-153 combined with a targeting chelant, ^{153}Sm-EDTMP (Lexidronam® or Quadramet®) is the radioisotope compound currently used in veterinary medicine. ^{153}Sm-EDTMP has an affinity for hydroxyapatite within bone and binds at sites of increased osteoblastic activity such as osteoblastic primary bone tumors. A tumor-to-normal bone ratio greater than 4:1 on scintigraphy is the standard criteria used to select patients for whom ^{153}Sm-EDTMP treatment is considered suitable. The ^{153}Sm-EDTMP compound decays by β- and γ-emissions where the β-component is therapeutic and the γ-component permits imaging of the distribution of the radiopharmaceutical within the patient through the use of a standard planar γ camera. ^{153}Sm-EDTMP has the attractive features of a short physical half-life (reducing isolation time), low tissue penetration with minimal bone marrow toxicity, and no liver or other soft tissue uptake. Several small case series report the use of ^{153}Sm-EDTMP in dogs with naturally occurring bone tumors (Aas et al., 1999; Barnard et al., 2007). Because the agent localizes in bone, adverse effects include myelosuppression (mild, reversible thrombocytopenia and neutropenia) and "flare" reactions in which bone pain is temporarily worsened. A group at the University of Missouri has recently evaluated ^{153}Sm combined with an alternative chelant, DOTMP, in a small number of cases. ^{153}Sm-DOTMP has shown equal targeting in comparison to ^{153}Sm-EDTMP but at an equivalent dosing scheme has the advantage of no hematological toxicity in the six patients treated (Selting et al., 2011). Significant barriers to the use of ^{153}Sm in veterinary patients exist, including the need for specialized containment facilities and licensure, which may prevent widespread implementation of radiopharmaceuticals. ^{153}Sm-EDTMP therapy is currently available at The Veterinary Medicine and Teaching Hospital of Missouri, and Veterinary Specialty Center, Buffalo Grove, IL (see an up-to-date list of radiation therapy facilities at http://www.vetcancersociety.org/include/pdf/radiation-facilities.pdf).

End-of-Life Management

Management of cancer pain in the veterinary patient must include a dialogue between the owner and the veterinarian about QOL as well as death. Euthanasia is a valid therapeutic tool in the management of progressive and intractable pain in veterinary patients, but it is not one that is applied easily in most situations. Many owners have questions about timing and fear making the "wrong" decision. The veterinarian managing a terminal patient must be prepared to handle a wide range of physical, financial, and emotional issues. At present, the role of the companion animal has developed to include beloved pet and family member, emotional and social support, as well as physical support for those with special needs. When euthanasia or death occurs, these expanded companion animal roles may lead to a more profound experience of loss. The grieving process is an individual experience, making it essential to be supportive, permitting clients to grieve in a manner we may not understand. Clients may also need encouragement to speak openly with children.

Veterinarians must perform many functions during the course of treatment and palliative care of the oncology patient: (1) listening to the goals, fears, and contextual experience of the owners; (2) demonstrating awareness of the difficult nature of the situation—reflective listening and empathy can help build trust between the client and the veterinarian; (3) guiding the owners through the expected course of the disease and helping them define an appropriate QOL for the patient; and (4) providing a peaceful and dignified release from suffering through appropriate methods of euthanasia. Veterinarians have an inordinate amount of pressure to provide for patients, especially those under protracted care. Attention should be given to the internal struggles that may ensue, should compassion fatigue arise.

The hospice movement originated in the late 1960s driven by the advocacy of Dame Cicely Saunders (Oransky, 2005), who recognized that once a disease was considered terminal, many human patients were forced out of the care of the medical establishment and left to suffer without systematic support. She established the first medical hospice that focused on palliative care of the whole patient in an attempt to control distressing symptomatology while also managing the psychosocial aspects of dying for the patient and the patient's family. These ideas are quite applicable to veterinary medicine, with the focus on QOL over quantity of life, and extension of psychological support and resources to the human family members. The American Veterinary Medical Association's established guidelines for hospice care are available at: http://www.avma.org/products/hab/hospice.asp and hospice care is discussed further in Chapter 40.

SUMMARY

Unrelieved pain is a major cause of suffering in patients with cancer. Veterinarians managing cancer patients must be vigilant about monitoring for and providing relief from pain, whether caused by the neoplastic process itself or coincidental in nature. Providing adequate management of pain is central to oncological care and will improve the QOL of the animal patient.

REFERENCES

Aas, M., Moe, L., Gamlem, H., Skretting, A., Ottesen, & N., Bruland, O.S. (1999) Internal radionuclide therapy of primary osteosarcoma in dogs, using 153Sm-ethylene-diamino-tetramethylene-phosphonate (EDTMP). *Clinical Cancer Research*, 5(10S), 3148s–3152s.

Abbo, L.A., Ko, J.C., Maxwell, L.K., et al. (2008) Pharmacokinetics of buprenorphine following intravenous and oral transmucosal administration in dogs. *Veterinary Therapeutics*, 9(2), 83–93.

Afsharimani, B., Cabot, P., & Parat, M.O. (2011) Morphine and tumor growth and metastasis. *Cancer Metastasis Review*, 30(2), 225–238.

Ahmed, N., Hansen, V.N., Harrington, K.J., Nutting, C.M. (2009) Reducing the risk of xerostomia and mandibular osteoradionecrosis: the potential benefits of intensity modulated radiotherapy in advanced oral cavity carcinoma. *Medical Dosimetry*, 34(3), 217–224.

American Association of Oral and Maxillofacial Surgeons (AAOMS) (2009) Position Paper on Bisphosphonate-Related Osteonecrosis of the Jaw.Update Available at: http://www.aaoms.org/docs/position_papers/bronj_update.pdf (accessed July 10, 2011).

Ananthan, S. (2006) Opioid ligands with mixed μ/δ opioid receptor interactions: an emerging approach to novel analgesics. *The American Association Pharmaceutical Scientists Journal*, 8(1), e118–e125.

Aragon, C.L., Read, M.R., Gaynor, J.S., et al. (2009) Pharmacokinetics of an immediate and extended release oral morphine formulation utilizing the spheroidal oral drug absorption system in dogs. *Journal of Veterinary Pharmacology and Therapeutics*, 32(2), 129–136.

Bamigbade, T.A., Davidson, C., Langford, R.M., Barnhart, M.D., Wilson, D., & Papich, M.G. (1997) Actions of tramadol, its enantiomers and principal metabolite, O-desmethyltramadol, on serotonin (5-HT) efflux and uptake in the rat dorsal raphe nucleus. *British Journal of Anaesthesia*, 79(3), 352–356.

Barnard, S.M., Zuber, R.M., & Moore, A.S. (2007) Samarium Sm 153 lexidronam for the palliative treatment of dogs with primary bone tumors: 35 cases (1999-2005). *Journal of the American Veterinary Medical Association*, 230(12), 1877–1881.

Bateman, K.E., Catton, P.A., Pennock, P.W., & Kruth, S.A. (1994) 0-7-21 radiation therapy for the palliation of advanced cancer in dogs. *Journal of Veterinary Internal Medicine*, 8(6), 394–399.

Bjordal, J.M., Bensadoun, R.J., Tunèr, J., Frigo, L., Gjerde, K., & Lopes-Martins, R.A. (2011) A systematic review with meta-analysis of the effect of low-level laser therapy (LLLT) in cancer therapy-induced oral mucositis. *Supportive Care in Cancer*, 19(8), 1069–1077.

Burr, D.B. & Allen, M.R. (2009) Mandibular necrosis in beagle dogs treated with bisphosphonates. *Orthodontics & Craniofacial Research*, 12(3), 221–228.

Cameron, D., Fallon, M., & Diel, I. (2006) Ibandronate: its role in metastatic breast cancer. *Oncologist*, 11(1S), 27–33.

Carati, C.J., Anderson, S.N., Gannon, B.J., & Piller, N.B. (2003) Treatment of postmastectomy lymphedema with low-level laser therapy: a double blind, placebo-controlled trial. *Cancer*, 98(6), 1114–1122.

Carsten, R.E., Hellyer, P.W., Bachand, A.M., & LaRue, S.M. (2008) Correlations between acute radiation scores and pain scores in canine radiation patients with cancer of the forelimb. *Veterinary Anaesthesia & Analgesia*, 35(4), 355–362.

Cashmore, R.G., Harcourt-Brown, T.R., Freeman, P.M., Jeffery, N.D., & Granger, N. (2009) Clinical diagnosis and treatment of suspected neuropathic pain in three dogs. *Australian Veterinary Journal*, 87(1), 45–50.

Catbagan, D.L., Quimby, J.M., Mama, K.R., Rychel, J.K., & Mich, P.M. (2011) Comparison of the efficacy and adverse effects of sustained-release buprenorphine hydrochloride following subcutaneous administration and buprenorphine hydrochloride following oral transmucosal administration in cats undergoing ovariohysterectomy. *American Journal of Veterinary Research*, 72(4), 461–466.

Chew, D.J., Buffington, C.A., Kendall, M.S., DiBartola, S.P., & Woodworth, B.E. (1998) Amitriptyline treatment for severe recurrent idiopathic cystitis in cats. *Journal of the American Veterinary Medical Association*, 213(9), 1282–1286.

Collen, E.B. & Mayer, M.N. (2006) Acute effects of radiation treatment: skin reactions. *Canadian Veterinary Journal*, 47(9), 931–935.

Collins, S., Sigtermans, M.D., Dahan, A., Zuurmond, W.W., & Perez, R.S. (2010) NMDA receptor antagonists for the treatment of neuropathic pain. *Pain Medicine*, 11(11), 1726–1742.

Coomer, A., Farese, J., Milner, R., Liptak, J., Bacon, N., & Lurie, D. (2009) Radiation therapy for canine appendicular osteosarcoma. *Veterinary and Comparative Oncology*, 7(1), 15–27.

Davis, J.L., Posner, L.P., & Elce, Y. (2007) Gabapentin for the treatment of neuropathic pain in a pregnant horse. *Journal of the American Veterinary Medical Association*, 231(5), 755–758.

de Vries, F., Setakis, E., & van Staa, T.P. (2010) Concomitant use of ibuprofen and paracetamol and the risk of major clinical safety outcomes. *British Journal of Clinical Pharmacology*, 70(3), 429–438.

Dharmshaktu, P., Tayal, V., & Kalra, B.S. (2012) Efficacy of antidepressants as analgesics: a review. *Journal of Clinical Pharmacology*, 52(1), 6–17.

Dickinson, B.D., Head, C.A., Gitlow, S., & Osbahr, A.J. III. (2010) Maldynia: pathophysiology and management of neuropathic and maladaptive pain– a report of the AMA Council on Science and Public Health. *Pain Medicine*, 11(11), 1635–1653.

Egger, C.M., Glerum, L.E., Allen, S.W., & Haag, M. (2003) Plasma fentanyl concentrations in awake cats and cats undergoing anesthesia and ovariohysterectomy using transdermal administration. *Veterinary Anaesthesia & Analgesia*, 30(4), 229–236.

Egger, C.M., Duke, T., Archer, J., & Cribb, P.H. (1998) Comparison of plasma fentanyl concentrations by using three transdermal fentanyl patch sizes in dogs. *Veterinary Surgery*, 27(2), 159–166.

Eguchi, K. (2010) Development of palliative medicine for cancer patients in Japan: From isolated voluntary effort to integrated multidisciplinary network. *Japanese Journal of Clinical Oncology*, 40(9), 870–875.

Fan, T.M., Charney, S.C., de Lorimer, L.P., et al. (2009) Double blind placebo-controlled trial of adjuvant pamidronate with palliative radiotherapy and intravenous doxorubicin for canine appendicular osteosarcoma bone pain. *Journal of Veterinary Internal Medicine*, 23(1), 152–160.

Fan, T.M., de Lorimer, L.P., Charney, S.C., & Hintermeister, J.G. (2005) Evaluation of intravenous pamidronate administration in 33 cancer-bearing dogs with primary or secondary bone involvement. *Journal of Veterinary Internal Medicine*, 19(1), 74–80.

Fan, T.M., de Lorimer, L.P., Garrett, L.D., & Lacoste, H.I. (2008) The bone biologic effects of zoledronate in healthy dogs and dogs with malignant osteolysis. *Journal of Veterinary Internal Medicine*, 22(2), 380–387.

Fan, T.M., de Lorimer, L.P., O'Dell-Anderson, K., Lacoste, H.I., & Charney, S.C. (2007) Single-agent pamidronate for palliative therapy of canine appendicular osteosarcoma bone pain. *Journal of Veterinary Internal Medicine*, 21(3), 431–439.

Farese, J.P., Milner, R., Thompson, M.S., et al. (2004) Stereotactic radiosurgery for treatment of osteosarcomas involving the distal portions of the limbs in dogs. *Journal of American Veterinary Association*, 225(10), 1567–1572.

Farrelly, J., Denman, D.L., Hohenhaus, A.E., Patnaik, A.K., & Bergman, P.J. (2004) Hypofractionated radiation therapy of oral melanoma in five cats. *Veterinary Radiology & Ultrasound*, 45(1), 91–93.

Fleming, J.M., Creevy, K.E., & Promislow, D.E.L. (2011) Mortality in North American dogs from 1984 to 2004: an investigation into age-, size-, and breed-related causes of death. *Journal of Veterinary Internal Medicine*, 25(2), 187–198.

Foley, P.L., Liang, H., & Crichlow, A.R. (2011) Evaluation of a sustained-release formulation of buprenorphine for analgesia in rats. *Journal of the American Association for Laboratory Animal Science*, 50(2), 198–204.

Frigo, L., Luppi, J.S., Favero, G.M., et al. (2009) The effect of low-level laser irradiation (In-Ga-Al-AsP - 660 nm) on melanoma in vitro and in vivo. *BMC Cancer*, 9, 404.

Garrett, L., Bigio, A., Schmit, J., et al. (2011) in *2011 Proceedings of the Veterinary Cancer Society, Personal communication*, Albuquerque, New Mexico.

Ghosh, N., Chaki, R., Mandal, V., & Mandal, S.C. (2010) COX-2 as a target for cancer chemotherapy. *Pharmacological Reports*, 62, 233–244.

Giorgi, M., Meizler, A., & Mills, P.C. (2012) Pharmacokinetics of the novel atypical opioid tapentadol following oral and intravenous administration in dogs. *Veterinary Journal*, 194(3), 309–313.

Goblirsch, M., Lynch, C., Mathews, W., Manivel, J.C., Mantyh, P.W., & Clohisy, D.R. (2005) Radiation treatment decreases bone cancer pain through direct effect on tumor cells. *Radiation Research*, 164(4), 400–408.

Goblirsch, M.J., Zwolak, P.P, & Clohisy, D.R. (2006) Biology of bone cancer pain. *Clinical Cancer Research*, 12(20), 6231–6235.

Gottschalk, A., Sharma, S., Ford, J., Durieux, M.E., & Tiouririne, M. (2010) Review article: the role of the perioperative period in recurrence after cancer surgery. *Anesthesia & Analgesia*, 110(6), 1636–1643.

Green, E.M., Adams, W.M., & Forrest, L.J. (2002) Four fraction palliative radiotherapy for osteosarcoma in 24 dogs. *Journal of the American Animal Hospital Association*, 38(5), 445–451.

Harland, L., Stell, A., & Costard, S. (2011) Investigation of pet owners' baseline knowledge of cancer therapies for dogs and cats and factors that might affect their decision to pursue treatment options. *Clinicians Brief*, 9(7), 68.

Hartrick, C.T. & Rozek, R.J. (2011) Tapentadol in pain management: a μ-opioid receptor agonist and noradrenaline reuptake inhibitor. *CNS Drugs*, 25(5), 359–70.

Hoskin, P.J., Stratford, M.R., Folkes, L.K., Regan, J., & Yarnold, J.R. (2000) Effect of local radiotherapy for bone pain on urinary markers of osteoclast activity. *The Lancet*, 355, 1428–1429.

Ide, S., Minami, M., Ishihara, K., Uhl, G.R., Sora, I., & Ikeda, K. (2006) Mu opioid receptor-dependent and independent components in effects of tramadol. *Neuropharmacology*, 51(3), 651–658.

Khan, Z., Khan, N., Tiwari, R.P., Sah, N.K., Prasad, G.B., & Bisen, P.S. (2011) Biology of Cox-2: an application in cancer therapeutics. *Current Drug Targets*, 12(7), 1082–1093.

Knapp, D.W., Richardson, R.C., Chan, T.C., et al. (1994) Piroxicam therapy in 34 dogs with transitional cell carcinoma of the urinary bladder. *Journal of Veterinary Internal Medicine*, 8(4), 273–278.

Knapp-Hoch, H.M., Fidel, J.L., Sellon, R.K., & Gavin, P.R. (2009) An expedited palliative radiation protocol for lytic or proliferative lesions of appendicular bone in dogs. *Journal of the American Animal Hospital Association*, 45(1), 24–32.

KuKanich, B. (2010) Pharmacokinetics of acetaminophen, codeine, and the codeine metabolites morphine and codeine-6-glucuronide in healthy Greyhound dogs. *Journal of Veterinary Pharmacology and Therapeutics*, 33(1), 15–21.

KuKanich, B., Lascelles, B.D., Aman, A.M., et al. (2005a) The effects of inhibiting cytochrome P450 3A, p-glycoprotein, and gastric acid secretion on the oral bioavailability of methadone in dogs. *Journal of Veterinary Pharmacology & Therapeutics*, 28(5), 461–466.

KuKanich, B., Lascelles, B.D., & Papich, M.G. (2005b) Pharmacokinetics of morphine and plasma concentrations of morphine-6-glucuronide following morphine administration to dogs. *Journal of Veterinary Pharmacology and Therapeutics*, 28(4), 371–376.

KuKanich, B. & Papich, M.G. (2011) Pharmacokinetics and antinociceptive effects of oral tramadol hydrochloride administration in Greyhounds. *American Journal of Veterinary Research*, 72(2), 256–262.

LaDue, T. & Klein, M.K. (2001) Toxicity criteria of the veterinary radiation oncology group. *Veterinary Radiology and Ultrasound*, 42(5), 475–476.

Lascelles, B.D.X., Gaynor, J.S., Smith, E.S., et al. (2008) Amantadine in a multimodal analgesic regimen for alleviation of refractory osteoarthritis pain in dogs. *Journal of Veterinary Internal Medicine*, 22(1), 53–59.

Lawrence, J.A., Forrest, L.J., Turek, M.M., et al. (2010) Proof of principle of ocular sparing in dogs with sinonasal tumors treated with intensity-modulated radiation therapy. *Veterinary Radiology and Ultrasound*, 51(5), 561–570.

Lin, J.H., Duggan, D.E., Chen, I.W., & Ellsworth, R.L. (1991) Physiological disposition of alendronate, a potent anti-osteolytic bisphosphonate, in laboratory animals. *Drug Metabolism and Disposition*, 19(5), 926–932.

Listing, M., Reisshauer, A., Krohn, M., et al. (2009) Massage therapy reduces physical discomfort and improves mood disturbances in women with breast cancer. *Psychooncology*, 18(12), 1290–1299.

Lynch, S., Savary-Bataille, K., Leeuw, B., & Argyle, D.J. (2011) Development of a questionnaire assessing health-related quality-of-life in dogs and cats with cancer. *Veterinary and Comparative Oncology*, 9(3), 172–182.

Mallet, C., Barrie, D.A., Ermund, A., et al. (2010) TRPV1 in brain is involved in acetaminophen-induced antinociception. *PLoS One*, 5(9), e12748.

Mallet, C., Daulhac, L., Bonnefont, J., et al. (2008) Endocannabinoid and serotonergic systems are needed for acetaminophen-induced analgesia. *Pain*, 139(1), 190–200.

Mastrocinque, S. & Fantoni, D.T. (2003) A comparison of preoperative tramadol and morphine for the control of early postoperative pain in canine ovariohysterectomy. *Veterinary Anaesthesia and Analgesia*, 30(4), 220–228.

Mattia, C. & Coluzzi, F. (2009) What anesthesiologists should know about paracetamol (acetaminophen). *Minerva Anesthesiologica*, 75(11), 644–653.

McEntee, M.C., Page, R.L., Novotney, C.A., et al. (1993) Palliative radiotherapy for canine appendicular osteosarcoma. *Veterinary Radiology & Ultrasound*, 34(5), 367–370.

McMillan, S.K., Boria, P., & Moore, G.E. (2011) Antitumor effects of deracoxib treatment in 26 dogs with transitional cell carcinoma of the urinary bladder. *Journal of the American Veterinary Medical Association*, 239(8), 1084–1089.

Mehl, M.L., Withrow, S.J., Seguin, B., et al. (2001) Spontaneous regression of osteosarcoma in four dogs. *Journal of American Veterinary Association*, 219(5), 614–617.

Mehlisch, D.R., Aspley, S., Daniels, S.E., & Bandy, D.P. (2010) Comparison of the analgesic efficacy of concurrent ibuprofen and paracetamol with ibuprofen or paracetamol alone in the management of

moderate to severe acute postoperative dental pain in adolescents and adults: a randomized, double-blind, placebo-controlled, parallel-group, single-dose, two-center, modified factorial study. *Clinical Therapeutics*, 32(5), 882–895.

Mercadante, S. (1997) Malignant bone pain: pathophysiology and treatment. *Pain*, 69, 1–18.

Moreira, L. & Castells, A. (2010) Cyclooxygenase as a target for colorectal cancer chemoprevention. *Current Drug Targets*, 12(13), 1888–1894.

Morris, M.J., Pandit-Taskar, N., Carrasquillo, J., et al. (2009) Phase I study of samarium-153 lexidronam with docetaxel in castration-resistant metastatic prostate cancer. *Journal of Clinical Oncology*, 27(15), 2436–2442.

Naing, A., Stephen, S.K., Frenkel, M., et al. (2011) Prevalence of complementary medicine use in a phase 1 clinical trials program: the MD Anderson Cancer Center Experience. *Cancer*, 117(22), 5142–5150.

Norrbrink, C. & Lundeberg, T. (2009) Tramadol in neuropathic pain after spinal cord injury: a randomized, double-blind, placebo-controlled trial. *Clinical Journal of Pain*, 25(3), 177–184.

Oransky, I. (2005) Dame Cicely Mary Strode Saunders. *Lancet*, 366(9486), 628.

Ouellet, M. & Percival, M.D. (2001) Mechanism of acetaminophen inhibition of cyclooxygenase isoforms. *Archives of Biochemistry and Biophysics*, 387(2), 273–280.

Paley, C.A., Johnson, M.I., Tashani, O.A., & Bagnall, A.M. (2011) Acupuncture for cancer pain in adults. *Cochrane Database of Systematic Reviews*, (1), CD007753.

Pepek, J.M., Willett, C.G., Wu, Q.J., Yoo, S., Clough, R.W., & Czito, B.G. (2010) Intensity-modulated radiation therapy for anal malignancies: a preliminary toxicity and disease outcomes analysis. *International Journal of Radiation Oncology, Biology, Physics*, 78(5), 1413–1419.

Prescott, D. (2010) VRTOG Survey on RT Protocols (2010) Abstract. in *The Proceedings of the 2010 American College of Veterinary Radiation Oncology Annual Meeting*, Asheville, North Carolina.

Pypendop, B.H. & Ilkiw, J.E. (2008) Pharmacokinetics of tramadol, and its metabolite O-desmethyl-tramadol, in cats. *Journal of Veterinary Pharmacology and Therapy*, 31(1), 52–59.

Pypendop, B.H., Siao, K.T., & Ilkiw, J.E. (2009) Effects of tramadol hydrochloride on the thermal threshold in cats. *American Journal of Veterinary Research*, 70(12), 1465–1470.

Quintero, J., Dooley, D.J., Pomerleau, F., Huettl, P., & Gerhardt, G.A. (2011) Amperometric measurement of glutamate release modulation by gabapentin and pregabalin in rat neocortical slices: role of voltage-sensitive Ca2+ {alpha}2{delta}-1 subunit. *Journal of Pharmacology and Experimental Therapeutics*, 338(1), 240–245.

Ramirez, O. III, Dodge, R.K., Page, R.L., et al. (1999) Palliative radiotherapy of appendicular osteosarcoma in 95 dogs. *Veterinary Radiology & Ultrasound*, 40(5), 517–522.

Ratanatharathorn, V., Powers, W.E., & Temple, H.T. (2004) Palliation of bone metastasis, in *Principles and Practice of Radiation Oncology*, 4th edn (eds C.A. Perez, L.W. Brady, E.C. Halperin, et al.), Williams & Wilkins, Philadelphia, pp. 2385–2404.

Ripamonti, C., Fagnoni, E., Campa, T., Seregni, E., Maccauro, M., & Bombardieri, E. (2007) Incident pain and analgesic consumption decrease after samarium infusion: a pilot study. *Supportive Care in Cancer*, 15(3), 339–342.

Robertson, S.A., Taylor, P.M., & Sear, J.W. (2003) Systemic uptake of buprenorphine by cats after oral mucosal administration. *Veterinary Record*, 152(22), 675–678.

Robinson, D.R. & Gebhart, G.F. (2008) Inside information: the unique features of visceral sensation. *Molecular Interventions*, 8(5), 242–253.

Roelofs, A.J., Thompson, K., Gordon, S., & Rogers, M.J. (2006) Molecular mechanisms of action of bisphosphonates: current status. *Clinical Cancer Research*, 12(20 Suppl.), 6222s–6230s.

Roqué, M., Martinez-Zapata, M.J., Scott-Brown, M., Alonso, P. (2011) Radioisotopes for metastatic bone pain. *Cochrane Database of Systematic Reviews*, 6(7), CD003347.

Rostom, A., Dube, C., Wells, G., et al. (2002) Prevention of NSAID-induced gastroduodenal ulcers. *Cochrane Database of Systematic Reviews*, 4, CD002296.

Roy, I., Fortin, A., & Larochelle, M. (2001) The impact of skin washing with water and soap during breast irradiation: a randomized study. *Radiotherapy and Oncology*, 58(3), 333–339.

Salazar, V., Dewey, C.W., Schwark, W., et al. (2009) Pharmacokinetics of single-dose oral pregabalin administration in normal dogs. *Veterinary Anaesthesia and Analgesia*, 36(6), 574–580.

Sartor, O., Reid, R.H., Bushnell, D.L., Quick, D.P., & Ell, P.J. (2007) Safety and efficacy of repeat administration of samarium Sm-153 lexidronam to patients with metastatic bone pain. *Cancer*, 109(3), 637–643.

Savides, M.C., Oehme, F.W., Nash, S.L., & Leipold, H.W. (1984) The toxicity and biotransformation of single doses of acetaminophen in dogs and cats. *Toxicology and Applied Pharmacology*, 74(1), 26–34.

Schröder, W., Tzschentke, T.M., Terlinden, R., et al. (2011) Synergistic interaction between the two mechanisms of action of tapentadol in analgesia. *Journal of Pharmacology and Experimental Therapeutics*, 337(1), 312–320.

Selting, K.A., Lattimer, J.C., Ketring, J.R., et al. (2011) in *The 2011 Proceedings of The American College of Veterinary Radiology, Personal Communication,* Albuquerque, New Mexico.

Shaver, S.L., Robinson, N.G., Wright, B.D., Kratz, G.E., & Johnston, M.S. (2009) A multimodal approach to management of suspected neuropathic pain in a prairie falcon (*Falco mexicanus*). *Journal of Avian Medicine and Surgery*, 23(3), 209–213.

Shrestha, B., Reed, J.M., Starks. P.T., et al. (2011) Evolution of a major drug metabolizing enzyme defect in the domestic cat and other felidae: phylogenetic timing and the role of hypercarnivory. *PLoS ONE*, 6(3), e18046.

Siegel, R., Ward, E., Brawley, O., & Jemal, A. (2011) The impact of eliminating socioeconomic and racial disparities on premature cancer deaths. *CA: A Cancer Journal for Clinicians*, 61(4), 212–236.

Sorenmo, K.U., Goldschmidt, M.H., Shofer, F.S., et al. (2004) Evaluation of cyclooxygenase-1 and cyclooxygenase-2 expression and the effect of cyclooxygenase inhibitors in canine prostatic carcinoma. *Veterinary and Comparative Oncology*, 2(1), 13–23.

Sturgeon, M., Wetta-Hall, R., Hart, T., Good, M., & Dakhil, S. (2009) Effects of therapeutic massage on the quality of life among patients with breast cancer during treatment. *Alternative & Complementary Medicine*, 15(4), 373–380.

Thrall, D.E., & LaRue, S.M. (1995) Palliative radiation therapy. *Seminars in Veterinary Medicine & Surgery (Small Animal)*, 10(3), 205–208.

Tzschentke, T.M., Christoph, T., Kogel, B., et al. (2007) (-)-(1R,2R)-3-(3-dimethylamino-1-ethyl-2-methyl-propyl)-phenol hydrochloride (tapentadol HCl): a novel mu-opioid receptor agonist/norepinephrine reuptake inhibitor with broad-spectrum analgesic properties. *The Journal of Pharmacology and Experimental Therapeutics*, 323(1), 265–276.

Vakaet, L. & Boterberg, T. (2004) Pain control by ionizing radiation of bone metastasis. *International Journal of Developmental Biology*, 48, 599–604.

Valverde, A. (2008) Epidural analgesia and anesthesia in dogs and cats. *Veterinary Clinics of North America Small Animal Practice*, 38(6), 1205–1230.

van den Beuken-van Everdingen, M.H., de Rijke, J.M., Kessels, A.G., Schouten, H.C., van Kleef, M., & Patijn, J. (2007) High prevalence of pain in patients with cancer in a large population-based study in The Netherlands. *Pain*, 132(3), 312–320.

Veldeman, L., Madani, I., Hulstaert, F., De Meerleer, G., Mareel, M., & De Neve, W. (2008) Evidence behind use of intensity-modulated radiotherapy: a systematic review of comparative clinical studies. *Lancet Oncology*, 9(4), 367–375.

Voscopoulos, C. & Lema, M. (2010) When does acute pain become chronic? *British Journal of Anaesthesia*, 105(Suppl. 1), 69–85.

Weinstein, J. I., Payne, S., Poulson, J.M., & Azuma, C. (2009) Use of force plate analysis to evaluate the efficacy of external beam radiation to alleviate osteosarcoma pain. *Veterinary Radiology & Ultrasound*, 50(6), 673–678.

Wiseman-Orr, M.E., Scott, E.M., Reid, J., & Nolan, A.M. (2006) Validation of a structured questionnaire as an instrument to measure chronic pain in dogs on the basis of effects on health-related quality of life. *American Journal of Veterinary Research*, 67, 1826–1836.

Wong, R. & Wiffen, P.J. (2002) Bisphosphonates for the relief of pain secondary to bone metastases. *Cochrane Database of Systematic Reviews*, (2):CD002068.

Yaksh, T.L., Dirig, D.M., Conway, C.M., Svensson, C., Luo, Z.D., & Isakson, P.C. (2001) The acute antihyperalgesic action of nonsteroidal, anti-inflammatory drugs and release of spinal prostaglandin E2 is mediated by the inhibition of constitutive spinal cyclooxygenase-2 (COX-2) but not COX-1. *Journal of Neuroscience*, 21(16), 5847–5853.

Yazbek, K.V.B. & Fantoni, D.T. (2005) Validity of a health-related quality-of-life scale for dogs with signs of pain secondary to cancer. *Journal of the American Veterinary Medical Association*, 226(8), 1354–1358.

Recognition and Treatment of Pain in the Small Animal Critical Care Patient

Jane Quandt

Pain management is a fundamental part of patient care, including care of the critically ill animal. However, critically ill animals pose a challenge when assessing pain. A careful examination is required to determine if sympathetic activation is a result of noxious stimulation or if it is a response to factors such as stress, metabolic or acid–base disturbances, hypovolemia, or severe anemia (Hellyer, 2002). Analgesia may be withheld during the initial patient examination to fully assess neurological, cardiovascular, and respiratory functions but, conversely, analgesia may be required during the initial examination if the animal is too painful and therefore difficult or unsafe to handle (Hellyer, 2002). Analgesia may also be withheld in animals that are hypothermic, obtunded, or unconscious, but as the animal warms and regains consciousness analgesia may become necessary (Hellyer, 2002).

CONSEQUENCES OF PAIN IN CRITICALLY ILL PATIENTS

The negative consequences of pain are well established. Pain may result in physiological and psychological consequences that can lead to significant morbidity and mortality (Joshi & Ogunnaike, 2005). The stress response to pain activates the autonomic nervous system resulting in endocrine, metabolic, and inflammatory changes (Joshi & Ogunnaike, 2005). Untreated pain contributes to morbidity and mortality by resulting in immunosuppression, delayed wound healing and infection, tachycardia, increased myocardial oxygen demand, decreased cerebrovascular autoregulation, increased intracranial pressure, and increased catabolism (Rose et al., 2011). Unrelieved pain may induce atelectasis due to reduced movement of the diaphragm and chest wall, particularly when thoracic or upper abdominal pain is present, and can worsen pulmonary function and lead to respiratory failure (Rose et al., 2011). Pain also impairs the ability to rest and sleep (Rose et al., 2011). Inadequate treatment of animals in pain may lead to chronic persistent pain syndromes (Mathews & Hansen, 2003; Joshi & Ogunnaike, 2005; Hansen, 2008; Rose et al., 2011). Sustained nociception can trigger central sensitization, which can lead to subsequent development of hyperalgesia and allodynia (Chapter 2), intensifying pain and creating more challenges for

achieving adequate pain relief (Hansen, 2008). The critically ill patient is not able to cope with the metabolic and energy demands of a disease if they are also dealing with untreated pain (Hellyer, 2002). Thus, effective analgesia makes therapeutic sense (Holden & Hammond, 2007). Providing analgesia improves the ability to rest, improves immune function, improves mobility, decreases the stress response, and improves survival (Hellyer, 2002).

RECOGNITION OF PAIN IN THE CRITICALLY ILL PATIENT

Assessing pain in critically ill animals is difficult, as it may not be possible to determine which indicators are related to pain, which are due to physiological derangements, and which are due to the stress of being in ICU. Intensive care patients frequently experience anxiety, agitation, and restlessness (Gelinas et al., 2004). Pain is often undertreated in human patients who are critically ill, and there is concern that pain is not managed appropriately in sedated patients because sedation may be used to manage agitated and restless patients, and painful patients may go untreated (Cade, 2008; Pasero et al., 2009). This may also occur in animal ICU patients. Sedatives should only be used once pain has been ruled out as the cause of clinical signs (Walden & Carrier, 2009).

Other hurdles to effective pain management in critically ill patients can include ICU order sheets that do not list pain as a condition to be monitored and treated, and the number of painful manipulations required in the care of unstable critically ill patients (Rose et al., 2011). Thus, the critically ill patient needs an ICU team that is motivated to provide effective pain relief (Gelinas et al., 2011). Checklists may be a way to implement the regular assessment and treatment of pain signs. The pain scores and when to give an analgesic should be noted on ICU order sheets; and this should include assessment of the level of pain during procedures such as feeding tube placement and peripheral and central IV catheter placement.

Clinical Signs of Pain

Behavioral observations are a key component in determining if an animal is in pain. Frequently, normal behavioral responses to pain

Pain Management in Veterinary Practice, First Edition. Edited by Christine M. Egger, Lydia Love and Tom Doherty.
© 2014 John Wiley & Sons, Inc. Published 2014 by John Wiley & Sons, Inc.

are obscured in the critically ill animal, and it requires more vigilant monitoring to detect and manage pain in these patients.

Signs of pain may include abnormal postures or positions as the animal tries to become comfortable. This may include reduced movement or tensing to guard the painful site. These animals will not rest or sleep comfortably (MacIntire et al., 2012). Painful animals may be less tolerant of nursing manipulation and respond with splinting of the body, striking, crying, or biting when a painful area is touched (Hellyer, 2002; MacIntire et al., 2012). A dog or cat that is falling asleep standing up or propped against the cage wall is painful (Hellyer, 2002). In human patients, facial expression is commonly used as a pain indicator. Behaviors that nurses considered indicative of pain in human patients were grimacing, vocalization, and wincing (Rose et al., 2011). This may be difficult to interpret in veterinary patients, but anxious, "worried" expressions as well as a disinterested expression (e.g., "staring off into space"), grimacing, ears flattened against the head, shivering or shaking, or appearing obtunded have been described in painful veterinary patients (Hellyer, 2002; MacIntire et al., 2012). Excessive salivation may indicate nausea, but can also indicate pain, and painful animals may have a decreased appetite. Head pressing or head banging may be seen with abdominal pain (Hellyer, 2002).

Pain assessment of the cat can be difficult, as this species may not be as demonstrative as dogs when in pain. When determining if a cat is painful, posture, orientation in the cage, facial expression, loss of normal behavior, and response to palpation of the surgery site should be evaluated (Robertson, 2008). A cat that is hunched with its head hung low, sitting quietly, not seeking attention, eyelids half-closed, or that resents being handled, is likely to be experiencing pain (Robertson, 2008). The painful cat will tend to sit in the back of the cage.

Besides the animal's demeanor, it is also important to consider the degree of tissue injury, any underlying disease processes, overall health status, and the animal's ability to demonstrate pain behaviors, when deciding if a specific behavior is pain related.

Pain Assessment Tools in the ICU

The first step in providing adequate pain relief is performing a systematic and consistent assessment and documentation of pain (Arif-rahu & Grap, 2010). Unfortunately, there is no universally accepted scoring system or tool for use in pain management in animals. A critical-care pain observation tool for pain assessment or management in an ICU for nonverbal critically ill human adults has been developed (Gelinas et al., 2011). The before and after implementation study showed that there were positive effects on pain assessment and management once the nursing staff had become trained in the use of the scale, and that education about pain assessment should include the proper use of analgesics and sedatives. The use of a valid pain scale was found to aid the nurses in discriminating pain from other causes such as anxiety. The categories for assessment in the critical care pain observation tool included facial expression, body movements, compliance with the ventilator if intubated, vocalization in nonintubated patients, and muscle tension. Three facial expressions were described: relaxed neutral, tense, and grimacing.

Pain scoring systems have been developed for use in the dog and the cat, but these scoring systems are usually used to assess post-surgical pain and may be difficult to implement in ICU patients. A similar scale could be developed for critically ill animals based on

the Colorado veterinary acute pain scale, which has a separate scale for the dog and the cat (Shaffran, 2008) (see Chapters 20 and 22). The categories in this scoring system include psychological and behavioral factors, response to palpation, and body tension. A multidimensional pain assessment tool should also include measurements of physiological indicators (e.g., heart rate, blood pressure, and respiratory rate) given the multifaceted nature of pain (Walden & Carrier, 2009).

Regardless of the scoring system used, the patient should initially be observed at rest in order to obtain a baseline score, and observed again during procedures such as turning and bandage changing to detect associated behavioral changes in response to pain. Assess the pain systematically, every 3–4 hours, or as indicated by pain scores. Evaluate muscle tension when the patient is at rest and during manipulation. Evaluate the patient before administering analgesics and again at the time of expected peak analgesic effects to see if the analgesic treatment was effective (Walden & Carrier, 2009).

MANAGEMENT OF PAIN IN THE CRITICALLY ILL PATIENT

Prevention is the first step of pain management (Walden & Carrier, 2009). Simple strategies such as grouping blood draws and other diagnostic procedures to reduce the number of exposures to needle sticks or other invasive techniques over the course of the day can be very helpful (Walden & Carrier, 2009). If multiple blood draws are necessary, consider placing a central IV line to minimize repeated venipuncture (Walden & Carrier, 2009). Orders to treat pain during rest and during procedures should be written. For example, a simple way to provide local analgesia for IV catheter placement would be the use of EMLA® cream (EMLA Cream Astra Zeneca) or liposomal lidocaine cream (LMX® 4% Ferndale Laboratories Michigan) placed on the site 20 minutes prior to catheter placement. Premedication with an analgesic and possibly a sedative prior to any invasive procedure will help to alleviate discomfort (Walden & Carrier, 2009; Rose et al., 2011).

Whenever possible, have skilled personnel perform procedures, as multiple failed attempts can dramatically increase the pain experienced by the patient (Walden & Carrier, 2009).

Preemptive or preventative analgesia should be used whenever possible. A test dose of an analgesic may be given when it is not clear if the animal is experiencing pain, and the response should be monitored (Hellyer, 2002; MacIntire et al., 2012). A more comfortable relaxed animal would support the diagnosis of pain and the need for continued analgesia (MacIntire et al., 2012). It is important to provide analgesic therapy on a regular schedule rather than waiting for pain to return before treating. Allowing pain to return or persist without alleviation can result in stimulation of the nociceptive pathways that may lead to hyperalgesia and reduced efficacy of analgesics (MacIntire et al., 2012).

Nonpharmacological Treatments for Pain

Nonpharmacological pain management techniques can be very effective. In human infants, blanket swaddling was effective at reducing the heart rate and negative facial expressions during heel sticks for blood sampling; and skin-to-skin contact during painful procedures reduced pain scores (Walden & Carrier, 2009). Environmental modifications, such as reduced lighting and noise levels, help to minimize stress during procedures and allow recovery post-procedure without an ongoing source of stressful stimuli (Walden & Carrier, 2009). Similar techniques should be used with animal patients, including minimizing noise levels and providing a clean, dry, and warm cage. Fear and anxiety can exacerbate pain, and animals housed in an ICU away from their owners are often fearful and anxious (Shaffran, 2008). A favorite blanket or toy placed with the animal may help alleviate distress (Shaffran, 2008). If the condition allows, frequent visits by the owner may reassure the pet. Animals with disabilities such as blindness or deafness need special consideration such as frequent reassuring touches. A comforting hand and soothing voice can lessen stress and make pain assessment easier (Shaffran, 2008). The animal's cage should be made a "safe zone" in that, whenever possible, all noxious procedures should be done away from the cage (Shaffran, 2008).

Pharmacological Treatment of Pain in the ICU

Providing analgesia to the critically ill patient can consist of a variety of techniques including locoregional techniques, continuous rate infusions, and multimodal analgesia.

LOCOREGIONAL TECHNIQUES

Local anesthetics (Chapter 6) can be used in local and regional blocks to provide analgesia without systemic sedative effects. Animals that have a chest tube placed for the treatment of pleural disease will experience pain from the presence of the chest tube and any underlying tissue trauma. Interpleural analgesia can be provided via administering lidocaine or bupivacaine through the chest tube or an intravenous catheter inserted into the chest. This will provide analgesia of 3–6 hours duration (Gaynor & Mama, 2002). Animals that have had thoracic surgery or have suffered fractured ribs will benefit from an intercostal nerve block, and this should decrease splinting and improve ventilation (Gaynor & Mama, 2002; Quandt & Lee, 2009).

Dogs with pancreatitis can be difficult to manage on systemic agents alone, and peritoneal and/or interpleural application of bupivacaine will provide additional analgesia (Lemke & Dawson, 2000); however, absorption will be limited if there is significant peritoneal or pleural fluid (Quandt & Lee, 2009).

Patients with injury or pain emanating from the caudal half of the body or the thorax will benefit from an epidural. Local anesthetics and opioids are commonly used, and epidural morphine can provide analgesia of 12–24 hours duration (Torske & Dyson, 2000). For long-term analgesia, an epidural catheter can be placed and this allows for repeated drug injections or a continuous rate infusion of appropriate analgesics (Torske & Dyson, 2000; Egger & Love, 2009; Quandt & Lee, 2009).

CONSTANT RATE INFUSIONS

Constant rate infusions (CRIs) (Table 28.1) of analgesic agents allow for steady-state plasma concentrations and more consistent analgesia. In human ICUs, the use of CRIs for sedation and

Table 28.1. Constant rate infusions (CRIs) commonly administered to intensive care patients

Drug	LD and CRI rate	Reference
Butorphanol	LD: 0.1 mg/kg IV CRI: 0.03–0.4 mg/kg/h IV	Quandt & Lee, 2009
Dexmedetomidine (medetomidine)	LD: 1 µg/kg IV CRI: 1–5 µg/kg/h IV	Quandt & Lee, 2009
Fentanyl	LD in dogs: 2 µg/kg IV CRI in dogs: 2–5 mg/kg/h LD in cats: 1 µg/kg IV CRI in cats: 1–4 µg/kg/h	Quandt & Lee, 2009
Ketamine	LD: 0.5 mg/kg IV CRI: 2 µg/kg/min IV	Wagner et al., 2002
Lidocaine	LD: 1–2 mg/kg IV CRI: 2–3 mg/kg/h IV Not recommended for use in cats	Quandt & Lee, 2009
Morphine	LD: 0.15–0.5 mg/kg slow IV to avoid histamine release CRI: 0.1–1 mg/kg/h IV	Quandt & Lee, 2009
Morphine–lidocaine–ketamine infusion	Morphine: 3.3 µg/kg/min Lidocaine: 50 µg/kg/min Ketamine: 10 µg/kg/min Mix 10 mg of morphine sulfate, 150 mg of 2% lidocaine, and 30 mg of ketamine into a 500 mL bag of lactated Ringer's solution. CRI: 10 mL/kg/h	Muir et al., 2003
Remifentanil	LD: 3 µg/kg IV CRI: 0.1–0.3 µg/kg/min	(Anagnostou et al., 2011); Allweiler et al., 2007; Brosnan et al., 2009

LD, loading dose.

analgesia is common. In one study, hypnotic-based sedation consisting of midazolam and/or propofol was compared to analgesic-based sedation with remifentanil (Park et al., 2007). The endpoint was the relief of pain and a hypnotic agent was given only if required to achieve patient comfort. Thirty-seven percent of patients given remifentanil did not require a hypnotic agent, and significantly more patients in the hypnotic group required additional analgesia (Park et al., 2007). That study suggests that patients benefit more from adequate analgesia than sedation with a hypnotic, and this is likely to be true in veterinary medicine.

Remifentanil, a μ-agonist (Chapter 4), has been used in dogs as a CRI to provide analgesia (Anagnostou et al., 2011). The advantage of this opioid over other opioids is that it is metabolized by ester hydrolysis with renal excretion and does not require hepatic metabolism. It has an ultrashort duration of action and is only effective when given as a CRI (Anagnostou et al., 2011). This is an advantage for the ICU patient with impaired hepatic function but in need of analgesia, and the use of a CRI of short acting remifentanil would allow for titration to effect.

Morphine and fentanyl are commonly used as CRIs but do require some hepatic metabolism. An advantage to using opioids is that their effect can be reversed with naloxone, if necessary. Adjunctive agents that can be used as CRIs include lidocaine, ketamine, and dexmedetomidine. These agents can be used individually or in combination. The combination of more than one agent allows for a synergistic effect for antinociception while decreasing adverse effects because lower doses are used. Combinations of fentanyl and lidocaine or morphine–lidocaine–ketamine are commonly used. Lidocaine should be used cautiously, if at all, in the cat because it has cardiovascular depressant effects that would be of concern in the critically ill feline (Pypendop & Ilkiw, 2005). Syringe pump delivery of CRIs is preferred for more accurate dosing (Quandt & Lee, 2009).

SUMMARY

Critical care patients pose a challenge when assessing pain as sympathetic stimulation could be due to pain, anxiety, or a number of physiological derangements. Control of pain in the critically ill patient is paramount, however, as untreated pain contributes to morbidity and mortality by resulting in sympathetic stimulation, immunosuppression, increased catabolism, and delayed wound healing and infection. Successful control of pain in these patients often requires a preemptive and multimodal approach.

REFERENCES

Allweiler, S., Brodbelt, D.C., Borer, K., Hammond, R.A., & Alibhai, H.I. (2007) The isoflurane-sparing and clinical effects of a constant rate infusion of remifentanil in dogs. *Veterinary Anaesthesia and Analgesia*, 34, 388–393.

Anagnostou, T.L., Kazakos, G.M., Sawas, I., Papazoglou, L.G., Rallis, T.S., & Raptopoulos, D. (2011) Remifentanil/isoflurane anesthesia in five dogs with liver disease undergoing liver biopsy. *Journal of American Animal Hospital Association*, 47, e103–e109.

Arif-Rahu, M. & Grap, M.J. (2010) Facial expression and pain in the critically ill non-communicative patient: state of science review. *Intensive and Critical Care Nursing*, 26, 343–352.

Brosnan, R.J., Pypendop, B.H., Siao, K.T., & Stanley, S.D. (2009) Effects of remifentanil on measures of anesthetic immobility and analgesia in cats. *American Journal Veterinary Research*, 70, 1065–1071.

Cade, C.H. (2008) Clinical tools for the assessment of pain in sedated critically ill adults. *British Association of Critical Care Nurses, Nursing in Critical Care*, 13, 288–297.

Egger, C. & Love, L. (2009) Local and regional anesthesia techniques, Part 4: Epidural anesthesia and analgesia. *Veterinary Medicine*, http://veterinarymedicine.dvm360.com/vetmed/Medicine/Local-and-regional-anesthesia-techniques-Part-4-Ep/ArticleStandard/Article/detail/632170 (accessed July 12, 2013).

Gaynor, J.S. & Mama, K.R. (2002) Local and regional anesthetic techniques for alleviation of perioperative pain, in: *Handbook of Veterinary Pain Management,* 2nd edn (eds J.S. Gaynor & W.W. Muir), Mosby Elsevier, St. Louis, MO, pp. 261–280.

Gelinas, C., Fortier, M., Viens, C., Fillion, L., & Puntillo, K. (2004) Pain assessment and management in critically ill intubated patients: a retrospective study. *American Journal of Critical Care*, 13, 126–135.

Gelinas, C., Arbour, C., Michaud, C., Vaillant, F., & Desjardins, S. (2011). Implementation of the critical-care pain observation tool on pain assessment/management nursing practices in an intensive care unit with nonverbal critically ill adults: a before and after study. *International Journal of Nursing Studies*, 48, 1495–1504.

Hellyer, P.W. (2002) Pain management, in *The Veterinary ICU Book* (eds W.E. Wingfield & M.R. Raffe), Teton NewMedia, Jackson, WY, pp. 68–85.

Hansen, B. (2008) Analgesia for the critically ill dog or cat: an update. *Veterinary Clinics of North America Small Animal Practice*, 38(6):1353–1363.

Holden, D.J. & Hammond, R. (2007) Anaesthesia and analgesia for the critical patient, in *Manual of Canine and Feline Emergency and Critical Care*, 2nd edn (eds L. King & R. Hammond), British Small Animal Veterinary Association Cheltenham, UK, pp. 261–270.

Joshi, G.P. & Ogunnaike, B.O. (2005) Consequences of inadequate postoperative pain relief and chronic persistent postoperative pain. *Anesthesiology Clinics of North America*, 23(1):21–36.

Lemke, K.A. & Dawson, S.D. (2000) Local and regional anesthesia. *Veterinary Clinics of North America Small Animal Practice*, 30(4), 839–857.

MacIntire, D.K., Drobatz, K.J., Haskins, S.C., et al. (2012) Anesthetic protocols for short procedures, in *Manual of Small Animal Emergency and Critical Care Medicine*, 2nd edn (eds D.K. MacIntire, K.J. Drobatz, S.C. Haskins, et al.) pp 38–54. Wiley Blackwell.

Mathews, K. & Hansen, B. (2003) Consequences of Pain, *Proceedings of 9th IVECCS Symposium*. New Orleans, LA, pp. 79–82.

Muir, W.W., Wiese, A.J., & March, P.A. (2003) Effects of morphine, lidocaine, ketamine, and morphine–lidocaine–ketamine drug combination on minimum alveolar concentration in dogs anesthetized with isoflurane. *American Journal of Veterinary Research*, 64(9), 1155–1160.

Park, G., Lane, M., Rogers, S., & Bassett, P. (2007). A comparison of hypnotic and analgesic based sedation in a general intensive care unit. *British Journal of Anaesthesia*, 98, 76–82.

Pasero, C., Puntillo, K., Li, D., et al. (2009) Structured approaches to pain management in the ICU. *Chest*, 135, 1665–1672.

Pypendop, B.H., & Ilkiw, J.E. (2005) Assessment of the hemodynamic effects of lidocaine administered IV in isoflurane-anesthetized cats. *American Journal of Veterinary Research*, 66, 661–668.

Quandt, J.E. & Lee, J.A. (2009) Analgesia and constant rate infusions, in: *Small Animal Critical Care Medicine* (eds D.C. Silverstein & K. Hopper), Saunders Elsevier, St. Louis, MO, pp. 710–716.

Robertson, S.A. (2008) Behaviors suggestive of postoperative pain in cats. *Veterinary Medicine*, 103(12), 652–653.

Rose, L., Haslam, L., Dale, C., et al. (2011) Survey of assessment and management of pain for critically ill adults. *Intensive and Critical Care Nursing*, 27, 121–128.

Shaffran, N. (2008) Pain management: the veterinary technician's perspective, *Veterinary Clinics of North America Small Animal Practice Update on Management of Pain*, 38(6):1415–1428.

Torske, K.E. & Dyson, D.H. (2000) Epidural analgesia and anesthesia, *Veterinary Clinics of North America Small Animal Practice Management of Pain*, 30(4):859–874.

Walden, M. & Carrier, C. (2009) The Ten Commandments of pain assessment and management in preterm neonates, *Critical Care Nursing Clinics North America*, 21(2):235–252.

Wagner, A.E., Walton, J.A., Hellyer, P.W., Gaynor, J.S., & Mama, K.R. (2002) Use of low doses of ketamine administered by constant rate infusion as an adjunct for postoperative analgesia in dogs. *Journal of the American Veterinary Medicine Association*, 221(1), 72–75.

29
Recognition and Assessment of Pain in Horses

Emma Love

IDENTIFICATION OF PAIN IN HORSES

It is essential to be able to recognize and assess pain in horses in order to determine when intervention is required, and to establish the efficacy of administered analgesics. Unfortunately, it is extremely difficult to directly measure pain, which is a complex subjective and dynamic experience. In people verbal self-reporting of pain is considered the "gold standard," as pain is unique to each individual.

Similar to the situation in young children who are unable to report their pain experience, pain assessment in animals presents clinicians with a considerable challenge. The clinician has to observe the animal and interpret signs that may indicate the type and degree of pain and distress that the individual animal is experiencing. There are marked species, breed, and individual variations in behavior, and environmental and physical factors also influence animals' willingness and ability to express signs of pain. The type of pain (e.g., physiological, inflammatory, or chronic) and location (e.g., abdominal or musculoskeletal) significantly affects the signs exhibited by horses. In addition, horses may experience more than one type of pain simultaneously. Acute abdominal pain often results in dramatic and easily identifiable signs including rolling, flank watching, kicking at the abdomen, and violent behavior such as striking and kicking. In contrast, an older horse suffering from osteoarthritis may demonstrate more subtle signs such as weight loss resulting from reduced food intake, reduced spontaneous locomotor activity, loss of muscle mass, and mild lameness—all of which are relatively nonspecific and are often attributed to the aging process.

Housing ponies individually, in pairs, or in groups could potentially influence behaviors associated with pain through a number of mechanisms. Interaction with other horses is important to maintain social bonds; and separation of horses, as may occur in clinical situations, may lead to abnormal behavior (VanDierendonck et al., 2009). This could potentially influence pain behaviors and make interpretation of pain behaviors more difficult. Maintaining ponies in small groups is not a perfect solution either. It has been suggested that mice housed in pairs show empathy in response to observation of the pain-related distress in their cage mate (Langford et al., 2006). Empathy in horses has not been investigated.

Pain Scoring Systems

Ashley et al. (2005) suggested that the advantages of using a defined pain scoring system include:

- The ability to objectively monitor progress and response to treatment.
- Increased awareness among the staff (or owners) involved in the care of the animal about the importance of monitoring for pain and analgesic efficacy.
- Consistency in the evaluation of individual animals. The ideal pain scoring system should be linear, weighted, sensitive to pain type, breed- and species-specific, and easy to interpret with excellent intra- and interobserver agreement.

The development of pain scales for use in horses lags behind the progress made in the fields of human and small animal pain management. In people who can self-report their pain, a number of pain scoring systems are used, including simple descriptive scales (SDSs), numerical rating scales (NRSs), visual analog scales (VASs) and multidimensional pain scales. These have been adapted for use in horses, and modifications of the SDS, NRS, and VAS have been used in clinical studies and case reports evaluating analgesics (Jochle, 1989; Jochle et al., 1989; Valverde et al., 1990; Johnson et al., 1993; Walker, 2007). The main disadvantage of these pain scales is that they are based on subjective assessments. In addition, only limited validation of the scoring systems has been performed in horses and attention has been focused on acute pain, with almost no work performed to address the significant issue of chronic pain. The inherent variability in pain assessment using these systems may be less of a concern if a single trained observer performs all assessments in an individual horse.

The SDS, NRS, and VAS are one-dimensional scales that assess the intensity of the pain, and do not take into account the pain that is multidimensional, with emotional and cognitive effects. In an attempt to get a more complete view of the pain that the animal is suffering, the VAS has been extended to incorporate dynamic and interactive components (DIVAS) (Lascelles et al., 1995). The DIVAS scale has been used in horses and is relatively simple to adopt in practice.

Initially, the demeanor of the animal is assessed from a remote position. The horse's demeanor may range from excited and violent to moribund, and, in addition to being influenced by the type of pain and the horse's emotional state, demeanor may be significantly influenced by the primary disease process. If appropriate, the horse is encouraged to walk out of or around the stable. It is important to touch the horse in nonpainful areas to accustom the horse to the observer's touch, and then the area of interest should be gently palpated while the observer closely assesses the horse's responses. Although interaction with the horse should improve assessment of pain quantification, it is still subjective and observer dependent.

Food and Water Consumption

Monitoring food and water consumption is important and can be included in a global pain assessment. Dental pain may manifest itself as a reluctance to eat or difficulty masticating food. The position of the food and water buckets should be considered, as horses with thoracic limb, neck, or back pain may be unwilling to bear weight on their forelimbs and lower the head to eat and drink.

Mechanical Threshold Testing

The advantages, disadvantages, and potential clinical applications of mechanical threshold testing in horses have recently been reviewed by Love et al. (2011). Pressure algometry has been used to quantify the pressure required to elicit a withdrawal or avoidance response in horses with experimentally induced back (Haussler & Erb, 2006) and thoracic limb (Haussler et al., 2007) pain. This technique involves the application of pressure perpendicular to the surface of the skin, at a constant rate, until a behavioral avoidance reaction is observed. At this point, the application of pressure is stopped and the value is recorded as the threshold. Pressure algometry has the potential to be a useful way of monitoring responses to treatment in horses with naturally occurring musculoskeletal disease, with the caveats that the operator receive comprehensive and frequent training (De Heus et al., 2010).

Hoof testers are routinely used in clinical practice to identify areas of pain in the foot, although assessment of the degree of force required to produce a response is usually subjective. The British Veterinary Association Animal Welfare Foundation has funded a study that developed and validated hoof testers modified to enable measurement of the pressure applied to the hoof during the application. The full results have not yet been published, but the use of these modified hoof testers could play an important role in monitoring the response to treatment in horses with acute and chronic laminitis.

Wound sensitivity in small animals has been assessed using a palpometer (Slingsby et al., 2001). This device quantifies the pressure required to elicit a withdrawal response during palpation of wounds, and has been used in studies investigating the analgesic efficacy of treatments after elective surgery (Slingsby et al., 2001). This technique could easily be adapted for use in horses, although the temperament of the animal and site of the wound will influence whether the wound can be palpated safely. Assessment of a site remote from the wound is important so that the animal's response to touch can be ascertained. Fear or anxiety may influence the animal's response to wound palpation, and horses may learn to respond to palpation as soon as pressure is applied.

Objective measurement of mechanical thresholds could potentially be incorporated into pain assessment protocols and deserves further investigation.

Behavioral Assessment of Pain

Behavioral assessment and heart rate are reported to be the two most commonly used factors influencing pain assessment and subsequent analgesic administration to horses (Price et al., 2002). Unfortunately, objective measures such as heart rate, heart rate variability, and hormonal responses do not appear to correlate with subjective assessment of pain in the horse (Raekallio et al., 1997; Rietmann et al., 2004). Behavior is recognized as the most sensitive and specific way of assessing pain in other animal species (Molony & Kent, 1997; Houlton et al., 1998). Behaviors exhibited by horses with a range of potentially painful conditions or after surgery have not yet been comprehensively evaluated (Ashley et al., 2005; Valverde & Gunkel, 2005), but progress has been made recently. Signs that have been traditionally thought to indicate pain in horses include: rolling; restlessness; agitation; kicking at the abdomen; head-lowering; repeatedly looking at a body part (Figure 29.1); vocalization; rigid posture; uneven weightbearing; sweating; bruxism; increased jaw tone; flared nostrils; and muscle fasciculation. After the horse has been observed from a distance it is then approached, and its response and willingness to interact with the observer are noted. In the clinical setting, factors such as transportation, hospitalization, fasting, and anesthetic and analgesic drugs may alter behavior, and the effects of these factors should be considered when assessing potential pain-related behaviors.

The importance of facial expression has been recognized, for many years, as a marker of pain in man, and is thought to reflect both the intensity and emotional components of pain (Prkachin, 2009). The use of facial expressions to detect and quantify pain in animals is a novel area of research, although, anecdotally, owners often report that they can tell if their horse is in pain by looking at its face. In mice, facial expressions based on photographs taken in the presence and absence of a painful stimulus have been used to create a three-point Mouse Grimace Scale (Langford et al., 2010). The

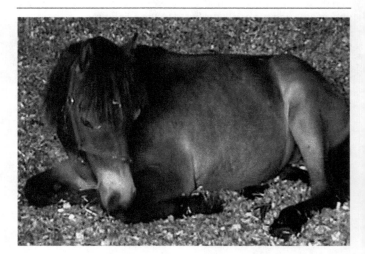

Figure 29.1. A pony postcastration looking round at his surgical site when recumbent.

British Veterinary Association Animal Welfare Foundation Norman Hayward Fund is currently underwriting a project to investigate the horse "pain face."

ORTHOPEDIC PAIN

Evaluation via the video of activity budgets (time spent exhibiting defined behaviors) in horses after arthroscopic surgery has been performed to determine the specific behavioral indices for inclusion in future pain scoring systems (Price et al., 2003). Compared with the control horses that did not undergo anesthesia and surgery, the horses that underwent arthroscopy spent less time exploring their environment and walking around, and restlessness and weight shifting were observed. Horses in the operated group spent less time at the front of the stable, although this finding was not statistically significant. Observation of continuous video footage has the advantage that the horses may exhibit behaviors they would not demonstrate in the presence of an observer, and it may be a sensitive method of detecting changes in behavior, although, at present, such technologies are impractical outside of a research setting (Price et al., 2003).

The reproducibility, specificity, and sensitivity of several parameters selected from a review by Ashley et al. (2005) have been established in the development of a composite orthopedic pain scale in horses (Bussieres et al., 2008). The authors identified several behavioral parameters which they considered to merit further investigation including posture, pawing at the floor, head movement, kicking at the abdomen, and response to palpation of an injured area (Bussieres et al., 2008). The results of that study also suggested that noninvasive measurement of blood pressure was a specific and sensitive parameter for the assessment of orthopedic pain. This appears to be the only physiological measurement that is potentially useful in assessing pain, whereas heart and respiratory rate changes did not predict the severity of the pain.

Recently, the analgesic efficacy of intra-articular morphine in a lipopolysaccharide synovitis model was evaluated using three different scoring systems: lameness, on an eight-point ordinal scale; a composite measure pain scale (CMPS); and a VAS (Lindegaard et al., 2010). The CMPS was based on six behavioral categories, with up to four ranked levels indicating no pain to severe pain. The categories were: gross pain behaviors (tooth-grinding, lip-curling, pawing, sweating) scored from absent to continuous; weight bearing scored from normal weight bearing to no weight bearing; head position scored from above the withers (or eating) to below the withers; location in stall, varying from at the stall door watching the environment to standing in the middle, facing back or standing in the back; response to door opening, varying from moving toward the door to no response; and response to the approach of observer varying from moving toward the observer with ears forward to not moving with ears back. An overall subjective pain score was also assigned, ranging from no apparent pain through to severe orthopedic pain. Inter-observer agreement on the CMPS was good and better than for the visual analog scale. The CMPS did have a low sensitivity for mild pain, although it may be useful for the detection and monitoring of severe pain in clinical cases.

A modified composite pain scale has been used to monitor the progress of an individual horse with severe hoof pain (Dutton et al., 2009). The pain scale used in that case was based on a pain scoring system for dogs (Morton et al., 2005) and the Obel laminitis pain scale which is a four-point ordinal scale based on the degree of lameness and responses to lifting of the leg by an observer (Obel, 1948). The case report highlights that although there is currently no fully validated robust pain scoring system for horses, modified scoring systems can be used to aid recognition of changing pain states and to guide analgesic treatment.

ABDOMINAL PAIN

Behavioral signs associated with severe abdominal pain are often dramatic and easily detected by owners. Potential indicators of postoperative pain in horses following emergency laparotomy for the surgical management of colic have been described (Pritchett et al., 2003). Compared with horses that did not undergo any procedure and horses that underwent anesthesia (for MRI) only, horses that had surgery spent less time moving around the stall. They also demonstrated some "pain-related" behaviors such as the Flehmen response, flank gestures, kicking at the abdomen, and stretching the body, although the time spent performing these active pain behaviors was significantly less than in the preoperative phase. Increased plasma cortisol and heart rate were also found in the surgical group, although these may not be specific for pain and require interpretation in light of the clinical picture. A subsequent study by the same research group concluded that the heart rate is not a sensitive indicator of pain following exploratory laparotomy (Sellon et al., 2004).

CASTRATION

Castration is a very commonly performed husbandry procedure in horses, and, using an anthropomorphic approach, could be assumed to result in at least moderate pain. Despite this, the requirement for administration of analgesia to horses following castration has been debated within the literature, with some authors asserting that the procedure is not painful and that provision of analgesia is "unwarranted sympathy". A survey of UK equine veterinary surgeons indicated that only 36.9% of horses undergoing castration routinely receive analgesics postoperatively (Price et al., 2005). This could potentially be due to difficulties in assessing and quantifying pain, but could also be due to limited opportunities to observe the horses postoperatively. Castration is often performed in the field or as an outpatient procedure, and analgesia in the immediate postoperative period may be adequate until the effects of the sedatives and local anesthesia used to facilitate the surgery wane.

The analgesic effects of butorphanol have been studied in ponies undergoing castration under a brief general anesthetic (acepromazine, detomidine, ketamine plus or minus butorphanol) (Love et al., 2009). Pain was assessed subjectively from 1 hour until 24 hours, postoperatively using a DIVAS. Only one of the 20 ponies did not require additional analgesia. Behavioral signs that were observed and interpreted as being associated with pain included: weight shifting; reluctance to walk and a stiff hind limb gait; bruxism; low head carriage; increased reaction to gentle pressure on the caudal abdomen compared with gentle pressure on the neck; lack of grooming behavior; and absence of interaction with other ponies and the observer (Figure 29.2). These behaviors were ameliorated by the administration of butorphanol, suggesting that they were related to pain (Love et al., 2009).

A VAS and NRS have been used to investigate the analgesic effects of butorphanol and phenylbutazone in horses undergoing castration. The highest pain scores were recorded at 4 and 8 hours after surgery and mean 24 hour VAS scores were significantly greater (more pain) for day 2 compared with days 3 and 4, and

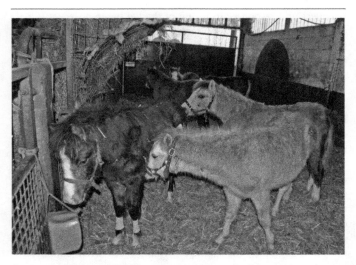

Figure 29.2. Ponies 6 hours after castration. The darker colored pony had separated himself from the herd, was not interested in interacting with other ponies or the observer, had a low head carriage, and a tense jaw. He was reluctant to move and walked with a stiff pelvic limb gait. His demeanor, willingness to interact, and gait improved after administration of flunixin meglumine.

significantly greater on day 3 than 4. This suggests that pain intensity decreases over time, although studies are needed to indicate how long analgesics are required after routine castration, and whether there are any long-term consequences of inadequate pain control in the perioperative period.

Differences in eyelid and lip position have been observed following castration (Love, 2009). Preoperatively, eyes were described as "open" most of the time and the lower lip "drooping," whereas postoperatively, the eyes appeared to be "semiclosed" with the lips "closed." It is possible that these features resulted from an increase in facial muscle tone, possibly as a result of pain, and this merits further investigation.

SUMMARY

The assessment of pain in horses is an active area of research, and recent advances hold promise for the development of a pain assessment tool in this species. The use of a multifactorial approach to pain assessment is likely to be more successful than focusing on an individual characteristic. At present, accurate pain assessment in horses is a challenge, but involving all members of the health care team and implementing a standardized approach to assessing individual animals has the potential to improve pain recognition and management and, thereby, to significantly improve the welfare of horses.

REFERENCES

Ashley, F.H., Waterman-Pearson, A.E., & Whay, H.R. (2005) Behavioural assessment of pain in horses and donkeys: application to clinical practice and future studies. *Equine Veterinary Journal*, 37, 565–575.

Bussieres, G., Jacques, C., Lainay, O., et al. (2008) Development of a composite orthopaedic pain scale in horses. *Research in Veterinary Science*, 85, 294–306.

De Heus, P., Van Oossanen, G., Van Dierendonck, M.C., & Willem, B. (2010) A pressure algometer is a useful tool to objectively monitor the effect of diagnostic palpation by a physiotherapist in Warm blood horses. *Journal of Equine Veterinary Science*, 30, 310–321.

Dutton, D.W., Lashnits, K.J., & Wegner, K. (2009) Managing severe hoof pain in a horse using multimodal analgesia and a modified composite pain score. *Equine Veterinary Education*, 21, 37–43.

Haussler, K.K. & Erb, H.N. (2006) Pressure algometry for the detection of induced back pain in horses: a preliminary study. *Equine Veterinary Journal*, 38, 76–81.

Haussler, K.K., Hill, A.E., Frisbie, D.D., & McIlwraith, C.W. (2007) Determination and use of mechanical nociceptive thresholds of the thoracic limb to assess pain associated with induced osteoarthritis of the middle carpal joint in horses. *American Journal of Veterinary Research*, 68, 1167–1176.

Houlton, L.L., Scott, E.M., Nolan, A.M., Reid, J., Welsh, E., & Flaherty, D. (1998) Comparison of three methods used for assessment of pain in dogs. *Journal of the American Veterinary Medicine Association*, 212, 61–66.

Jochle, W. (1989) Field trial evaluation of detomidine as a sedative and analgesic agent in horses with colic. *Equine Veterinary Journal Supplement*, 7, 117–120.

Jochle, W., Moore, J.N., Brown, J., et al. (1989) Comparison of detomidine, butorphanol, flunixin meglumine and xylazine in clinical cases of equine colic. *Equine Veterinary Journal Supplement* 7, 111–116.

Johnson, C.B., Taylor, P.M., Young, S.S., & Brearley, J.C. (1993) Postoperative analgesia using phenylbutazone, flunixin or carprofen in horses. *Veterinary Record*, 133, 336–338.

Langford, D.J., Crager, S.E., Shehzad, Z., et al. (2006) Social modulation of pain as evidence for empathy in mice. *Science*, 312, 1967–1970.

Langford, D.J., Bailey, A.L., Chanda, M.L., et al. (2010) Coding of facial expressions of pain in the laboratory mouse. *Nature Methods*, 7, 447–449.

Lascelles, B.D.X., Cripps, P., Mirchandani, S., & Waterman, A.E. (1995) Carprofen as an analgesic for postoperative pain in cats: dose titration and assessment of efficacy in comparison to pethidine hydrochloride. *Journal of Small Animal Practice*, 36, 535–541.

Lindegaard, C., Thomsen, M.H., Larsen, S., & Andersen, P.H. (2010) Analgesic efficacy of intra-articular morphine in experimentally induced radiocarpal synovitis in horses. *Veterinary Anaesthesia and Analgesia*, 37, 171–185.

Love, E.J. (2009) Advances in the objective evaluation of pain and analgesic efficacy in horses. PhD Thesis. University of Bristol.

Love, E.J., Murrell, J, Whay, H.R. (2011) Thermal and mechanical nociceptive threshold testing in horses: a review. *Veterinary Anaesthesia and Analgesia*, 38(1), 3–14.

Love, E.J., Taylor, P.M., Clark, C., Whay, H.R., & Murrell, J. (2009) Analgesic effect of butorphanol in ponies following castration. *Equine Veterinary Journal*, 41, 552–556.

Molony, V. & Kent, J.E. (1997) Assessment of acute pain in farm animals using behavioral and physiological measurements. *Journal of Animal Science*, 75, 266–272.

Morton, C.M., Reid, J., Scott, E.M., Holton, L.L., & Nolan, A.M. (2005) Application of a scaling model to establish and validate an interval level pain scale for assessment of acute pain in dogs. *American Journal of Veterinary Research*, 66, 2154–2166.

Obel, N. (1948) Studies on the Histopathology of Acute Laminitis. Thesis. Almqvist and Wilcsells Bottrykeri Ab Uppsala.

Prkachin, K.M. (2009) Assessing pain by facial expression: facial expression as nexus. *Pain Research & Management*, 14, 53–58.

Price, J., Catriona, S., Welsh, E.M., & Waran, NK. (2003) Preliminary evaluation of a behaviour-based system for assessment of postoperative pain in horses following arthroscopic surgery. *Veterinary Anaesthesia and Analgesia*, 30, 124–137.

Price, J., Eager, R.A., Welsh, E.M., & Waran, N.K. (2005) Current practice relating to equine castration in the UK. *Research in Veterinary Science*, 78, 277–280.

Price, J., Marques, J.M., Welsh, E.M., & Waran, N.K. (2002) Pilot epidemiological study of attitudes towards pain in horses. *Veterinary Record*, 151, 570–575.

Pritchett, L.C., Ulibarri, C., Roberts, M.C., Robert, K S., & Debra, C.S. (2003) Identification of potential physiological and behavioral indicators of postoperative pain in horses after exploratory celiotomy for colic. *Applied Animal Behaviour Science*, 80, 31–43.

Raekallio, M., Taylor, P.M., & Bloomfield, M. (1997) A comparison of methods for evaluation of pain and distress after orthopaedic surgery in horses. *Journal of Veterinary Anaesthesia*, 24, 17–20.

Rietmann, T.R., Stauffacher, M., Bernasconi, P., Auer, J.A., & Weishaupt, M.A. (2004) The association between heart rate, heart rate variability, endocrine and behavioural pain measures in horses suffering from laminitis. *Journal of Veterinary Medicine Series a-Physiology Pathology Clinical Medicine*, 51, 218–225.

Sellon, D.C., Roberts, M.C., Blikslager, A.T., Ulibarri, C., & Papich, M.G. (2004) Effects of continuous rate intravenous infusion of butorphanol on physiologic and outcome variables in horses after celiotomy. *Journal of Veterinary Internal Medicine*, 18, 555–563.

Slingsby, L.S., Jones, A., & Waterman-Pearson, A.E. (2001) Use of a new finger-mounted device to compare mechanical nociceptive thresholds in cats given pethidine or no medication after castration. *Research in Veterinary Science*, 70, 243–246.

Valverde, A. & Gunkel, C.I. (2005) Pain management in horses and farm animals. *Journal of Veterinary Emergency and Critical Care*, 15, 295–307.

Valverde, A., Little, C.B., Dyson, D.H., & Motter, C.H. (1990) Use of epidural morphine to relieve pain in a horse. *Canadian Veterinary Journal-Revue Veterinaire Canadienne*, 31, 211–212.

VanDierendonck, M.C., de Vries, H., Schilder, M.B.H., Colenbrander, B., Þorhallsdóttir, A.G., & Sigurjónsdóttir, H. (2009) Interventions in social behaviour in a herd of mares and geldings. *Applied Animal Behaviour Science*, 116, 67–73.

Walker, A.F. (2007) Sublingual administration of buprenorphine for long-term analgesia in the horse. *Veterinary Record*, 160, 808–809.

30

Treatment of Acute and Chronic Pain in Horses

Bernd Driessen and Laura Zarucco

Pain therapy in the horse is in its infancy and lags far behind developments in human medicine (Muir, 2010a). There are many reasons for this, including misconceptions, such as the long-held belief that effective analgesia is detrimental to tissue healing; incomplete understanding of the neurobiological mechanisms producing pain and the neuropathophysiological consequences of persistent nociception/pain; difficulties in reliably assessing the intensity and duration of nociception/pain; and the continued struggle to find effective analgesic drugs and treatment regimens/techniques for acute and persistent pain without causing adverse outcomes (Taylor et al., 2002). Recent surveys among equine practitioners indicate that a majority of veterinarians consider their knowledge of analgesic therapy in horses to be moderate at best, and that multiple barriers to optimal management of pain in horses continue to exist, including skepticism toward newly marketed drugs and more sophisticated techniques developed for improved pain management in horses (Price et al., 2002; Hubbell et al., 2010; Dujardin & van Loon, 2011). What follows is an overview of therapeutic modalities currently described for treatment of pain in horses.

CLASSIFICATION OF EQUINE PAIN AND ITS RELEVANCE TO PAIN THERAPY

The International Association for the Study of Pain (IASP) has defined pain as an "unpleasant sensory and emotional experience" in a conscious subject. More appropriately for horses, pain may be described as "an aversive sensory and emotional experience representing awareness by the animal of damage or threat to the integrity of its tissues" (Molony & Kent, 1997). Systems of pain classification have been used to direct analgesic therapy or to describe efficacy of therapeutic interventions. Common pain descriptors denote anatomical origin such as superficial somatic (i.e., cutaneous), deep somatic (i.e., musculoskeletal), or visceral pain; site of impulse generation such as nociceptors (nociceptive pain) versus injured peripheral and central afferents discharging uncontrolled impulses (nonnociceptive or neuropathic pain); intensity (mild, moderate, or severe pain); and duration (acute vs. chronic). However, from a therapeutic standpoint, those classifications are not particularly meaningful. For example, none of the analgesic agents available

today has been shown to be exclusively effective toward pain of somatic, visceral, or neuropathic origin.

Separating acute from chronic pain is also challenging. According to the taxonomy of the IASP, chronic pain is defined by a duration of more than 3 months (Merskey, 1986). Therefore, acute pain covers a long period of time during which many neurophysiological and pathological processes occur simultaneously (Woolf & Salter, 2000). As nociceptive input continues and becomes persistent, central sensitization goes through increasingly longer-lasting, irreversible, and pathological stages.

MULTIMODAL PAIN THERAPY (BALANCED ANALGESIA)

Opinion polls conducted during the past decade among North American and European equine practitioners have revealed that veterinarians continue to rely primarily on nonsteroidal anti-inflammatory drugs (NSAIDs) for pain therapy in horses (Price et al., 2002; Hubbell et al., 2010; Dujardin & van Loon, 2011). During the same period, a fundamental shift in perioperative and chronic pain management has taken place in human medicine. Advancements in the understanding of the complex physiology and pathophysiology of pain (Chapter 2) have led to widespread implementation of a new strategy, often referred to as *multimodal* or *balanced analgesia* as opposed to the traditional *unimodal* pain therapy (Carr, 2001; Elvir-Lazo & White, 2010). Multimodal analgesia involves the administration of a combination of drugs with different pharmacological mechanisms of action, and often includes systemic and local (or regional) techniques of administration, and may include complementary modalities of pain treatment (Table 30.1). Given the manifold mechanisms and dynamic neuronal processes involved in generation and aggravation of the pain experience in humans and animals, it is not reasonable to assume that, in horses suffering from moderate to severe pain as a result of major tissue trauma and/or inflammation, monotherapy will produce adequate analgesia and long-term pain relief (Lemke, 2004; Muir, 2005; Taylor, 2005; Driessen & Zarucco, 2007). Rather, different analgesic agents and techniques should be employed and tailored to the specific situation of the individual horse, with continuation for

Pain Management in Veterinary Practice, First Edition. Edited by Christine M. Egger, Lydia Love and Tom Doherty.
© 2014 John Wiley & Sons, Inc. Published 2014 by John Wiley & Sons, Inc.

Table 30.1.   Components of multimodal analgesia in the horse

Anti-inflammatory treatment	Systemic analgesia	Local/regional anesthesia and analgesia	Complementary therapies

Nonsteroidal anti-inflammatory drugs (NSAIDs)	Opioids
	α-2 agonists
	Local anesthetics (including IV lidocaine)
	Nonconventional therapeutics
	– Butylscopolamine
	– Ketamine
	– α₂δ ligands
	    – Gabapentin
	    – Pregabalin
		Peripheral nerve blocks using topical, infiltration, perineural, intra-articular administration techniques:
		– Local anesthetics
		– Ketamine
		– Morphine
		– α-2 agonists
		Local intravenous administration (intravenous regional analgesia; Bier block)
		– Lidocaine 1–2%
		– Mepivacaine 1–2%
		Epidural anesthesia/analgesia
		– Local anesthetics
		– Opioids
		– α-2 agonists
		Local capsaicin or resiniferatoxin application
			Acupuncture
			Electroacupuncture
			Physical therapy
			Chiropractic

a minimum of 3 days after routine elective surgical procedures, and as long as required based on pain assessment (Lemke, 2004; Driessen & Zarucco, 2007). The purpose of multimodal analgesia is to choose drugs and techniques that target different sites within the somato- and viscerosensory neural conduit that act synergistically, thereby achieving the six main goals listed in Table 30.2 (Livingston, 2006). Multimodal pain therapy allows integration of complementary modalities of treatment such as chiropractic, physical therapy, or acupuncture, where and whenever appropriate, and allows new drugs and techniques of pain treatment to be

included as they become available. Whatever pharmacological or other approach is chosen in an individual multimodal analgesic protocol, the ultimate objective is to achieve optimum pain control, while at the same time minimizing the risk of adverse responses to pain therapy.

Continuous Rate Infusions in Horses

Intravenous continuous rate infusion (CRI) of analgesic drugs like opioids, α-2 agonists, lidocaine, or ketamine (Table 30.3) is frequently applied in equine anesthesia as part of a partial

Table 30.2.   Drugs and treatment modalities used to achieve main goals of *multimodal* analgesia

Goal	Treatment
Blockade of nociceptive signal generation in primary afferent terminals	Tissue infiltration with local anesthetics
Suppression of primary hyperalgesia	Nerve blocks with local anesthetic agents, systemic NSAIDs, or opioids
Blockade of nociceptive signal conduction, thereby preventing/inhibiting development of secondary hyperalgesia	Nerve blocks with local anesthetics or TRPV-1 agonists (e.g., capsaicin, RTX)
Inhibition of spinal nociceptive signal transmission and inhibition of secondary hyperalgesia	Epidural or intrathecal administration of – Local anesthetics, opioids, α-2 agonists – Intrathecal TRPV-1 agonist RTX application Systemic administration of opioids, α-2 agonists, ketamine, NSAIDs, antiepileptic drugs (e.g., gabapentin, pregabalin)
Inhibition/decrease of the pain experience by interference with cerebral nociceptive signal processing	Systemic lidocaine, opioids, α-2 agonists, ketamine, NSAIDs, antiepileptic drugs
Restoration of homeostasis and normal function	All treatment modalities

TRPV-1, transient receptor potential channel vanilloid subfamily member 1; RTX, resiniferatoxin.

Table 30.3. Drugs commonly used for systemic analgesia via continuous rate infusion (CRI)[a]

Drug class	Drug	IV Bolus loading dose (mg/kg)	IV CRI rate (mg/kg/h)
Opioids	Morphine	0.05–0.15 (up to 0.3)	0.1–0.4
	Butorphanol	0.02	0.013–0.024
	Fentanyl	0.00028–0.005	0.0004–0.008
α-2 agonists	Xylazine	0.2–1.0	1.0 (up to 4.0)
	Detomidine	0.006–0.04	0.007–0.036
	Medetomidine	0.003–0.01	0.0015–0.0036
	Dexmedetomidine	0.003–0.005	0.00075–0.0018
	Romifidine	0.01–0.04	0.1–0.4
Local anesthetics	Lidocaine	1.3–2.5 (over 10–15 min)	1.8–3.0
Dissociative anesthetics	Ketamine	none or 1.0–2.3 (over 30–40 min)	0.003–0.018 or 0.4–1.5
	With lidocaine	none or 1.0	0.2

Higher CRI rates typically used intraoperatively, lower CRI rates typically used in the nonanesthetized horse or when combined with other drugs listed in the table. Doses and CRI rates are based on references quoted in the text.

intravenous anesthetic (PIVA) protocol (i.e., a combination of one or more analgesic agents with a low dose of inhalational anesthetic for balanced anesthesia) or in total intravenous anesthesia (TIVA) (Bettschart-Wolfensberger & Larenza, 2007; Caulkett, 2007; Staffieri & Driessen, 2007; Auckburally & Flaherty, 2011). Intravenous CRI of potent analgesic/sedative agents, such as α-2 agonists alone or in conjunction with opioids, is also commonly used for surgical procedures in the standing sedated horse (Muir, 1981; Hubbell et al., 2010). In these situations, those drugs are usually administered in conjunction with local or regional anesthesia to control short periods of acute pain and facilitate surgery.

Continuous infusion of analgesic drugs is indicated in animals with persistent moderate to severe pain, in order to provide more consistent and durable analgesia, while at the same time minimizing adverse effects that may occur with bolus administration of high doses (Sellon et al., 2002; Sellon et al., 2004; Driessen et al., 2010). A CRI of analgesic medication(s) should supply a sufficient amount of analgesic drugs to provide adequate pain relief during most of the day, requiring additional drug administration only when breakthrough pain occurs. This, however, implies frequent or continuous monitoring of the horse. Ideally, breakthrough pain medication is tailored to individual episodes of peak pain, which may vary substantially in duration and intensity, and is composed of either boluses of analgesic drugs that are being already infused and/or additional therapeutics that synergistically enhance the analgesic efficacy of the currently administered drugs. Lidocaine and butorphanol CRIs have been used with variable satisfaction in horses suffering from gastrointestinal discomfort after colic surgery or intestinal disease such as large colon impactions. Opioids (e.g., morphine, methadone, butorphanol), α-2 agonists (e.g., detomidine, medetomidine, dexmedetomidine), or ketamine alone or in conjunction with lidocaine have been administered via CRI to horses with persistent musculoskeletal pain such as with long-bone fracture and repair, arthrodesis, septic joint or septic tendon sheath treatment, cellulitis, or hoof-wall resection in laminitic horses (Driessen & Zarucco, 2007; Driessen et al., 2010).

Complementary Modalities for Pain

Complementary modalities of pain therapy are probably most frequently applied in animals suffering from thoracolumbar or lumbosacral pain. They include acupuncture/electroacupuncture (Martin & Klide, 1991; Xie et al., 1996; Ridgway, 2005), chiropractic/manipulative therapy (Haussler, 2009), physical therapy (Chapter 12), and mesotherapy (Allan et al., 2010). Details of some of these techniques are addressed elsewhere in this textbook.

SYSTEMIC ANALGESICS USED IN THE EQUINE PATIENT

The drugs most commonly administered systemically to treat pain in horses belong to four different pharmacological classes: NSAIDs, opioids, α-2 agonists, and local anesthetics. The basic pharmacology of these drug classes has been addressed in preceding chapters. The following review will therefore highlight new developments within each class, and discuss new experimental data as they relate to pain therapy in the horse. In recent years, the pharmacological armamentarium available to treat more severe and persistent pain in the equine has been expanded by drugs that can be grouped together as nontraditional analgesics and which includes antiepileptic drugs and NMDA receptor antagonists. These drugs, and their use in equine pain management, will be addressed separately. Table 30.4 lists doses for individual pain therapeutics that have been reported in the horse. The interested reader may also consult recently published comprehensive reviews of common pain therapeutics in the equine species (Baller & Hendrickson, 2002; Bennett & Steffey, 2002; Daunt & Steffey, 2002; Goodrich & Nixon, 2006; Driessen, 2007; Clutton, 2010; Doherty & Seddighi, 2010; Driessen et al., 2010; Muir, 2010c; Robertson & Sanchez, 2010; Valverde, 2010; Van Weeren & de Grauw, 2010).

Nonsteroidal Anti-inflammatory Drugs

Inflammation accompanies nearly every tissue insult to some degree, but can also occur as a primary disease entity. Pain is one

Table 30.4. Drugs commonly used for systemic analgesia

Pharmacological class	Drug	Dose (mg/kg)	Route of administration	Dosing interval (hours)
NSAIDs	Phenylbutazone	2.2–4.4	IV, PO	12–24
	Flunixin meglumine	0.2–1.1	IV, PO	8–12
	Dipyrone (Metamizole)	10–20	IV, IM	8–12
	Acetylsalicylic acid (Aspirin)	5–20	PO	24–48
	Naproxen	5 (10)	IV (PO)	Initial slow IV bolus, then PO dose once daily
	Ketoprofen	2.0–2.5	IV, IM	24
	Carprofen	0.7–1.4	IV, PO	24
	Meloxicam	0.6	IV	24
	Etodolac	10–20	IV, IM, PO	12–24
	Eltenac	0.5–1.0	IV	24
	Vedaprofen	1–2	IV, PO	12–24
		0.1	PO, IV	12
	Firocoxib	1–2	IV	24
		2	PO	
Opioids	Morphine	0.1–0.2	IV, IM	4–6
	Methadone	0.1–0.2	IV, IM	4–6
	Butorphanol	0.01–0.4	IV, IM	2–4
	Buprenorphine	0.005–0.02	IV, IM	6–8
	Fentanyl	Three 10 mg patches (100 μg/h)	Transdermal	48–72
α-2 agonists	Xylazine	0.2–1.0	IV, IM	0.3–1.0
	Detomidine	0.01–0.04	IV, IM	1–2
	Medetomidine	0.005–0.007	IV, IM	1–4
	Dexmedetomidine	0.0025–0.0035	IV, IM	1–4
	Romifidine	0.04–0.08	IV, IM	4
Local anesthetics	Lidocaine	1.3–2.3 (loading dose)	IV	CRI: 3 mg/kg/hour
Nonconventional drugs	Butylscopolamine	0.2–0.3 (once)	IV	4–6
	Ketamine	0.2–0.5	IV, IM	6–8
	Gabapentin	20–40	PO	

Routes of drug administration: IV, intravenous; IM, intramuscular; NSAIDs, nonsteroidal anti-inflammatory drugs; PO, per os. Dosages are based on references quoted in the text.

of the most significant clinical manifestations of inflammation, and treatment with NSAIDs (Chapter 5) continues to be the mainstay of pain therapy in the horse (Table 30.4).

Hyperalgesia typically accompanies inflammation, and is produced by mediator substances released in response to tissue injury and repair (Woolf & Salter, 2000; Muir, 2005; Goodrich & Nixon, 2006). Among the key players in hyperalgesia are prostaglandins (PGs), formed via the action of cyclooxygenase (COX) enzymes. Released locally in the injured or inflamed tissue, PGs contribute to sensitization of peripheral nociceptors, and PGs in the dorsal horn of the spinal cord contribute to the accelerated and amplified response of secondary afferents to nociceptive input from the periphery (central sensitization), thereby augmenting, and possibly changing, the quality of pain perception (Svensson & Yaksh, 2002; Coutaux et al., 2005; Yaksh, 2006).

During the past decade, novel NSAIDs that preferentially (meloxicam, etodolac) or highly selectively (firocoxib) inhibit

COX-2 have become available for use in horses. Initially expected to be therapeutically superior, this view has been challenged both in human and veterinary medicine (Simon, 1998). The long-held belief that inhibition of the COX-1 isoenzyme causes the many adverse effects associated with use of NSAIDs, such as gastrointestinal ulceration and hemorrhage, coagulopathy, and nephropathy, and that inhibition of COX-2 was thought to be primarily responsible for the anti-inflammatory and analgesic actions of these agents, has proven to be untrue (Divers, 2008; Blikslager, 2009). New laboratory data indicate that suppression of inflammation-evoked central nociceptive activity and hyperalgesia by NSAIDs may, however, be related to their selectivity for COX isoforms. The COX-2 isoform seems to be primarily involved in the initiation, but not necessarily the maintenance, of nociceptive spinal neuron activation, which may largely depend on COX-1 (Urdaneta et al., 2009). In contrast, in the absence of any extensive peripheral inflammation, spinally initiated hyperalgesia has been shown to be mediated exclusively by constitutive COX-2, likely localized within the spinal cord dorsal horn. This argues for the prescription of selective COX-2 inhibitors as antihyperalgesic agents under circumstances of inflammation-independent central nociceptive sensitization (Yaksh et al., 2001). In principle, inflammation is the common pathological characteristic of tissue trauma, and hence the trigger for increased spinal sensory nerve excitability in the majority of musculoskeletal and visceral disease conditions of the horse. Therefore, these laboratory findings suggest that the continued use of nonselective or even COX-1 preferential NSAIDs as potentially more effective candidates for analgesic therapy is not only justified but may even be warranted. Unfortunately, clinical studies in horses investigating the analgesic efficacy of NSAIDs with different COX-1/COX-2 selectivity ratios under different conditions of trauma and inflammation and during different phases of the disease process are very sparse. Therefore, at this point, it is too early to draw definite conclusions as to which NSAIDs, under which circumstances, are better suited for equine pain therapy. For the time being, all currently available NSAIDs listed in Table 30.4 should be considered appropriate for the treatment of mild to severe, acute, persistent, or chronic pain in the horse. They may differ in potency and therapeutic efficacy depending upon the underlying disease process for which they are being prescribed, pharmacokinetic characteristics resulting in variable tissue uptake and residence times, their efficacy in inhibiting COX isoenzymes at peripheral and central sites, type of cytokine production, mechanisms other than COX inhibition contributing to their anti-inflammatory and antinociceptive/analgesic actions, and their analgesic versus anti-inflammatory effect profile. For example, Owens et al. (1995) compared the therapeutic efficacy of phenylbutazone (PBZ) and ketoprofen (Ketofen®) in laminitic horses with chronic hoof pain. While the recommended therapeutic doses of PBZ (4.4 mg/kg) and ketoprofen (2.2 mg/kg) were roughly equivalent in their efficacy to provide analgesia and decrease lameness, a 3.6 mg/kg dose of ketoprofen (a PBZ equimolar dose) produced a greater reduction in lameness, presumably due to a greater antinociceptive activity. Interestingly, the stereoisomers of ketoprofen are also known to exert antinociceptive actions through mechanisms other than COX inhibition. The R(-)-enantiomer of ketoprofen suppresses tactile allodynia via a yet to be defined mechanism of action, and the S(+)-enantiomer produces analgesia through mechanisms involving serotoninergic pathways at the spinal and supraspinal levels (Ossipov et al., 2000; Diaz-Reval et al., 2004). In addition, ketoprofen has been demonstrated to exert antihyperalgesic activity in dairy cows suffering from unilateral hindlimb lameness (Whay et al., 2005). In a clinical trial of acute equine joint synovitis, PBZ was superior to ketoprofen in the treatment of the acute joint inflammation (Owens et al., 1996a). Thus, one may conclude that ketoprofen may not be consistently superior to other nonselective NSAIDs, even though, in general, it provides good-to-excellent analgesia for musculoskeletal pain (Goodrich & Nixon, 2006). Unfortunately, ketoprofen is restricted to parenteral administration given its extremely low oral bioavailability, which somewhat limits its use for long-term therapy (Goodrich & Nixon, 2006).

FLUNIXIN MEGLUMINE

Flunixin meglumine (Banamine®, Finadyne®), a nonselective COX inhibitor, is known for its much lower toxicity compared to PBZ (Trillo et al., 1984). In horses with abdominal pain, the drug usually produces good analgesia when administered IV at a dose of 1 mg/kg. Therefore, flunixin meglumine is still the most commonly used NSAID in horses with gastrointestinal discomfort (Zimmel, 2003); however, the agent has been shown to impair epithelial restitution, and hence recovery of intestinal barrier function, following ischemic bowel injury, an adverse response that has not been observed with more COX-2 selective agents such as etodolac, deracoxib, and firocoxib (Campbell & Blikslager, 2000; Tomlinson & Blikslager, 2005; Letendre et al., 2008; Cook et al., 2009).

The efficacy of flunixin meglumine in reducing lameness (Houdeshell & Hennessy, 1977) and providing long-lasting postoperative analgesia (Johnson et al., 1993), and its capacity to inhibit PGE$_2$ synthesis in synovial membranes (Moses et al., 2001), have been documented in the equine species. However, clinically the drug does not seem to be more efficacious than PBZ. Erkert et al. (2005), applying a force plate analysis system to evaluate the analgesic efficacy of flunixin meglumine and PBZ at clinically used doses in horses with navicular syndrome, found that both NSAIDs exhibited similar analgesic effects. What these data indicate, however, is that flunixin meglumine may be appropriate not only for animals suffering from pain of visceral or soft tissue origin, but also for horses afflicted by musculoskeletal pain, particularly those more susceptible (i.e., geriatric horses, ponies, foals, and those with compromised vascular, hemodynamic, renal, or hepatic function) to the adverse effects of NSAIDs with a more narrow therapeutic index such as PBZ. Flunixin meglumine is not recommended for intramuscular administration.

CARPROFEN

Carprofen (Rimadyl®) was developed for use in dogs in an attempt to identify NSAIDs with superior anti-inflammatory efficacy, yet reduced gastrointestinal toxicity. Widely used in small animal practice because of its preferential COX-2 activity in these species, carprofen lacks COX-2 selectivity in the equine (Brideau et al., 2001; Beretta et al., 2005). Although its mode of action in the horse has not yet been fully elucidated, it probably also includes COX-independent mechanisms. Overall, carprofen exerts only minimal COX inhibition both in vitro and in vivo, yet tends to accumulate in inflamed tissues and exudates similar to other NSAIDs (Goodrich & Nixon, 2006), making it a candidate for pain therapy. In fact, at doses of 0.7 mg/kg IV or 1.4 mg/kg orally (twice the recommended dose), it exhibits analgesic effects in horses under experimental and clinical conditions (Johnson et al., 1993). Furthermore, experimental evidence has accumulated demonstrating that carprofen may have beneficial effects on proteoglycan metabolism of equine chondrocytes, and protect articular cartilage from inflammatory damage, thus creating a distinct therapeutic niche for this drug in the treatment of osteoarthritis, despite its narrow therapeutic index (Goodrich & Nixon, 2006).

MELOXICAM

Meloxicam (Metacam®), at a concentration that in vitro inhibits 50% of COX enzyme activity (IC$_{50}$), is a far more selective COX-2 inhibitor than flunixin meglumine or PBZ in the horse; however, at higher concentrations COX-1 is increasingly inhibited (Beretta et al., 2005). A dose of 0.6 mg/kg meloxicam produces anti-inflammatory and analgesic effects in ponies and horses, including alleviation of lameness and reduced production of heat, protein, lactic dehydrogenase, leukocyte numbers, PGE$_2$, thromboxane B$_2$ (TXB$_2$), bradykinin, and Substance P at the sites of inflammation

(Lees et al., 1991; Toutain & Cester, 2004; De Grauw et al., 2009). Pharmacokinetic data for meloxicam in the equine have been determined, and indicate that a once-daily dose of meloxicam of 0.6 mg/kg is appropriate, and that bioavailability is close to 100% after oral administration, regardless of the feeding status (Lees et al., 1991; Toutain & Cester, 2004; Sinclair et al., 2006).

ETODOLAC

Etodolac (Etogesic®) is an NSAID that is four times more selective for COX-2 compared to COX-1 (Davis et al., 2007). Though licensed only for the treatment of osteoarthritis in humans and dogs, repeated positive drug testing results in race horses indicate the agent is also used in the equine. The agent has been investigated in the horse in search of an NSAID with less severe (especially gastrointestinal) adverse effects than flunixin meglumine. *In vitro* data suggest that etodolac selectively inhibits production of certain (e.g., PGE_2 and PgI_2) but not all prostanoids (e.g., TXA_2) in ischemic injured equine jejunum (Campbell & Blikslager, 2000). In contrast, flunixin meglumine at an equivalent concentration fully inhibits synthesis of all prostanoids. These findings were associated with superior recovery of intestinal barrier function in etodolac-treated tissues. Furthermore, etodolac was shown to be less deleterious to colonic mucosa compared with flunixin (Campbell et al., 2002), and has fewer adverse effects on colonic motility when compared to the nonselective COX inhibitor indomethacin (Van Hoogmoed et al., 2002).

Etodolac, given orally every 12 or 24 hours to horses at a dose of 23 mg/kg, provides musculoskeletal analgesia (Morton et al., 2005; Symonds et al., 2006). The drug is very effective in the horse, particularly when compared with humans, and more efficacious than flunixin meglumine or PBZ (Beretta et al., 2005; Davis et al., 2007b). The pharmacokinetic properties of etodolac have been reported (Davis et al., 2007b). Doses of 20 mg/kg administered once or twice daily IV or orally have been used clinically in horses that had shown prior gastrointestinal toxicity from other NSAIDs (PBZ, flunixin meglumine), and no overt toxicity was noted (Davis et al., 2007b). This coincides with the report of Symonds et al. (2006) who did not observe signs of toxicity in clinical trials following oral doses of 23 mg/kg either once or twice a day over a period of 3 days.

ELTENAC

Eltenac (Toxline®) is an acetic acid derivative. Although not extensively studied, there is evidence that eltenac is an efficacious NSAID in horses when used at recommended doses. In randomized, placebo-controlled, double-blinded studies, a 1 mg/kg IV dose significantly improved pain-related lameness and postoperative wound swelling (Prügner et al., 1991; Goodrich et al., 1998). Eltenac (0.5 mg/kg) is also as effective as flunixin meglumine (1.1 mg/kg) in relieving pain and inflammation in experimentally induced equine carpitis (Hamm et al., 1997). MacKay et al. (2000) demonstrated significant antiendotoxic activity of eltenac (0.5 mg/kg IV) in experimental horses; thus, potentially providing clinical benefit in horses with endotoxemia similar to that demonstrated for flunixin meglumine. In addition, the effects of eltenac are long lasting, with a dosing interval of once every 24 hours recommended for most conditions. The pharmacokinetic profile of eltenac has been examined in horses (Dyke et al., 1998). It has a short plasma half-life

of between 1.7 and 3 hours, and a small volume of distribution (~0.2 L/kg). Unlike PBZ, there was no indication of accumulation in plasma after 4 days of repeated IV administration (0.5 mg/kg). The safety of eltenac (0.5 mg/kg) in horses appears to be similar to other commonly used NSAIDs (Goodrich et al., 1998). However, higher doses (1.5 and 2.5 mg/kg IV) administered daily for 15 days caused dose-dependent signs of toxicity.

VEDAPROFEN

Vedaprofen (Quadrisol®) is structurally related to ketoprofen and carprofen (Lees et al., 1999). It is approved in Europe for the horse for treatment of inflammation and pain associated with musculoskeletal disorders and soft tissue lesions (traumatic injuries and surgical trauma), as well as for relief of pain associated with colic. In a recent field trial, 96 horses with radiographic evidence of osteoarthritis and clinically diagnosed lameness received vedaprofen treatment (initially 2 mg/kg orally and then 1 mg/kg orally twice daily) for 2 weeks. Of the horses treated with vedaprofen, 56% showed improvement with respect to lameness, and 33% showed improvement with respect to pain upon limb manipulation (Koene et al., 2010). In ponies, vedaprofen (1.1–3.0 mg/kg IV) reversed, in a dose-dependent fashion, the inhibition of intestinal contractile activity observed in the ileum following endotoxin challenge, and also abolished systemic effects on respiratory and cardiovascular functions, body temperature, and hematocrit (Renault et al., 2003). The drug is available both in gel form for oral administration and as an injectable solution for IV administration. It has pharmacokinetic and pharmacodynamic properties very similar to ketoprofen (Lees et al., 1999).

FIROCOXIB

Firocoxib is by far the most COX-2-selective NSAID approved for control of osteoarthritis-related pain and inflammation in the horse (McCann et al., 2002). The paste formulation (Equioxx®) is administered orally at a dose of 0.1 mg/kg. A formulation for intravenous administration is also available.

Pharmacokinetic studies indicate an average bioavailability of 79% and an average elimination half-life of approximately 30–40 hours after oral and IV administration (Kvaternick et al., 2007; Lettendre et al., 2008). Doucet et al. (2008) compared the efficacy and safety of oral firocoxib (0.1 mg/kg per day) and PBZ (4.4 mg/kg per day) in 253 horses with naturally occurring osteoarthritis. By day 14, horses that were treated with firocoxib improved significantly more than animals treated with PBZ with regard to pain scores during manipulation or palpation, joint circumference score, and range of motion score; however, there was no difference between groups in overall lameness or joint swelling scores. No direct treatment-related adverse effects were detected during the trial. In a recent study, the analgesic effects of increasing doses of firocoxib were tested in 64 horses with chronic lameness due to osteoarthritis (Back et al., 2009). Force plate measurements revealed that increasing the dose of the COX-2 inhibitor from 0.1 to 0.25 mg/kg did not produce any better outcome. Finally, the field trial by Koene et al. (2010) demonstrated that firocoxib (0.1 mg/kg per day PO) was significantly more efficacious than vedaprofen. Of the horses receiving firocoxib, 65% displayed improvement in lameness and 44% showed improvement with respect to pain on manipulation after 2 weeks of treatment.

In horses with ischemic bowel injury, firocoxib may offer significant advantages over flunixin meglumine, as the drug seems to better support postischemic intestinal epithelial recovery (Cook et al., 2009), coinciding with the effect of other more selective COX-2 inhibitors (Marshall & Blikslager, 2011). Hilton et al. (2011) examined the distribution of orally administered flunixin meglumine (1.1 mg/kg per day) and firocoxib (0.1. mg/kg per day) in horses with healthy eyes, and found that the COX-2 inhibitor penetrates the aqueous humor better than flunixin meglumine. Firocoxib may, therefore, be considered for the treatment of horses with inflammatory ophthalmic diseases. The risk of developing adverse effects is similar to that of a nonselective NSAID.

Opioids

Opioids (Table 30.4) (Chapter 4) are generally indicated for moderate to severe pain (Martin, 1983; Inturrisi, 2002). However, their analgesic efficacy in horses compared to other species is less well defined, especially when used at common clinical doses. At high doses (i.e., ≥0.1 mg/kg) that have supporting experimental and clinical evidence for antinociceptive or analgesic efficacy (see Bennett & Steffey, 2002; Clutton, 2010 for detailed reviews), butorphanol, methadone, or morphine may provoke central excitatory responses and undesirable locomotor activity, requiring their combination with sedatives such as acepromazine or α-2 agonists (Clark & Clark, 1999; Bennett & Steffey, 2002; Driessen, 2007; Clutton, 2010; Knych et al., 2013). When combined with phenothiazines such as acepromazine, opioids produce a state of neuroleptanalgesia or in higher doses one of neuroleptanesthesia, characterized by an indifference of the animal to its environment and potent analgesia. In addition, these opioids decrease gastrointestinal motility and can cause colonic impaction (Roger et al., 1985; Boscan et al., 2006), which may limit their long-term use in animals with persistent pain. However, pain itself can promote the development of ileus and postoperative gastrointestinal complications (colic) are caused by a multitude of factors (Clutton, 2010).

Combining lower doses of μ-opioid agonists with low doses of α-2 agonists (preferably in the form of a CRI) may achieve the desired level of analgesia by making use of the well-described synergism between the two drug classes, while avoiding profound CNS stimulatory effects of the opioids and adverse hemodynamic effects of α-2 agonists. However, impaired intestinal motility caused by opioids and α-2 agonists (Sasaki et al., 2000) remains a concern with long-term treatment. Whether opioids elicit less CNS stimulatory effects, and are more effective in horses experiencing pain as a result of a naturally occurring disease compared to pain from experimental noxious stimulation (Clutton, 2010) is controversial, as any scientific evidence for this claim is lacking.

Controlled trials in human patients revealed efficacy of opioids against peripheral neuropathic pain and some components of central neuropathic pain (Finnerup et al., 2005; Dworkin et al., 2007). However, there is also laboratory animal and human clinical evidence that long-term use of μ-opioid agonists, such as morphine, can trigger the development of a state of opioid-induced hyperalgesia (OIH), whereby a subject receiving opioids for the treatment of pain may actually become more sensitive to pain (Angst, 2006; Silverman, 2009). This potentially profound adverse effect should be considered when prescribing long-term opioid therapy in horses, even if the mechanisms leading to OIH and its clinical relevance are still being debated and the phenomenon is not described in horses (Fishbain, 2009).

BUTORPHANOL

Butorphanol (Torbugesic®), a κ-opioid receptor agonist and μ-opioid receptor antagonist, is probably the most widely used opioid in equine species. Kalpravidh et al. (1984a, 1984b) studied the antinociceptive effects of IV butorphanol (0.05–0.4 mg/kg) against experimentally induced superficial and visceral pain in horses and ponies. Analgesic effects of butorphanol in horses were dose-related and lasted 15–90 minutes, and a dose of 0.2 mg/kg IV was considered to provide optimal analgesia (Kalpravidh et al., 1984a). In ponies, an IV dose of 0.2 mg/kg of butorphanol provided good effect against visceral nociception for a period of 4 hours; however, in ponies and in horses it was accompanied by adverse behavioral effects (Kalpravidh et al., 1984b). In accordance with those findings, IV butorphanol at a dose of 0.1 mg/kg did not produce satisfactory analgesia in a clinical cohort of colicky horses (Jöchle et al., 1989). The drug's relatively short half-life after IV and IM bolus administration and low bioavailability after IM administration (37%), limits its use as an analgesic in clinical practice, and calls for frequent drug administration (at least every 1–3 hours) or a CRI (13–25 μg/kg/h) to achieve the clinically effective plasma concentrations of 10 ng/mL or greater (Sellon et al., 2001, 2004, 2008). The most recent pharmacokinetic study was performed by Knych et al. (2012) in 10 horses that were given IV butorphanol at a dose of 0.1 mg/kg. Using a highly sensitive analytical chemistry technique (limit of detection 0.01 ng/mL) the authors found an average elimination half-life of 5.9 ± 1.5 hours (3.8–8.1 hours); however, butorphanol plasma concentrations declined within 2 hours to below the 10 ng/mL mark.

Scientific evidence for analgesic efficacy of single-dose butorphanol administration at doses commonly applied in the clinical setting (5–30 μg/kg) is missing (Bennett & Steffey, 2002; Driessen, 2007; Clutton, 2010). Unlike other domestic species, administration of butorphanol and other opioids (e.g., morphine, fentanyl) to horses does not consistently reduce dose requirements for inhalational anesthetics (Bennett & Steffey, 2002; Bettschart-Wolfensberger & Larenza, 2007; Auckburally & Flaherty, 2011). A recent clinical study in horses undergoing a balanced anesthetic regimen including isoflurane and a CRI of medetomidine revealed that addition of a butorphanol CRI (25 μg/kg/h) did not further reduce the inhalational anesthetic requirements (Bettschart-Wolfensberger et al., 2011), corroborating similar previous observations with administration of morphine in xylazine- or halothane-anesthetized horses (Bennett et al., 2004). The meaning of these inconsistent findings with respect to whether systemically administered opioids mediate any clinically relevant antinociceptive/analgesic action in the horse remains unclear.

TRANSDERMAL FENTANYL PATCHES

Transdermal administration of fentanyl (Duragesic®), a potent but very short-acting synthetic μ-opioid receptor agonist, does not consistently alleviate musculoskeletal pain (Wegner et al., 2002; Thomasy et al., 2004). If fentanyl patches were to be used as part of multimodal pain management one should probably apply as many patches as necessary to achieve plasma fentanyl concentrations generally considered to be analgesic in other species (≥ 1 ng/mL) (Orsini et al., 2006) (Table 30.4).

BUPRENORPHINE

Buprenorphine (Buprenex®) is a partial μ-opioid agonist and κ-opioid antagonist, which is thought to have a ceiling effect in horses, though data supporting this assumption have not been reported (Bennett & Steffey, 2002). When applied as a sole analgesic agent in horses, measurable antinociception has been reported to occur at doses of 10 μg/kg or greater, but significant excitement, hemodynamic stimulation, and long-lasting reduction in gastrointestinal motility were noted as well (Carregaro et al., 2007; Davis et al., 2011). Walker (2007) reported a case of a filly with severe head and neck trauma that was administered buprenorphine (6 μg/kg every 12 hours) for 5 days via the sublingual/buccal mucosal route of administration. The drug provided clinically effective analgesia, when given twice daily, without provoking signs of excitement or toxicity. Signs of GI distress were not noted.

Davis et al. (2011) determined the pharmacokinetic profile of buprenorphine after IV and IM administration (5 μg/kg) to six horses. They described an elimination half-life of 3.6 ± 3.9 hours (1.4–13.3 hours) after IV administration, and a bioavailability after IM injection of the same dose of 65 ± 17% (51–88%) in four of the six horses.

In conclusion, it appears unrealistic to expect systemic opioids to effectively contribute to pain relief in the equine, unless drugs like butorphanol, methadone, and morphine are dosed markedly higher than currently used in clinical practice. Only clinical experience will tell how much accompanying sedation is required, in animals with moderate to severe pain, to attenuate excitatory behavioral responses to these drugs, and to what extent gastrointestinal complications will occur.

α-2 Adrenoceptor Agonists

α-2 agonists (Chapter 7) are among the most commonly used analgesics in equine practice. They provide analgesia primarily through spinal and supraspinal mechanisms, although peripheral mechanisms may contribute (Daunt & Steffey, 2002; Valverde, 2010).

Three α-2 agonists are currently licensed in North America and in Europe for use in horses: xylazine (Rompun®), detomidine (Dormosedan®), and romifidine (Sedivet®). In addition, **medetomidine** (Domitor®) and dexmedetomidine (Dexdomitor®) have been administered off-label to horses. Potent analgesic effects have been reported in numerous equine studies (e.g., Muir & Robertson, 1985; Brunson & Majors, 1987; Kamerling et al., 1988; Jöchle, 1989; Jöchle et al., 1989; Chambers et al., 1993; Owens et al., 1996b; Naylor et al., 1997; Moens et al., 2003; Figueiredo et al., 2005; Spadavecchia et al., 2005; Wagner et al., 2011); however, marked sedation and centrally mediated muscle relaxation frequently accompany antinociceptive effects, complicating assessment of drug-induced analgesia.

Many of the characteristics of the individual α-2 agonists, with respect to duration of action and degree of sedation and analgesia produced, can be explained by differences in receptor binding specificity and affinity, as well as in pharmacokinetic properties. The α-2: α-1 selectivity ratios for xylazine, detomidine, and medetomidine/

dexmedetomidine are 160, 260, and 1620, respectively (Virtanen et al., 1988). For romifidine, Ki values (expressing the affinity of a ligand to a receptor) at α-1 adrenoceptors (rat neocortex) of 241 nM and at α-2 receptors (human α-2A in transfected cells) of 9.4 nM have been reported (Virtanen, 2010, personal communication), revealing an α-2:α-1 selectivity ratio of only 26. Furthermore, it should be noted that the compound is only a partial agonist at both α-1 and α-2 receptors (Virtanen, 2010, personal communication). Among all α-2 agonists, medetomidine and dexmedetomidine are by far the most α-2 selective compounds available in clinical practice. In the lower-dose range (<5 μg/kg), both drugs exhibit less pronounced α-1-mediated effects on the circulatory system in horses (Yamashita et al., 2000).

In the equine, the plasma elimination half-lives of α-2 agonists indicate a distinctly longer duration of drug action for romifidine (≈138 minutes) compared to xylazine (≈50 minutes), medetomidine (≈51 minutes), dexmedetomidine (≈23 minutes), and detomidine (≈30–71 minutes) (Garcia-Villar et al., 1981; Dyer et al., 1987; Salonen et al., 1989; Bettschart-Wolfensberger et al., 1999; Grimsrud et al., 2009; Wojtasiak-Wypart et al., 2012). All α-2 agonists can be used as a single IV or IM dose. As Table 30.4 indicates, the dosing range is quite broad, with higher doses tending to produce longer duration of effect, but also causing more adverse effects. The pharmacokinetic data support the administration of α-2 agonists in the form of CRIs (Table 30.3). This mode of application not only allows better titration to clinical endpoints with less risk of severe adverse effects, but also provides prolonged periods of consistent analgesia and/or sedation. For example, after an IV loading dose of 6–9 μg/kg of detomidine, a CRI of 0.4–0.6 μg/kg/min is initiated, which then is successively decreased every 15–30 minutes by up to 50% until an adequate degree of analgesia and sedation can be maintained (Wilson et al., 2002). Likewise, medetomidine or dexmedetomidine can be infused after a loading dose of 2–5 and 1.0–2.5 μg/kg, respectively, starting at a rate of 0.4–0.6 and 0.1–0.3 μg/kg/min, respectively, and then successively be reduced in 10–15 minute intervals until eventually reaching a CRI rate of 0.0125–0.025 and 0.025–0.050 μg/kg/min, respectively. Because of their potent analgesic properties, CRIs of α-2 agonists have become a popular component of balanced anesthesia, balanced analgesia, and TIVA protocols (Bettschart-Wolfensberger & Larenza, 2007; Caulkett, 2007; Staffieri & Driessen, 2007; Auckburally & Flaherty, 2011).

All α-2 agonists produce a significant decrease in cardiac output, an initial increase followed by a decrease in blood pressure, bradycardia, decreased gastric emptying, and long-lasting reduction in gut motility (large intestines > small intestines) upon repeated, continuous and/or higher-dose administration (Merritt et al., 1998; Doherty et al., 1999; Sasaki et al., 2000; Freeman & England, 2001; Freeman et al., 2002; Sutton et al., 2002; Elfenbein et al., 2009; Wojtasiak-Wypart et al., 2012). This must be taken into consideration, particularly in the immediate postoperative/postanesthetic period when residual anesthetic drug effects are still prevailing or when these drugs are repeatedly or continuously administered for treatment of persistent pain in the awake horse. Furthermore, the prominent cardiovascular and CNS depressant effects limit the extent to which α-2 agonists can be employed in pain management for horses with colic signs that may already be suffering from compromised gastrointestinal perfusion. In addition, profound analgesia as a result of repetitive or continued α-2 agonist administration carries the risk of postponing a necessary surgical intervention for lack of display of sufficiently severe signs of pain and discomfort signifying a worsening of the underlying pathophysiological disease process. Caution must be exercised particularly with longer-acting agents.

Local Anesthetics

SYSTEMIC LIDOCAINE

The clinical use of systemic lidocaine (Chapter 6) for pain treatment in humans was first reported more than half a century ago (Mao & Chen, 2000), and during the past decade IV lidocaine has gained much popularity in equine practice. Current understanding of how the local anesthetic affects pain in equine species remains unclear (Valverde & Gunkel, 2005; Driessen, 2005; Doherty & Seddighi, 2010).

Intravenous lidocaine must be administered as a CRI (Table 30.3) due to its short elimination half-life (79 ± 41 minutes; Feary et al., 2005). In horses, a loading dose of 1.3–1.5 mg/kg, administered slowly IV over 3–15 minutes, followed by a CRI of 50–100 µg/kg/min is most commonly used (Valverde & Gunkel, 2005; Driessen, 2007; Doherty & Seddighi, 2010). Doherty and Frazier (1998) reported the anesthetic-sparing effect of systemic lidocaine in halothane-anesthetized ponies; reduction ranged from 30–70% depending upon infusion dose and corresponding plasma concentrations (2.1–7.0 µg/mL). Anesthetic sparing effects of 20–25% have been observed with lidocaine infusion in horses undergoing inhalational anesthesia with either isoflurane or sevoflurane for elective orthopedic or emergency abdominal surgeries (Dzikiti et al., 2003; Driessen, 2005). These studies suggested, but did not prove, the possibility of an analgesic action of lidocaine in the horse. Likewise, an electroencephalographic (EEG) study in ponies undergoing castration during halothane anesthesia and receiving a CRI of lidocaine provided indirect evidence of a centrally mediated antinociceptive action (Murrell et al., 2005). The local anesthetic suppressed those EEG activities that were identified earlier in these ponies as indicative of noxious stimulation during castration. Another study by Robertson et al. (2005) produced inconclusive data. The authors conducted a randomized, blinded crossover study with saline to determine whether a bolus dose of lidocaine (2 mg/kg) followed by infusion (50 µg/kg/min) increased skin thermal or duodenal and colorectal distension pressure thresholds that produced discomfort in awake horses. At the relatively low plasma concentrations (0.7–1.2 µg/mL) measured, sustained antinociceptive activity was recorded against heat (somatic), but not viscero-mechanical stimuli. Other data regarding the immediate analgesic effect of lidocaine on naturally occurring pain in animals or human patients are also inconsistent, and this may be in part due to certain nociceptive mechanisms and pathways not being targeted by lidocaine, and highly variable drug plasma concentrations among subjects (Mao & Chen, 2000; Driessen, 2007; Gormsen et al., 2009).

Higher infusion rates, at least in awake animals, carry the risk of cardio- and neurotoxicity (Meyer et al., 2001). Plasma concentrations achieved during long-term infusion vary widely among horses, and may accumulate over time (Feary et al., 2005; Robertson et al., 2005; Feary et al., 2006; De Solis & McKenzie, 2007; Dickey et al., 2008); monitoring of plasma concentrations (via a lidocaine ELISA kit; Neogen Corporation, Lansing, MI 48912, USA) is ideal, not only to avoid toxicity but also to ensure that concentrations known to reduce nociceptive behaviors in experimental animals (approximately 1.2–2.1 µg/mL; Mao & Chen, 2000; Robertson et al., 2005) are being achieved.

Information from laboratory animal investigations indicates that any potential antinociceptive action of IV lidocaine is far more complex than previously thought. Besides its well-studied local anesthetic actions (i.e., Na^+ channel blockade) in the peripheral and central nervous systems, lidocaine also exerts multiple other mechanisms of action that may target the spinal and supraspinal nociceptive systems (Woolf & Wiesenfeld-Hallin, 1985; Ness, 2000; Lauretti, 2008). Laboratory animal and controlled clinical trials in humans have found that IV lidocaine suppresses the development of peripheral hyperalgesia as well as central nociceptive sensitization and allodynia (Mao & Chen, 2000; Attal et al., 2004; Lauretti, 2008). Its efficacy as an analgesic and antineuropathic agent has recently been demonstrated in adult patients suffering from chronic pain with tactile hyperalgesia and/or mechanical allodynia for more than 3 months as a result of a peripheral nerve injury (Gormsen et al., 2009). In that trial, IV lidocaine failed to produce any alleviation of spontaneous pain from an acute nerve injury, but significantly reduced evoked pain. Nonetheless, it has been reported that systemic lidocaine may inhibit acute spontaneous pain (Mao & Chen, 2000; Attal et al., 2004).

In addition to its analgesic and antihyperalgesic/antineuropathic properties described above, lidocaine also has inflammation-modifying effects and has been shown to protect tissues against ischemic and reperfusion injury in various species including the horse (Doherty & Seddighi, 2010; Robertson & Sanchez, 2010), which may impact nociceptive mechanisms and pain perception.

Nontraditional Systemic Pain Therapeutics

BUTYLSCOPOLAMINE

Butylscopolamine (N-butylscopolammonium bromide [Buscopan®]) is an anticholinergic agent with spasmolytic properties that has been used in equine practice in Europe for many decades, and has obtained FDA approval for treatment of abdominal pain associated with spasmodic colic, flatulent colic, and simple impactions in horses. By inhibiting intestinal smooth muscle contraction, the drug ablates gastrointestinal peristalsis and, thus, suppresses pain responses to bowel distension. The potent spasmolytic, and thus analgesic, efficacy of butylscopolamine has been demonstrated both under experimental and clinical conditions (Keller & Faulstich, 1985; Roelvink et al., 1991; Boatwright et al., 1996; Bertone, 2002; Luo et al., 2006; Sanchez et al., 2008). The drug takes effect in less than a minute after IV administration (0.2–0.3 mg/kg), and does not last much longer than 30 minutes. In experimental horses, Keller (1986) provoked intestinal paralysis with intravenous administration of 0.4 mg/kg doses at intervals of 2 hours, with return of normal intestinal function 6–8 hours after the last injection. Colic was not induced by doses of 0.2 mg/kg injected 4 times at intervals of 2 hours, however. Of some concern, however, are the hemodynamic responses to butylscopolamine administration. In adult, noncolicky horses an IV dose of the drug (0.3 mg/kg) causes an immediate significant increase in heart rate that lasts for up to 50 minutes, and is accompanied by a significant increase in arterial blood pressure lasting for about 25 minutes

(Morton et al., 2011). If an α-2 agonist, such as xylazine, is given simultaneously, the sudden rise in arterial blood pressures is even more pronounced. Therefore, to avoid further hemodynamic complications, and also erroneous assessment of the animal with regard to pain evaluation, surgical decision making, and prognostication (Morton et al., 2011) these cardiovascular effects should be considered carefully when administering butylscopolamine to colicky horses with existing markedly increased heart rates.

Antihyperalgesic and Antineuropathic Pain Therapeutics

Ketamine

Persistent peripheral sensory nerve stimulation with ongoing nociceptive input to the spinal cord leads to activation of the NMDA receptor, a voltage- and ligand-gated ion channel complex on the postsynaptic membrane in spinal cord dorsal horn neurons. Activation of spinal NMDA receptors is a key step in both initiation and maintenance of activity-dependent central sensitization, and NMDA receptor antagonists have been shown experimentally to prevent and reverse the hyperexcitability of secondary afferent neurons that occurs soon after intense, repeated, or sustained nociceptive signal input to the dorsal horn (Giordano, 2001; Latremoliere & Woolf, 2009; Woolf, 2011). Once activated, NMDA receptors allow a rapid inward current of Ca^{2+} ions, which in turn activates a cascade of intracellular events, including the phosphorylation of NMDA receptors, subsequently causing a change in their activity and density, and thereby contributing to postsynaptic hyperexcitability (Latremoliere & Woolf, 2009).

The pharmacology of the dissociative anesthetic ketamine (Ketavet®), a racemic mixture of two stereoisomers (S- and R-enantiomers), has been addressed in detail in a preceding chapter (Chapter 8) and elsewhere (Muir, 2010c). Besides being a noncompetitive antagonist at NMDA receptors, the drug interacts with opioid and central muscarinic receptors, central voltage-gated calcium channels, and activates descending monoaminergic inhibitory pathways, all contributing to its well-known analgesic effect at higher doses (Berti et al., 2009). Based on those mechanisms, ketamine exhibits additive or synergistic effects with traditional analgesics such as opioids, NSAIDs, local anesthetics, and α-2 agonists and, as a result, reduces overall dose requirements for those analgesic drugs (De Kock & Lavand'homme, 2007).

At low doses (3–18 µg/kg/h), ketamine seems to have specific selectivity for postsynaptic NMDA receptors in the dorsal horn of the spinal cord (Berti et al., 2009). It is believed that binding of ketamine to its receptor site is greatly facilitated when the NMDA receptor is in its open state, because the high-affinity binding site is located within the channel pore. Interestingly, the more potent S-ketamine binds with an approximately four times greater affinity than R-ketamine to the receptor (Visser & Schug, 2006). Because prolonged afferent nociceptive signaling elicits sustained activation of spinal NMDA receptors, it has been proposed that low-dose ketamine will preferentially bind to those activated receptors, thereby inhibiting or reversing development of central hyperalgesia. Consequently, perioperative low-dose ketamine infusion might not be considered as an analgesic treatment in the traditional sense, but rather as an antihyperalgesic/antiallodynic modality in multimodal analgesia for patients at risk of developing chronic maladaptive pain after major tissue damage (Visser & Schug, 2006; Berti et al., 2009; Suzuki, 2009).

Clinical effects of subanesthetic (not low-dose) ketamine infusion (400 and 800 µg/kg/h) have been studied in awake horses (Fielding et al., 2006). During or after a 12-hour infusion, no obvious analgesic effects could be demonstrated, and no signs of excitement or significant changes in measured physiological variables occurred. A CRI of 400–1500 µg/kg/h has been used safely in conscious horses (Lankveld et al., 2006). Although with those infusion regimens the measured plasma ketamine concentrations were about 10 times lower than concentrations (2–4 µg/mL) associated with objectively measured acute antinociceptive effects in isoflurane-anesthetized ponies (Knobloch et al., 2006; Levionnois et al., 2010), they were within or above the range of plasma

Table 30.5. Drugs used for local and regional anesthesia/analgesia and reported concentrations and doses. Dosages are based on references quoted in the text

Duration of action	Drug	Route of administration	Onset of action	Comments
Short (60–90 min)	Procaine 1–2%	Topical	Slow	Vasoconstrictive properties
	Proparacaine 0.5%	Topical	Rapid	Used primarily in ophthalmology
Intermediate (90–240 min)	Lidocaine 1–2%	SQ, infiltration, epidural, spinal, perineural, intra-articular	Fast	
	Mepivacaine 1–2%		Fast	
Long (180–360 min)	Bupivacaine 0.5–0.75% or less	SQ, infiltration, epidural, spinal, perineural, intra-articular	Intermediate	Vasoconstrictive action at lower concentrations; less motor blockade effect
	Ropivacaine 0.2–1.0% or less		Fast	
Long (>240 min)	Lidocaine 2% plus Bupivacaine 0.5–0.75%	SQ, infiltration, perineural	Fast	
Very short (5–15 min)	Ketamine 1–2%	Perineural	Fast	

concentrations (0.02–0.12 µg/mL) at which ketamine has been shown to produce acute antinociceptive effects in awake ponies (Peterbauer et al., 2008), and antihyperalgesic activity in other animal models and human patients (Berti et al., 2009). Matthews et al. (2004) administered ketamine via infusion (400 and 800 µg/kg/h) for up to 5 days in eight horses with osteomyelitis, septic joint disease, burns, or colic in a search for analgesic effects. Responses to ketamine varied substantially, with some animals showing no or only slight improvement of pain signs, while others appeared to be markedly more comfortable within 6–12 hours of the start of drug

infusion. Likewise, the analgesic effects of ketamine in humans in states of persistent pain are inconsistent, particularly in patients suffering from hyperalgesia and neuropathic pain (Hocking & Cousins, 2003; Collins et al., 2010). Thus, in horses, as in humans, low-dose ketamine infusion may be considered an adjunctive or second- or third-tier medication for treatment of persistent pain. Whether the S-enantiomer should be preferred for long-term pain therapy in the equine because of its higher affinity to NMDA receptors and fewer behavioral side effects as compared to R-ketamine has to be determined (Muir, 2010c). At plasma concentrations of

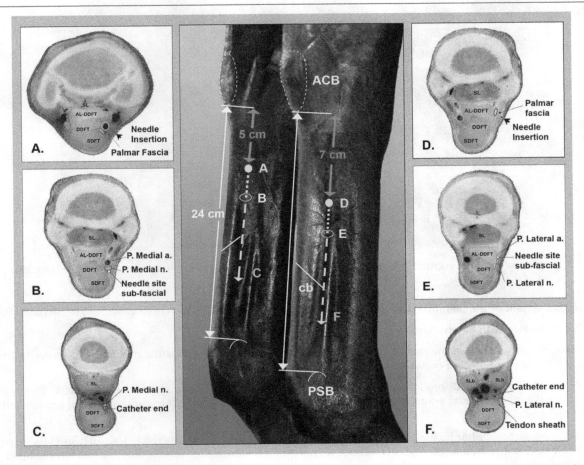

Figure 30.1. Continuous peripheral nerve blocks (CPNBs) along the palmar nerves can be performed with the horse standing, crossed-tied, or restrained in stocks in a quiet, clean area or in an operating room. Adequate sedation is typically required for CPNB catheter placement and the lower forelimbs need to be clipped and the skin surgically prepared prior to CPNB needle and catheter placement. It is essential to carefully identify the anatomical landmarks and needle placement locations. A, D = needle entry points and are approximately 5 and 7 cm from the distal margin of the accessory carpal bone (ACB); A–B, D–E = intended path for subcutaneous tunneling of the needle/catheter; B, E = subfascial needle insertion sites; B–C, E–F = intended path for subfascial placement of needle/catheter; cb, communicating branch between medial and lateral palmar nerves; A, B, C, D, E, F cross-sections = cross-sectional anatomy at the corresponding levels of the metacarpus; PSB, proximal sesamoid bone; double-arrow white lines (i.e., 24 cm) = distal margin ACB to proximal margin PSB distance measurements to estimate the needle insertion points A (20% of ACB–PSB) and D (30% of ACB–PSB). Once key landmarks have been identified, the skin, subcutaneous tissue, and palmar nerves should be properly anesthetized for subsequent CPNB catheter insertion (Figure 30.2) as well as for the intended tunneling path of the catheter. The skin and subcutaneous tissues are usually infiltrated with 4–5 mL of mepivacaine 2% at each estimated needle insertion site using a 25G needle. The injection for cutaneous anesthesia should be shallow and in a line extending dorsally to allow for subsequent tunneling of the CPNB catheter. A perineural palmar block is subsequently performed 2 cm distally, above the communicating branch, with additional 4 mL of mepivacaine 2% on each side using 25G needles.

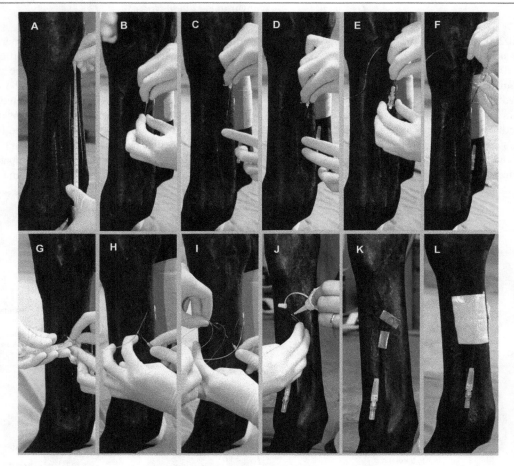

Figure 30.2. Step-by-step illustration of left lateral palmar CPNB needle/catheter placement technique (see also Figure 30.1).

A. Measurement of the distance between accessory carpal bone and the proximal sesamoid bone (ACB–PSB).

B. Perforate skin with a hypodermic needle (16G, 2.5 cm).

C. Advance under manual palpation a Tuohy–Schliff needle (18G, 8.9 cm) subcutaneously parallel to the skin for 2–2.5 cm (bevel pointing outward).

D. Redirect needle by ~20° medially and —under manual palpation— penetrate the palmar fascia, slowly advancing the needle distally for its entire length until its tip reaches a point distal to the communicating branch and proximal to the digital sheath.

E. Insert the catheter after flushing the needle with 0.5 mL of heparinized saline (HEP-SAL; 10 IU/mL) using a threading assist device attached to the hub of the needle (pink) and advance the catheter beyond the needle tip (11–12 cm).

F. Withdraw needle back to the skin level, while simultaneously advancing the catheter; carefully remove needle avoiding any withdrawal of the catheter and then adjust length.

G. Check for accidental intravascular placement, patency (1–2 mL heparinized saline), injection pressure <20 psi [1.4 bar]), and location with a small bolus of HEP-SAL under ultrasound (US) imaging; then adjust length of the inserted portion of the catheter to 8–11 cm (based on individual metacarpal anatomy measurements) to avoid excessive curling of the distal catheter tip under the palmar fascia.

H. Insert 16G hypodermic needle as a guiding tool palmar-proximally for 2–3 cm in the subcutis.

I. Feed the free (proximal) ending of catheter retrograde through 16G hypodermic needle to allow for skin tunneling of the catheter; after passage of the catheter, remove the needle and seal the skin insertion point with liquid bandage.

J. and K. Shorten the catheter to the appropriate length and thread it into a clamp-style Luer lock connector with cap; fix the resulting skin bridge formed by the catheter loop and the catheter where it exits the skin tunnel to the skin using butterfly-shaped sterile duct tape (Nextcare™ [3M]) and cyanoacrylate glue.

L. Apply a small sterile dressing and bandage.

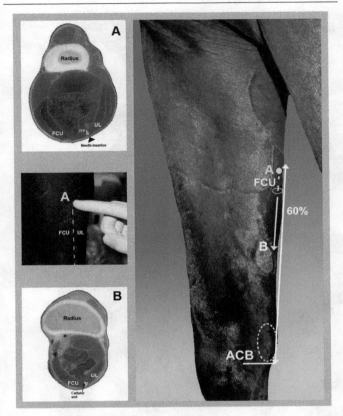

Figure 30.3. Continuous peripheral nerve block (CPNB) of the ulnar nerve can also be performed with the horse standing, as described for the palmar CPNB technique (see legend to Figure 30.1). For the ulnar CPNB technique it is essential to carefully identify the anatomical landmarks and needle placement locations. In order to obtain a good anatomical orientation, the ulnar nerve and needle skin insertion site (A) are identified on the caudal aspect of the proximal antebrachium between the flexor carpi ulnaris (FCU) and the ulnaris lateralis (UL) muscles at ~60% of the measured antebrachium length (from the accessory carpal bone (ACB) to the proximal lateral tuberosity of the radius). A, B: Anatomical cross-sectional areas of the antebrachium.

0.02–0.03 μg/mL, the racemic mixture of ketamine exhibited significant antinociceptive activity in awake ponies, while the S-enantiomer did not (Peterbauer et al., 2008).

ANTINEUROPATHIC PAIN THERAPEUTICS

Neuropathic (neurogenic) pain has been defined as pain arising as a direct consequence of a lesion or disease affecting the somatosensory system (Treede et al., 2008). Postmortem findings in horses afflicted by chronic laminitis suggest that neuropathic pain exists in the equine species (Jones et al., 2007; Yaksh, 2010). Unlike in human medicine where guidelines for diagnosis and grading of neuropathic (as opposed to nonneuropathic) pain are published and widely accepted (Cruccu & Truini, 2009; Haanpaa et al., 2011), no such guidelines have been developed in veterinary medicine; and,

thus, one may only speculate about the prevalence of neuropathic pain in equine and other domestic animal species.

Evidence-based guidelines for the pharmacological treatment of neuropathic pain, though not completely uniform, have been broadly published in the human medical literature (Dworkin et al., 2007; Moulin et al., 2007; O'Connor & Dworkin, 2009; McGeeney, 2009; Bohlega et al., 2010; De Leon-Casasola, 2011). All recent guidelines recommend certain antidepressants (i.e., tricyclic antidepressants and dual [i.e., serotonin and norepinephrine] reuptake inhibitors), drugs that have not been tested in the equine species, and calcium channel $\alpha_2\delta$ ligands (gabapentin, pregabalin) as first-line treatments for patients with neuropathic pain. Topical lidocaine is recommended for patients with localized peripheral neuropathies (e.g., postherpetic neuralgia). Controlled release opioid analgesics and tramadol, which are not useful for the horse because of pharmacokinetic properties, are recommended as second-line treatments that can be considered for first-line use in selected clinical circumstances. Other medications that generally could be used for therapy are considered third- or fourth-line treatments, and include certain other antidepressant and antiepileptic medications, topical capsaicin, mexiletine (Na^+-channel blocker), as well as NMDA receptor antagonists.

Calcium Channel $\alpha_2\delta$-ligands The anticonvulsant drugs, gabapentin and pregabalin, bind with high affinity to the $\alpha_2\delta$-1 subunit of voltage-gated calcium channels in the spinal cord and brain (Taylor, 2004; Maneuf et al., 2006; Dworkin et al., 2007). As a result, neuronal calcium currents are inhibited, ultimately causing a change in the release of neurotransmitters such as glutamate, GABA, norepinephrine, and Substance P; these actions account for much of the analgesic activity of these compounds (Dixit & Bhargava, 2002; Sills, 2006). The expression of the $\alpha_2\delta$-1 subunit has been shown in experimental neuropathic pain models to increase in chronic pain states, both in afferent sensory neurons and in the spinal cord dorsal horn (Luo et al., 2001; Newton et al., 2001). This correlates well with the observation that gabapentin exerts analgesic properties primarily in sensitized or hyperalgesic states (Harding et al., 2005; Maneuf et al., 2006; Arendt-Nielsen et al., 2007). More recently, gabapentin and pregabalin have been used clinically in humans to treat a variety of neuropathic and acute pain states, and to reduce early postsurgical pain, but with variable success (Galluzzi, 2005; Finnerup et al., 2005; Dworkin et al., 2007; Gilron, 2007; O'Connor & Dworkin, 2009; McGeeney, 2009; Zhang et al., 2011). These drugs appear especially effective in patients with paroxysmal pain (lancinating/shooting pain), brush-induced allodynia, and cold-induced allodynia/hyperalgesia, in whom they significantly lower pain scores (Ripamonti & Dickerson, 2001). Laboratory animal data suggest that the $\alpha_2\delta$-ligands also have activity against OIH (Van Elstraete et al., 2008).

Documented therapeutic use in horses refers only to oral administration of gabapentin (Neurontin®) in two animals which were thought to exhibit signs of neuropathic pain, one in conjunction with acute femoral nerve injury postsurgery, and one with a history of white line disease and chronic laminitis (Davis et al., 2007a; Dutton et al., 2009). Lacking information on pharmacokinetic properties of the drug in the equine at that time, gabapentin doses were extrapolated from use in other species (2.5 mg/kg at intervals of 8, 12, or 24 hours [Davis et al., 2007]; 2.0–3.3 mg/kg at intervals of 8 or 12 hours [Dutton et al., 2009]). In the meantime, two studies

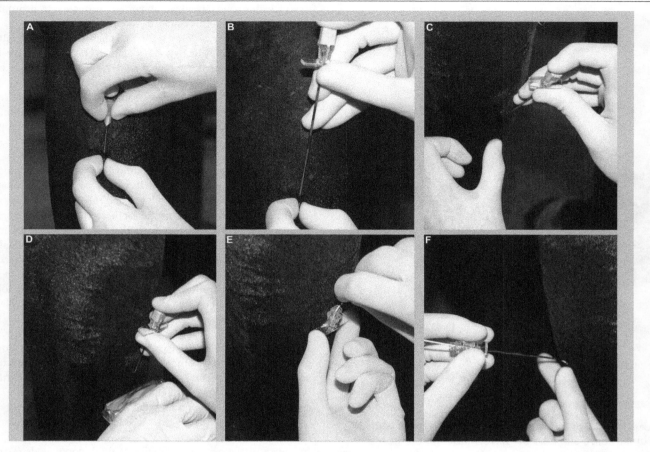

Figure 30.4. Step-by-step illustration of ulnar CPNB needle/catheter placement technique (see also Figure 30.3).

A. Perforate skin with a hypodermic needle (16G, 2.5 cm).

B. First advance a Tuohy–Schliff needle (17G, 8.9 cm) subcutaneously parallel to the skin for 2–2.5 cm (bevel pointing outward).

C. Then redirect needle ~20° medially and penetrate the fascia antebrachii.

D. Advance the needle distally under ultrasound (US) guidance with the probe at ~50° (out of line; short-axis view) for its entire length, that is, close and parallel to the ulnar nerve.

E. Insert the catheter after flushing the needle with 0.5 mL of heparinized saline (HEP-SAL; 10 IU/mL) using a threading assist device and advance beyond the needle tip (11–12 cm).

F. Withdraw needle back to the skin level, while simultaneously advancing the catheter. Carefully remove needle, avoiding any withdrawal of the catheter, and then adjust catheter length. Check for accidental intravascular placement, patency (1–2 mL HEP-SAL, injection pressure <20 psi [1.4 bar]), and location with a small bolus of HEP-SAL under US imaging.

G. Secure the catheter with the stabilization (anchoring) device by threading the catheter through posts on the crescent pad that is attached with cyanoacrylate glue and sutures to the skin.

H. Adjust catheter length and check again for correct placement of catheter.

I. Insert the 17G Tuohy needle subcutaneously disto-proximally using it as a guiding tool for subsequent subcutaneous tunneling of the catheter.

J. Feed the free (proximal) ending of the catheter retrograde through the 17G Tuohy needle.

K. Apply a butterfly-shaped sterile duct tape (Nextcare™ [3M]) to the proximal end of the catheter and secure it to the skin with cyanoacrylate glue. Thread the catheter into a snap lock Luer connector with cap.

L. Apply a small sterile dressing and bandage.

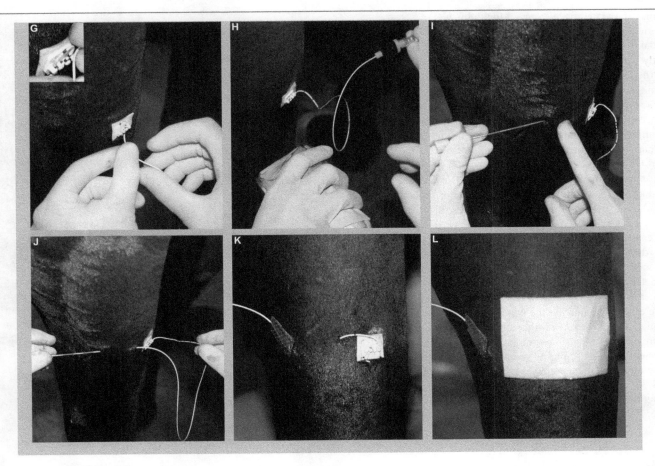

Figure 30.4. (*Continued*)

have been conducted in horses investigating the drug's pharmacokinetic properties as well as behavioral and cardiovascular parameters after IV and oral administration (Dirikolu et al., 2008; Terry et al., 2010). After IV (over 30 minutes) and oral administration of gabapentin (20 mg/kg), the median elimination half-lives were 8.5 and 7.7 hours, respectively, corresponding well with data in other species (Terry et al., 2010). After IV administration, plasma gabapentin concentrations remained above 3–4 µg/mL for approximately 15 hours, that is, plasma concentrations associated with analgesic effects in adult human volunteers (Eckhardt et al., 2000). In the horse, oral bioavailability of gabapentin is poor (~16%), and therefore plasma gabapentin concentrations decreased below the analgesic concentration threshold much more rapidly than after IV drug administration (i.e., within 2–3 hours). Neither route of gabapentin administration was associated with effects on heart rate, rhythm, or blood pressure, nor pronounced central nervous effects (Terry et al., 2010). In the human, in which gabapentin is characterized by an oral bioavailability of at least twice that in the horse, therapy for neuropathic pain usually entails three oral doses of 15–60 mg/kg of gabapentin per day (Moulin et al., 2007; O'Connor & Dworkin, 2009; Bohlega et al., 2010). It is, therefore, reasonable to predict that oral gabapentin should be administered at a dose of at least 20 mg/kg three or more times daily to obtain a clinically relevant analgesic effect against neuropathic pain.

LOCOREGIONAL ANESTHESIA AND ANALGESIA

The neuropathophysiological processes leading to the development of central hyperalgesia, neuropathic pain, and allodynia are primarily triggered by increased spontaneous firing activity in ascending sensory nerve fibers during the first 4–5 days following peripheral nerve injuries (Xie et al., 2005; Reuben & Buvanendran, 2007). Experimental evidence, and clinical experiences in human medicine, indicate that not only acute, but also persistent pain with development of central hyperalgesia, are obliterated by no other treatment modality as effectively as locoregional anesthesia and analgesia aimed at interrupting or diminishing impulse trafficking from the site of tissue injury to the CNS (Finnerup et al., 2005; Xie et al., 2005; McGeeney, 2009; Reuben & Buvanendran, 2007). These techniques may include wound infiltration or intra-articular injections with local anesthetics and opioids—topical local anesthetic application using 5% lidocaine patches (Lidoderm®); single, repetitive, or continuous peripheral nerve blocks; and epidural or intrathecal anesthesia and analgesia. It is beyond the scope of this chapter to provide a comprehensive review of the many locoregional anesthesia techniques that have been employed in the horse. Local anesthetics commonly used are listed in Table 30.5 and discussed in Chapter 6. Interested readers may consult other texts for more details (e.g., Skarda et al., 2009).

Continuous Peripheral Nerve Blockade

Continuous peripheral nerve blockade (CPNB) is a treatment modality that has long been used in human medicine, and is currently widely applied in orthopedic and trauma surgery (Boezaart, 2006). The technique entails continuous or intermittent low-dose administration of local anesthetics via catheters placed along or in close proximity to peripheral nerves, thus providing persistent pain control while reducing the need for systemic medications. Techniques for percutaneous placement of catheters close to the palmar nerves in the standing, sedated horse were recently developed (Figure 30.1 and 30.2), and provide a method for repeated or continuous perineural administration of low concentrations of local anesthetic solutions (e.g., bupivacaine or ropivacaine 0.125–0.5%) over a period of multiple days (Zarucco et al., 2007; Driessen et al., 2008a; Zarucco et al., 2010; Watts et al., 2011). The therapy can continue for longer periods by exchanging catheters every 4–8 days. With these techniques, significant analgesia can be obtained in horses with pain that is poorly responsive or even refractory to traditional systemic pain therapy. These techniques further offer the advantage of determining the intensity of the analgesic effect by adjusting the concentration of the local anesthetic solution and/or the rate of drug administration to a desired level of comfort without causing complete sensory blockade. The CPNB catheters can also be placed proximally on the thoracic limb close to the ulnar and median nerves (Zarucco et al., 2008) (Figure 30.3, 30.4, 30.5, and 30.6). These techniques may then provide significant reduction of pain perception in the entire distal forelimb (Driessen et al., 2008b).

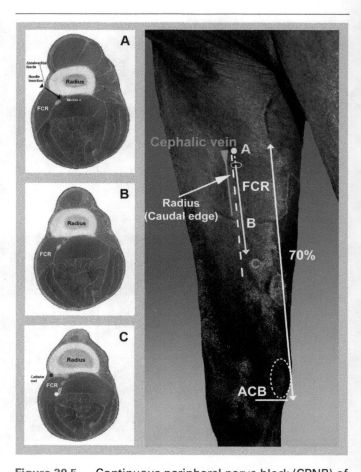

Figure 30.5. Continuous peripheral nerve block (CPNB) of the median nerve can also be performed with the horse standing, as described for the palmar CPNB technique (see legend to Figure 30.1). For the median CPNB technique it is essential to carefully identify the anatomical landmarks and needle placement locations. In order to obtain a good anatomical orientation, the median nerve and needle skin insertion site (A) are identified on the medial side of the proximal antebrachium just caudal to the cephalic vein between the caudal edge of the radius and the cranial margin of flexor carpi radialis (FCR) muscle. The needle entry point for the median nerve is located on the medial side of the proximal antebrachium just caudal to the cephalic vein between the cranial margin of the FCR and the caudal edge of the radius at a distance ~70% of the measured antebrachium length (from accessory carpal bone (ACB) to the proximal lateral tuberosity of the radius). A, B, C: Anatomical cross-sectional areas of the antebrachium.

CAUDAL EPIDURAL ANALGESIA

In horses experiencing severe pain due to lesions in their pelvic limb(s), caudal epidural (sacrococcygeal or first intercoccygeal space) administration of analgesics such as opioids (e.g., morphine 0.05–0.2 mg/kg; methadone 0.1 mg/kg), α-2 agonists (e.g., xylazine 0.17 mg/kg; detomidine 20–40 μg/kg; medetomidine 2–5 μg/kg) or a combination thereof with or without low doses of local anesthetic (e.g., bupivacaine or ropivacaine 0.125–0.25%) provides long-term pain control (Natalini & Driessen, 2007; Natalini, 2010). Unlike local anesthetics and α-2 agonists, morphine is characterized by slow onset of action (1–2 hours) but long duration of effect (3–8 hours). To allow repeated drug administration, placement of an epidural catheter that is advanced from the sacrococcygeal or first intercoccygeal space up to 30 cm cranially is recommended (Natalini & Driessen, 2007; Natalini, 2010) (Figure 30.7). Medications may be administered as intermittent boluses (15–30 mL per average adult horse) or as an infusion (0.5–3.0 mL/h). When administered with saline in total volumes of 50–70 mL epidurally, opioids (e.g., morphine 0.05–0.2 mg/kg; methadone 0.1 mg/kg) spread far enough cranially to reach the thoracic and cervical segments of the spinal cord (Hendrickson et al., 1998; Bellei et al., 2009). Therefore, these opioids may also inhibit nociception originating from organs and tissues within the pelvic, abdominal, and thoracic cavities, abdominal and chest walls, as well as thoracic limbs and hence can complement other locoregional techniques such as intercostal nerve blocks, intrapleural regional anesthesia, or peripheral nerve blocks.

TRPV1 Receptor Agonists (Capsaicin, Resiniferatoxin)

The transient receptor potential cation channel, subfamily V, member 1 (TRPV1) is a membrane ion channel that, in most species, is highly expressed in sensory neurons of the dorsal root and trigeminal ganglia giving rise to the A δ and C fibers of the primary nociceptive afferents (Grimm et al., 2011; Xia et al., 2011). The TRPV1, also referred to as vanilloid receptor, is a polymodal cation

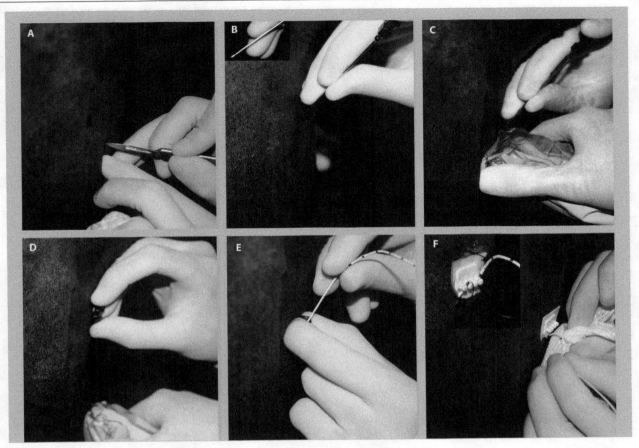

Figure 30.6. Step-by-step illustration of median CPNB needle/catheter placement technique (see also Figure 30.5).

A. Perforate skin with a no. 11 blade scalpel.

B. First advance straight bulb-end infusion needle with stylet (1.2 mm ID, 10 cm) through the skin and fascia antebrachii.

C. Then under ultrasound (US) imaging in the short axis view (out-of-line) redirect the needle by ∼30–40°.

D. Under US guidance advance the needle between the proximal margin of the flexor carpi radialis muscle (FCR) and the caudal edge of the radius distally, rotate the probe 90° (in line with the needle) and continue advancing the needle along the median nerve.

E. After withdrawal of the stylet and flushing the needle with 1.0 mL of heparinized saline (HEP-SAL; 10 IU/mL) insert the catheter into the needle hub and advance it beyond the needle tip (15–16 cm). Withdraw the needle back to skin level, while simultaneously advancing the catheter, and carefully remove it, avoiding any withdrawal of the catheter.

F. Secure the catheter with the stabilization (anchoring) device by threading the catheter through posts on the crescent pad that is attached with cyanoacrylate glue and sutures to the skin.

G. Check for accidental intravascular placement, and correct location in near vicinity of the median nerve using US imaging.

H. Check for patency by injecting a small bolus (2–3 mL HEP-SAL, injection pressure < 20 psi [1.4 bar]) under US imaging.

I. Insert a Tuohy–Schliff needle (17G, 8–9 cm) subcutaneously caudo-cranially using it as a guiding tool for subsequent subcutaneous tunneling of the catheter.

J. Feed the free (proximal) ending of the catheter retrograde through the 17G needle.

K. Apply a butterfly-shaped sterile duct tape (Nextcare™ [3M]) to the proximal end of the catheter and secure it to the skin with cyanoacrylate glue. Thread the catheter into a snap lock Luer connector with cap.

L. Apply a small sterile dressing and bandage.

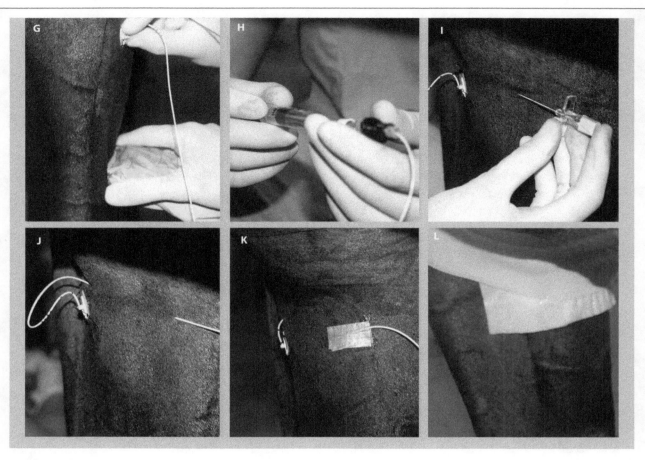

Figure 30.6. (*Continued*)

channel and is involved in sensory signaling, ranging from thermal and mechanical nociception to vision, taste, olfaction, touch, and osmosensation. The TRPV1 has been identified in horses (DaCunha et al., 2008).

Current thoughts are that peripheral perineural (i.e., remote from the neuronal perikarya in the dorsal root ganglia) administration of TRPV1 agonists, such as capsaicin or resiniferatoxin (RTX), initially produces nociceptor depolarization, and hence pain, as a result of TRPV1 channel activation. However, receptor desensitization, accompanied by long-term but reversible blockade of a portion of nociceptive afferent fibers within peripheral nerves, subsequently ensues (Winter et al., 1990; Neubert et al., 2008; Wong & Gavva, 2009). Therefore, treatment with TRPV1 agonists may serve as a method for regional pain control in situations in which traditional pain therapy fails.

Studies in laboratory animals indicate that perineural capsaicin and RTX application produces significant inhibition of inflammatory nociception (including hyperalgesia) that is dose and time dependent, without changing proprioceptive sensations and motor control. Using a range of mechanical and thermal algesic tests, investigators found that the most sensitive measure following perineural RTX administration was inhibition of inflammatory hyperalgesia (Winter et al., 1990; Neubert et al., 2008). Recovery studies

showed that physiological sensory function can return as early as 2 weeks post-RTX or capsaicin treatment; however, immunohistochemical examination of the dorsal root ganglion revealed a partial, but significant, reduction in the number of the TRPV1-positive neurons.

While the use of RTX in horses has not yet been described, the effects of local administration of capsaicin in the equine have been reported (Seino et al., 2003). Compared to no treatment, one time topical application of capsaicin ointment (Equi-Block® containing capsaicin 0.25%) over the medial and lateral palmar digital nerves significantly attenuated signs of pain in a reversible model of severe (nonweight bearing) foot lameness. This effect lasted for up to 4 hours. Some horses initially displayed an episode of increased pain sensation, likely due to the initial agonistic action of capsaicin on TPRV-1 receptors described above. This response can likely be obliterated by prior perineural local anesthetic drug infiltration proximal to the site of capsaicin application. Berardinelli et al. (2003) injected 8% capsaicin solution along the medial and lateral palmar nerves in horses to study whether selective deafferentiation of sensory fibers (A δ and C fibers) in the distal part of the forelimb would alter the muscle fiber composition in the muscles of the same limb. Indeed, eliminating sensory input to the CNS by perineural injection of capsaicin along the palmar nerves caused a shift in the

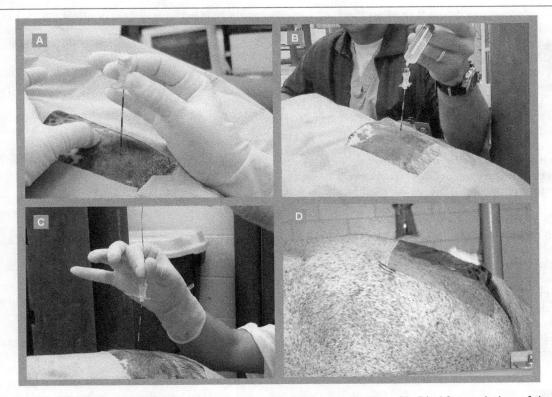

Figure 30.7. Step-by-step illustration of caudal epidural catheterization technique (A–D). After sedation of the horse, epidural catheterization is performed using a similar technique as for caudal (i.e., intercoccygeal) epidural injection (Skarda et al., 2009). Various epidural trays or kits are suitable for use in horses (e.g., Perifix® epidural catheter set, B. Braun Medical, Inc., Bethlehem, PA, USA; TheraCath® epidural catheter, Arrow International, Reading, PA, USA, the latter providing exceptionally long-term patency). For catheter placement an epidural Huber point (Tuohy) needle should be used instead of a spinal needle. This needle design has a slight curve on the end which aids in catheter directional placement and is more blunted at the end so less likely to sever the catheter than a regular spinal needle. The skin should be clipped, surgically prepared, and covered with surgical sterile drapes or clear plastic adhesive drape (Bioclusiv® transparent dressing) to avoid catheter contamination (A). A disposable sterile or reusable 17G or 18G 7.5 cm epidural Tuohy needle (Reusable technique needle, Tuohy, thin wall, Becton Dickinson Inc., Franklin Lakes, NJ, USA) is used to penetrate the epidural space (A). After confirmation of successful epidural puncture (B), a 19G or 20G epidural catheter is introduced through the needle up to the desired length (C). Generally for injections in the sacral area, 2–4 cm of catheter is advanced cranially from the needle tip. Catheters have length marks that indicate how far the catheter has been advanced into the epidural space. Usually the catheter should be inserted no more than 30 cm into the epidural space to avoid catheter kink. The authors prefer using a spring-wire reinforced catheter, 19G, 91.4 cm (TheraCath®) that facilitates introduction and rarely kinks. After the needle is removed, the catheter is wrapped with a butterfly tape that is then sutured to the skin. A bacterial filter may be attached to the catheter connector. The site of catheter penetration should be covered with iodine paste and the region covered with sterile dressings and gauze sponges and an adhesive clear plastic dressing (D). After each drug injection the catheter should be flushed with sterile 0.9% saline. Any presence of blood in the catheter suggests vascular catheterization, which should be ruled out before catheter use. Epidural catheters elicit inflammatory reactions that may become uncomfortable and increase risks of contamination. Catheter care includes daily inspection and flushing with saline or heparinized (10 IU/mL) saline and skin cleaning with antiseptic solution.

muscle fiber composition from fast (type II) to slow contracting (type I) fibers, within 120 days posttreatment, in the flexor carpi radialis (FCR) muscle, which is responsible for the flexor activity in the front limb. This indicates that long-term deafferentiation of sensory nerve fibers produces a plastic remodeling of the CNS and indirectly influences motor neuron activity enhancing their tonic discharge. More equine studies with capsaicin and RTX are warranted before the risks and long-term success of local treatment

with these TRPV1 ligands in animals suffering from persistent pain can be assessed.

SUMMARY

Currently available experimental and clinical data in a wide variety of species indicate that moderate to severe pain, particularly if persistent, may trigger a cascade of events that drives the somatosensory nervous system into a state of nociceptive hyperactivity with abnormal impulse processing, rendering the animal eventually minimally or unresponsive to classic anti-inflammatory drug treatment. Thus, appreciating this maladaptive pain state as the product of complex neuropathological processes affecting both the peripheral and central somatosensory nervous systems is crucial when devising a treatment plan, since any state of acute pain has the potential to progress to a maladaptive form. Effective analgesic therapy for moderate to severe pain calls, from the outset, for a multimodal approach that involves a combination of agents with different pharmacological mechanisms of action targeting different sites within the nociceptive system, and requires both systemic and local/regional drug administration. Multimodal pain management should be tailored to the particular situation in each individual horse, and not be limited to traditional pharmacological approaches but rather involve other modalities such as chiropractic techniques, mesotherapy, physical therapy, and acupuncture, whenever indicated. Nonetheless, most, if not all, information about therapeutic strategies are derived from observations in human patients and laboratory animal experimentation, thus successfully managing horses afflicted by acute or persistent pain continues to be a prodigious task. Yet, the equine veterinarian should not be discouraged, but take up this challenge. After all, horses, as all other living subjects, are entitled to freedom from pain, injury, and disease (Muir, 2010b).

REFERENCES

Allan, A.K., Johns, S., & Hyman, S.S. (2010) How to diagnose and treat back pain in the horse. *Proceedings of the American Association of Equine Practitioners*, 56, 384–388.

Angst, M.S. (2006) Opioid-induced hyperalgesia: a qualitative systematic review. *Anesthesiology*, 104, 570–587.

Arendt-Nielsen, L., Brøndum Frøkjær, J., Staahl, C., et al. (2007) Effects of gabapentin on experimental somatic pain and temporal summation. *Regional Anesthesia and Pain Medicine*, 32, 382–388.

Attal, N., Rouaud, J., Brasseur, L., et al. (2004) Systemic lidocaine in pain due to peripheral nerve injury and predictors of response. *Neurology*, 62, 218–225.

Auckburally, A. & Flaherty, D. (2011) Use of supplemental intravenous anaesthesia/analgesia in horses. *In Practice*, 33, 334–339.

Back, W., MacAllister, C.G., Heel, M.C.V., et al. (2009) The use of force plate measurements to titrate the dosage of a new COX-2 inhibitor in lame horses. *Equine Veterinary Journal*, 41, 309–312.

Baller, L.S. & Hendrickson, D.A. (2002) Management of equine orthopedic pain. *Veterinary Clinics of North America - Equine Practice*, 18, 117–131.

Bellei, M.H., Kerr, C., Johnson, R., et al. (2009) Pharmacokinetics of epidural morphine in awake and isoflurane-anesthetized horses. *Veterinary Anaesthesia and Analgesia*, 36, 14.

Bennett, R.C. & Steffey, E.P. (2002) Use of opioids for pain and anesthetic management in horses. *Veterinary Clinics of North America - Equine Practice*, 18, 46–60.

Bennett, R.C., Steffey, E.P., Kollias-Baker, C., et al. (2004) Influence of morphine sulfate on the halothane sparing effect of xylazine hydrochloride in horses. *American Journal Veterinary Research*, 65, 519–526.

Berardinelli, P., Barazzoni, A.M., Russo, V., et al. (2003) Selective deafferentation of hand cutaneous territory is followed by changes in fibre type distribution of a forearm muscle in the horse. *Archives Italiennes de Biologie*, 141, 19–25.

Beretta, C., Garavaglia, G., & Cavalli, M. (2005) COX-1 and COX-2 inhibition in horse blood by phenylbutazone, flunixin, carprofen and meloxicam: an in vitro analysis. *Pharmacological Research*, 52, 302–306.

Berti, M., Baciarello, M., Troglio, R., et al. (2009) Clinical uses of low–dose ketamine in patients undergoing surgery. *Current Drug Targets*, 10, 707–715.

Bertone, J.J. (2002) Clinical field efficacy and safety study of Buscopan in horses. *Proceedings of the American Association of Equine Practitioners*, 48, 370–374.

Bettschart-Wolfensberger, R. & Larenza, M.P. (2007) Balanced anesthesia in the equine. *Clinical Techniques in Equine Practice*, 6, 104–110.

Bettschart-Wolfensberger, R., Clarke, K.W., Vainio, O., et al. (1999) Pharmacokinetics of medetomidine in ponies and elaboration of a medetomidine infusion regime which provides a constant level of sedation. *Research in Veterinary Sciences*, 67, 41–46.

Bettschart-Wolfensberger, R., Dicht, S., Vullo, C., et al. (2011) A clinical study on the effect in horses during medetomidine–isoflurane anaesthesia, of butorphanol constant rate infusion on isoflurane requirements, on cardiopulmonary function and on recovery characteristics. *Veterinary Anaesthesia and Analgesia*, 38, 186–194.

Blikslager, A. (2009) Role of NSAIDs in the management of pain in horses. Proceedings of the American Association of Equine Practitioners' Focus Meeting on the foot, Raleigh, NC, pp. 218–223.

Boatwright, C.E., Fubini, S.L., Grohn, Y.T., et al. (1996) A comparison of N-butylscopolammonium bromide and butorphanol tartrate for analgesia using a balloon model of abdominal pain in ponies. *Canadian Journal Veterinary Research*, 62, 65–68.

Boezaart, A.P. (2006) Perineural infusion of local anesthetics. *Anesthesiology*, 104, 872–880.

Bohlega, S., Alsaadi, T., Amir, A., et al. (2010) Guidelines for the pharmacological treatment of peripheral neuropathic pain: expert panel recommendations for the Middle East region. *Journal of International Medical Research*, 38, 295–317.

Boscan, P., Van Hoogmoed, L.M., Farver, T.B., et al. (2006) Evaluation of the effects of the opioid agonist morphine on gastrointestinal tract function in horses. *American Journal Veterinary Research*, 67, 992–997.

Brideau, C., Van Staden, C., & Chan, C.C. (2001) In vitro effects of cyclooxygenase inhibitors in whole blood of horses, dogs, and cats. *American Journal Veterinary Research*, 62, 1755–1760.

Brunson, D.B. & Majors, L.J. (1987) Comparative analgesia of xylazine, xylazine/morphine, xylazine/butorphanol, and xylazine/nalbuphine in the horse, using dental dolorimetry. *American Journal Veterinary Research*, 48, 1087–1091.

Campbell, N.B. & Blikslager, A.T. (2000) The role of cyclooxygenase inhibitors in repair of ischemic-injured jejunal mucosa in the horse. *Equine Veterinary Journal*, 32(S32), 59–64.

Campbell, N.B., Jones, S.L., & Blikslager, A.T. (2002) The effects of cyclooxygenase inhibitors on bile-injured and normal equine colon. *Equine Veterinary Journal*, 34, 493–498.

Carr, B.D. (2001) The development of national guidelines for pain control: synopsis and commentary. *European Journal of Pain*, 5(Suppl. A), 91–98.

Carregaro, A.B., Luna, S.P., Mataqueiro, M.I., et al. (2007) Effects of buprenorphine on nociception and spontaneous locomotor activity in horses. *American Journal Veterinary Research*, 68, 246–250.

Caulkett, N. (2007) Equine field anesthesia and sedation. *Large Animal Veterinary Rounds*, 7(9), 6.

Chambers, J.P., Livingston, A., Waterman, A.E. et al. (1993) Analgesic effects of detomidine in thoroughbred horses with chronic tendon injury. *Research in Veterinary Science*, 54, 52–56.

Clark, J.O. & Clark, T.P. (1999) Analgesia. *Veterinary Clinics of North America - Equine Practice*, 15, 705–723.

Clutton, R.E. (2010) Opioid analgesia in horses. *Veterinary Clinics Equine*, 26, 493–514.

Collins, S., Sigtermans, M.J., Dahan, A., et al. (2010) NMDA receptor antagonists for the treatment of neuropathic pain. *Pain Medicine*, 11, 1726–1742.

Cook, V.L., Meyer, C.T., Campbell, N.B., et al. (2009) Effect of firocoxib or flunixin meglumine on recovery of ischemic-injured equine jejunum. *American Journal Veterinary Research*, 70, 992–1000.

Coutaux, A., Adam, F., Willer, J.C. et al. (2005) Hyperalgesia and allodynia: peripheral mechanism. *Joint Bone Spine*, 72, 359–371.

Cruccu, G. & Truini, A. (2009) Tools for assessing neuropathic pain. *PLoS Medicine/Public Library of Science*, 6, e1000045, http://www.plosmedicine.org (last accessed November 7, 2011).

DaCunha, A.F., Chirgwin, S.R., Stokes, A.M., et al. (2008) Quantitative expression of the TRPV-1 Gene in central and peripheral nervous tissue in horses. *International Journal of Applied Research in Veterinary Medicine*, 6, 15–23.

Daunt, D.A. & Steffey, E.P. (2002) Alpha-2 adrenergic agonists as analgesics in horses. *Veterinary Clinics of North America – Equine Practice*, 18, 39–46.

Davis, J.L., Messenger, K.M., LaFevers, D.H., et al. (2011) Pharmacokinetics of intravenous and intramuscular buprenorphine in the horse. *Journal of Veterinary Pharmacology and Therapeutics*, 35, 52–58.

Davis, J.L., Papich, M.G., Morton, A.J., et al. (2007a) Pharmacokinetics of etodolac in the horse following oral and intravenous administration. *Journal of Veterinary Pharmacology and Therapeutics*, 30, 43–48.

Davis, J.L., Posner, L.P., & Elce, Y. (2007b) Gabapentin for the treatment of neuropathic pain in a pregnant horse. *Journal of the American Veterinary Medical Association*, 231, 755–758.

De Grauw, J.C., van de Lest, C.H., Brama, P.A., et al. (2009) In vivo effects of meloxicam on inflammatory mediators, MMP activity and cartilage biomarkers in equine joints with acute synovitis. *Equine Veterinary Journal*, 41, 693–699.

De Kock, M.F. & Lavand'homme, P.M. (2007) The clinical role of NMDA receptor antagonists for the treatment of postoperative pain. *Best Practice & Research Clinical Anaesthesiology*, 21, 85–98.

De Leon-Casasola, O. (2011) New developments in the treatment algorithm for peripheral neuropathic pain. *Pain Medicine*, 12(Suppl. 3), S100–S108.

De Solis, C.N. & McKenzie, H.C. 3rd (2007) Serum concentrations of lidocaine and its metabolites MEGX and GX during and after prolonged intravenous infusion of lidocaine in horses after colic surgery. *Journal of Equine Veterinary Science*, 27, 398–404.

Diaz-Reval, M.I., Ventura-Martinez, R., Deciga-Campos, M., et al. (2004) Evidence for a central mechanism of action of S-(+)-ketoprofen. *European Journal of Pharmacology*, 483, 241–248.

Dickey, E.J., McKenzie, H.C. 3rd, Brown, K.A., et al. (2008) Serum concentrations of lidocaine and its metabolites after prolonged infusion in healthy horses. *Equine Veterinary Journal*, 40, 348–352.

Dirikolu, L., Dafalla, A., Ely, K.J., et al. (2008) Pharmacokinetics of gabapentin in horses. *Journal of Veterinary Pharmacology and Therapeutics*, 31, 175–177.

Divers, T.J. (2008) COX inhibitors: making the best choice for the laminitic case. *Journal of Equine Veterinary Science*, 28, 367–369.

Dixit, R.K. & Bhargava, V.K. (2002) Neurotransmitter mechanisms in gabapentin antinociception. *Pharmacology*, 65, 198–203.

Doherty, D.J. & Frazier, D.L. (1998) Effect of intravenous lidocaine on halothane minimum alveolar concentration in ponies. *Equine Veterinary Journal*, 30, 300–303.

Doherty, T.J., Andrews, F.M., Provenza, M.K., et al. (1999) The effect of sedation on gastric emptying of a liquid marker in ponies. *Veterinary Surgery*, 28, 375–379.

Doherty, T.J. & Seddighi, M.R. (2010) Local anesthetics as pain therapy in horses. *Veterinary Clinics Equine*, 26, 533–549.

Doucet, M.Y., Bertone, A.L., Hendrickson, D., et al. (2008) Comparison of efficacy and safety of paste formulations of firocoxib and phenylbutazone in horses with naturally occurring osteoarthritis. *Journal of the American Veterinary Medical Association*, 232, 91–97.

Driessen, B. (2005) Intravenous lidocaine infusion in balanced anaesthesia for abdominal surgery: update and clinical experiences. *Pferdeheilkunde*, 21, 133–141.

Driessen, B. (2007) Pain: systemic and local/regional drug therapy. *Clinical Techniques in Equine Practice*, 6, 135–144.

Driessen, B., Bauquier, S.H., & Zarucco, L. (2010) Neuropathic pain management in chronic laminitis. *Veterinary Clinics Equine*, 26, 315–337.

Driessen, B., Scandella, M., & Zarucco, L. (2008a) Development of a technique for continuous perineural blockade of the palmar nerves in the distal equine thoracic limb. *Veterinary Anaesthesia and Analgesia*, 35, 432–448.

Driessen, B. & Zarucco, L. (2007) Pain: from diagnosis to effective treatment. *Clinical Techniques in Equine Practice*, 6, 126–134.

Driessen, B., Zarucco, L., Scandella, M., et al. (2008b) Antinociceptive efficacy of continuous perineural blockade of median and ulnar nerves in the equine forelimb. Proceedings of the Association of Veterinary Anaesthetists' Meeting, October 14–18, 2008, Barcelona, Spain.

Dujardin, C.L.L. & van Loon, J.P.A.M. (2011) Pain recognition and treatment in the horse: a survey of equine veterinarians in the Netherlands and Belgium. *Tijdschrift voor Diergenees-kunde*, 136, 715–722.

Dutton, D.W., Lashnits, K.J., & Wegner, K. (2009) Managing severe hoof pain in a horse using multimodal analgesia and a modified composite pain score. *Equine Veterinary Education*, 21, 37–43.

Dworkin, R.H., O'Connor, A.B., Backonja, M., et al. (2007) Pharmacologic management of neuropathic pain: evidence-based recommendations. *Pain*, 132, 237–251.

Dyer, D.C., Hsu, W.H., & Lloyd, W.E. (1987) Pharmacokinetics of xylazine in ponies: influence of yohimbine. *Archives Internationales de Pharmacodynamie et de Thérapie*, 289, 5–10.

Dyke, T.M., Sams, R.A., Thompson, K.G., et al. (1998) Pharmacokinetics of multiple-dose administration of eltenac in horses. *American Journal Veterinary Research*, 59, 1447–1450.

Dzikiti, T.B., Hellebrekers, L.J., & van Dijk, P. (2003) Effects of intravenous lidocaine on isoflurane concentration, physiological parameters, metabolic parameters and stress-related hormones in horses undergoing surgery. *Journal of Veterinary Medicine (Series A)*, 50, 190–195.

Eckhardt, K., Ammon, S., Hofmann, U., et al. (2000) Gabapentin enhances the analgesic effect of morphine in healthy volunteers. *Anesthesia and Analgesia*, 91, 185–191.

Elfenbein, J.R., Sanchez, L.C., Robertson, S.A., et al. (2009) Effect of detomidine on visceral and somatic nociception and duodenal motility in conscious adult horses. *Veterinary Anaesthesia and Analgesia*, 36, 162–172.

Elvir-Lazo, O.L. & White, P.F. (2010) The role of multimodal analgesia in pain management after ambulatory surgery. *Current Opinion in Anaesthesiology*, 23, 697–703.

Erkert, R.S., MacAllister, C.G., Payton, M.E., et al. (2005) Use of force plate analysis to compare the analgesic effects of intravenous administration of phenylbutazone and flunixin meglumine in horses with navicular syndrome. *American Journal Veterinary Research*, 66, 284–288.

Feary, D.J., Mama, K.R., Thomasy, S.M., et al. (2006) Influence of gastrointestinal tract disease on pharmacokinetics of lidocaine after intravenous infusion in anesthetized horses. *American Journal Veterinary Research*, 67, 317–322.

Feary, D.J., Mama, K.R., Wagner, A.E., et al. (2005) Influence of general anaesthesia on pharmacokinetics of intravenous lidocaine infusion in horses. *American Journal Veterinary Research*, 66, 574–580.

Fielding, C.L., Brumbaugh, G.W., Matthews, N.S., et al. (2006) Pharmacokinetics and clinical effects of a subanesthetic continuous rate infusion of ketamine in awake horses. *American Journal Veterinary Research*, 67, 1484–1490.

Figueiredo, J.P., Muir, W.W., Smith, J., et al. (2005) Sedative and analgesic effects of romifidine in horses. *The International Journal of Applied Research in Veterinary Medicine*, 3, 249–258.

Finnerup, N.B., Otto, M., McQuay, H.J., et al. (2005) Algorithm for neuropathic pain treatment: an evidence based proposal. *Pain*, 118, 289–305.

Fishbain, D.A.A. (2009) Do opioids induce hyperalgesia in humans? An evidence-based structured review. *Pain Medicine*, 10, 829–839.

Freeman, S.L., Bowen, I.M., Bettschart-Wolfensberger, R., et al. (2002) Cardiovascular effects of romifidine in the standing horse. *Research in Veterinary Science*, 72, 123–129.

Freeman, S.L. & England, G.C. (2001) Effect of romifidine on gastrointestinal motility, assessed by transrectal ultrasonography. *Equine Veterinary Journal*, 33, 570–576.

Garcia-Villar, R., Toutain, P.L., Alvinerie, M., et al. (1981) The pharmacokinetics of xylazine hydrochloride: an interspecific study. *Journal of Veterinary Pharmacology and Therapeutics*, 4, 87–92.

Galluzzi, K.E. (2005) Management of neuropathic pain. *Journal of the American Osteopathic Association*, 105, S12–S19.

Gilron, I. (2007) Gabapentin and pregabalin for chronic neuropathic and early postsurgical pain: current evidence and future directions. *Current Opinion in Anaesthesiology*, 20, 456–472.

Giordano, J. (2001) The neurobiology of pain, in *Pain Management: A Practical Guide for Clinicians*, 6th edn (ed. R.S. Weiner), CRC Press, Boca Raton, FL, pp. 1089–1100.

Goodrich, L.R., Furr, M.O., Robertson, J.L., & Warnick, L.D. (1998) A toxicity study of eltenac, a nonsteroidal anti-inflammatory drug, in horses. *Journal of Veterinary Pharmacology and Therapeutics*, 21(1), 24–33.

Goodrich, L.R. & Nixon, A.J. (2006) Medical treatment of osteoarthritis in the horse - a review. *Veterinary Journal*, 171, 51–69.

Gormsen, L., Finnerup, N.B., Almqvist, P.M., et al. (2009) The efficacy of the AMPA receptor antagonist NS1209 and lidocaine in nerve injury pain: a randomized, double-blind, placebo-controlled, three-way crossover study. *Anesthesia and Analgesia*, 108, 1311–1319.

Grimm, C., Aneiros, E., & de Groot, M. (2011) Dissecting TRPV1: lessons to be learned. *Channels*, 5, 201–204.

Grimsrud, K.N., Mama, K.R., Thomasy, S.M., et al. (2009) Pharmacokinetics of detomidine and its metabolites following intravenous

and intramuscular administration in horses. *Equine Veterinary Journal*, 41, 361–365.

Haanpaa, M., Attal, N., Backonja, M., et al. (2011) NeuPSIG guidelines on neuropathic pain assessment. *Pain*, 152, 14–27.

Harding, L.M., Kristensen, J.D., & Baranowski, A.P. (2005) Differential effects of neuropathic analgesics on wind-up-like pain and somatosensory function in healthy volunteers. *The Clinical Journal of Pain*, 21, 127–132.

Haussler, K.K. (2009) Review of manual therapy techniques in equine practice. *Journal of Equine Veterinary Science*, 29, 849–869.

Hendrickson, D.A., Southwood, L.L., Lopez, M.J., et al. (1998) Cranial migration of different volumes of new-methylene blue after caudal epidural injection in the horse. *Equine Practice*, 20, 12–14.

Hilton, H.G., Magdesian, K.G., Groth, A.D., et al. (2011) Distribution of flunixin meglumine and firocoxib into aqueous humor of horses. *Journal of Veterinary Internal Medicine*, 25, 1127–1133.

Hocking, G. & Cousins, M.J. (2003) Ketamine in chronic pain management: an evidence-based review. *Anesthesia and Analgesia*, 97, 1730–1739.

Houdeshell, J.W. & Hennessy, P.W. (1977) A new non-steroidal, anti-inflammatory analgesic for horses. *The Journal of Equine Medicine and Surgery*, 1, 57–63.

Hubbell, J.A.E., Saville, W.J.A., & Bednarski, R.M. (2010) The use of sedatives, analgesic and anaesthetic drugs in the horse: an electronic survey of members of the American Association of Equine Practitioners (AAEP). *Equine Veterinary Journal*, 42, 487–493.

Inturrisi, C.E. (2002) Clinical pharmacology of opioids for pain. *Clinical Journal of Pain*, 18(Suppl), S3–S13.

Jöchle, W. (1989) Field trial evaluation of detomidine as a sedative and analgesic agent in horses with colic. *Equine Veterinary Journal*, 7(Suppl), 117–120.

Jöchle, W., Moore, J.N., Brown, J., et al. (1989) Comparison of detomidine, butorphanol, flunixin meglumine, and xylazine in clinical cases of equine colic. *Equine Veterinary Journal*, 7(Suppl), 111–116.

Johnson, C.B., Taylor, P.M., Young, S.S., et al. (1993) Postoperative analgesia using phenylbutazone, flunixin or carprofen in horses. *Veterinary Record*, 133, 336–338.

Jones, E., Vinuela-Fernandez, I., Eager, R.A., et al. (2007) Neuropathic changes in equine laminitis pain. *Pain*, 132, 321–331.

Kalpravidh, M., Lumb, W.V., Wright, M., et al. (1984a) Analgesic effects of butorphanol in horses: dose-response studies. *American Journal of Veterinary Research*, 45, 211–216.

Kalpravidh, M., Lumb, W.V., Wright, M., et al. (1984b) Effects of butorphanol, flunixin, levorphanol, morphine, and xylazine in ponies. *American Journal of Veterinary Research*, 45, 217–223.

Kamerling, S.G., Cravens, W.M., & Bagwell, C.A. (1988) Objective assessment of detomidine-induced analgesia and sedation in the horse. *European Journal of Pharmacology*, 151, 1–8.

Keller, H. (1986) Induction of intestinal paralysis by a large dose of Buscopan (scopolamine butylbromide) in the horse. *Tierärztliche Umschau*, 41, 266–268.

Keller, H. & Faulstich, A. (1985) Treatment of colic in the horse with Buscopan (hyoscine butylbromide with dipyrone). *Tierärztliche Umschau*, 40, 581–584.

Knobloch, M., Portier, C.J., Levionnois, O.L., et al. (2006) Antinociceptive effects, metabolism and disposition of ketamine in ponies under target-controlled drug infusion. *Toxicology & Applied Pharmacology*, 216, 373–386.

Knych, H.K., Casbeer, H.C., McKemie, D.S., et al. (2013) Pharmacokinetics and pharmacodynamics of butorphanol following intravenous administration to the horse. *Journal of Veterinary Pharmacology and Therapeutics*, 36(1), 21–30.

Koene, M., Goupil, X., Kampmann, C., et al. (2010) Field trial validation of the efficacy and acceptability of firocoxib, a highly Selective Cox-2 inhibitor, in a group of 96 lame horses. *Journal of Equine Veterinary Science*, 30, 237–243.

Kvaternick, V., Pollmeier, M., Fischer, J., et al. (2007) Pharmacokinetics and metabolism of orally administered firocoxib, a novel second generation coxib, in horses. *Journal of Veterinary Pharmacology and Therapeutics*, 30, 208–217.

Lankveld, D.P.K., Driessen, B., Soma, L.R., et al. (2006) Pharmacodynamic effects and pharmacokinetic profile of a long-term continuous rate infusion of racemic ketamine in healthy conscious horses. *Journal of Veterinary Pharmacology and Therapeutics*, 29, 477–488.

Latremoliere, A. & Woolf, C.J. (2009) Central sensitization: a generator of pain hypersensitivity by central neural plasticity. *The Journal of Pain*, 10, 895–926.

Lauretti, G.R. (2008) Mechanisms of analgesia of intravenous lidocaine. *Revista Brasileira de Anestesiologia*, 58, 280–286.

Lees, P., May, S.A., Hoeijmakers, M., et al. (1999) A pharmacodynamic and pharmacokinetic study with vedaprofen in an equine model of acute nonimmune inflammation. *Journal of Veterinary Pharmacology and Therapeutics*, 22, 96–106.

Lees, P., Sedgwick, A.D., Higgins, A.J., et al. (1991) Pharmacodynamics and pharmacokinetics of meloxicam in the horse. *British Veterinary Journal*, 147, 97–108.

Lemke, K.A. (2004) Understanding the pathophysiology of perioperative pain. *Canadian Veterinary Journal*, 45, 405–413.

Letendre, L.T., Tessman, R.K., McClure, S.R., et al. (2008) Pharmacokinetics of firocoxib after administration of multiple consecutive daily doses to horses. *American Journal of Veterinary Research*, 69, 1399–1405.

Levionnois, O.L., Menge, M., & Thormann, W. (2010) Effect of ketamine on the limb withdrawal reflex evoked by transcutaneous electrical stimulation in ponies anaesthetised with isoflurane. *The Veterinary Journal*, 186, 304–311.

Livingston, A. (2006) Physiological basis of pain management, in *Manual of Equine Anesthesia & Analgesia* (eds T. Doherty & A. Valverde), Blackwell, Oxford, UK, pp. 293–300.

Luo, T., Bertone, J.J., Greene, H.M., et al. (2006) A comparison of N-butylscopolammonium and lidocaine for control of rectal pressure in horses. *Veterinary Therapeutics*, 7, 243–248.

Luo, Z.D., Chaplan, S.R., Higuera, E.S., et al. (2001) Upregulation of dorsal root ganglion $\alpha 2\delta$ calcium channel subunit and its correlation with allodynia in spinal nerve-injured rats. *Journal of Neuroscience*, 21, 1868–1875.

MacKay, R.J., Daniels, C.A., Bleyaert, H.F. et al. (2000) Effect of eltenac in horses with induced endotoxaemia. *Equine Veterinary Journal*, 32, 26–31.

Maneuf, Y.P., Luo, Z.D., & Lee, K. (2006) $\alpha 2\delta$ and the mechanism of action of gabapentin in the treatment of pain. *Seminars in Cell and Developmental Biology*, 17, 565–570.

Mao, J. & Chen, L.L. (2000) Systemic lidocaine for neuropathic pain relief. *Pain*, 87, 7–17.

Marshall, J.F. & Blikslager, A.T. (2011) The effect of nonsteroidal anti-inflammatory drugs on the equine intestine. *Equine Veterinary Journal*, 43, 140–144.

Martin, B.B. & Klide, A.M. (1991) Acupuncture for the treatment of chronic back pain in 200 horses. *Proceedings of the American Association of Equine Practitioners*, 37, 593–601.

Martin, W.R. (1983) Pharmacology of opioids. *Pharmacological Reviews*, 35, 283–323.

Matthews, N.S., Fielding, C.I., & Swineboard, E. (2004) How to use a ketamine constant rate infusion in horses for analgesia. *Proceedings of the American Association of Equine Practitioners*, 37, 1431.

McCann, M.E., Andersen, D.R., Brideau, C., et al. (2002) In vitro activity and in vivo efficacy of a novel COX-2 inhibitor in the horse. *Journal of Veterinary Internal Medicine*, 16, 355.

McGeeney, B.E. (2009) Pharmacological management of neuropathic pain in older adults: an update on peripherally and centrally acting agents. *Journal of Pain and Symptom Management*, 38(Suppl), S15–S27.

Merritt, A.M., Burrow, J.A., & Hartless, C.S. (1998) Effect of xylazine, detomidine, and a combination of xylazine and butorphanol on equine duodenal motility. *American Journal Veterinary Research*, 59, 619–623.

Merskey, H. (1986) Classification of chronic pain. Descriptions of chronic pain syndromes and definitions of pain terms. *Pain*, 3(Suppl), S1–S225.

Meyer, G.A., Lin, H.C., Hanson, R.R., et al. (2001) Effects of intravenous lidocaine overdose on cardiac electrical activity and blood pressure in the horse. *Equine Veterinary Journal*, 33, 434–437.

Moens, Y., Lanz, F., Doherr, M.G., et al. (2003) A comparison of the antinociceptive effects of xylazine, detomidine and romifidine on experimental pain in horses. *Veterinary Anaesthesia and Analgesia*, 30, 183–190.

Molony, V. & Kent, J.E. (1997) Assessment of acute pain in farm animals using behavioural and physiological measurements. *Journal of Animal Sciences*, 75, 266–272.

Morton, A.J., Campbell, N.B., Gayle, J.M., et al. (2005) Preferential and nonselective cyclooxygenase inhibitors reduce inflammation during lipopolysaccharide-induced synovitis. *Research in Veterinary Sciences*, 78, 189–192.

Morton, A.J., Varney, C.R., Ekiri, A.B., et al. (2011) Cardiovascular effects of N-butylscopolammonium bromide and xylazine in horses. *Equine Veterinary Journal*, 43(Suppl), 117–122.

Moses, V.S., Hardy, J., Bertone, A.L., et al. (2001) Effects of anti-inflammatory drugs on lipopolysaccharide-challenged and -unchallenged equine synovial explants. *American Journal Veterinary Research*, 62, 54–60.

Moulin, D.E., Clark, A.J., Gilron, I., et al. (2007) Pharmacological management of chronic neuropathic pain – Consensus statement and guidelines from the Canadian Pain Society. *Pain Research & Management*, 12, 13–21.

Muir, W.W. (1981) Drugs used to produce standing chemical restraint in horses. *Veterinary Clinics of North America – Large Animal Practice*, 3, 17–44.

Muir, W.W. (2005) Pain therapy in horses. *Equine Veterinary Journal*, 37, 98–100.

Muir, W.W. (2010a) Preface – Pain in horses: physiology, pathophysiology, and therapeutic implications. *Veterinary Clinics Equine*, 26, xi–xii.

Muir, W.W. (2010b) Pain: mechanisms and management in horses. *Veterinary Clinics Equine*, 26, 467–480.

Muir, W.W. (2010c) NMDA receptor antagonists and pain: ketamine. *Veterinary Clinics Equine*, 26, 565–578.

Muir, W.W. & Robertson, J.T. (1985) Visceral analgesia: effects of xylazine, butorphanol, meperidine, and pentazocine in horses. *American Journal of Veterinary Research*, 46, 2081–2084.

Murrell, J.C., White, K.L., Johnson, C.B., et al. (2005) Investigation of the EEG effects of intravenous lidocaine during halothane anaesthesia in ponies. *Veterinary Anaesthesia and Analgesia*, 32, 212–221.

Natalini, C.C. (2010) Spinal anesthetics and analgesics in the horse. *Veterinary Clinics Equine*, 26, 551–564.

Natalini, C.C. & Driessen, B. (2007) Epidural and spinal anesthesia and analgesia in the equine. *Clinical Techniques in Equine Practice*, 6, 144–115.

Naylor, J.M., Garven, E., & Fraser, L. (1997) A comparison of romifidine and xylazine in foals: the effects on sedation and analgesia. *Equine Veterinary Education*, 9, 329–334.

Ness, T. (2000) Intravenous lidocaine inhibits visceral nociceptive reflexes and spinal neurons in the rat. *Anesthesiology*, 92, 1685–1691.

Neubert, J.K., Mannes, A.J., Karai, L.J., et al. (2008) Perineural resiniferatoxin selectively inhibits inflammatory hyperalgesia. *Molecular Pain*, 4, 3. Open access journal, doi:10.1186/1744-8069-4-3

Newton, R.A., Bingham, S., Case, P.C., et al. (2001) Dorsal root ganglion neurons show increased expression of the calcium channel $\alpha 2\delta$-1 subunit following partial sciatic nerve injury. *Molecular Brain Research*, 95, 1–8.

O'Connor, A.B. & Dworkin, R.H. (2009) Treatment of neuropathic pain: an overview of recent guidelines. *The American Journal of Medicine*, 122(Suppl), S22–S32.

Orsini, J.A., Moate, P.J., Kuersten, K., et al. (2006) Pharmacokinetics of fentanyl delivered transdermally in healthy adult horses – variability among horses and its clinical implications. *Journal of Veterinary Pharmacology and Therapeutics*, 29, 539–546.

Ossipov, M.H., Jerussi, T.P., Ren, K., et al. (2000) Differential effects of spinal (R)-ketoprofen and (S)-ketoprofen against signs of neuropathic pain and tonic nociception: evidence for a novel mechanism of action of (R)-ketoprofen against tactile allodynia. *Pain*, 87, 193–199.

Owens, J.G., Kamerling, S.G., Stanton, S.R., et al. (1995) Effects of ketoprofen and phenylbutazone on chronic hoof pain and lameness in the horse. *Equine Veterinary Journal*, 27, 296–300.

Owens, J.G., Kamerling, S.G., Stanton, S.R., et al. (1996a) Effects of pretreatment with ketoprofen and phenylbutazone on experimentally induced synovitis in horses. *American Journal Veterinary Research*, 57, 866–874.

Owens, J.G., Kamerling, S.G., Stanton, S.R., et al. (1996b) Evaluation of detomidine-induced analgesia in horses with chronic hoof pain. *Journal of Pharmacology & Experimental Therapeutics*, 278, 179–184.

Peterbauer, C., Larenza, P.M., Knobloch, M., et al. (2008) Effects of a low dose infusion of racemic and S-ketamine on the nociceptive withdrawal reflex in standing ponies. *Veterinary Anaesthesia and Analgesia*, 35, 414–423.

Price, J., Marques, J.M., Welsh, E.M., et al. (2002) Pilot epidemiology study of attitude towards pain in horses. *Veterinary Record*, 151, 570–575.

Prügner, W., Huber, R., & Luhmann, R. (1991) Eltenac, a new anti-inflammatory and analgesic drug for horses: clinical aspects. *Journal of Veterinary Pharmacology & Therapeutics*, 14, 193–199.

Renault, A., Gerring, E.L., & Baker, S. (2003) Comparative study on the use of vedaprofen and flunixin in an endotoxin-induced ileus model in horses. *Bulletin de la Societe Veterinaire Pratique de France*, 87, 138–144.

Reuben, S.S. & Buvanendran, A. (2007) Preventing the development of chronic pain after orthopaedic surgery with preventive multimodal analgesic techniques. *Journal of Bone and Joint Surgery*, 89, 1343–1358.

Ridgway, K.J. (2005) Diagnosis and treatment of equine musculo-skeletal pain. The role of complementary modalities: acupuncture and chiropractic. *Proceedings of the American Association of Equine Practitioners*, 51, 403–408.

Ripamonti, C. & Dickerson, E.D. (2001) Strategies for the treatment of cancer pain in the new millennium. *Drugs*, 61, 955–977.

Robertson, S.A. & Sanchez, L.C. (2010) Treatment of visceral pain in horses. *Veterinary Clinics of North American - Equine*, 26, 603–617.

Robertson, S.A., Sanchez, L.C., Merritt, A.M., et al. (2005) Effect of systemic lidocaine on visceral and somatic nociception in conscious horses. *Equine Veterinary Journal*, 37, 122–127.

Roelvink, M.E., Goossens, L., Kalsbeek, H.C., et al. (1991) Analgesic and spasmolytic effects of dipyrone, hyoscine-N-butylbromide and a combination of the two in ponies. *Veterinary Record*, 129, 378–380.

Roger, T., Bardon, T., & Ruckebusch, Y. (1985) Colonic motor responses in the pony: relevance of colonic stimulation by opiate antagonists. *American Journal Veterinary Research*, 46, 31–36.

Salonen, J.S., Vaha-Vahe, T., Vainio, O., et al. (1989) Single-dose pharmacokinetics of detomidine in the horse and cow. *Journal of Veterinary Pharmacology and Therapeutics*, 12, 65–72.

Sanchez, C.L., Elfenbein, J.R., & Robertson, S.A. (2008) Effect of acepromazine, butorphanol, or N-butylscopolammonium bromide on visceral and somatic nociception and duodenal motility in conscious horses. *American Journal Veterinary Research*, 69, 579–585.

Sasaki, N., Yoshihara, T., & Hara, S. (2000) Difference in the motile reactivity of jejunum, cecum, and right ventral colon to xylazine and medetomidine in conscious horses. *Journal of Equine Science*, 11, 63–68.

Seino, K.K., Foreman, J.H., Greene, S.A., et al. (2003) Effects of topical perineural capsaicin in a reversible model of equine foot lameness. *Journal of Veterinary Internal Medicine*, 17, 563–566.

Sellon, D.C., Monroe, V.L., Roberts, M.C., et al. (2001) Pharmacokinetics and adverse effects of butorphanol administered by single intravenous injection or continuous intravenous infusion in horses. *American Journal Veterinary Research*, 62, 183–189.

Sellon, D.C., Papich, M.G., Palmer, L., et al. (2008) Pharmacokinetics of butorphanol in horses after intramuscular injection. *Journal of Veterinary Pharmacology and Therapeutics*, 32, 62–65.

Sellon, D.C., Roberts, M.C., Blikslager, A.T., et al. (2002) Continuous butorphanol infusion for analgesia in the postoperative colic horse. *Veterinary Surgery*, 48, 244–246.

Sellon, D.C., Roberts, M.C., Blikslager, A.T., et al. (2004) Effects of continuous rate intravenous infusion of butorphanol on physiologic and outcome variables in horses after celiotomy. *Journal of Veterinary Internal Medicine*, 18, 461–462.

Sills, G.J. (2006) The mechanisms of action of gabapentin and pregabalin. *Current Opinion in Pharmacology*, 6, 108–113.

Silverman, S.M. (2009) Opioid induced hyperalgesia: clinical implications for the pain practitioner. *Pain Physician*, 12, 679–684.

Simon, L.S. (1998) Biology and toxic effects of nonsteroidal anti-inflammatory drugs. *Current Opinions in Rheumatology*, 10, 153–158.

Sinclair, M.D., Mealey, K.L., Matthews, N.S., et al. (2006) Comparative pharmacokinetics of meloxicam in clinically normal horses and donkeys. *American Journal Veterinary Research*, 67, 1082–1085.

Skarda, R.T., Muir, W.W., & Hubbell, J.A.E. (2009) Local anesthetic drugs and techniques, in *Equine Anesthesia*, 2nd edn (eds W.W. Muir & J.A.E. Hubbell), Saunders-Elsevier, St. Louis, MO, pp. 210–242.

Spadavecchia, C., Arendt-Nielsen, L., Andersen, O.K., et al. (2005) Effect of romifidine on the nociceptive withdrawal reflex and temporal summation in conscious horses. *American Journal of Veterinary Research*, 66, 1992–1998.

Staffieri, F. & Driessen, B. (2007) Field anesthesia in the equine. *Clinical Techniques in Equine Practice*, 6, 111–119.

Sutton, D.G.M., Preston, T., Christley, R.M., et al. (2002) The effects of xylazine, detomidine, acepromazine and butorphanol on equine solid phase gastric emptying rate. *Equine Veterinary Journal*, 34, 486–492.

Suzuki, M. (2009) Role of N-methyl-D-aspartate receptor antagonists in postoperative pain management. *Current Opinion in Anaesthesiology*, 22, 618–622.

Svensson, C.I. & Yaksh, T.L. (2002) The spinal phospholipase-cyclooxygenase-prostanoid cascade in nociceptive processing. *Annual Reviews of Pharmacology and Toxicology*, 42, 553–583.

Symonds, K.D., MacAllister, C.G., Erkert, R.S., et al. (2006) Use of force plate analysis to assess the analgesic effects of etodolac in horses with navicular syndrome. *American Journal Veterinary Research*, 67, 557–561.

Taylor, C.P. (2004) The biology and pharmacology of calcium channel $\alpha 2$-δ proteins. *CNS Drug Reviews*, 10, 183–188.

Taylor, P.M. (2005) Pharmacological approaches to pain management in the horse. *Proceedings of the American Association of Equine Practitioners*, 51, 398–402.

Taylor, P.M., Pascoe, P.J., & Mama, K.R. (2002) Diagnosing and treating pain in the horse. Where are we today? *Veterinary Clinics of North America: Equine Practice*, 18, 1–19.

Terry, R., McDonnell, S.M., van Eps, A.W., et al. (2010) Pharmacokinetic profile and behavioral effects of gabapentin in the horse. *Journal of Veterinary Pharmacology and Therapeutics*, 33, 485–494.

Thomasy, S.M., Slovis, N., Maxwell, L.K., et al. (2004) Transdermal fentanyl combined with non-steroidal anti-inflammatory drugs for analgesia in horses. *Journal of Veterinary Internal Medicine*, 18, 550–554.

Tomlinson, J.E. & Blikslager, A.T. (2005) Effects of cyclooxygenase inhibitors flunixin and deracoxib on permeability of ischaemic-injured equine jejunum. *Equine Veterinary Journal*, 37, 75–80.

Toutain, P.L. & Cester, C.C. (2004) Pharmacokinetic-pharmacodynamic relationships and dose response to meloxicam in horses with induced arthritis in the right carpal joint. *American Journal Veterinary Research*, 65, 1533–1541.

Treede, R.D., Jensen, T.S., Campbell, J.N., et al. (2008) Neuropathic pain: redefinition and a grading system for clinical and research purposes. *Neurology*, 70, 1630–1635.

Trillo, M.A., Soto, G., & Gunson, D.E. (1984) Flunixin toxicity in a pony. *Equine Practice*, 6, 21–29.

Urdaneta, A., Siso, A., Urdaneta, B., et al. (2009) Lack of correlation between the central anti-nociceptive and peripheral anti-inflammatory effects of selective COX-2 inhibitor parecoxib. *Brain Research Bulletin*, 80, 56–61.

Valverde, A. (2010) Alpha-2 agonists as pain therapy in horses. *Veterinary Clinics Equine*, 26, 515–532.

Valverde, A., Gunkel, C., Doherty, T.J., Giguère, S., & Pollak, A.,S. (2005) Effect of a constant rate infusion of lidocaine on the quality of recovery from sevoflurane or isoflurane general anaesthesia in horses. *Equine Veterinary Journal*, 37(6), 559–564.

Van Elstraete, A.C., Sitbon, P., Mazoit, J.X., et al. (2008) Gabapentin prevents delayed and long-lasting hyperalgesia induced by fentanyl in rats. *Anesthesiology*, 108, 484–494.

Van Hoogmoed, L.M., Snyder, J.R., & Harmon, F.A. (2002) *In vitro* investigation of the effects of cyclooxygenase-2 inhibitors on contractile activity of the equine dorsal and ventral colon. *American Journal Veterinary Research*, 63, 1496–1500.

Van Weeren, P.R. & de Grauw, J.C. (2010) Pain in osteoarthritis. *Veterinary Clinics Equine*, 26, 619–642.

Virtanen, R., Savola, J.M., Saano, V., et al. (1988) Characterization of the selectivity, specificity and potency of medetomidine as an α_2-adrenoceptor agonist. *European Journal of Pharmacology*, 150, 9–14.

Visser, E. & Schug, S.A. (2006) The role of ketamine in pain management. *Biomedicine & Pharmacotherapy*, 60, 341–348.

Wagner, A.E., Mama, K.R., Contino, E.K., et al. (2011) Evaluation of sedation and analgesia in standing horses after administration of xylazine, butorphanol, and subanesthetic doses of ketamine. *Journal of the American Veterinary Medical Association*, 238, 1629–1633.

Walker, A.F. (2007) Sublingual administration of buprenorphine for long-term analgesia in the horse. *Veterinary Record*, 160, 808–809.

Watts, A.E., Nixon, A.J., & Reesink, H.L. (2011) Continuous peripheral neural blockade to alleviate signs of experimentally induced severe forelimb pain in horses. *Journal of the American Veterinary Medical Association*, 238, 1032–1039

Wegner, K., Franklin, R.P., Long, M.T., et al. (2002) How to use fentanyl transdermal patches for analgesia in horses. *Proceedings of the American Association of Equine Practitioners*, 48, 291–294.

Whay, H.R., Webster, A.J.F., & Waterman-Pearson, A.E. (2005) Role of ketoprofen in the modulation of hyperalgesia associated with lameness in dairy cattle. *Veterinary Record*, 157, 729–733.

Wilson, D.V., Bohart, G.V., Evans, A.T., et al. (2002) Retrospective analysis of detomidine infusion for standing chemical restraint in 51 horses. *Veterinary Anaesthesia and Analgesia*, 29, 54–57.

Winter, J., Dray, A., Wood, J.N., et al. (1990) Cellular mechanism of action of resiniferatoxin: a potent sensory neuron excitotoxin. *Brain Research*, 520, 131–140.

Wojtasiak-Wypart, M., Soma, L.R., Rudy, J.A., et al. (2012) Pharmacokinetic profile and pharmacodynamic effects of romifidine hydrochloride in the horse. *Journal of Veterinary Pharmacology and Therapeutics*, 35(5), 478–488.

Wong, G.Y. & Gavva, N.R. (2009) Therapeutic potential of vanilloid receptor TRPV1 agonists and antagonists as analgesics: recent advances and setbacks. *Brain Research Reviews*, 60, 267–277.

Woolf, C.J. (2011) Central sensitization: implications for the diagnosis and treatment of pain. *Pain*, 152, S2–S15.

Woolf, C.J. & Salter, M.W. (2000) Neuronal plasticity: increasing the gain in pain. *Science*, 288, 1765–1768.

Woolf, C.J. & Wiesenfeld-Hallin, Z. (1985) The systemic administration of local anaesthetics produces a selective depression of C-afferent fibre evoked activity in the spinal cord. *Pain*, 23, 361–374.

Xia, R., Dekermendjian, K., Lullau, E., et al. (2011) TRPV1: a therapy target that attracts the pharmaceutical interests. *Advances in Experimental Medicine & Biology*, 704, 637–665.

Xie, H.S., Asquith, R.L., & Kivipelto, J. (1996) A review of the use of acupuncture for treatment of equine back pain. *Journal of Equine Veterinary Science*, 16, 285–290.

Xie, W., Strong, J.A., Mei, J.T., et al. (2005) Neuropathic pain: early spontaneous afferent activity is the trigger. *Pain*, 116, 243–256.

Yaksh, T.L. (2006) Central pharmacology of nociceptive transmission, in *Wall & Melzack's Textbook of Pain*, 5th edn (eds S.B. McMahon

& M. Koltzenburg), Elsevier Churchill-Livingstone, Philadelphia, PA, pp. 371–414.

Yaksh, T.L. (2010) The pain state arising from the laminitic horse: insights into future analgesic therapies. *Journal of Equine Veterinary Science*, 30, 79–82.

Yaksh, T.L., Dirig, D.M., Conway, C.M., et al. (2001) The acute anti-hyperalgesic action of nonsteroidal, anti-inflammatory drugs and release of spinal prostaglandin E2 is mediated by the inhibition of constitutive spinal cyclooxygenase-2 (COX-2) but not COX-1. *Journal of Neuroscience*, 21, 5847–5853.

Yamashita, K., Tsubakishita, S., Futaok, S., et al. (2000) Cardiovascular effects of medetomidine, detomidine and xylazine in horses. *Journal of Veterinary Medical Science*, 62, 1025–1032.

Zarucco, L., Driessen, B., Scandella, M., et al. (2007) Continuous perineural block of the palmar nerves: a new technique for pain relief in the distal equine forelimb. *Clinical Techniques in Equine Practice*, 6, 154–164.

Zarucco, L., Driessen, B., Scandella, M., et al. (2010) Sensory nerve conduction and nociception in the equine lower forelimb during perineural bupivacaine infusion along the palmar nerves. *Canadian Journal Veterinary Research*, 74, 305–313.

Zarucco, L., Scandella, M., Seco, O., et al. (2008) Ultrasound-guided technique for continuous ulnar and median nerve blockade in the horse. *Veterinary Surgery*, 37, E34.

Zhang, J., Ho, K-Y., & Wang, Y. (2011) Efficacy of pregabalin in acute postoperative pain: a meta-analysis. *British Journal of Anaesthesia*, 106, 454–462.

Zimmel, D.N. (2003) How to manage pain and dehydration in horses with colic. *Proceedings of the American Association of Equine Practitioners*, 49, 127–131.

31
Recognition and Assessment of Pain in Ruminants

Kevin J. Stafford

It is widely accepted that mammals feel pain, and much is understood about the physiology of pain. Pain is, however, a subjective experience, and the manner in which an animal actually experiences pain may never be known. This chapter will review the behavioral, physiological, and other responses which have been identified as useful parameters in identifying pain in cattle, sheep, and goats.

RECOGNITION AND ASSESSMENT OF PAIN IN RUMINANTS

Interest in the experience of pain in ruminants is long standing among farmers. Animals in pain may be more dangerous to handle than pain-free individuals. Cows with acute painful mastitis kick out in response to palpation, and cattle being dehorned will attempt to escape, and may lash out in self-defense. Although veterinarians have had access to sedatives and anesthetics, particularly local anesthetics, to assist in pain prevention during surgical procedures and facilitate surgical activity, interest in pain management has been stymied until a few decades ago by the lack of suitable systemic analgesics for use in ruminants. The advent of α-2 agonists in the 1970s and nonsteroidal anti-inflammatory drugs (NSAIDs) in the 1980s stimulated interest in the assessment and alleviation of pain in ruminants and encouraged veterinarians to use analgesics when undertaking surgical procedures or when treating painful conditions (Laven et al., 2009). Moreover, the desire to alleviate pain in ruminants used for research has prompted the use of effective analgesics during research activities.

Clinically, veterinarians are limited to using overt behaviors and specific clinical signs when identifying and assessing pain, and evaluation may be influenced by previous experience and empathy for the afflicted animal. Clinical evaluation of posture and gait may be sufficient to identify the pain experienced by a cow with acute lameness (Figure 31.1). Similarly, the response of a cow with acute mastitis to udder palpation is obvious and diagnostic. The behavior of a weanling calf during amputation dehorning is also an obvious indication of pain, as is the elimination of such signs by use of local anesthesia. Thus, at a certain level of severity, pain in ruminants can be identified easily because an animal is unable to hide the experience of pain or the physical insult causing the pain may interfere with normal function (e.g., lameness).

It is hypothesized, however, that because adult ruminants are unlikely to be assisted by a conspecific there is no advantage in indicating the experience of pain overtly, particularly as it may make the animal more obvious to predators. The presence of a predator, moreover, may further inhibit the expression of behavior indicative of pain or illness. Thus, the presence of a human or a dog may reduce or minimize the expression of pain-related behaviors. However, pain-related behaviors that act in self-defense, prevent ongoing injury, assist in convalescence, or act to relieve pain (Stafford & Mellor, 2002) may be useful. It is possible, for example, that because a cow will defend a calf that is being injured, overt expression of pain by the calf may be advantageous. These hypotheses need to be tested further across species.

The age of an animal may influence its experience of and responses to pain. Moreover, the response to pain may be influenced by individual characteristics as is seen in humans. As an example, the cortisol response to tail docking in calves is generally small but in some calves the response is much greater than in others, suggesting that some individuals experienced more intense pain (Petrie et al., 1996).

The methods used to assess pain in animals can be crudely divided into animal-based or human-based techniques. In the animal-based methods, specific behaviors or physiological responses that occur during or after a painful experience are used to identify pain and to assess its severity (Flecknell, 2000). Human-based methods to identify and gauge pain utilize human interpretation of animal behavior, empathy, and opinion regarding the likely severity of the animal's experience. Human-based assessment techniques may use scales such as a visual analog scale (VAS) or numerical rating systems (NRS) (Spretcher et al., 1997; Staffieri et al., 2009) or pain assessment protocols using specific behaviors to evaluate pain (Thornton & Waterman-Pearson, 1999). In addition, nociceptive threshold responses can be used to assess an animal's sensitivity to different painful stimuli, and are used to investigate chronic pain in animals (Thornton & Waterman-Pearson, 1999).

SOURCES OF PAIN IN RUMINANTS

Ruminants experience pain in many different contexts, including that arising from injury and specific disease entities or that

Pain Management in Veterinary Practice, First Edition. Edited by Christine M. Egger, Lydia Love and Tom Doherty.
© 2014 John Wiley & Sons, Inc. Published 2014 by John Wiley & Sons, Inc.

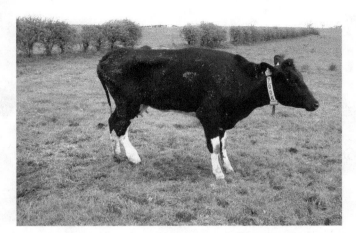

Figure 31.1.   A cow with obvious signs of lameness.

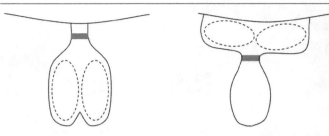

Figure 31.3.   Castration and "short scrotum" of lambs using a rubber ring (in blue). See text for further explanation.

caused by husbandry. The two most important diseases of dairy cattle—lameness due to a number of hoof conditions (sole bruising, white line disease, laminitis) and acute mastitis—are painful, but cattle experience many other disease conditions that probably cause pain, including arthritis, lumpy jaw (actinomycosis), hardware disease, pleuritis, bloat, urolithiasis, dystocia, and wounds and injuries (Parkinson et al., 2010). The arched back, reluctance to move, and grunting of cattle with traumatic reticuloperitonitis are certainly suggestive of pain. Cattle are castrated, dehorned or disbudded, branded and, in some countries, they are tail docked, ear tagged or marked, or have nose rings or loops placed (Stafford & Mellor, 2010). All of these procedures are probably painful. It can be assumed that many other surgical procedures commonly carried out on cattle (abdominal surgery, claw amputation, ear tagging, liver biopsy) are painful, but the specific pain-related behaviors caused by such surgical procedures have not yet been identified.

Sheep experience pain due to many different diseases and procedures. Footrot (Figure 31.2), foot abscess, and external myiasis, which are common conditions (West et al., 2009), undoubtedly cause pain, as do the standard husbandry procedures such as

castration, tail docking, mulesing, and ear tagging or marking. Mulesing is the removal of skin from the perineal area in lambs to reduce the incidence of flystrike. The cuts which may occur during shearing and crutching are surely painful, as are injuries that may occur during oral dosing. Some dental problems are almost certainly painful.

Lambs may be castrated, tail docked, ear tagged, or clipped, often called "marking" in countries such as New Zealand or Australia. In the latter country, Merino lambs may be mulesed at the same time. Depending on farm production practices, lambs may not be castrated or may be subject to a condition called "short scrotum," when a castration ring is placed below the testes such that the distal scrotum becomes necrotic and falls off (Figure 31.3). In short-scrotum lambs the testes are pushed up against the abdominal wall and these lambs are generally infertile. Growth rates are similar to those of intact rams, but as the scrotum is absent the lambs are cleaner when presented for slaughter. This procedure is common in New Zealand where about 20% of male lambs are castrated, 40% are left intact, and 40% are made to have a "short scrotum."

Goats are subjected to some of the same husbandry procedures that cattle and sheep experience—disbudding, castration, and ear tagging or marking—though much less research on pain associated with these procedures has been conducted in this species.

PARAMETERS FOR ASSESSING PAIN

The clinical tools for the identification of pain in ruminants include observation of posture, movement, and other behaviors, palpation of specific tissues or organs, listening for specific pain-related sounds, and assessment of clinical signs (respiration rate, heart rate, rectal temperature).

The physiological parameters used to identify and assess pain and whether it has been alleviated include changes in plasma stress hormones, particularly total plasma cortisol, heart rate, blood pressure, rectal and skin temperature, and brain electrical activity (Table 31.1). Plasma cortisol concentrations can change in response to many different stressors, and it is most useful if used in experimental protocols. Immunological responses have been used as parameters of pain, but appear limited in their clinical usefulness (Fisher, 2002). Weight gain or weight loss have been used as crude parameters to determine the severity of husbandry experiences, such as dehorning adult cattle (Fisher, 2002; Stafford & Mellor, 2005a). The speed of wound healing and adverse effects of different husbandry procedures are also used as crude indicators of what the

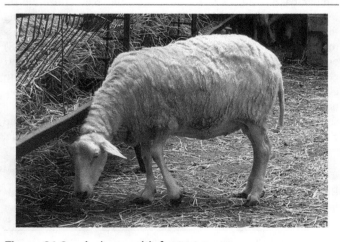

Figure 31.2.   A sheep with footrot.

Table 31.1. Some parameters used to identify and assess pain in ruminants

Physiological
Heart rate variability (Grondahl-Nielson et al., 1999)
Respiratory rate (Heinrich et al., 2009)
Rectal temperature (Marti et al., 2010)
Blood pressure (Peers et al., 2002)
Eye temperature infrared thermography (Stewart et al., 2010)
EEG activity (Gibson et al., 2007)

Biochemical
Cortisol concentrations (McMeekan et al., 1998a, 1998b)
ACTH response (Marti et al., 2010)
Adrenaline and noradrenaline concentrations
(Mellor et al., 2002)
Endorphins (Shutt et al., 1988)

Immunological response
Keyhole limpet hemocyanin (antigen) induced Interferon-γ
production (Ting et al., 2003)

Behavior
Behaviors (Dinniss et al., 1999; McMeekan et al., 1999)
Avoidance behavior (Stafford et al., 1996)
Pain threshold (Whay et al., 1997)
Weight gain (Fisher et al., 1996)
Wound healing (Stafford & Mellor, 2005b)
Visual analog scales (Welsh et al., 1993)
Numerical rating scale (Welsh et al., 1993)

animal may be experiencing with regard to pain. VASs and NRSs have been used in ruminants (Welsh et al., 1993).

Research into pain and its alleviation in ruminants has identified specific responses to pain by comparing the responses of animals subjected to a husbandry practice with or without effective anesthesia and analgesia with nontreated (control) animals. It is thought that behaviors in animals subjected to the procedure without analgesia that are absent in animals that receive effective pain relief or nontreated animals, are indicative of pain. This is a circular argument, but given that animals in pain will self-administer an analgesic (Danbury et al., 2000) and, thence behave differently, it is an acceptable and intuitive position. Much less work has been done in comparing the responses of animals following veterinary procedures, such as abdominal surgery (Stafford et al., 2006), with and without analgesia, but analgesics are often used after such procedures on the premise that it is best, when in doubt, to use an analgesic. The research on assessing and alleviating pain during and after husbandry procedures has allowed scientists to identify effective analgesic protocols that can be used under other circumstances. For example, attempts to alleviate the pain caused by dehorning using scientific protocols allow identification of effective analgesics and their duration of effect (Stafford & Mellor, 2005a).

In veterinary medicine, a group of generic behaviors are generally considered to be indicative of pain and illness. These include inappetance, decreased gastrointestinal motility, inactivity, and isolation. Specific behavioral responses (vocalization, escape, self-defense) have been identified during particular procedures and in response to particular diagnostic procedures (e.g., palpation).

Research on laboratory rats and rabbits subjected to abdominal surgery has identified behaviors indicative of pain that are useful in a clinical context (Roughan & Flecknell, 2001). The research on ruminants has focused on husbandry procedures and the parameters identified, especially the particular behaviors, and may or may not be useful in other contexts. Ear flicking, for example, may relate specifically to dehorning, disbudding, or ear damage and infection, and may not be present in other painful circumstances. The behaviors recorded in the minutes and hours after an animal experiences a husbandry procedure, such as castration, are much less overt than those that occur during the procedure, and become even less obvious as time passes (Marti et al., 2010).

The assessment or measurement of pain using behavior in a clinical setting is difficult, and clinicians often use empathy and imagination to place a value on the severity of the pain. Empathy is a useful human facility, but it is influenced by gender, age, and past experience; individuals may either over- or underdiagnose pain and its severity (Laven et al., 2009).

Even in an experimental setting, using behavior to compare the pain caused by different procedures is problematic. As an example, after ring castration lambs are restless (they stand up and lie down frequently) and after surgical castration lambs lie in unusual postures. These different behaviors might suggest different intensities of pain, but it is not possible to identify which behavior is indicative of the greater pain. In fact, the plasma cortisol responses to the two procedures suggest that acute pain is greater with surgical castration in lambs (Mellor & Stafford, 2000).

INDICATORS OF PAIN IN CATTLE

The generic signs of illness and pain identified in cattle include inactivity, inappetance, reduced rumination, and isolation. Display of other behaviors related to pain may be particular to the individual condition, and may include shallow breathing, arched back, and straining. Bruxism is thought to indicate abdominal pain. The pain caused by acute mastitis can be identified by the cow's response to palpation of the udder and her gait; adduction of the hind limbs is common.

Lameness in cows due to hoof disorders results in a change in gait which is indicative of dysfunction either with or without pain. There was good correlation between an NRS of locomotion and reduced daily activity as recorded by a pedometer (O'Callaghan et al., 2003). Gait changes may be quite subtle at the start of lameness (Table 31.2), but become very obvious as the condition progresses until cows may be unwilling to stand or to move. Severe lameness may result in pathological pain when the cows become hyperresponsive to stimuli that would normally be considered insignificant (Whay et al., 1998; Laven et al., 2008).

The responses of calves to disbudding by cautery, caustic paste, or amputation during and after the procedure have been described in detail (Stafford & Mellor, 2005a). During cautery disbudding, calves struggle violently (rearing, falling down, jerking their heads) (Taschke & Folsch, 1993; Graf & Senn, 1999; Grondahl-Nielson et al., 1999), and in the following 4 hours they head shake, stand up and lie down frequently, kick out with their hind legs, and show increased grooming and rubbing and less rumination. These changes in behavior are eliminated or reduced by effective local anesthesia, and thus appear to be indicative of pain. During the administration of caustic disbudding paste there are no obvious

Table 31.2. Gait evaluation in dairy cows

Lameness score	Description
1. Normal	Stands and walks with level back; normal gait
2. Mild lameness	Stands with level back but when walks back arched
3. Moderate lameness	Arched back when standing and walking; short stride in one or more limbs
4. Severe lameness	Arched back always present Gait slow and deliberate Cow favors one or more hooves
5. Extreme lameness	Unwilling to bear weight on one or more limbs

Source: Spretcher et al., 1997.

behaviors indicative of pain, but soon afterward calves show head rubbing and shaking, inert lying, decreased grooming, and restlessness, and this continues for up to 4 hours (Morisse et al., 1995; Stilwell et al., 2009). During amputation dehorning, calves struggle to escape, and afterward they engage in tail shaking, head shaking, ear flicking, and reduced grazing and rumination (Sylvester et al., 2004). They lie down more, groom less, and scratch more against the pen fittings than do control calves (McMeekan et al., 1999; Stafford et al., 2000). Between 24 and 48 hours after amputation dehorning, calves feed and ruminate less than control animals (Stafford, personal observation). Amputation dehorning of large cattle without local anesthesia is dangerous as they struggle violently to escape. Their behavior after dehorning is likely to be similar to that of young cattle.

Tail docking of dairy heifers may be carried out on young animals when they are being disbudded or later when they are in late pregnancy or beginning to lactate. In young calves, docking by rubber ring evoked tail shaking, restlessness, and vocalization during the first 2 hours after placement, and some calves also kicked up their hind legs and attempted to mouth their tails (Petrie et al., 1995). Rubber ring docking in calves caused a more severe response than docking by cautery, and the former licked their tails for up to 5 days after docking (Tom et al., 2002). Older cattle tail swish in the hours following docking, and in cows there was a decline in milk yield for 3 to 7 days following rubber ring docking (Elliott, 1969).

Most male calves are castrated, and if this is done surgically or by Burdizzo without local anesthesia, the animals will struggle and kick out with their hind legs. Two hours after surgical castration, calves moved about much less than those not castrated or calves castrated chemically or by Burdizzo; this reduced activity was still seen 2 days later (Macaulay et al., 1986). In the afternoon following surgical castration, animals stamped their feet and swished their tails and grazed less than control animals (Fisher et al., 2001). Rubber ring castration caused lifting of hind legs, turning head toward the flanks, slow movement of the tail, and abnormal posture for some weeks after the procedure, suggesting ongoing pain (Molony et al., 1995). Surgical castration caused greater reduction in weight than Burdizzo castration, but wounds from the former healed more quickly (Fisher et al., 1996).

Hot branding is painful and cattle may vocalize (Watts & Stookey, 1999), tail flick, kick, fall, and attempt to escape (Schwartzkopf-Genswein et al., 1997a) during the procedure. Vocalization may be a useful indicator of pain when the effects of very painful procedures are being assessed, but the propensity of cattle to vocalize differs among breeds or types (Watts & Stookey, 2001). Freeze branding is probably less acutely painful than hot branding, but the response to branded tissue palpation was similar in hot- and freeze-branded cattle 1 and 7 days after branding (Schwartzkopf-Genswein et al., 1997b).

Beef calves may be castrated, dehorned, and ear marked or tagged at one time, often at weaning around 6 months of age. The behaviors observed during and after disbudding, dehorning, castration, and docking have much in common and are often intuitive, but may be contradictory. For example, in some situations cattle are inactive and in others they are restless. These differences have been associated with different types of damage or different tissues being damaged as illustrated below in lambs.

The physiological responses to common husbandry procedures in cattle have been described in detail (Stafford & Mellor, 2005a, 2005b). The common parameter used in research is the change in plasma cortisol concentrations. The plasma cortisol response to cautery disbudding in the hours following treatment is less than the response to amputation dehorning (Figure 31.4), which suggests that the former is less painful (Stafford & Mellor, 2005a). It is also less than the response to chemical disbudding. The different types of amputation dehorning (saw, embryotomy wire, shears, scoop) all evoke a similar cortisol response and, therefore, probably produce a similar experience of pain. The plasma cortisol response to amputation dehorning is eliminated by effective use of local anesthesia, but after the effect wears off there is an increase in plasma cortisol concentrations, which is indicative of pain. This delayed response can be eliminated by using an NSAID. Interestingly, cauterizing the wound under local anesthetic has a similar effect.

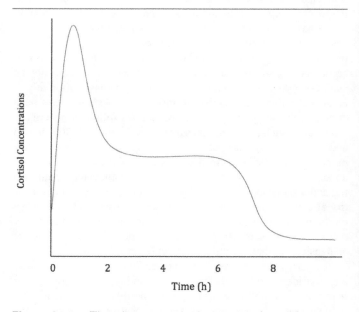

Figure 31.4. The plasma cortisol response (y-axis) to amputation dehorning in Friesian calves.

The plasma cortisol response to different methods of castration suggests that castration by Burdizzo causes less pain than surgical castration or castration by rubber ring or band (Stafford & Mellor, 2005b). Local anesthesia eliminates the cortisol response to ring or band castration and, by inference, the acute pain caused by these procedures, but needs to be combined with an NSAID to eliminate the cortisol response to surgical or Burdizzo castration.

The heart rate, cortisol response, and epinephrine response show that hot iron branding is more painful than freeze branding (Lay et al., 1992; Schwartzkopf-Genswein et al., 1997b). These physiological parameters are generally not useful clinically for identifying pain and its severity. The many behaviors listed above (tail flicking, ear flicking, etc.) may be used to identify pain but, apart from being a rough guide that suggests that vocalization and violent attempts to escape during a procedure infer severe pain, the other behaviors have not been "titrated" as parameters to measure the degree of pain being experienced. Moreover, as all these behaviors also occur in pain-free animals, their presence cannot be used as an indicator of pain.

INDICATORS OF PAIN IN SHEEP

Sheep are a timid prey species and unlikely to advertise that they are compromised; thus, one would expect overt signs of pain only after seriously painful procedures or experiences. Moreover, unlike cattle and goats, sheep tend to remain silent rather than vocalizing during painful procedures.

The behavioral responses of sheep (Table 31.3) after painful husbandry practices have been identified and assessed by teams of researchers in Scotland and New Zealand.

When lambs are subjected to docking, castrating, and mulesing they are held either manually or in a frame, and they may not have much opportunity to show pain-related behavior beyond some limited movement. After these procedures are carried out and lambs are released, they show specific behaviors which have been identified as being pain-related.

In the 60 minutes or so after rubber ring castration and docking, lambs stand up and lie down frequently. This behavior is more common in lambs docked at 21 or 42 days of age than at 5 days, and is more common after ring treatment than surgical castration and docking (Table 31.4; Lester et al., 1996; Molony & Kent, 1993). In addition, lambs castrated and docked by rubber ring engaged in more abnormal lying postures (lying with hindlimbs extended) and more kicking and rolling than after surgical castration and docking. Abnormal standing (kicking, stamping, walking backwards, walking on knees) was also seen after castration and docking by ring and surgery, but especially after the former (Molony & Kent, 1993). In contrast, the incidence of abnormal standing was seen to decrease earlier in lambs castrated by ring than those castrated surgically but the latter showed less abnormal lying (Lester et al., 1996). One week old lambs gambolled less after ring castration, and four- to six-week-old lambs lay down for a shorter time period, and spent more time lying in abnormal postures (Thornton & Waterman-Pearson, 2002).

There is considerable variation in the pain-related behavior of individual lambs after castration and docking, and this makes the identification and quantification of pain in individual animals difficult. To assess pain more effectively, Thornton and Waterman-Pearson (1999) combined active behaviors, response to an observer,

Table 31.3. Behaviors recorded in sheep during and after castration and docking by rubber ring

Behavior	Description
Restlessness	Standing up and lying down
Rolling	Rolling side to side without standing; half rolls
Jumping	Leap forward using bunny hops
Foot stamping/kicking	Front or hind limb lifted and then stamped or kicked
Easing quarters	One quarter eased
Tail wagging	Side to side movement
Head turning	Movement of head beyond shoulders
Vocalization	Bleats
Lip curl	Curling of upper or both lips away from teeth
Teat seeking	Teat seeking
Trembling	Trembling of torso or limbs but not ears
Normal lying	Ventral with legs tucked in
Abnormal lying—ventral	Ventral with hind legs extended, or scrotal area off ground
Abnormal lying—lateral	Lateral with one shoulder on ground, hind legs extended
Normal standing	Standing, walking or playing without abnormalities
Statue standing	Standing with hind limbs apart and further back than normal
Abnormal standing	Unsteady, backward, on knees, hops, circling, leaning, falling

Source: Molony et al., 2002.

Table 31.4. Restlessness scores (mean ± SEM) for the 60 minutes after castration with or without docking (number of times lamb stood up or lay down)

Parameter	Score
Control handling	3.1 (1)
Docking by hot iron	2.5 (1.4)
Docking using cold knife	3.0 (1.3)
Castration surgically	4.6 (1.6)
Castration and docking surgically	2.0 (0.7)
Castration by ring & docking by hot iron	73 (8)
Castration by ring	77 (9)
Docking by ring	100 (20)
Short scrotum and docking by ring	111 (18)
Castration and docking by ring	148 (14)

Source: Lester et al., 1996.

and response to scrotal palpation in a combined VAS to compare the pain caused by a number of castration techniques with and without analgesia. A castration clamp combined with a rubber ring, when compared to a rubber ring alone, reduced the active pain behaviors and the response to observers but not the scrotal palpation response. The scrotal palpation response pain persisted in the lambs for several days after castration by ring or ring and clamp.

Surgical castration caused increased nociceptive thresholds for 7 hours after treatment, but ring castration did not. The authors suggest that this period of hypoalgesia could be due to stress-induced analgesia (Thornton & Waterman-Pearson, 1999). Vocalization resulted from application of a Burdizzo in some lambs (Molony et al., 1997), and can be taken as a good indicator of severe immediate pain, as suggested for cattle.

Mulesed lambs stood hunched and walked less than untreated lambs in the hours after the surgery (Paull et al., 2008). The abnormal postures seen in lambs after castration, mulesing, and docking are not seen frequently in pain-free lambs, and are thus useful indicators of pain and its severity (Molony et al., 1997).

The plasma cortisol response to castration and docking of lambs has been extensively studied (Mellor & Stafford, 2000). The response is greater for surgical castration than ring, clamp, or ring plus clamp castration (Figure 31.5). Similarly, surgical docking causes a greater cortisol response than ring docking. Rubber ring docking produced a much greater cortisol response than docking by cautery (Graham et al., 1997).

Lameness due to footrot is a painful condition in sheep, and there may be a close correlation between the observed lameness score, foot pathology, pain severity, and nociceptive thresholds (Table 31.5) (Ley et al., 1995). Acute footrot and foot abscessation is easily identified, as the affected sheep often graze in a kneeling posture. Efforts to quantify the chronic pain caused by footrot have been made using VASs and NRSs (Welsh et al., 1993). Ley et al. (1991)

Table 31.5. A scoring system used to assess lameness and pathology in sheep with footrot

Lameness score	Pathology
0. Normal movement	0. Normal foot
1. Occasional limping	1. Damage to foot, no smell
2. Lift foot when stand, use in movement	2. Swollen and hot
3. Carry foot and lame on movement	3. Swollen, hot, and broken hoof
4. Carry foot all the time	4. As for 3, plus suppuration and smell
5.	5. As for 4, plus sensitive tissues exposed

Add two scores to get range of 0–9; 1–5, mild and 6–9, severe lameness.
Source: Ley et al., 1992.

suggested that the relationship between plasma cortisol, prolactin, and vasopressin may be a useful index of chronic pain in lame sheep, as may plasma concentrations of adrenaline and noradrenaline (Ley et al., 1992). Sheep affected with footrot showed lower response thresholds to mechanical stimuli than control (unaffected) animals (Ley et al., 1989). Repeated administration of flunixin over 3 days increased the threshold to noxious mechanical stimulation in sheep affected by footrot (Welsh & Nolan, 1995), suggesting that the mechanical response threshold may be a useful tool in assessing chronic pain in lame animals.

INDICATORS OF PAIN IN GOATS

Goats are more vocal animals than sheep or cattle. Less information about behavioral responses to painful conditions is available for goats than sheep or cattle, though Staffieri et al. (2009) investigated perioperative analgesic protocols. These workers modified a detailed NRS for goats based on one produced by Shafford et al. (2004) for sheep. The scale rated comfort, movement, and flock behavior, and added the scores.

During cautery disbudding, kids struggled and afterward vocalized and kicked out (Alvarez et al., 2009; Alvarez & Gutierrez, 2010). After castration by rubber ring, one-day-old kids lay down either laterally or ventrally with their neck extended for up to 60 minutes. By 90 minutes they were lying ventrally and asleep, where they remained for the following 150 minutes (Mellor et al., 1991). Kids commonly hide and wait for their mother to return and feed them, unlike lambs, which follow their mother all the time. This may explain the difference in the behavior of kids and lambs after castration.

SUMMARY

The identification, assessment, and alleviation of pain in farm animals are basic veterinary and animal husbandry activities. The identification of acute severe pain is often simple, but less severe and chronic pain syndromes may not be easy to identify. Furthermore,

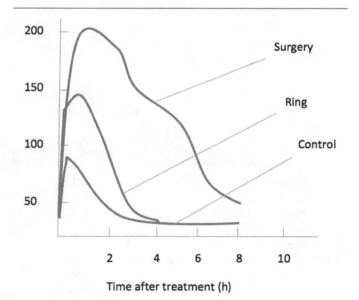

Figure 31.5. The plasma cortisol response (y-axis) to castration by surgery and rubber ring in lambs (adapted from Mellor & Stafford, 2000).

detailed assessment may be impossible beyond simple categorization, such as severe, moderate, and minor. Using a mix of behavior, clinical signs, physiological responses, and empathy, most veterinarians can estimate how severe the pain an animal experiences is, but this assessment may be inaccurate. Much work needs to be done to improve our ability to assess pain in ruminants.

This quantification will be furthered by utilizing developments in remote monitoring technology to measure movement (e.g., pedometers), activity, and physiological parameters. Techniques such as infrared thermography measurements may also provide a useful clinical tool when combined with heart rate to assess pain in animals (Stewart et al., 2010). Equipment that facilitates the collection of behavioral and physiological data and the analysis of such data will improve our assessment of pain, as will the ongoing developments in analgesics.

REFERENCES

Alvarez, L. & Gutierrez, J. (2010) A first description of the physiological and behavioral responses to disbudding in goat kids. *Animal Welfare*, 19, 55–59.

Alvarez, L., Nava, R.A., Ramirez, A., Ramirez, E., & Gutierrez, J. (2009) Physiological and behavioral alterations in disbudded goat kids with and without local anaesthesia. *Applied Animal Behaviour Science*, 117, 190–196.

Danbury, T.C., Weeks, C.A., Chambers, J.P., Waterman-Pearson, A.E., & Kestin, S.C. (2000) Self-selection of the analgesic drug carprofen by lame broiler chickens. *The Veterinary Record*, 146, 307–311.

Dinniss, A.S., Stafford, K.J., Mellor, D.J., Bruce, R.A., & Ward, R.N. (1999) The behaviour pattern of lambs after castration using a rubber ring and/or a castration clamp with or without local anaesthesia. *New Zealand Veterinary Journal*, 47, 198–203.

Elliott, R.E.W. (1969) The effect of tail amputation on the milk yield of cows. *New Zealand Veterinary Journal*, 17, 89.

Fisher, A.D. (2002) Pain – its effects on immune function and growth in animals. *Proceedings of the New Zealand Society of Animal Production*, 62, 363–367.

Fisher, A.D., Crows, M.A., Alonso de la Varga, M.E., & Enright, W.J. (1996). Effect of castration method and the provision of local anaesthesia on plasma cortisol, scrotal circumference, growth and feed intake of beef bulls. *Journal of Animal Science*, 74, 2336–2343.

Fisher, A.D., Knight, T.W., Cosgrove, G.P., et al. (2001) Effects of surgical or banding castration on stress responses and behavior of bulls. *Australian Veterinary Journal*, 79, 279–284.

Flecknell, P. (2000) Recognition and assessment of pain in animals, in *Pain: Its Nature and Management in Man and Animals* (eds E.J.L. Soulsby & D. Morton), The Royal Society of Medicine Press, London, UK, pp. 63–68.

Gibson, T.J., Johnson, C.B., Stafford, K.J., Mitchinson, S.L., & Mellor, D.J. (2007) Validation of the acute electroencephalographic response of calves to noxious stimulus with scoop dehorning. *New Zealand Veterinary Journal*, 55, 152–157.

Graf, B. & Senn, M. (1999) Behavioral and physiological responses of calves to dehorning by heat cauterisation with or without local anaesthesia. *Applied Animal Behaviour Science*, 62, 153–171.

Graham, M.J., Kent, J.E., & Molony, V. (1997) Effects of four analgesic treatments on the behavioral and cortisol responses of 3-week-old lambs to tail docking. *The Veterinary Journal*, 153, 87–97.

Grondahl-Nielson, C., Simonsen, H.B., Damkjer Lund, J., & Hesselholt, M. (1999) Behavioral, endocrine and cardiac responses in young calves undergoing dehorning without and with the use of sedation and analgesia. *The Veterinary Journal*, 158, 14–20.

Heinrich, A., Duffield, T., Lissemore, K.D., Squires, E.J., & Millman, S.T. (2009) The impact of meloxicam on postsurgical stress associated with cautery dehorning. *Journal of Dairy Science*, 92, 540–547.

Laven, R.A., Huxley, J.N., Whay, H.R., & Stafford, K.J. (2009) Results of a survey of attitudes of dairy veterinarians in New Zealand regarding painful procedures and conditions in cattle. *New Zealand Veterinary Journal*, 57, 215–220.

Laven, R.A., Lawrence, K.E., Weston, J.F., Dowson, K.R., & Stafford, K.J. (2008) Assessment of duration of the pain response associated with lameness in dairy cows and the influence of treatment. *New Zealand Veterinary Journal*, 56, 210–217.

Lay, D.C. Jr., Friend, T.H., Randel, R.D., Bowers, C.L., Grissom, K.K., & Jenkins, O.C. (1992) Behavioral and physiological effects of freeze or hot-iron branding on crossbred cattle. *Journal of Animal Science*, 70, 330–336.

Lester, S.J., Mellor, D.J., Holmes, R.J., Ward, R.N., & Stafford, K.J. (1996) Behavioural and cortisol responses of lambs to castration and tailing using different methods. *New Zealand Veterinary Journal*, 44, 45–54.

Ley, S.J., Livingston, A., & Waterman, A.E. (1989) The effect of chronic clinical pain on thermal and mechanical thresholds in sheep. *Pain*, 39, 353–357.

Ley, S.J., Livingston, A., & Waterman, A.E. (1991) Effects of chronic lameness on the concentrations of cortisol, prolactin and vasopressin in the plasma of sheep. *The Veterinary Record*, 129, 45–47.

Ley, S.J., Livingston, A., & Waterman, A.E. (1992) Effects of clinically occurring chronic lameness in sheep on the concentrations of plasma noradrenaline and adrenaline. *Research in Veterinary Science*, 53, 122–125.

Ley, S.J., Waterman, A.E., & Livingston, A. (1995) A field study of the effect of lameness on mechanical nociceptive thresholds in sheep. *The Veterinary Record*, 137, 85–87.

Macaulay, A.S., Friend, T.H., & LaBore, J.M. (1986) Behavioral and physiological responses of dairy calves to different methods of castration. *Journal of Animal Science*, 63, 166.

Marti, S., Velarde, A., de la Torre, J.L., et al. (2010) Effects of ring castration with local anaesthesia and analgesia in Holstein calves at 3 months of age on welfare indicators. *Journal of Animal Science*, 88, 2789–2796.

McMeekan, C.M., Mellor, D.J., Stafford, K.J., Bruce, R.A., Ward, R.N., & Gregory, N.G. (1998a) Effects of local anaesthesia of 4 to 8 hours duration on the acute cortisol response to scoop dehorning in calves. *Australian Veterinary Journal*, 76, 281–285.

McMeekan, C.M., Stafford, K.J., Mellor, D.J., Bruce, R.A., Ward, R.N., & Gregory, N.G. (1998b) Effects of regional analgesia and/or a non-steroidal anti-inflammatory analgesic on the acute cortisol response to dehorning in calves. *Research in Veterinary Science*, 64, 147–150.

McMeekan, C., Stafford, K.J., Mellor, D.J., Bruce, R.A., Ward, R.N., & Gregory, N.G. (1999) Effects of a local anaesthetic and a non-steroidal anti-inflammatory analgesic on the behavioral responses of calves to dehorning. *New Zealand Veterinary Journal*, 47, 92–96.

Mellor, D.J. & Stafford, K.J. (2000) Acute castration and/or tailing distress and its alleviation in lambs. *New Zealand Veterinary Journal*, 48, 33–43.

Mellor, D.J., Molony, V., & Robertson, I.S. (1991) Effects of castration on behavior and plasma cortisol concentrations in young lambs, kids and calves. *Research in Veterinary Science*, 51, 149–154.

Mellor, D.J., Stafford, K.J., & Todd, S.E. (2002) A comparison of catecholamine and cortisol responses of young lambs and calves to painful husbandry procedures. *Australian Veterinary Journal*, 80, 228–233.

Molony, V. & Kent, J.E. (1993) Behavioral responses of lambs of three ages in the first three hours after three methods of castration and tail docking. *Research in Veterinary Science*, 55, 234–245.

Molony, V., Kent, J.W., & McKendrick, I.J. (2002) Validation of a method for assessment of an acute pain in lambs. *Applied Animal Behaviour Science*, 76, 215–238.

Molony, V., Kent, J.E., & Robertson, I.S. (1995) Assessment of acute and chronic pain after different methods of castration of calves. *Applied Animal Behaviour Science*, 46, 33–48.

Molony, V., Kent, J.E., Hosie, B.D., et al. (1997) Reduction in pain suffered by lambs at castration. *The Veterinary Journal*, 153, 205–213.

Morisse, J.P., Cotte, J.P., & Huonnic, D. (1995) Effect of dehorning on behavior and plasma cortisol responses in young calves. *Applied Animal Behaviour Science*, 43, 239–247.

O'Callaghan, K.A., Cripps, P.J., Downham, D.Y., et al. (2003) Subjective and objective assessment of pain and discomfort due to lameness in dairy cows. *Animal Welfare*, 12, 605–610.

Parkinson, T.J., Vermunt, J.J., & Malmo, J. (2010) *Diseases of Cattle in Australasia*, Published by the NZVA Foundation for continuing education, Palmerston North, New Zealand.

Paull, D.R., Lee, C., Atkinson, S.J., et al. (2008) Effects of meloxicam or telfenamic acid administration on the pain and stress response of Merino lambs to mulesing. *Australian Veterinary Journal*, 86, 303–311.

Peers, A., Mellor, D.J., Wintour, E.M., et al. (2002) Blood pressure, heart rate, hormonal and other acute responses to rubber ring castration plus tailing of lambs. *New Zealand Veterinary Journal*, 50, 56–62.

Petrie, N., Mellor, D.J., Stafford, K.J., et al. (1996) Cortisol responses of calves to two methods of tail docking used with or without local anaesthetic. *New Zealand Veterinary Journal*, 44, 4–8.

Petrie, N., Stafford, K.J., Mellor, D.J., Bruce, R.A., & Ward, R.N. (1995) The behavior of calves tail docked with a rubber ring used with or without local anaesthetic. *Proceedings of the New Zealand Society of Animal Production*, 55, 58–60.

Roughan, J.V. & Flecknell, P.A. (2001) Behavioral effects of laparotomy and analgesic effects of ketoprofen and carprofen in rats. *Pain*, 90, 65–70.

Schwartzkopf-Genswein, K.S., Stookey, J.M., & Welford, R. (1997a) Behavior of cattle during hot-iron and freeze branding and the effects on subsequent handling ease. *Journal of Animal Science*, 75, 2064–2072.

Schwartzkopf-Genswein, K.S., Stookey, J.M., dePassille, A.M. & Rushen, J. (1997b) Comparison of hot-iron and freeze branding on cortisol levels and pain sensitivity in beef cattle. *Canadian Journal of Animal Science*, 77, 369–374.

Shafford, H.L., Hellyer, P.W., & Turner, A.S. (2004) Intra-articular lidocaine plus bupivicaine in sheep undergoing stifle arthrotomy. *Veterinary Anaesthesia and Analgesia*, 31, 20–26.

Shutt, D.A., Fell, L.R., Connell, R., & Bell, A.K. (1988) Stress responses in lambs docked and castrated surgically or by application of rubber rings. *Australian Veterinary Journal*, 65, 5–7.

Spretcher, D.J., Hostetler, D.E., & Kaneene, J.B. (1997) A lameness scoring system that uses posture and gait to predict dairy cattle reproductive performance. *Theriogenology*, 47, 1179–1187.

Staffieri, F., Driessen, B., Lacitignola, L., & Crovace, A. (2009) A comparison of subarachnoid buprenorphine or xylazine as an adjunct to lidocaine for analgesia in goats. *Veterinary Anaesthesia and Analgesia*, 36, 502–511.

Stafford, K.J. & Mellor, D.J. (2002) Monitoring pain in animals using behavior. *Proceedings of the New Zealand Society of Animal Production*, 62, 355–358.

Stafford, K.J. & Mellor, D.J. (2005a) Dehorning and disbudding distress and its alleviation in calves. *The Veterinary Journal*, 169, 337–349.

Stafford, K.J. & Mellor, D.J. (2005b) The welfare significance of the castration of cattle: a review. *New Zealand Veterinary Journal*, 53, 271–278.

Stafford, K.J. & Mellor, D.J. (2010) Painful husbandry procedures in livestock and poultry, in *Improving Animal Welfare; A Practical Approach* (ed. T. Grandin), CABI, Wallingford, UK, pp. 88–114.

Stafford, K.J., Chambers, J.P., Sylvester, S.P., et al. (2006) Stress caused by laparoscopy and its alleviation. *New Zealand Veterinary Journal*, 54, 109–113.

Stafford, K.J., Mellor, D.J., Ward, R.N., Bruce, R.A., & Ward, R.N. (2000) Behavioral responses of calves to amputation dehorning with or without local anaesthetic. *Proceedings of the New Zealand Society of Animal Production*, 60, 234–236.

Stafford, K.J., Sporenberg, J., West, D.M., Vermunt, J.J., Petrie, N., & Lawoko, C.R. (1996). The effects of electroejaculation on aversive behavior and plasma cortisol in rams. *New Zealand Veterinary Journal*, 44, 95–98.

Stewart, M., Verkerk, G.A., Stafford, K.J., Schaefer, A.L., & Webster, J.R. (2010) Noninvasive assessment of autonomic activity for evaluation of pain in calves using surgical castration as a model. *Journal of Dairy Science*, 93, 3602–3609.

Stilwell, G., Campos de Carvalho, R., Lima, M.S., & Broom, D.M. (2009) Effect of caustic paste disbudding, using local anaesthesia with and without analgesia, on behavior and cortisol of calves. *Applied Animal Behaviour Science*, 116, 35–44.

Sylvester, P., Stafford, K.J., Mellor, D.J., Bruce, R.A., & Ward, R.N. (2004) Behavioral responses of calves to amputation dehorning with or without local anaesthetic. *Australian Veterinary Journal*, 82, 697–700.

Taschke, A. & Folsch, D. (1993) Belastungen von Kalbern durch die thermische enthornung ohne Betaubung. *Landwirtschaft Schweiz Bund*, 6, 340–344.

Thornton, P.D. & Waterman-Pearson, A.E. (1999) Quantification of pain and distress responses to castration in young lambs. *Research in Veterinary Science*, 66, 107–118.

Thornton, P.D. & Waterman-Pearson, A.E. (2002) Behavioral responses to castration in lambs. *Animal Welfare*, 11, 203–212.

Ting, S.T.L., Earley, B., & Crowe, M.A. (2003) Effects of repeated ketoprofen administration during surgical castration of bulls on cortisol, immunological function, feed intake, growth and behavior. *Journal of Animal Science*, 81, 1253–1264.

Tom, E.M., Rushen, J., Duncan, I.J.H., & de Passille, A.M. (2002) Behavioral, health and cortisol response of young calves to tail docking using a rubber ring or docking iron. *Canadian Journal of Animal Science*, 82, 1–9.

Watts, J.M. & Stookey, J.M. (1999) Effects of restraint and branding on rates and acoustic parameters of vocalisation in beef cattle. *Applied Animal Behaviour Science*, 62, 125–135.

Watts, J.M. & Stookey, J.M. (2001) The propensity of cattle to vocalise during handling and isolation is affected by phenotype. *Applied Animal Behaviour Science*, 74, 81–95.

Welsh, E.M. & Nolan, A.M. (1995) Effect of flunixin meglumine on the thresholds to mechanical stimulation in healthy and lame sheep. *Research in Veterinary Science*, 58, 61–66.

Welsh, E.M., Gettinby, G., & Nolan, A.M. (1993) Comparison of a visual analogue scale and a numerical rating scale for assessment of lameness, using sheep as a model. *American Journal of Veterinary Research*, 54, 976–983.

West, D.M., Bruere, A.N., & Ridler, A.N. (2009) *The Sheep: Health, Disease and Production*, VetLearn, Palmerston North, New Zealand.

Whay, H.R., Waterman, A.E., & Webster, A.J.F. (1997) Associations between locomotion, claw lesions and nociceptive threshold in dairy heifers during the peri-partum period. *The Veterinary Journal*, 154, 155–161.

Whay, H.R., Waterman, A.E., Webster, A.J.F., & O'Brien, J.K. (1998) The influence of lesion type on the duration of hyperalgesia associated with hindlimb lameness in dairy cattle. *The Veterinary Journal*, 156, 23–29.

32

Treatment of Acute and Chronic Pain in Ruminants

Alexander Valverde

Pain management is a major issue in ruminant practice because many husbandry procedures thought to improve productivity and safety, such as castration and dehorning, are commonly performed with minimal or no analgesia. An increased awareness of ruminant welfare issues has led to more extensive use of analgesic drugs and techniques to decrease pain and distress.

PAIN RECOGNITION AND ASSESSMENT IN RUMINANTS

An in-depth discussion of pain assessment in ruminants is presented in Chapter 31. It is important to emphasize that pain recognition is difficult and depends on an individual animal's variation from normal behavior. Among herd animals, behavior may be affected by social interactions as well as the evolutionary benefit of stoicism in prey species to mask illness and weakness. In addition, observers often interpret pain based on their personal experiences, and this may result in subjective and erroneous assessments.

Current surveys of practitioners indicate that cesarean section, claw amputation, omentopexy, and mastitis are considered to be the most painful conditions in adult cattle. Fracture of a distal limb and repair of umbilical herniorrhaphy are considered to be the most painful conditions in calves (Watts & Clarke, 2000; Whay & Huxley, 2005; Huxley & Whay, 2006; Hewson et al., 2007; Kielland et al., 2009).

Pain in ruminants is often not treated effectively due to difficulties in detection of pain-related behaviors, assessors with limited knowledge of pain-related behaviors, and a lack of cost-effective analgesics. Most available analgesic drugs have a short duration of action and a risk of adverse effects, such as sedation in the case of α-2 agonists, in addition to a withdrawal period (Whay & Huxley, 2005; Huxley & Whay, 2006; Hewson et al., 2007).

In North America, withdrawal periods for opioids vary between 2 and 4 days for milk and meat; for α-2 agonists, between 2 and 3 days for milk and 3 and 5 days for meat; for local anesthetics, less than 1 day for milk and meat; for nonsteroidal anti-inflammatory drugs (NSAIDs), 1–3 days for milk and 3–7 days for meat; and for ketamine, 2 days for milk and 3 days for meat. Similar withdrawal times are recommended in countries in Europe, the United

Kingdom, and Australia and New Zealand; an exception is xylazine's 14 day withdrawal time for meat in the United Kingdom (Valverde & Doherty, 2008a).

Another factor leading to inadequate treatment of pain in ruminants is delaying elective surgery, such as castration or dehorning, until the animal is older, which usually results in more tissue trauma and pain. This is often due to poor herd management and/or a lack of practitioner interest in pain management (Huxley & Whay, 2006).

ANALGESIC DRUGS USED IN RUMINANTS

Opioids, α-2 agonists, local anesthetics, ketamine, and NSAIDs are administered either alone or in various combinations to control pain. Routes of administration include the intravenous (IV), intramuscular (IM), epidural, local infiltration, transdermal, and intraarticular.

Opioids

The mode of action of opioids is described in detail in Chapter 4. Recommended opioid doses for ruminants are presented in Table 32.1.

Factors that constrain the use of opioids in ruminants under farming conditions include their schedule classification for controlled substances, and the preference among practitioners for drugs such as NSAIDs, α-2 agonists, and local anesthetics. Compared with other species, there is little information about the use of opioids for analgesia in ruminants, and their clinical use is usually as a component of anesthetic combinations rather than individual use for analgesic purposes. Opioids are, however, effective for many types of pain, not just perioperative pain.

SYSTEMIC USE OF OPIOIDS IN RUMINANTS

Evidence for the efficacy of opioids in ruminants comes from pain models using cutaneous thermal and mechanical stimulation in sheep and cattle. Butorphanol, fentanyl, buprenorphine, and meperidine in sheep and morphine in cattle have proven to be effective analgesics for thermal noxious stimulation when administered intravenously (Nolan et al., 1987a, 1988, Waterman et al. 1990, 1991a, 1991b; Machado-Filho et al., 1998). Fentanyl, and

Pain Management in Veterinary Practice, First Edition. Edited by Christine M. Egger, Lydia Love and Tom Doherty.
© 2014 John Wiley & Sons, Inc. Published 2014 by John Wiley & Sons, Inc.

Table 32.1.   Opioids commonly used in ruminants

Drug	Dose (mg/kg, unless indicated otherwise)	Route	Duration of analgesia (h)	Species
Morphine	0.05–0.5	IM, IV	1–6	Sheep, goats, cattle
	0.1	EPI	6–12	Sheep, goats, cattle
	0.01	IT		Sheep, goats
Buprenorphine	0.0015– 0.006	IM, IV	1–4	Sheep
	0.005	IT	4–6	Goats
Fentanyl	0.01	IM, IV	1–2	Sheep, goats, cattle
	50 μg/h	TRA	5–12	Goats
Meperidine	5	IM	0.25–0.5	Sheep, goats, cattle
Butorphanol	0.05–0.2	IM, IV	1–3	Sheep, goats, cattle

Source: Nolan et al., 1987a; Nolan et al., 1988; Waterman et al., 1990; Waterman et al., 1991a; Waterman et al., 1991b; Pablo, 1993; Hendrickson et al., 1996; Machado-Filho et al., 1998; Carroll et al., 1999; Doherty et al., 2002; George, 2003; Doherty et al., 2004; Fierheller et al., 2004; Staffieri et al., 2009; George, 2003

IM, intramuscular; IV, intravenous; EPI, epidural; IT, intrathecal; TRA, transdermal patch.

to a lesser extent, meperidine were effective when administered intravenously to sheep when a pressure (mechanical) stimulus was applied (Nolan et al., 1988; Waterman et al., 1990).

IV administered morphine (2 mg/kg) decreased the minimum alveolar concentration (MAC) of isoflurane by approximately 30% in goats (Doherty et al., 2004), whereas butorphanol (0.05–0.1 mg/kg IV) induced variable individual changes and no overall change in MAC (Doherty et al., 2002).

EPIDURAL ADMINISTRATION OF OPIOIDS

Epidurally administered morphine (0.1 mg/kg) has been used clinically in goats and cattle. Morphine is administered at the sacrococcygeal or first intercoccygeal space in cattle, and at the lumbosacral space in goats and sheep. Analgesia of 6–12 hours' duration has been achieved after abdominal surgery, hind limb amputation, and other painful musculoskeletal conditions (Pablo, 1993; Hendrickson et al., 1996; George, 2003; Valverde & Doherty, 2008b). Epidural administration of nonlipid soluble opioids, such as morphine or hydromorphone, provides a longer duration of analgesia than systemic administration. Epidural administration of lipid soluble opioids, such as fentanyl or butorphanol, does not result in a longer duration of analgesia than systemic administration; therefore, they provide no advantage by this route, unless administered as a CRI.

INTRATHECAL ADMINISTRATION OF OPIOIDS

Intrathecal (subarachnoid) injection may occur when drugs are administered at the lumbosacral space in small ruminants, due to the presence of the meninges at that anatomical level. Intrathecal doses of opioids should be no more than one-tenth of the epidural dose to avoid toxicity (Valverde, 2008). Signs of toxicity include pruritus, ataxia, and erratic motor activity (Wagner et al., 1996; Valverde, 2008).

Intrathecal administration of buprenorphine (5 μg/kg) combined with lidocaine (2 mg/kg) provided better and longer-lasting analgesia than xylazine (0.05 mg/kg) combined with lidocaine (2 mg/kg) in the first 24 hours after stifle surgery in goats (Staffieri et al., 2009).

INTRA-ARTICULAR ADMINISTRATION OF MORPHINE

Intra-articular administration of morphine is effective in other species (rats, dogs, horses, humans) for the relief of pain resulting from inflammatory processes of the joint (Day et al., 1995; Nagasaka et al., 1996; Sammarco et al., 1996; Kizilkaya et al., 2005; Lindegaard et al., 2010). The recommended dose (0.05–0.1 mg/kg) is diluted with sterile saline (5–15 mL) according to the joint size. Either a preservative-free or preservative-containing morphine preparation can be used.

TRANSDERMAL ADMINISTRATION OF OPIOIDS

Fentanyl patches (50 μg/h) placed on the neck region in goats (40 kg body weight) resulted in bioavailability that exceeded 100% due to recycling of the highly lipid soluble fentanyl through the ruminosalivary cycle (Carroll et al., 1999). This high degree of bioavailability may result in the occurrence of adverse affects, such as dysphoria, respiratory depression, inappetance, excessive sedation, and ileus. Another disadvantage of transdermal fentanyl administration is that peak plasma concentrations are not achieved until 8–18 hours after application (Carroll et al., 1999), and therapeutic plasma concentrations may not be achieved on all occasions due to technical problems with patch placement. Careful monitoring for adverse effects and adequacy of analgesia is required.

α-2 Agonists

The sedative and analgesic properties of this pharmacological group make them popular as analgesics for surgical patients. α-2 adrenergic receptors are located supraspinally and spinally. A detailed description of these receptors and α-2 agonists is found in Chapter 7.

Commonly used α-2 agonists in ruminants include xylazine, detomidine, medetomidine, dexmedetomidine, and romifidine (Table 32.2). Unfortunately, analgesia is accompanied by adverse effects including sedation, bradycardia, vasoconstriction, hypertension and/or hypotension, decreased cardiac output, increased respiratory resistance, decreased lung compliance, hypoxemia, and hypercapnia, and these drugs should not be used in animals that are hypovolemic or have cardiorespiratory compromise (Doherty et al.,

Table 32.2. α-2 agonists commonly used in ruminants

Drug	Dose (mg/kg)	Route	Duration of analgesia (h)	Species/comments
Xylazine	0.05–0.2	IM, IV	1–4	Sheep, goats, cattle
	0.025–0.1	EPI		Sheep, goats, cattle Paresis/ataxia is common
	0.025–0.1	IT		Sheep, goats, cattle Paresis/ataxia is common
Detomidine	0.003–0.01	IM, IV	1–4	Sheep, goats, cattle
	0.04	EPI		Cattle
	0.01	IT		Sheep
Romifidine	0.003–0.02	IM, IV	1–4	Sheep, goats, cattle
	0.05	EPI		Cattle
	0.05	IT		Goats
Medetomidine	0.005–0.01	IM, IV	1–4	Sheep, goats, cattle
	0.01–0.03	EPI		Goats, cattle

Source: St. Jean et al., 1990; Aithal et al., 1996; Scott & Gessert, 1997; Lin et al., 1998; Mpanduji et al., 1999; Prado et al., 1999; Mpanduji et al., 2000; Ting et al., 2003; Chevalier et al., 2004; Meyer et al., 2007; Condino et al., 2010.

IM, intramuscular; IV, intravenous; EPI, epidural; IT, intrathecal.

1986; Doherty et al., 1987; Kutter et al., 2006; Kästner et al., 2006; Rioja et al., 2008). Sheep are predisposed to pulmonary edema from the release of inflammatory mediators from pulmonary intravascular macrophages in response to α-2 agonists (Celly et al., 1997). Xylazine increases myometrial tone in the gravid uterus of the cow, goat, and sheep during late gestation (LeBlanc et al., 1984; Jansen et al., 1984; Sakamoto et al., 1996; Hodgson et al., 2002). Medetomidine is reported to increase intrauterine pressure in goats (Sakamoto et al., 1997). Detomidine appears to have a lesser effect on uterine electrical activity in the cow (Jedruch & Gajewski, 1986). In the fetus, α-2 agonists decrease heart rate, increase blood pressure, and decrease PaO_2 (Sakamoto et al., 1996; Sakamoto et al., 1997). Because of the increase in uterine contractions and the negative effects on the fetus, caution is advised with the use of α-2 agonists during the last trimester of pregnancy.

SYSTEMIC ADMINISTRATION OF α-2 AGONISTS

Evidence for the analgesic efficacy of α-2 agonists in ruminants comes from pain models using cutaneous thermal, electrical, and mechanical stimulation after IV or IM administration of these drugs. Analgesia after α-2 agonist administration may last for 60–90 minutes (Nolan et al., 1987b; Grant & Upton, 2001).

EPIDURAL ADMINISTRATION OF α-2 AGONISTS

Epidural administration of α-2 agonists at the sacrococcygeal or first intercoccygeal space in cattle and sheep or at the lumbosacral space in sheep and goats, results in analgesia. Ultimately, absorption into the circulation results in clinically important depression of the cardiorespiratory and central nervous systems, similar to systemic administration of these drugs. Epidural doses are similar to systemic doses (Table 32.2).

After epidural administration of α-2 agonists, analgesia is more profound in the hind limbs, perineum, and abdomen. Systemic absorption may also result in generalized analgesia and sedation (Aithal et al., 1996; Mpanduji et al., 1999; Mpanduji et al., 2000; Condino et al., 2010).

Epidural xylazine can induce complete sensory blockade, and has been used to perform cesarean section in sheep (Scott & Gessert, 1997). Calves administered xylazine (0.1 mg/kg) at the first coccygeal or sacrococcygeal space developed analgesia to needle pricking of the navel, flank, and hind limb for at least 95 minutes, and were able to regain the standing position in less than 95 minutes (Meyer et al., 2007). A combination of romifidine (0.05 mg/kg) and morphine (0.1 mg/kg) administered at the first coccygeal space provided analgesia in cattle for up to 12 hours against a noxious electrical stimulus applied to the flank (Fierheller et al., 2004). Paresis is common with epidurally administered xylazine (Aminkov & Hubenov, 1995; Aithal et al., 1996; Scott & Gessert, 1997; Ting et al., 2003; Meyer et al., 2007) but not with other α-2 agonists. A case of hind limb paralysis in a goat after lumbosacral epidural medetomidine was most likely the result of iatrogenic trauma to the spinal cord during the injection, because other goats that were given two or three times the dose did not develop complications (Mpanduji et al., 2000). In cattle, demyelination of lumbar spinal cord segments and irreversible paralysis was reported after the administration of xylazine epidurally in three cows (George, 2003).

INTRATHECAL ADMINISTRATION OF α-2 AGONISTS

Intrathecal injection at the lumbosacral space is easy to perform in small ruminants. Intrathecal administration has been reported for xylazine in sheep, goats, and calves; romifidine in goats; and detomidine in sheep (Aithal et al., 2001; Amarpal et al., 2002; Haerdi-Landerer et al., 2005; DeRossi et al., 2005; Staffieri et al., 2009; Condino et al., 2010) (Table 31.2).

In goats, intrathecal administration of xylazine (0.1 mg/kg) provided analgesia caudal to the last rib, as assessed by response to pricking the skin and muscle with a hypodermic needle, and motor blockade persisted for almost 90 minutes (DeRossi et al., 2005). The duration of analgesia doubled when a smaller dose of xylazine (0.05 mg/kg) was combined with lidocaine (1.25 mg/kg); however, motor blockade persisted for almost 120 minutes (DeRossi et al., 2005). Xylazine (0.05 mg/kg) combined with lidocaine (2 mg/kg) provided adequate anesthesia during stifle surgery in goats and adequate analgesia for 24 hours (Staffieri et al., 2009).

In calves, intrathecal administration of xylazine (0.025 mg/kg) and lidocaine (0.1 mg/kg) at the lumbosacral space provided complete antinociception to pinprick to the level of the umbilicus for 45 minutes, and to the level of the cranial abdomen for 15 minutes (Condino et al., 2010). Intrathecal administration of romifidine (0.05 mg/kg) provided moderate analgesia of the abdomen, perineum, and hind limbs for 60 minutes in goats (Aithal et al., 2001; Amarpal et al., 2002); whereas, romifidine (0.05 mg/kg) and ketamine (2.5 mg/kg) resulted in complete analgesia of the same anatomical areas, but was accompanied by severe ataxia Aithal et al., 2001).

In sheep, intrathecal administration of detomidine (0.01 mg/kg) or xylazine (0.05 mg/kg) induced antinociception to electrical stimulation of the skin over the pastern of the hind limbs. The analgesia from xylazine was more complete and of longer duration (2 hours vs. 1 hour), but induced more ataxia than did detomidine (Haerdi-Landerer et al., 2005).

Local Anesthetics

The most commonly used local anesthetics include lidocaine, bupivacaine, ropivacaine, and mepivacaine (Table 32.3). Local anesthetics prevent depolarization of nociceptors by blocking sodium channels. Local anesthetics block sensory (A-δ and C fibers), motor (A-α fibers), and sympathetic (β fibers) nerve fibers. Lidocaine and mepivacaine provide fast onset (5–10 minutes) but short duration (1–2 hours) of anesthesia and analgesia. Bupivacaine and ropivacaine have a longer onset (10–20 minutes) but, due to greater protein binding, have the longest duration (4–6 hours) of action. A detailed description of local anesthetic pharmacology can be found in Chapter 6.

TOXICITY OF LOCAL ANESTHETICS

Toxicity manifests differently in conscious versus anesthetized individuals. Toxic doses cause initial depressive effects that are quickly followed by excitatory effects in conscious animals, including seizure activity and cardiac dysrhythmias, followed by death in later stages. The depressive cardiovascular effects occur in anesthetized animals at twice the toxic doses for conscious animals, and death is less likely to occur (Copeland et al., 2008).

IV doses of bupivacaine (2 mg/kg) and ropivacaine (3 mg/kg), injected over 3 minutes, caused death from seizure activity and pulseless ventricular tachycardia in 3 out of 11 and 2 out of 13 conscious sheep, respectively; however, no fatalities occurred when the same doses were administered to halothane-anesthetized sheep (Copeland et al., 2008). IV doses of lidocaine (7 mg/kg) were well tolerated in halothane-anesthetized and conscious sheep (Copeland et al., 2008). Bupivacaine should never be given intravenously because of its cardiotoxicity.

SYSTEMIC ADMINISTRATION OF LIDOCAINE

IV lidocaine provides systemic analgesia through several mechanisms of action that include inhibitory actions on primary afferent A-δ and C fiber-evoked responses and spinal dorsal horn neurons; increased intraspinal release of acetylcholine through agonistic actions on presynaptic muscarinic and nicotinic receptors; actions on spinal strychnine-sensitive glycine receptors; reduction of postsynaptic depolarization from N-methyl-D-aspartic acid (NMDA)

and neurokinin receptors; and attenuation of tissue damage induced by inflammatory endothelial and vascular cytokines (Biella & Sotgiu, 1993; Nagy & Woolf, 1996; Abelson & Höglund, 2002; De Klaver et al., 2003; Ness & Randich, 2006).

In goats, a lidocaine infusion of 0.1 mg/kg/min, preceded by a loading dose of 2.5 mg/kg, decreased the MAC of isoflurane by 18%, and potentiated the effect of ketamine (1.5 mg/kg loading dose and 0.05 mg/kg/min) on MAC by an additional 20% (Doherty et al., 2007). In sheep, infusions of lidocaine and ketamine decreased the dose of isoflurane by 23% in clinical cases (Raske et al., 2010).

LOCAL INFILTRATION OF LOCAL ANESTHETICS

Local anesthetics can be administered by perineural injection, infiltration at nerve endings in the skin, and injection into a peripheral vein for IV regional anesthesia. These techniques provide complete anesthesia of the area supplied by the infiltrated nerves, and are described below and in Table 32.4. It is important to aspirate prior to injection to avoid inadvertent IV administration.

Analgesia of the Eye and Nasal Structures

For corneal analgesia, local anesthetic drops, such as proparacaine or tetracaine, placed on the cornea will provide relief of pain during removal of foreign bodies and during diagnostic procedures in the presence of corneal ulcers. For analgesia of the globe to facilitate enucleation of the eye, a retrobulbar block or a Peterson block can be performed with lidocaine and/or bupivacaine to cause blockade of the oculomotor, trochlear, abducens, ophthalmic, and maxillary nerves. An infraorbital block desensitizes nasal structures.

Anesthesia for Dehorning

Anesthesia for dehorning can be achieved by blockade of the cornual branch of the zygomaticotemporal nerve in calves; however, for complete blockade in adult cattle it is necessary to block the infratrochlear nerve, and blockade of the cervical nerves that supply the caudal area of the horn base is necessary for a cosmetic dehorning procedure. In goats, it is necessary to block the cornual branch of the zygomaticotemporal nerve and the infratrochlear nerve (Figure 32.1).

Anesthesia of the Flank

Flank anesthesia can be achieved by employing a line block, an inverted "L" block, a proximal or distal paravertebral block of T13, L1, and L2 (and occasionally L3) (Figure 32.2), or an epidural block. For either paravertebral block, local anesthetic volumes of 15–25 mL per nerve (divided between the dorsal and ventral branches) and 2–3 mL per nerve (divided) are efficacious in adult cattle and in calves or small ruminants, respectively. Blockade of the ventral branch of each nerve usually requires 3–4 times the volume required to block the dorsal branch. Similar volumes of local anesthetic can be used for the line or inverted "L" block. These volumes correspond to an approximate dose of 3.6 mg/kg of lidocaine 2% or 0.9 mg/kg of bupivacaine 0.5% in a 500 kg adult cow or a 50 kg calf or small ruminant, well below toxic doses.

Intravenous Regional Anesthesia (Bier Block)

The IV regional or Bier block is performed by injecting lidocaine into a catheter placed in a distal limb vein, while a tourniquet is applied proximal to the catheter. The volume of lidocaine injected

Table 32.3. Local anesthetics, NSAIDs, and ketamine for analgesic use in ruminants

Drug	Dose (mg/kg, unless indicated otherwise)	Route	Duration of analgesia (h)	Species/comments
Lidocaine	2.5	IV	1	Sheep, goats, cattle
	0.05–0.1 mg/kg/min	IV	Duration of infusion	Sheep, goats, cattle
	0.1–1	EPI (S1–Cc1 or Cc1–Cc2)	1–2	Sheep, goats, cattle Higher doses and volumes will block more rostral dermatomes.
	8–12	High Caudal EPI	2	Calves injected at the sacrococcygeal space for abdominal block Paresis of <4 h
	0.04–0.08	IT	1–2	Sheep, goats, cattle
	3 mL	EPI L1–L2	3	Cattle undergoing standing flank surgery 1 mL of xylazine 2% combined with the lidocaine
	<3	IVR	1–2	Sheep, goats, cattle
	40 mg	IA	3–7	Sheep Combined with 10 mg of bupivacaine
Bupivacaine	1.5–1.9	EPI	3–4	Goats Paresis of >4 h
	0.05	EPI	2–4	Cattle
Ketoprofen	3	IM, IV, SC	24	Cattle
Flunixin	1.5–2.2	IV, SC	12–24	Sheep, goats, cattle
Meloxicam	0.5	IM	24	Cattle
Carprofen	1.4	IV, SC	24	Cattle
Phenylbutazone	2–4	IV	24	Cattle, sheep Prohibited in dairy cows >20 months old.
Ketamine	0.1–0.8	IM, IV	1–2	Sheep, goats, cattle
	0.5–2.5	EPI	1–2	Sheep, goats, cattle Ataxia is common.
	2.5	IT	1–2	Goats Marked ataxia

Source: Trim, 1989; Aithal et al., 1996; Hendrickson et al., 1996; Mpanduji et al., 1999; Aithal et al., 2001; Stafford et al., 2002; Lee et al., 2003; Stafford et al., 2003; Ting et al., 2003; Doherty et al., 2004; Milligan et al., 2004; Shafford et al., 2004; DeRossi et al., 2005; Lee & Yamada, 2005; Guedes et al., 2006; Pang et al., 2006; Doherty et al., 2007; Meyer et al., 2007; Currah et al., 2009; Stewart et al., 2009; Duffield et al., 2010; Heinrich et al., 2010; Raske et al., 2010.

Cc, coccygeal vertebrae; IM, intramuscular; IV, intravenous; EPI, epidural; IT, intrathecal; EPI L1–L2, epidural at the L1–L2 space; IVR, intravenous regional; IA, intra-articular; SC, subcutaneous; S1, sacrum.

is based on the size of the limb and the location of the tourniquet; 30–50 mL of lidocaine in adult ruminants and 5–10 mL in small ruminants is typical. Sedation and lateral recumbency facilitate the technique. An IV catheter is placed in the distal vein of the limb after placement of a tourniquet proximal to the location of the catheter. The pressure of the tourniquet should exceed the animal's systolic blood pressure, and should be maintained throughout the surgical procedure in order to prevent arterial flow and drainage of the lidocaine from the limb. The limb distal to the catheter will

become completely anesthetized until the tourniquet is removed. The surgical procedure should be completed within 60–90 minutes to avoid excessive tissue hypoxia from the tourniquet. Bupivacaine should not be used for this block to avoid rapid systemic absorption of IV bupivacaine if the tourniquet unexpectedly loosens.

Epidural Analgesia
Epidural administration of local anesthetics has the potential for blocking sensory fibers (desired effect), motor fibers (undesired

Table 32.4. Description of local anesthetic blocks used in ruminants

Block	Anatomical area	Landmarks/description	Drug/dose
Retrobulbar or four-point	Eye, eyelids, muscles adjacent to the eye –Optic nerve –Oculomotor nerve –Trochlear nerve –Trigeminal nerve –Abducens nerve –Facial nerve	18 or 20 gauge, 3 inch needle in adult cattle 20 or 22 gauge, 1.5 inch needle in calves and small ruminants –Needle is inserted into the back of the orbit at 12:00, 3:00, 6:00, and 9:00 positions. –Avoid the eye by curving the needle and penetrate the orbital septum for drug injection.	Lidocaine 5–10 mL per site in adult cattle 1–3 mL per site in calves and small ruminants
Peterson and eyelid	Eye –Optic nerve –Oculomotor nerve –Trigeminal nerve Eyelid –Auriculopalpebral (facial nerve)	18 or 20 gauge, 5 inch needle in adult cattle 20 or 22 gauge, 1.5 or 2.5 inch needle in calves and small ruminants –Needle is inserted perpendicular to the notch between the zygomatic arch and supraorbital process until it reaches the coronoid process of the mandible, then directed cranially to bypass the coronoid process until it strikes bone behind the eye. –Insert the needle subcutaneously along the caudal border of the zygomatic arch for 2–3 inches to desensitize the auriculopalpebral nerve. Alternatively, infiltrate the eyelids along their circumference.	Lidocaine Eye: 15–20 mL in adult cattle 3–7 mL in calves and small ruminants Eyelid: 5–10 mL in adult cattle 2–3 mL in calves and small ruminants
Cornual	Horn –Cornual branch of zygomaticotemporal nerve –Cornual branch of infratrochlear nerve –Second cervical nerve	20 or 22 gauge, 1.5 inch needle –Needle is inserted along the lateral edge of the frontal bone, between the lateral canthus of the eye and lateral base of the horn, 1inch in front of the base of the horn, to block the zygomaticotemporal nerve. –Needle is inserted halfway between the medial canthus of the eye and medial base of the horn to block the infratrochlear nerve. –Needle is inserted between the base of the ear and the caudal aspect of the base of the horn to block the second cervical nerve.	Lidocaine Zygomaticotemporal nerve: 5–10 mL in adult cattle 1–3 mL in calves and small ruminants Infratrochlear nerve: 5 mL in adult cattle 1–3 mL in calves and small ruminants Second cervical nerve: 5–10 mL in adult cattle 1–3 mL in calves Not necessary in goats
Proximal paravertebral	Flank –T13, L1, L2, (±L3) spinal nerves	20 gauge, 3.5 inch needle in adult cattle 20 gauge, 1.5 inch needle in calves or small ruminants –A 14 gauge, 1.5 inch needle is inserted perpendicular to the skin, 2 inches lateral to spinous process to serve as a guide for longer needle in adult cattle. –20 gauge needle is inserted through the guide needle in adult cattle or without the guide needle in calves and small ruminants until it strikes the cranial edge of the transverse process behind the nerve to be blocked (e.g., L3 transverse process for L2 spinal nerve), then the needle is walked off cranially until it penetrates the intertransverse ligament to block the ventral branch. –Needle is withdrawn to the level of the ligament to block the dorsal branch.	Lidocaine 20 mL for ventral branch and 5 mL for dorsal branch in adult cattle 2–4 mL for ventral branch and 1 mL for dorsal branch in calves and small ruminants

(continued)

Table 32.4. (*Continued*)

Block	Anatomical area	Landmarks/description	Drug/dose
Distal paravertebral	Flank –T13, L1, L2, (± L3) spinal nerves	20 gauge, 3.5 inch needle in adult cattle 20 gauge, 1.5 inch needle in calves or small ruminants –Needle is inserted perpendicular and ventral to the lateral distal edge of the transverse processes of L1, L2, and L4 to block the ventral branches of the T13, L1, and L2 spinal nerves, respectively. –Needle is withdrawn and redirected dorsal to the transverse process to block the dorsal branches.	Lidocaine 10–20 mL for ventral branch and 5 mL for dorsal branch in adult cattle 2–4 mL for ventral branch and 1 mL for dorsal branch in calves and small ruminants
Intravenous regional (Bier block)	Limb	20 or 22 gauge, 1 or 1.5 inch catheter or butterfly –Place a tourniquet above the anatomical area of interest to prevent leakage or blood flow to the restricted area. Prior exsanguination of the limb is not mandatory, but it prevents leakage of the local anesthetic into the systemic circulation as a result of increased venous pressure. –Place the catheter or butterfly in a vein below the tourniquet and above the area of interest and inject slowly the local anesthetic. –Maximum tourniquet time of 1 h –Release the tourniquet slowly (1–2 min) once the surgical procedure is completed.	Lidocaine 30–40 mL in adult cattle 10–20 mL in calves or small ruminants
Sacrococcygeal or intercoccygeal epidural	Skin and viscera included in middle sacral area, skin and adjacent tissue of perineum and inner aspect of thigh, tail	20 or 22 gauge, 1 or 1.5 inch needle –Needle is inserted perpendicular in the sacrococcygeal or first intercoccygeal space. –With the animal in standing or sternal position it is possible to verify proper location of the needle by filling the hub with saline or local anesthetic before it penetrates the flavum ligament, and once the needle is placed in the epidural space the fluid will run down the hub due to the negative pressure in the space.	Lidocaine or bupivacaine 0.01–0.02 mL/kg Morphine 0.1 mg/kg
Lumbosacral epidural (L6–S1)	Abdomen and pelvic area	18 or 20 gauge, 5 inch needle in adult cattle 20 or 22 gauge, 1 or 1.5 inch needle in calves or small ruminants –Needle is inserted perpendicular in the lumbosacral space, located slightly caudal to a line that joins the cranial border of the ilial crest. –The spinal cord is present at this level and subarachnoid injection should be avoided with epidural doses. –Recumbency is common from motor blockade.	Lidocaine or bupivacaine 0.1–0.3 mL/kg
Lumbosacral intrathecal	Abdomen and pelvic area	As for lumbosacral epidural but penetrating the arachnoid membrane	Lidocaine or bupivacaine 0.002–0.004 mL/kg

Source: Skarda & Tranquilli, 2007; Valverde & Doherty, 2008b.

effect leading to paresis, ataxia, and recumbency), and sympathetic fibers (undesired effect causing hypotension). The degree of blockade induced by local anesthetics depends on the volume and concentration (total mass) of the anesthetic.

Larger volumes and greater concentrations of local anesthetics are more likely to result in motor paralysis and sympathetic blockade because they result in more rostral spread of the drug (Lee et al., 2005) and a greater total mass of drug. Injection of methylene blue dye at the first intercoccygeal space at volumes of 5, 10, or 20 mL in cattle weighing approximately 500 kg resulted in rostral spread to the sixth (L6), fourth (L4), and first (L1) lumbar vertebra, respectively. A group of younger cattle (400 kg) injected with 0.1 mL/kg of methylene blue had rostral spread to the first sacral vertebra (Lee et al., 2005).

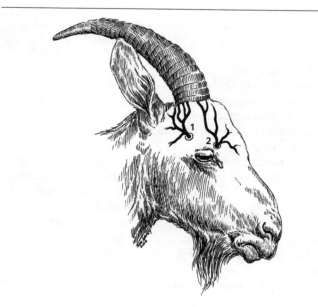

Figure 32.1. Locations for nerve block for dehorning an adult goat. The cornual branch of the zygomaticotemporal is blocked behind the root of the supraorbital process (1) and the cornual branch of the infratrochlear nerve is blocked at the dorsomedial margin of the orbit (2) (Table 32.4). (Valverde & Doherty, 2008b)

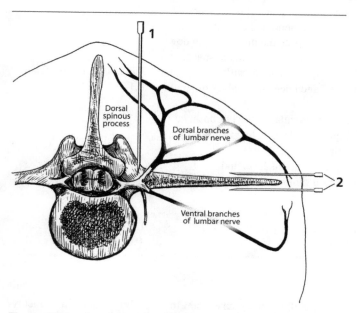

Figure 32.2. Locations for proximal (1) and distal (2) paravertebral blocks involving dorsal and ventral branches of T13, L1, and L2 (and occasionally L3) (Table 32.4). (Valverde & Doherty, 2008b)

Lidocaine (2%) at doses of 0.2–0.4 mg/kg (0.01–0.02 mL/kg) administered epidurally at the first intercoccygeal space or sacrococcygeal space in cattle and small ruminants is effective for perineal analgesia, and does not cause excessive ataxia or paralysis. This lack of ataxia is supported by examination of the segments stained by methylene blue, which indicates that there is minimal involvement of motor innervation to the limb. Lidocaine (0.6 mg/kg) with 1:100,000 epinephrine injected into the sacrococcygeal space (0.03 mL/kg) has been used in 10–13-week-old calves for standing castration (Currah et al., 2009).

The combination of lidocaine (0.4 mg/kg) with xylazine (0.05 mg/kg) administered at the first intercoccygeal space in 13-month-old bulls was effective in allowing castration to be performed in standing animals and decreasing pain-associated responses; however, sedation and paresis developed shortly after and persisted for 40–200 minutes (Ting et al., 2003), possibly due to systemic absorption of xylazine and a synergistic drug effect.

High caudal epidural anesthesia, with a combination of either lidocaine or procaine at 10–12 mg/kg (0.5–0.6 mL/kg) and xylazine (0.1 mg/kg), injected at the first intercoccygeal or sacrococcygeal space in 57 kg calves, allowed umbilical surgery to be performed (Meyer et al., 2007). Lidocaine alone at 8 mg/kg provided analgesia to needle pricking of the navel, flank, and hind limb for 95 minutes, although it was less intense at the navel; calves were able to remain standing without support at 4 hours postinjection (Meyer et al., 2007).

In small ruminants, lumbosacral injection is commonly performed and facilitates the spread of the anesthetic to cause blockade of the hind limb and caudal abdomen. Small doses of epidural bupivacaine and ropivacaine can induce sensory anesthesia with minimal impairment of motor function; however, most studies in small ruminants have used doses greater than 1.5 mg/kg, which results in recumbency. Epidural bupivacaine (1.9 mg/kg) in goats results in longer-lasting analgesia than does lidocaine (4 mg/kg) with 1:100,000 epinephrine for flank laparotomies; however, the onset of analgesia is longer (up to 40 minutes) and goats are unable to stand for at least 11 hours due to hind limb motor blockade (Trim, 1989).

Epidural administration of bupivacaine (1.5 mg/kg) or morphine (0.1 mg/kg) administered at the lumbosacral space provided better analgesia than saline after abdominal surgery in goats (Hendrickson et al., 1996). Time to standing was a minimum of 6 hours for the bupivacaine group and less than 1 hour in the morphine and saline groups.

An alternative method to the paravertebral block is described using an epidural injection at the L1–L2 space of fixed volumes of 1 mL of 2% xylazine and 3 mL of 2% lidocaine in adult cattle (450–800 kg) for standing flank surgery. This technique provided analgesia for as long as 3 hours (Lee & Yamada, 2005). Sedation, due to systemic absorption, is common when xylazine is used epidurally in this fashion.

Intrathecal Administration of Local Anesthetics

Intrathecal injection of local anesthetics is used less frequently than the epidural route in cattle and small ruminants. It can be performed at the lumbosacral space in cattle and small ruminants.

Lidocaine (1.25–2 mg/kg) has been combined with xylazine (0.05 mg/kg) to provide analgesia in goats in a needle prick model and also after stifle surgery. At these doses of lidocaine, motor blockade, and hypotension are common (DeRossi et al., 2005; Staffieri et al., 2009). Based on the greater bioavailability of local anesthetics when injected into the intrathecal space versus the epidural space (Clément et al., 1999), a substantially smaller dose should be used to avoid adverse effects. For example, if the epidural coccygeal dose of lidocaine is 0.2–0.4 mg/kg, then 0.04–0.08 mg/kg is satisfactory for intrathecal administration.

In calves, the intrathecal injection of a combination of xylazine (0.025 mg/kg) and lidocaine (0.1 mg/kg) at the lumbosacral space resulted in analgesia of the umbilical area for 45 minutes (Condino et al., 2010). In adult cattle, intrathecal injection at the lumbosacral space using a catheter introduced through a Tuohy needle and advanced 60 cm to the midthoracic area for injection of 1.5–2 mL of 2% lidocaine (0.06–0.08 mg/kg in a 500 kg cow) is described. This resulted in bilateral desensitization of spinal segments T9–L3, and allowed flank surgery (Skarda & Tranquilli, 2007).

Intra-Articular Administration of Local Anesthetics

Local anesthetics have been used intra-articularly in sheep undergoing stifle surgery. A combination of lidocaine (40 mg) and bupivacaine (10 mg) has been recommended, with administration of the lidocaine into the joint before the start of surgery, due to its fast onset of action, and the administration of bupivacaine after joint closure due to its longer duration of action (3–7 hours) (Shafford et al., 2004). In goats, 0.75 mg/kg of bupivacaine (0.5%) administered intra-articularly before stifle arthrotomy provided 78–100 minutes of analgesia, but was not effective in the postoperative period. Postoperative administration reduced periarticular hyperalgesia initially, but no reduction in postoperative analgesia requirements was achieved when compared to a control group and the group that received preoperative bupivacaine (Krohm et al., 2011).

Nonsteroidal Anti-Inflammatory Drugs

Nonsteroidal anti-inflammatory drugs are used frequently by veterinarians because of their ease of parenteral administration, their duration of action, and their potent anti-inflammatory and analgesic actions (Watts & Clarke, 2000; Whay & Huxley, 2005; Hewson et al., 2007). The pharmacology of NSAIDs is described in detail in Chapter 5. The most commonly used NSAIDs in ruminants are flunixin meglumine, ketoprofen, aspirin, meloxicam, and carprofen. Dosages and routes of administration of NSAIDs are outlined in Table 32.3. Phenylbutazone is prohibited by the FDA in dairy cattle 20 months of age or older due to its prolonged half-life, and the risk of toxicity to humans from its metabolites (Haskell et al., 2003).

SYSTEMIC USE OF NSAIDS

The preemptive use of NSAIDs in combination with local anesthetic techniques and sedative/analgesic drugs is common during general anesthesia and procedures under sedation, and positive effects have been demonstrated in several studies. However, flunixin (1.5 mg/kg IV) had no effect on the MAC of isoflurane in goats and did not potentiate the effects of morphine (Doherty et al., 2004).

Ketoprofen (3 mg/kg IV, IM, or SC) or meloxicam (0.5 mg/kg IM) combined with a lidocaine cornual nerve block in young calves was better at decreasing the cortisol response, and calves had fewer pain-associated behaviors than those treated with xylazine (0.1 mg/kg IM) or a placebo and a lidocaine cornual nerve block (Stafford et al., 2003; Milligan et al., 2004; Stewart et al., 2009;

Duffield et al., 2010; Heinrich et al., 2010). Ketoprofen (3 mg/kg IV) was more effective than epidural xylazine (0.05 mg/kg) combined with lidocaine (0.4 mg/kg) in decreasing the inflammatory responses associated with castration in 13-month-old bulls (Ting et al., 2003). In calves younger than 4 months of age undergoing castration, ketoprofen (3 mg/kg IV) and intratesticular lidocaine, but not lidocaine alone, blocked the cortisol response (Stafford et al., 2002).

Carprofen (1.4 mg/kg, SC) or flunixin (2.2 mg/kg, SC) in combination with an epidural block with lidocaine (0.44 mL/kg), in 25-week-old calves undergoing castration, resulted in lower cortisol concentrations in the postoperative period than placebo and epidurally treated calves. The effects of carprofen were longer lasting than were those of flunixin (Stilwell et al., 2008). Flunixin (2.2 mg/kg IV) and an epidural block with lidocaine with 1:100,000 epinephrine (0.06 mg/kg) was effective in providing pain relief for up to 8 hours after castration in calves (Currah et al., 2009). Carprofen (1.4 mg/kg IV) decreased plasma cortisol concentration and inflammatory responses associated with castration in 22-week-old bulls (Pang et al., 2006).

Intrathecal NSAIDs

The actions of NSAIDS are, in part, spinally mediated and involve the blockade of prostaglandin production elicited by greater influx of extracellular calcium when NMDA receptors are activated (Lizarraga et al., 2008). Intrathecal administration of ketoprofen or ketamine (an NMDA antagonist) or their combination prevented the development of NMDA-induced mechanical hypersensitivity after intrathecal NMDA in sheep, but had no hypoalgesic effect if prior intrathecal NMDA was not administered (Lizarraga et al., 2008). Other NSAIDs, such as phenylbutazone, salicylic acid, and tolfenamic acid, also failed to show a hypoalgesic effect after intrathecal administration, although ketoprofen and tolfenamic acid have a hypoalgesic effect when given IV (Lizarraga & Chambers, 2006; Lizarraga et al., 2008). Nevertheless, the use of NSAIDs by this route is experimental and, at this time, is not recommended for clinical use.

Ketamine

Ketamine has analgesic properties at subanesthetic doses through antagonism of the NMDA receptor, decreasing postsynaptic excitability and long-term potentiation. This prevents the relay of nociceptive impulses from the periphery to the brain, and decreases the establishment of hyperalgesic states (Himmelseher & Durieux, 2005).

SYSTEMIC ADMINISTRATION OF KETAMINE

In calves undergoing castration, those receiving IV xylazine (0.05 mg/kg) and ketamine (0.1 mg/kg) had lower cortisol concentrations and fewer behavioral changes than placebo-treated calves. The authors suggest that low doses of xylazine and ketamine prior to castration may offer an efficacious and cost-effective way to improve analgesia for castration, and can be combined with local anesthetic techniques (Coetzee et al., 2010). Ketamine doses of 0.1–0.8 mg/kg (IV, IM) have been used in other species (Wagner et al., 2002; Fielding et al., 2006, and are not associated with the adverse effects on motor activity and behavior seen with anesthetic doses.

EPIDURAL ADMINISTRATION OF KETAMINE

The epidural administration of ketamine has been reported in cattle, sheep, goats, and buffalo (Table 32.3) (Aithal et al., 1996; Lee et al., 2003; Singh et al., 2005; Guedes et al., 2006). In cattle, ketamine (0.5 mg/kg, 1 mg/kg, and 2 mg/kg, diluted to 5 mL, 10 mL, and 20 mL, respectively) administered at the first intercoccygeal space caused dose-dependent analgesia for a maximum period of 1 hour. Sedation was not observed, although ataxia was present with the higher doses (Lee et al., 2003). In sheep undergoing orthopedic surgery, ketamine (1 mg/kg, diluted to a total volume of 7–9 mL) administered at the lumbosacral space decreased the degree of lameness and prolonged the time for administration of rescue analgesia from 3.3 hours in the control group to 5 hours in ketamine-treated sheep (Guedes et al., 2006). In goats, ketamine (2.5 mg/kg) administered at the lumbosacral space prevented the response to perineal pinprick for 5–20 minutes. In contrast, combining ketamine with xylazine (0.05 mg/kg) extended the duration of analgesia for up to 1 hour (Aithal et al., 1996). In the goats receiving ketamine alone ataxia, but not sedation, was generally present by 5 minutes after ketamine administration and was most severe within 15 minutes, whereas goats that were given the ketamine and xylazine combination developed ataxia (for up to 60 minutes) and sedation (for up to 45 minutes) (Aithal et al., 1996). Considering its relatively short duration of action and adverse effects (ataxia) the epidural route may not be practical for ketamine administration.

INTRATHECAL ADMINISTRATION OF KETAMINE

The intrathecal administration of ketamine (2.5 mg/kg) in combination with romifidine (0.05 mg/kg) provided complete analgesia of the tail, perineum, and hind limbs in goats, but was accompanied by marked ataxia (Aithal et al., 2001).

SUMMARY

Great strides have been made in our ability to recognize and treat pain in ruminants. A variety of analgesics, including opioids, NSAIDs, local anesthetics, and ketamine, administered by a variety of routes, including IV, IM, per os, subcutaneously, epidurally, intrathecally, or perineurally, can be used to provide effective preemptive, multimodal analgesia to ruminants.

REFERENCES

Abelson, K.S. & Höglund, A.U. (2002) Intravenously administered lidocaine in therapeutic doses increases the intraspinal release of acetylcholine in rats. *Neuroscience Letters*, 317, 93–96.

Aithal, H.P., Pratap, A.K., & Singh, G.R. (1996) Clinical effects of epidurally administered ketamine and xylazine in goats. *Small Ruminant Research*, 24, 55–64.

Aithal, H.P., Amarpal, Kinjavdekar, P., Pawde, A.M., & Pratap, K. (2001) Analgesic and cardiopulmonary effects of intrathecally administered romifidine or romifidine and ketamine in goats (Capra hircus). *Journal of the South African Veterinary Association*, 72, 84–91.

Amarpal, Kinjavdekar, P., Aithal, H.P., Pawde, A.M., & Pratap, K. (2002) Analgesic, sedative and haemodynamic effects of spinally administered romifidine in female goats. *Journal of Veterinary Medicine. A, Physiology, Pathology, Clinical Medicine*, 49, 3–8.

Aminkov, B.J. & Hubenov, H.D. (1995) The effect of xylazine epidural anaesthesia on blood gas and acid-base parameters in rams. *British Journal of Anaesthesia*, 151, 579–585.

Biella, G. & Sotgiu, M.L. (1993) Central effects of systemic lidocaine mediated by glycine spinal receptors: an iontophoretic study in the rat spinal cord. *Brain Research*, 603, 201–206.

Carroll, G.L., Hooper, R.N., Boothe, D.M., Hartsfield, S.M., & Randoll, L.A. (1999) Pharmacokinetics of fentanyl after intravenous and transdermal administration in goats. *American Journal of Veterinary Research*, 60, 986–991.

Celly, C.S., McDonell, W.N., Young, S.S., & Black, W.D. (1997) The comparative hypoxaemic effect of four α_2 adrenoceptor agonists (xylazine, romifidine, detomidine and medetomidine) in sheep. *Journal of Veterinary Pharmacology and Therapeutics*, 20, 464–471.

Chevalier, H.M., Provost, P.J., & Karas, A.Z. (2004) Effect of caudal epidural xylazine on intraoperative distress and post-operative pain in Holstein heifers. *Veterinary Anaesthesia and Analgesia*, 31, 1–10.

Clément, R., Malinovsky, J.M., Le Corre, P., et al. (1999) Cerebrospinal fluid bioavailability and pharmacokinetics of bupivacaine and lidocaine following intrathecal and epidural administrations in rabbits using microdialysis. *Journal of Pharmacology and Experimental Therapeutics*, 289, 1015–1021.

Coetzee, J.F., Gehring, R., Tarus-Sang, J., & Anderson, D.E. (2010) Effect of sub-anesthetic xylazine and ketamine ('ketamine stun') administered to calves immediately prior to castration. *Veterinary Anaesthesia and Analgesia*, 37, 566–578.

Condino, M.P., Suzuki, K., & Taguchi, X. (2010) Antinociceptive, sedative and cardiopulmonary effects of subarachnoid and epidural xylazine-lidocaine in xylazine-sedated calves. *Veterinary Anaesthesia and Analgesia*, 37, 70–78.

Copeland, S.E., Ladd, L.A., Gu, X.Q., & Mather, L.E. (2008) The effects of general anesthesia on the central nervous and cardiovascular system toxicity of local anesthetics. *Anesthesia and Analgesia*, 106, 1429–1439.

Currah, J.M., Hendrick, S.H., & Stookey, J.M. (2009) The behavioral assessment and alleviation of pain associated with castration in beef calves treated with flunixin meglumine and caudal lidocaine epidural anesthesia with epinephrine. *Canadian Veterinary Journal*, 50, 375–382.

Day, T.K., Pepper, W.T., Tobias, T.A., Flynn, M.F., & Clarke, K.M. (1995) Comparison of intra-articular and epidural morphine for analgesia following stifle arthrotomy in dogs. *Veterinary Surgery*, 24, 522–530.

De Klaver, M.J, Buckingham, M.G, & Rich, G.F. (2003) Lidocaine attenuates cytokine-induced cell injury in endothelial and vascular smooth muscle cells. *Anesthesia and Analgesia*, 97, 465–470.

DeRossi, R., Junqueira, A.L., & Beretta, M.P. (2005) Analgesic and systemic effects of xylazine, lidocaine and their combination after subarachnoid administration in goats. *Journal of the South African Veterinary Association*, 76, 79–84.

Doherty, T.J., Will, W.A., Rohrbach, B.W., & Geiser, D.R. (2004) Effect of morphine and flunixin meglumine on isoflurane minimum alveolar concentration in goats. *Veterinary Anaesthesia and Analgesia*, 31, 97–101.

Doherty, T.J., Rohrbach, B.W., & Geiser, D.R. (2002) Effect of acepromazine and butorphanol on isoflurane minimum alveolar concentration in goats. *Journal of Veterinary Pharmacology and Therapeutics*, 25, 65–67.

Doherty, T.J., Pascoe, P.J., McDonell, W.N., & Monteith, G. (1986) Cardiopulmonary effects of xylazine and yohimbine in laterally recumbent sheep. *Canadian Journal of Veterinary Research*, 50, 517–521.

Doherty, T.J., Ballinger, J.A., McDonell, W.N., Pascoe, P.J., & Valliant, A.E. (1987) Antagonism of xylazine induced sedation by idazoxan in calves. *Canadian Journal of Veterinary Research*, 51, 244–248.

Doherty, T., Redua, M.A., Queiroz-Castro, P., Egger, C., Cox, S.K., & Rohrbach, B.W. (2007) Effect of intravenous lidocaine and ketamine on the minimum alveolar concentration of isoflurane in goats. *Veterinary Anaesthesia and Analgesia*, 34, 125–131.

Duffield, T.F., Heinrich, A., Millman, S.T., DeHaan, A., James, S., & Lissemore, K. (2010) Reduction in pain response by combined use of local lidocaine anesthesia and systemic ketoprofen in dairy calves dehorned by heat cauterization. *Canadian Veterinary Journal*, 51, 283–288.

Fielding, C.L., Brumbaugh, G.W., Matthews, N.S., Peck, K.E., & Roussel, A.J. (2006) Pharmacokinetics and clinical effects of a subanesthetic continuous rate infusion of ketamine in awake horses. *American Journal of Veterinary Research*, 67, 1484–1490.

Fierheller, E.E., Caulkett, N.A., & Bailey, J.V. (2004) A romifidine and morphine combination for epidural analgesia of the flank in cattle. *Canadian Veterinary Journal*, 45, 917–923.

George, L.W. (2003) Pain control in food animals, in *Recent advances in anesthetic management of large domestic animals* (ed. Steffey, E.P.), International Veterinary Information Service (www.ivis.org), A0615.1103, Ithaca, NY (accessed November 2010).

Grant, C. & Upton, R.N. (2001) The anti-nociceptive efficacy of low dose intramuscular xylazine in lambs. *Research in Veterinary Science*, 70, 47–50.

Guedes, A.G.P., Pluhar, E., Daubs, B.M., & Rudé, E.P. (2006) Effects of preoperative epidural administration of racemic ketamine for analgesia in sheep undergoing surgery. *American Journal of Veterinary Research*, 67, 222–229.

Haerdi-Landerer, M.C., Schlegel, U., & Neiger-Aeschbacher, G. (2005) The analgesic effects of intrathecal xylazine and detomidine in sheep and their antagonism with systemic atipamezole. *Veterinary Anaesthesia and Analgesia*, 32, 297–307.

Haskell, S.R.R., Gehring, R., Payne, M.A., Webb, A.I., Baynes, R.E., & Riviere, J.E. (2003) Update on FARAD food animal drug withholding recommendations. *Journal of the American Veterinary Medical Association*, 223, 1277–1278.

Heinrich, A., Duffield, T.F., Lissemore, K.D., & Millman, S.T. (2010) The effect of meloxicam on behavior and pain sensitivity of dairy calves following cautery dehorning with a local anesthetic. *Journal of Dairy Science*, 93, 2450–2457.

Hendrickson, D.A., Kruse-Elliot, K.T., & Broadstone, R.V. (1996) A comparison of epidural saline, morphine, and bupivacaine for pain relief after abdominal surgery in goats. *Veterinary Surgery*, 25, 83–87.

Hewson, C.J., Dohoo, I.R., Lemke, K.A., Barkema, H.W. (2007) Canadian veterinarians' use of analgesics in cattle, pigs and horses in 2004 and 2005, *Canadian Veterinary Journal*, 48, 155–164.

Himmelseher, S. & Durieux, M.E. (2005) Ketamine for perioperative pain management. *Anesthesiology*, 102, 211–220.

Hodgson, D.S., Dunlop, C.I., Chapman, P.L., & Smith, J.A. (2002) Cardiopulmonary effects of xylazine and acepromazine in pregnant cows in late gestation. *American Journal of Veterinary Research*, 63, 1695–1699.

Huxley, J.N. & Whay, H.R. (2006) Current attitudes of cattle practitioners to pain and the use of analgesics in cattle. *The Veterinary Record*, 159, 662–668.

Jansen, C.A., Lowe, K.C., & Nathaielsz, P.W. (1984) The effect of xylazine on intrauterine activity, fetal and maternal oxygenation, cardiovascular function and fetal breathing. *American Journal of Obstetrics and Gynecology*, 148, 386–390.

Jedruch, J. & Gajewski, Z. (1986) The effect of detomidine hydrochloride dormosedan on the electrical activity of the uterus in cows. *Acta Veterinaria Scandinavica, Supplementum* 82, 189–192.

Kästner, S.B.R., Kutter, A.P.N., von Rechenberg, B., & Bettschart-Wolfensberger, R. (2006) Comparison of two pre-anesthetic medetomidine doses in isoflurane anaesthetized sheep. *Veterinary Anaesthesia and Analgesia*, 33, 8–16.

Kielland, C., Skjerve, E., & Zanella, A.J. (2009) Attitudes of veterinary students to pain in cattle. *The Veterinary Record*, 165, 254–258.

Kizilkaya, M., Yildirim, O.S., Ezirmik, N., Kursad, H., & Karsan, O. (2005) Comparisons of analgesic effects of different doses of morphine and morphine plus methylprednisolone after knee surgery. *European Journal of Anaesthesiology*, 22, 603–608.

Krohm, P., Levionnois, O., Ganster, M., Zilberstein, L., & Spadavecchia, C. (2011) Antinociceptive activity of pre- versus post-operative intra-articular bupivacaine in goats undergoing stifle arthrotomy. *Veterinary Anaesthesia and Analgesia*, 38, 363–373.

Kutter, A.P., Kästner, S.B., Bettschart-Wolfensberger, R., & Huhtinen, M. (2006) Cardiopulmonary effects of dexmedetomidine in goats and sheep anaesthetised with sevoflurane. *The Veterinary Record*, 159, 624–629.

LeBlanc, M.M., Hubbell, J.A., & Smith, H.C. (1984) The effects of xylazine hydrochloride on intrauterine pressure in the cow. *Theriogenology*, 21, 681–690.

Lee, I., Yamagishi, N., Oboshi, K., Ayukawa, Y., Sasaki, N., & Yamada, H. (2005) Distribution of new methylene blue injected into the caudal epidural space in cattle. *The Veterinary Journal* 169, 257–261.

Lee, I. & Yamada, H. (2005) Epidural administration of fixed volumes of xylazine and lidocaine for anesthesia of dairy cattle undergoing flank surgery. *Journal of the American Veterinary Medical Association*, 227, 781–784.

Lee, I., Yoshiuchi, T., Yamagishi, N., et al. (2003) Analgesic effect of caudal epidural ketamine in cattle. *Journal of Veterinary Science*, 4, 261–264.

Lin, H.C., Trachte, E.A., DeGraves, F.J., Rodgerson, D.H., Steiss, J.E., & Carson, R.L. (1998) Evaluation of analgesia induced by epidural administration of medetomidine to cows. *American Journal of Veterinary Research*, 59, 162–167.

Lindegaard, C., Gleerup, K.B., Thomsen, M.H., Martinussen, T., Jacobsen, S., & Andersen, P.H. (2010) Anti-inflammatory effects of intra-articular administration of morphine in horses with experimentally induced synovitis. *American Journal of Veterinary Research*, 71, 69–75.

Lizarraga, I., Chambers, J.P., & Johnson, C.B. (2008) Prevention of N-methyl-D-aspartate-induced mechanical nociception by intrathecal administration of ketoprofen and ketamine in sheep. *Anesthesia and Analgesia*, 107, 2061–2067.

Lizarraga, I. & Chambers, J.P. (2006) Involvement of opioidergic and α_2-adrenergic mechanisms in the central analgesic effects of non-steroidal anti-inflammatory drugs in sheep. *Research in Veterinary Science*, 80, 194–200.

Machado-Filho, L.C., Hurnik, J.F., & Ewing, K.K. (1998) A thermal threshold assay to measure the nociceptive response to morphine sulphate in cattle. *Canadian Journal of Veterinary Research*, 62, 218–223.

Meyer, H., Starke, A., Kehler, W., & Rehage, J. (2007) High caudal epidural anaesthesia with local anaesthetics or alpha(2)-agonists in calves. *Journal of Veterinary Medicine. A, Physiology, Pathology, Clinical Medicine*, 54, 384–389.

Milligan, B.N., Duffield, T., & Lissemore, K. (2004) The utility of ketoprofen for alleviating pain following dehorning in young dairy calves. *Canadian Veterinary Journal*, 45, 140.

Mpanduji, D.G., Mgasa, M.N., Bittegeko, S.B., & Batamuzi, E.K. (1999) Comparison of xylazine and lidocaine effects for analgesia and cardiopulmonary functions following lumbosacral epidural injection in goats, *Zentralblatt fürr Veterinärmedizin. Reihi A*, 46, 605–611.

Mpanduji, D.G., Bittegeko, S.B.P., Mgasa, M.N., & Batamuzi, E.K. (2000) Analgesic, behavioural and cardiopulmonary effects of epidurally injected medetomidine (Domitor) in goats, *Journal of Veterinary Medicine. A, Physiology, Pathology, Clinical Medicine*, 47, 65–72.

Nagasaka, H., Awad, H., & Yaksh, T.L. (1996) Peripheral and spinal actions of opioids in the blockade of the autonomic response evoked by compression of the inflamed knee joint. *Anesthesiology*, 85, 808–816.

Nagy, I. & Woolf, C.J. (1996) Lignocaine selectively reduces C fibre-evoked neuronal activity in rat spinal cord in vitro by decreasing N-methyl-D-aspartate and neurokinin receptor-mediated post-synaptic depolarizations; implications for the development of novel centrally acting analgesics. *Pain*, 64, 59–70.

Ness, T.J. & Randich, A. (2006) Which spinal cutaneous nociceptive neurons are inhibited by intravenous lidocaine in the rat? *Regional Anesthesia and Pain Medicine*, 31, 248–253.

Nolan, A., Livingston, A., & Waterman, A.E. (1987a) Investigation of the antinociceptive activity of buprenorphine in sheep. *British Journal of Anaesthesia*, 92, 527–533.

Nolan, A., Livingston, A., & Waterman, A.E. (1987b) Antinociceptive actions of intravenous alpha 2-adrenoceptor agonists in sheep. *Journal of Veterinary Pharmacology and Therapeutics*, 10, 202–209.

Nolan, A., Waterman, A.E., & Livingston, A. (1988) The correlation of the thermal and mechanical antinociceptive activity of pethidine hydrochloride with plasma concentrations of the drug in sheep. *Journal of Veterinary Pharmacology and Therapeutics*, 11, 94–102.

Pablo, L.S. (1993) Epidural morphine in goats after hindlimb orthopedic surgery. *Veterinary Surgery*, 22:307–310.

Pang, W.Y., Earley, B., Sweeney, T., & Crowe, M.A. (2006) Effect of carprofen administration during banding or burdizzo castration of bulls on plasma cortisol, in vitro interferon-gamma production, acute-phase proteins, feed intake, and growth. *Journal of Animal Science*, 84, 351–359.

Prado, M.E., Streeter, R.N., Mandsager, R.E., Shawley, R.V., & Claypool, P.L. (1999) Pharmacologic effects of epidural versus intramuscular administration of detomidine in cattle. *American Journal of Veterinary Research*, 60, 1242–1247.

Raske, T.G., Pelkey, S., Wagner, A.E., & Turner, A.S. (2010) Effect of intravenous ketamine and lidocaine on isoflurane requirement in sheep undergoing orthopedic surgery. *Lab Animal*, 39, 76–79.

Rioja, E., Kerr, C.L., Enouri, S.S., & McDonell, W.N. (2008) Sedative and cardiopulmonary effects of medetomidine hydrochloride and xylazine hydrochloride and their reversal with atipamezole hydrochloride in calves. *American Journal of Veterinary Research*, 69, 319–329.

Sakamoto, H., Misumi, K., Nakama, M., & Aoki, Y. (1996) The effects of xylazine on intrauterine pressure, uterine blood flow, maternal and fetal cardiovascular and pulmonary function in pregnant goats. *The Journal of Veterinary Medical Science*, 58, 211–217.

Sakamoto, H., Kirihara, H., Fujiki, M., Miura, N., & Misumi, K. (1997) The effects of medetomidine on maternal and fetal cardiovascular

and pulmonary function, intrauterine pressure and uterine blood flow in pregnant goats. *Experimental Animals*, 46, 67–73.

Sammarco, J.L., Conzemius, M.G., Perkowski, S.Z., Weinstein, M.J., Gregor, T.P., & Smith, G.K. (1996) Postoperative analgesia for stifle surgery: A comparison of intra-articular bupivacaine, morphine, or saline. *Veterinary Surgery*, 25:59–69.

Scott, P.R. & Gessert, M.E. (1997) Evaluation of extradural xylazine injection for cesarean operation in ovine dystocia cases. *Veterinary Journal*, 154, 63–67.

Shafford, H.L., Hellyer, P.W., & Turner, A.S. (2004) Intra-articular lidocaine plus bupivacaine in sheep undergoing stifle arthrotomy. *Veterinary Anesthesia and Analgesia*, 31, 20–26.

Singh, V., Amarpal, Kinjavdekar, P., Aithal, H.P., & Pratap, K. (2005) Medetomidine with ketamine and bupivacaine for epidural analgesia in buffaloes. *Veterinary Research Communications*, 29, 1–18.

Skarda, R.T. & Tranquilli, W.J. (2007) Local and regional anesthetic and analgesic techniques: ruminants and swine. In: *Lumb & Jones' Veterinary Anesthesia and Analgesia*, 4th edn (eds W.J. Tranquilli, J.C. Thurmon, & K.A. Grimm), Blackwell Publishing, Ames, IA, pp. 643–681.

Staffieri, F., Driessen, B., Lacitignola, L., & Crovace, A. (2009) A comparison of subarachnoid buprenorphine or xylazine as an adjunct to lidocaine for analgesia in goats. *Veterinary Anaesthesia and Analgesia*, 36, 502–511.

Stafford, K.J., Mellor, D.J., Todd, S.E., Bruce, R.A., & Ward, R.N. (2002) Effects of local anaesthesia or local anaesthesia plus a nonsteroidal anti-inflammatory drug on the acute cortisol response of calves to five different methods of castration. *Research in Veterinary Science*, 73: 61–70.

Stafford, K.J., Mellor, D.J., Todd, S.E., Ward, R.N., & McMeekan, C.M. (2003) The effect of different combinations of lignocaine, ketoprofen, xylazine and tolazoline on the acute cortisol response to dehorning in calves. *New Zealand Veterinary Journal*, 51, 219–226.

Stilwell, G., Lima, M.S., & Broom, D.M. (2008) Effects of nonsteroidal anti-inflammatory drugs on long-term pain in calves castrated by use of an external clamping technique following epidural anesthesia. *American Journal of Veterinary Research*, 69(6), 744–750

St. Jean, G., Skarda, R.T., Muir, W.W., & Hoffsis, G.F. (1990) Caudal epidural analgesia induced by xylazine administration in cows. *American Journal of Veterinary Research*, 51, 1232–1236.

Stewart, M., Stookey, J.M., Stafford, K.J., et al. (2009) Effects of local anesthetic and a non-steroidal antiinflammatory drug on pain response of dairy calves to hot-iron dehorning. *Journal of Dairy Science*, 92, 1512–1519.

Ting, S.T., Earley, B., Hughes, J.M., & Crowe, M.A. (2003) Effect of ketoprofen, lidocaine local anesthesia, and combined xylazine and lidocaine caudal epidural anesthesia during castration of beef cattle on stress responses, immunity, growth, and behavior. *Journal of Animal Science*, 81, 1281–1293.

Trim, C.M. (1989) Epidural analgesia with 0.75% bupivacaine for laparotomy in goats. *Journal of the American Veterinary Medical Association* 194, 1292–1296.

Valverde, A. (2008) Epidural analgesia and anesthesia in dogs and cats. *Veterinary Clinics of North America Small Animal Practice*, 38, 1205–1230.

Valverde, A. & Doherty, T.J. (2008a) Pain management in cattle and small ruminants, in *Current Veterinary Therapy Food Animal Practice*, 5th edn (eds D. Anderson & M. Rings), , Saunders, St. Louis, MO, pp. 534–542.

Valverde, A. & Doherty, T. (2008b) Anesthesia and analgesia of ruminants. In: *Anesthesia and Analgesia in Laboratory Animals*, 2nd edn (eds R. Fish, PJ. Danneman, M. Brown, & A. Karas), Academic Press, San Diego, CA, pp. 385–412.

Wagner, A.E., Dunlop, C.I. & Turner, A.S. (1996) Experiences with morphine injected into the subarachnoid space in sheep. *Veterinary Surgery*, 25, 256–260.

Wagner, A.E., Walton, J.A., Hellyer, P.W., Gaynor, J.S., & Mama, K.R. (2002) Use of low doses of ketamine administered by constant rate infusion as an adjunct for postoperative analgesia in dogs. *Journal of the American Veterinary Medical Association*, 221, 72–75.

Waterman, A.E., Livingston, A., & Amin, A. (1990) The antinociceptive activity and respiratory effects of fentanyl in sheep. *Journal of the Association of Veterinary Anaesthesia*, 17, 20–23.

Waterman, A.E., Livingston, A., & Amin, A. (1991a) Analgesic activity and respiratory effects of butorphanol in sheep. *Research in Veterinary Science*, 51, 19–23.

Waterman, A.E., Livingston, A., & Amin, A. (1991b) Further studies on the antinociceptive activity and respiratory effects of buprenorphine in sheep. *Journal of Veterinary Pharmacology and Therapeutics*, 14, 230–234.

Watts, S.A. & Clarke, K.W. (2000) A survey of bovine practitioners attitudes to pain and analgesia in cattle, *Cattle Practice*, 8, 361–362.

Whay, H.R. & Huxley, J.N. (2005) Pain relief in cattle: a practitioner's perspective. *Cattle Practice*, 13, 81–85.

33
Recognition and Treatment of Pain in Camelids

Tamara Grubb

Although the recognition and treatment of pain in small-animal species has rapidly improved over the last decade, and many analgesic drugs and techniques are available to treat large-animal species, pain management techniques remain underutilized (Hewson et al., 2007). Specific studies in camelids are not available, but it can be presumed that their pain is also undertreated, and factors contributing to inadequate pain management are probably similar to those in other farm species. These factors include the lingering belief that animals, particularly farm animals, do not feel pain; the difficulty of recognizing pain in large animals; the perceived economic impact of pain management; the lack of knowledge of analgesic techniques and drugs available to treat pain in large animals; and the fear of adverse effects from those drugs and techniques (Hewson et al., 2007; Fajt et al., 2011). Most of these factors are easily overcome with proper education, and it is the author's hope that information in this chapter will aid in providing appropriate analgesia for camelids.

RECOGNITION OF PAIN

As with other prey species, camelids tend to hide signs of pain. Pain behavior can be subtle, vague, and infrequently demonstrated, so any change in behavior should be carefully investigated. Mild-to-moderate pain can lead to anorexia, lethargy, excessive time spent in recumbency, avoidance of contact, and abnormal stance. Signs specific to abdominal pain include kicking or looking at the abdomen, and tenesmus. More severe colic can lead to clearly recognizable signs of pain, and may include violent movements like rolling and thrashing. Bruxism, tachycardia, and tachypnea can occur with pain of any degree and from any source. Unfortunately, pain-scoring systems utilized in small animals (Holton et al., 1998) and in small ruminants (Fitzpatrick et al., 2006) have not yet been adapted to camelids.

ANALGESIC DRUGS AND TECHNIQUES

As with most veterinary species, analgesics commonly used for the treatment of acute pain in camelids include nonsteroidal anti-inflammatory drugs (NSAIDs), opioids, local anesthetics, and α-2 agonists. The use of ketamine as an analgesic has also been reported. In addition to specific drugs, analgesic techniques like locoregional

analgesia, delivery of drugs by constant rate infusion (CRI), and nonpharmacological therapies should be considered as part of a multimodal analgesic plan.

Nonsteroidal Anti-inflammatory Drugs

Because NSAIDs (Chapter 5) alleviate pain and decrease inflammation they are an excellent choice for the treatment of many painful conditions in camelids. NSAIDs typically used in camelids include flunixin meglumine, phenylbutazone, and ketoprofen. Other NSAIDs that have been used anecdotally in camelids include aspirin, carprofen, etodolac, and topical sodium diclofenac (Table 33.1).

NSAIDs can be administered by a variety of routes including IV, SC, and PO. Unlike some drugs administered to ruminants, NSAIDs tend to be readily absorbed from the GI tract in camelids. Gastrointestinal ulceration is the most common adverse effect of NSAIDs in large-animal species, and third compartment ulcers have been suspected in camelids being treated with NSAIDs. However, stress is the most common cause of the third compartment ulceration in camelids (Smith et al., 1994), and pain and hospitalization for painful procedures, such as surgery, can increase stress; thus, withholding NSAIDs because of fear of inducing ulceration is not recommended. Nevertheless, because of the potential for ulceration during the treatment with NSAIDs, concurrent administration of cimetidine has been recommended (Fowler, 1989). Oral omeprazole may not be effective in protecting against gastrointestinal ulceration because 6 days of oral administration, at doses up to 12 mg/kg, failed to produce plasma drug concentrations associated with clinical efficacy in camelids (Poulson et al., 2005). Although NSAID-mediated adverse effects occur in all species, therapy-limiting adverse effects are uncommon when the drugs are used in suitable patients at appropriate dosages.

FLUNIXIN MEGLUMINE

The pharmacokinetics of flunixin meglumine after IV administration have been described in the llama (Navarre et al., 2001b). The recommended IV dose is 0.5–1.0 mg/kg, once to twice daily (Fowler, 1989; Miesner, 2009). Oral flunixin meglumine granules have been used anecdotally at the same dose. Based on the author's experience this dose can be used for 7–10 days after orthopedic procedures without adverse effects.

Table 33.1. Nonsteroidal anti-inflammatory drugs (NSAIDs) used in camelids. The species listed in this table are the species in which published references or personal recommendations are available for dosing. However, this is not meant to imply that the drugs are not used in other camelid species.

Drug/species	Dose/Route/Frequency	References
Flunixin meglumine—llama	0.5–1.0 mg/kg IV q12–24h	Miesner, 2009; Fowler, 1989
Phenylbutazone—llama	2–4 mg/kg IV or PO q24–48h	Navarre et al., 2001c
Ketoprofen—llama	1–2 mg/kg IM or SC, q12–24h	Navarre et al., 2001a
Etodolac	5 mg/kg PO, q24–48h	David E. Anderson, DVM, personal communication
Meloxicam—llama	0.5–1.0 mg/kg PO q24–48h	David E. Anderson, DVM, personal communication

PHENYLBUTAZONE

The pharmacokinetics of oral and IV phenylbutazone have been described in the llama (Navarre et al., 2001c). Phenylbutazone has a long half-life in camelids, and the most commonly used dose is 2–4 mg/kg IV or PO once daily or every other day. The bioavailability of orally administered phenylbutazone is 70% in llamas (Navarre et al., 2001c).

KETOPROFEN

The pharmacokinetics of IV ketoprofen have been described in the llama (Navarre et al., 2001a). There are no published pharmacokinetics, but a dose of 1–2 mg/kg IM or SC once to twice daily is commonly used in camelids.

ETODOLAC

Etodolac has been used in llamas and alpacas at 5 mg/kg, PO, once daily or every other day (David E. Anderson, DVM, personal communication, 2010).

MELOXICAM

Meloxicam has been administered orally to llamas at 0.5–1.0 mg/kg PO once daily or every other day (David E. Anderson, DVM, personal communication, 2010).

Opioids

Opioids (Chapter 4) should be considered if the patient is experiencing moderate-to-severe pain. The advantages of opioids, used at appropriate dosages, include moderate-to-profound analgesia with minimal or no adverse cardiovascular or respiratory effects, and reversibility with naloxone or naltrexone. Furthermore, opioids are inexpensive and can be administered by a variety of routes including PO, IM, IV, SC, epidurally, intra-articularly, transdermally, and by CRI (Table 33.2).

The disadvantages of opioids include their relatively short duration of action when compared with the duration of pain from most procedures or injuries (emphasizing the need for multimodal analgesia), the possibility of causing excessive sedation in some camelids or excitement in nonpainful camelids (rare), and the potential to contribute to ileus in some circumstances (e.g., large doses or long duration of administration). However, in most instances, the benefits of opioids outweigh the risks, especially because the adverse effects (as well as the desirable effects) of opioids are reversible. Bias against opioids has arisen because much of the research on the adverse effects of this drug class has been done in nonpainful animals and, intriguingly, opioids cause more adverse effects in nonpainful animals than in painful animals.

BUTORPHANOL

Butorphanol is the most commonly used opioid in camelids. Butorphanol produces mild sedation when administered at 0.02–0.2 mg/kg IV, IM, or SC (Fowler, 1989; Riebold, 1996; Garcia-Pereira et al., 2006). Butorphanol is most commonly used at a dose of 0.05–0.1 mg/kg IM or IV (Abrahamsen, 2009) or 0.1–0.3 mg/kg IV, IM, or SC (Miesner, 2009). Butorphanol-mediated sedation is fairly predictable, and most camelids given the butorphanol alone will tolerate restraint and handling, but will not become recumbent or tolerate moderately to severely painful procedures. As with other species, all opioids can cause behavioral changes, especially when IV is administered rapidly and/or at high dosages. Sedation is fairly common; however, excitement and "prancing" have been reported (Carroll et al., 2001). These effects seem to be mild and brief at normal clinical dosages, but if the effects are exaggerated or prolonged, excitement can be controlled with the concurrent administration of an α-2 agonist or with the administration of an opioid antagonist.

The pharmacokinetics of butorphanol have been described (Carroll et al., 2001) and, as with other species, indicate that butorphanol may only provide analgesia of brief duration, especially when administered IV. The half-life is approximately 15 minutes after IV administration and approximately 60 minutes after IM administration of 0.1 mg/kg. This duration of analgesia may be appropriate for the relief of mild pain of short duration but is not appropriate for most postsurgical or post-trauma pain. The duration and intensity of analgesia is improved when multimodal analgesia is utilized and, for that reason, butorphanol is commonly administered with an α-2 agonist, NSAID, and/or local anesthetic. Also, repeat dosages (Riebold, 1996; Abrahamsen, 2009; Miesner, 2009) or a CRI (Abrahamsen, 2009) can be administered to extend the duration of analgesia. The CRI published dose (0.022 mg/kg/h) (Abrahamsen, 2009) has been found by the author to be effective for intraoperative and immediate postoperative pain with no adverse effects.

BUPRENORPHINE

Because it has a longer duration of action, buprenorphine may be a better choice than butorphanol for pain relief in camelids. However, the sedation provided by buprenorphine is not as predictable as butorphanol-mediated sedation, and rarely can invasive or noxious procedures be performed on camelids treated with buprenorphine alone. As with all opioids, excitement or agitation can occur in

Table 33.2. Opioids used in camelids. The species listed in this table are the species in which printed references or personal recommendations are available for dosing. However, this is not meant to imply that the drugs are not used in other camelid species.

Drug/species	Dose/route/frequency	References
Butorphanol	0.02–0.2 mg/kg IV, IM, or SQ	Fowler, 1989; Riebold, 1996;
Llama and alpaca		Garcia-Pereira et al., 2006
	0.1 mg/kg IV or IM	Carroll et al., 2001
	0.05–0.1 mg/kg IM or IV	Abrahamsen, 2009
	0.1–0.3 mg/kg IV, IM, or SC	Miesner, 2009
Buprenorphine	0.002–0.01 mg/kg IM or IV	Gunkel, 2009
Morphine	0.25 mg/kg IV every 4 hours	Uhrig et al., 2007
Llama and alpaca	0.05–0.1 mg/kg IV or IM	Abrahamsen, 2009
	0.1–0.5 mg/kg IM	Garcia-Pereira et al., 2006
	0.1 mg/kg IM every 4 hours	Riebold, 1996; Abrahamsen, 2009
	(moderate-to-severe pain)	
Fentanyl	One 50 mcg/h patch per 30–50kg	Miesner, 2009
Llama	Four 75 mcg/h patches per adult llama	Grubb et al., 2005
Alpaca	0.002 mg/kg IV bolus	Larenza et al., 2008
Tramadol—llama	2 mg/kg IV, IM	Cox et al., 2011

nonpainful patients. The half-life of 0.05 mg/kg of buprenorphine is 3 hours after IM administration and 2 hours after IV administration (Gunkel, 2009; Hanselmann et al., 2009). Buprenorphine is almost 100% bioavailable after IM administration, and plasma concentrations are measureable within 2 minutes of injection (Hanselmann et al., 2009). The clinical dose range is 0.002–0.01 mg/kg (Gunkel, 2009) IV or IM. As with other opioids, greater dosages can cause sedation (more common in painful animals) or agitation (more common in nonpainful animals) but may provide a longer duration of action. Buprenorphine appears to have minimal impact on gastrointestinal function in camelids. Buprenorphine is considerably more expensive than pure μ agonists such as morphine.

MORPHINE

Morphine is now used routinely in camelids because it produces moderate-to-profound analgesia of roughly 4 hours duration, and is the most cost-effective of the opioids. Although the pharmacokinetics of morphine in the llama indicate that a dose of 0.25 mg/kg IV every 4 hours might be necessary to provide effective analgesia (Uhrig et al., 2007), the more commonly used doses of 0.05–0.1 mg/kg IV or IM (Abrahamsen, 2009) or 0.1–0.5 mg/kg IM (Garcia-Pereira et al., 2006) appear to be clinically effective. For prolonged, moderate-to-severe pain, morphine at 0.1 mg/kg IM every 4 hours provides adequate analgesia and causes minimal-to-no adverse effects (Riebold, 1996; Abrahamsen, 2009). Another advantage of morphine is its versatility, as it can be used PO, IV, IM, as a CRI, epidurally, and intra-articularly. Although most veterinarians feel that morphine provides effective analgesia in camelids there is some disagreement (Miesner, 2009).

Because morphine is a more effective opioid, the likelihood of adverse effects, such as ileus, might be expected to be greater than with butorphanol or buprenorphine. However, the dose can be fairly easily titrated "to effect" and, if necessary, adverse effects of the drug can be reversed and analgesia can be addressed by other means. At low dosages (e.g., 0.1 mg/kg), adverse effects are minimal to

nonexistent. However, because decreased GI motility is the most likely complication in camelids receiving opioids, GI motility and fecal output (volume and moisture content) should be monitored frequently (Abrahamsen, 2009).

FENTANYL

Fentanyl has been administered to camelids transdermally, as an IV bolus, or as a CRI. Transdermal patches can be used for the treatment of postoperative and trauma pain that is moderate to severe in intensity (Miesner, 2009). The application of four 75 mcg/h fentanyl patches provides consistent, sustained serum fentanyl concentrations without sedation in adult llamas (Grubb et al., 2005). However, the serum concentration of fentanyl that provides analgesia in llamas is not known, and the presumption of analgesia from this study is based on the serum concentration of fentanyl that provides analgesia in other species. Because of the thickness of a camelid's skin, patches should be placed on the medial side of the brachium or in other areas where the skin is thinner. A single 50 mcg/h fentanyl patch has been recommended for patients weighing 30–50 kg (Miesner, 2009). Fentanyl has been used as IV boluses and as CRIs (Larenza et al., 2008). The duration of action of a single IV bolus of fentanyl is approximately 20 minutes, and its effect can be extended by the use of a CRI.

TRAMADOL

The pharmacokinetics of injectable tramadol in llamas has been described after IM and IV administration of 2.0 mg/kg (Cox et al., 2011). The bioavailability of IM tramadol was $110 \pm 21\%$. The half-life of tramadol administered IM or IV to llamas was comparable to the half-life in other species. The intermediate metabolite (M1) was detected and its half-life was extremely long (10.4 hours after IV administration and 7.7 hours after IM administration). In humans, M1 is responsible for a major portion of tramadol-mediated analgesia. Thus, when compared to the effects of tramadol in other species, injectable tramadol may produce a moderate-to-prolonged period of analgesia in llamas. Intravenous tramadol caused a brief period of ataxia in one llama (Cox et al., 2011), and IV doses should be administered very slowly. The pharmacokinetics of oral tramadol (2 mg/kg) has not been described in camelids but has been described in goats (de Sousa et al., 2008). It appears to have a fairly short half-life after oral administration, and there was no measurable M1 in goats. This is similar to the pharmacokinetic data described in other domestic species and, if this holds true for camelids, it would mean that oral tramadol may produce analgesia, but the duration would most likely be short and the intensity of analgesia limited. However, because the pharmacokinetics of injectable tramadol in the llama was not equivalent to the pharmacokinetics in the goat, extrapolation of oral data may not be accurate.

α-2 Agonists

The α-2 agonists (Table 33.3) (Chapter 7) are used primarily for their sedative effects, yet this class of drugs also produces analgesia that is mild to moderate in intensity and duration. Xylazine is the most commonly used α-2 agonist in camelids, but the use of dexmedetomidine and medetomidine is increasing. Dexmedetomidine and medetomidine are better analgesics than xylazine as they have greater α-2:α-1 receptor binding ratios, and analgesia from α-2 agonists is mediated at the α-2 receptor.

Adverse effects of α-2 agonists include bradycardia, increased cardiac work (because of the α-2 mediated vasoconstriction and increased afterload), and decreased GI motility. These effects are short-lived and have minimal clinical significance in healthy patients. However, α-2 agonists should not be used in patients with cardiovascular disease or in conditions that cause impairment of the cardiovascular system (e.g., hypovolemia, shock). The effects (positive and adverse) of α-2 agonists are reversible with the α-2 antagonists, yohimbine, tolazoline, and atipamezole.

XYLAZINE

Reported sedative dosages of xylazine in camelids range from 0.1–0.66 mg/kg IV to 0.25–0.9 mg/kg IM (Riebold et al., 1989). The sedative response to α-2 agonists is dose-dependent and smaller dosages result in light-to-moderate sedation, whereas higher dosages often result in very deep sedation marked by recumbency and lack of response to noxious stimuli. Llamas administered doses of 0.1–0.2 mg/kg IV become sedate but generally not recumbent (Riebold, 1996), and a dose of 0.3–0.6 mg/kg IV will produce profound sedation and recumbency of 30–45 minutes duration (Riebold et al., 1989). Alpacas are generally less sensitive than llamas to the effects of α-2 agonists; thus the higher end of the dosage range is used for sedation and analgesia (Abrahamsen, 2009). As occurs in other species, the sedative effects of the α-2 agonists probably last longer than the analgesic effects (Abrahamsen, 2009). Commonly used dosages include 0.1–0.3 mg/kg IV, IM, or SC for both llamas and alpacas (Miesner, 2009) or, for standing sedation and analgesia, 0.1–0.15 mg/kg IV and 0.2–0.3 mg/kg IM in alpacas and 0.075–0.1 mg/kg IV and 0.15–0.2 mg/kg IM in llamas (Abrahamsen, 2009).

MEDETOMIDINE AND DEXMEDETOMIDINE

Medetomidine has been used to produce sedation and analgesia in llamas at dosages of 0.01–0.03 mg/kg IM (Waldridge et al., 1997), but doses of 0.04–0.08 mg/kg IM or IV have also been reported (Fowler, 1989). The analgesic effects of dexmedetomidine have not

Table 33.3. α-2 agonists used in camelids. The species listed in this table are the species in which printed references or personal recommendations are available for dosing. However, this is not meant to imply that the drugs are not used in other species.

Drug/species	Dose/route/ frequency/ comments	References
Xylazine Llamas Alpacas	0.1–0.2 mg/kg IV (sedation)	Riebold, 1996 Riebold et al., 1989
	0.3–0.6 mg/kg IV (profound sedation and recumbency)	Abrahamsen, 2009
	0.075–0.1 mg/kg IV (sedation)	Abrahamsen, 2009
	0.15–0.2 mg/kg IM or SQ (sedation)	
	0.22–0.33 mg/kg IV (recumbency)	
	0.44–0.66 mg/kg IM or SQ (recumbency)	
	0.1–0.15 mg/kg IV (sedation)	
	0.2–0.3 mg/kg IM or SQ (sedation)	
	0.33–0.44 mg/kg IV (recumbency)	
	0.66–0.88 mg/kg IM o SQ (recumbency)	
Medetomidine llamas	0.01–0.03 mg/kg IM	Waldridge et al., 1997
	0.05–0.15 mg/kg IV	Fowler, 1989
	0.04–0.08 mcg/kg IM or IV	

been reported in camelids, but the anesthetic effects of dexmedetomidine and ketamine are similar to those of medetomidine and ketamine (Gadeyne et al., 2010).

Opioid/α-2 Agonist Combinations

A combination of an opioid and an α-2 agonist will provide analgesia of greater intensity and longer duration than either drug alone. Any opioid can be combined with any α-2 agonist, but the most typical combination is xylazine and butorphanol (Riebold et al., 1989; Riebold, 1996; Garcia-Pereira et al., 2006; Abrahamsen, 2009; Miesner, 2009). Combinations of medetomidine or dexmedetomidine with butorphanol, buprenorphine, or morphine would also be effective. Generally, the lower end of the dose range is used for each drug.

Constant Rate Infusions (CRIs)

CRIs of analgesic drugs (Table 33.4) are an excellent way to manage prolonged perioperative pain, medical pain (e.g., painful abdomen), and pain due to trauma.

Drugs that are useful for CRIs in camelids include fentanyl, hydromorphone, morphine, butorphanol, ketamine, lidocaine,

Table 33.4. Constant rate infusions used in camelids for delivery of analgesic drugs

Drug	Loading dose	Infusion rate	References
Lidocaine	1.0 mg/kg IV	50 mcg/kg/min	Abrahamsen, 2009 and Authors' experience
Butorphanol	0.05–0.1 mg/kg IV or IM	0.02 mg/kg/h	Abrahamsen, 2009 and Author's experience
Fentanyl	0.002 mg/kg IV	0.01 mg/kg/h	Larenza et al., 2008
Morphine	0.1 mg/kg IM or SLOWLY IV	0.02 mg/kg/h	Abrahamsen, 2009
Ketamine	For anesthetized patients, use 1–3 mg/kg ketamine as induction bolus. Loading dose not reported for conscious patients.	40 mcg/kg/min (use lower doses in awake camelids and titrate to effect)	Schlipf et al., 2009

α-2 agonists, and a myriad of combinations of these drugs. Of these drugs, only fentanyl (Larenza et al., 2008), ketamine (Larenza et al., 2008; Abrahamsen, 2009; Schlipf et al., 2009), morphine (Abrahamsen, 2009), and butorphanol (Abrahamsen, 2009) have been described in camelids, but almost all of them have been used in camelids. More complex CRIs (e.g., "trifusion," a combination of lidocaine, ketamine, and an opioid) have also been described in camelids (Abrahamsen, 2009).

Local Anesthetics and Local Anesthetic Techniques

Sensory blockade using local anesthetics (e.g., lidocaine, mepivacaine, bupivacaine) (Chapter 6) is an effective, efficient, and economical way to provide profound analgesia. Local anesthetics can be used in a variety of local and regional techniques including ocular, mandibular, maxillary, testicular, brachial plexus, Bier, intercostal, paravertebral, and epidural blocks. Local anesthetics can also be used topically in creams or patches and can be delivered through infusion or "soaker" catheters buried in incisions or wounds. Lidocaine can also be administered IV as a CRI (Table 33.4). Opioids and α-2 agonists can be combined with local anesthetics for locoregional analgesia, particularly in the epidural space.

A description of some of the locoregional techniques currently used in camelids is provided in the following section. Not all of the techniques described here have been documented for use in camelids but many (e.g., the field, oral, testicular, and epidural blocks) are used extensively in camelid practice and have been used by the author. If not described in the literature for camelids, most of the techniques listed here have at least been described in the literature for sheep and goats (Skarda, 2007a) (see descriptions in Chapter 32), and the techniques are similar among sheep, goats, and camelids. Whenever possible, specific camelid references are listed.

Lidocaine and bupivacaine are the most commonly used local anesthetic drugs in camelids. To avoid toxicity, the total maximal dose of local anesthetics is 4 mg/kg lidocaine or 2 mg/kg bupivacaine, for all blocks. The duration of blockade is 1–1.5 hours with lidocaine and 3–4 hours with bupivacaine.

TESTICULAR BLOCKS

Castrations performed with local anesthetic blockade (Figure 33.1) result in less stress for the patient (Dinniss et al., 1997; Haga & Ranheim, 2005). This is true for standing procedures performed under sedation as well as castrations performed under general anesthesia (Portier et al., 2009). A testicular block is easy to perform,

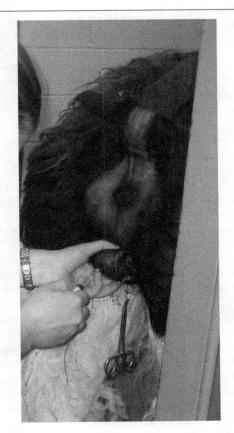

Figure 33.1. A testicular block is easy to perform, inexpensive, and provides both intraoperative and postoperative analgesia. (see text for technique) Photo courtesy of Drs. Jessie Ziegler and Colleen McCoy.

inexpensive, and provides both intraoperative and postoperative analgesia. Using a 20-gauge, 1.5 inch needle and syringe, insert the needle into the body of the testicle and inject local anesthetic (2–5 mL) until the testicle is turgid. Repeat with the other testicle. Local anesthetic injected into the testicle is rapidly distributed into the spermatic cord (Cottrell & Molony, 1995; Ranheim et al., 2005), and may be more effective than injections into the spermatic cord (Dinniss et al., 1997), although spermatic cord injections have

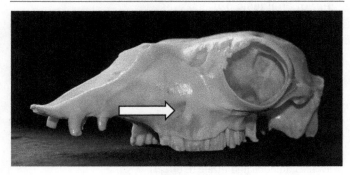

Figure 33.2. The infraorbital foramen is indicated by the arrow. The direction that the arrow is pointing is the direction that the needle should be inserted when blocking the infraorbital nerve (see text for technique).

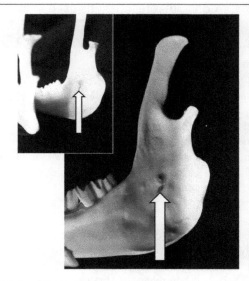

Figure 33.3. The mandibular foramen is indicated by the arrow. The direction that the arrow is pointing is the direction that the needle should be inserted when blocking the mandibular nerve. The inset photo emphasizes the location of the foramen on the lingual side of the mandible (see text for technique).

been used to provide analgesia in sedated llamas undergoing castration (Miesner, 2009). With either technique, desensitization of the skin does not occur, and this can be provided by injection of local anesthetic along the scrotal incision site (Dinniss et al., 1997).

ORAL BLOCKS

The infraorbital nerve is blocked by injecting 1–3 mL of local anesthetic into or immediately rostral to the infraorbital foramen (Figure 33.2), which is identified as a depression 1–3 cm (depending on the size of the camelid) directly above the premolars. To block the maxillary nerve, a 1.5–4.0 inch needle is inserted percutaneously along the ventral border of the zygomatic process approximately 0.5–1.5 cm caudal to the lateral canthus of the eye. Direct the needle medially and slightly cranially (in an angle that would draw an imaginary line with the premolars on the opposite side of the head) until it hits the bone. Withdraw the needle 1–5 mm, aspirate and inject 1–4 mL of local anesthetic.

The mandibular nerve can be blocked at the mandibular foramen (Figure 33.3) located on the lingual side of the mandible directly dorsal to the most prominent portion of the most caudoventral aspect of the mandible and immediately rostral to the ventral curve of the ramus. Insert a 1.5–4.0 inch needle extraorally and perpendicular to the ventral border of the mandible at the point just described. Advance the needle, keeping it close to the bone (it should be felt "scraping" the bone) so that it does not exit the oral mucosa, which would result in deposition of the local anesthetic into the oral cavity. Inject when the needle tip is approximately at a mid-mandible location.

The mental nerve is blocked by the injection of 1–3 mL of local anesthetic into or immediately rostral to the mental foramen, which is located 2–3 cm caudal to the incisors and is palpable on the labial side of the mandible.

INTERDIGITAL BLOCK AND ABAXIAL NERVE BLOCK

Sensory blockade of a portion of the foot can be achieved with an interdigital block (Miesner, 2009) (Figure 33.4). A 1–1.5 inch 18- or 20-gauge needle is inserted into the dorsal interdigital space at the junction of the two digits. The needle should be held parallel to the coronary band and directed toward the heel to a depth that places the needle tip just under the skin of the heel. The needle should then be slowly withdrawn while injecting 5–10 mL of lidocaine or

bupivacaine, aspirating occasionally to avoid intravenous injection. In addition, the abaxial nerves can be palpated on the medial and lateral aspects of the fetlock and desensitized with 2–3 mL of lidocaine injected around each nerve (Miesner, 2009). These two blocks performed together will provide complete anesthesia of the foot.

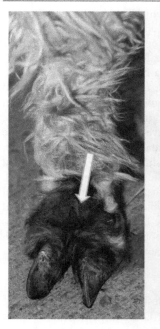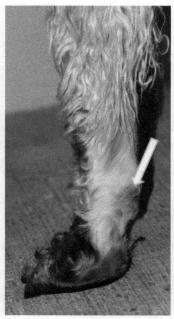

Figure 33.4. Interdigital and abaxial nerve blocks will provide complete anesthesia to the foot (see text for technique).

INTRAVENOUS REGIONAL ANESTHESIA

Intravenous regional anesthesia or the "Bier block" is a technique that provides regional anesthesia using an IV injection of lidocaine, and the block has been described for use in camelids (Miesner, 2009). Refer to the chapter on ruminant analgesia for technique.

INTRA-ARTICULAR BLOCK

Morphine (0.1 mg/kg), with or without local anesthetic drugs (1–4 mL lidocaine or bupivacaine), is commonly used for intra-articular analgesia. Ideally, local anesthetics are injected into the joint prior to surgery for pre-emptive and intraoperative analgesia, and local anesthetics and/or morphine are injected immediately after closure of the joint capsule for postoperative analgesia.

EPIDURALS

The injection of drugs into the epidural space is used to provide analgesia to the hind limbs, perineum and tail, udder, prepuce, and caudal portion of the abdomen with its associated structures (e.g., bladder, vagina, uterus, intestines). Depending on the location and volume of the injection, analgesia may extend up to the thorax and the forelimb. Complications from epidurals are rare, and the main "complication" is the failure to achieve adequate blockade. To prevent more serious complications, such as abscess and/or hematoma formation, the epidural space should not be pierced if there is dermatitis at the site of the injection or if the patient has platelet or clotting factor disorders, particularly with lumbosacral injection.

Drugs can be injected at either the lumbosacral space (LS) or the sacrococcygeal or first intracoccygeal space. Injection at the LS is slightly more difficult, although relatively easier in camelids than many other species because the landmarks can be readily palpated. Drugs injected into the LS generally have a more cranial spread, thus providing a more cranial distribution of analgesia. This injection site is recommended for abdominal pain, and is the most common site used for rear limb pain. For perineal pain and minor reproductive procedures, the sacrococcygeal or first intracoccygeal site is appropriate. Drugs used in the epidural space include opioids, local anesthetics, α-2 agonists, and ketamine.

Epidural Opioids

Although the efficacy of opioid epidurals is somewhat controversial in cattle (Anderson & Muir, 2005), they appear to be effective in camelids (Garcia-Pereira et al., 2006; Miesner, 2009) for analgesia lasting approximately 12 hours, without causing motor dysfunction (Miesner, 2009). Preservative-free morphine is the gold standard for epidural injections, but regular morphine is used routinely with no evidence that the preservative (formaldehyde) causes adverse effects. The dose of morphine in camelids is similar to that used in other species (0.1 mg/kg diluted to a total volume of 1 mL/4.5 kg with sterile water, saline, or a local anesthetic). The time to onset of analgesia for epidurally injected morphine is typically 30–45 minutes. To avoid any delay in analgesia, due to the slow onset of the opioid effect, a local anesthetic or an α-2 agonist is often combined with the morphine. The combination of romifidine (50 mcg/kg) and morphine (0.1 mg/kg) resulted in a 10-minute onset and 12-hour duration of analgesia when administered epidurally to cattle (Fierheller et al., 2004). Sedation is expected in some patients following the epidural administration of opioids (Pablo, 1993).

Epidural Local Anesthetics

Local anesthetic drugs may be used alone or in combination with opioids or α-2 agonists. Lidocaine (2–4 mg/kg) and bupivacaine (1–2 mg/kg) are the two most common local anesthetics used epidurally. Approximate duration of action of lidocaine and bupivacaine in the epidural space is 90 minutes and 4 hours, respectively, making bupivacaine a better choice for prolonged pain treatment (Miesner, 2009). Because local anesthetic drugs block motor and sensory nerves, lidocaine or bupivacaine injected into the epidural space can cause loss of motor control of the rear limbs. This occurs frequently when local anesthetics are injected at the lumbosacral junction, and is likely to occur when large volumes (>1–2 mL depending on the size of the camelid) of local anesthetics are injected at the sacrococcygeal junction. Smaller doses of local anesthetics injected at the sacrococcygeal junction are unlikely to cause loss of motor function or recumbency, although ataxia may occur. Motor blockade is usually not a problem in camelids because these species generally do not panic if they lose pelvic limb motor function. However, patients that do lose pelvic limb motor function should be placed in sternal recumbency until they can ambulate. If the animal attempts to stand before it has regained full motor function, restraint should be used to keep it recumbent; otherwise, the animal should be supported in the standing position with the rear limbs hobbled together. Local anesthetic drugs used alone in the epidural space provide satisfactory conditions for most surgeries of the perineum and tail, and for minor reproductive procedures (Bennett et al., 1998; Brogliatti et al., 2000; Saltet et al., 2000).

Epidural α-2 Agonists

α-2 agonists administered into the epidural space will prolong the duration of local anesthetic-mediated analgesia. Lidocaine (0.22 mg/kg) combined with xylazine (0.17 mg/kg) has an analgesic onset time of approximately 3 minutes, and duration of approximately 6 hours (Grubb et al., 1993).

Injecting 20 mg of xylazine plus 1 mL of 2% lidocaine into the caudal epidural space of an adult llama provides analgesia with minimal motor dysfunction (Miesner, 2009). Although analgesia is fairly profound with this technique, neither lidocaine alone nor a xylazine/lidocaine combination administered into the caudal epidural space provided adequate analgesia for castration of alpacas (Padula, 2005). In that study, an injection of lidocaine into the spermatic cord was required to obtain adequate analgesia to complete the surgery. As with epidurally administered morphine, epidurally administered α-2 agonists cause sedation in some patients. Furthermore, systemic absorption of the α-2 agonist can lead to negative cardiovascular effects and, thus, should only be used in healthy camelids.

Epidural Ketamine

Ketamine has also been used in the epidural space in camelids, although the dose was not reported (Miesner, 2009). Reported dosages range from 1 mg/kg of ketamine used alone in sheep to 2.5 mg/kg used with α-2 agonists in goats. A similar dosage range was used in adult cattle, and provided an analgesic onset of 5–6 minutes and a duration of 17–62 minutes, with ataxia but no sedation at the higher dosages (Miesner, 2009). Although the response in camelids is unknown, it is likely they would respond similarly.

Technique for Lumbosacral Injection of Analgesic Drugs

- The injection can be performed with the patient standing or in sternal or lateral recumbency.

- Palpate the wings of the ilium and draw a line that crosses mid-line between the two wings. The site where the line crosses the midline should be the approximate location of the LS. This should be confirmed by palpation of the dorsal spinous processes of the lumbar vertebrae immediately cranial (tall dorsal lumbar spinous process) and caudal (short dorsal sacral spinous process) to a distinctly palpable space.
- This area should be clipped free of hair and surgically scrubbed.
- An epidural needle (generally 22-G, 2–3 inch) should be positioned in the center of the LS ON MIDLINE at a 45° angle from the line made by the spinal column. Some veterinarians prefer to start with the needle exactly perpendicular to the spinal column. Both techniques are appropriate and will not change the success rate since the needle will be used to "walk" into the space if bone is encountered.
- The needle should be slowly inserted through the skin. Once the needle penetrates the skin, the stylet can be removed and a drop of saline can be placed in the hub of the needle if the "hanging drop" assessment is to be used.
- The needle should be advanced until a "pop" is felt (as the needle passes through the interarcuate ligament) or the fluid from the "hanging drop" is aspirated into the epidural space.
- Often, bone is encountered and the needle must be redirected and "walked" off of the vertebrae into the space. In this case, the entry into the canal is determined by a change in depth of the needle as the needle is "walked" off of the bone and into the canal.
- The needle may be caudal or cranial to the space, so "walking" should occur in each direction.
- Neither the "pop" nor the aspiration of the fluid from the "hanging drop" occur every time an epidural is successful, but the depth difference after "walking off" the bone is fairly definitive.
- Once the appropriate location has been reached, aspirate and then slowly inject the analgesic drug(s) into the epidural space (the drugs should flow easily if the needle placement is correct).
- If CSF is aspirated at the LS junction then only one-fourth of the injection volume should be administered, as this is an intrathecal injection.
- The needle is removed when the injection is completed.

Technique for Sacrococcygeal or Intracoccygeal Injection

This block is generally performed in the standing patient but can be done in patients in sternal or lateral recumbency.

- The sacrococcygeal or first intracoccygeal space is located by "pumping" the tail up and down while palpating over the spinal column for an identifiable articulation at the base of the tail.
- Once the site is identified, the procedure should progress as described for the lumbosacral injection. The main difference is that CSF fluid will not be present this far caudally.

Epidural Catheters

Epidural catheters can be inserted at either the lumbosacral or the sacrococcygeal sites although the lumbosacral site is used more commonly. Epidural catheters can be used for repeated administration of drugs when treating pain in the caudal portion of the patient that is expected to last for several days. Catheters inserted aseptically and covered with a sterile bandage have been left in place for up to 2 weeks (Miesner, 2009).

Nonpharmacological Treatment of Pain

Treatment of pain should not be limited to the use of pharmaceuticals, and many nonpharmacological analgesic modalities are available. However, the efficacy of these modalities is not supported by scientific studies, and selection of a nonpharmacological modality should be based on the evidence of effect. Acupuncture is commonly used in camelids, but no studies have been published to date. The use of acupuncture has been described for analgesia in goats (Liu et al., 2009), sheep (Bossut et al., 1986), and cattle (Kim et al., 2004). The use of physical therapy has been described for cattle (Kumar et al., 1980) and goats (Khol & Licka, 2007), and massage therapy has been described for cattle (Kumar et al., 1980). It is likely that these modalities would have similar effects in camelids.

SUMMARY

Untreated pain has a negative medical impact on the patient, and is ethically unacceptable if it impacts the patient's welfare. Although pain can be difficult to assess in camelids, one can anticipate that if a procedure causes pain in a human then it must cause some degree of pain in an animal, because all mammals have the same neuroanatomical pain pathways. Analgesic treatment plans should be based on the expected intensity and duration of pain. A myriad of drugs and techniques are available to treat pain and most of the drugs are relatively inexpensive and the techniques are easy to perform.

REFERENCES

Abrahamsen, E.J. (2009) Chemical restraint, anesthesia, and analgesia for camelids. *Veterinary Clinics of North America Food Animal Practice*, 25(2), 455–494.

Anderson, D.E. & Muir, W.W. (2005) Pain management in cattle. *Veterinary Clinics of North America Food Animal Practice*, 21(3), 623–635.

Bennett, J., Kennel, A., & Stanhope, C.R. (1998) Surgical correction of an acquired vaginal stricture in a llama, using a carbon-dioxide laser. *Journal American Veterinary Medical Association*, 212(9), 1436–1437.

Bossut, D.F., Stromberg, M.W., & Malven, P.V. (1986) Electro-acupuncture-induced analgesia in sheep: measurement of cutaneous pain thresholds and plasma concentrations of prolactin and beta-endorphin immunoreactivity. *American Journal Veterinary Research*, 47(3), 669–676.

Brogliatti, G.M., Palasz, A.T., Rodriguez-Martinez, H., Mapletoft, R.J., & Adams, G.P. (2000) Transvaginal collection and ultrastructure of llama (Lama glama) oocytes. *Theriogenology*, 54(8), 1269–1279.

Carroll, G.L., Boothe, D.M., Hartsfield, S.M., Martinez, E.A., Spann, A.C., & Hernandez, A. (2001) Pharmacokinetics and pharmacodynamics of butorphanol in llamas after intravenous and intramuscular administration. *Journal American Veterinary Medical Association*, 219(9), 1263–1267.

Cottrell, D.F. & Molony, V. (1995) Afferent activity in the superior spermatic nerve of lambs–the effects of application of rubber castration rings. *Veterinary Research Communications*, 19(6), 503–515.

Cox, S., Martin-Jimenez, T., VanAmstel, S. & Doherty, T. (2011) Pharmacokinetics of intravenous and intramuscular tramadol in llamas. *Journal Veterinary Pharmacology and Therapeutics* 34(3), 259–264.

deSousa, A.B., Santos, A.C., Schramm, S.G., et al. (2008) Pharmacokinetics of tramadol and o-desmethyltramadol in goats after intravenous and oral administration. *Journal Veterinary Pharmacology and Therapeutics* 31(1), 45–51.

Dinniss, A.S., Mellor, D.J., Stafford, K.J., Bruce, R.A., & Ward, R.N. (1997) Acute cortisol responses of lambs to castration using a rubber ring and/or a castration clamp with or without local anaesthetic. *New Zealand Veterinary Journal*, 45(3), 114–121.

Fajt, V.R., Wagner, S.A., & Norby, B. (2011) Analgesic drug administration and attitudes about analgesia in cattle among bovine practitioners in the United States. *Journal American Veterinary Medical Association* 238(6), 755–767.

Fierheller, E.E., Caulkett, N.A., & Bailey, J.V. (2004) A romifidine and morphine combination for epidural analgesia of the flank in cattle. *Canadian Veterinary Journal*, 45(11), 917–923.

Fitzpatrick, J., Scott, M., & Nolan, A. (2006) Assessment of pain and welfare in sheep. *Small Ruminant Research*, 62(1–2), 55–61.

Fowler, M.E. (1989) Anesthesia, in: *Medicine and Surgery of American Camelids* (ed M.E. Fowler), Iowa State University Press, Ames, IA, pp. 51–63.

Gadeyne, C., Schauvliege, S., Ven, S., Marcilla, M.G., & Gasthuys, F. (2010) Comparison of medetomidine-ketamine and dexmedetomidine-ketamine anaesthesia in llamas. *Veterinary Anaesthesia and Analgesia*, 37(3), 84.

Garcia-Pereira, F.L., Greene, S.A., McEwen, M-M., & Keegan, R. (2006) Analgesia and anesthesia in camelids. *Small Ruminant Research*, 61(2–3), 227–233.

Grubb, T.L., Gold, J.R., Schlipf, J.W., Craig, A.M., Walker, K.C., & Riebold, T.W. (2005) Assessment of serum concentrations and sedative effects of fentanyl after transdermal administration at three dosages in healthy llamas. *American Journal of Veterinary Research*, 66(5), 907–909.

Grubb, T.L., Riebold, T.W., & Huber, M.J. (1993) Evaluation of lidocaine, xylazine, and a combination of lidocaine and xylazine for epidural analgesia in llamas. *Journal American Veterinary Medical Association*, 203(10), 1441–1444.

Gunkel, C.I. (2009) *Buprenorphine and other Intra-op and Post-op Analgesics in Camelids. Proceedings international camelid health conference.* Corvallis, OR.

Haga, H.A., & Ranheim, B. (2005) Castration of piglets: the analgesic effects of intratesticular and intrafunicular lidocaine injection. *Veterinary Anaesthesia and Analgesia*, 32(1), 1–9.

Hanselmann, R., Mosley, C.I., Mosley, C.M., et al. (2009) *Pharmacokinetics of Buprenorphine in Alpacas (Lama Pacos) After Intravenous and Intramuscular Administration, Proceedings world congress veterinary anesthesia*, Glasgow, Scotland, pp. 61.

Hewson, C.J., Dohoo, I.R., Lemke, K.A., & Barkema, H.W. (2007) Canadian veterinarians' use of analgesics in cattle, pigs, and horses in 2004 and 2005. *Canadian Veterinary Journal*, 48(2), 155–164.

Holton, L.L., Scott, E.M., Nolan, A.M., Reid, J., Welsh, E., & Flaherty, D. (1998) Comparison of three methods used for assessment of pain in dogs. *Journal American Veterinary Medical Association*, 212(1), 61–66.

Khol, J.L., & Licka, T.F. (2007) Closed reduction of coxofemoral luxation in a goat: case report. *Acta Veterinaria Hungary*, 55(3), 301–308.

Kim, D.H., Cho, S.H., Song, K.H., et al. (2004) Electroacupuncture analgesia for surgery in cattle. *American Journal Chinese Medicine*, 32(1), 131–140.

Kumar, R., Prasad, B., Kohli, R.N., & Singh, J. (1980) Repair of femoral and humeral fractures in adult cattle. *Modern Veterinary Practice*, 61(6), 535–537.

Larenza, M.P., Zanolari, P., & Jäggin-Schmucker, N. (2008) Balanced anesthesia and ventilation strategies for an alpaca (*Lama pacos*) with an increased anesthetic-risk. *Schweizer Archiv für Tierheilkunde*, 150(2), 77–81.

Liu, D.M., Zhou, Z.Y., Ding, Y., et al. (2009) Physiologic effects of electroacupuncture combined with intramuscular administration of xylazine to provide analgesia in goats. *American Journal Veterinary Research*, 70(11), 1326–1332.

Miesner, M.D. (2009) *Field Anesthesia Techniques in Camelids. Proceedings 81st western veterinary conference*, Las Vegas, NV.

Navarre, C.B., Ravis, W.R., Campbell, J., Nagilla, R., Duran, S.H., & Pugh, D.G. (2001a) Stereoselective pharmacokinetics of ketoprofen in llamas following intravenous administration. *Journal Veterinary Pharmacology and Therapeutics*, 24(3), 223–226.

Navarre, C.B., Ravis, W.R., Nagilla, R., et al. (2001b) Pharmacokinetics of flunixin meglumine in llamas following a single intravenous dose. *Journal Veterinary Pharmacology and Therapeutics*, 24(5), 361–364.

Navarre, C.B., Ravis, W.R., Nagilla, R., Simpkins, A., Duran, S.H., & Pugh, D.G. (2001c) Pharmacokinetics of phenylbutazone in llamas following single intravenous and oral doses. *Journal Veterinary Pharmacology Therapeutics*, 24(3), 227–231.

Pablo, L.S. (1993) Epidural morphine in goats after hind limb orthopedic surgery. *Veterinary Surgery*, 22(4), 307–310.

Padula, A.M. (2005) Clinical evaluation of caudal epidural anaesthesia for the neutering of alpacas. *Veterinary Record*, 156(19), 616–617.

Portier, K.G., Jaillardon, L, Leece, E.A., & Walsh, C.M. (2009) Castration of horses under total intravenous anaesthesia: analgesic effects of lidocaine. *Veterinary Anaesthesia and Analgesia*, 36(2), 173–179.

Poulsen, K.P., Smith, G.W., Davis, J.L., & Papich, M.G. (2005) Pharmacokinetics of oral omeprazole in llamas. *Journal Veterinary Pharmacology and Therapeutics*, 28(6), 539–543.

Ranheim, B., Haga, H.A., & Ingebrigtsen, K. (2005) Distribution of radioactive lidocaine injected into the testes in piglets. *Journal Veterinary Pharmacology and Therapeutics*, 28(5), 481–483.

Riebold, T.W. (1996) Ruminants, in: *Lumb and Jones' Veterinary Anesthesia*, 3rd edn (eds J.C. Thurmon, W.J. Tranquilli, & G.J. Benson), Williams and Wilkins, Baltimore, pp. 610–626.

Riebold, T.W., Kaneps, A.J., & Schmotzer, W.B. (1989) Anesthesia in the llama. *Veterinary Surgery*, 18(5), 400–404.

Saltet, J., Dart, A.J., Dart, CM, & Hodgson, D.R. (2000) Ventral midline caesarean section for dystocia secondary to failure to dilate the cervix in three alpacas. *Australian Veterinary Journal*, 78(5), 326–328.

Schlipf, J., Eaton, K., Fulkerson, P., et al. (2009) *Constant Rate Infusion of Ketamine in Alpacas Reduces Minimal Alveolar Concentration Values For Isoflurane. Proceedings American college veterinary anesthesia*, Chicago, IL.

Skarda, R.T. (2007a) Local and regional anesthetic and analgesic techniques: ruminants and swine, in: *Lumb and Jones' Veterinary Anesthesia*, 4th edn. (eds W.J. Tranquilli, J.C. Thurmon, & K.A. Grimm), Blackwell Publishing, Ames, IA, pp. 643–682.

Smith, B.B., Pearson, E.G., & Timm, K.I. (1994) Third compartment ulcers in the llama. *Veterinary Clinics of North America Food Animal Practice*, 10(2), 319–330.

Uhrig, S.R., Papich, M.G., KuKanich, B., et al. (2007) Pharmacokinetics and pharmacodynamics of morphine in llamas. *American Journal Veterinary Research*, 68(1), 25–34.

Waldridge, B.M., Lin, H.C., De Graves, F.J., & Pugh, D.G. (1997) Sedative effects of medetomidine and its reversal by atipamizole in llamas. *Journal American Veterinary Medical Association*, 211(12), 1562–1565.

34

Recognition and Treatment of Pain in Pet Pigs

Kristie Mozzachio and Valarie V. Tynes

RECOGNIZING PAIN IN PIGS

Pain recognition in pet pigs can be challenging. Pigs are stoic animals, but are also a prey species inclined to mask signs of illness, weakness, pain, or vulnerability until they can no longer compensate. Signs of pain can be subtle, and recognizing these signs depends on careful observation, a basic knowledge of normal swine behavior, and common sense. Studies documenting signs of pain in pigs have been mostly limited to the pain associated with common management practices in commercial swine, such as tail docking, teeth clipping, and castration. More recently, the use of a global scale to assess pain and the effects of analgesics has been reported for miniature swine used in laboratory research (Harvey-Clark et al., 2000; Reyes et al., 2002). With some caution, much can be extrapolated from these data and applied to the pet pig.

When a pig is initially presented it is critical to rely on the owner's knowledge and experience of the pet's behavior. A pig's behavior in the clinical setting is likely to be very different from its behavior at home. An observant owner will be the first to recognize the subtle changes in behavior that suggest something is wrong. At this stage, the pig might appear perfectly normal on physical examination, but even small changes in behavior may indicate pain or discomfort and, in some cases, may suggest which body system to examine more closely.

Clinical Signs Suggestive of Pain

Several recognizable indicators of pain, distress, or illness in pigs are similar to those observed in other species (Table 34.1). However, one should also remember that every pig is an individual, and sensitivity to pain may vary depending on age, gender, and personality, as well as the duration and severity of the pain.

Decreased food intake, as well as less time spent eating, has been well documented in painful or ill swine of all ages (McGlone & Hellman, 1988; Harvey-Clark et al., 2000; Escobar et al., 2007). Decreased food intake may be a subtle sign in commercial swine kept in groups; however, for most pet pigs, individual meals are fed and consumed rapidly and completely upon presentation. Any pet pig that completely stops eating should be assumed to be in serious pain or distress until proven otherwise. Not all ill or painful pigs stop eating, but all pigs that stop eating are likely to be suffering. In one study of postoperative pain in pigs, a return to eating was considered the best predictor of adequate pain control (Malavasi et al., 2006).

Decreased activity is an important sign of pain or discomfort in an animal like the pig that normally spends a large part of its day foraging and exploring. Studies in swine of all types demonstrated that ill or painful pigs are less active (McGlone et al., 1993; Harvey-Clark et al., 2000; Taylor et al., 2001; Hay et al., 2003; Escobar et al., 2007). They may spend more time recumbent and demonstrate a reluctance to move or change position (Harvey-Clark et al., 2000). This may, however, be dependent upon where the source of pain is; pigs that underwent laryngeal transplantation consistently demonstrated an unwillingness to lie down when they were in pain (Murison et al., 2009).

Changes in posture, such as a pig standing with its back hunched, can be an important sign of pain or distress (Figure 34.1). Pigs with forelimb arthritis frequently stand in a hunched position with more weight on the pelvic limbs. Lying and rising may be more painful than simply standing in a position in which pressure on the sore limb or limbs can be relieved. Pigs in pain may also be stiff, tremble, or isolate themselves from other pigs (Hay et al., 2003) and people. Pigs with visceral pain may kick at the abdomen or may shift repeatedly when lying down, suggesting that they cannot get comfortable.

Changes in ambulation can be suggestive of pain, and are of particular importance when dealing with aged pigs. Arthritis is one of the most common problems in the geriatric pig, and the chronic pain associated with this condition often leads to the decision to euthanize the pet (see further discussion of arthritis in chronic pain section).

Lip smacking and teeth grinding can also be the signs of pain or distress in pigs. However, because teeth grinding is a common behavior in some pigs it may be difficult to determine whether the pig is bored, agitated, or in physical pain or distress. The client's knowledge of the pig's normal behavior will again be critical in making that determination. If the pig has never performed the behavior, and suddenly begins grinding its teeth, then this should be considered a sign that something is wrong. Teeth grinding is generally considered to be more an indicative of gastrointestinal pain, although evidence for this is mainly anecdotal. Lip smacking is also a normal behavior, and is often demonstrated as a threat or warning to unfamiliar pigs or people. Additionally, lip smacking

Pain Management in Veterinary Practice, First Edition. Edited by Christine M. Egger, Lydia Love and Tom Doherty.

Table 34.1. Clinical signs associated with pain in pigs

Behavioral changes
- Decreased food intake
- Decreased activity levels
- Remaining isolated from others
- Kicking at the abdomen
- Trembling
- Lip smacking, teeth grinding, "teeth champing"
- Rapid tail wagging or tail "flicking"
- Increased irritability and/or aggression
- High pitched vocalizations, squealing, screaming, staccato grunting

Changes in posture/ambulation
- Carpal walking (walking on knees)
- Standing with a hunched posture
- Persistent sitting and reluctance to lie down
- Frequent shifting of position when recumbent
- Difficulty rising and/or lying down
- Limping

Table 34.2. Normal physiological values for miniature pigs

Parameter	Values
Respiratory rate (breaths/min)	25–60 (piglets under 26 weeks) 13–18 (Adults)
Heart rate (beats/min)	75–250 (piglets under 26 weeks) 70–80 (adults)
Rectal temperature	37.6–39 C (99.7–102.2 F)
Life expectancy	15–18 years

that leads to the development of large quantities of frothy foam in and around the mouth is a normal behavior for a pig that is anticipating food. Again, differentiating between normal and abnormal may be difficult and is dependent on owner observation. Studies on commercial piglets (Noonan et al., 1994; Lewis et al., 2005) have demonstrated increased "teeth champing" in the hours after piglets' teeth are clipped, suggesting that this behavior may be particularly related to mouth pain or discomfort. Therefore, any unusual manipulations of the mouth, teeth, lips, or tongue that persist for more than a few minutes should be investigated.

Tail wagging is a normal behavior for the pet pig and may occur almost constantly when not sleeping. However, the slow, relaxed, rhythmic wagging of a pig grazing or exploring is very different from the agitated flicking tail of a pig in pain. The pig in pain will flick the tail in a rapid, irregular manner, and the tail, along with the entire body posture, will be held more stiffly. These alterations can be very subtle but, with practice, one can learn to recognize the difference, and most observant pet owners will be able to differentiate relaxed tail wagging from the agitated tail flicking of a painful pig. Tail flicking has been well documented in piglets as a sign of pain (Noonan et al., 1994; Hay et al., 2003; Lewis et al., 2005), and latencies to tail flicking have been used by researchers to assess pigs' sensitivities to pain (Rushen & Ladewig, 1991).

Increased irritability and aggression can be a sign of pain or discomfort in some pigs (Harvey-Clark et al., 2000; Murison et al., 2009).

Increased heart and respiratory rate (Table 34.2) have been associated with pain in most species. Although these parameters may indicate pain in pigs, when used alone they may lead to inaccurate pain assessment, particularly because complicating factors such as stress may alter these parameters in a nonpainful animal (Murison et al., 2009). Thus, cardiopulmonary parameters should be considered part of a multifactorial pain assessment.

Vocalization can be helpful when determining if a pig is in distress or experiencing pain or discomfort. Pigs are notoriously vocal and produce a large, complex range of sounds. Some experience is needed to ascertain whether a pig is hungry, scared, agitated, or painful, although the owner's experience with, and knowledge of, the pet can again be extremely useful. The frequency, amplitude, pitch, tone, and duration of pig vocalizations, including squeals and screams, tend to increase with pain or distress (Marx et al., 2003). Piglets restrained and castrated without anesthesia demonstrate significantly higher pitched calls that are more frequent and of longer duration than piglets that are restrained and not castrated (White et al., 1995; Weary et al., 1998; Taylor & Weary, 2000; Taylor et al., 2001). Staccato grunts are commonly heard when a pig is distressed, but may also be produced when a pig is simply irritable or hungry.

Recognition of Chronic Pain in Pigs

Potential causes of chronic pain, such as neoplasia or severe infectious or degenerative processes, are often discovered late in the course of the disease and typically lead to euthanasia. Arthritis is a primary example of a chronic pain condition in the pet pig.

Pigs with chronic pain exhibit many of the same signs as pigs with acute pain (Table 34.1). Chronic pain does not typically lead to loss of appetite, although changes in feeding habits may be noted by the owner, including the desire to eat foods other than the regular feed, slow ingestion of a meal, or leaving small amounts of

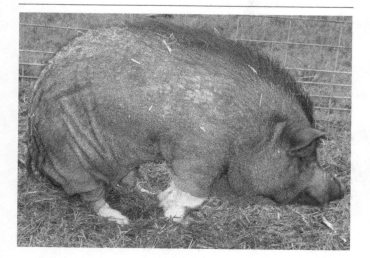

Figure 34.1. Geriatric pig exhibiting the typical "hunched" posture associated with end-stage arthritis. This posturing is often mistaken for constipation.

feed in the bowl. Changes in ambulation (slower pace, occasional limping) or alteration of urination and defecation habits (toileting close to the sleeping area, urinating or defecating less frequently) may be observed. Evidence of urination or defecation in or near the sleeping quarters is a foreboding sign as pigs are fastidious, and an unwillingness to ambulate to the normal toileting area is a strong indication that quality of life is poor. More subtle behavioral changes such as increased time spent sleeping, decreased grazing or sunbathing are other common indicators.

Arthritis occurs to some extent in the majority of pet pigs. Radiographic signs are visible as early as 2 years of age, although clinical signs are highly variable and do not correlate well with radiographic abnormalities. The elbow, distal limb joints (metacarpals, metatarsals, phalanges) and spine are typically affected, and larger joints such as the shoulder and coxofemoral joints are often spared. Arthritic pigs may initially demonstrate difficulty rising in the morning, and a stiffness that decreases with movement throughout the day. Lameness is typically associated with a forelimb, and is usually unilateral, but may be shifting. Decreased roaming, exploring, and grazing are common signs. In addition, arthritic pigs may frequently seek out warm, sunny locations for resting. More severe signs include ambulation in a kneeling position ("carpal walking") (Figure 34.2). This is a natural position for some wild pigs, but in the miniature domestic pig it often indicates pain due to arthritis. Persistent "carpal walking" in the pet pig is strongly suggestive of significant forelimb arthritis.

Other signs that are indicative of severe arthritic pain include sleeping for most of the day, spending the majority of time in one area, such as the shelter or sleeping area, and a hunched posture that is often mistaken for constipation. The range of motion of the elbow joints is often markedly decreased, and even carpal walking may be impossible. Valgus deformity and enlargement of the elbow joint are commonly observed in advanced cases.

TREATMENT OF ACUTE PAIN IN PET PIGS

Acute pain, such as surgical pain, is generally easier to treat than chronic pain but requires a pre-emptive and multimodal approach. The expected degree and duration of pain can be predicted based on the age and weight of the animal, type and duration of surgery, traumatic insult, disease, and wound location and size. For example, castration or skin mass removal would be expected to be less painful than more invasive surgeries such as laparotomy (e.g., for ovariohysterectomy) or fracture repair. Uterine tumors and tooth (tusk) abscessation are two common conditions in pigs that are associated with moderate-to-severe pain. Uterine tumors, primarily leiomyomas, are extremely common in pet pigs and the incidence increases with age (Mozzachio et al., 2004). An affected pig typically presents with an enlarged abdomen and, despite the potential for massive tumor size, the animal generally does not appear to be overtly painful. Subtle indicators may include frequent recumbent body shifting as the pig attempts to get comfortable. When recognized by the attending clinician, curative ovariohysterectomy can be performed. Common sense dictates that the large incision, extensive manipulation of internal organs, and long duration of surgery lead to a greater degree of pain and a longer recovery period than would be expected with a routine spay; and thus requires careful planning for analgesia pre-, intra- and postoperatively.

In older males, abscessation of the canines (tusks), typically the mandibular teeth, is a common problem (pers. obs.; Duchess Fund database) (Figure 34.3). An affected animal typically presents

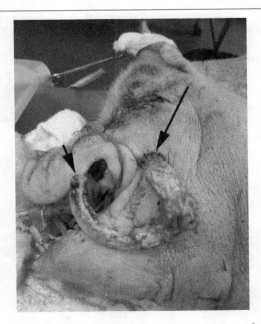

Figure 34.3. Geriatric male following extraction of an abscessed left mandibular tusk. Note the size and shape of the tusk relative to the jaw of the pig; only the tip (short arrow) protruded into the oral cavity while the remainder was embedded within the ramus of the mandible. There is extensive remodeling of the tooth leading to a highly irregular surface that complicated surgical extraction. Sutures visible just above the tusk (long arrow) mark the surgical incision required to access the tooth root.

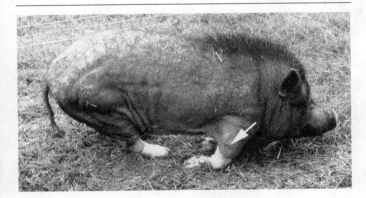

Figure 34.2. A geriatric pig with end-stage arthritis attempting to ambulate via "carpal walking." Arthritic changes in the elbows have resulted in severe limitations to range of motion of the joint as evidenced by the position of the forelimbs. The carpus is flexed but the elbow joint (arrow) cannot be positioned to allow this pig to fully "kneel." Despite the severity of arthritis, this pig had a significant return to mobility for several years with daily medication. However, a lack of response to medication at this stage should warrant euthanasia.

with recurring abscesses of the chin or neck area and may not exhibit overt signs of pain, have few or no abnormalities on oral examination, and have no difficulty eating. However, radiographs, computed tomography (CT), or magnetic resonance imaging often reveal substantial bone lysis because the mandibular tusk root in the pig extends at least half the length of the ramus. Obviously, a condition involving extreme bone lysis, infection, and requiring much surgical manipulation would be expected to produce a high degree of pain postoperatively.

Analgesics Used to Treat Acute Pain in Pigs

OPIOIDS

Pure μ-agonists, such as fentanyl, and partial agonists, such as buprenorphine, are efficacious in the pig (Swindle, 1986; Smith & Swindle, 2008) (Chapter 4) (Table 34.3). The only commercially available buprenorphine formulations are 0.3 mg/mL solutions, making administration impractical considering the volume needed for most pigs; however, more concentrated compounded formula-

tions have been used experimentally (Rodriguez et al., 2001). There is no report of the use of buprenorphine patches in pigs. Fentanyl can be used in pigs as a bolus injection, IM or IV, but it has a short half-life. Fentanyl can be administered as a constant rate infusion (CRI) in the perioperative period or for moderate to severe pain. Analgesic doses in pigs are not known, although its minimum alveolar concentration (MAC)-sparing effect is less in pigs than other species (Moon et al., 1995).

Transdermal Fentanyl Patches

Transdermal fentanyl patches (12.5 or 25 μg/h) (Chapter 9) have been used successfully in pet pigs (27–82 kg), and can be efficacious for as long as 3 days (pers. obs.; Harvey-Clark et al., 2000; Malavasi et al., 2006). Transdermal absorption has been demonstrated in several research studies (Harvey-Clark et al., 2000; Malavasi et al., 2005), and uptake may be similar to that of humans because pigs, like humans, have a direct musculocutaneous arterial blood supply (Daniel & Williams, 1973; Harvey-Clark et al., 2000). Because absorption is dependent on the area of contact, covering

Table 34.3. Dosages for some common analgesics in pigs

Drug	Dose and route	Reference
Opioids		
Hydromorphone	0.1–0.2 mg/kg IV q2h	Papich, 2007
	0.2 mg/kg SC or IM q4–6h	
Oxymorphone	0.1–0.2 mg/kg IV, SC, or IM	Papich, 2007
	Redose at 0.05–0.1 mg/kg q1–2h	
Fentanyl	0.02–0.05 mg/kg IV or IM PRN	(Love, personal experience)
	0.02–0.1 mg/kg/h IV CRI	
Morphine	0.2 mg/kg SC or IM q4h	Heard, 1993
Buprenorphine	0.01–0.05 mg/kg IV, SC, or IM q6–12h	Flecknell, 1996
Butorphanol	0.2–0.4 mg/kg IV, SC, or IM q2–4h	Papich, 2007
Pentazocine	2–5 mg/kg IV, SC, or IM q4h	Heard, 1993
Tramadol	2–4 mg/kg PO q6–24h	Mozzachio, personal experience
		Papich, Extrapolated from canine dose, personal communication
NSAIDs		
Flunixin meglumine	1.1 mg/kg IV, SC, or IM q12–24h	Mozzachio, personal experience
Carprofen	2.2 mg/kg SC q12h	(Love, personal experience)
	4.4 mg/kg q24h	
Ketoprofen	3 mg/kg IV, SC, or IM q24h	Flecknell, 1996; Mozzachio, personal experience
	1 mg/kg PO q24h	
Meloxicam	0.4 mg/kg IM q24h	Papich, 2007; Flecknell, 1996; Mozzachio, personal experience; Papich, Extrapolated from canine dose, personal communication
	0.1 mg/kg PO q24h	
Phenylbutazone	4–8 mg/kg PO q12h	Heard, 1993
	4 mg/kg IV q24h	
Aspirin (enteric coated)	10 mg/kg PO q6–8h	Heard, 1993
Ibuprofen	10 mg/kg PO q6–8h	Extrapolated from human dose
Etodolac	10–15 mg/kg PO q24h	Papich, 2007
Corticosteroids		
Dexamethasone	0.01–0.04 mg/kg IV or IM q24h	Mozzachio, personal experience
Prednisone	0.5–1 mg/kg PO q12–24h initially, then tapering to q48h	Papich, 2007

a portion of the adhesive surface of a patch will decrease the dose delivered (Papich, 2007); however, absorption can be highly variable (Malavasi et al., 2005, 2006; Papich, 2007). In the authors' experience, the patches appear to be efficacious and are primarily employed for more intense pain, prolonged pain, or cases where injectable or oral analgesics are not an option. Pigs are not amenable to handling and restraint, and the need for multiple injections is stressful unless an intravenous catheter can be maintained for drug delivery. Additionally, stress has been demonstrated to at least partially obviate the analgesic effects of many drugs (Harvey-Clark et al., 2000; Ugarte & O'Flaherty, 2005). Fentanyl patches larger than 25 µg/h may cause paradoxical excitation and agitation (pers. obs.); however, research studies have typically employed 50 µg/h patches (Harvey-Clark et al., 2000; Malavasi et al., 2005, 2006) and have suggested that doses less than 50 µg/h are not reliably efficacious (Harvey-Clark et al., 2000), although this is not consistent with the authors' observations. The literature in pigs reports no adverse effects, such as inappetance, respiratory depression, hypoxemia, or dysphoria, as may occur with the use of other opioids (Harvey-Clark et al., 2000; Malavasi et al., 2005), but inappetance has been observed by the authors.

The fentanyl patch is particularly useful for preoperative analgesia for major surgeries, such as uterine tumor removal or tusk extraction, when applied at least 12 hours prior to surgery, and may be complemented, as needed, with other analgesics. Maximum serum concentrations in pigs have been consistently measured at approximately 24 hours post application (Malavasi et al., 2006). The sharp bristles that remain in the skin after clipping the hair may hamper application and absorption. Direct contact between the patch and the skin must be maintained to allow absorption, and disruption of contact has been reported as a cause of failure to produce analgesia (Harvey-Clark et al., 2000; Riviere & Papich, 2001; Malavasi et al., 2005). The interscapular area or behind-the-ear area have been reported to be suitable application sites (Harvey-Clark et al., 2000; Riviere & Papich, 2001; Malavasi et al., 2005, 2006); however, skin thickness, subcutaneous adipose tissue, and difficulties in maintenance of patch-to-skin contact have been the issues with those sites. Based on the authors' clinical experience, the leg (i.e., the "meaty" part below the elbow, knee, or tarsal joints) is the recommended application site, as the hair is sparser, softer, and the patch is easily kept in place by a light, nonocclusive leg wrap. Placing the patch on the leg will also avoid exposure of the patch to a heat source during surgery or recovery, which could unintentionally increase drug absorption and result in overdose (see manufacturer insert/label). Pigs are not flexible animals, and do not have the ability to easily chew at or remove the patch, so the chance of accidental ingestion is unlikely unless the patch falls off. The owner can easily maintain the patch at home, although it should be prescribed with caution if there are small children in the household, as accidental ingestion has resulted in fatalities in children.

NONSTEROIDAL ANTI-INFLAMMATORY DRUGS
Nonsteroidal anti-inflammatory drugs (NSAIDs) (Chapter 5) are useful for perioperative pain control, but potential negative effects on renal blood flow have limited their use in pre-emptive surgical analgesia. NSAID-induced gastrointestinal adverse effects, such as ulceration, are generally related to repeated use and are not an important consideration in limited perioperative administration. In one study in pigs, meloxicam was found to only minimally and transiently alter renal blood flow, and ketoprofen had more profound effects (Junot et al., 2008). Pre-emptive preoperative NSAID use is best coupled with fluid therapy and monitoring of blood pressure during anesthesia to reduce adverse effects, and should always be employed with caution. After anesthetic recovery, NSAID use is warranted, safe, and effective for most surgical procedures.

α-2 AGONISTS
It should be noted that although α-2 agonists (Chapter 7) have sedative and analgesic properties in most species, and appear to work well in pigs in combination with other drugs, they can produce considerable negative cardiovascular effects (Gómez de Segura et al., 1997; Papich, 2007), limiting their use to the perioperative setting in healthy patients.

Epidural Analgesia and Local Nerve Blocks
Local anesthetics (Chapter 6), (e.g., lidocaine or bupivicaine), opioids (e.g., morphine), and α-2 agonists (e.g., detomidine) (Malavasi et al., 2006; Papich, 2007) can provide analgesia via epidural administration for abdominal, pelvic, perineal, and hindlimb surgery and via several other local nerve block techniques. Parenteral morphine can be diluted with local anesthetic (lidocaine or bupivicaine) or sterile saline to a total volume of 1 mL/5.0–7.5 kg body weight, not exceeding 0.2 mL/kg, although preservative-free morphine (0.1 mg/mL) can be used. The landmarks and techniques in pigs are similar to those in dogs (Egger & Love, 2009d). Other local nerve blocks can be employed in pigs for indications similar to those in other species (Egger & Love, 2009a, 2009b, 2009c, 2009d). For example, a mandibular nerve block is effective for mandibular tusk extraction and a soaker catheter could be useful for a large wound.

ANALGESICS FOR CHRONIC PAIN

There are a number of effective oral medications employed for chronic pain in pet pigs. Arthritis is extremely common and long-term pain management is required for this insidious, progressive, and incurable disease. The medication regimen must be carefully monitored and adjusted, as needed, to keep the animal comfortable with a minimum of adverse effects. Dosages of analgesics in the pet pig are typically extrapolated from other species if no data are available for pigs. As many organ systems in the pig, including the gastrointestinal tract, bear remarkable similarity to humans (Bode et al., 2010; Minipig Research Forum, 2010), doses employed in humans may be effective.

NSAIDs
The anti-inflammatory properties of NSAIDs help provide analgesia in pigs with arthritis and other painful inflammatory processes. Common doses for use in pigs are in Table 34.3. Many of the drug dosages listed are extrapolated from other species and based on clinical experience.

In arthritic patients, a multimodal drug combination consisting of an anti-inflammatory drug and analgesics of other classes are often employed, with adjustments made to keep the pig comfortable using the fewest medications, lowest dosages, and least frequent dosing intervals. Some pigs only require treatment for "flare-ups," such as those caused by acute injury, hoof overgrowth, or damp, humid, or cold weather. Other pigs require daily medication for the remainder of their lives, as discontinuation may lead to such severe clinical signs that euthanasia may be warranted. Risks versus benefits must be determined, and in end-stage arthritis benefits typically outweigh potential complications. Quality of life must be assessed and given the highest priority.

Complications of NSAID use are similar to those in other species. For example, NSAIDs have the potential to produce GI upset, including rare but possibly fatal bleeding from gastric ulcers. However, it should be noted that pigs have few problems with NSAIDs and, not only are antemortem adverse effects very rarely reported, numerous necropsies performed on geriatric pigs treated long-term with NSAIDs (i.e., high-dose daily treatment for 3–5 years) have provided no evidence of gastrointestinal ulceration or gastric hemorrhage (A. Wilbers, pers. obs.; personal communication). NSAIDs are best administered with food, and gastrointestinal protectants may be given in conjunction (e.g., famotidine, omeprazole), especially if other stress factors (e.g., hospitalization, illness) are involved. Combination products such as Ascriptin® (aspirin buffered with Maalox, Novartis) are another alternative.

Over-the-counter aspirin, administered orally at the labeled dose for humans, is often the first medication employed when clinical signs of arthritis pain manifest. For long-term use, buffered aspirin may decrease the likelihood of gastrointestinal problems. Maintenance therapy for an arthritic pig might include daily aspirin, ibuprofen, naproxen, etodolac, meloxicam, or other NSAIDs (Table 34.3). During severe flare-ups, a course of prednisone, after discontinuing the NSAID for several days, may alleviate signs until the pig can return to the normal regimen of pain medication. Other analgesics, such as tramadol or gabapentin may need to be added during the washout period and until NSAID administration can be resumed.

Tramadol

Oral tramadol is reported to be very effective in pigs, and although the half-life is approximately 4–6 hours in humans (Payne et al., 2002; Grond & Sablotzki, 2004), pigs seem to do well with once to twice daily administration, and a greater frequency may cause undesirable effects such as lethargy. In advanced severe arthritis, tramadol and an NSAID may be given in combination. Individual pigs have variable responses to tramadol, thus the owner must be vigilant in observing for efficacy versus sedation, and the dose should be adjusted accordingly.

Adjunctive Treatment of Arthritis in Pigs

Alleviation of arthritis pain is an art, and the goal is to adjust medication(s) to achieve maximum efficacy at the lowest dose, at the least frequent intervals, with cessation of medications, if possible, during periods of minimal clinical signs (e.g., during warm, dry weather). Prevention or reduction of arthritis pain may also be achieved by providing a warm, dry environment with a raised floor to prevent contact with cold or damp surfaces; providing traction, such as rubber mats or throw rugs with rubber backing; and avoidance of stairs or inclines, as even the slightest incline may present a formidable obstacle to an arthritic pig.

In addition to analgesic and anti-inflammatory medications, daily glucosamine/chondroitin sulfate supplementation can improve overall joint health, and may even be administered as a dietary supplement long before clinical signs manifest. Although nutriceutical efficacy is backed by minimal research, supplementation has been anecdotally reported by owners to have dramatic effects. An initial glucosamine dose of 12 mg/kg and a chondroitin sulfate dose of 3.8 mg/kg, q12h for 4 weeks is recommended (Papich, 2007), followed by 4 mg/kg glucosamine and 1.3 mg/kg of chondroitin sulfate, q12h, for maintenance.

There is more information available on the use of NSAIDs and opioids in pigs than for other drug classes, but pigs are likely to be responsive to other drugs such as gabapentin, amitriptyline, and amantadine (Chapter 8). Doses for pigs are frequently extrapolated from other species (especially dogs).

DRUG WITHDRAWAL TIMES

One important consideration in food animals with the use of any drug is withdrawal time. Although these pigs are pets, and owners may be offended at the suggestion of pet pigs as a food source, the porcine is considered a food animal species although its legal classification as "exotic" has allowed this unique pet to be maintained in areas that otherwise prohibit farm animals. Medical records, including discharge instructions as well as prescription labels, should include mention of drug withdrawal times. Additionally, drugs illegal for use in food animals should not be used in pet pigs as legal action may be taken if such use is reported. Although a rare event, pet pigs occasionally enter the food chain. Up-to-date data is maintained by the Food Animal Residue Avoidance & Depletion Program (FARAD) and can be accessed online at http://www.farad.org/.

SUMMARY

Recognition of pain in pigs is challenging because pigs are a stoic prey species. Reliance on the owner to detect changes in behavior is critical, and it should be assumed that conditions which humans identify as painful are likely to be so for pigs as well. Strategic preemptive and multimodal analgesic therapy is essential to the proper medical and surgical care of pet pigs and a variety of medications, including opioids and NSAIDs, as well as management strategies, can be used to achieve this goal.

ACKNOWLEDGMENTS

The authors deeply appreciate the valuable input and reviews of this manuscript provided by Drs. Jonathan Bergmann, Kristen Messenger, and Arlen Wilbers.

REFERENCES

Bode, G., Forster, R., Ellegaard, L., & van der Laan, J.W.; Steering Group of the RETHINK Project. (2010) The RETHINK project–minipigs as models for the toxicity testing of new medicines and chemicals: an impact assessment. *Journal of Pharmacological and Toxicological Methods*, 62(3), 158–159.

Daniel, R.K. & Williams, H.B. (1973) The free transfer of skin flaps by microvascular anastomoses. An experimental study and a reappraisal *Plastic and Reconstructive Surgery*, 52, 16–31.

Duchess Fund database, http://www.portec.com.au/thepig/petpig/duchessfund/index.htm (accessed August 1, 2013)

Egger, C. & Love, L. (2009a) Local and regional anesthesia techniques, Part 1: overview and five simple techniques. *Veterinary Medicine*, Advanstar Communications, http://veterinarymedicine.dvm360.com/vetmed/Anesthesia/Local-and-regional-anesthesia-techniques/ArticleStandard/Article/detail/575560 (accessed July 16, 2013)

Egger, C. & Love, L. (2009b) Local and regional anesthesia techniques, Part 2: stifle, intercostal, intrapleural, and forelimb techniques. *Veterinary Medicine*, Advanstar Communications, http://veterinarymedicine.dvm360.com/vetmed/Medicine/Local-and-regional-anesthesia-techniques-Part-2-St/ArticleStandard/Article/detail/585255 (accessed July 16, 2013)

Egger, C. & Love, L. (2009c) Local and regional anesthesia techniques, Part 3: blocking the maxillary and mandibular nerves. *Veterinary Medicine*, Advanstar Communications, http://veterinarymedicine.dvm360.com/vetmed/Medicine/Local-and-regional-anesthesia-techniques-Part-3-Bl/ArticleStandard/Article/detail/601619 (accessed July 16, 2013)

Egger, C. & Love, L. (2009d) Local and regional anesthesia techniques, Part 4: epidural anesthesia and analgesia. *Veterinary Medicine*, Advanstar Communications, http://veterinarymedicine.dvm360.com/vetmed/Medicine/Local-and-regional-anesthesia-techniques-Part-4-Ep/ArticleStandard/Article/detail/632170 (accessed July 16, 2013)

Escobar, J., Van Alstine, W.G., Baker, D.H., & Johnson, R.W. (2007) Behaviour of pigs with viral and bacterial pneumonia. *Applied Animal Behavior Science*, 105, 42–50.

Gómez de Segura, I.A., Tendillo, F.J., Mascías, A., Santos, M., Castillo-Olivares, J.L., & Steffey, E.P. (1997) Actions of xylazine in young swine. *American Journal of Veterinary Research*, 58(1), 99–102.

Grond, S. & Sablotzki, A. (2004) Clinical pharmacology of tramadol. *Clinical Pharmacokinetics*, 43(13), 879–923.

Harvey-Clark, C.J., Gilespie, K., & Riggs, K.W. (2000) Transdermal fentanyl compared with parenteral buprenorphine in post-surgical pain in swine: a case study. *Laboratory Animals*, 34, 386–398.

Hay, M., Vulin, A., Génin, S., Sales, P., & Prunier, A. (2003) Assessment of pain induced by castration in piglets: behavioral and physiological responses over the subsequent 5 days. *Applied Animal Behavior Science*, 82, 201–218.

Heard, D. J. (1993) Principles and techniques of anesthesia and analgesia for exotic practice. *Veterinary Clinics of North America Small Animal Practice*, 23, 1301–1327.

Junot, S., Troncy, E., Keroack, S., et al. (2008) Renal effect of meloxicam versus ketoprofen in anaesthetized pseudo-normovolaemic piglets. *Canadian Journal of Physiologic Pharmacology*, 86(1–2), 55–63.

Lewis, E., Boyle, L.A., Lynch, P.B., Brophy, P., & O'Doherty, J.V. (2005) The effect of two teeth resection procedures on the welfare of piglets in farrowing crates. Part 1. *Applied Animal Behavior Science*, 90, 233–249.

Malavasi, L.M., Augustsson, H., Jensen-Waern, M., & Nyman, G. (2005) The effect of transdermal delivery of fentanyl on activity in growing pigs. *Acta Veterinaria Scandinavica*, 46, 149–157.

Malavasi, L.M., Nyman, G., Augustsson, H., Jacobson, M., & Jensen-Waern, M. (2006) Effects of epidural morphine and transdermal fentanyl analgesia on physiology and behavior after abdominal surgery in pigs. *Laboratory Animals*, 40, 16–27.

Marx, G., Horn, T., Thielebein, J., Knubel, B. & von Borell, E. (2003) Analysis of pain related vocalizations in young pigs. *Journal of Sound and Vibration*, 266, 687–698.

McGlone, J.J. & Hellman, J.M. (1988) Local and general anesthetic effects on behavior and performance of two- and seven-week-old castrated and uncastrated piglets. *Journal of Animal Science*, 66, 3049–3058.

McGlone, J.J., Nicholson, R.I., Hellman, J.M., & Herzog, D.N. (1993) The development of pain in young pigs associated with castration and attempts to prevent castration-induced behavioral changes. *Journal of Animal Science*, 71, 1441–1446.

Minipig Research Forum (2010) various presentations, Minipigresearchforum.org (accessed August 1, 2013).

Moon, P.F., Scarlett, J.M., Ludders, J.W., Conway, T.A., & Lamb, S.V. (1995) Effect of fentanyl on the minimum alveolar concentration of isoflurane in swine. *Anesthesiology*, 83(3), 535–542.

Mozzachio, K., Linder, K., & Dixon, D. (2004) Uterine smooth muscle tumors in potbellied pigs (Sus scrofa) resemble human fibroids: a potential animal model. *Toxicologic Pathology*, 32(4), 402–407.

Murison, P.J., Jones, A., Mitchard, L., Burt, R., & Birchall, M.A. (2009) Development of perioperative care for pigs undergoing laryngeal transplantation: a case series. *Laboratory Animals*, 43, 338–343.

Noonan, C.J., Rand, J.S., Priest, J., Ainscow, J. & Blackshaw, J.K. (1994) Behavioural observations of piglets undergoing tail docking, teeth clipping and ear notching. *Applied Animal Behavior Science*, 39, 203–213.

Papich, M.G. (2007) *Saunders Handbook of Veterinary Drugs*, 2nd edn, Saunders Elsevier, St. Louis, MO.

Payne, K.A., Roelofse, J.A., & Shipton, E.A. (2002) Pharmacokinetics of oral Tramadol drops for postoperative pain relief in children aged 4–7 years–a pilot study. *Anesthesia Progress*, 49, 109–112.

Reyes, L., Tinworth, K.D., Li, K.M., Yau, D.F., Waters, & K.A. (2002) Observer-blinded comparison of two nonopioid analgesics for postoperative pain in piglets. *Pharmacology, Biochemistry and Behavior*, 73, 521–528.

Riviere, J.E. & Papich, M.G. (2001) Potential and problems of developing transdermal patches for veterinary applications. *Advanced Drug Delivery Reviews*, 50, 175–203.

Rodriguez, N.A., Cooper, D.M., & Risdahl, J.M. (2001) Antinociceptive activity of and clinical experience with buprenorphine in swine. *Contemporary Topics in Laboratory Animal Science*, 40, 17–20.

Rushen, J. & Ladewig, J. (1991) Stress induced hypoalgesia and opioid inhibition of pigs' responses to restraint. *Physiology and Behavior*, 50, 1093–1096.

Smith, A.J. & Swindle, M.M. (2008) Anesthesia and analgesia in swine, in *Anesthesia and Analgesia in Laboratory Animals*, 2nd edn (eds R.E. Fish, M.J. Brown, P.J. Danneman, & A. Karas), Academic Press, Waltham, MA, pp. 424–425.

Swindle, M.M. (1986) Surgery and anesthesia, in *Swine in Biomedical Research* (ed. M.E. Tumbleson), Plenum Press, New York, pp. 233–433.

Taylor, A.A. & Weary, D.M. (2000) Vocal responses of piglets to castration: identifying procedural sources of pain. *Applied Animal Behavior Science*, 70, 17–26.

Taylor, A.A., Weary, D.M., Lessard, M., & Braithwaite, L. (2001) Behavioural responses of piglets to castration: the effect of piglet age. *Applied Animal Behavior Science*, 73, 35–43.

Ugarte, C.E. & O'Flaherty, K.O. (2005) The use of a medetomidine, butorphanol and atropine combination to enable blood sampling in young pigs. *New Zealand Veterinary Journal*, 53(4), 249–252.

Weary, D.M., Braithwaite, L.A., & Fraser, D. (1998) Vocal response to pain in piglets. *Applied Animal Behavior Science*, 56, 161–172.

White, R.G., DeShazer, J.A., Tressler, C.J., et al. (1995) Vocalization and physiological response of pigs during castration with or without a local anesthetic. *Journal of Animal Science*, 73, 381–386.

35

Recognition and Assessment of Pain in Small Exotic Mammals

Lesa Thompson

Exotic species of small mammals are regularly seen in veterinary practice, and their owners expect the same level of care and analgesia as is provided for cats and dogs. Although it is generally accepted that larger mammalian species suffer pain and that analgesia should be provided, veterinarians are hesitant to administer analgesics to small mammals. In a questionnaire of clinicians in the United Kingdom, only 21% gave rabbits and rodents postoperative analgesia compared to 50–70% for dogs and cats (Capner et al., 1999; Lascelles et al., 1999). Postulated reasons for the lack of provision of analgesia included problems in recognizing pain in small mammals and a lack of knowledge regarding suitable analgesics for these species.

All mammalian species have the physiological capability to experience pain. The undesirable effects of pain extend beyond local discomfort for the patient and include adverse systemic changes such as inflammation, sympathetic nervous system activation, negative effects on the cardiovascular system, and suppression of the immune system. These systemic effects may slow the animal's recovery and adversely affect prognosis. Caregivers should assume that the patient is experiencing pain if a condition known to be painful in humans is present or if surgery or trauma has occurred. This chapter aims to familiarize the reader with the subtle signs demonstrated by small exotic mammals experiencing pain.

CHALLENGES IN ASSESSING PAIN IN SMALL MAMMALS

Three major factors contribute to difficulty in detection of pain in these species.

- These animals are very small and may have a tendency to hide, making clinical assessment difficult;
- Caregivers may not be familiar with the normal appearance and behavior of the species in question;
- Many of these species will mask signs of discomfort, and any behavioral changes will be subtle.

The normal behavior of small exotic species may present special difficulties. For example, some rodents can vocalize outside the normal hearing range of humans (Dobromylskyj et al., 2000); thus, abnormal vocalization relating to pain may not even be detectable by the animal's caregivers (Cuomo et al., 1988). Several small mammals, including rats, hamsters, and gerbils, are nocturnal (Dobromylskyj et al., 2000), and their relative inactivity during normal working hours makes monitoring difficult. In addition, an animal's behavior may be altered when an observer is present (Dobromylskyj et al., 2000). For example, rabbits and guinea pigs may become immobile when viewed by a human caregiver. Many small mammal species, including rabbits, guinea pigs, rats, and mice, are social, and normal behavior involves interaction with conspecifics in their enclosure. Social species may react differently to pain when in groups or housed singly and, in some, for example rabbits and rodents, the presence of pain in an individual may alter group dynamics (Kohn et al., 2007). Knowledge of such normal behavior is invaluable when assessing for abnormalities that may indicate pain is present. Because many animals behave differently in novel environments with unfamiliar caregivers, the animal's owner should be questioned regarding abnormal behaviors that the animal is exhibiting in the home environment.

The cause of pain may also affect the clinical signs. Acute, highly intense pain is likely to result in different physiological and behavioral changes compared to low-grade, chronic pain (Kohn et al., 2007). Many indicators have been described for acute pain, but the animal with chronic pain has likely compensated gradually and the behavioral changes may be very subtle. Not unexpectedly, pain tolerance and pain behaviors vary among species, among strains, among individuals, and in the same individual under different circumstances.

Stress, distress, and pain are overlapping sensations and there are no agreed-upon objective measures to reliably detect pain and rate its severity in small mammals (Kohn et al., 2007). Although physiological parameters, such as heart rate and respiratory rate, may increase with pain they can be influenced by variables such as restraint and handling (Harcourt-Brown & Baker, 2001; Miller & Richardson, 2011). Blood pressure and body temperature may also fluctuate with pain and/or stress (Kohn et al., 2007). Monitoring the animal's response after administration of analgesics may be required to confirm the link between pain and the changes noted.

Pain Management in Veterinary Practice, First Edition. Edited by Christine M. Egger, Lydia Love and Tom Doherty.
© 2014 John Wiley & Sons, Inc. Published 2014 by John Wiley & Sons, Inc.

RECOGNITION AND ASSESSMENT OF PAIN IN SMALL MAMMALS

Recognition and assessment of pain requires that several factors, including species, breed, strain, age, gender, individual behaviors, and environment be considered. Because objective data are lacking for many species, recognition of pain in small exotic mammals requires practice (KuKanich, 2011). Many research studies use small exotic mammals as test subjects, and clinicians can learn a lot about pain behaviors and response to analgesics from information gleaned in such situations (Livingston & Chambers, 2000). Frequently, it is the absence of normal behavior that indicates pain; for example, loss of appetite, decreased alertness, mobility, and grooming, and poor body condition (Kohn et al., 2007).

Clinical examination of the animal is a critical part of pain assessment. If the animal has undergone surgery, behavior "before and after" can be compared; it is vital to record baseline behavior prior to a procedure and before giving an analgesic drug. Monitoring at regular intervals will allow the clinician to become familiar with the patient, assess the efficacy of analgesics, and follow trends. The frequency of checks can be tapered as pain subsides and/or analgesics take effect. It is most useful if the same observer performs all pain assessments (Price et al., 1994). If a composite measures score is to be used, a panel of observed behaviors is scored. Each behavior is given a weighted value—often between 1 and 5—and the sum of values creates an overall pain score, with a greater score suggesting a greater degree of pain. Certain criteria may be given greater weight, such as a score of 10 for vocalization on palpation or for self-trauma (Kohn et al., 2007).

The patient should first be observed without being disturbed. Most normal animals are inquisitive and will explore a new environment, whereas animals in pain may not (Flecknell, 1998). Spontaneous activity may be decreased in animals suffering pain (Morton & Griffith, 1985; Dobromylskyj et al., 2000). Lethargy is commonly seen but is not specific for pain. Social animals may also interact less with conspecifics in their group and isolate themselves when in pain.

A full clinical examination should then be performed to help localize a painful region, detect comorbidities, and detect other signs of pain. Animals in pain may be hypersensitive to touch and apprehensive about handling (Kohn et al., 2007). Clinicians should be familiar with examination of normal individuals of the species before attributing clinical signs to pain. For example, normal rabbits become immobile when handled and guinea pigs may vocalize loudly before tensing musculature and becoming immobile (Flecknell, 1998). Vocalizing may indicate the presence of pain in some species, but is more likely with acute or severe pain. The pattern and pitch of vocalization may be different from normal alarm calls (Flecknell, 1998).

Changes in temperament may be seen with pain. The animal may become more aggressive or passive. Aggression is more likely when the patient is approached or handled (Flecknell, 1998). Restlessness may be seen on some occasions (Hawkins, 2006). Animals may seem distanced from their environment, with a silent demeanor and eyes half-closed (Lichtenberger & Ko, 2007). Many small exotic mammals in pain do not respond positively to human presence or contact, particularly restraint. Owners may report a subtle change in response to petting or attention (Lichtenberger & Ko, 2007).

A reduction in appetite is commonly seen in animals in pain, particularly rabbits and rodents (Dobromylskyj et al., 2000). It can be difficult to detect this decreased food intake in animals that are fed *ad libitum*. The simplest method of detecting hyporexia is by daily weight monitoring, but it can also be useful to weigh food to determine intake. Weight loss can be rapid in these small patients, and accurate digital scales should be used to ensure changes are identified. Weighing the animal regularly should also aid in detection of gastrointestinal motility disturbances (which can be particularly severe in rabbits and guinea pigs). Some individuals may have altered feeding behavior with altered mastication, selection of certain foodstuffs, or hyporexia, especially if dental or gastrointestinal discomfort is present (Flecknell, 1998). Similarly, small mammals in pain may have reduced water intake. Water intake should also be monitored by comparing the volumes offered and consumed. Decreased food and water intake could also be due to a reduced willingness to move to the water and food receptacles due to musculoskeletal pain or to oral discomfort; thus, water and food should be placed within easy reach of the animal.

Decreased food and water intake may result in reduced fecal and urine output, although constipation may also be present. Gut motility should be monitored frequently as animals in pain may have decreased motility. This is particularly notable in rabbits. Some analgesics, particularly opioids, can affect intestinal transit time.

Animals may guard body parts that are painful (Hawkins, 2006). The animal may have an abnormal posture during locomotion, such as back arching in rats or a raised tail position in mice (Roughan & Flecknell, 2001b; Miller & Richardson, 2011). The spine may be hunched and/or abdominal musculature tensed to protect the abdomen. Any painful body part may be guarded or, alternatively, animals may bite or scratch the region. Animals in pain may over groom painful sites, potentially resulting in self-mutilation (Vos et al., 1998; Hawkins, 2006), or may groom less (Wright & Woodson, 1990). A decrease in grooming will result in poor, unkempt, and ruffled coat condition or obvious soiling of the coat. Piloerection may be present, and the coat will have a "bristly" or "spikey" appearance.

SPECIES-SPECIFIC SIGNS OF PAIN (TABLE 35.1)

Rabbits

Pain causes stress in rabbits, as in other species, and has several effects on the animal that should be considered. Chronic stress may induce cardiomyopathy, and acute heart failure and death may be caused by massive catecholamine release (Weber & Van der Walt, 1975). The glucocorticoids released with stress may also increase gastric acidity and cause ulceration, affect colonic motility and cecotrophy, reduce renal blood flow and urine output, and suppress the immune system (Kaplan & Smith, 1935; Cheeke, 1987; Lebas et al., 1997; Harcourt-Brown, 2002). Anecdotally, painful rabbits have been reported to go into shock and die despite having nonfatal illness (Barter, 2011). In this species in particular, fear and anxiety may play a role in increased pain perception.

The normal breathing pattern for rabbits is rapid and shallow; however, they may squeal and change to a deep breathing pattern with decreased respiratory rate and pronounced flaring of the nares if in severe pain (Johnston, 2005). It is thought that this response may be due to fear (Brown, 1997; Dobromylskyj et al., 2000). Severe acute pain may also be associated with epiphora and serous nasal discharge (Figure 35.1) (Johnston, 2005).

A normal rabbit is a quiet animal that may appear anxious but inquisitive when in unfamiliar surroundings (Johnston, 2005).

Table 35.1. Behaviors associated with pain in small mammals

Species	Clinical signs of pain	Species	Clinical signs of pain
Rabbits	Squealing	Rats	Pale (in albinos), squinting eyes
	Deep breathing pattern with decreased respiratory rate and flaring of nares		Porphyrin staining around eyes and nares
	Epiphora		Reduced intake of food and water
	Serous nasal discharge		Twitching, horizontal stretching, back arching, abdominal writhing or pressing abdomen, falling or staggering, poor gait
	Hiding		
	Remaining immobile	Mice	Reduced spontaneous activity
	Rapid uncontrolled locomotion during handling		Reduced exploratory behaviors
	Avoidance of raising rump, e.g., to urinate		Isolation from cage mates
	Reduced grooming		Increased aggressiveness when handled
	Anorexia		Reduced grooming
	Reduced water intake (may be polydipsic with dental disease)		Piloerection
			Hunched posture
	Gastrointestinal disturbance—lack of cecotrophy, "pseudo-diarrhea", true diarrhea, reduced fecal output		Pale (in albinos), squinting eyes
			Changes in facial expression
			Reduced intake of food and water
	Dehydration		Twitching, flinching, writhing
	Bruxism	Guinea pigs	Reduced responsiveness
	"Inactive pain behavior"—twitching, wincing, staggering, flinching, pressing abdomen, slow postural adjustments, shuffling		Aggression towards cage mates
			May vocalize less, e.g., silent when handled
			Changes in facial expression
	Altered posture or gait, altered or reduced locomotion		Anorexia
			Reduced grooming
	Licking painful area	Ferrets	Reduced general activity
Rodents in general	Vocalization, sometimes abnormal pitch		Disinterest in exploration of novel environments
	Decrease in normal exploratory behaviors		Remaining curled in a ball
	Increase in sleeping and time spent stationary		Hiding
	Abnormally aggressive when handled		Exhibiting aggression if disturbed
	Immobility, but may try to escape when restrained		Apathy in usually aggressive individuals
	Bruxism		Vocalizations of differing pitch and pattern
	Polyphagia of bedding		Absence of normal posture
	Loss of appetite and thirst		Hunched abdominal posture
	Gastrointestinal disturbance		Altered gait, lameness
	Self-mutilation		Reduced grooming
	Piloerection		Aversion to external palpation
	Lack of grooming		Reduced appetite
	Excessive grooming, licking, biting, or scratching		Bruxism
	Hunched posture		Ipsilateral tongue protrusions with dental pain
	Guarding painful body part		Half-closed eyelids
	Twitching, abdominal contractions, back arching, or belly pressing		Restricted or labored breathing patterns
Rats	Reduced spontaneous activity		Trembling/shivering despite normal body temperature
	Repeated abrupt short movements during resting		Focal muscle fasciculations
	Increased aggressiveness when handled		Rubbing incision site
	Reduced grooming		Bristle or "bottle brush" tail
	Piloerection		

Rabbits in pain tend to hide in a corner, in a box, under bedding, or in a food receptacle (Dobromylskyj et al., 2000). Although they may react when handled, they may remain immobile in the enclosure. Some painful individuals may have periods of rapid uncontrolled locomotion during handling. Normal rabbits raise their rump to urinate and rear up to accept treats or investigate a novel item, and

painful rabbits may avoid these activities (Figure 35.2). Other normal behaviors, such as grooming, may be decreased, resulting in an unkempt coat.

Rabbits normally graze continuously, and anorexia is one of the first signs of pain in this species. Water intake may also be decreased. Changes in appetite, thirst, and body weight are useful,

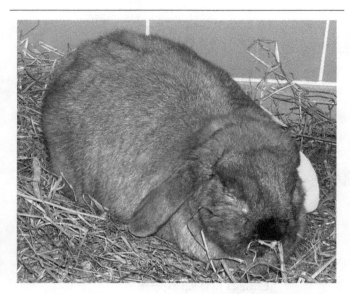

Figure 35.1. Epiphora and a depressed attitude may be associated with pain in rabbits.

though not specific, indicators for pain (Liles & Flecknell, 1992; Shavit et al., 2005; Wheat & Cooper, 2009).

Rabbits perform cecotrophy by consuming soft pellets directly from the anal region, and this is a normal physiological process to enable a "second pass" and digestion/reabsorption of various nutrients from the gastrointestinal tract. Rabbits in pain may not perform this process, particularly if they have vertebral, limb, or abdominal pain restricting movement or oral discomfort making prehension painful. If cecotrophy is not performed, the rabbit may show signs of "pseudo-diarrhea", with the accumulation of cecotrophs at the perianal region.

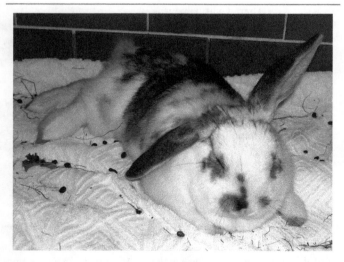

Figure 35.2. Inability to perform normal locomotion or raise the rump during urination may indicate pain in rabbits, such as in this rabbit with a tibial fracture and urine staining of rear legs.

Gastrointestinal dysfunction is common in rabbits in pain, especially if they have a reduced appetite or a low-fiber diet, and could result in reduced fecal output. Reduced gastrointestinal motility and ileus are associated with decreased reabsorption of water and electrolytes from the colon leading to dehydration. Prevention of this potentially fatal condition includes supportive care with prokinetics, assisted feeding, and maintenance of normal hydration.

Bruxism (teeth grinding) may be seen in rabbits with abdominal or dental pain (Dobromylskyj et al., 2000; Johnston, 2005). Although some animals in pain may have reduced thirst, rabbits with dental disease may be polydipsic secondary to anorexia associated with oral pain (O'Malley, 2005).

General behavioral indicators of pain in rabbits are similar to those in many species of small animals. "Inactive pain behavior" is considered the most useful indicator of pain (Leach et al., 2009), and includes such behavior as twitching, wincing, staggering, flinching, pressing of the abdomen, slow postural adjustments, and shuffling. In the study by Leach et al. (2009), movement, rearing, grooming, exploring, and interaction was reduced in painful animals. Rabbits in pain may have altered posture or gait and altered or reduced locomotion, usually to protect painful areas (Flecknell & Morton, 1991). For example, rabbits with acute foot pain exhibited sudden movements, limping, abnormal posture, licking of the area, and vocalization (Farabollini et al., 1988). When the dominant animal was affected, behavior of group members changed.

Rodents

Rodents are often housed in groups and this, combined with their small size, may make detection of behavioral changes difficult. Group-housed animals are less likely to display signs of pain in an attempt to maintain their social status (Kohn et al., 2007). Rats, hamsters, and gerbils are nocturnal and normally inactive during the day; thus, assessment of pain is more difficult because observations are usually conducted during the daytime.

Most pain studies in rodents have been conducted in laboratory animals. Although information obtained from these studies is useful, population differences between laboratory and companion animals should be considered. For example, pet rodents frequently have concurrent disease and are often geriatric.

Rodents in pain have certain similarities to other species, including rabbits (Dobromylskyj et al., 2000). They may vocalize, sometimes at an abnormal pitch, and be abnormally aggressive if handled. They may be immobile, except during restraint when they may try to escape. Some rodents exhibit bruxism with abdominal pain (Hawkins, 2006). Rodents with pain-induced distress may show polyphagia of bedding and self-mutilation (Kohn et al., 2007).

A loss of appetite and thirst in rodents in pain predisposes them to hypoglycemia and dehydration (Miller & Richardson, 2011). Guinea pigs and hamsters are coprophagic and this may cease when the animal is painful (see comments above regarding cecotrophy in rabbits). As in rabbits, the herbivorous species guinea pigs and chinchillas are highly susceptible to gastrointestinal disturbance, including ileus (Longley, 2008).

Rodents in pain may present with an abnormal appearance due to lack of grooming, piloerection, hunched posture, and, in rats, porphyrin staining (Miller & Richardson, 2011). A painful area may be groomed excessively, licked, bitten, or scratched (Figure 35.3). Guarding of a painful body part may alter the animal's body position or posture.

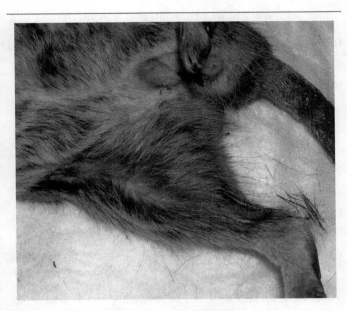

Figure 35.3. Self-mutilation may be seen in painful rodents, such as on the hindlimb of this degu.

Changes in behavior that may be related to pain include a decrease in normal exploratory behaviors such as walking, sniffing, and rearing. Conversely, sleeping and time spent stationary may increase. Specific changes in behavior may help localize the region of pain. For example, twitching, abdominal contractions, back arching, or belly pressing are associated with abdominal discomfort. Painful rodents often vocalize when handled, particularly if a painful region is palpated; however, guinea pigs may vocalize less.

Rats

Signs of pain in rats include reduced grooming, piloerection, reduced spontaneous activity, pale (in albinos) squinting eyes with porphyrin staining, increased aggressiveness when handled, and decreased intake of food and water (Kohn et al., 2007). Reduced grooming or hypersecretion by the Harderian gland with resulting chromodacryorrhea occurs in stressed rats (Hebel & Stromberg, 1986; Harkness & Wagner, 1995). This results in deposition of the red porphyrin pigment periocularly and at the nares. This is not pathognomonic for discomfort, but is seen in rats with reduced grooming due to pain.

After abdominal surgery rats display twitching, stretching, back arching, abdominal writhing, falling or staggering, and poor gait (Roughan & Flecknell, 2001a, 2003). They may press their abdomen to the ground and have repeated abrupt short movements during rest (Dobromylskyj et al., 2000). These behaviors are subtle, and back arching and abdominal pressing require close observation to detect (Roughan & Flecknell, 2001a, 2001b).

Mice

The most common signs of pain in mice are reduced grooming, piloerection, reduced spontaneous activity, hunched posture, pale (in albinos) squinting eyes, isolation from cage mates, increased aggressiveness when handled, and reduced intake of food and water (Karas et al., 2001; Goecke et al., 2005). Significant behavioral changes after abdominal surgery in mice include twitching, flinching, and writhing (Wright-Williams, 2007; Dickinson et al., 2009; Miller & Richardson, 2011). Concurrently, general exploratory behaviors such as walking, rearing, and sniffing are reduced. Laboratory studies have detected changes in facial expression including orbital tightening, nose or cheek bulges, and changes in ear and whisker position after pain has been induced (Langford et al., 2010).

Guinea Pigs

Guinea pigs normally squeal when handled, but tend to be silent when in pain. Studies suggest that guinea pigs may also demonstrate changes in facial expression or aggression to cage mates when experiencing acute pain (Svendsen, 1991). Reduced water and food intake, activity, grooming, and responsiveness may be seen in guinea pigs with chronic pain (Svendsen, 1991).

Ferrets

Ferrets are unique among the small mammals as they are carnivores and predatory. Their normal and pain-induced behaviors are thus much different than those of herbivores. Normal ferrets are mischievous and gregarious even in unfamiliar surroundings (Johnston, 2005). They will actively investigate a novel environment; however, ferrets also spend up to 70% of the day sleeping, interspersed with short periods of activity (Jha et al., 2006; Thurber et al., 2008). As in other species, physiological changes are difficult to assess, and behavioral signs of pain in ferrets are nonspecific and can be very subtle. Caregivers should be vigilant in observing for small changes in behavior. For example, one study demonstrated that ipsilateral tongue protrusions were the most significant behavioral change noted with tooth pain (Chattipakorn et al., 2002).

Signs of pain in common with other small mammals include reduced general activity and exploration of novel environments, altered gait, including lameness and stiff movements, hiding from the observer, reduced grooming with resulting unkempt coat, reduced drinking and appetite, particularly with gastrointestinal or dental pain, and aversion to external palpation (Brown, 1997; Pollock, 2007; Lichtenberger & Ko, 2007; van Oostrom et al., 2011). Bruxism may accompany abdominal pain. One study describing behavioral changes in ferrets after abdominal surgery noted restricted or labored breathing patterns, trembling, and rubbing the incision site (Sladky et al., 2000).

Ferrets in pain prefer to remain curled in a ball (Johnston, 2005). Normally friendly animals may exhibit aggression, such as teeth baring and biting, if disturbed. Conversely, apathy may be seen in individuals that are usually aggressive (van Oostrom et al., 2011). It is normal for interacting ferrets to vocalize, but vocalizations of differing pitch and pattern may be present in painful animals.

Ferrets normally have a hunched back, and the absence of this posture may indicate pain (van Oostrom et al., 2011). Other signs may include shivering, despite normal body temperature, bristle or "bottle brush" tail due to piloerection, half-closed eyelids, focal muscle fasciculations, and general disinterest in their surroundings. Vocalization during handling may be high-pitched or low grunts. As with other small mammals reduced appetite, bruxism, and a hunched abdominal posture may be associated with visceral pain in ferrets.

SUMMARY

Diagnosis of pain can be difficult in small mammals due to lack of clinician familiarity with normal species behavior, small size of the patients and their inclination to hide, and the tendency of prey species to minimize overt signs of pain to avoid predation. Small mammals possess the same anatomy and physiology of pain pathways as larger mammals, so one should expect that procedures or disease painful for a large mammal are also painful for a small exotic mammal. The clinician must be familiar with normal behavior for the species and carefully observe the animal closely for pain. The ability to recognize pain will also enable the clinician to reassess and monitor the patient's response to analgesics and the requirement for further treatment. If in doubt, animal welfare considerations suggest that analgesia should be provided.

REFERENCES

Barter, L.S. (2011) Rabbit analgesia. *Veterinary Clinics of North America: Exotic Animals*, 14, 93–104.

Brown, S.A. (1997) Clinical techniques in domestic ferrets. *Seminars in Avian and Exotic Pet Medicine*, 6, 75–95.

Capner, C.A., Lascelles, B.D., & Waterman-Pearson, A.E. (1999) Current British veterinary attitudes to perioperative analgesia for dogs. *The Veterinary Record*, 145, 95–99.

Chattipakorn, S.C., Sigurdsson, A., Light, A.R., Narhi, M., & Maixner, W. (2002) Trigeminal c-Fos expression and behavioral responses to pulpal inflammation in ferrets. *Pain*, 99, 61–69.

Cheeke, P.R. (1987) Nutrition-disease interrelationships, in *Rabbit Feeding and Nutrition* (ed. P.R. Cheeke), Academic Press, Orlando, FL, pp. 176–197.

Cuomo, V., Cagiano, R., De Salvia, M.A., Maselli, M.A., Renna, G., & Racagni, G. (1988) Ultrasonic vocalization in response to unavoidable aversive stimuli in rats: effects of benzodiazepines. *Life Sciences*, 43(6), 485–491.

Dickinson, A.L., Leach, M.C., & Flecknell, P.A. (2009) The analgesic effects of oral paracetamol in two strains of mice undergoing vasectomy. *Laboratory Animal*, 43(4), 357–361.

Dobromylskyi, P., Flecknell, P.A., Lascelles, B.D., Livingston, A., Taylor, P., & Waterman-Pearson, A. (2000) Pain assessment, in *Pain Management in Animals* (eds P. Flecknell & A. Waterman-Pearson), WB Saunders, London, pp. 53–80.

Farabollini, F., Giordano, G., & Carli, G. (1988) Tonic pain and social behavior in male rabbits. *Behavioral Brain Research*, 31(2), 169–175.

Flecknell, P.A. (1998) Analgesia in small mammals. *Seminars in Avian and Exotic Pet Medicine*, 7(1), 41–47.

Flecknell, P.A. & Morton, D.B. (1991) Use of animals in research. *The Veterinary Record*, 128(22), 531.

Goecke, J.C., Awad, H., Lawson, J.C., & Boivin, G.P. (2005) Evaluating postoperative analgesics in mice using telemetry. *Comparative Medicine*, 55, 37–44.

Harcourt-Brown, F. (2002). The rabbit consultation and clinical techniques, in *Textbook of Rabbit Medicine* (ed. F Harcourt-Brown), Butterworth Heinemann, Oxford, pp. 52–93.

Harcourt-Brown, F. & Baker, S.J. (2001) Parathyroid hormone, haematological and biochemical parameters in relation to dental disease and husbandry in pet rabbits. *Journal of Small Animal Practice*, 42, 130–136.

Harkness, J.E. & Wagner, J.E. (1995) Biology and husbandry – the rat, in *The Biology and Medicine of Rabbits and Rodents*, 4th edn (eds J.E. Harkness & J.E. Wagner), Williams & Wilkins, Baltimore, pp. 65–73.

Hawkins, M.G. (2006) The use of analgesics in birds, reptiles, and small exotic mammals. *Journal of Exotic Pet Medicine*, 15(3), 177–192.

Hebel, R. & Stromberg, M.W. (1986) Sensory organs, in *Anatomy and Embryology of the Laboratory Rat* (eds R. Hebel & M.W. Stromberg), Biomed Verlag, Worthsee, Germany, pp. 218–223.

Jha, S.K., Coleman, T., & Frank, M.G. (2006) Sleep and sleep regulation in the ferret (*Mustela putorius furo*). *Behavioral Brain Research*, 172, 106–113.

Johnston, M.S. (2005) Clinical approaches to analgesia in ferrets and rabbits. *Seminars in Avian and Exotic Pet Medicine: Anesthesia and Analgesia*, 14(4), 299–355.

Kaplan, B.L. & Smith, H.W. (1935) Excretion of inulin, creatinine, xylose and urea in the normal rabbit. *American Journal of Physiology*, 113, 354–360.

Karas, A.Z., Gostyla, K., Aronovitz, M., et al. (2001) Diminished body weight and activity patterns in mice following surgery: implications for control of postprocedural pain/distress in laboratory animals. *Contemporary Topics in Laboratory Animal Science*, 40, 83–87.

Kohn, D.F., Martin, T.E., Foley, P.L., et al. ACLAM (American College of Laboratory Animal Medicine) Task Force Members (2007) Guidelines for the assessment and management of pain in rodents and rabbits. *Journal of the American Association of Laboratory Animal Sciences*, 46(2), 97–108.

KuKanich, B. (2011) Clinical interpretation of pharmacokinetic and pharmacodynamic data in zoologic companion animal species. *Veterinary Clinics of North America: Exotic Animals*, 14, 1–20.

Langford, D.J., Bailey, A.L., Chanda, M.L., et al. (2010) Coding of facial expressions of pain in the laboratory mouse. *Nature Methods*, 7, 447–452.

Lascelles, B.D.X., Capner, C.A., & Waterman-Pearson, A.E. (1999) Current British veterinary attitudes to perioperative analgesia for cats and small mammals. *The Veterinary Record*, 145, 601–604.

Leach, M.C., Allweiler, S., Richardson, C., Roughan, J.V., Narbe, R., & Flecknell, P.A. (2009) Behavioural effects of ovariohysterectomy and oral administration of meloxicam in laboratory housed rabbits. *Research in Veterinary Science*, 87(2), 336–347.

Lebas, F., Coudert, P., de Rochambeau, H., Thébault, R.G. (1997) Nutrition and feeding, in *The Rabbit: Husbandry*, Health and Production No 2, FAO United Nations, Rome, pp. 19–36.

Lichtenberger, M. & Ko, J. (2007) Anesthesia and analgesia for small mammals and birds. *Veterinary Clinics of North America: Exotic Animals*, 10, 293–315.

Liles, J.H. & Flecknell, P.A. (1992) The effects of buprenorphine, nalbuphine and butorphanol alone or following halothane anaesthesia on food and water consumption and locomotor movement in rats. *Laboratory Animal*, 26(3), 180–189.

Livingston, A. & Chambers, P. (2000) The physiology of pain, in *Pain Management in Animals* (eds P. Flecknell & A. Waterman-Pearson), WB Saunders, London, pp. 9–19.

Longley, L.A. (2008) Rodent anaesthesia, in *Anaesthesia of Exotic Pets* (ed. L.A. Longley), Elsevier, Edinburgh, pp. 59–84.

Miller, A.L. & Richardson, C.A. (2011) Rodent analgesia. *Veterinary Clinics of North America: Exotic Animals*, 14, 81–92.

Morton, D.B. & Griffith, P.H.M. (1985) Guidelines on the recognition of pain, distress and discomfort in experimental animals and an hypothesis for assessment. *The Veterinary Record*, 116, 431–436.

O'Malley, B. (2005) Rabbits, in *Clinical Anatomy and Physiology of Exotic Species: Structure and Function of Mammals, Birds, Reptiles, and Amphibians* (ed. B. O'Malley), Elsevier Saunders, Edinburgh, pp. 173–195.

Pollock, C. (2007) Emergency medicine of the ferret. *Veterinary Clinics of North America: Exotic Animals*, 10, 463–500.

Price, D.D., Bush, F.M., Long, S., & Harkins, S.W. (1994). A comparison of pain measurement characteristics of mechanical visual analogue and simple numerical rating scales. *Pain*, 56, 217–226.

Roughan, J.V. & Flecknell, P.A. (2001a) Behavioural effects of laparotomy and analgesic effects of ketoprofen and carprofen in rats. *Pain*, 90, 65–74.

Roughan, J.V. & Flecknell, P.A. (2001b) Effects of surgery and analgesic administration on spontaneous behaviour in singly housed rats. *Research in Veterinary Science*, 69, 283–288.

Roughan, J.V. & Flecknell, P.A. (2003) Evaluation of a short duration behavior-based post-operative pain scoring system in rats. *European Journal of Pain*, 7, 397–406.

Shavit, Y., Fish, G., Wolf, G., et al. (2005) The effects of perioperative pain management techniques on food consumption and body weight after laparotomy in rats. *Anesthesia and Analgesia*, 101(4), 1112–1116.

Sladky, K.K., Horne, W.A., Goodrowe, K.L., Stoskopf, M.K., Loomis, M.R., & Harms, C.A. (2000) Evaluation of epidural morphine for postoperative analgesia in ferrets (*Mustela putorius furo*). *Contemporary Topics in Laboratory Animal Science*, 39, 33–38.

Svendsen, P. (1991) Pain expression in different laboratory animal species. *Scandinavian Journal of Laboratory Animal Science*, 18(4), 135–140.

Thurber, A., Jha, S.K., Coleman, T., & Frank, M.G. (2008) A preliminary study of sleep ontogenesis in the ferret (*Mustela putorius furo*). *Behavioral Brain Research*, 189, 41–51.

van Oostrom, H., Schoemaker, N.J., & Uilenreef, J.J. (2011) Pain management in ferrets. *Veterinary Clinics of North America: Exotic Animals*, 14, 105–116.

Vos, B.P., Hans, G., & Adriaensen, H. (1998) Behavioral assessment of facial pain in rats: face grooming patterns after painful and non-painful sensory disturbances in the territory of the rat's infraorbital nerve. *Pain*, 76(1–2), 173–178.

Weber, H.W. & Van der Walt, J.J. (1975) Cardiomyopathy in crowded rabbits. *Recent Advances in the Study of Cardiac Structure and Metabolism*, 6, 471–477.

Wheat, N.J. & Cooper, D.M. (2009) A simple method for assessing analgesic requirements and efficiency in rodents. *Laboratory Animal*, 38(7), 246–247.

Wright, E.M. Jr. & Woodson, J.F. (1990) Clinical assessment of pain in laboratory animals, in *The Experimental Animal in Biomedical Research* (eds B.E. Rollin & M.L. Kesel), CRC Press, Boca Raton, FL, p. 205.

Wright-Williams, S.L. (2007) Behavior-based assessment of postoperative pain in laboratory mice [PhD Thesis].

36
Treatment of Pain in Small Exotic Mammals

Cheryl B. Greenacre

The education of practitioners and researchers about the importance of recognizing pain and providing analgesia, and the species-specific information that has recently become available to aid in the recognition of pain, have led to increased use of analgesics in small mammals (Coulter et al., 2009, 2011). Pain management can be improved by providing analgesics pre-, intra-, and postoperatively, offering multimodal analgesia, and increasing the use of NSAIDs (Coulter et al., 2009, 2011). Clinical procedures expected to cause minimal to mild pain in small mammals include venous catheter insertion, superficial lymphadenectomy, and vasectomy; mild to moderate pain can be expected with minor laparotomy incisions, orchidectomy, and ovariohysterectomy; and moderate to severe pain is expected to be associated with procedures such as major laparotomy or organ incision, thoracotomy, burns, trauma, and orthopedic surgery (Kohn et al., 2007).

The recognition of pain in small mammals is described in detail in Chapter 35. Recognition of pain is particularly difficult in small mammals due to the fact that most small mammals are prey species and, thus, may hide their pain (Mayer, 2007). An example of an objective pain assessment system for small mammals is a behavior-based pain scoring system in rats that provides an easily learned method for objectively rating postoperative pain (Roughan & Flecknell, 2003, 2004). For a nominal fee, a video is available for instant download to train individuals to recognize pain in rats after abdominal surgery (http://www.digires.co.uk/product/pain-assessment-in-the-rat). Unfortunately, an objective pain assessment tool is not yet available for other small exotic companion mammals, and the practitioner is limited to the observation of certain behaviors (e.g., anorexia or lack of grooming) and/or anthropomorphism (a human would ask for pain relief in a similar situation), which may or may not be useful for pain assessment in small mammals. In fact, anorexia is not part of the rat immediate postoperative pain assessment tool. Once pain is recognized or suspected, it must be treated, and the following information, organized by drug instead of by species, is provided to help the practitioner choose the appropriate pain relief protocol for a given species and situation.

In this chapter, the scientific literature regarding the alleviation of pain in small mammals, including pets and laboratory animals, will be summarized. Much anecdotal information exists in the pet animal literature, and much information that does not translate to use in pet animals is in the laboratory animal literature; thus, a distinction will be made, whenever possible, to include usable scientific information, and identify anecdotal information as such. The term "small mammal" refers to rabbits, ferrets, and rodents (rats, mice, hamsters, gerbils, chinchillas, and guinea pigs). All drugs used in exotic companion mammals are off-label, except sulfaquinoxaline for treating rabbits with coccidiosis, and specific rabies and distemper vaccines for ferrets.

SUPPORTIVE CARE AND HUSBANDRY

Alleviating pain in small mammals is an integral part of patient care. Essential to this end is the treatment of concurrent disease, attention to hydration status, minimization of stress, and provision of other types of supportive care. The treatment of small mammals can be challenging, and the following should be considered when providing supportive care:

- Handling to check weight, temperature, pulse, respiration, GI sounds, and surgical incisions, and to change substrate, should be minimized, and done in a way to reduce stress.
- Animals that are easily stressed, for example, rabbits, may benefit from the use of a low dose of a sedative, such as midazolam.
- The patient should be weighed daily, using a sensitive gram scale, to assess intake of food and water and losses through urine and feces, and to allow accurate dosing.
- The patient should have access to fresh water *ad libitum*. If the patient is painful it may not be able to ambulate; thus, water should be easily accessible from a bowl or a sipper bottle. Rabbits require approximately 100–150 mL/kg of water daily, which is more than most animals (Mader, 2004). A 2 kg rabbit drinks as much water in a day as a 10 kg dog.
- Those species that ferment ingesta in the cecum, such as the rabbit, guinea pig, and chinchilla, should have their gastrointestinal motility monitored and recorded at least twice daily. A baseline should be obtained before noxious stimulation and before the patient is given sedatives or analgesics. A rabbit should have approximately 4 to 8 gut sounds per minute. If motility is not normalized after rehydration and oral syringe feeding of a

Pain Management in Veterinary Practice, First Edition. Edited by Christine M. Egger, Lydia Love and Tom Doherty.
© 2014 John Wiley & Sons, Inc. Published 2014 by John Wiley & Sons, Inc.

specially made critical care formula[1] for rabbits, motility enhancing drugs (prokinetics), such as cisapride or metoclopramide, may be indicated. Gastrointestinal stasis can lead to dysbiosis, diarrhea, and death, due to overgrowth of gram negative and anaerobic bacteria.

- Prey species should be housed in a different room than predator species. Stress and distress can occur in prey species if they smell or hear a predatory species, such as a ferret or a barking dog.
- Ensure that the animals are housed at the appropriate ambient temperature for the species. Most small mammals require 12 hours of light and 12 hours of dark daily.
- The enclosure substrate should provide stable, nonslippery footing, allow urine and feces to drain away from the patient, not cause irritation or allergies, and preferably be a product the animal is accustomed to at home.
- Prey species prefer to have a place to hide, and a simple cardboard box usually suffices for this purpose. Even a predator species, such as a ferret, prefers to hide under a towel.

GUIDELINES FOR TREATMENT OF PAIN IN SMALL MAMMALS

Because of advancements in laboratory animal medicine, some detailed scientific information is available regarding the effects of analgesics in small mammals. Most information is derived from studies in the rat, including pharmacokinetic (PK) and pharmacodynamic (PD) studies, standard pain models (e.g., tail-flick and hot-plate tests), and standardized methods of assessing pain (Roughan & Flecknell, 2003, 2004). One PD study performed in male rats ($n = 62$) and mice ($n = 61$) determined the relative magnitude and duration of analgesia of several opioids using the standard hot-plate test and the tail-flick test (Gades et al., 2000) (Table 36.1).

The recommendations from that study included the use of morphine every 2–3 hours for severe pain, the use of butorphanol every 1–2 hours for mild pain of short duration, and the use of buprenorphine every 6–8 hours in rats and every 3–5 hours in mice for mild to moderate pain of longer duration (Gades et al., 2000). Interestingly, the dose of buprenorphine and butorphanol found to be analgesic in mice was more than double the analgesic dose for rats, underscoring the need to utilize species-specific doses. In addition, the analgesic doses in the study were greater than the doses published in a well-referenced and commonly used companion exotic animal formulary (Ness, 2005).

Species differences exist in the metabolism of various drugs. For example, rabbits rapidly metabolize tramadol into five or more metabolites as compared to dogs and humans that produce only one metabolite, and in which tramadol has a longer duration of action. Strain differences also exist, and there are significant differences among mice strains in their response to morphine (Semenova et al., 1995). Thus, whenever possible, drug doses should be based on PK/PD studies in the specific species. In addition, because most studies are performed on healthy animals, the health status of the patient should always be considered when choosing drug dosages, and it is important to evaluate the response of the individual animal to the drug. Patients should be regularly assessed for pain, degree of sedation, and maintenance of normal GI motility and appetite.

[1.] Critical Care Regular or Fine Grind, Oxbow Hay Company, Nebraska.

ANALGESICS USED IN SMALL MAMMALS

Opioids

A survey of diplomats of the American College of Laboratory Animal Medicine reported that opioids were the most frequently used analgesics in biomedical studies using laboratory animals (Hubbell & Muir, 1996). Opioids (Chapter 4) include pure μ-agonists such as morphine, oxymorphone, hydromorphone, meperidine, and fentanyl; partial agonists such as buprenorphine; and agonist/antagonists such as butorphanol, pentazocine, and nalbuphine. Butorphanol and buprenorphine exhibit a ceiling effect, such that increasing doses do not result in increased analgesia, but may increase the duration of analgesia (Barter, 2011). Tramadol is a weak μ-opioid agonist, but can have significant analgesic efficacy due to its inhibition of norepinephrine and serotonin uptake (Souza & Cox, 2011).

Opioids are efficacious analgesics for mild to severe pain, depending on the class of opioid used, and they can be used as part of a balanced analgesic protocol. Pre-emptive use of opioids is recommended. Conscious rabbits given pre-emptive buprenorphine exhibited fewer signs of visceral pain than those given intra- or postoperative buprenorphine at the same dose, using a colonic distension model (Shafford & Schadt, 2008a).

Opioids can cause significant adverse effects in mammals, including decreased gastrointestinal motility, sedation, and respiratory depression (Barter, 2011). Multiple studies evaluating isolated rabbit and guinea pig intestine have demonstrated that μ- and κ-opioid agonists inhibit motility by activating receptors on enteric neurons and intestinal muscle cells (Shahbazian et al., 2002; Cosola et al., 2006; Barter, 2011). If ileus develops post opioid administration in rabbits it needs to be addressed quickly and intensively with appropriate fluid therapy and oral syringe feeding of a high fiber critical care type formula made for rabbits (Barter, 2011). μ-Agonist opioids can cause moderate to marked sedation in rabbits, especially at high doses or if given to sick rabbits (Barter, 2011). μ-Opioid agonists can cause respiratory depression in small mammals (Barter, 2011). Buprenorphine (approximately 0.02 mg/kg) decreased mean respiratory rate from 252 to 39 and from 306 to 90 breaths per minute when administered IV or SC, respectively, to eight awake, young, healthy rabbits (Shafford & Schadt, 2008b). This study also showed a mean increase in the $PaCO_2$ and alveolar–arterial oxygen gradient, and a mean decrease in PaO_2 (Shafford & Schadt, 2008b). Another study showed significant decreases in respiratory rates and PaO_2 compared to the saline control group and the baseline respiratory rates, in six healthy 1–3-year-old rabbits administered buprenorphine (0.03 mg/kg), butorphanol (0.3 mg/kg), midazolam (2.0 mg/kg), midazolam (2.0 mg/kg) and buprenorphine (0.03 mg/kg), and midazolam (2.0 mg/kg) and butorphanol (0.3 mg/kg), intramuscularly (Schroeder & Smith, 2011). Butorphanol, buprenorphine, or midazolam alone resulted in mild sedation for 30–60 minutes, whereas the combination of midazolam and butorphanol resulted in moderate sedation for 60–90 minutes, and the combination of midazolam and buprenorphine resulted in marked sedation lasting 90–120 minutes (Schroeder & Smith, 2011). Therefore, careful monitoring of respiratory rate and depth is necessary when using opioids in rabbits and guinea pigs, especially those that are ill or have respiratory compromise. Supplemental oxygen may be necessary in some cases.

Table 36.1. Magnitude and duration (hours) of analgesic effect of various opioids given subcutaneously to male rats ($n = 62$) and mice ($n = 61$) using the standard hot-plate test and the tail-flick test for evaluation

Drug	Dose (mg/kg)	Species	Relative magnitude of effect	Duration
Butorphanol	2	Rat	Least	1–2 h
Butorphanol	5	Mouse	Least	1–2 h
Buprenorphine	0.5	Rat	Intermediate	6–8 h
Buprenorphine	2	Mouse	Greatest	2–3 h
Morphine	10	Mouse	Greatest	2–3 h

Source: Gades et al., 2000.

Recommended doses for opioids in small mammals are listed in Table 36.2.

MORPHINE

Morphine is a μ-receptor agonist that provides rapid onset, dose-dependent analgesia and is used to treat moderate to severe pain in mammals, but is rarely used clinically in rabbits due to its adverse effects. Research using a thermal stimulus model showed morphine to be an effective analgesic in rabbits, but its adverse effects included sedation, respiratory depression, and decreased gastrointestinal motility (Barter, 2011). Morphine use in ferrets is associated with nausea, ileus, and vomiting, even at very low doses and, thus, it is not commonly used in ferrets (Van Oostrom et al., 2011

OXYMORPHONE

Oxymorphone is a μ-opioid agonist that is more potent than morphine. Few studies have reported the use of oxymorphone in small mammals, but its use has been described in rabbits (Barter, 2011) and ferrets (Van Oostrom et al., 2011). One study comparing the metabolism and urinary excretion of oxymorphone in humans, rats, guinea pigs, rabbits, and dogs found that oxymorphone was less extensively metabolized in the rabbit compared with other species, and that the rabbit excreted far more free oxymorphone in the urine (31.7% compared to ≤10% in other species) (Cone et al., 1983). Duration of oxymorphone's analgesic action in ferrets is thought to be 6–8 hours (Van Oostrom et al., 2011).

HYDROMORPHONE

Little information is available regarding the clinical use of hydromorphone in small mammals, and doses are generally not listed in most formularies. One study evaluated the pharmacokinetics and bioavailability of hydromorphone administered via various routes in the rabbit, but pharmacodynamic information is not available (Chang et al., 1988). Oral absorption was poor, but the intranasal and transdermal routes (inner ear pinna) have good absorption rates (Chang et al., 1988).

FENTANYL

Fentanyl is a very potent, short-acting, μ-opioid agonist. Fentanyl doses are described for some small mammals (Table 36.2). It is critical to titrate to the lowest dose possible to achieve adequate analgesia, and the patient should be observed closely for respiratory depression and provided with supplemental oxygen if necessary. When using fentanyl at higher doses, particularly if combined with sedatives, be prepared to tracheally intubate and provide positive pressure ventilation (Barter, 2011). Rabbits given an IM combination of medetomidine (0.02 mg/kg), fentanyl (0.02 mg/kg), and midazolam (1.0 mg/kg) experienced transient apnea that necessitated endotracheal intubation (Henke et al., 2005).

Transdermal Fentanyl Patches and Fentanyl Continuous Rate Infusion

Peak plasma fentanyl concentrations of 1.11 ng/mL were obtained at 24 hours in rabbits with transdermal fentanyl patches (25 μg/h) applied immediately after clipping the hair. Rapid hair regrowth in some rabbits slowed absorption and resulted in plasma fentanyl concentrations that were not detectable within 24 hours. Peak fentanyl concentrations of 6.70 ng/mL were reported at 12 hours after using a depilatory cream prior to patch application. This rapid initial increase in plasma concentrations resulted in moderate sedation for 12 hours and decreased respiratory rate for 24 hours; arterial blood gas results were not reported, thus, adequacy of ventilation could not be assessed (Foley et al., 2001), however, using the depilatory cream is not recommended. A recent study reported better postoperative pain management with the use of fentanyl patches (12.5 μg/h) applied to a shaved neck region for 72 hours, as opposed to 24 hours of application, in 16 adult female rabbits undergoing surgery for an aneurism model (Sherif et al., 2011).

Use of a fentanyl CRI in ferrets has been described for intraoperative and postoperative pain relief or in cases of severe, acute trauma (Johnston, 2005; Lichtenberger & Ko, 2007; Van Oostrom et al., 2011). Again, frequent reassessment of pain, analgesia, and adverse effects is mandatory.

BUPRENORPHINE

Buprenorphine is a partial μ-agonist with a slow onset and comparatively long duration of action, and is thought to have fewer adverse effects compared to pure μ-agonists. It is the opioid of choice for mild to moderate pain of prolonged duration (Gades et al., 2000; Roughan & Flecknell, 2002; Kohn et al., 2007).

Buprenorphine can cause pica, especially in rats (Miller & Richardson, 2011). Buprenorphine is commonly used in rabbits due to its efficacy for treating moderate pain, its long duration of action, and presumed lesser incidence of adverse effects compared to morphine, but experimental evidence of its efficacy is lacking (Barter, 2011). A study in rabbits reported decreased respiratory rate, mildly increased arterial CO_2 partial pressures, and mild hypoxemia, after IV administration of about 0.02 mg/kg buprenorphine (Shafford & Schadt, 2008a; Barter, 2011). After IV or SC administration of buprenorphine (about 0.02 mg/kg) the respiratory rate decreased by

Table 36.2.   Opioid doses for various small mammals from references listed below the table. All doses are IM or SC

Species/drug	Dose; frequency
Morphine	
Ferret	[a]0.2–5 mg/kg, q2–6h
Rabbit	1.2–10 mg/kg, 2–5 mg/kg, q3–4h
Guinea pig	2–10 mg/kg, q4h; 2–5 mg/kg, q4h
Gerbil and hamster	2–5 mg/kg, 2–4 h
Rat and mouse	2–5 mg/kg, q2–4h; 2.5 mg/kg, q4h; 10 mg/kg, q2–3h
Oxymorphone	
Ferret	0.05–0.2 mg/kg; 0.05–0.2 mg/kg, q6–8h
Rabbit	0.05–2.0 mg/kg; 0.1–0.3 mg/kg, q3–4h
Guinea pig, chinchilla, gerbil, hamster, rat, mouse	0.2–0.5 mg/kg
Fentanyl	
Ferret	1–4 µg/kg/h continuous rate infusion, 1–3 µg/kg loading dose
Rabbit	7 µg/kg IV
	Transdermal patch 12.5–25 µg/h, q72h
Meperidine	
Ferret	5–10 mg/kg, q2–4h
Rabbit	5–10 mg/kg, q2–3h
Guinea pig, gerbil, hamster, rat, mouse	10–20 mg/kg
Buprenorphine	
Ferret	0.01–0.05 mg/kg, q8–12h; 0.004–0.05 mg/kg, q6–12h; 0.02–0.03 mg/kg, q4–6h
Rabbit	0.01–0.05 mg/kg, q8–12h; 0.02–0.1 mg/kg, q6h
Guinea pig	0.01–0.03 mg/kg[b], 0.05–0.1 mg/kg, q8–12h; 0.05 mg/kg, q8–12h; 0.03–0.05 mg/kg[b]
Chinchilla	0.05–0.1 mg/kg, q8–12h; 0.01–0.05 mg/kg, q6–12h
Gerbil	0.01–0.2 mg/kg, q8h; 0.01–0.05 mg/kg[b]
Hamster	0.01–0.5 mg/kg; 0.01–0.05 mg/kg[b]
Rat	0.02–0.5 mg/kg, q6–12h; 0.5 mg/kg, q6–8h; 0.01–0.05 mg/kg, q8–12h;
Mouse	0.02–0.05 mg/kg[b]; 0.1–0.25 mg/kg PO, q8–12h
	0.05–2.5 mg/kg, q6–12h; 0.05–0.1 mg/kg, q12h
Butorphanol	
Ferret	0.05–0.4 mg/kg; 0.1–0.5 mg/kg, q2–12h; 0.2–0.3 mg/kg, q2–4h[b]
Rabbit	0.1–1 mg/kg; 0.1–0.5 mg/kg, q12h; 0.2 mg/kg, q2–4h[b]
Guinea pig	0.2–2 mg/kg; 1–2 mg/kg, q4h; 0.2–0.3 mg/kg, q2–4h[b]
Chinchilla	0.2–2 mg/kg; 0.2–2 mg/kg, q24h; 0.2–0.3 mg/kg, q2–4h[b]
Gerbil and hamster	0.2–0.5 mg/kg; 0.2 mg/kg, q2–4h[b]
Rat and mouse	0.2–2 mg/kg; 1–2 mg/kg, q4h; 2 mg/kg, q1–2h; 0.5–1 mg/kg, q2–4h[b]
Pentazocine	
Ferret	5–10 mg/kg, IM, q4h
Rabbit	5–10 mg/kg, IM, q2–4h
Guinea pig, gerbil, hamster, rat, mouse	10 mg/kg, SC, q2–4h
Tramadol	
Ferret	10 mg/kg, PO, q24h
Rabbit	[c]10 mg/kg, PO, q12–24h
Mouse and rat	5 mg/kg, SC

Sources: Gades et al., 2000; Gamble and Morrisey, 2005; Hernandez-Divers, 2005; Ness, 2005; Kohn et al., 2007; Barter, 2011; Miller and Richardson, 2011; Van Oostrom et al., 2011. IM = intramuscular; IV = intravenous; PO = per os; SC = subcutaneous.

[a]Vomiting reported at 0.1 mg/kg.

[b]Author's usual starting dose.

[c]Author does not use tramadol alone in rabbits as PK studies indicate that therapeutic concentrations are not reached at doses as high as 11 mg/kg PO.

85% and 71%, respectively, at all time points (10 and 22 minutes for IV, and 30, 60, and 90 minutes for SC) (Shafford & Schadt, 2008b). The $PaCO_2$ was significantly greater than baseline at 30, 60, and 90 minutes after SC administration (Shafford & Schadt, 2008b). Anecdotally, the duration of effect of buprenorphine in rabbits is thought to be about 6 hours. Although some studies suggest that measurable plasma concentrations are present for up to 12 hours (Barter, 2011), the analgesic plasma concentration in rabbits is unknown. Unlike morphine, buprenorphine alone does not cause overt sedation in healthy rabbits, but buprenorphine (0.03 mg/kg) in combination with midazolam (2.0 mg/kg) caused marked sedation lasting 90–120 minutes (Barter, 2011; Schroeder & Smith, 2011). In healthy awake rabbits, pre-emptive buprenorphine (0.06 mg/kg IV) attenuated the increase in arterial blood pressure due to acute colorectal distention (Shafford & Schadt, 2008a).

The use of buprenorphine in ferrets is commonly reported. It is described as having a long duration of action and may have profound sedative effects at the higher doses (Van Oostrom et al., 2011).

Butorphanol

Butorphanol is a mixed agonist/antagonist opioid with antagonist activity at the μ-receptor, but strong agonist activity at the κ-receptor, through which it provides analgesia. In rats and mice, butorphanol is used for mild pain of short duration and dosed every 1–2 hours (Gades et al., 2000). In rabbits, butorphanol is recommended for mild to moderate pain of short duration (2–3 hours) (Barter, 2011). In ferrets, butorphanol use is commonly described and, anecdotally, the duration of action is short compared with buprenorphine (Van Oostrom et al., 2011).

Pentazocine, Meperidine, and Nalbuphine

Anecdotal pentazocine and meperidine doses (Table 36.2) are described in the literature, but there are no experimental studies describing their effects in small mammals. Nalbuphine is a κ-opioid agonist that is rarely used clinically in small mammals. A study in rabbits, utilizing the paw pressure test as a pain model, reported the median analgesic dose to be 8.4 mg/kg of nalbuphine (Hu et al., 1996). Another study reported that the elimination half-life of nalbuphine (10 mg/kg IV bolus) in rabbits increased significantly with age (Ho et al., 1995). In a study evaluating eight different strains of inbred rats, no analgesic effect was observed with nalbuphine at 1 mg/kg IV (Avsaroglu et al., 2007).

Tramadol

Tramadol is a weak μ-opioid agonist that also provides analgesia by inhibiting the uptake of norepinephrine and serotonin in the central nervous system. An advantage of tramadol is a reduced adverse effect profile compared to μ-agonist opioids. Most animals, including humans and dogs, produce one active metabolite, designated M1 or O-tramadol, adding to its analgesic efficacy. A few studies have been conducted in small mammals. In rabbits, a pharmacokinetic study reported that after oral administration of tramadol (11 mg/kg), the measured plasma concentration of M1 rapidly decreased to a concentration considered nontherapeutic in humans (Souza et al., 2008; Souza & Cox, 2011). In addition, in an isoflurane MAC study, IV tramadol (4.4 mg/kg) caused a significant, but clinically unimportant, reduction of isoflurane MAC in rabbits (Egger et al., 2009). Based on the pharmacokinetic and

MAC studies, the authors believe that tramadol should not be used alone in rabbits for pain relief, despite anecdotal reports to the contrary (Souza & Cox, 2011). Although doses of tramadol for ferrets are published, they are not based on scientific data in ferrets (Van Oostrom et al., 2011) and further study is needed. A study in rats given varying doses (1 to 25 mg/kg) of intraperitoneal tramadol reported delayed responses to thermal or ischemic noxious stimuli, suggesting analgesia, but the higher doses caused decreased motor function (Loram et al., 2007). A study compared the analgesic effects of tramadol, tramadol and gabapentin, or buprenorphine in rats, and reported that tramadol alone provided insufficient analgesia, and that buprenorphine, and to a lesser extent tramadol with gabapentin, provided relief of thermal hyperalgesia and normalized weight bearing, but was not efficacious against mechanically induced hyperalgesia (McKeon et al., 2011).

Anti-inflammatory Medications

Nonsteroidal anti-inflammatory drugs (NSAIDs) (Table 36.3) act centrally and peripherally to produce analgesia. Commonly used NSAIDs include meloxicam, ketoprofen, carprofen, and flunixin meglumine. The NSAIDs are useful for mild to moderate inflammatory pain and can be used as part of a multimodal analgesic protocol. Use of NSAIDS with an opioid may better address analgesia by acting at different parts of the pain pathway, and reduce adverse effects by allowing reduction of the dose of each drug (Kohn et al., 2007). Reported adverse effects of NSAIDs include gastric irritation or ulceration and renal dysfunction. Because of the protective effect of prostaglandins on renal perfusion in the face of hypovolemia and/or hypotension, the author recommends that NSAIDs be given as the animal is recovering from anesthesia. If blood pressure is monitored and hypotension treated, NSAIDs can be given pre-emptively. When prescribing any NSAID for long-term use, BUN and creatinine should be monitored, especially in geriatric animals. Chronic progressive nephropathy (CPN) is the most important kidney disease in aged rats, and is the most common cause of death in many strains of rats, especially Sprague-Dawley and F344 strains (Hrapkiewicz & Medina, 2007). Rats, especially male rats, can experience chronic progressive nephropathy starting at 6 months of age, with clinically significant loss of renal function by age 1.5 years; thus, NSAIDs should be used cautiously and only with close monitoring in rats.

Meloxicam

Meloxicam is one of the most commonly used NSAIDs in small mammals. A study of meloxicam in New Zealand white rabbits reported no clinically observable adverse effects and no significant changes in serum biochemistry after 5 days of oral administration at 1.5 mg/kg (Turner et al., 2006).

Meloxicam alone was not adequate to control pain after an ovariohysterectomy in rabbits, and coadministration of an opioid was required (Leach et al., 2009). In the author's practice, rabbits are usually given buprenorphine preoperatively followed by meloxicam after isoflurane is discontinued. Buprenorphine is usually administered every 4 hours pending reassessment of the patient's pain, appetite, and GI motility.

Miscellaneous NSAIDS

Many other NSAIDs are available for use in veterinary species and suggested doses are listed in Table 36.3. Although ibuprofen

Table 36.3. Nonsteroidal anti-inflammatory drug doses for various small mammals

Species/drug	Dose; frequency[a]
Meloxicam	
Ferret	0.1–0.2 mg/kg SC/PO, q24h; 0.2 mg/kg SC or 0.3 mg/kg PO, q24h[b]
Rabbit	0.2 mg/kg SC, q24h or 0.1–0.3 mg/kg PO, q24h
Guinea pig	0.3–0.5 mg/kg SC, q24h or 0.5–1.5 mg/kg PO, q24h
Gerbil	0.1–0.3 mg/kg SC, q24h; 0.2–0.3 mg/kg SC/PO, q24h
Hamster	0.1–0.3 mg/kg SC/PO, q24h; 0.2–0.3 mg/kg SC/PO[b]; 0.3 mg/kg PO, q24h
Rat	0.2–0.3 mg/kg SC/PO[b]
Mouse	1–2 mg/kg SC/PO; 1.0 mg/kg SC/PO, q12–24h; 0.5–1.0 mg/kg SC/PO[b]
	5 mg/kg SC/PO, q24h; 0.2–0.3 mg/kg SC/PO[b]
Carprofen	
Ferret	1 mg/kg PO, q12–24h; 1–4 mg/kg SC/PO, q24h; 4 mg/kg PO, q24h[b]
Rabbit	2–4 mg/kg SC, q24h or 1–2.2 mg/kg PO, q12h; 4 mg/kg SC, q24h or 2–4 mg/kg PO, q12–24h; 2 mg/kg PO, q24h[b]
Guinea pig	1–4 mg/kg SC, q12–24h; 4 mg/kg SC, q12–24h[b]
Chinchilla	4 mg/kg SC, q24h; 1–2 mg/kg SC, q24h[b,c];
Rat	1.5–10 mg/kg PO, q12h or 5 mg/kg SC, q24h; 5 mg/kg SC; or 1–5 mg/kg PO, q12–24h; 2.0 mg/kg SC[b]
Mice	5 mg/kg SC, q12–24h
Ketoprofen	
Ferret	1 mg/kg SC/PO, q24h; 1–5 mg/kg SC/PO, q24h
Rabbit	1–3 mg/kg SC, q24h; 1 mg/kg SC, q24h[b]
Guinea pig	1 mg/kg SC, q12–24h[b]
Chinchilla	1 mg/kg SC, q12–24h[b]
Gerbil, hamster	5 mg/kg SC/PO, q24h
Rat, mouse	5 mg/kg SC/PO, q24h
Flunixin meglumine	
Ferret	0.3–2 mg/kg SC, q12–24h; 0.3–2 mg/kg SC/PO, q12–24h
Rabbit	0.3–2 mg/kg SC, q12–24h; 1 mg/kg SC, q24h[b]
Guinea Pig	1–5 mg/kg SC, q12–24h; 2.5 mg/kg; 1 mg/kg SC, q24h[b]
Chinchilla	1–3 mg/kg SC, q12–24h; 1 mg/kg SC, q24h[b]
Rat	1.1–2.5 mg/kg SC, q12–24h; 2.5 mg/kg; 1 mg/kg SC; q24h[b]
Mouse	2.5 mg/kg SC, q12–24h

Sources: Gades et al., 2000; Gamble and Morrisey, 2005; Hernandez-Divers, 2005; Ness, 2005; Barter, 2011; Miller and Richardson, 2011; Van Oostrom et al., 2011. PO = per os; SC = subcutaneous.

[a]Author uses lower doses in older, especially male, rats due to high incidence of chronic progressive nephropathy.

[b]Author's usual starting dose.

[c]Anecdotally, the author has seen anorexia with higher doses.

doses are available for rats and guinea pigs, the author does not recommend using ibuprofen in small mammals. Death from acute ibuprofen toxicosis has been described in a ferret that presented for vomiting and depression after ingesting an unknown amount of ibuprofen (Cathers et al., 2000). Although there are published doses of acetaminophen for rodents and rabbits, and aspirin for rabbits and ferrets, the author has seen several cases of toxicity from administration by well-meaning owners, and therefore recommends careful dosing. Available doses are anecdotal and not based on specific experimental study. A study in rats using a hind paw incisional model reported that buprenorphine (0.025, 0.05, and 0.1 mg/kg SC), fentanyl (0.01 and 0.1 mg/kg IP), and flunixin meglumine (1.1 and 2.5 mg/kg SC) significantly decreased mechanical sensitivity, but acetaminophen (100 and 300 mg/kg PO) did not (St A Stewart & Martin, 2003).

Local Anesthetics

Local anesthetics can be administered topically, locally or regionally around specific nerves, epidurally, or spinally. They can be combined with opioids (e.g., morphine 0.1 mg/kg) to increase efficacy and prolong duration of analgesia. All of the local and regional nerve blocks described for cats and dogs can be performed in small mammals. An advantage of using local or regional analgesia is that there are fewer systemic effects, such as decreased gut motility. Local anesthetics do, however, have a narrow therapeutic index, and because of the size of most small mammals, careful, accurate weighing and dosage calculations are critical. The author recommends a dose of 2 mg/kg of lidocaine or 1 mg/kg of bupivacaine in small mammals. It is recommended that local anesthetics be diluted 1:2 to 1:4 prior to administration to avoid overdosage with concentrated solutions.

The literature has many descriptions of how to place epidural catheters in laboratory animals including guinea pigs, rabbits, and ferrets. A study in pregnant guinea pigs described placing a 27 gauge epidural catheter in the L3–4 intervertebral space and administering bupivacaine. Histopathological examination showed most catheters were properly placed, but some were inadvertently placed in the intrathecal space resulting in severe CNS depression from intrathecal injection of drug, and some catheters had penetrated the spinal cord (Eisele et al., 1994). A study of epidural morphine (0.1 mg/kg) for ovariohysterectomy in ferrets demonstrated attenuation of pain when compared with a saline control (Sladky et al., 2000; Eshar & Wilson, 2010). Epidural use of morphine (0.1 mg/kg) has been described in rabbits (Barter, 2011). Lidocaine at 0.2 mL/kg (2% solution) epidurally provided a rapid onset (1–3 minutes) and a significant duration (30–40 minutes) of analgesia in rabbits (Doherty et al., 1995; Barter, 2011). Epidural bupivacaine has not been well studied in rabbits (Barter, 2011).

New methods of providing analgesia with local anesthetics are currently being studied. A recent study reported better pain relief in ferrets undergoing acute, experimentally induced hernia repair when bupivacaine-impregnated small intestinal submucosa was incorporated into the surgical site as compared to hernia repair with nonimpregnated small intestinal submucosa (Johnson et al., 2011). Bupivacaine-impregnated foam infiltrated into acute hernia incisions in rabbits produced no adverse effects (Richard et al., 2011).

CHRONIC PAIN

Chronic pain is difficult to alleviate. Long-term use of opioids in any animal that ferments ingesta in the cecum (rabbit, guinea pig, chinchilla) may induce ileus. Long-term use of NSAIDs is also problematic due to gastric and renal adverse effects, although use of gastric protectants and an explanation of the risks, adverse effects, and clinical signs of adverse effects to owners can make longer-term use possible. Other modalities such as acupuncture or acupressure have also been used. Much research into neuropathic pain in laboratory animal models exists, and may form the basis for extrapolation to control of chronic pain states in clinical settings. One study compared the activity of various anticonvulsants (oxycarbazepine, carbamazepine, lamotrigine, and gabapentin) in a model of neuropathic pain induced by partial sciatic nerve ligation in rats and guinea pigs (Fox et al., 2003). A single oral dose of gabapentin (100 mg/kg) in rats and guinea pigs was minimally efficacious against mechanical hyperalgesia, but repeated doses produced 70% and 90% increases in response thresholds in rats and guinea pigs, respectively (Fox et al., 2003). A single dose of gabapentin provided significant dose-related reversal of tactile allodynia in the rat (Fox et al., 2003). Oxycarbazepine and carbamazepine had no effect in this model in rats, but was efficacious in guinea pigs. Lamotrigine produced only slight inhibition of tactile allodynia in the rat (100 mg/kg), and none in the guinea pig (Fox et al., 2003). This study highlights profound species differences that need to be taken into consideration prior to administering analgesics to small mammals.

SUMMARY

More species-specific analgesia studies, better pain models, and better methods of assessing pain are needed for clinicians to provide species appropriate drugs, doses, and dosing intervals. Given the information currently available, the best approach is to individualize treatment and continually reassess the patient.

REFERENCES

Avsaroglu, H., van der Sar, A.S., van Lith, H.A., van Zutphen, L.F., & Hellebrekers, L.J. (2007) Differences in response to anaesthetics and analgesics between inbred rat strains. *Laboratory Animal*, 41(3), 337–344.

Barter, L.S. (2011) Rabbit analgesia, in *Analgesia and Pain Management, Veterinary Clinics of North America: Exotic Animal Practice*, vol. 14 (ed. J. Paul-Murphy), W.B. Saunders, pp. 93–104.

Cathers, T.E., Isaza, R., & Oehme, F. (2000) Acute ibuprofen toxicosis in a ferret. *Journal of the American Veterinary Medical Association*, 216(9), 1426–1428, 1412.

Chang, S.F., Moore, L., & Chien, Y.W. (1988) Pharmacokinetics and bioavailability of hydromorphone: effect of various routes of administration. *Pharmaceutical Research*, 5(11), 718–721.

Cone, E.J., Darwin, W.D., Buchwald, W.F., & Gorodetzky, C.W. (1983) Oxymorphone metabolism and urinary excretion in human, rat, guinea pig, rabbit, and dog. *Drug Metabolism and Disposition*, 11(5), 446–450.

Cosola, C., Albrizio, M., Guaricci, A.C., et al. (2006) Opioid agonist/antagonist effect of naloxone in modulating rabbit jejunum contractility in vitro. *Journal of Physiology and Pharmacology*, 57(3), 439–449.

Coulter, C.A., Flecknell, P.A., & Richardson, C.A. (2009) Reported analgesic administration to rabbits, pigs, sheep, dogs and non-human primates undergoing experimental surgical procedures. *Laboratory Animal*, 43(3), 232–238.

Coulter, C.A., Flecknell, P.A., Leach, M.C., & Richardson, C.A. (2011) Reported analgesia administration to rabbits undergoing experimental surgical procedures. *British Medical College Veterinary Research*, 7, 12.

Doherty, M.M., Hughes, P.J., & Korzniak, N.V. (1995) Prolongation of lidocaine induced epidural anesthesia by medium molecular weight hyaluronic acid formulation: pharmacodynamic and pharmacokinetic studies in the rabbit. *Anesthesia and Analgesia*, 80(4), 740–746.

Egger, C.M., Souza, M.J., Greenacre, C.B., Cox, S.K., & Rohrbach, B.W. (2009) Effect of intravenous administration of tramadol hydrochloride on the minimum alveolar concentration of isoflurane in rabbits. *American Journal of Veterinary Research*, 70, 945–949.

Eisele, P.H., Kaaekuahiwi, M.A., Canfield, D.R., Golub, M.S., & Eisele, Jr., J.H. (1994) Epidural catheter placement for testing of obstetrical analgesics in female guinea pigs. *Laboratory Animal Science*, 44(5), 486–490.

Eshar, D. & Wilson, J. (2010) Epidural anesthesia and analgesia in ferrets. *Laboratory Animal*, 39(11), 339–340.

Foley, P.L., Henderson, A.L., Bissonette, E.A., Wimer, G.R., Feldman, S.H., et al. (2001) Evaluation of fentanyl transdermal patches in rabbits: blood concentrations and physiological response. *Comparative Medicine*, 51(3), 239–244.

Fox, A., Gentry, C., Patel, S., Kesingland, A., & Bevan, S. (2003) Comparative activity of the anticonvulsants oxycarbazepine, carbamazepine, lamotrigine and gabapentin in a model of neuropathic pain in the rat and guinea pig. *Pain*, 105(1–2), 355–362.

Gades, N.M., Danneman, P.J., Wixson, S.K., & Tolley, E.A. (2000) The magnitude and duration of the analgesic effect of morphine, butorphanol, and buprenorphine in rats and mice. *Contemporary Topics in Laboratory Animal Science*, 39(2), 8–13.

Gamble, C. & Morrisey, J.K. (2005) Ferrets, in *Exotic Animal Formulary*, 3rd edn (ed. J.W. Carpenter), Elsevier, St. Louis, MO, pp. 447–478.

Henke, J., Astner, S., Brill, T., Eissner, B., Busch, R., & Erhardt, W. (2005) Comparative study of three intramuscular anesthetic combinations (medetomidine/ketamine, medetomidine/fentanyl/midazolam and xylazine/ketamine in rabbits. *Veterinary Anesthesia and Analgesia*, 32(5), 261–270.

Hernandez-Divers, S.J. (2005) Rabbits, in *Exotic Animal Formulary*, 3rd edn (ed. J.W. Carpenter), Elsevier, St. Louis, MO, pp. 410–446.

Ho, S.T., Wang, J.J., Hu, O.Y., & Hu, T.M. (1995) The effect of aging on the pharmacokinetics of nalbuphine in rabbits. *Biopharmaceutical Drug Disposition*, 16(8), 695–703.

Hrapkiewicz, K. & Medina, L. (eds) (2007) *Clinical Laboratory Medicine—An Introduction*, 3rd edn, Blackwell Publishing, Ames, IA.

Hu, O.Y., Ho, S.T., Wang, J.J., & Lee, S.C. (1996) Paw pressure test in the rabbit: a new animal model for the study of pain. *Acta Anaesthesiology Sinica*, 34(1), 1–8.

Hubbell, J.A. & Muir, W.W. (1996) Evaluation of a survey of the diplomates of the American College of Laboratory Animal Medicine on use of analgesic agents in animals used in biomedical research. *Journal of the American Veterinary Medical Association*, 209(5), 918–921.

Johnson, B.M., Ko, J.C., Hall, P.J., Saunders, A.T., & Lantz, G.C. (2011) Analgesic effect of bupivacaine eluting porcine small intestinal submucosal (SIS) in ferrets undergoing acute abdominal hernia defect surgery. *Journal of Surgical Research*, 167(2), e403–e412.

Johnston, M.S. (2005) Clinical approaches to analgesia in ferrets and rabbits. *Seminars in Avian and Exotic Pet Medicine*, 14, 229–235.

Kohn, D.F., Martin, T.E., Foley, P.L., et al. (2007) Guidelines for the assessment and management of pain in rodents and rabbits. *Journal of the American Association of Laboratory Animal Science*, 46(2), 97–108.

Leach, M.C., Allweiler, S., Richardson, C., Roughan, J.V., Narbe, R., & Flecknell, P.A. (2009) Behavioural effects of ovariohysterectomy and oral administration of meloxicam in laboratory housed rabbits. *Research Veterinary Science*, 87(2), 336–347.

Lichtenberger, M. & Ko, J. (2007) Anesthesia and analgesia for small mammals and birds. *Veterinary Clinics of North America: Exotic Animal Practice*, 10, 293–315.

Loram, L.C., Mitchell, D., Skosana, M., & Fick, L.G. (2007) Tramadol is more effective than morphine and amitriptyline against ischaemic pain but not thermal pain in rats. *Pharmacological Research*, 56(1), 80–85.

Mader, D.R. (2004) Rabbits—basic approach to veterinary care, in *Ferrets, Rabbits, and Rodent—Clinical Medicine and Surgery*, 2nd edn (eds K.E. Quesenberry & J.W. Carpenter), Saunders, St. Louis, MO, pp. 147–154. basic approach to veterinary care Ferrets, Rabbits, and Rodent—Clinical Medicine and Surgery

Mayer, J. (2007) Use of behavior analysis to recognize pain in small mammals. *Laboratory Animal*, 36(6), 43–48.

McKeon, G.P., Pacharinsak, C., Long, C.T., et al. (2011) Analgesia effects of tramadol, tramadol-gabapentin, and buprenorphine in an incisional model of pain in rats (*Rattus norvegicus*). *Journal of American Association of Laboratory Animal Scientists*, 50(2), 192–197.

Miller, A.L. & Richardson, C.A. (2011) Rodent analgesia, in *Analgesia and Pain Management, Veterinary Clinics of North America: Exotic Animal Practice*, vol. 14 (ed. J. Paul-Murphy), W.B. Saunders, pp. 81–92.

Ness, R.D. (2005) Rodents, in *Exotic Animal Formulary*, 3rd edn (ed. J.W. Carpenter), Elsevier, St. Louis, MO, pp. 377–410.

Richard, B.M., Ott, L.R., Haan, D., et al. (2011) The safety and tolerability evaluation of DepoFoam bupivacaine (bupivacaine extended-release liposome injection) administered by incision wound infiltration in rabbits and dogs. *Expert Opinion in Investigational Drugs*, 20(10), 1327–1341.

Roughan, J.V. & Flecknell, P.A. (2002) Buprenorphine: a reappraisal of its antinociceptive effects and therapeutic use in alleviating postoperative pain in animals. *Laboratory Animal*, 36(3), 322–343.

Roughan, J.V. & Flecknell, P.A. (2003) Evaluation of a short duration behavior-based post-operative pain scoring system in rats. *European Journal Pain*, 7, 397–406.

Roughan, J.V. & Flecknell, P.A. (2004) Behaviour-based assessment of the duration of laparotomy-induced abdominal pain and the analgesic effects of carprofen and buprenorphine in rats. *Behavioral Pharmacology*, 15, 461–472.

Schroeder, C.A. & Smith, L.J. (2011) Respiratory rates and arterial blood-gas tensions in healthy rabbits given buprenorphine, butorphanol, midazolam, or their combinations. *Journal of the American Association for Laboratory Animal Science*, 50(2), 205–211.

Semenova, S., Kuzmin, A., & Zvartau, E. (1995) Strain differences in the analgesic and reinforcing action of morphine in mice. *Pharmacology Biochemical Behavior*, 50, 17–21.

Shafford, H.L. & Schadt, J.C. (2008a) Effect of buprenorphine on the cardiovascular and respiratory response to visceral pain in conscious rabbits. *Veterinary Anesthesia and Analgesia*, 35(4), 333–340.

Shafford, H.L. & Schadt, J.C. (2008b) Respiratory and cardiovascular effects of buprenorphine in conscious rabbits. *Veterinary Anesthesia and Analgesia*, 35(4), 326–332.

Shahbazian, A., Heinemann, A., Schmidhammer, H., Beubler, E., Holzer-Petsche, U., & Holzer, P. (2002) Involvement of mu- and kappa-, but not delta-, opioid receptors in the peristaltic motor depression caused by endogenous and exogenous opioids in the guinea pig intestine. *British Journal of Pharmacology*, 135(3), 741–750.

Sherif, C., Marbacjer, S., Erhardt, S., & Fandino, J. (2011) Improved microsurgical creation of venous pouch arterial bifurcation aneurisms in rabbits. *American Journal of Neuroradiology*, 32(1), 165–169.

Sladky, K.K., Horne, W.A., Goodrowe, K.L., Stoskopf, M.K., Loomis, M.R., & Harms, C.A. (2000) Evaluation of epidural morphine for postoperative analgesia in ferrets (*Mustela putorius furo*). *Contemporary Topics in Laboratory Animal Science*, 39(6), 33–38.

Souza, M.J. & Cox, S.K. (2011) Tramadol use in zoologic medicine, in *Analgesia and Pain Management, Veterinary Clinics of North America: Exotic Animal Practice*, vol. 14 (ed. J. Paul-Murphy), W.B. Saunders, pp. 117–130.

Souza, M.J., Greenacre, C.B., & Cox, S.K. (2008) Pharmacokinetics of orally administered tramadol in domestic rabbits (*Oryctolagus cuniculus*). *American Journal of Veterinary Research*, 69(8), 979–982.

St A Stewart, L. & Martin, W.J. (2003) Evaluation of postoperative analgesia in a rat model of incisional pain. *Contemporary topics in Laboratory Animal Medicine*, 42(1), 28–34.

Turner, P.V., Chen, H.C., & Taylor, W.M. (2006) Pharmacokinetics of meloxicam in rabbits after single and repeated oral dosing. *Comparative Medicine*, 56(1), 63–67.

Van Oostrom, H., Schoemaker, N.J., & Uilenreef, J.J. (2011) Pain management in ferrets, in *Analgesia and Pain Management, Veterinary Clinics of North America: Exotic Animal Practice*, vol. 14, issue 1, (ed. J. Paul-Murphy), W.B. Saunders, pp. 105–116.

37
Recognition and Treatment of Pain in Birds

Karen L. Machin

Birds (class Aves) are a highly diverse group with almost 10,000 species inhabiting ecosystems from the Arctic to Antarctica. With such a range in behavior, size, and structure, it is difficult to devise a consistent set of criteria to assess pain. Therefore, practitioners must be familiar with the normal behavior of the species with which they work. Information about the behavior of birds in pain is limited, and has been derived from only a handful of species from the anseriforme (e.g., ducks and geese); columbiforme (e.g., pigeons and doves); falconiforme (e.g., hawks and eagles); galliforme (e.g., chickens); and psittaciforme (e.g., parrots) orders (Necker, 1973; Gottschaldt et al., 1982; Hughes, 1990a; Paul-Murphy, 1999a; Hocking et al. 2005; Souza et al., 2009). Some extrapolation among species is necessary until more species-specific information becomes available. In addition to differences in behavior there may also be interspecies variation in neuroanatomical structure and physiology. Finally, genetic differences that influence individual responses to pain and/or analgesics have been identified in chickens (Hughes, 1990a).

Perception of pain allows an animal to minimize its exposure to potentially harmful stimuli. Birds have the anatomical and physiological components to respond appropriately to painful stimuli, have endogenous mechanisms to modulate the pain experience (Reiner et al., 1984), and respond to analgesic strategies with modified behavioral responses (Paul-Murphy, 1999b). Birds often do not display overt signs of pain because prey species are less likely to manifest pain-associated behavior that may attract the attention of predators (Livingston, 2002). It is, therefore, advisable to treat for pain in birds when dealing with any condition known to be painful in humans (Flecknell, 1994). If the procedure or injury involves tissue damage and/or the bird demonstrates changes in posture (guarding), temperament (aggressive or passive), appetite, or activity level, the veterinarian should assume that the bird is in pain (Jenkins, 1993).

PAIN PATHWAYS IN BIRDS

The physiology of pain (Chapter 2) involves peripheral and central processes, including the detection and transmission of noxious information and the modulation and perception of this information (Kanjhan, 1995). The anatomy and physiology of pain is covered in depth in chapter 2, and information specific to birds is presented here.

Peripheral Nervous System

Several types of nociceptors have been identified in birds. Mechanothermal receptors are polymodal nociceptors that respond to thermal ($>40°C$) and mechanical stimulations, and have been identified in pigeons (Kitchell et al., 1959; Necker & Reiner, 1980), ducks (Leitner & Roumy, 1974), and chickens (McKeegan & Philbey, 2012). Conduction along nerve fibers is relatively slow, and is likely comparable to mammalian unmyelinated C fibers. An increase in stimulus magnitude results in an increase in the number of responses (Gentle, 1989, 1991).

Nociceptors identified in birds are similar to those found in mammals but there are a few differences. These receptors appear to be less sensitive to cold than the corresponding receptors in mammals (Leitner & Roumy, 1974). The threshold of heat nociceptors tends to be higher in avian species compared to mammals and this is not surprising, as body and skin temperature are higher ($41–42°C$) in birds (Necker & Reiner, 1980). However, when comparing the physiological responses of nociceptors found in the chicken with those found in mammals, discharge patterns and receptive field size are very similar (Beitel & Dubner, 1976; Holloway et al., 1980).

Central Nervous System

As in mammals, pain signals in birds are transmitted from peripheral receptors to several areas of the midbrain and forebrain via multiple ascending spinal pathways (Argoff, 2011). The spinal cord dorsal horn of chickens is arranged into six side-by-side laminae, which can be distinguished on the basis of cell size and distribution, whereas other species (e.g., pigeons) demonstrate dorsoventral organization (Wild et al., 2010). Nociceptive information is transmitted to lamina I and outer lamina II of the dorsal horn via Aδ and C primary afferent fibers (Willis, 2006). In birds, the distribution of the neurons in the dorsal horn is similar to that of the nociceptive spinothalamic tract cells in the monkey (Willis, 1979) and the cat (Jones et al., 1985), and these neurons receive input from substance P (SP)-containing axon terminals (Otsuka & Yanagisawa, 1990). A study examining the 2-[^{125}I]iodomelatonin-binding sites in chicken spinal cord suggests that melatonin may also be important in the transmission of pain sensation, as the distribution of [^{125}I]iodomelatonin within the dorsal gray horn was similar to that of SP and opiate receptors (Pang, 1997).

Pain Management in Veterinary Practice, First Edition. Edited by Christine M. Egger, Lydia Love and Tom Doherty.
© 2014 John Wiley & Sons, Inc. Published 2014 by John Wiley & Sons, Inc.

Little is known about the modulation of pain in birds, but endogenous opioids have been identified in the central nervous system (CNS) (Reiner et al., 1989; Csillag et al., 1990). Endogenous opioids are inhibitory neurotransmitters with receptor subtypes (μ, κ, and δ) distributed throughout the CNS in vertebrates (Sheehan, 2009). Birds possess μ, δ, and κ opioid receptors. The effect of μ and κ agonists in pigeons appears to be similar to mammals (Concannon et al., 1995). Pigeons can be trained to distinguish the difference between μ agonists, κ agonists, and saline (Wessinger et al., 2011). Autoradiographic studies of the forebrain of pigeons show a predominance of κ receptors in comparison to mammals (Mansour et al., 1988; Reiner et al., 1989), but μ and κ agonists are analgesic in this species (Concannon et al., 1995). Species differences in response to opioid analgesics may be related to the variation in distribution of opioid receptor subclasses amongst species (Csillag et al., 1990). While a predominance of κ receptors has been demonstrated in pigeons (Reiner et al., 1989), there are no studies in other species. To make the assumption that all birds have more κ opioid receptors than other classes of opioid receptors cannot be justified, especially as μ opioids are also capable of producing analgesia in birds (Machin, 2005). In a study evaluating the effects of μ and κ agonists on the minimum anesthetic concentration of isoflurane in chickens, both agonists decreased the minimum anesthetic concentration in a dose-dependent manner (Concannon et al., 1995), suggesting that both receptor types are important in pain modulation and/or sedation. Opioid receptors are detectable in chick embryos and are concentrated in areas that are thought to play key roles in sensory input processing and memory (Csillag et al., 1990). The proportion of receptors may vary with age (Csillag et al., 1990). The distribution of β-endorphin and enkephalin-like immunoreactivity within the avian telencephalon is similar to that of a mammal (Reiner et al., 1984). Broiler breeding male chickens with degenerative joint disease affecting the hip walk more slowly when given an injection of naloxone, demonstrating that the endogenous opioid system modulates nociception and perception in avian species (Hocking, 1994).

PAIN-ASSOCIATED BEHAVIORS IN BIRDS

Recognition of pain and anxiety in animals is critical for appropriate analgesic selection and relief of pain and suffering. Birds demonstrate a relationship between activation of nociceptors and behavioral and/or physiological evidence of pain (Gentle & Tilston, 1999; Livingston, 2002). Acute pain, lasting from seconds to days, is adaptive, having a protective role to prevent or limit tissue damage (Shaver et al., 2009), and is accompanied by increased heart and respiratory rates and blood pressure (Gentle, 1991). Chronic pain is maladaptive as it causes a chronic state of discomfort and distress (Shaver et al., 2009) because pain lasts beyond the expected healing time (Cheng, 2006).

In response to acute pain, birds may display fight-or-flight responses including escape reactions and vocalization, and/or lack of escape attempts and tonic immobility (Gentle, 1991; Gentle & Tilston, 1999). Immobility in reaction to a noxious stimulus is termed the conservation-withdrawal response, and has been studied most in chickens with the use of noxious cutaneous thermal stimulation that produces a crouching or tonic immobility (crouched posture with the head drawn into the body and the eyes partially or fully closed) (Gentle, 1989). This response is a complex behavioral reaction to aversive traumatic events that continue to occur despite the animal's attempts to reduce or eliminate the events (Gentle & Hill, 1987, Gentle, 1989; Hughes, 1990b). It is characterized by suppression of the righting reflex without the evidence of loss of central processing, and it may last from a few seconds to several hours. It is thought to be an antipredator behavior, and procedures that increase fear prolong the immobility reaction (Gentle, 1989). Change in behavior from the fight-or-flight response to tonic immobility may be related to learned helplessness.

Inappetence and weight loss are nonspecific signs of pain (Gentle & Hill, 1987). Piloerection or a "puffed up" appearance can be associated with illness or pain. Grooming behavior may be decreased (Gentle & Tilston, 1999) but over-grooming, feather picking, and self-mutilation are also seen in chronic pain states (Shaver et al., 2009). Mutual grooming or aggression among birds that live in social groups or segregation of the individual from the flock can also indicate pain (Hawkins & Paul-Murphy, 2011). Reluctance to use an affected limb or unwillingness to move (Gentle & Corr, 1995) and wound-guarding behavior are seen with both acute and chronic pain (Shaver et al., 2009).

Electrical (Bardo & Hughes, 1978), mechanical, and thermal noxious stimuli (Hothersall et al., 2011) have been used to study acute pain responses in gallinaceous birds. Conscious African gray parrots (*Psittacus erithacus erithacus* and *P. erithacus timneh*) looked down at their feet or chewed on the wire in response to an electrical stimulus, but large individual variation in responses prevented meaningful quantitative assessment of temperature threshold (Paul-Murphy, 1999a).

Humans with chronic neuropathic pain report abnormal sensation or hypersensitivity of the affected area including paresthesias (i.e., skin crawling sensations or tingling), spontaneous ongoing pain, and shooting, electric shock-like sensations (Baron et al., 2010). Self-mutilation is not uncommon in mammalian neuropathic pain models (Zhang et al., 2008). Beak trimming is commonly performed in commercial operations, especially on layers and turkeys, but may also be performed on ducks and quail. Partial beak amputation in the chicken involves cutting and cautery and results in full-thickness burns, the formation of neuromas by damaged and regenerating nerve fibers, and spontaneous neural discharge (Breward & Gentle, 1985). The initial pain experienced results from massive discharge of the injured nerve fibers and lasts approximately 15 seconds. A painless phase follows, and this phase may last for several hours (Gentle, 1991). Normal beak usage is observed for approximately 6 hours after amputation, and may be related to a sudden lack of normal afferent input from the beak as a result of injured nerves being incapable of transmitting information from the injured periphery, activation of large mechanoreceptive axons stimulating spinal interneurons to suppress the nociceptive signal, and/or endogenous analgesia activation (Cheng, 2006). By 24 hours after amputation, however, chickens were less mobile, unwilling to peck at the environment, and had decreased food and water intake (Duncan et al., 1991). Birds treated topically with analgesics (bupivacaine and dimethyl sulphoxide [isobutalone]) had higher feeding and pecking rates than untreated birds following partial beak amputation (Gentle et al., 1991; Glatz et al., 1992).

In 16-week-old laying hens, partial beak amputation resulted in guarding behavior and hyperalgesia, with significant reduction in environmental pecking, preening, beak wiping, and head shaking for 6 weeks after surgery (Duncan et al., 1989). Another study reported inactivity for as long as 56 weeks after surgery (Eskeland, 1977). Altered food intake and reduced weight gain and egg production also occur with chronic pain associated with beak trimming (Gentle, 1982; Duncan et al., 1989).

Consequences of beak trimming depend on the age at which the procedure is performed. In older birds, although beaks heal rapidly, there is scar tissue and neuroma development leading to chronic pain states (Breward & Gentle, 1985; Gentle, 2011). In young birds, there is rapid healing and an absence of scar tissue or neuroma formation (Gentle et al., 1997; Gentle, 2011). In one study where chicks were trimmed using infrared technology at one day of age, there were no behavioral indications of pain from 1 to 6 weeks (Gentle & McKeegan, 2007). However, other studies have demonstrated reduced feed intake, reduced activity, and beak guarding in the first week after trimming (Gentle et al., 1997; Marchant-Forde et al., 2008). The method of beak trimming may also impact the length of time that pain-related behaviors are present, although both hot-blade trimming (Gentle et al., 1997) and infrared trimming (Marchant-Forde et al., 2008) significantly impacted production.

TREATMENT OF PAIN IN BIRDS

Controlling pain involves pharmacological, physical, environmental, and behavioral management (Wright et al., 1985). The contribution of proper husbandry and nonpharmacological methods of analgesia should not be overlooked. Environmental modification with appropriate choice and location of perches, bedding, food, and water will make a patient more comfortable. A dry, warm, quiet, nonstressful environment is essential (Clyde & Paul-Murphy, 2000).

Preventative Analgesia
Injury can induce prolonged changes in CNS function, influencing responses to subsequent afferent inputs and contributing to chronic pain states (Katz, 2001; Pogatzki-Zahn & Zahn, 2006). Central sensitization can be prevented by timely administration of effective analgesic agents for a sufficient duration (Katz, 2001; Pogatzki-Zahn & Zahn, 2006).

Analgesia Produced Through Changes in Attention
Behavioral responses to pain are complex, but pain-coping behavior can be influenced by changes in the motivational state of the animal. When placed in a novel environment, painful birds can appear normal and alert because attentional mechanisms are occupied with exploring a new physical and/or social environment (Gentle & Tilston, 1999). In chickens, changes in attention produced a significant reduction in lameness during an experimentally induced tonic pain stimulus from sodium urate synovitis (Wylie & Gentle, 1998; Gentle & Tilston, 1999). Hypoalgesia was produced by diversion of attention in situations designed to increase feeding motivation or motivation to explore (Wylie & Gentle, 1998; Gentle & Tilston, 1999). Complete analgesia or marked hypoalgesia was observed in birds deprived of food for 16 hours and then given access to food after induction of sodium urate synovitis. This analgesia could be completely reversed by naloxone, suggesting that it is opioid mediated (Wylie & Gentle, 1998). Distraction- and attention-focusing strategies have been used to help human patients cope with chronic

low-level pain. Coping is based on the cognitive action of switching attention; thus, when patients were fully engaged in a task they were not processing pain at the same time (Eccleston, 1995).

Sensorial saturation is a multisensorial procedure used to comfort human infants involving tactile (massage), auditory (speaking to the infant gently), visual (eye contact), and gustative (sweet solution on the tongue) stimulation (Bellieni et al., 2012). Similar techniques can be used in pet birds to provide temporary comfort. Tactile (stroking, gentle massage; assuming the bird enjoys being touched), auditory (speaking gently), visual (introduction of a toy or object), and gustative (offering of a sugar solution) stimuli can be used to comfort a bird that is in pain. It is important to keep in mind that the absence of pain-related behavior does not necessarily indicate an absence of pain. Regardless, owners should be encouraged to try this when pain is present.

Analgesics Used in Birds

OPIOIDS
Opioids (Chapter 4) have been used as analgesics in avian species with variable and conflicting results (Bardo & Hughes, 1978; Hughes, 1990b; Concannon et al., 1995; Paul-Murphy, 1999b). A dearth of published information concerning efficacy and safety of opioids in avian species has delayed widespread clinical adoption. Adverse effects, such as excessive sedation and respiratory depression are uncommon, and can be readily reversed with naloxone or naltrexone; however, analgesia will also be reversed (Pascoe, 2000).

Initial studies in chickens using high doses (200 mg/kg) of morphine produced analgesia to a toe pinch test (Schneider, 1961); however, more recent studies demonstrate morphine analgesia at much lower doses (5–30 mg/kg) using alternative nociceptive tests (Bardo & Hughes, 1978; Fan et al., 1981). Chickens can be trained to associate color with the presence of analgesic agents in their food. Lame chickens select food with the highest dose of morphine when given food with three different doses of morphine (8.6, 49, and 430 mg/kg). Chickens without lameness also showed an obvious preference for morphine, perhaps for its euphoric effect (Pickup et al., 1997). Genetic factors play an important role in determining sensitivity to opioid analgesic effects. In domestic fowl, morphine can produce either hypoalgesia or hyperalgesia during thermal and chemical nociceptive testing, depending upon the dose used and the strain of fowl tested (Hughes, 1990b, Hughes & Sufka, 1991). Hyperalgesia in domestic fowl is strain dependent and naloxone sensitive (Hughes, 1990a, 1990b, Hughes et al., 1992; Sufka & Hughes, 1992), and is mediated primarily by μ-receptor activation at CNS loci (Sufka et al., 1991; Hughes et al., 1992).

Fentanyl is a potent μ agonist that is rarely used in birds because it is very short acting (Pascoe, 2000). In red tailed hawks fentanyl continuous rate infusions dose-dependently reduced the minimum anesthetic concentration of isoflurane by up to 55%, with minimal cardiovascular changes (Pavez et al., 2011). In white cockatoos (*Cacatua alba*), fentanyl, 0.02 mg/kg administered subcutaneously, produced significant analgesia in some birds but is not recommended because of the large volume required and the hyperactivity it causes in some birds (Hoppes et al., 2003).

Buprenorphine is a partial μ agonist that is generally reserved for treating mild-to-moderate pain (Pascoe, 2000). Buprenorphine has a strong affinity for the μ receptor, thus it is difficult to reverse.

Its main advantage in mammals is that it can have a long duration of action (6–12 hours). The duration of action in birds is unknown. Buprenorphine has been reported to be clinically effective in birds, but in African gray parrots large doses produced no significant analgesic effect (Paul-Murphy, 1999b). Buprenorphine displays an inverted U-shaped dose–response curve, with supraclinical doses resulting in reduced analgesic effects (Pascoe, 2000).

Butorphanol is a synthetic opioid agonist–antagonist that is a weak antagonist at the μ receptor but a strong agonist at the κ receptor. It is often considered the analgesic of choice, given that birds may have a higher proportion of κ receptors compared to mammals (Reiner et al., 1989). The effect of butorphanol on isoflurane-sparing was studied in parrots. Butorphanol decreased the minimum anesthetic concentration of isoflurane by 25% and 11% in cockatoos and African gray parrots, respectively, but did not significantly change the isoflurane minimum anesthetic concentration in blue-fronted Amazon parrots (Curro et al., 1994, 1994). Likewise, butorphanol decreased the minimum anesthetic concentration of sevoflurane in guinea fowl, and, although increasing the dose of butorphanol further decreased the minimum anesthetic concentration for sevoflurane, the effect was small and of short duration (Escobar et al., 2012). Minimum anesthetic concentration-sparing studies should be interpreted cautiously because these effects may be related to sedation as well as analgesia (Dohoo, 1990; Reim & Middleton, 1995).

Riggs et al., (2008) examined the pharmacokinetics of butorphanol in red-tailed hawks (*Buteo jamaicensis*) and great horned owls (*Bubo virginianus*) and suggested that butorphanol should be given every 2–4 hours. In Hispaniolan amazon parrots (*Amazona ventralis*), butorphanol should be administered IV or IM at a dose of 5 mg/kg every 2–3 hours, and oral administration is not recommended because of poor bioavailability (Guzman, 2011a). In another study, butorphanol plasma concentrations remained above the minimum effective concentration for analgesia in broiler chickens for 2 hours (Singh et al., 2011). Butorphanol has minimal respiratory effects as it produces an increase in respiratory frequency with a decrease in tidal volume and no significant change in minute ventilation (Curro, 1994).

Liposome-encapsulated butorphanol provided analgesia and detectable serum butorphanol concentrations for up to 5 days in Hispaniolan parrots (Sladky et al., 2006). In green-cheeked conures (*Pyrrhura molinae*) a microcrystalline sodium urate injection into the tibiotarsal–tarsometatarsal joint induced temporary, self-resolving arthritic pain, which was used to evaluate the analgesic efficacy of liposome-encapsulated butorphanol (Paul-Murphy et al., 2009a). Analgesia was evaluated with the use of a capacitance meter adapted to measure the weight load of the pelvic limb in conures. In that study, a significant difference from time zero was detected during the first 6 hours (Paul-Murphy et al., 2009a), compared to differences detected for 26 hours in Hispaniolan parrots (Paul-Murphy et al., 2009b). This illustrates the variability among species regarding the behavioral response to arthritic pain and analgesic treatment.

Nalbuphine is a κ agonist and μ antagonist, similar to butorphanol, and may provide appropriate analgesia to those species that have a predominance of κ receptors. In studies in parrots in which the efficacy of nalbuphine was measured as an increase in thermal threshold, 12.5 mg/kg IM was effective for 3 hours (Guzman et al., 2011b; Keller et al., 2011).

Tramadol is a weak μ agonist that also has serotonergic and noradrenergic effects. It can be administered orally and is inexpensive (Souza et al., 2009). A pharmacokinetic study in bald eagles (*Haliaeetus leucocephalus*) suggests that a dose of 5 mg/kg orally would produce analgesia for approximately 12 hours (Souza et al., 2009). The authors of a pharmacokinetic study in red-tailed hawks predict that an oral dose of 15 mg/kg will result in plasma tramadol concentrations in the range found to be analgesic in humans for 5–6 hours after administration, although more than twice a day dosing may be excessively stressful for the bird (Souza et al., 2011). In peafowl (*Pavo cristatus*), 7.5 mg/kg, per os, produced plasma concentrations of the active metabolite O-desmethyltramadol that were higher than the minimum effective analgesia concentration in humans for 12 hours (Black et al., 2010).

A pharmacodynamic study evaluating the antinociceptive effects of tramadol on thermal thresholds in Hispaniolan Amazon parrots found that a dose of 30 mg/kg, per os, resulted in thermal antinociception for about 6 hours (Sanchez-Migallon Guzman et al., 2012). A companion pharmacokinetic study in Hispaniolan Amazon parrots found that mean plasma tramadol concentrations were >100 ng/mL, the plasma concentration associated with analgesia in humans, for 2–4 hours after IV administration of 5 mg/kg and for 6 hours after an oral dose of 30 mg/kg (Souza et al., 2012). Further studies are required.

CORTICOSTEROIDS

Corticosteroids (Chapter 5) reduce pain by reducing inflammation. Betamethasone is a potent steroidal anti-inflammatory drug that reduces pain associated with degenerative hip disorders in adult male turkeys (Duncan et al., 1989), and has been used to decrease inflammation in uric acid-induced joint pain in chickens (Hocking, 2001). Polydypsia, polyphagia, polyuria, and immunosuppression may be seen at anti-inflammatory doses, thus making nonsteroidal anti-inflammatory drugs (NSAIDs) preferable in most situations (Clyde & Paul-Murphy, 2000).

NONSTEROIDAL ANTI-INFLAMMATORY DRUGS

Although NSAIDs (Chapter 5) have been used in avian species with some success, renal toxicity has occurred (Klein et al., 1994). Oriental white-backed vultures (*Gyps bengalensis*) died of renal failure after ingestion of tissues of dead livestock containing diclofenac (Meteyer et al., 2005). Ketoprofen, in combination with isoflurane or propofol and bupivacaine, also produced renal lesions that ultimately resulted in death (Mulcahy et al., 2003). A more recent toxicity study in broiler chickens compared diclofenac with ketoprofen (Mohan et al., 2012). Ketoprofen-treated birds did not show any adverse clinical signs and no significant increase in concentration of creatinine, uric acid, alanine aminotransferase, and aspartate aminotransferase when compared with birds receiving diclofenac. Gross and microscopic examination of kidney and liver showed normal organ architecture. Thus, it was concluded that ketoprofen at the dose of 3 mg/kg administered IM daily for 5 days was nontoxic to broiler chickens. As in mammals, maintaining hydration when using NSAIDs may aid in the prevention of renal morbidity (Hassan et al., 2011). Flunixin meglumine at 5 mg/kg IM into the pectoral muscles of mallard ducks (*Anas platyrhynchos*) produced necrotic lesions at the site of administration (Machin et al., 2001).

Pharmacokinetic studies with broiler chickens indicate that peak plasma concentrations of carprofen are reached between 1 and

2 hours after subcutaneous administration. In a preliminary pharmacodynamic study, a subcutaneous dose of 1 mg/kg of carprofen raised mechanical pressure thresholds for at least 90 minutes (McGeown et al., 1999). Plasma concentrations of NSAIDs likely do not reflect physiological or pharmacodynamic activity (Owen et al., 1995), as NSAIDs are weak acids (Landoni & Lees, 1995) and highly protein bound, and tend to accumulate in areas of inflammation (Lees et al., 2004). Because NSAIDs may produce effects longer than that would be predicted from their actual plasma concentrations, plasma thromboxane B concentrations may be a better estimate of duration of drug action. In mallard ducks, flunixin meglumine (5 mg/kg) and ketoprofen (5 mg/kg) suppressed thromboxane B concentrations for up to 12 hours, possibly suggesting that their therapeutic effect may last that long (Machin et al., 2001), but further studies are necessary. Unfortunately, pharmacokinetic data cannot be extrapolated among species (Baert & De Backer, 2003).

Lame chickens preferentially selected food with carprofen at three doses (3.4, 34.3, and 343.0 mg/kg) compared to food without analgesics (Danbury et al., 2000). However, healthy chickens showed an aversion to the highest dose, which may reflect an aversive taste or the occurrence of adverse effects such as nausea (Danbury et al., 2000). In another study, carprofen (1 mg/kg subcutaneously) increased the speed and walking ability of rapidly growing broiler chickens with chronic lameness (McGeown et al., 1999). In contrast, in an arthritis model in parrots evaluating carprofen alone and carprofen in combination with liposomal-encapsulated butorphanol, 3 mg/kg of carprofen did not provide analgesia or improve analgesia provided by the butorphanol (Paul-Murphy et al., 2009b). However, opioids and NSAIDs are generally considered more effective when delivered in combination (multimodal analgesia) (Corletto, 2007).

In parrots, flunixin meglumine did not produce an isoflurane-sparing effect at 4 mg/kg IM (Curro, 1994). NSAIDs have not been shown to have an isoflurane-sparing effect in mammals. The recommended dose range of flunixin is 1–10 mg/kg (Ritchie et al., 1994); however, there are no experimental data available to confirm analgesic doses. Ketoprofen administered at 5 mg/kg IM in mallard ducks demonstrated analgesic efficacy, but the onset of action was 30 minutes (Machin & Livingston, 2002). Phenylbutazone applied topically to the beak of chickens resulted in maintenance of pretrimming feed intake values over the first 24 hours after the procedure (Glatz et al. 1992).

Parrots with experimentally induced arthritis given 0.05, 0.1, 0.5, or 1.0 mg/kg of meloxicam IM every 12 hours had improved weight bearing with 1.0 mg/kg of meloxicam (Cole et al., 2009). Administration of 0.5 mg/kg of meloxicam was not sufficient for postoperative orthopedic pain control in pigeons, but 2 mg/kg every 12 hours for 9 days provided quantifiable analgesia, as assessed by weight bearing (Desmarchelier et al., 2012). Meloxicam was used at 0.5 mg/kg once daily in a case report of external skeletal fixation to repair a tarsometatarsal fracture in a Harris hawk (*Parabuteo unicinctus*) (Hoybergs et al., 2008).

α-2 ADRENERGIC AGONISTS

As in mammals, drugs with adrenergic activity can modulate avian nociception as well as perception of pain. α-2 receptor activation can produce sedation, anxiolysis, analgesia, and anesthetic-sparing effects (Maze & Tranquilli, 1991). α-2 agonists, such as xylazine and dexmedetomidine (Chapter 7), may cause abnormal motor movement, decreased ventilation, hypothermia, sedation, hypersalivation, and adverse cardiovascular effects including arrhythmias and hypo- and hypertension (Samour et al., 1984; Milne, 1991). Although inclusion of α-2 agonists can be useful for premedication in a balanced anesthesia protocol for painful procedures (e.g., combined with ketamine and an opioid), postoperative administration of α-2 agonists is not typically used for analgesia in avian species because of the negative cardiovascular effects and the potential for excessive sedation. Atipamezole, a highly potent, competitive antagonist at centrally and peripherally located α-2 adrenoceptors will quickly reverse any adverse effects; however, desired effects such as sedation and analgesia will also be reversed (Virtanen et al., 1989).

KETAMINE

Even at low doses, ketamine may contribute to analgesia and antihyperalgesia by preventing NMDA receptor-mediated central sensitization. Therefore, ketamine is useful for both pre-emptive and postoperative analgesia, and it may even abolish hypersensitivity once it is established (Lamont et al., 2000). Ketamine as a sole agent does not provide adequate analgesia for laparotomies or orthopedic surgery (Lamont et al., 2000).

The ability of ketamine to inhibit NMDA receptor-mediated changes thought to sensitize CNS nociceptive pathways makes it useful for lessening hyperalgesia, allodynia, and spontaneous pain associated with chronic neuropathic pain (Qian et al., 1996). Ketamine (0.5 mg/kg IM daily) was successfully used with gabapentin (11 mg/kg PO q12h) and low-level laser therapy (<5 mW, 630–680 nm, 5 second application per site) in a prairie falcon with suspected neuropathic pain (Shaver et al., 2009).

LOCAL ANESTHETICS

Local anesthetics (e.g., lidocaine, bupivacaine) provide analgesia by preventing depolarization of Na^+ channels and resultant conduction of pain impulses (Chapter 6). Administration of local anesthesia before tissue trauma can significantly reduce postoperative pain by preventing central sensitization (Clyde & Paul-Murphy, 2000). Local nerve blockade before nerve transection during amputation can decrease the prevalence of "phantom limb" pain in humans (Coderre et al., 1993). Although local anesthesia is sufficient for pain relief, it does not reduce the stress induced by physical restraint and handling of an awake bird, so sedation or general anesthesia may also be necessary. The toxic dose of bupivacaine in birds is 2.7–3.3 mg/kg (Hocking et al., 1997). It is recommended that the lidocaine dose not exceed 4 mg/kg in birds as seizures and cardiac arrest can result with overdose (Paul-Murphy & Ludders, 2001). Chickens receiving high IV doses of bupivacaine (2.7–3.3 mg/kg) showed signs of distress immediately after injection and signs of toxicity, including recumbency with outstretched legs and drowsiness (Hocking et al., 1997). Adverse cardiac effects occur at high plasma concentrations and are associated with prolonged PR and QRS intervals and shortened QT intervals. Overdose of local anesthesia can result in depression, drowsiness, ataxia, nystagmus, muscle tremors, hypotension, and death (Lemke & Dawson, 2000).

Topical application of bupivacaine to the beak stump of chickens after hot-blade amputation allowed maintenance of pretrimming feed intake values over the first 4 hours after the procedure (Glatz et al., 1992). In an acute synovitis model, intra-articular injection of sodium urate produced inflammatory changes including joint swelling, increased joint temperature, and sensitization of the joint capsule receptors lasting at least 3 hours (Gentle et al., 1997; Hocking et al.,1997; Gentle et al. 1999). Intra-articular bupivacaine increased feeding, pecking, and standing behaviors while the proportion of time spent resting declined. Birds treated with bupivacaine (2 mg/kg) were indistinguishable from animals in the nonarthritic control group (Hocking et al., 1997).

More recently, brachial plexus blocks have been investigated in chickens (Figueiredo et al., 2008) and mallard ducks (Brenner et al., 2010). Although the region of the brachial plexus was relatively easy to identify, both studies found variable results and incomplete blockade. More research is necessary to determine the appropriate approach, and volume and concentration of local anesthetic (Figueiredo et al., 2008; Brenner et al., 2010). In mammals, lidocaine is shorter acting (60–120 minutes) compared to bupivacaine (240–360 minutes) (Lemke & Dawson, 2000).

SUMMARY

Pain perception in birds is likely analogous to that of mammals, and invasive and painful procedures should always be accompanied by appropriate analgesia and anesthesia. When choosing an analgesic for an avian patient, the practitioner should consider the level of pain and treat appropriately, as they would in mammalian species. Pharmacological intervention is important but physical, environmental, and behavioral management should not be overlooked (Clyde & Paul-Murphy, 2000). As with mammals, understanding pain pathways and applying a multimodal, pre-emptive approach to pain management in birds will benefit the patient. Likewise, identifying pain-related behaviors is important so that patients can be evaluated and re-evaluated. Pain evaluation and management are inextricably linked.

Although avian pain management is in its infancy, research and clinical studies demonstrate benefit from the use of opioids, corticosteroids, and NSAIDs, as well as other analgesics such as α-2 agonists, ketamine, and local anesthetics. Assessment of analgesic efficacy is extremely important, as the dosage and choice of analgesic may vary widely among species and individuals. The information given in this chapter is meant to be used as a guide for treatment of pain in avian species. Clearly, there is a need for further clinical investigations and both successes and failures should be reported in the veterinary literature to expand the limited information available.

REFERENCES

Argoff, C. (2011) Mechanisms of pain transmission and pharmacologic management. *Current Medical Research and Opinion*, 27, 2019–2031.

Baert, K. & De Backer, R. (2003) Comparative pharmacokinetics of three non-steroidal anti-inflammatory drugs in five bird species. *Comparative Biochemistry and Physiology C-Toxicology & Pharmacology*, 134, 25–33.

Bardo, M.T. & Hughes, R.A. (1978) Shock-elicited flight response in chickens as an index of morphine analgesia. *Pharmacology Biochemistry and Behavior*, 9, 147–149.

Baron, R., Binder, A., & Wasner, G. (2010) Neuropathic pain: diagnosis, pathophysiological mechanisms, and treatment. *Lancet Neurology*, 9, 807–819.

Beitel, R.E. & Dubner, R. (1976) Response of unmyelinated (C) polymodal nociceptors to thermal stimuli applied to monkeys face. *Journal of Neurophysiology*, 39, 1160–1175.

Bellieni, C.V., Tei, M., Coccina, F., & Buonocore, G. (2012) Sensorial saturation for infants' pain. *Journal of Maternal, Fetal and Neonatal Medicine*, 25, 79–81.

Black, P.A., Cox, S.K., Macek, M., Tieber, A., & Junge, R.E. (2010) Pharmacokinetics of tramadol hydrochloride and its metabolite O-desmethyltramadol in peafowl (*Pavo cristatus*). *Journal of Zoo and Wildlife Medicine*, 41, 671–676.

Brenner, D.J., Larsen, R.S., Dickinson, P.J., Wack, R.F., Williams, D.C., & Pascoe, P.J. (2010) Development of an avian brachial plexus nerve block technique for perioperative analgesia in mallard ducks (*Anas platyrhynchos*). *Journal of Avian Medicine and Surgery*, 24, 24–34.

Breward, J. & Gentle, M.J. (1985) Neuroma formation and abnormal afferent nerve discharges after partial beak amputation (beak trimming) in poultry. *Experientia*, 41, 1132–1134.

Cheng, H. (2006) Morphopathological changes and pain in beak trimmed laying hens. *World's Poultry Science Journal*, 62, 41–52.

Clyde, V.L., Paul-Murphy, J., & Bonagura, J.D. (2000) Avian analgesia, in *Kirks Current Veterinary Therapy XIII: Small Animal Practice*, (ed. J.D. Bonagura), WB Saunders, Philadelphia, pp. 1126–1128.

Coderre, T.J., Katz, J., Vaccarino, A.L., & Melzack, R. (1993) Contribution of central neuroplasticity to pathological pain: review of clinical and experimental evidence. *Pain*, 52, 259–285.

Cole, G.A., Paul-Murphy, J., Krugner-Higby, L., et al. (2009) Analgesic effects of intramuscular administration of meloxicam in Hispaniolan parrots (Amazona ventralis) with experimentally induced arthritis. *American Journal of Veterinary Research*, 70, 1471–1476.

Concannon, K.T., Dodam, J.R., & Hellyer, P.W. (1995) Influence of a mu-opioid and kappa-opioid agonist on isoflurane minimal anesthetic concentration in chickens. *American Journal of Veterinary Research*, 56, 806–811.

Corletto, F. (2007) Multimodal and balanced analgesia. *Veterinary Research Communications*, 31, 59–63.

Csillag, A., Bourne, R.C., & Stewart, M.G. (1990) Distribution of mu, delta, and kappa opioid receptor binding sites in the brain of the one-day-old domestic chick (*Gallus domesticus*): an in vitro quantitative autoradiographic study. *Journal of Comparative Neurology*, 302, 543–551.

Curro, T.G. (1994) *Evaluation of the Isoflurane-Sparing Effects of Butorphanol and Flunixin in Psittaciformes.* Proceedings of the Association of Avian Veterinarians Conference, September, Reno, NV, pp. 17–19.

Curro, T.G., Brunson, D.B., & Paul-Murphy, J. (1994a) Determination of the ED50 of isoflurane and evaluation of the isoflurane-sparing effects of butorphanol in cockatoos (*Cacatua* spp). *Veterinary Surgery*, 23, 429–433.

Danbury, T.C., Weeks, C.A., Chambers, J.P., Waterman-Pearson, A.E., Kestin, S.C. (2000) Self-selection of the analgesic drug carprofen by lame broiler chickens. *Veterinary Record*, 146, 307–311.

Desmarchelier, M., Troncy, E., Fitzgerald, G., & Lair, S. (2012) Analgesic effects of meloxicam administration on postoperative orthopedic pain in domestic pigeons (*Columba livia*). *American Journal of Veterinary Research*, 73, 361–367.

Dohoo, S.E. (1990) Isoflurane as an inhalational anesthetic agent in clinical practice. *Canadian Veterinary Journal*, 31, 847–850.

Duncan, I.J., Slee, G.S., Seawright, E., & Breward, J. (1989) Behavioural consequences of partial beak amputations (beak trimming) in poultry. *British Poultry Science*, 30, 479–488.

Duncan, I.J., Beatty, E.R., Hocking, P.M., & Duff, S.R. (1991) Assessment of pain associated with degenerative hip disorders in adult male turkeys. *Research in Veterinary Science*, 50, 200–203.

Eccleston, C. (1995) The attentional control of pain: methodological and theoretical concerns. *Pain*, 63, 3–10.

Escobar, A., Valadao, C.A., Brosnan, R.J., et al. (2012) Effects of butorphanol on the minimum anesthetic concentration for sevoflurane in guineafowl (*Numida meleagris*). *American Journal of Veterinary Research*, 73, 183–188.

Eskeland, B. (1977) Behaviour as an indicator of welfare in hens under different systems of management, population-density, social-status and by beak trimming. *Meldinger Fra Norges Landbrukshogskole*, 56, 2–20.

Fan, S.G., Shutt, A.J., & Vogt, M. (1981) The importance of 5-hydroxytryptamine turnover for the analgesic effect of morphine in the chicken. *Neuroscience*, 6, 2223–2227.

Figueiredo, J.P., Cruz, M.L., Mendes, G.M., Marucio, R.L., Riccó, C.H., & Campagnol, D. (2008) Assessment of brachial plexus blockade in chickens by an auxiliary approach. *Veterinary Anaesthesia and Analgesia*, 35, 511–518.

Flecknell, P.A. (1994) Refinement of animal use–assessment and alleviation of pain and distress. *Laboratory Animals*, 28, 222–231.

Gentle, M.J. (1989) Cutaneous sensory afferents recorded from the nervus intramandibularis of *Gallus gallus var domesticus*. *Journal of Comparative Physiology A-Sensory Neural and Behavioral Physiology*, 164, 763–774.

Gentle, M.J. (1991) The acute effects of amputation on peripheral trigeminal afferents in *Gallus gallus var domesticus*. *Pain*, 46, 97–103.

Gentle, M.J. (2011) Pain issues in poultry. *Applied Animal Behaviour Science*, 135, 252–258.

Gentle, M.J. & Corr, S.A. (1995) Endogenous analgesia in the chicken. *Neuroscience Letters*, 201, 211–214.

Gentle, M.J. & Hill, F.L. (1987) Oral lesions in the chicken: behavioral responses following nociceptive stimulation. *Physiology & Behavior*, 40, 781–783.

Gentle, M.J. & McKeegan, D.E. (2007) Evaluation of the effects of infrared beak trimming in broiler breeder chicks. *Veterinary Record*, 160, 145–148.

Gentle, M.J. & Tilston, V.L. (1999) Reduction in peripheral inflammation by changes in attention. *Physiology & Behavior*, 66, 289–292.

Gentle, M.J., Hocking, P.M., Bernard, R., & Dunn, L.N. (1999) Evaluation of intra-articular opioid analgesia for the relief of articular pain in the domestic fowl. *Pharmacology Biochemistry and Behavior*, 63, 339–343.

Gentle, M.J., Hughes, B.O., Fox, A., & Waddington, D. (1997) Behavioural and anatomical consequences of two beak trimming methods in 1- and 10-day-old domestic chicks. *British Journal of Poultry Science*, 38, 453–463.

Gentle, M.J., Hughes, B.O., Hubrecht, R.C. (1982) The effect of beak trimming on food-intake, feeding-behaviour and body-weight in adult hens. *Applied Animal Ethology*, 8, 147–159.

Gentle, M.J., Hunter, L.N., & Waddington, D. (1991) The onset of pain related behaviors following partial beak amputation in the chicken. *Neuroscience Letters*, 128, 113–116.

Glatz, P.C., Murphy, L.B., & Preston, A.P. (1992) Analgesic therapy of beak-trimmed chickens. *Australian Veterinary Journal*, 69, 18.

Gottschaldt, K.M., Fruhstorfer, H., Schmidt, W., & Kräft, I. (1982) Thermosensitivity and its possible fine-structural basis in mechanoreceptors in the beak skin of geese. *Journal of Comparative Neurology*, 205, 219–245.

Guzman, D.S.M., Flammer, K., Paul-Murphy, J.R., Barker, S.A., & Tully, T.N Jr. (2011a) Pharmacokinetics of butorphanol after intravenous, intramuscular, and oral administration in Hispaniolan Amazon parrots (*Amazona ventralis*). *Journal of Avian Medicine and Surgery*, 25, 185–191.

Guzman, D.S.M., KuKanich, B., Keuler, N.S., Klauer, J.M., & Paul-Murphy, JR. (2011b) Antinociceptive effects of nalbuphine hydrochloride in Hispaniolan Amazon parrots (*Amazona ventralis*). *American Journal of Veterinary Research*, 72, 736–740.

Hassan, K., Khazim, K., Hassan, F., & Hassan, S. (2011) Acute kidney injury associated with metamizole sodium ingestion. *Renal Failure*, 33, 544–547.

Hawkins, M.G. & Paul-Murphy, J. (2011) Avian analgesia. *Veterinary Clinics of North America Exotic Animal Practice*, 14, 61–80.

Hocking, P.M. (1994) Assessment of the welfare of food restricted male broiler breeder poultry with musculoskeletal disease. *Research in Veterinary Science*, 57, 28–34.

Hocking, P.M., Gentle, M.J., Bernard, R., & Dunn, L.N. (1997) Evaluation of a protocol for determining the effectiveness of pretreatment with local analgesics for reducing experimentally induced articular pain in domestic fowl. *Research in Veterinary Science*, 63, 263–267.

Hocking, P.M., Robertson, G.W., Gentle, M.J. (2001) Effects of anti-inflammatory steroid drugs on pain coping behaviours in a model of articular pain in the domestic fowl. *Research in Veterinary Science*, 71(3), 161–166.

Hocking, P.M., Robertson, G.W., & Gentle, M.J. (2005) Effects of non-steroidal anti-inflammatory drugs on pain-related behaviour in a model of articular pain in the domestic fowl. *Research in Veterinary Science*, 78, 69–75.

Holloway, J.A., Trouth, C.O., Wright, L.E., & Keyser, G.F. (1980) Cutaneous receptive-field characteristics of primary afferents and dorsal horn in the avian (*Gallus domesticus*). *Experimental Neurology*, 68, 477–488.

Hoppes, S., Flammer, K., Hoersch, K., Papich, M.,& Paul-Murphy, J. (2003) Disposition and analgesic effects of fentanyl in white cockatoos (*Cacatua alba*). *Journal of Avian Medicine and Surgery*, 17, 124–130.

Hothersall, B., Caplen, G., Nicol, C.J., et al. (2011) Development of mechanical and thermal nociceptive threshold testing devices in unrestrained birds (broiler chickens). *Journal of Neuroscience Methods*, 201, 220–227.

Hoybergs, Y., Bosmans, T., Risselada, M., & Van Caelenberg, A. (2008) General anesthesia for the surgical repair of a tarsometatarsal fracture in a Harris's Hawk (*Parabuteo unicinctus*). *Vlaams Diergeneeskundig Tijdschrift*, 77, 309–314.

Hughes, R.A. (1990a) Codeine analgesic and morphine hyperalgesic effects on thermal nociception in domestic fowl. *Pharmacology Biochemistry and Behavior*, 35, 567–570.

Hughes, R.A. (1990b) Strain-dependant morphine-induced analgesic and hyperalgesic effects on thermal nociception in domestic fowl (*Gallus gallus*). *Behavioral Neuroscience*, 104, 619–624.

Hughes, R.A. & Sufka, K.J. (1991) Morphine hyperalgesic effects on formalin test in domestic fowl (*Gallus gallus*). *Pharmacology Biochemistry and Behavior*, 38, 247–251.

Hughes, R.A., Bowes, M. & Sufka, K.J. (1992) Morphine hyperalgesic effects on developmental changes in thermal nociception and respiration in domestic fowl (*Gallus gallus*). *Pharmacology Biochemistry and Behavior*, 42, 535–539.

Jenkins, J. (1993) Postoperative care of the avian patient. *Seminars in Avian and Exotic Pet Medicine* 2, 97–102.

Jones, M.W., Hodge, C.J., Apkarian, A.V., & Stevens, R.T. (1985) A dorsolateral spinothalamic pathway in the cat. *Brain Research*, 335, 188–193.

Kanjhan, R. (1995) Opioids and pain. *Clinical and Experimental Pharmacology and Physiology*, 22, 397–403.

Katz, J. (2001) Pre-emptive analgesia: importance of timing. *Canadian Journal of Anaesthesia*, 48, 105–114.

Keller, D.L., Guzman, D.S.M., Klauer, J.M., et al. (2011) Pharmacokinetics of nalbuphine hydrochloride after intravenous and intramuscular administration to Hispaniolan Amazon parrots (*Amazona ventralis*). *American Journal of Veterinary Research*, 72, 741–745.

Kitchell, R.L., Strom, L., & Zotterman, Y. (1959) Electophysiological studies of thermal and taste reception in chickens and pigeons. *Acta Physiologica Scandinavica*, 46, 133–151.

Klein, P.N., Charmatz, K., & Langenberg, J. (1994) *The Effect of Flunixin Meglumine (Banamine®) on the Renal Function in Northern Bobwhite (Colinus virginianus): An Avian Model*. Proceedings of the American Association of Zoo Veterinarians and Association of Reptilian and Amphibian Veterinarians Annual Conference, October, Pittsburg, PA, pp. 128–131.

Lamont, L.A., Tranquilli, W.J., & Mathews, K.A. (2000) Adjunctive analgesic therapy. *Veterinary Clinics of North America Small Animal Practice*, 30, 805–813.

Landoni, M.F. & Lees, P. (1995) Comparison of the anti-inflammatory actions of flunixin and ketoprofen in horses applying PK/PD modeling. *Equine Veterinary Journal*, 27, 247–256.

Lees, P., Landoni, M.F., Giraudel, J., & Toutain, P.L. (2004) Pharmacodynamics and pharmacokinetics of nonsteroidal anti-inflammatory drugs in species of veterinary interest. *Journal of Veterinary Pharmacology and Therapeutics*, 27, 479–490.

Leitner, L.M. & Roumy, M. (1974) Thermosensitive units in tongue and skin of ducks. *Pflugers Archives*, 346, 151–155.

Lemke, K.A. & Dawson, S.D. (2000) Local and regional anesthesia. *Veterinary Clinics of North America Small Animal Practice*, 30, 839–857.

Livingston, A. (2002) Ethical issues regarding pain in animals. *Journal of the American Veterinary Medical Association*, 221, 229–233.

Machin, K.L. (2005) Controlling avian pain. *Compendium on Continuing Education for the Practicing Veterinarian*, 27, 299–309.

Machin, K.L. & Livingston, A. (2002) Assessment of the analgesic effects of ketoprofen in ducks anesthetized with isoflurane. *American Journal of Veterinary Research*, 63, 821–826.

Machin, K.L., Tellier, L.A., Lair, S., & Livingston, A. (2001) Pharmacodynamics of flunixin and ketoprofen in mallard ducks (*Anas platyrhynchos*). *Journal of Zoo and Wildlife Medicine*, 32, 222–229.

Mansour, A., Khachaturian, H., Lewis, M.E., Akil, H., & Watson, S.J. (1988) Anatomy of CNS opioid receptors. *Trends in Neuroscience*, 11, 308–314.

Marchant-Forde, R.M., Fahey, A.G., & Cheng, H.W. (2008) Comparative effects of infrared and one-third hot-blade trimming on beak topography, behavior, and growth. *Poultry Science*, 87, 1474–1483.

Maze, M. & Tranquilli, W. (1991) Alpha-2 adrenoceptor agonists: defining the role in clinical anesthesia. *Anesthesiology*, 74, 581–605.

McGeown, D., Danbury, T.C., Waterman-Pearson, A.E., & Kestin, S.C. (1999) Effect of carprofen on lameness in broiler chickens. *Veterinary Record*, 144, 668–671.

McKeegan, D.E.F. & Philbey, A.W. (2012) Chronic neurophysiological and anatomical changes associated with infra-red beak treatment and their implications for laying hen welfare. *Animal Welfare*, 21, 207–217.

Meteyer, C.U., Rideout, B.A., Gilbert, M., Shivaprasad, H.L., & Oaks, J.L. (2005) Pathology and proposed pathophysiology of diclofenac poisoning in free-living and experimentally exposed oriental white-backed vultures (*Gyps bengalensis*). *Journal of Wildlife Diseases*, 41, 707–716.

Milne, B. (1991) Alpha-2 agonists and anesthesia. *Canadian Journal of Anaesthesia*, 38, 809–813.

Mohan, K., Jayakumar, K., Narayanaswamy, H.D., Manafi, M., & Pavithra, B.H. (2012) An initial safety assessment of hepatotoxic and nephrotoxic potential of intramuscular ketoprofen at single repetitive dose level in broiler chickens. *Poultry Science*, 91(6), 1308–1314.

Mulcahy, D.M., Tuomi, P., & Larsen, R.S. (2003) Differential mortality of male spectacled eiders (*Somateria fischeri*) and king eiders (*Someteria spectabilis*) subsequent to anesthesia with propofol, bupivacaine, and ketoprofen. *Journal of Avian Medicine and Surgery*, 17, 117–123.

Necker, R. (1973) Temperature sensitivity of thermoreceptors and mechanoreceptors on beak of pigeons. *Journal of Comparative Physiology*, 87, 379–391.

Necker, R. & Reiner, B. (1980) Temperature-sensitive mechanoreceptors, thermoreceptors in the feathered skin of pigeons. *Journal of Comparative Physiology*, 135, 201–207.

Otsuka, M. & Yanagisawa, M. (1990) Pain and neurotransmitters. *Molecular Neurobiology*, 10, 293–302.

Owen, J.G., Kamerling, S.G., & Barker, S.A. (1995) Pharmacokinetics of ketoprofen in healthy horses and horses with acute synovitis. *Journal of Veterinary Pharmacology and Therapeutics*, 18, 187–195.

Pang, C.S., Tang, P.L, Song, Y., et al. (1997) Differential inhibitory effects of melatonin analogs and three naphthalenic ligands on 2-[125I]iodomelatonin binding to chicken tissues. *Journal of Pineal Research*, 23(3), 148–155.

Pascoe, P.J. (2000) Opioid analgesics. *Veterinary Clinics of North America Small Animal Practice*, 30, 757–772.

Paul-Murphy, J. & Ludders, J.W. (2001) Avian analgesia. *Veterinary Clinics of North America Exotic Animal Practice*, 4, 35–45.

Paul-Murphy, J.R., Brunson, D.B., & Miletic, V. (1999a) Analgesic effects of butorphanol and buprenorphine in conscious African grey parrots (*Psittacus erithacus erithacus* and *Psittacus erithacus timneh*). *American Journal of Veterinary Research*, 60, 1218–1221.

Paul-Murphy, J.R., Brunson, D.B., & Miletic, V. (1999b) A technique for evaluating analgesia in conscious perching birds. *American Journal of Veterinary Research*, 60, 1213–1217.

Paul-Murphy, J.R., Krugner-Higby, L.A., Tourdot, R.L., et al. (2009a) Evaluation of liposome-encapsulated butorphanol tartrate for alleviation of experimentally induced arthritic pain in green-cheeked conures (*Pyrrhura molinae*). *American Journal of Veterinary Research*, 70, 1211–1219.

Paul-Murphy, J.R., Sladky, K.K., Krugner-Higby, L.A., et al. (2009b) Analgesic effects of carprofen and liposome-encapsulated butorphanol tartrate in Hispaniolan parrots (*Amazona ventralis*) with experimentally induced arthritis. *American Journal of Veterinary Research*, 70, 1201–1210.

Pavez, J.C., Hawkins, M.G., Pascoe, P.J., Knych, H.K., & Kass, P.H. (2011) Effect of fentanyl target-controlled infusions on isoflurane minimum anaesthetic concentration and cardiovascular function in red-tailed hawks (*Buteo jamaicensis*). *Veterinary Anaesthesia and Analgesia*, 38, 344–351.

Pickup, H.E., Cassidy, A.M., Danbury, T.C., Weeks, C.A., Waterman, A.E. & Kestin, S.C. (1997) Self selection of an analgesic by broiler chickens. *British Poultry Science Journal*, 38, S12–S13.

Pogatski-Zahn, E.M., & Zahn, P.K. From preemptive to preventive analgesia. (2006) *Current Opinions in Anaesthesiology.* 19(5), 551–555.

Qian, J., Brown, S.D., & Carlton, S.M. (1996) Systemic ketamine attenuates nociceptive behaviors in a rat model of peripheral neuropathy. *Brain Research,* 715, 51–62.

Reim, D.A. & Middleton, C.C. (1995) Use of butorphanol as an anesthetic adjunct in turkeys. *Laboratory Animal Science,* 45, 696–698.

Reiner, A., Brauth, S.E., Kitt, C.A., & Quirion, R. (1989) Distribution of mu, delta, and kappa opiate receptor types in the forebrain and midbrain of pigeons. *Journal of Comparative Neurology,* 280, 359–382.

Reiner, A., Davis, B., & Brecha, N. (1984) The distribution of enkephalin like immunoreactivity in the telencephalon of the adult and developing domestic chicken. *Journal of Comparative Neurology,* 228, 245–262.

Riggs, S.M., Hawkins, M.G., Craigmill, A.L., Kass, P.H., Stanley, S.D., & Taylor, I.T. (2008) Pharmacokinetics of butorphanol tartrate in red-tailed hawks (*Buteo jamaicensis*) and great horned owls (*Bubo virginianus*). *American Journal of Veterinary Research,* 69, 596–603.

Ritchie, B.W., Harrison, G.J., & Harrison, L.R. (1994) *Avian Medicine: Principles and Applications,* Wingers Publishing, Lake Worth, FL.

Samour, J.H., Jones, D.M., Knight, J.A., & Howlett, J.C. (1984) Comparative studies of the use of some injectable anesthetic agents in birds. *Veterinary Record,* 115, 6–11.

Sanchez-Migallon Guzman, D., Souza, M.J., Braun, J.M., Cox, S.K., Keuler, N.S., & Paul-Murphy, J.R. (2012) Antinociceptive effects after oral administration of tramadol hydrochloride in Hispaniolan Amazon parrots (*Amazona ventralis*). *American Journal of Veterinary Research,* 73(8), 1148–1152.

Schneider, C. (1961) Effects of morphine-like drugs in chicks. *Nature,* 191, 607–608.

Shaver, S.L., Robinson, N.G., Wright, B.D., Kratz, G.E., & Johnston, M.S. (2009) A multimodal approach to management of suspected neuropathic pain in a prairie falcon (*Falco mexicanus*). *Journal of Avian Medicine and Surgery,* 23, 209–213.

Sheehan, M.H. (2009) Opiate processes in poultry. *Archives of Medical Science,* 5, 626–636.

Singh, P.M., Johnson, C., Gartrell, B., Mitchinson, S., & Chambers, P. (2011) Pharmacokinetics of butorphanol in broiler chickens. *Veterinary Record,* 168, 588–591.

Sladky, K.K., Krugner-Higby, L., Meek-Walker, E., Heath, T.D., & Paul-Murphy, J. (2006) Serum concentrations and analgesic effects of liposome-encapsulated and standard butorphanol tartrate in parrots. *American Journal of Veterinary Research,* 67, 775–781.

Souza, M.J., Martin-Jimenez, T., Jones, M.P., & Cox, S.K. (2009) Pharmacokinetics of intravenous and oral tramadol in the bald eagle (*Haliaeetus leucocephalus*). *Journal of Avian Medicine and Surgery,* 23, 247–252.

Souza, M.J., Martin-Jimenez, T., Jones, M.P., & Cox, S.K. (2011) Pharmacokinetics of oral tramadol in red-tailed hawks (*Buteo jamaicensis*). *Journal of Veterinary Pharmacology and Therapeutics,* 34(1), 86–88.

Souza, M.J., Sanchez-Migallon Guzman, D., Paul-Murphy, J.R., & Cox, S.K. . (2012) Pharmacokinetics after oral and intravenous administration of a single dose of tramadol hydrochloride to Hispaniolan Amazon parrots (*Amazona ventralis*). *American Journal of Veterinary Research,* 73(8), 1142–1147.

Sufka, K.J. & Hughes, R.A. (1992) Time-dependant codeine hypoalgesia and hyperalgesia in domestic fowl. *Pharmacology Biochemistry and Behavior,* 41, 349–353.

Sufka, K.J., Hughes, R.A., & Giordano, J. (1991) Effects of selective opiate antagonists on morphine-induced hyperalgesia in domestic fowl. *Pharmacology Biochemistry and Behavior,* 38, 49–54.

Virtanen, R., Savola, J.M., & Saano, V. (1989) Highly selective and specific antagonism of central and peripheral alpha-2-adrenoceptors by atipamezole. *Archives Internationales De Pharmacodynamie Et De Therapie,* 297, 190–204.

Wessinger, W.D., Li, M., & McMillan, D.E. (2011) Drug discrimination in pigeons trained to discriminate among morphine, U50488, a combination of these drugs, and saline. *Behavioural Pharmacology,* 22, 468–479.

Wild, J.M., Krützfeldt, N.O., & Altshuler, D.L. (2010) Trigeminal and spinal dorsal horn (dis)continuity and avian evolution. *Brain, Behavior, and Evolution,* 76(1), 11–19.

Willis, W.D. (1979) Studies of the spinothalamic tract. *Texas Reports on Biology and Medicine,* 38, 1–45.

Willis, W.D. (2006) The somatosensory system, with emphasis on structures important for pain. *Brain Research Reviews,* 55, 297–313.

Wright, E.M., Marcella, K.L., Woodson, J.F. (1985) Animal pain and control. *Laboratory Animal,* 14, 20–36.

Wylie, L.M. & Gentle, M.J. (1998) Feeding-induced tonic pain suppression in the chicken: reversal by naloxone. *Physiology & Behavior,* 64, 27–30.

Zhang, S.H., Blech-Hermoni, Y., Faravelli, L., & Seltzer, Z. (2008) Ralfinamide administered orally before hind paw neurectomy or postoperatively provided long-lasting suppression of spontaneous neuropathic pain-related behavior in the rat. *Pain,* 139, 293–305.

Recognition and Treatment of Pain in Reptiles, Amphibians, and Fish

Lysa Pam Posner and Sathya K. Chinnadurai

Anesthesia and analgesia in ectotherms is a rapidly developing field, though much of the currently available information is anecdotal. Due to the difficulty of assessing pain in reptiles and amphibians and the paucity of literature, many potentially painful conditions are untreated or inappropriately treated. In a survey of members of the Association of Reptile and Amphibian Veterinarians, 98% of responding veterinarians stated that they believe reptiles feel pain; however, only 39% reported using analgesics in the majority of cases (Read, 2004). This survey also highlighted a lack of concern among reptile owners about the potential for pain and the need for analgesia. Veterinarians who feel that there is inadequate information about pain management in reptiles and amphibians may be less likely to emphasize analgesia to their clients.

PRESENCE OF A PAIN PATHWAY

A common excuse for not using analgesia in reptiles, amphibians, and fish is that these species do not have the neuroanatomic pathways sufficient for pain perception. While it is true that these animals possess a neuroanatomy that is different from mammals, all three groups possess nociceptors, an ascending neural pathway, and a higher brain center that is the primary target for that information (Machin, 2001; Sneddon, 2009a). All three groups show learned aversive behavior (Machin, 2001; Dunlop et al., 2006), and have descending modulatory pathways (Xia & Haddad, 2001; Brasel et al., 2008; Sneddon, 2009a). There is little doubt in the authors' minds that all animals in these groups experience pain and should, therefore, be treated with analgesics for situations that would be considered painful in mammals.

CONSEQUENCES OF PAIN

There is a large body of evidence that continued activation of the pain pathway produces clinically relevant physiological changes and increases morbidity and mortality (Stadler et al., 2004). Conversely, good pain management has been shown to decrease morbidity and mortality in humans and animals (Lun Tsui et al., 1997; Sellon et al., 2004). Activation of the pain pathway enhances the sympathetic nervous system and causes release of norepinephrine

(NE). The increase in NE results in an increase in cardiac output with a concurrent increase in myocardial work and oxygen demand; an increase in carbon dioxide production and work of breathing; a decrease in GI motility; and activation of the renin–angiotensin–aldosterone system, resulting in increased sodium and water retention. Additionally, increased production of cortisol impairs immunological and healing functions. The decrease in morbidity and mortality afforded by adequate pain management is probably due to the attenuation of metabolic demands and return of normal parasympathetic function. Most relevant research has been conducted in mammals; however, specific physiological responses have been documented in some species of fish (Roques et al., 2010) and, based on anatomy, it is reasonable to apply these findings to reptiles, amphibians, and other species of fish.

REPTILES AND AMPHIBIANS

As reptiles and amphibians grow in popularity as pet species, veterinarians must increase their knowledge of the diseases affecting these animals. The clinician must also be knowledgeable about the natural history of the patient's species when assessing its health, pain, and behavior. Reptile and amphibian taxa demonstrate diversity in behavior, environmental needs, anatomy, and physiology, and it is easy to make misguided extrapolations across species.

The configuration and sensitivity of the nociceptive pathways may vary with species to suit different evolutionary niches. For example, snakes possess cutaneous mechanoreceptors that can sense subtle vibrations from prey or shifting substrate but, because they possess few thermoreceptors, will allow themselves to be burned by heating elements in a cage (Proske, 1969; Mader, 2006). Such behavior often leads to the misconception that a reptile cannot feel pain or detect noxious stimuli, when the stimulus in question is vastly different from those to which the species is adapted.

Behavioral Components of Pain in Reptiles and Amphibians
Recognizing pain requires interaction of the clinician and the owner, and familiarity with the normal behavior of the given species and individual animal. Reptiles and amphibians can be very stoic patients from a clinician's perspective, and a poor understanding of

Pain Management in Veterinary Practice, First Edition. Edited by Christine M. Egger, Lydia Love and Tom Doherty.
© 2014 John Wiley & Sons, Inc. Published 2014 by John Wiley & Sons, Inc.

normal behaviors may hinder the assessment of an animal's pain status. The stress of captivity may make recognition and assessment of pain more difficult because the patient's fear of the clinician and hospital setting will cloud interpretation of normal behavior. In addition, prey species are adept at masking pain and stress responses. Furthermore, social animals, such as many anurans (e.g., frogs, toads), will not exhibit normal behavior when separated from conspecifics.

Injured or painful iguanas may be lethargic, hunch their backs, and hide. They may also become very aggressive and begin biting and whipping the tail. The authors have found that, without adequate analgesia, many iguanas become aggressive and resistant to handling postceliotomy. Some lizard and chelonian species with painful medical conditions, such as fractures or intestinal obstructions, will hold their heads elevated with the neck extended for long periods (Mayer & Bradley Bays, 2006). Many reptiles will recoil from a brief noxious stimulus and hide, but similar reactions are seen with sudden movement and sounds. Amphibians may respond to a focal stimulus by rubbing their skin with their forelimbs. This behavior is commonly seen with chemical irritants (Stevens, 2008). In addition, sick or distressed amphibians and chameleons will change color.

Inappetence may be a clinical sign of pain, though this sign can be extremely difficult to detect and interpret in reptiles. Reptiles may undergo periods of prolonged anorexia due to normal seasonal changes, housing at inappropriate temperatures, or being offered unsuitable food items. In addition, reptiles can go for prolonged periods of time without eating and maintain body weight, making it difficult for the clinician to notice, without a detailed history. Captive animals routinely fail to feed after excessive handling, changes in environment, and changes in diet type. Many reptile owners will fail to notice inappetence in their pets that normally only eat once or twice per month.

Many reptile and amphibian species are secretive, and their normal behavior involves hiding under substrate or in a hide box. This may make it difficult for the owner to assess the animal daily. Sick or injured animals may spend more time out of a hide box, or be unwilling to move around the enclosure to hide. Chelonians with either acute or chronic pain may spend much of their time hidden or retracted into their shells. Many reptile species are sedentary in captivity and difficult to assess in their enclosures; thus, lameness may also be missed by owners.

Sources of Pain

Pain can originate from a number of processes. Acute trauma, such as shell fractures, lacerations, and bites from prey or cage mates, may be common and straightforward to diagnose, but more subtle chronic problems may go unnoticed. Spondylosis and osteomyelitis of the spine occur frequently in aging reptiles. These conditions are often multifactorial in origin, but result in decreased mobility and pain, and may go undetected for months until there is obviously decreased function or when radiographs are taken for another reason (Mader & Stein, 2006). Upon diagnosis, chronic management of this pain is necessary using pharmacological treatment and environmental adjustments. Conditions such as coelomitis (peritonitis) are considered to be extremely painful in mammals, which often present acutely for pain. In reptiles, such conditions may go unnoticed until the animal is moribund, and pain management should be implemented while the animal is being stabilized with appropriate fluids and antibiotics.

As mentioned previously, very sensitive mechanoreceptors are found in the skin of snakes. The chelonian shell, once thought to be an inert protective structure, may also be an important sensory organ. Turtles are able to detect subtle stimuli such as scratching and tapping of the shell, and can discern the location of the stimulus (Rosenberg, 1986). This suggests a fine degree of sensation on the surface of the shell, and trauma or infection of the shell is likely to result in pain. Articular gout occurs in reptiles fed diets high in animal protein, and may be related to inadequate hydration. Poorly soluble monosodium urate crystals precipitate out of the blood into joints, and granulomas form around the crystals. Humans report debilitating pain with articular gout. Treatment for articular gout in reptiles is prolonged and often incomplete, highlighting the need for multimodal analgesia in these patients.

Reptile-specific painful conditions include thermal burns from heat sources, because these animals often lie on a heat source until tissue sloughing has occurred. Addressing these burns can be tricky. The animal has obviously not responded to the thermal stimulus of the heat rock, but may respond when the damaged skin is being treated and debrided, indicating different responses to different noxious stimuli (Mader, 2006).

Experimental Studies

The clear difference in response to different types of noxious stimuli highlights the difficulty in assessing pain (or nociception) in an experimental setting. Recent antinociceptive studies in reptiles have utilized hindlimb thermal withdrawal latency, reduction of the minimum anesthetic concentration (MAC) of isoflurane, and electrostimulation, to assess the efficacy of certain drugs (Mosley et al., 2003; Greenacre et al., 2006; Sladky et al., 2007; Sladky et al., 2008). In addition, one study examined postoperative physiological variables such as heart rate, blood pressure, and cortisol concentrations (Olesen et al., 2008). As with mammals, a single experimental stimulus cannot simulate all painful stimuli, and the results of analgesia studies must be carefully interpreted and applied to each clinical patient.

Assessing the Quality of Life

Quality of life determination in reptiles and amphibians is extremely challenging. Many animals continue to eat and ambulate with injuries that would render a human incapacitated. Given the slow healing rate of many ectotherms, treatment and resolution of a disease condition must be extended, and the provision of adequate analgesia during that time must be strongly considered. When dealing with injured or sick wildlife, the likelihood of full return to function should also be considered. In some cases, the potential for prolonged pain is so high that humane euthanasia is the only ideal treatment.

DRUG CHOICES FOR REPTILES (TABLE 38.1)

Opioids

Some of the most exciting recent discoveries in the field of reptile analgesia have involved opioid analgesics. Response to opioids suggests that μ opioid receptors are present and functional in multiple species, including crocodilians, chelonians, and frogs (Kanui & Hole, 1992; Stevens et al., 1996; Sladky et al., 2007).

Table 38.1. Analgesics in Reptile Species

Drug	Reptile species	Dose	Comments	Data type	Reference
Opioids					
Morphine	Red-eared sliders	1.5 mg/kg IM	Respiratory depression	Ex	Sladky et al., 2007
	Corn snakes	Up to 40 mg/kg	Uncertain analgesic effect	Ex	Sladky et al., 2008
	Bearded dragons	10–20 mg/kg IM		Ex	Sladky et al., 2008
	Green iguana	1 mg/kg IM		Ex	Greenacre et al., 2006
Butorphanol	Ball python	5 mg/kg	No analgesic effect	Ex	Olesen et al., 2008
	Red-eared sliders	Up to 28 mg/kg	No analgesic effect	Ex	Sladky et al., 2007
	Bearded dragons	Up to 28 mg/kg	No analgesic effect	Ex	Sladky et al., 2008
Fentanyl	Prehensile tailed skinks	1cm^2 of a 25 µg/h TD patch	Effects not reported	PK	Gamble, 2008
Buprenorphine	Red-eared sliders	0.05 mg/kg SC in forelimbs	Effects not reported	PK	Kummrow et al., 2008
NSAIDs					
Ketoprofen	Green iguana	2 mg/kg IV or IM	Effects not reported	PK	Tuttle et al., 2009
Meloxicam	Green iguana	0.2 mg/kg PO, SC, IM, IV; q48h	Effects not reported	PK (IV, PO) A (SC, IM)	Hernandez-Divers et al., 2010
	Ball python	0.3 mg/kg IM	No analgesic effect	Ex	Olesen et al., 2008

Reported dosages of analgesic drugs in reptiles based on prospective studies. Note that pharmacokinetic studies (PK) alone do not demonstrate analgesic effect.

PK, pharmacokinetic; A, anecdotal; Ex, experimental trial.

Traditionally, severe pain in reptiles has been treated with the kappa agonist butorphanol because of the literature stating its efficacy in birds (Schumacher & Yelen, 2006). Recent literature has critically evaluated the efficacy of butorphanol in chelonians, snakes, and lizards. In a MAC reduction model, butorphanol failed to decrease the MAC of isoflurane in green iguanas (Mosley et al., 2003). Using a thermal withdrawal latency model, even high doses of butorphanol (up to 28 mg/kg IM) did not affect time to withdrawal for 24 hours post injection in freshwater turtles, whereas high- (6.5 mg/kg IM) and low-dose morphine (1.5 mg/kg IM) increased thermal thresholds for >24 hours post injection. Maximal effect was seen at 8 hours for both dosages. High-dose morphine only exceeded low-dose morphine during the first 4 hours, and the difference was insignificant after 8 hours (Sladky et al., 2007).

High doses of morphine (10 and 20 mg/kg) increased thermal thresholds for >24 hours post injection in bearded dragons, and the maximal effect was recorded between 2 and 8 hours for both dosages. For snakes, only a very high dose of butorphanol (20 mg/kg) altered thermal withdrawal latency, again with peak effect at 8 hours. Inconsistent results with morphine in corn snakes precluded usable conclusions. The authors recommend 10–20 mg/kg morphine in bearded dragons, and do not make a recommendation for corn snakes (Sladky et al., 2008).

The potential for respiratory depression with opioids is high. Butorphanol and morphine at high doses severely impaired ventilation in turtles (Sladky et al., 2007). The authors recommend administering IM morphine 1–2 hours prior to a painful procedure to allow for peak efficacy, and to allow the clinician to assess the sedation and respiratory depression caused by the drug prior to inducing general anesthesia. The authors have noted prolonged apnea in patients after general anesthesia when morphine was administered

intraoperatively, and have had to administer naloxone to reverse the respiratory depression. This is not ideal, as the analgesia is also reversed.

The ideal dosing regimen for morphine in reptiles is unknown, as there are probably species differences and differences in the level of analgesia needed for different disease processes. Currently, there is no evidence that butorphanol is analgesic in any reptile species at any studied dose. Pharmacokinetic data are available for two other µ opioid agonists, buprenorphine in red-eared sliders (Kummrow et al., 2008) and transdermal fentanyl in prehensile-tailed skinks (Gamble, 2008). Based on the promising pharmacokinetic data, both of these drugs have potential for use in reptiles but must be evaluated with an experimental pain model.

Local Anesthetics

Local anesthetics have been used extensively for wound debridement, biopsy collection, and abscess drainage in reptiles, but studies on efficacy and toxicity are lacking. Directed local anesthesia (1 mg/kg of 2% mepivicaine), with the aid of a nerve locator, has been used for mandibular nerve blocks in a number of crocidilian species (Wellehan et al., 2006). Perineural application of local anesthetic to any nerve will provide anesthesia and analgesia to the area innervated by the nerve; thus, good knowledge of neuroanatomy will help guide placement of local anesthetic blocks in reptiles, chelonians, and amphibians.

Nonsteroidal Anti-inflammatory Drugs

Multiple nonsteroidal anti-inflammatory drugs (NSAIDs) are widely used in reptiles without experimental evidence of efficacy. The pharmacokinetic behavior of IV and IM ketoprofen has been evaluated in green iguanas (Tuttle et al., 2009). Meloxicam and

Table 38.2.   Analgesics in amphibian species

Drug	Amphibian species	Dose	Side Effects	Data type	Reference
Opioids					
Morphine	Northern Leopard Frog	30–100 mg/kg	None reported	Ex	Pezalla, 1983
Fentanyl	Northern Leopard Frog	1 mg/kg SC	None reported	Ex	Stevens, 1996
Alpha-2 agonists					
Dexmedetomidine	Northern Leopard Frog	120 mg/kg SC	None reported	Ex	Brenner et al., 1994

Reported dosages of analgesic drugs in amphibians based on prospective studies. Note that pharmacokinetic studies (PK) alone do not demonstrate the analgesic effect.

PK, pharmacokinetic; A, anecdotal; Ex, experimental trial.

ketoprofen are widely used in reptiles with no reported adverse effects (Hernandez-Divers et al., 2010; Carpenter et al., 2005). The only study evaluating the analgesic effects of meloxicam in snakes showed no effect on postoperative cortisol, heart rate, or blood pressure in ball pythons (Olesen et al. 2008).

ANALGESIC DRUG CHOICES IN AMPHIBIANS (TABLE 38.2)

The biochemical properties of amphibian skin allow interesting opportunities and challenges for medication. Any topical drug applied to an amphibian should be considered to have some degree of systemic uptake. This increases the risk for systemic toxicity with topical analgesics, such as local anesthetics, but it also allows for ease of drug administration.

Opioids

In amphibians, withdrawal latencies to multiple stimuli were increased with systemic and spinal administration of morphine, as well as numerous endogenous opioids, and this effect was reversible with naloxone (Stevens et al., 1996; Willenbring & Stevens, 1995). Endogenous opioid production in frogs is downregulated during hibernation and cold, and hibernating amphibians may demonstrate decreased pain tolerance (Suckow et al., 1999). In laboratory settings, μ agonists such as morphine (30–100 mg/kg IM, SC, or topically), provide analgesia that peaks at 60–90 minutes, with minimal reported adverse effects. The seemingly high doses of morphine administered to frogs typically do not result in depression of CNS or motor function, and feeding behavior and normal activity are maintained. Chronic administration of opioids to frogs has resulted in a decreased response to the opioid over time, suggesting the development of tolerance (Stevens et al., 1996).

α-2 Agonists

α-2 agonists have been investigated in a number of experimental studies in amphibians. Dose-dependent analgesia has been noted with dexmedetomidine, and the analgesic effects are reversible with atipamezole. Interestingly, subcutaneously administered dexmedetomidine provides analgesia in amphibians similar to that which would be expected in mammals, but without notable sedation (Brenner et al., 1994).

FISH

Teleost (bony) fish are common pets, aquarium inhabitants, and research subjects, but analgesia in fish has rarely been investigated. Pharmacokinetic data exists on many analgesic drugs, but there is little information on the pharmacodynamic properties of these drugs. Furthermore, dosing intervals are almost impossible to extrapolate, regardless of existing pharmacokinetic data, due to huge variability among species; for example, trout clear morphine approximately twice as fast as flounder (Newby et al., 2006). Regardless of the species variability, teleost fish would need less frequent dosing than mammals, as the half-life ($t_{1/2}$) of morphine was ~34 hours and ~14 hours in flounder and trout, respectively (Newby et al., 2006).

Recognition of Pain in Fish

Assessment of pain in fish is challenging due to the lack of clear pain-related behaviors, and the difficulty in acquiring physiological parameters such as heart rate. Nonspecific parameters including gilling rate, height in the water column, or appetite have been used as indirect markers of pain and discomfort. Although those parameters might be demonstrated in fish in pain, they are not specific for pain. Caution should be used when interpreting scientific studies, as many assess safety but not analgesia.

Sources of Pain in Fish

Fish possess extensive peripheral nociceptors, a large proportion of which are located in the head (Sneddon, 2009a). It is therefore reasonable to assume that lesions or injuries, which would be considered painful in mammals, should also be considered painful for fish. Surgical incisions, extensive skin lesions (chemical, infectious, wounds), and trauma to the mouth (e.g., from a fishhook) should all be considered painful, and fish should be provided adequate analgesia.

ANALGESIC DRUG CHOICES IN FISH (TABLE 38.3)

Opioids

Fish possess mu, kappa, and delta opioid receptors (Sneddon, 2009a). Presently, only the μ and kappa receptors are manipulated clinically in any species. Morphine is the μ opioid agonist that has been most widely studied in fish. There is extensive pharmacokinetic evaluation of morphine in many species, but only a few that indicate morphine reduces nociception in fish (Sneddon, 2003; Jones et al., 2012; Ward et al., 2012). In a recent dose–response study in rainbow trout, the response (movement of the fins or tail) to a noxious stimulus (electrical shock to the face region) was monitored before and after a dose of morphine was administered

Table 38.3.   Analgesics in fish species

Drug	Fish species	Dose	Data type	Reference
Opioids				
Morphine	Winter flounder *Pseudopleuronectes americanus*	40 mg/kg IP	Ex	Newby et al., 2006
Morphine	Rainbow trout *Oncorhynchus mykiss*	30 mg/kg	Ex	Sneddon et al., 2003
Morphine	Sarasa comet goldfish *Carassius auratus*	10, 20, 40 mg/kg IM	Ex	Ward, 2009
Morphine	Winter flounder *Pseudopleuronectes americanus*	40 mg/kg IP	PK	Newby et al., 2006
Morphine	Rainbow trout *Oncorhynchus mykiss*	40 mg/kg IP	PK	Newby et al., 2006
Butorphanol	Koi carp *Cyprinus carpio*	0.4 mg/kg IM	Ex	Harms et al., 2005
NSAIDs				
Ketoprofen	Koi carp *Cyprinus carpio*	2 mg/kg IM	A	Harms et al., 2005
Ketoprofen	Sarasa comet goldfish *Carassius auratus*	0.05–2 mg/kg IM	Ex	Ward et al., 2012

Reported dosages of analgesic drugs in fish in prospective studies. Note that pharmacokinetic studies (PK) alone do not demonstrate analgesic effect.

PK, pharmacokinetic; A, anecdotal; Ex, experimental trial.

intraperitoneally. The ED50 for morphine was 6.7 ± 0.8 mg/kg and the corresponding plasma morphine concentration was 4.1 ± 1.5 mg/L (Jones et al., 2012).

Butorphanol is commonly used in fish; however, there are few analgesic studies and, to the authors' knowledge, only one that indicates butorphanol reduces pain-associated behaviors in fish (Harms et al., 2005).

α-2 Agonists

α-2 adrenergic receptors have been identified in the brain of zebrafish (Ampatzis et al., 2008). They mediate sedation (Ruuskanen et al., 2005), as they do in other species, but there is little objective evidence regarding analgesia in fish.

NSAIDs

Although teleost fish possess an inflammatory pathway, and NSAIDs decrease inflammatory markers (Harms et al., 2005), there is conflicting evidence as to whether NSAIDs provide analgesia to fish (Harms et al., 2005; Ward et al., 2012). However, the authors routinely use ketoprofen in fish after painful procedures.

NONPHARMACOLOGICAL PAIN MANAGEMENT

Pain management does not end at pharmacological manipulation of the patient. Adjunctive therapy can provide pain relief and minimize further tissue damage; for example, stabilization of shell fractures may decrease discomfort due to mobile bone fragments (Figure 38.1).

Reptiles and amphibians should be kept within their species preferred optimal temperature zone. When ectotherms are kept at inappropriate ambient temperatures wound healing is delayed and drug pharmacokinetics are unpredictable (Mader & Stein, 2006).

Hypothermia has been used as a means of immobilization for reptiles and is believed, by some, to provide adequate analgesia for painful procedures. Any desensitization that occurs with hypothermia is reversed when the patient is returned to its normal body temperature. There is no evidence of lasting analgesia, and the detrimental effect on wound healing and immune competence have

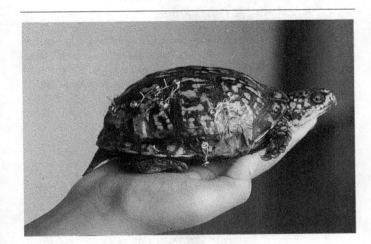

Figure 38.1.   Adjunctive therapy can provide pain relief and minimize further tissue damage; for example, stabilization of shell fractures may decrease discomfort due to mobile bone fragments.

rendered hypothermia an outdated and inadequate means of anesthesia or analgesia, and is not recommended by the authors.

SUMMARY

Reptiles, amphibians and fish have the neuroanatomy necessary to perceive pain. Additionally, they possess descending modulatory pathways and express behavioral changes that would be indicative of pain in mammals. It is, therefore, logical to conclude that these species experience pain and should be provided analgesia when appropriate. Treatment of pain in reptiles, amphibians, and fish should be specific for the animal in question, and care should be taken when trying to extrapolate drug efficacy or dose.

REFERENCES

Ampatzis, K., Kentouri, M., & Dermon, C.R. (2008) Neuronal and glial localization of alpha(2A)-adrenoceptors in the adult zebrafish (*Danio rerio*) brain. *Journal of Comparative Neurology*, 508, 72–93.

Brasel, C.M., Sawyer, G.W., & Stevens, C.W. (2008) A pharmacological comparison of the cloned frog and human mu opioid receptors reveals differences in opioid affinity and function. *European Journal of Pharmacology*, 599, 36–43.

Brenner, G., Klopp, A., Deason, L., & Stevens, C.W. (1996) Analgesic potency of alpha adrenergic agents after systemic administration in amphibians. *Journal of Pharmacology and Experimental Therapeutics*, 270, 540.

Carpenter, J., Mashima, T., & Rupiper, D. (2005) *Exotic animal formulary*, Elsevier Saunders, Philadelphia, PA.

Dunlop, R., Millsopp, S., & Laming, P. (2006) Avoidance learning in goldfish (*Carassius auratus*) and trout (*Oncorhynchus mykiss*) and implications for pain perception. *Applied Animal Behaviour Science*, 97, 255–271.

Gamble, K. (2008) Transdermal fentanyl plasma concentrations in prehensile-tailed skinks (*Corucia zebrata*). *Journal of Herpetological Medicine and Surgery*, 18, 81–85.

Greenacre, C., Takle, G., & Schumacher, J. (2006) Comparative antinociception of morphine, butorphanol, and buprenorphine versus saline in the green iguana (*Iguana iguana*), using electrostimulation. *Journal of Herpetological Medicine and Surgery*, 16, 88–92.

Harms, C.A., Lewbart, G.A., Swanson, C.R., Kishimori, J.M., & Boylan, S.M. (2005) Behavioral and clinical pathology changes in koi carp (*Cyprinus carpio*) subjected to anesthesia and surgery with and without intra-operative analgesics. *Comparative Medicine*, 55, 221–226.

Hernandez-Divers, S., McBride, M., Koch, T., et al. (2010) Single-dose oral and intravenous pharmacokinetics of meloxicam in the green iguana (*Iguana iguana*). *American Journal of Veterinary Research*, 71(11), 1277–1283.

Jones, S.G., Kamunde, C., Lemke, K., & Stevens, E.D. (2012) The dose-response relation for the antinociceptive effect of morphine in a fish, rainbow trout. *Journal of Veterinary Pharmacology and Therapeutics*, 35, 563–570

Kanui, T. & Hole, K. (1992) Morphine and pethidine antinociception in the crocodile. *Journal of Veterinary Pharmacology and Therapeutics*, 15, 101.

Kummrow, M. S., Tseng, F., Hesse, L., & Court, M. (2008) Pharmacokinetics of buprenorphine after single-dose subcutaneous administration in red-eared sliders (Trachemys scripta elegans). *Journal of Zoo and Wildlife Medicine*, 39, 590–595.

Lun Tsui, S., Law, S., Fok, M., et al. (1997) Postoperative analgesia reduces mortality and morbidity after esophagectomy. *The American Journal of Surgery*, 173, 472–478.

Machin, K. L. (2001) Fish, amphibian, and reptile analgesia. *Veterinary Clinics of North America Exotic Animal Practice*, 4, 19–33.

Mader, D. (2006). Thermal burns, in *Reptile Medicine and Surgery*, Saunders Elsevier Inc., St. Louis, MO, 916–923.

Mader, D. & Stein, G. (2006). *Reptile Medicine and Surgery*, Saunders Elsevier Inc., St. Louis, MO.

Mayer, J. & Bradley Bays, T. (eds) (2006). Reptile behavior, in *Exotic Pet Behavior: Birds, Reptiles, and Small Mammals*. Saunders Elsevier Inc., St. Louis, MO.

Mosley, C., Dyson, D., & Smith, D. (2003). Minimum alveolar concentration of isoflurane in green iguanas and the effect of butorphanol on minimum alveolar concentration. *Journal of the American Veterinary Medical Association*, 222, 1559–1564.

Newby, N.C., Mendonca, P.C., Gamperl, K., & Stevens, E.D. (2006) Pharmacokinetics of morphine in fish: winter flounder (Pseudopleuronectes americanus) and seawater-acclimated rainbow trout (Oncorhynchus mykiss). *Comparative Biochemistry and Physiology C Toxicology Pharmacology*, 143, 275–283.

Olesen, M.G., Bertelsen, M.F., Perry, S.F., & Wang, T. (2008) Effects of preoperative administration of butorphanol or meloxicam on physiologic responses to surgery in ball pythons. *Journal of the American Veterinary Medical Association*, 233, 1883–1888.

Pezalla, P.D. (1983) Morphine-induced analgesia and explosive motor behavior in an amphibian. *Brain Research*, 273, 297–305.

Proske, U. (1969) Vibration-sensitive mechanoreceptors in snake skin. *Experimental Neurology*, 23, 187–194.

Read, M. (2004) Evaluation of the use of anesthesia and analgesia in reptiles. *Journal of the American Veterinary Medical Association*, 224, 547–552.

Roques, J.A., Abbink, W., Geurds, F., van de Vis, H., Flik, G. (2010) Tailfin clipping, a painful procedure: studies on Nile tilapia and common carp. *Physiology & Behavior*, 101(4), 533–540.

Rosenberg, M. (1986) Carapace and plastron sensitivity to touch and vibration in the tortoise (*Testudo hermanni* and *T. graeca*). *Journal of Zoology*, 208, 443–455.

Ruuskanen, J.O., Peitsaro, N., Kaslin, J.V., Panula, P., & Scheinin, M. (2005) Expression and function of alpha-adrenoceptors in zebrafish: drug effects, mRNA and receptor distributions. *Journal of Neurochemistry*, 94, 1559–1569.

Schumacher, J. & Yelen, T. (2006) Anesthesia and analgesia, in *Reptile Medicine and Surgery*, (ed. D.R. Mader), Saunders Elsevier Inc., St Louis, MO, pp. 442–452.

Sellon, D.C., Roberts, M.C., Blikslager, A.T., Ulibarri, C., & Papich, M.G. (2004) Effects of continuous rate intravenous infusion of butorphanol on physiologic and outcome variables in horses after celiotomy. *Journal of Veterinary Internal Medicine*, 18, 555–563.

Sladky, K.K., Kinney, M.E., & Johnson, S.M. (2008) Analgesic efficacy of butorphanol and morphine in bearded dragons and corn snakes. *Journal of the American Veterinary Medical Association*, 233, 267–273.

Sladky, K.K., Miletic, V., Paul-Murphy, J., Kinney, M.E., Dallwig, R.K., & Johnson, S.M. (2007) Analgesic efficacy and respiratory effects of butorphanol and morphine in turtles. *Journal of the American Veterinary Medical Association*, 230, 1356–1362.

Sneddon, L.U. (2003) The evidence for pain in fish: the use of morphine as an analgesic. *Applied Animal Behaviour Science*, 83, 153–162.

Sneddon, L.U. (2009a). Pain perception in fish: indicators and endpoints. *ILAR Journal*, 50, 338–342.

Stadler, M., Schlander, M., Braeckman, M., Nguyen, T., & Boogaerts, J.G. (2004) A cost-utility and cost-effectiveness analysis of an acute pain service. *Journal of Clinical Anesthesia*, 16, 159–167.

Stevens, C. (2008) Nonmammalian models for the study of pain, in *Sourcebook of Models for Biomedical Research* (ed. P.M. Conn), Humana Press Inc., Totowa, NJ, pp. 341–352.

Stevens, C., Klopp, A., & Facello, J. (1994) Analgesic potency of mu and kappa opioids after systemic administration in amphibians. *Journal of Pharmacology and Experimental Therapeutics*, 269, 1086.

Suckow, M., Terril, L., Grigdesby, C., & March, P.A. (1999) Evaluation of hypothermia-induced analgesia and influence of opioid antagonists in Leopard frogs (*Rana pipiens*). *Pharmacology Biochemistry and Behavior*, 63, 39–43.

Tuttle, A.D., Papich, M., Lewbart, G.A., Christian, S., Gunkel, C., & Harms, C.A. (2009) Pharmacokinetics of ketoprofen in the green iguana (*Iguana iguana*) following single intravenous and intramuscular injections. *Journal of Zoo and Wildlife Medicine*, 37, 567–570.

Ward, J.L., McCartney, S.P., Chinnadurai, S.K., & Posner, L.P. (2012) Development of a minimum-anesthetic-concentration depression model to study the effects of various analgesics in goldfish (Carassius auratus). *Journal of Zoo and Wildlife Medicine,* 43(2):214–222.

Wellehan, J., Gunkel, C., Kledzik, D., Robertson, S.A., & Heard, D.J. (2006) Use of a nerve locator to facilitate administration of mandibular nerve blocks in crocodilians. *Journal of Zoo and Wildlife Medicine*, 37, 405–408.

Willenbring, S. & Stevens, C.W. (1995) Thermal, mechanical and chemical peripheral sensation in amphibians: opioid and adrenergic effects. *Life Sciences*, 58, 125–133.

Xia, Y. & Haddad, G.G. (2001) Major difference in the expression of delta- and mu-opioid receptors between turtle and rat brain. *Journal of Comparative Neurology*, 436, 202–210.

Section 5
Incorporating Pain Management into Your Practice and Hospice and Palliative Care

Pain Management in Veterinary Practice, First Edition. Edited by Christine M. Egger, Lydia Love and Tom Doherty.
© 2014 John Wiley & Sons, Inc. Published 2014 by John Wiley & Sons, Inc.

39
Integrating Pain Management into Veterinary Practice

Robin Downing

The veterinary profession has begun to make pain management a priority, and in 2007 the American Animal Hospital Association (AAHA) and the American Association of Feline Practitioners (AAFP) copublished pain management guidelines for dogs and cats. The AAHA/AAFP pain management guidelines for dogs and cats advocate that patients be evaluated for pain at each visit to the veterinarian, no matter the reason for the visit. The AAHA Standards for Accreditation (2011) mandate that pain assessment be performed on every patient and the result recorded in the medical record (www.aahanet.org).

Veterinary practitioners and healthcare team members have an obligation to look for, recognize, assess, prevent, and treat pain in animals, and this needs to become part of the culture of the veterinary practice. Pain should be considered the fifth vital sign, after temperature, pulse, respiratory rate, and blood pressure, and every veterinary patient should be evaluated for pain every time it is examined. When pain assessment tools are chosen, every member of the veterinary team must be trained in their use. Even team members who will not routinely evaluate patients for pain or whose jobs do not include technical patient interactions (e.g., client care specialists) must understand how pain is assessed. A consistent message from the team is essential to achieving client compliance (AAHA, 2003).

Effective pain prevention and management strategies benefit all parties in the veterinary caregiving equation. The patient benefits by escaping the suffering and physical detriments of the pain experience, and the patient and the pet owner benefit through enhancement of the human–animal bond. Pain management makes animals less likely to strike out, enhancing safety for the veterinary healthcare team. Improved patient comfort provides tangible rewards to members of the team, including improved job satisfaction and morale, pride in one's education and work, and pride in fulfilling the obligations of the veterinarian's oath.

BUILDING INFRASTRUCTURE AND CREATING CULTURE

Pain management is good medicine and good medicine is good business. The key to successfully integrating pain management strategies and practices is to create infrastructure that identifies pain recognition and management as priorities of the practice. Creating the systems that support pain management takes planning and demands strategic thinking, but the rewards are far-reaching. The details of pain recognition and specific pain management tools and strategies may be found elsewhere in this text and in the recommended readings and references listed at the end of this chapter.

Make a Plan
Planning is critical to the success of integrating pain management into a veterinary practice, and to succeed fiscally it is necessary to develop a business plan. The focus of the practice (companion animal, mixed practice, equine, exotics, food, and fiber species) will determine which products, equipment, and supplies are most appropriate. Effective pain management protocols mandate the inclusion of opioid analgesics and other controlled substances; thus, storage and record-keeping procedures that are in alignment with legal requirements must be in place. Understanding that pain is best managed from a multimodal perspective, a complement of adjunctive treatments, for example, medications, nutritional products, disease-modifying agents, and nutraceuticals, should be available. It may be desirable to add certain technologies to assist in delivering comprehensive pain management services, for example, therapeutic laser, electroacupuncture, or physical therapy.

Choose Appropriate Pain Scoring Tools
Pain scoring provides the opportunity to track trends during treatment, gauges the success of the treatment plan, and provides the opportunity to fine-tune the pain management protocol. Pain scoring tools should be chosen to aid in assessing patient pain in various contexts, including the outpatient wellness examination, the postsurgical setting, and the chronic pain patient (e.g., osteoarthritis). The ideal pain scoring system is user-friendly, validated in the target species, and overcomes interobserver differences.

Although validated pain scoring options in veterinary species are limited, it is critical not to be immobilized by the lack of a perfect pain scoring instrument; veterinary healthcare team members must start somewhere in scoring pain in their patients. Something as simple as a 0–10 scale (10 = the worst possible pain)

Pain Management in Veterinary Practice, First Edition. Edited by Christine M. Egger, Lydia Love and Tom Doherty.
© 2014 John Wiley & Sons, Inc. Published 2014 by John Wiley & Sons, Inc.

pain scoring is adequate for many practice situations. Colorado State University has developed interactive acute pain scales, available online at: (http://csuanimalcancercenter.org/anesthesia-pain-management), that are easily applied to dogs and cats in a busy clinical setting (Hellyer et al., 2006a, 2006b).

Develop Pain Management Protocols

Pain management protocols should be developed for acute and chronic pain patients to provide structure, focus, and continuity of care. Acute pain management protocols should include a designated pain scoring system for acute pain; consistent quantification of pain using the designated scoring system (i.e., what constitutes a 3/10 or a 7/10); provision of pre-emptive, multimodal pain management; and a plan for frequency of reassessment and how breakthrough pain will be handled. Patients should be reassessed frequently in the immediate postoperative period in order to fine-tune the pain management protocol. Assessment should be active, involving palpation of the area near the surgical site as well as interaction with the patient. Chronically painful patients require a different set of pain management templates and protocols than those needed by patients experiencing acute pain. These patients can be difficult to treat and also need to be regularly reassessed to allow for fine-tuning of pain management strategies.

Training

Training must target three distinct groups: veterinarians in the practice, the veterinary healthcare team, and clients. Fortunately, excellent training is available for veterinarians and veterinary technicians in the form of recently written textbooks, online seminars and webinars, and live training events. In addition to the more formal training opportunities, in-house training is a critical component of success in integrating pain management into everyday practice. Regular team meetings, during which a single and specific aspect of pain management is discussed, is a great place to start. For instance, the practice's perioperative balanced analgesic protocol may serve as the focus for a meeting to review current techniques, assess efficacy and patient comfort, and make appropriate modifications. Another example is the education of the team in the use of the chosen pain scoring systems for acute and chronic pain. Through on-site training, the variability among pain observers can be significantly minimized.

Clients, too, must be trained in the basic principles of pain recognition and management and the strategies applied to painful patients, so that they may appreciate how their animals will benefit. In order to enhance communication with clients, everyone on the healthcare team must be adequately trained to present pain management plans, once developed by the veterinarian, and be capable of appropriate support and follow-up with clients. This enhances the practice's credibility, reinforcing to clients that the practice team has their animal's best interest at heart.

Build Awareness

There is really no better way to make pain management a priority than to practice pain assessments on every animal that is presented. By evaluating every patient, members of the veterinary healthcare team become comfortable with the response of a normal, non-painful animal during an examination, thus enhancing their ability to recognize those animals that are painful.

It is important to be cognizant of the commonly encountered medical conditions and procedures that have an easily overlooked

Table 39.1. Unexpected, unintentional, and often overlooked causes of pain

Abdominocentesis
Abscessation
Acute renal failure
Anal sac infection or rupture
Bandage changes
Cancer
Corneal disease
Glaucoma
Hemorrhagic gastroenteritis
IV catheter placement
Megacolon
Obstipation
Oral tumors
Osteoarthritis
Otitis
Pancreatitis
Paraneoplastic syndrome
Pulmonary edema
Pleural effusion
Pleuritis
Resorptive lesions—teeth
Restraint of a painful patient
Stomatitis
Thoracocentesis
Urinary catheterization
Urinary obstruction
Wound management

Adapted from American Animal Hospital Association, American Association of Feline Practitioners, AAHA/AAFP Pain Management Guidelines Task Force Members, et al. (2007) AAHA/AAFP pain management guidelines for dogs and cats. *Journal of the American Animal Hospital Association*, 43, 235–248.

pain component, and to raise awareness of these issues among all members of the practice (Table 39.1). The next step is to implement strategies to prevent discomfort and relieve existing pain. For example, restraint of animals with osteoarthritis or musculoskeletal pain for radiographic positioning on hard radiology tables can be very uncomfortable, and a small intravenous (IV) dose of a full μ-agonist opioid or buprenorphine may be enough to decrease the pet's anxiety and to prevent acute pain as a result of positioning and handling. The addition of a sedative, such as an α-2 agonist, unless contraindicated, provides additional sedation, analgesia, and anxiolysis. Another commonly ignored source of discomfort is IV catheter placement, which can be made less unpleasant with the application of EMLA® (2.5% prilocaine/2.5% lidocaine) cream to the shaved catheter site under an occlusive bandage 15 to 20 minutes prior to catheter placement.

Implementation

The most effective way to become good at a particular technique or skill is to use it; however, trying to change too many things at once can lead to frustration and failure. Effectively integrating pain management into a veterinary practice is best accomplished systematically. Identify particular aspects on which to focus, rank these accordingly, and create specific plans to address them. For example, expanding and enhancing perioperative pain management makes an excellent first focus. A practical way to develop a compassion-driven perioperative, pre-emptive pain management strategy for surgical patients is to consider all the small steps included in the most commonly performed routine surgical procedures, for example, ovariohysterectomy or castration, and identify the times during the procedure when pain could be induced. Next, determine what can be done to prevent pain at those specific times. Finally, practice those pain preventive procedures and assess the results.

Once the routine surgical procedures have been modified to include expanded pain management options, the less routine procedures should be addressed; particularly orthopedic surgery or major soft tissue procedures that are often performed on patients that are compromised in some way (e.g., exploratory laparotomy, amputation, or large tumor removal). Many of these procedures warrant more advanced pain management techniques, such as epidurals, continuous rate infusions, and regional nerve blocks.

Chronically Painful Patients

Once a veterinary practice commits to assessing every patient for pain at every visit many conditions associated with pain are discovered. Because animals are so adept at continuing activities of daily living in spite of discomfort, painful pets may present without client knowledge of their pain. It is critical to ask open-ended questions to allow clients to give "clues" that may lead to pain identification. Client comments that raise suspicion about the possibility of pain include:

- "He's getting old"
- "She's slowing down"
- "We've had to shorten our walks"
- "He doesn't jump up on the couch anymore"
- "She's not grooming herself as well" (cats)

These animals require a more careful assessment specifically for pain. It is critical to identify all the sites at which the pet is painful, and determine, to the greatest degree possible, where the primary issue resides. Remember that chronically painful animals may also present with acute pain.

For the animal with chronic pain, it is critical to maintain ongoing contact with the owners and conduct frequent assessments once a pain management strategy is initiated. Each chronically painful patient is unique in its presentation, progression, and needs. The nature of chronic pain is that it changes over time. Many of the conditions that lead to chronic pain are progressive, for example, osteoarthritis, and that means there is a high probability for chronic pain to escalate. Likewise, most chronic pain patients are older and may suffer from or develop concomitant disease. The veterinary healthcare team must remain alert to changes in chronically painful patients that may seem to have nothing to do with the patient's pain issues. In order to best address chronic pain, the patient must be kept in good health with appropriate management of all comorbidities. A chronic pain protocol template that includes plans for the timing of pain reassessments and adjustments to the pain plan should be implemented.

Because managing chronic pain is complex, the veterinary healthcare team must do everything possible to assist the client with implementation and compliance. One strategy for maximizing the client's ability to provide the prescribed care is to schedule the next reassessment before the client leaves. This ensures continuity and consistency in the necessary modifications of the pain management protocol. A second strategy is to provide the client with tools that help them to remember to give medications, supplements, and food in precise amounts and on a precise schedule. "Pill minders" help clients remember to give medications and prevent confusion when there is more than one caregiver in the home, and tracking forms and checklists can be provided to ensure that treatments are provided according to the schedule.

FORMAL CERTIFICATION IN PAIN MANAGEMENT

As of this writing, there is a formal credentialing process available in veterinary pain management. The International Veterinary Academy of Pain Management (IVAPM) (www.ivapm.org) has developed the Certified Veterinary Pain Practitioner (CVPP) certification program to assist veterinary healthcare team members in the process of building and expanding their ability to effectively serve painful patients. Because the majority of advanced certification or credentialing available in veterinary medicine is oriented toward individuals involved in academic or specialty practice, the CVPP credential was developed specifically for the primary care practice. The IVAPM training program and the CVPP certification are open to veterinarians and licensed veterinary technicians in the primary care setting where the majority of veterinary patients receive care. Pain is an everyday event in veterinary practice, thus, it is in the primary care setting that effective pain management strategies have the potential to create the most significant impact on the everyday lives of animals. Veterinary medical professionals who have completed animal-specific training, such as canine or equine rehabilitation or animal chiropractic, may also pursue CVPP designation.

The details of certification will evolve over time, but the core requirements are fairly straightforward. The candidate must be engaged in full-time practice for a number of years, submit letters of recommendation, complete a minimum number of continuing education hours in veterinary pain management, demonstrate competency in specific pain management related skills, submit digital images of the pain management drugs and equipment available in their practice settings, take a standardized multiple-choice examination, and submit two relevant case reports.

The CVPP certification was developed in order to accomplish several goals:

- Emphasize the importance of effective pain management for every patient in general veterinary practice.
- Encourage networking with colleagues positioned to support expansion of pain management strategies.
- Provide encouragement to all practitioners to pursue expanded pain management protocols in their practices.
- Provide guidance, by way of a skill list, recommended reading, and approved pain management-oriented continuing education courses, for specific strategies a practice may utilize to expand and enhance pain management offerings to patients.

Supporting one or more member(s) of the veterinary healthcare team to pursue the CVPP credential enhances pain management practice-wide, and encourages the practice team to keep control of pain at the forefront for all patients.

Independent of the CVPP credential, the IVAPM provides members with access to resources that allow any practice to improve its standard of pain care, including interaction with other like-minded professionals via online discussion forums. Membership in the IVAPM, by definition, raises the standard of pain management care in any veterinary practice.

SUMMARY

Pain prevention, identification, and treatment must be accomplished for every patient. It is critical to educate pet owners about behaviors or behavior changes that are commonly associated with pain and painful conditions, but client education is only one of the steps that must be taken. There must be a deep, abiding, lasting, and ongoing commitment throughout the practice to look for and find pain in its many presentations, and to manage it appropriately.

The key to success in integrating pain management into any veterinary practice is to start—start somewhere, start small, start with surgical pain, start with osteoarthritis patients, and start by learning pain assessment. Pain management is an ongoing and evolving process, a journey rather than a destination; start with small steps and put one piece after another in place. The path you build will lead to rewarding outcomes.

ONLINE RESOURCES

American Animal Hospital Association: www.aahanet.org

International Veterinary Academy of Pain Management: www.ivapm.org

Veterinary Anesthesia and Analgesia Support Group: www.vasg.org

REFERENCES

American Animal Hospital Association, American Association of Feline Practitioners, AAHA/AAFP Pain Management Guidelines Task Force Members, et al. (2007) AAHA/AAFP pain management guidelines for dogs and cats. *Journal of the American Animal Hospital Association*, 43, 235–248.

American Animal Hospital Association (2003) *The Path to High Quality Care*, AAHA Press, Denver, CO.

Hellyer, P.W., Uhrig, S.R., & Robinson, N.G. (2006a). *Colorado State University Acute Pain Scale – Canine*, Fort Collins, CO.

Hellyer, P.W., Uhrig, S.R., & Robinson, N.G. (2006b). *Colorado State University Acute Pain Scale – Feline*, Fort Collins, CO.

40
Pain Management in Hospice and Palliative Care

Keri Jones

Veterinarians frequently interact with clients who have high expectations for the provision of end-of-life care for their pets. Most owners value quality over quantity of life for their pet (Oyama et al., 2008) and, in the absence of good quality of life (QOL), may elect to end their pet's suffering through euthanasia. QOL refers to the level of pleasant and unpleasant feelings in one's life (Hancock et al., 2004; McMillan, 2005). The intensity of the feeling dictates the degree of influence on QOL. Major contributing factors to QOL include pain, social relationships, mental stimulation, health, food intake, and stress (McMillan, 2005). There are many new tools to help our patients maintain a good QOL, and it is our ethical duty to do so, and we no longer need to be limited to a "treat or euthanize" mentality (Monti, 2000). Palliative and hospice care allow pets to be kept comfortable while preparing their human families for the approaching death of their animal.

PALLIATIVE CARE

Palliative care refers to the treatment of clinical signs of a disease without the intent of curing the disease (Hellyer et al., 2007; Downing, 2011). The aim of palliative care is to achieve the best possible QOL through relief of suffering and restoration of functional capacity, regardless of life expectancy (Forrow & Smith, 2004). Human palliative care patients are happier, more mobile, have less pain, and live longer than those not receiving palliative care (Temel et al., 2010). Most palliative care patients have limited life expectancy due to one or more morbidities. An excellent reference by Shearer, (2011) regarding the benefits of palliative and hospice care is available.

HOSPICE CARE

Hospice is a type of palliative care that addresses end-of-life issues in terminally ill patients. In humans, hospice designation determines service availability, home care, and third party payment (Gazelle, 2007). Fortunately, medical coding and third party payment do not dictate service availability in veterinary patients, so a strict hospice designation is unnecessary. Thus, in animal patients the term hospice typically indicates a short life expectancy (days to

months) and that preparation for death should be underway. Client education is an important part of the process, and emotional and spiritual support for the family should be included (AVMA, 2001; 2008; AAH-ABV.org, 2011).

There are concerns among veterinarians that pet hospice and palliative care may contribute to animal suffering if it is carried out by well-meaning laypeople not trained in recognition and treatment of animal suffering (Nolen, 2007). Such a situation may delay or prevent euthanasia of the suffering patients. Simply providing care and hygiene for a dying pet is not hospice care, and does not ensure good QOL. Frequent veterinary assessments and a dynamic treatment regimen ensure that hospice meets its goal of a "good death" (Osborne, 2009).

Hospice and palliative care treatments are primarily delivered on an outpatient basis. Outpatient treatment allows pets to spend time with their families in a comfortable low-stress environment, preserving the human–animal bond. However, episodic decompensation may mean that hospital services are needed occasionally. These may include hospitalization for palliative surgery, radiation, or delivery of intravenous fluids or injectable medications. Some clinics may provide medical day care while owners are at work (Villalobos, 2008), but the goal should always be to have the pets return home when they are comfortable and stable.

PAIN, SUFFERING, AND QUALITY OF LIFE IN PALLIATIVE CARE

People and pets are often undertreated for pain at the end of their lives (Meier et al., 2006; Villalobos & Kaplan, 2007). Knowing that it is likely that our terminal patients are experiencing pain (Meier et al., 2006), veterinarians should treat for pain rather than assuming comfort when complaint behavior is absent. Palliative care is based on a short-term benefit to the patient, and pain medications should never be discontinued out of fear of long-term sequelae (Good et al., 2005). In addition, although we have come to focus on the relief of physical pain in veterinary patients, all forms of suffering, including that caused by emotional states, should be addressed in palliative care patients (McMillan, 2003; Downing, 2011; Villalobos, 2011).

Pain Management in Veterinary Practice, First Edition. Edited by Christine M. Egger, Lydia Love and Tom Doherty.
© 2014 John Wiley & Sons, Inc. Published 2014 by John Wiley & Sons, Inc.

Sources of Pain in Palliative Care Patients

The type(s) and sources of pain should be identified when evaluating a pet. Pain can be acute or chronic, adaptive or maladaptive, physical or psychological, central or peripheral, somatic or visceral, and more than one type of pain may be present. Adaptive pain involves stimulation of nociceptive pathways, and subsequent modulation and perception of the noxious stimulus. Maladaptive pain may occur without a noxious stimulus, and generally produces an exaggerated perception of pain (Borsook, 2011; Downing, 2011; McGreavy et al., 2011). Hyperalgesia and allodynia are very common in hospice and palliative care patients, and involve anatomical and physiological alterations in nociceptive processing, making a multimodal approach to pain essential (Davis, 2010).

Besides the pain caused by the underlying disease(s), palliative care patients often have other sources of pain. Dental pain is extremely common in older pets, and pet owners and veterinarians often do not pursue dental care in geriatric pets out of fear of the risks associated with anesthesia (Hollstrum, 2005). An accelerated cleaning procedure addressing the worst areas and extracting loose teeth under a balanced anesthetic protocol, with meticulous monitoring and supportive care, will increase comfort and decrease the opportunities for sepsis. If anesthesia must be avoided, the patient may be placed on pulse antibiotic therapy to control infection and dysphagia (Jones et al., 2011).

Osteoarthritis affects a large percentage of geriatric dogs and cats (Hardie et al., 2002; Kerwin, 2010; Rychel, 2010; Slingerland et al., 2011). Even those pets with mild osteoarthritic pain have decreased activity levels and decreased opportunity for social interaction. When severe or prolonged, the resulting muscle atrophy can cause weakness, and the patient may not be able to stand or ambulate. These changes, particularly in larger dogs, create a downward spiral to euthanasia (Burns, 2006). A multimodal approach to treating osteoarthritic patients is most beneficial. Appropriate analgesic therapy together with weight management, acupuncture, therapeutic lasers, and rehabilitation exercises help patients maintain QOL by helping them remain ambulatory (Robinson, 2009; Marshall et al., 2010; Downing, 2011).

Discomfort and Suffering

Suffering may be of a physical or emotional nature (McMillan, 2000). In the Senior Care Guidelines published by the American Animal Hospital Association in 2005, determination of suffering is made by the evaluation of *hunger, thirst, discomfort, pain, injury, disease, fear, distress, and freedom to express normal behavior* (Epstein et al., 2005). All of these should be evaluated regularly in the palliative care patient.

The clinical signs that affect QOL, but which are not overtly painful, may influence decisions about palliative care and euthanasia. Digestive discomfort, dyspnea, pruritus, thermoregulatory difficulty, incontinence, blindness, and cognitive dysfunction are examples of conditions that cause discomfort, and which should be addressed (Linek & Favrot, 2010; Villalobos, 2011). The inability to breathe normally produces extreme anxiety, fear, and suffering. If respiratory distress is not controllable with medications and interventions, such as thoracocentesis and drainage of pleural fluid and oxygen therapy, euthanasia should be discussed with the owner. Opioids may be useful in relieving the sensation of air hunger in pets that are unable to effectively oxygenate (Bruera

et al., 1993). Benzodiazepines may relieve anxiety in these patients (Jordan, 1982).

Gastrointestinal dysfunction causes discomfort, and gastrointestinal obstruction should be relieved surgically if the pet is not to be euthanized right away. Oral feeding of obstructed patients may cause more discomfort and should be discontinued. Liquid diets may pass if the obstruction is partial. Feeding tubes should only be used in patients that have an otherwise good QOL and are able to digest food without discomfort or pain. Constipation and diarrhea should be corrected whenever possible. Good hygiene and soothing creams may be helpful for irritated perineal tissues in pets with chronic diarrhea or urinary incontinence. Histamine blockers, promotility drugs, sucralfate, appetite stimulants, and antibiotics may be necessary for those pets with gastrointestinal disease that are still able to eat.

According to McMillan (2000), social bonds create a pleasant effect, and separation and isolation an unpleasant effect. Cognitive dysfunction does not cause physical pain but can severely impact QOL by changing social interaction with other pets and family members (Landsberg et al., 1998). It may also contribute to anxiety, aggression, house soiling, or other undesirable behaviors that may further isolate the patient. Oral selegiline, a monoamine oxidase (MAO) inhibitor, may be beneficial for these patients (Landsberg & Araujo, 2005; Landsberg, 2011). Pets with loss of bladder or bowel control or those that have diseases that produce an unpleasant odor may be confined away from the main living areas of the family (Linek & Favrot, 2010). This isolation may negatively affect their QOL and the human–animal bond. Other disabilities, such as paralysis or blindness, diminish a pet's opportunity to experience pleasurable activities (McMillan, 2005).

Quality of Life Assessment

Because the QOL encompasses so many factors it is difficult to quantify (Wojciechowska, 2005). An assessment tool, such as Alice Villalobos' HHHHHMM Scale (Figure 40.1), may help owners evaluate their pet more objectively (Villalobos, 2004), and is available at: www.veterinarypracticenews.com/images/pdfs/Quality_of_Life.pdf.

Veterinarians should discuss with owners the QOL of the pet in terms of what the patient does now versus what it did before the illness. Is the pet still greeting the owner at the door when he or she comes home? Does the pet still play with toys or other pets? Does the pet still chase squirrels or stalk bugs or is it just sleeping and eating? These discussions should be included in the medical record for future reference (Rollin, 2006).

It is also important to discuss with the owner the level of care they can and are willing to provide for the pet, given the issues likely to occur with the pet's illness. As the pet's advocate, the veterinarian must develop a treatment plan based on what the owners can afford, and can reasonably deliver based on their schedule and physical ability. Extensive treatments and medications may make owners feel like they are no longer their pet's best friend. Treatment plans should be tailored to what the individual pet and owner will tolerate, while maintaining the human–animal bond and QOL.

Simple changes in the living space can help pets maintain interaction with their family and a good QOL. Providing necessities such as food, water, and elimination areas on a single level of the home will help pets with ambulation difficulties. Rugs and runners on slippery floors will help large dogs to stand and walk. If the

Quality of Life Scale

(The HHHHHMM Scale)

Pet caregivers can use this Quality of Life Scale to determine the success of Pawspice care. Score patients using a scale of: 0 to 10 (10 being ideal).

Score	Criterion
0-10	**HURT** - Adequate pain control & breathing ability is of top concern. Trouble breathing outweighs all concerns. Is the pet's pain well managed? Can the pet breathe properly? Is oxygen supplementation necessary?
0-10	**HUNGER** - Is the pet eating enough? Does hand feeding help? Does the pet need a feeding tube?
0-10	**HYDRATION** - Is the pet dehydrated? For patients not drinking enough water, use subcutaneous fluids daily or twice daily to supplement fluid intake.
0-10	**HYGIENE** - The pet should be brushed and cleaned, particularly after eliminations. Avoid pressure sores with soft bedding and keep all wounds clean.
0-10	**HAPPINESS** - Does the pet express joy and interest? Is the pet responsive to family, toys, etc.? Is the pet depressed, lonely, anxious, bored or afraid?　Can the pet's bed be moved to be close to family activities?
0-10	**MOBILITY** - Can the pet get up without assistance? Does the pet need human or mechanical help (e.g., a cart)? Does the pet feel like going for a walk? Is the pet having seizures or stumbling? (Some caregivers feel euthanasia is preferable to amputation, but an animal with limited mobility yet still alert, happy and responsive can have a good quality of life as long as caregivers are committed to helping their pet.)
0-10	**MORE GOOD DAYS THAN BAD** - When bad days outnumber good days, quality of life might be too compromised. When a healthy human—animal bond is no longer possible, the caregiver must be made aware that the end is near. The decision for euthanasia needs to be made if the pet is suffering. If death comes peacefully and painlessly at home, that is okay.
*TOTAL	*A total over 35 points represents acceptable life quality to continue with pet hospice (Pawspice).

Figure 40.1. An assessment tool, such as Alice Villalobos' HHHHHMM Scale, may help owners evaluate their pet more objectively (Villalobos, 2004), and is available at www.veterinarypracticenews.com/images/pdfs/Quality_of_Life.pdf.

home's yard exit is not on ground level, a custom ramp may be helpful. Other useful recommendations for household changes are available in recent publications (Downing, 2011; Shearer, 2011).

Eating and drinking are often high on the list of activities owners use to assess their pet's condition. Well-hydrated patients are more comfortable, and can better maintain the bodily functions such as bowel motility and corneal lubrication. However, a point may be reached when continued hydration may be prolonging a poor QOL, and is no longer in the pet's best interest (Zerwekh, 2003; Lamers, 2011). This occurs when organ systems are failing, and the pet is no longer ambulatory, may be anorexic, and water consumption is declining despite dehydration. Advising owners that the process of gradual dehydration leads to comfortable sleep and coma can ease the client's fear of thirst in dying pets (Goodlin et al., 2006; Emanuel et al., 2010).

A similar situation may be true of food intake. While the digestive tract is functioning, eating contributes positively to a pet's QOL. However, when digestion or eating causes discomfort, encouraging food intake may be deleterious (Goodlin et al., 2006). Feeding tubes may be appropriate for cases in which the pet is hungry and has a good QOL but is unable to eat due to oral or esophageal disease. If the pet is anorexic due to systemic disease (as in renal failure), placement of a feeding tube may not be in the pet's best interest. Force feeding pets with terminal disease causes physical and mental distress, diminishes the human—animal bond, and is not recommended.

TREATING PAIN IN HOSPICE AND PALLIATIVE CARE PATIENTS

Traditional routes of administration of medication may be unavailable or suboptimal in palliative care patients; thus, the palliative care veterinarian must be creative when developing a treatment plan. Most oral medications can be compounded into flavored liquids for easier delivery. Some compounding pharmacies can make medications into chewable treats or transdermal gels and creams. Transdermal medications are easy to administer; however, because absorption is quite variable, monitoring for effectiveness is especially important. Clients can be taught to give injectable pain medications subcutaneously when other routes are unavailable or ineffective (Villalobos & Kaplan, 2007). Complete and accurate medical records are imperative when treating patients receiving multiple medications. Policies and procedures should be in place to ensure compliance with local and federal controlled substance dispensing regulations (Downing, 2011).

Almost all geriatric pets have some degree of organ dysfunction, but it is important not to undertreat pain in these patients out of fear of adverse effects. Abnormalities in blood tests, such as azotemia or increased bile acids, may help guide dosages and dosing intervals in these patients, but should not be a cause to discontinue needed pain control.

It is not uncommon to see a palliative care patient with three or more morbidities that must be treated concurrently, and allodynia and hyperalgesia are very common in patients that are aged or have been sick for a long time. Thus, although opioids are the cornerstone of treatment for many palliative care patients, multimodal therapies utilizing adjunct medications such as glucocorticoid and anabolic steroids, NSAIDs, local anesthetics, gabapentin, amantadine, and amitriptyline are more likely to be effective than monotherapy (Borsook, 2011; Downing, 2011; McGreavy et al., 2011). Careful monitoring is necessary when using polypharmacy in order to minimize adverse effects and ensure effective absorption and bioavailability of medications (Welsh & Fallon, 1998).

Palliative Surgery

If halting disease progression is not possible, palliative surgery may be more effective than medication for controlling pain. Amputation of appendicular osteosarcoma lesions removes the pain source and avoids the possibility of pathological fracture. Debulking ulcerated soft-tissue masses may allow the skin to heal. Excision of large inguinal or axillary lipomas may improve mobility. Obstruction of the gastrointestinal or urinary tract may be relieved in some cases by surgery or placement of stents (Gilson, 1998; Hume et al., 2006; Newman et al., 2009). Esophagostomy tubes may be helpful for feeding and medication of pets with painful oral lesions.

END-OF-LIFE CARE

Assisted Natural Death versus Euthanasia

The decision to euthanize a pet is a difficult one for many owners (McMillan, 2001). Pets may suffer needlessly, due to lack of veterinary management, if their owners are uncomfortable with euthanasia or simply wish for the pet to die naturally at home. The vast majority of patients with progressive incurable illness reach a point at which suffering cannot be relieved (Hancock et al., 2004), and a death that occurs without veterinary intervention is, in most cases, inhumane. An assisted natural death is defined as death that occurs without direct intervention by a veterinarian in terms of euthanasia, but does not exclude palliative care. It is ultimately the owner's decision whether the pet is to be euthanized, but it is the veterinarian's responsibility to make the animal as comfortable as possible in the period leading up to its death. Continued veterinary communication and monitoring is needed to ensure that the pet is not suffering. The client should be educated about the disease trajectory, what to expect as the pet's condition deteriorates, and which conditions need veterinary attention. Early discussion regarding euthanasia ensures proper communication and expectations for pet owners and the veterinary team. Ethical discussions on natural death and euthanasia are available on the American Association of Human-Animal Bond Veterinarians' website at www.aah-abv.org.

Proportionate Palliative Sedation

Proportionate palliative sedation is a relatively new concept in veterinary medicine, but it has been used extensively in human hospice situations (Lo & Rubenfeld, 2005; Shearer, 2011). This approach is recommended when the patient cannot be kept comfortable in a conscious state, and heavy sedation with analgesia is preferred while waiting for a natural death (Morita et al., 2002). This technique is based on the concept that an animal does not perceive pain while unconscious even though nociception may still be occurring (Robertson, 2002). A combination of opioids, midazolam, and phenobarbital has been used in dying human patients to relieve refractory discomfort (Lo & Rubenfeld, 2005), and comparable combinations can be used in animals.

Euthanasia Timing

When pain cannot be relieved, it is appropriate to again discuss euthanasia with the family members (Downing, 2011). Many owners need verification that they are making the correct decision regarding euthanasia, and it is important to answer questions in a nonjudgmental way. Correct timing of euthanasia is not a finite point in time, but rather a span of time dependent on the pet's QOL and the owner's preparedness. Some owners prefer euthanasia before the suffering occurs, and are willing to give up a few days or weeks with their pet to ensure this. Others prefer to have that extra time with their pet, provided medical issues are well controlled. In cases where a pet may acutely decompensate, a preneed referral letter to the emergency clinic may be helpful to ease the stress on the owner and provide the emergency staff with needed information (Shearer, 2011). In an emergency, the owners are under stress and may not recall important details. A brief outline of the pet's treatment plan as well as copies of recent blood work will help explain the pet's condition. Including owners' previously documented desires regarding further diagnostics and curative treatment versus palliation will help ensure that their wishes are honored if they are unable to think clearly.

Euthanasia

Historically, veterinarians have given a single injection of euthanasia solution to end a patient's life and suffering; however, because many pets are considered family members, extra sensitivity during euthanasia is needed. Providing a pre-euthanasia sedative and analgesic allows the patient and the owner some peaceful, comfortable, pain-free transition time. Many pet owners prefer that their pets' last moments not be on a stainless steel table or in a clinical setting; thus, home euthanasia is an excellent alternative. When euthanasia is performed in the hospital, a separate exam room or outdoor space may be made into a comfortable euthanasia area. Soft lighting, comfortable furniture, and a blanket or rug on the floor will allow owners and pets to be more relaxed. It is preferable to have a separate exit from this area so that clients do not have to leave through the reception area. Taking care of the necessary paperwork and payment in advance is recommended (Martin et al., 2004; Jones et al., 2011).

Educating clients about the euthanasia procedure itself and encouraging them to ask questions is recommended. Inform them as to which drugs will be administered and by which route, and how long it will take for death to occur. Clients should be advised that the eyes may not close at death, that agonal breathing or vocalization may occur, and that bladder and bowel control may be lost. Inquire as to which family members are to be present, and if children are to be present, take extra time to answer their questions regarding pet death. Client handouts with community resources such as pet loss help lines, pet loss groups, and online support should be made available.

Speak in a calm, quiet voice and touch the patient when approaching it for injection or IV catheter placement. Light touch reassures the pet and conveys compassion to the client. After sedation, and when the patient and client are comfortable, an experienced staff member should place an IV catheter to ensure uninterrupted venous access. This is done in the euthanasia area, whenever possible, to limit stress on the pet and the owner. EMLA® cream may be applied to the clipped area and covered with a bio-occlusive material 15–20 minutes prior to catheter placement to minimize patient discomfort. Injection of an induction dose of propofol immediately before the euthanasia solution will help prevent unwanted sequelae such as agonal breathing and vocalization. Dilute viscous euthanasia solutions with saline to ease injection through small gauge catheters.

Intravenous euthanasia injection in old or debilitated feline patients may be difficult and requires hair clipping and restraint. IP injection works very well in sedated feline patients, causes less stress than IV catheter placement, requires less restraint (the owner can often hold the patient), and patient response to the injection is minimal. In the author's experience, 4–5 mL of diluted euthanasia solution is adequate for IP injection in an average-sized cat. Injection just caudal to the last rib, high on the right side near the right kidney tends to yield good absorption, as does a ventral midline approach with the patient in lateral recumbency. Intraperitoneal injection produces a very gradual natural-appearing death, allowing the owners to hold their cat for the procedure, if desired. Death generally occurs within 10–15 minutes of injection.

For hypovolemic, hypotensive pets where venous access is not attainable, intracardiac injection may be the only route available.

AVMA guidelines for euthanasia advise performing intracardiac injection only in heavily sedated, unconscious, or fully anesthetized patients. This route is generally not recommended for client-present euthanasia. New AVMA guidelines for intrahepatic and intrarenal injection are expected in the near future.

After euthanasia the thorax is ausculted to verify death and the owner is gently informed that the animal has died. Allow owners the opportunity to spend time alone with their pet. Respectful private cremation with return of the ashes or burial options should be offered. Pet memorial services may be available in some areas.

SUMMARY

Advancements in veterinary diagnostics and treatments have allowed our patients to live longer than ever before, and it is our duty to ensure that the QOL is also good. The potential for prolongation of suffering is real, and it is our professional duty to acknowledge this and prevent it through education of veterinarians, veterinary technicians, and clients. There are many opportunities to improve the QOL of our patients, and many only require our time and minimal expense. Advocate for the pet and educate owners so that they may make the right choices for end-of-life care for their pet.

REFERENCES

American Association of Human-Animal Bond Veterinarians. (2011) *Hospice Care*, www.aah-abv.org (accessed July 15, 2013).

American Veterinary Medical Association (2008) *Guidelines for Veterinary Hospice Care*. [Online] Available at: www.avma.org/issues/policy/hospice_care.asp.

AVMA Panel on Euthanasia, 2000 Report of the AVMA Panel on Euthanasia. (2001) *Journal of the American Veterinary Medical Association*, 218(5), 669–696.

Borsook, D. (2011) Neurologic diseases and pain. *Brain, A Journal of Neurology*. Oxford University Press. 135(2), 320–344.

Bruera, E., MacEachern, T., Ripamonti, C., & Hanson, J. (1993) Subcutaneous morphine for dyspnea in cancer patients. *Annals of Internal Medicine*, 119(9), 906–907.

Burns, K. (2006) Research targets conditions of older cats and dogs. *Journal of the American Veterinary Medical Association*, 229(4), 479–496.

Davis, M. (2010) Recent advances in the treatment of pain. *F1000 Medicine Reports*, 2(63), doi: 10.3410/M2-63.

Downing, R. (2011) Pain management for veterinary palliative care and hospice patients, in *Veterinary Clinics of North America Small Animal Practice: Palliative Medicine and Hospice Care* (ed. T.S. Shearer), Saunders, Philadelphia, pp. 531–550.

Emanuel, L., Ferris, F., vonGunten, C., et al. (2010) The Last Hours of Living: Practical advice for Clinicians: Preparing for the Last Hours of Life. *Medscape Nurses*, www.medscape.com/viewarticle/716463_2 (accessed July 15, 2013).

Epstein, M., Kuehn, N.F., Landsberg, G., et al. (2005) AAHA senior care guidelines for dogs and cats. *Journal of the American Animal Hospital Association*, 41(2), 81–91.

Forrow, L. & Smith, H.S. (2004) Pain management in end of life: palliative care, in *Principles & Practice of Pain Medicine* 2nd edn (eds. C.A. Warfield & Z.H. Bajwah), McGraw-Hill, New York, pp. 492–502.

Gazelle, G. (2007) Understanding Hospice—an underutilized option for life's final chapter. *New England Journal of Medicine*, 357(4), 321–324.

Gilson, S.D. (1998) Principles of surgery for cancer palliation and treatment of metastasis. *Clinical Techniques in Small Animal Practice*, 13(1), 65–69.

Good, P.D., Ravenscroft, P.J., & Cavenaugh, J. (2005). Effects of opioids and sedatives on survival in an Australian inpatient palliative care population. *Internal Medicine Journal*, 35(9), 512–517.

Goodlin, S., (2006) Care near the end of life, in *Geriatric Medicine: an evidence-based approach,* 4th edn (eds. C. K. Cassel, R.M. Leipzig, H.J. Cohen, E.B. Larson, & D.E. Meier), Springer, New York, pp. 299–309.

Hancock, C.G., McMillan, F.D., & Ellenbogen, T.R. (2004) Owner services and hospice care, in *Geriatrics and Gerontology of the Dog and Cat*, 2nd edn (ed J.D. Hoskins), Saunders, St. Louis, MO pp. 5–17.

Hardie, E.M., Roe, S.C., & Martin, F.R. (2002) Radiographic evidence of degenerative joint disease in geriatric cats: 100 cases (1994–1997). *Journal of the American Veterinary Medical Association*, 220(5), 628–632.

Hellyer, P., Rodan, I., Brunt, J., et al. (2007) AAHA/AAFP Pain management guidelines for dogs and cats. *Journal of the American Animal Hospital Association*, 43(5), 235–248.

Hollstrum, S. E. (2005) Geriatric veterinary dentistry: medical and client relations and challenges, in *Veterinary Clinics of North America: Small Animal Practice* (ed. W. D. Fortney), Saunders, Philadelphia, pp. 699–712.

Hume, D.Z., Solomon, J.A., & Weisse, C.W. (2006) Palliative use of a stent for colonic obstruction caused by adenocarcinoma in two cats. *Journal of the American Veterinary Medical Association*, 228(3), 392–396.

Jones, K. L., Ellenbogen, T., Shanan, A., et al. (2011) Guidelines for Pain Management in Palliative and End-of-Life Care of Small Animals. *International Veterinary Academy of Pain Management*, www.ivapm.org (accessed July 15, 2013).

Jordan, C. (1982). Assessment of the effects of drugs on respiration. *British Journal of Anesthesia*, 54(7), 763–782.

Kerwin, S. (2010). Osteoarthritis in cats. *Topics in Companion Animal Medicine*, 25(4), 218–223.

Lamers, W. (2011) Nutrition and Hydration (End of Life). *Hospice Foundation of America*, www.hospicefoundation.org (accessed July 15, 2013).

Landsberg, G.M., Hunthausen, W., & Ackerman, L. (1998) Behavior problems in geriatric pets, in *Handbook of Behavior Problems of the Dog and Cat*, Butterworth Heinemann, Oxford, pp. 185–194.

Landsberg, G. & Araujo, J. (2005) Behavior problems in geriatric pets, in *Veterinary Clinics of North America: Small Animal Practice*. (ed. W. Fortney), Saunders, Philadelphia, pp. 675–698.

Landsberg, G.M., (2011) Clinical signs and management of anxiety, sleeplessness, and cognitive dysfunction in the senior pet. in *Veterinary Clinics of North America Small Animal Practice: Palliative Medicine and Hospice Care* (eds. T.S. Shearer), Saunders, Philadelphia, pp.565–590.

Linek, M. & Favrot, C. (2010) Impact of canine atopic dermatitis on the health-related quality of life of affected dogs and quality of life of their owners. *Veterinary Dermatology*, 21(5), 456–462.

Lo, B. & Rubenfeld, G. (2005) Palliative sedation in dying patients "we turn to it when everything else hasn't worked". *Journal of the American Medical Association*, 294(14), 1810–1816.

Marshall, W.G., Herman, A.W., Mullen, D., De Meyer, G., Baert, K., & Carmichael, S. (2010) The effect of weight loss on lameness in obese dogs with osteoarthritis. *Veterinary Research Communications*, 34(3), 241–253.

Martin, F., Ruby, K.L., Deking, T.M., & Taunton, AE. (2004) Factors associated with client, staff, and student satisfaction regarding small animal euthanasia procedures at a veterinary teaching hospital. *Journal of the American Veterinary Medical Association*, 224(11), 1774–1779.

McGreevy, K., Bottros, M., & Raja, S. (2011). Preventing chronic pain following acute pain: risk factors, preventive strategies, and their efficacy. *European Journal of Pain Supplements*, 5(2), 365–376.

McMillan, F. D. (2000) Quality of life in animals. *Journal of the American Veterinary Medical Association*, 216(12), 1904–1910.

McMillan, F.D. (2001) Rethinking euthanasia: death as an unintentional outcome. *Journal of the American Veterinary Medical Association*, 219(9), 1204–1206.

McMillan, F.D. (2003) A world of hurts–is pain special? *Journal of the American Veterinary Medical Association*, 223(2), 183–186.

McMillan, F.D., (2005) *Quality of Life in Animals*. Proceedings of the North American Veterinary Conference, January 8–12, 2005, Orlando, FL.

Meier, D.E. (2006) Old age and care near the end of life. in *Geriatric Medicine: an evidence-based approach,* 4th edn (eds. C.K. Cassel, R.M. Leipzig, H.J. Cohen, et al.), Springer, New York, pp. 281–285.

Monti, D. J., (2000) Pawspice an option for pets facing the end. *Journal of the American Veterinary Medical Association*, 217(7), 969.

Morita, T., Tsuneto, S., & Shima, Y. (2002) Definition of sedation for symptom relief: a systematic literature review and a proposal of operational criteria. *Journal of Pain and Symptom Management*, 24(4), 447–453.

Newman, R.G., Mehler, S.J., Beal, M.W., & Kitchell, B.E. (2009) Use of a balloon-expandable metallic stent to relieve malignant urethral obstruction in a cat. *Journal of the American Veterinary Medical Association*, 234(2), 236–239.

Nolen, R. S. (2007) Protecting pet hospice: growing popularity of pet hospices raises concerns of abuse. *Journal of the American Veterinary Medical Association*, 231(12), 1793–1794.

Osborne, M. (2009) Pet hospice movement gaining momentum. *Journal of the American Veterinary Medical Association*, 234(8), 998–999.

Oyama, M.A., Rush, J.E., O'Sullivan, L.M., et al. (2008) Perceptions and priorities of owners of dogs with heart disease regarding quality versus quantity of life for their pets. *Journal of the American Veterinary Medical Association*, 233(1), 104–108.

Robertson, S.A. (2002) What is pain? *Journal of the American Veterinary Medical Association*, 221(2), 202–205.

Robinson, N.G. (2009) Complimentary and alternative medicine for pain management in veterinary patients. in *Handbook of Veterinary Pain Management,* 2nd edn (eds. J.S. Gaynor & W.W. Muir), Mosby Elsevier, St. Louis, MO, pp. 301–329.

Rollin, B. (2006) Euthanasia and quality of life. *Journal of the American Veterinary Medical Association*, 228(7), 1014–1016.

Rychel, J. (2010). Diagnosis and treatment of osteoarthritis. *Topics in Companion Animal Medicine*, 25(1), 20–25.

Shearer, T. S. (2011) Pet hospice and palliative care protocols, in *Veterinary Clinics of North America Small Animal Practice: Palliative Medicine and Hospice Care* (ed. T.S. Shearer), Saunders, Philadelphia, pp. 507–518.

Slingerland, L., Hazelwinkel, H., Meij, B., et al. (2011). Cross-sectional study of the prevalence and clinical features of osteoarthritis in cats. *The Veterinary Journal*, 187, 304–309.

Temel, J.S., Greer, J.A., Muzikansky, M.A., et al. (2010) Early palliative care for patients with metastatic non-small-cell lung cancer. *New England Journal of Medicine*, 363(8), 733–742.

Villalobos, A., (2004) Quality of life scale helps make final call. www.veterinarypracticenews.com/images/pdfs/Quality_of_Life.pdf (accessed July 15, 2013).

Villalobos, A., & Kaplan, L. (2007) *Canine and Feline Geriatric Oncology: Honoring the Human-Animal Bond*, 1st edn. Blackwell Publishing, Ames, IA.

Villalobos, A., (2008) *"Pawspice" a Formal Pet Hospice Program.* Ontario VMA Conference speaker notes, www.pawspice.com (accessed July 15, 2013).

Villalobos, A. (2011). Quality-of-life assessment techniques for veterinarians, in *Veterinary Clinics of North America Small Animal Practice: Palliative Medicine and Hospice Care* (ed. T.S. Shearer), Saunders, Philadelphia, pp. 519–530.

Welsh, J., & Fallon, M. (1998) Palliative care, in: *Brocklehurst's Textbook of Geriatric Medicine and Gerontology,* 5th edn (eds R. Tallis, H. Fillit, & J.C. Brocklehurst), Churchill Livingstone, London, pp. 1583–1598.

Wojciechowska, J. I., (2005) Quality-of-life assessment in pet dogs. *Journal of the American Veterinary Medical Association*, 226(5), 722–728.

Zerwekh, J. (2003) End-of-life hydration—benefit or burden? *Nursing.* 33(2), 32hn1–32hn4.

Index

Note: Page number followed by f and t indicates figure and table respectively.

Pain Management in Veterinary Practice, First Edition. Edited by Christine M. Egger, Lydia Love and Tom Doherty.
© 2014 John Wiley & Sons, Inc. Published 2014 by John Wiley & Sons, Inc.

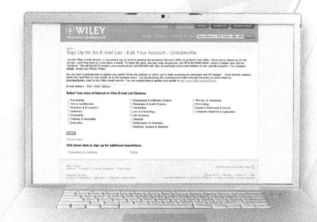
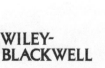